IAP Textbook of
TROPICAL DISEASES

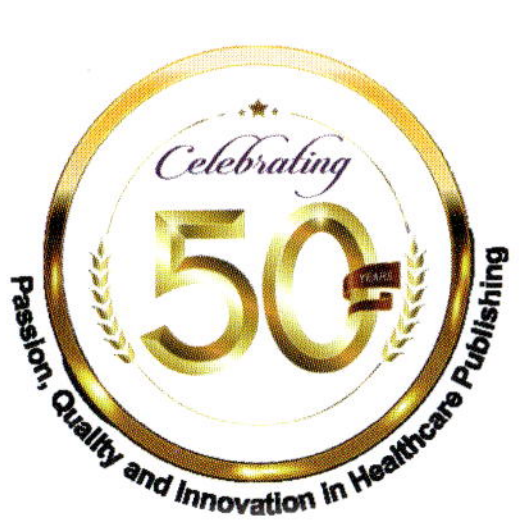

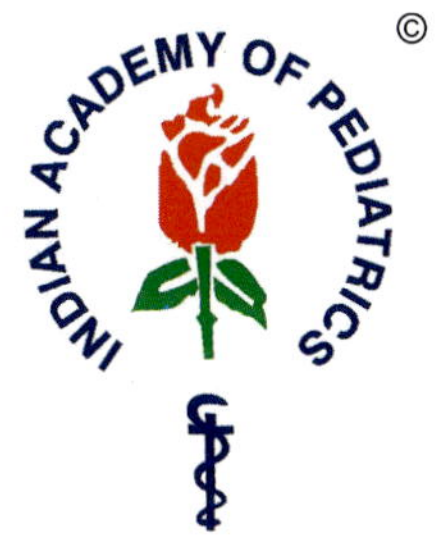

IAP Textbook of
TROPICAL DISEASES

Editor-in-Chief

Raju C Shah
MD DPed FIAP FRCPCH
Medical Director
Ankur Institute of Child Health, Ahmedabad
Former Professor and Head
Department of Pediatrics, GCS Medical College
Ahmedabad, Gujarat, India
President, 2005
Indian Academy of Pediatrics

Senior Academic Editors

Piyush Gupta
MD FNNF FIAP FAMS
Professor and Head
Department of Pediatrics, University College of Medical Sciences
New Delhi, India
President-Elect 2020
Indian Academy of Pediatrics

S Balasubramanian
MD DCH FIAP FRCPCH
Medical Director and Head
Department of Pediatrics and IAP IDC PID
Fellowship Coordinator
Kanchi Kamakoti CHILDS Trust Hospital
Chennai, Tamil Nadu, India

Academic Editors

Abhay K Shah
MD DPed FIAP
Senior Consultant Pediatrician
Children Hospital
Ahmedabad, Gujarat, India
Past President
IAP Infectious Diseases Chapter 2015

Jaydeep Choudhury
DNB MNAMS FIAP
Professor, Department of Pediatrics
Institute of Child Health
Kolkata, West Bengal, India
Chairperson
IAP Infectious Diseases Chapter 2020

Ashok Gupta
MD FIAP
Professor, Department of Pediatrics
Sawai Man Singh Medical College
Jaipur, Rajasthan, India
Executive Director
International Neonatology Association, Geneva, Switzerland

Forewords

Digant D Shastri, Bakul Jayant Parekh, Piyush Gupta

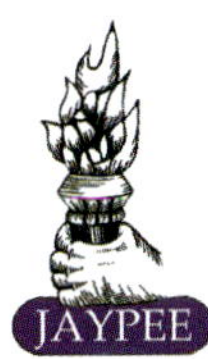

JAYPEE BROTHERS MEDICAL PUBLISHERS
The Health Sciences Publisher
New Delhi | London

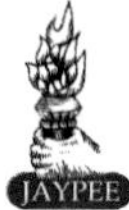 **Jaypee Brothers Medical Publishers (P) Ltd**

Headquarters

Jaypee Brothers Medical Publishers (P) Ltd
4838/24, Ansari Road, Daryaganj
New Delhi 110 002, India
Phone: +91-11-43574357
Fax: +91-11-43574314
E-mail: jaypee@jaypeebrothers.com

Overseas Office

JP Medical Ltd
83 Victoria Street, London
SW1H 0HW (UK)
Phone: +44 20 3170 8910
Fax: +44 (0)20 3008 6180
E-mail: info@jpmedpub.com

Website: www.jaypeebrothers.com
Website: www.jaypeedigital.com

IAP Textbook of Tropical Diseases

First Edition: **2020**

ISBN: 978-93-89776-33-1

Printed at: Samrat Offset Pvt. Ltd.

Contributors

Aakriti Gupta MSc
Research Scholar
Lady Irwin College
Delhi University
New Delhi, India

Aaradhana Singh MD
Associate Professor
Department of Pediatrics
University College of Medical Sciences
and Guru Teg Bahadur Hospital
New Delhi, India

Abhay K Shah MD DPed FIAP
Senior Consultant Pediatrician
Children Hospital
Ahmedabad, Gujarat, India
Past President
IAP Infectious Diseases Chapter 2015

Abhishek Paul DNB FICO
Department of Pediatric Ophthalmology
Medical Research Foundation
Sankara Nethralaya
Chennai, Tamil Nadu, India

Akash Bang MD DNB PGDMLS
Fellow
Division of Pediatric Critical Care
Additional Professor
Department of Pediatrics
All India Institute of Medical Sciences
Nagpur, Maharashtra, India

Alok Gupta MD (Ped) FIAP
Pediatrician and Counselor
Pediatric Specialties Clinic, Jaipur
Formerly Assistant Professor
Division of Pediatric Medicine
Mahatma Gandhi Medical College
and Hospital
Jaipur, Rajasthan, India

Amarnath Saran MBBS MD
Senior Resident
Department of Pediatrics
University College of Medical Sciences
and Guru Teg Bahadur Hospital
New Delhi, India

Amira M Khan DCH
Research Analyst
Centre for Global Child Health
The Hospital for Sick Children
Toronto, Canada

Anil Vasudevan MD
Professor and Head
Department of Pediatric Nephrology
St John's Medical College Hospital
Bengaluru, Karnataka, India

Aniruddha Ghosh MD DNB
Senior Resident
Department of Pediatrics
Institute of Child Health
Kolkata, West Bengal, India

Anitha P Moorkoth MD
Professor
Department of Microbiology
Government Medical College
Manjeri, Kerala, India

AR Karthick MD DNB
Assistant Professor
Department of Pediatrics
Madras Medical College
Chennai, Tamil Nadu, India

Arvind Shenoi MD DM (Neonatology)
Consultant
Neonatologist and Medical Director
Cloudnine Hospital
Bengaluru, Karnataka, India

Ashish Pradhan MD
Professor
Department of Pediatrics
Sikkim Manipal Institute of
Medical Sciences
Sikkim Manipal University
Sikkim, India

Ashok Gupta MD FIAP
Professor
Department of Pediatrics
Sawai Man Singh Medical College
Jaipur, Rajasthan, India
Executive Director
International Neonatology Association
Geneva, Switzerland

Ashok Rai MD PhD FIAP FIAMS FNNF FACI
Fellowship in Genetics
Hon IMA Professor and Faculty
Heritage Institute of Medical Sciences
Varanasi
Director
Indian Institute of Cerebral Palsy and
Handicapped Children
Varanasi, Uttar Pradesh India

Ashutosh V Yajurvedi
DCh (Fellowship in Neonatology)
Consultant Pediatrician
Yajurvedi Hospital
Solapur, Maharashtra, India

Ashwani K Sood MD FIAP
Professor and Head
Department of Pediatric Medicine
Indira Gandhi Medical College
Shimla, Himachal Pradesh, India
Member ACVIP 2018–19
Chair, Infectious Diseases Chapter
Indian Academy of Pediatrics, 2015

Atul Kulkarni MD
Associate Professor
Ashwini Rural Medical College
Solapur, Maharashtra, India

Bakul Jayant Parekh MD DCH
Head
Bakul Parekh Children's Hospital (BPCH)
and Multispecialty Tertiary Care Centre
Mumbai, Maharashtra, India

Baldev S Prajapati MD DPed FIAP MNAMS
Head and Professor
Department of Pediatrics
GCS Medical College, Hospital and
Research Centre, Ahmedabad
Aakanksha Children Hospital and
Postgraduate Institute
Ahmedabad, Gujarat, India

BD Bhatia MD DCH FICN FIAP FAMS FNNF
Emeritus Professor
Heritage Institute of Medical Sciences
Varanasi, Uttar Pradesh, India

Bhaskar Shenoy
MBBS MD (Ped) Dip in PID (UNSW) Cert. in Inf.
Control, Fellowship in Applied Nutrition (FAN)
Head, Department of Pediatrics
Chief
Division of Pediatric Infectious Diseases
Manipal Hospital
Bengaluru, Karnataka, India

Chabungbam Smilie MBBS
Resident
Department of Pediatrics
University College of Medical Sciences
and Guru Teg Bahadur Hospital
New Delhi, India

Deepak Pande MD (Ped) DCH
Consultant Pediatrician
Jamnagar, Gujarat, India

Dhanya Dharmapalan
MD PG Dip in PID (Oxford)
Consultant
Department of Pediatrics and
Pediatric Infectious Diseases
Apollo Hospitals
Navi Mumbai, Maharashtra, India

Dheeraj Shah MD FIAP MNAMS
Professor
Department of Pediatrics
University College of Medical Sciences
and Guru Teg Bahadur Hospital
New Delhi, India

Digant D Shastri MD (Ped) FIAP PGDHHM
CEO and Senior Pediatrician
Killol Children Hospital
Surat, Gujarat, India
President
Indian Academy of Pediatrics, 2019

Elizabeth KE
MBBS MD (Ped) PhD FIAP FRCPCH (London)
Professor and Head
Department of Pediatrics
Sree Mookambika Institute of
Medical Sciences
Kanyakumari, Tamil Nadu, India

Geeta M Govindaraj MD DCH DNB
Professor
Department of Pediatrics
Government Medical College
Kozhikode, Kerala, India

Geetha P MD
Additional Professor of Pediatrics
Government Medical College
Kozhikode, Kerala, India

Gibby Koshy
MBBS MTrop (Ped) MPH PhD FHEA FRSPH FRCPCH
(London)
Senior Public Health Specialist Advisor
Public Health England
Citizens Services Division
Phoenix House, Liverpool, UK

Hema Gupta Mittal MD
Senior Pediatrician
Department of Pediatrics
Dr RML Hospital and
Atal Bihari Vajpayee Institute
of Medical Sciences (ABVIMS)
New Delhi, India

Hema Jyoti Pahwa nee Bisht
MBBS MD
Consultant Pediatrician
Jayendra Child Care Clinic
Ghaziabad, Uttar Pradesh, India

Himali Meshram MD
Clinical Associate
Department of Pediatric GI and
Infectious Diseases
BJ Wadia Hospital for Children
Mumbai, Maharashtra, India

Hitesh Patel
MD Fellowship (Neonatology)
Neonatologist
NeoPlus ICU for Children
Surat, Gujarat, India

Ira Shah DPID (UK) MD DCH FCPS DNB (Ped)
Professor and Head
Department of Pediatric Infectious
Diseases and Pediatric GI, Hepatology
Nodal Officer
Pediatric DR-TB Center and
Pediatric HIV/ART Center
BJ Wadia Hospital for Children, Mumbai
Consultant in Pediatric Infectious
Diseases and Pediatric Hepatology
Nanavati Hospital
Mumbai, Maharashtra, India

Jaikrishan Mittal MD DM
Consultant Neonatologist
Neoclinic Children Hospital
Jaipur, Rajasthan, India

Janani Sankar DNB PhD MAMS
Senior Consultant
Department of Pediatrics
Kanchi Kamakoti CHILDS Trust Hospital
Chennai, Tamil Nadu, India

Jaydeep Choudhury DNB MNAMS FIAP
Professor
Department of Pediatrics
Institute of Child Health
Kolkata, West Bengal, India
Chairperson
IAP Infectious Diseases Chapter 2020

Jeeson C Unni MD
Senior Associate Consultant
Aster Medcity
Kochi, Kerala, India

Jijo Joseph John MD
Associate Professor
Department of Pediatrics
Believers Church Medical College
Hospital
Thiruvalla, Kerala, India

Jyoti Ranjan Behera MD
Assistant Professor
Department of Pediatrics
Kalinga Institute of Medical Sciences
Deemed to be university

K Dhanalakshmi DNB FIAP
Junior Consultant
Pediatric Infectious Diseases
Kanchi Kamakoti CHILDS Trust Hospital
Chennai, Tamil Nadu, India

Kamlesh Agarwal MBBS MD
Assistant Professor
Department of Pediatrics
SMS Medical College
Jaipur, Rajasthan, India

Kausik Mandal
MD (Ped) DM (Medical Genetics)
Associate Professor
Department of Medical Genetics
Sanjay Gandhi Postgraduate Institute of
Medical Sciences
Lucknow, Uttar Pradesh, India

Ketan Bharadva MD DCH FIAP
Director
NeoPlus ICU for Children
Masoom Children's Hospital
Surat, Gujarat, India
President
Indian Academy of Pediatrics-Infant and
Young Child Feeding (IAP-IYCF) Chapter
Convener
Human Milk Banking Association (India)

Ketan H Shah MD (Ped)
Practicing Pediatrician
Chief Pediatrician
Ketan Children Hospital
Surat, Gujarat, India

Kheya Ghosh Uttam DCH DNB
Associate Professor and In-Charge
Neonatal Intensive Care Unit
Institute of Child Health
Kolkata, West Bengal, India

Kiranpreet Kaur MBBS
Resident
Department of Pediatrics
University College of Medical Sciences
New Delhi, India

Krishna Mohan R
DNB Dip (Allergy and Asthma) MNAMS
Consultant Pediatrician
Department of Pediatrics
Government Taluk Hospital
Balussery, Kizhikade, Kerala
State Chairperson
Allergy and Applied Immunology
Chapter, IAP
Kerala, India

Kriti Mohan MD (Ped)
Associate Professor
Department of Pediatrics
All India Institute of Medical Sciences
Gorakhpur, Uttar Pradesh, India

Kumar Ankur MD DNB (Neonatology)
In-charge, NICU
Department of Neonatology
BLK Superspecialty Hospital
New Delhi, India

Lakshan Raj MD (Ped)
Fellowship in Pediatric Infectious Disease
Kanchi Kamakoti CHILDS Trust Hospital
Chennai, Tamil Nadu, India

Lalan Kumar Bharti MD (Ped) FNNF FIAP
Head
Department of Pediatrics
Jag Pravesh Chandra Hospital (JPCH)
New Delhi, India

Lokesh Saini MD DM (Pediatric Neurology)
Assistant Professor
Division of Pediatric Neurology
Department of Pediatrics
PGIMER, Chandigarh, India

Lokesh Tiwari MD DM
Associate Professor Head
Department of Pediatrics
All India Institute of Medical Sciences
Patna, Bihar, India

M Singaravelu
MD DCH DNB MNAMS FIAP
Professor
Department of Pediatrics
Sri Manakula Vinayagar Medical College
Puducherry, India

Madhu Singh MD
Lecturer
Department of Pediatrics
SN Medical College
Agra, Uttar Pradesh, India

Maharshi Trivedi MD DM
Resident
Department of Pediatric Oncology
Regional Cancer Centre
Thiruvananthapuram, Kerala

Mahesh A Mohite
MD DCH (Mumbai University)
Director
Sai Child Care Hospital, Navi Mumbai
Pediatric Intensivist
Bai Jerbai Wadia Hospital for Children
Mumbai, Maharashtra, India

Maheshwari
Senior Resident
Department of Pediatrics
SDM Medical College
Dharwad, Karnataka, India

Mamta Kumari MD (Ped)
Postgraduate Trainee
CSS College of Obstetrics, Gynecology
and Child Health
Kolkata, West Bengal, India

Manish Kumar MD
Assistant Professor
Department of Pediatrics
All India Institute of Medical Sciences
Rishikesh, Uttar Pradesh, India

Meenakshi Sesama MD
Senior Resident
Department of Pediatrics
University College of Medical Sciences
New Delhi, India

Meenakshi Swaminathan MS
Department of Pediatric Ophthalmology
Sankara Nethralaya, Medical Research
Foundation
Chennai, Tamil Nadu, India

Meet R Ramatri MDS (Pediatric Dentist)
Head, Department of Pedodontics and
Preventive Dentistry
Goenka Research Institute of Dental
Sciences
Gandhinagar, Gujarat, India

Mohit Vohra MBBS DNB (Ped)
Fellow in Neonatology, MHA
Consultant and Head
Department of Pediatrics, CKS Hospital
Jaipur, Rajasthan, India

Moinak Sen Sarma MD DM
Assistant Professor
Department of Pediatric Gastroenterology
Sanjay Gandhi Postgraduate Institute of
Medical Sciences
Lucknow, Uttar Pradesh, India

Mukul Tiwari MD DCH FIAP
Consultant Pediatrician
Department of Pediatrics
Apex Hospital, Gwalior
State President
Indian Medical Association
Madhya Pradesh, India

Narayanappa D MD FIAP
Professor
Department of Pediatrics
JSS Medical College
JSS Academy of Higher Education
and Research
Mysuru, Karnataka, India

Narmada S
MBBS DNB MRCPCH DAA PGDDN MBA
(Hosp Admin)
Consultant Pediatrician and Director
Department of Pediatrics
Nalam Medical Center and Hospital
Vellore, Tamil Nadu, India

Neelam Mohan
DNB MNAMS FPGH (UK) FIMSA FACG (USA) FIAP
FRCPCH (UK)
Director
Department of Pediatric Gastroenterology
Hepatology and Liver Transplantation
Medanta—The Medicity Hospital
Gurugram, Haryana, India

Nigam Prakash Narain
MD DCH PhD MRCP (UK) FRCPCH (UK)
Professor and Head (Retd)
Department of Pediatrics
Patna Medical College
Patna, Bihar, India

Niranjan Mohanty MD FIAP
Professor
Department of Pediatrics
Kalinga Institute of Medical Science
affiliated to KIIT University
(Deemed to be University)
Bhubaneswar, Odisha, India

Omar Irfan MD
Centre for Global Child Health
The Hospital for Sick Children
Toronto, Canada

Pallab Chatterjee DCH MD DNB FIAP
European Diplomate in Pediatric
Respiratory Medicine
Consultant Pediatrician
Columbia Asia Hospital
Kolkata, West Bengal, India

Payal Meshram MD
Assistant Professor
Department of Pediatrics
Mahatma Gandhi Institute of
Medical Sciences
Sewagram, Maharashtra, India

Pinky Meena MD
Senior Resident
Department of Pediatrics
University College of Medical Sciences
New Delhi, India

Piyali Bhattacharrya
DCH MD (Ped) FIAP FRCP (London)
Consultant Pediatrician
Department of Pediatrics
Sanjay Gandhi Postgraduate Institute of
Medical Sciences
Lucknow, Uttar Pradesh, India

Piyush Gupta MD FNNF FIAP FAMS
Professor and Head
Department of Pediatrics
University College of Medical Sciences
New Delhi, India
President-Elect 2020
Indian Academy of Pediatrics

Pooja Dewan MD MNAMS FIAP
Professor
Department of Pediatrics
University College of Medical Sciences
and Guru Tegh Bahadur Hospital
New Delhi, India

Prachi Jain MBBS
Postgraduate Student
Department of Pediatrics
University College of Medical Sciences
and Guru Tegh Bahadur Hospital
New Delhi, India

Preeti Malhotra MDA
Associate Professor
Department of Pediatrics
Sri Guru Ram Das Institute of
Medical Sciences
Amritsar, Punjab, India

Puneet Kumar MBBS MIAP
Owner-Consultant
Kumar Child Clinic
New Delhi, India

Purushothaman KK MD
Professor
Department of Pediatrics
Government Medical College
Thrissur, Kerala, India

Rahul Kadam
MBBS DNB Pediatrics, Fellowship in Neonatology
(FIAP)Lead Consultant
Department of Neonatology and Pediatrics
Yashoda Hospitals, Somajiguda
Hyderabad, Telangana, India

Rahul Patil MBBS DNB
Pediatrician
Sai Child Care Hospital
Navi Mumbai, Maharashtra, India

Rajal B Prajapati MD (Ped) DPed
Professor
Department of Pediatrics
Smt NHL Municipal Medical College
Ahmedabad, Gujarat, India

Rajani HS DCH DNB
Associate Professor
Department of Pediatrics
JSS Medical College
JSS Academy of Higher Education and
Research
Mysuru, Karnataka, India

Rajesh Kumar MBBS MD FCGP (Chennai)
Assistant Professor
Department of Pediatrics
Nalanda Medical College
Patna, Bihar, India

Rajesh Kumar Meena MD
Assistant Professor
Department of Pediatrics
University College of Medical Sciences
and Guru Tegh Bahadur Hospital
New Delhi, India

Rajeshwar Dayal
MD FAMS FIAP DNB DCH (London)
Professor and Head
Department of Pediatrics
Sarojini Naidu Medical College
Agra, Uttar Pradesh, India

Raju C Shah MD DPed FIAP FRCPCH
Medical Director
Ankur Institute of Child Health
Ahmedabad
Former Professor and Head
Department of Pediatrics
GCS Medical College
Ahmedabad, Gujarat, India
President, 2005
Indian Academy of Pediatrics

Ramachandran P MD (Ped) DNB (Ped)
Professor of Pediatrics and
Associate Dean (PG Studies)
Sri Ramachandra Medical College and
Research Institute
Sri Ramachandra Institute of Higher
Education and Research (SRIHER)
Chennai, Tamil Nadu, India

Ravi Sachan
MD MBA Fellowship in Neonatal and Perinatal
Medicine
Associate Professor
Division of Neonatology
University College of Medical Sciences
and Guru Teg Bahadur Hospital
New Delhi, India

Rekha Harish MD FIAP
Professor and Head
Department of Pediatrics
Hamdard Institute of Medical
Sciences and Research
New Delhi, India

Remesh Kumar R MD FIAP
Senior Consultant and HOD
Department of Pediatrics
Apollo Adlux Hospital
Cochin, Kerala India
Honorary Secretary General
Central IAP 2018 and 2019

Rhishikesh Thakre
DM (Neo) MD DNB DCH FCPS FIAP
Consultant Neonatologist
Neo Clinic and Hospital
Aurangabad, Maharashtra, India

Ritabrata Kundu MD
Professor
Department of Pediatric Medicine
Institute of Child Health
Kolkata, West Bengal, India

Rupa Banerjee DNB
Senior Resident
Department of Pediatric Surgery
Sir Gangaram Hospital
New Delhi, India

Rupal Dalal MD IBCLC
Adjunct Associate Professor
Department of CTARA, IIT B
Director of Health
Shrimati Malati Dahanukar Trust
Mumbai, Maharashtra, India

S Balasubramanian
MD DCH FIAP FRCPCH
Medical Director and Head
Department of Pediatrics and
IAP IDC PID
Fellowship Coordinator
Kanchi Kamakoti CHILDS Trust Hospital
Chennai, Tamil Nadu, India

Sachidananda Kamath
MBBS DCH MD
Medical Director and
Consultant Pediatrician
Welcare Hospital
Kochi, Kerala, India

Sahana M Srinivas
DNB DVD FRGUHS (Ped Dermatology)
Consultant Pediatric Dermatologist
Department of Pediatric Dermatology
Indira Gandhi Institute of Child Health
Bengaluru, Karnataka, India

Sandesh Guleria MD DM
Assistant Professor
Department of Pediatric Medicine
Indira Gandhi Medical College
Shimla, Himachal Pradesh, India

Sandipan Dhar MD DNB FRCP
Department of Pediatric Dermatology
Institute of Child Health
Kolkata, West Bengal, India

Sanjay Deshpande
DCH DNB Fellowship in Pediatric Diseases
Consultant
Department of Pediatrics and Pediatric
Infectious Diseases
Manipal Hospitals
Bengaluru, Karnataka, India

Sanjay Krishna Ghorpade MD
Director and Professor
Department of Pediatrics
Post Graduate Institute of Pediatrics
Niramay Hospital and Research Center
Satara, Maharashtra, India

Santosh T Soans MD FIAP
President IAP—2018
Founder President of OM Guild
Pediatrician and Intensivist
Professor and Head
AJ Institute of Medical Sciences and
Research Centre
Mangaluru, Karnataka, India

Sarika Gupta MD
Associate Professor
Department of Pediatrics
King George Medical College
Lucknow, Uttar Pradesh, India

Satish Tiwari MD LLB FIAP
Professor
Department of Pediatrics
Dr Panjabrao Deshmukh Memorial
Medical College
Amravati, Maharashtra, India

Shalu Jain DNB
Senior Resident
Department of Pediatrics
University College of Medical Sciences
and Guru Teg Bahadur Hospital
New Delhi, India

Shashi Kant Dhir MD DM
Associate Professor
Department of Pediatrics
Guru Gobind Singh Medical College
and Hospital
Faridkot, Punjab, India

Shilpa Aroskar MD (Ped)
Consultant Pediatrician
MGM Hospital
Navi Mumbai, Maharashtra, India

Shivan Kesavan MD (Ped)
Senior Resident
Pediatric Neurology Unit
Department of Pediatrics
Advanced Pediatrics Centre
Postgraduate Institute of Medical
Education and Research
Chandigarh, India

Shruthi TK MD IDPCCM
Associate Professor
Department of Pediatrics
Sri Ramachandra Medical College and
Research Institute, Sri Ramachandra
Institute of Higher Education and
Research (SRIHER)
Chennai, Tamil Nadu, India

Shyam Kukreja MD
Head
Department of Pediatrics
Max Super Speciality Hospital
New Delhi, India

Srinivas Murki
MD DM (Neonatology) DNB (Neonatology)
Consultant
Department of Neonatology
Paramitha Children's Hospital
Hyderabad, Telangana, India

Subhasish Bhattacharyya
DCH MD DNB MNAMS
Professor and Head
Department of Pediatrics
CSS College of Obstetrics, Gynecology
and Child Health, Kolkata
Former Professor and Head
College of Medicine and Sagore Dutta
Hospital, Kolkata
Former Professor and Program Director
Pediatric Centre of Excellence in
Pediatric HIV Care
Medical College and Hospital
Kolkata, West Bengal, India

Subramanya NK MD (Ped)
Vydehi Institute of Medical Sciences and
Research Center
Bengaluru, Karnataka, India

Sudip Dutta MD
Professor and Head
Department of Pediatrics
Sikkim Manipal Institute of
Medical Sciences
Sikkim Manipal University
Gangtok, Sikkim, India

Surender Singh Bisht
MBBS MD (Ped) DNB (Ped)
Senior Specialist and Incharge
Department of Neonatal ICU
Swami Dayanand Hospital
New Delhi, India

Swathi Kiran Shiri MD
Senior Resident
Department of Pediatric Nephrology
St John's Medical College Hospital
Bengaluru, Karnataka, India

Swathi Rao MD IAP
Fellow in Critical Care
Assistant Professor Incharge PICU
Department of Pediatrics
K.S Hegde medical academy
Mangaluru, Karnataka, India

Swati Kalra MD
Assistant Professor
Department of Pediatrics
Dr Baba Saheb Ambedkar Medical
College and Hospital
New Delhi, India

Tanu Singhal MD MSc
Consultant
Department of Pediatrics and
Infectious Diseases
Kokilaben Dhirubhai Ambani Hospital
and Medical Research Institute
Mumbai, Maharashtra, India

Tapisha Gupta MD
Senior Consultant
Department of Pediatrics
Max Super Speciality Hospital
New Delhi, India

Umesh Kapil MD
Former Professor and Head
Department of Gastroenterology and
Human Nutrition
All India Institute of Medical Sciences
New Delhi, India

Upendra Kinjawadekar MD DCH
Consultant Pediatrician and
Neonatologist
Department of Pediatrics
Kamlesh Mother and Child Hospital
Navi Mumbai, Maharashtra
Consultant Pediatrician
Apollo Hospitals
Navi Mumbai, Maharashtra, India

Uthaya Kumaran DCH MD (Ped)
Junior Consultant
Department of Neonatology
Cloudnine Hospital
Bengaluru, Karnataka, India

Varinder Singh MD FRCPCH
Director Professor
Department of Pediatrics
Lady Hardinge Medical College and
Associated Hospitals
Kalawati Saran Children's Hospital
New Delhi, India

Varun K Sharma
MD (Ped) Fellowship in Neonatology
The Royal College of Paediatrics and
Child Health, UK
Consultant Neonatologist
Neo Clinic Children Hospital
Jaipur, Rajasthan, India

Vijay Kulkarni MD
Professor and Head
Department of Pediatrics
SDM Medical College
Dharwad, Karnataka, India

Vijay Yewale MD DCH
Head
Department of Pediatrics
Apollo Hospitals
Navi Mumbai, Maharashtra, India

Vipin M Vashishtha MD FIAP
Director and Consultant Pediatrician
Mangla Hospital and Research Center
Bijnor, Uttar Pradesh, India

Viraraghavan VR
MD DM (Neonatology) DNB (Neonatology)
(LHMC, Delhi University, Delhi)
Neonatal Intensive Care Trainee
(Funded by Fredskorpset Norway)
(OUH, Oslo, Norway)
Consultant
Department of Neonatology
Nori Multi Speciality Hospital
Vijayawada, Andhra Pradesh, India

VP Goswami
DCH PGDAP MD Phd (CM) FIAP FNNF
Assistant Professor
MGM Medical College
Indore, Madhya Pradesh, India
President NNF-2019

Zulfiqar A Bhutta MD
Center of Excellence in Women
and Child Health
The Aga Khan University
Karachi, Pakistan

Foreword

Tropical diseases are those diseases that are prevalent in or unique to tropical and subtropical regions. The diseases are less prevalent in temperate climates, due in part to the occurrence of a cold season, which controls the insect population by forcing hibernation. However, even in 17th and 18th centuries, many tropical diseases were present in northern Europe and northern America before modern understanding of disease causation. The initial impetus for tropical medicine was to protect the health of colonial settlers, notably in India under the British Raj.

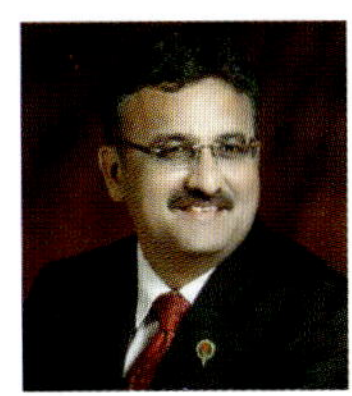

Even still in the 21st century, due to its geographic location, India is considered as a major hub of various tropical diseases. In view of the dynamic epidemiology of tropical diseases and emerging and re-emerging infections in the tropics, a comprehensive book on Tropical Diseases is a need of the time. Though there are many books available on tropical diseases, we definitely felt the void of a comprehensive book on tropical diseases from the Indian perspective. In view of these, as the President of the Indian Academy of Pediatrics (IAP), I had envisaged to bring out *IAP Textbook of Tropical Diseases* and I am happy to see the dream coming true.

I am sure that this comprehensive book will go a long way in helping to understand various aspects of Tropical Diseases in India. It will help our members and postgraduates in efficient and rational management of tropical diseases in the Indian context.

I am thankful to the editorial board of this book led by Drs Raju C Shah, Piyush Gupta, and S Balasubramanian. My sincere compliments and congratulations to all the contributors and all other members of the editorial board who have put in their sincere efforts to bring out this book and contribute in the IAP mission to disseminate knowledge through this book.

Digant D Shastri
President, 2019
Indian Academy of Pediatrics

Foreword

The world has seen a tremendous technology-driven change in the last couple of decades. Many things that were expensive and affordable only to the wealthiest people are now within the reach of the common man. The Internet, Mobile Phones, and Tablets have reduced the cost of communication nearly to zero. Ready access to knowledge is no longer the privilege of the few. Today, anybody can have ready access to the knowledge available online which would have taken us hours to find a few decades back. Also, the knowledge from across the globe is accessible right from the first day to each and every one, irrespective of the distance or amount of knowledge involved. Such is the impact of technology.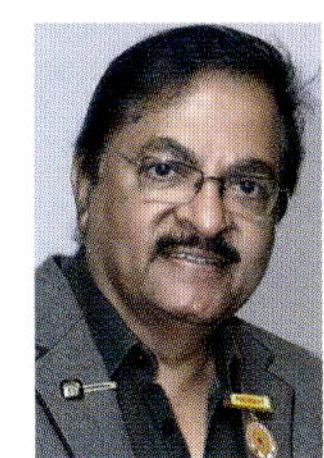

Technology is, however, not without its own limitations, one of the major ones being an explosion of online knowledge which may be often difficult to understand. In such a scenario, we must stick to the Gold standards of authors who keep on consistently giving great books year after year.

IAP Textbook of Tropical Pediatrics evolved out of various regimens of treatment developed in several pediatric wards. It was observed that busy pediatric departments, the quality of care tended to be better for daytime admissions as compared to night or during weekends. It became necessary to establish common standards of care for the guidance of interns and junior staff. These standards were further modified and simplified with experience. The facilities available for investigation and treatment are naturally better in teaching hospitals as compared to regional and district hospitals and healthcare centers. The various regimens were then further tried in these health institutions and modified in the lights of the comments received. This is an excellent book that provides essential details of several topics, relevant to a practicing pediatrician, in a lucid and easy-to-understand format.

It gives me great pleasure to write a Foreword to a book which has been edited by Dr Raju C Shah and his wonderful team. I can say that there is absolutely no compromise made to the science or the simplicity with which any pediatrician can understand the book.

I am certain that this book will be a great asset to all the practicing pediatricians and would like to take this opportunity to congratulate them on the Herculean task that they have managed together so easily once again. I would like to offer my best wishes to them and request the practicing pediatricians as well as postgraduate students to go through this manual completely from end to end so that they may derive maximum benefits from the hard work put in by Dr Raju C Shah and his entire team.

Thank you once again Sir for giving me such an honor. May you and your efficient and passionate team continue enriching our lives with your wisdom.

Bakul Jayant Parekh
National President, 2020
Indian Academy of Pediatrics

Foreword

By convention, the word "tropical" is defined as something related to the *tropics*—the warm, hot areas located between the *Tropic of Cancer* and the *Tropic of Capricorn*. These areas have some unique characteristics that make the people living there susceptible to certain diseases. The mean temperature remains above 18°C, regions are frost free, and sunlight remains intense. Thus, the tropics have either a wet season or a dry season. The conditions are ripe for the transmission of several infectious diseases; therefore, tropical areas are characterized by a higher morbidity and mortality as compared to the rest of the world.

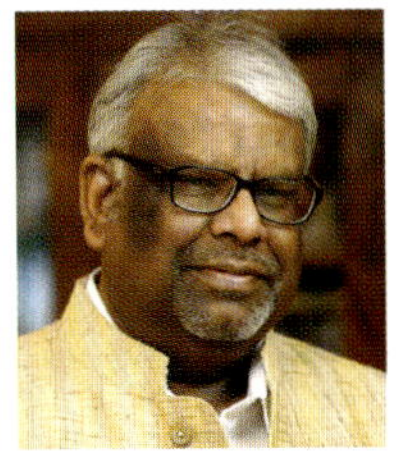

India's climate can be classified as a hot tropical country, except for a few northern and northeastern states, which have a cooler, more continental-influenced climate. Though the Tropic of Cancer—the boundary between the tropics and subtropics—passes through the middle of India, the bulk of the country can be regarded as climatically tropical. The climate can thus be classified as a typical tropical savanna or a tropical monsoon climate. It is thus, pertinent that we have a textbook devoted to the diseases that occur specifically in these climates.

I am happy to write a foreword for this unique venture by the Indian Academy of Pediatrics, conceptualized by Dr Digant D Shastri, President IAP 2019, and lead by Dr Raju C Shah with a team of able editors in Dr S Balasubramanian, Dr Abhay K Shah, Dr Jaydeep Choudhury, and Dr Ashok Gupta. I am also proud to be a part of this team as a Senior Academic Editor. The contents include not only infectious diseases typical of tropics but also other problems related to environment, nutrition, newborn health, and noncommunicable diseases. Tropical areas are also facing a double burden of diseases with diabetes, obesity, etc., being on the rise.

I am sure that the book will be equally useful to the practitioners, faculty, and students of pediatrics and will provide a new vision to look at these disorders. I am thankful to be given the honor of writing a few lines for this textbook of its own kind. Wishing all the best to the Academy and Editors for its thumping success.

Piyush Gupta MD FIAP FNNF FAMS
Professor and Head, Department of Pediatrics
University College of Medical Sciences and
Guru Teg Bahadur Hospital New Delhi, India
President-Elect, 2020
Indian Academy of Pediatrics

Preface

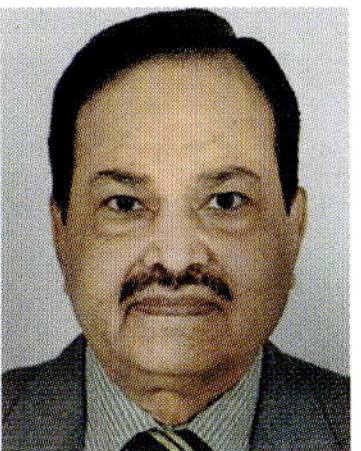

Last few decades have witnessed a rapid progress in medicine and technological advances in all the fields including Biological sciences. Most of the infectious diseases could be controlled or eliminated with good hygiene, antibiotics and vaccination in the developed world. The specialty of pediatrics has ripped benefits of further advances in preventive and therapeutic areas. This development made the biggest impact on morbidity and mortality of children in industrialized countries. As in all the fields, priorities in medicine have been dictated by power and economic dynamics for the ages. In spite of the global development impact seen in subtropical climate countries, the neglected tropical diseases can be shown to constitute a large burden on the health and economy of all the resource limited and poverty-stricken countries especially of the tropics including India. In the 21st century, in the new millennium, world leaders adopted 'The Millennium Declaration' and established Millennium Development Goals. However, the 'Neglected Tropical Diseases' were not part of such a program and did not benefit to an extent which was needed. The last few years we have witnessed emergence and re-emergence of many infectious diseases, not only in the tropics but also all over the world.

In the last decade, many books have been published on the infectious diseases and diseases affecting pediatric and adolescent population. There are also books on tropical diseases from other parts of the world, but not from resource-restricted countries. It was a felt need and rightly so President of Indian Academy of Pediatrics (IAP), Dr Digant D Shastri envisaged to publish the *IAP Textbook of Tropical Diseases* in the year 2020. His guidance and support were phenomenal.

We, the editorial board, has tried our best to make this book as comprehensive as possible with 14 sections which deals with different aspects of tropical diseases with special reference to India. We have tried to cover all the important topics, arranging them systematically starting from Epidemiology, Nutritional disorders, Neonatal problems, Infectious diseases (Bacterial, Viral, Parasitic and Protozoal and Fungal), Noncommunicable diseases, Pediatric subspecialties, Accidents and poisoning, Emergencies and intensive care, Environmental issues and certain neglected tropical diseases of our country.

We are fortunate to get authors who are experts and authorities in the subject and are from all over India. I on behalf of editorial team, thank all of them wholeheartedly because without their timely actions this book could not be published. I would like to mention name of Dr Zulfikar Bhutto from Pakistan and especially thank him for his contribution.

The editors of the book have worked as a team. They have put all their efforts and time to prepare the table of contents, select the authors, getting the manuscripts in the timeline, edit them and get the corrected proofs. They worked so meticulously and professionally that made my job very easy. I am so thankful to Drs Piyush Gupta, S Balasubramanian, Abhay K Shah, Jaydeep Choudhury and Ashok Gupta. I have no words to thank Dr Piyush Gupta whose expertise in editing the books and ever willing helping nature made my job easy and made me tension free especially in the last month of giving final shape to the book.

Our publishers M/s Jaypee Brothers Medical Publishers (P) Ltd, New Delhi, India and their staff under the leadership of Dr Savleen Kaur (Development Editor) are so good in their work with the utmost professional approach that our work of reminding authors, reediting after similarity check and proof reading became most easy and pleasant experience. Without this special team, probably this book would not have seen the light of the day.

Indian Academy of Pediatrics office and office bearers were always ready to help. President Dr Digant D Shastri has remained a constant source of guidance and support. He was like a backbone of the team. It was his vision that has come out as a book. Words are not enough to thank him. I am especially thankful to President-Elect Dr Bakul Jayant Parekh and Secretary General Dr Remesh Kumar R for time-to-time guidance and help.

We have kept practicing pediatricians and postgraduate students as target readers of this book and tried to design the book accordingly. Though we all have put our heart to bring out this book, but it is the reader's opinion which will matter the most. I request all the pediatricians and the postgraduates to give us feedback about the quality of the content and the need to improve in any of the facet of the book. We will be most happy to receive your reactions.

Raju C Shah

Contents

SECTION 4 — Bacterial and Rickettsial Infections

Section Editor: Abhay K Shah

SECTION 5 — Mycobacterial Infections
Section Editor: Abhay K Shah

SECTION 6 — Viral Infections
Section Editor: S Balasubramanian

SECTION 7 — Parasitic and Protozoal Infections/Infestations
Section Editor: Jaydeep Choudhury

ECTOPARASITES

SECTION 10 — Pediatric Subspecialties in Tropics
Section Editor: Raju C Shah

SECTION 11 — Accidents and Poisoning in the Tropics
Section Editor: Jaydeep Choudhury

Epidemiology of Tropical Diseases

Piyush Gupta

History of Tropical Pediatric Diseases

Raju C Shah

ANCIENT AFFLICTIONS OF STIGMA

All diseases that occur solely, or principally, in the tropics are Tropical Diseases as defined by the World Health Organization (WHO). A group of 13 conditions of the most common chronic infections and major disabling conditions occurring in the world's poorest people is called the neglected tropical diseases (NTDs). They are endemic in 149 countries. All these countries have differing populations and health regulations, political and legal arrangements, traditions and cultures, infrastructure and geographies as well as economies. Most of these diseases take toll of children especially those under 5 years as these diseases are not appreciated and diagnosed during this age. With progress in the areas of biology and evolution, the germ theory of disease explaining public health and hygiene, and increase in travel and exploration, historically, this led to the emergence of tropical medicine.[1]

As early as the 17th and 18th centuries, many European doctors were practicing in tropical countries such as India, the East Indies, the English West Indies (the "Sugar Islands") and later Africa, the western coast of which was widely termed the "white man's grave." Many of them had written monographs describing their experiences, with an outline of the disease pattern at these various locations which later came to be known as tropical diseases. From the 17th to 19th centuries in northern Europe and northern America, many infections which now fall under the category of "tropical" diseases were widely distributed.[2] During the Victorian era, smallpox, cholera, typhoid, plague, and typhus were major health hazards in Britain. Authors such as William Shakespeare (1564–1616) were well aware of malaria in England and John Bunyan (1628–1688) was well aware of the consumption (tuberculosis). During the 17th century, Thomas Sydenham (1624–1689) successfully used fever-tree bark (containing quinine) in the management of the "intermittent fevers." Descriptions of some of the NTDs such as leprosy, trachoma, schistosomiasis, guinea worm, and hookworm are found in the Bible, as well as in the writings of Hippocrates and other ancient texts. Such mentions are also seen in Talmud, *Papyrus Ebers* (c.1550 BC), and *Kahun papyrus* (c.1900 BC).[3] Some texts have mentioned about Joshua's curse and the abandonment of Jericho's walls attributed to schistosomiasis, while guinea worms (*Dracunculus medinensis*) are believed to be the "fiery serpents" that attacked the Israelites in the desert during their exodus from Egypt. These diseases were also termed as ancient affliction of stigma.

Since most of these so-called tropical diseases were prevalent in their own countries, European doctors laid emphasis on tropical medicine in many developing countries including India in the 17th and 18th centuries, more importantly due to military necessity. It has been believed by many that tropical medicine has originated during the period when the British Empire and Raj was expanding to more and more tropical countries.[1] To preserve the health of the British personnel, both when overseas and following return to Britain, the colonial rulers with a vested interest evolved the discipline. In the 19th century when the British Empire was expanding, tropical diseases caused high morbidity among "servants of the Raj." Joseph Chamberlain, Secretary of State for the Colonies, understood the necessity of training British doctors in this discipline of medicine. He considered that tropical medicine becomes a "colonial science" as was crucial to the realization of British economic and social imperialism.

The development of clinical parasitology following the work of Manson, Ross, and others, and superimposed on this complex backcloth, led to the inevitable genesis of "tropical medicine" as a formal discipline. The work on the role of mosquito in the transmission of malaria, which was carried out in India and was published by Ronald Ross in the year 1897 in the *British Medical Journal*, helped in boosting research by British doctors in specialty of tropical medicine. On October 2, 1899, the School of Tropical Medicine in London was set up as a result of these developments. There was a statement in the inaugural address that, "The school (of tropical medicine) strikes, and strikes effectively, at the root of the principal difficulty of most of our colonies—disease." Similarly in 1920 in India at Calcutta (now Kolkata) the British Raj established the first school of tropical medicine. Since low priority was given to tropical medicine in socioeconomically backward countries including India, with changing times the future of the discipline became uncertain.

In developed countries including Britain, the priority of tropical diseases lessened gradually as a result of the end of colonialism after the Second World War and certain other changes including change in priorities and financial crisis. Until the mid-20th century, due to improved hygiene and sanitation and better standards of living in these countries, infectious diseases including tropical diseases that dominated the burden of diseases showed a declining trend. In the 1940s and 1950s, with the advent of antibiotics, the whole scenario changed. Dr William H Stewart, US Surgeon General (1965–1969), a distinguished member of the US Public Health Services Corps, told *the US* Congress in 1967 that it was time to "close the book *on infectious diseases*, declare the *war against* pestilence *won*, and shift national resources to such chronic problems as cancer and heart *disease*." This created big impact; the discipline of tropical medicine, which had reached its peak during the British Raj, started losing its pride of place among the developed countries. A classic medical book in print since more than half a century, Davidson's *Principles and Practice of Medicine*, had a separate supplement on tropical diseases till the mid-1970s, which almost disappeared in the late 70s and 80s suggesting that these diseases were disappearing from western world. The Rockefeller Foundation in earlier time was supporting Schools of Public Health in developing countries, which in 1970s and 1980s started sponsoring Clinical Epidemiology Training Programs to make clinicians competent to carry out other and different clinical trials.

In developing regions of Africa, Asia, Central America, and South America, during this period, neglected infectious diseases were disproportionately affecting poor and marginalized populations; to focus on this, in 1975, at the WHO, the Special Programme for Research and Training in Tropical Diseases (TDR) was established. For this program, the WHO is the executing agency and is cosponsored by the United Nations Children's Fund, the United Nations Development Programme, the World Bank and the WHO.[4,5] In September 2000, to eliminate extreme poverty, hunger, and disease by 2015, world leaders at the United Nations adopted the Millennium Declaration, which established an ambitious set of eight millennium development goals. The sixth goal of this declaration, "to combat HIV-AIDS (human immunodeficiency virus infection–acquired immunodeficiency syndrome), malaria, and other diseases," specifically addresses some of the NTDs. Large-scale financial support such as the US President's Malaria Initiative and the Global Fund to Fight AIDS, Tuberculosis, and Malaria is all due to this initiative. To explain in terms of disease burden and human toll from the NTDs, it is better to use the disability-adjusted life year (DALY) as a metric. The NTDs account for approximately one-quarter of the global disease burden from malaria as well as HIV-AIDS when measured in DALYs (Murray, 1996). Recently new studies are pointing out the hidden morbidity and mortality of chronic infections with schistosomiasis, onchocerciasis, and other NTDs (King et al., 2005; Little et al., 2004; Hotez et al., 2004a) suggesting that even these high DALY figures are probably underestimates.

In December 2003, at an International Workshop in Berlin, for control and elimination of a group of neglected diseases, the WHO initiated a new approach, a paradigm shift.[6] This shift is to focus on strategy to an integrated response to the health needs of impoverished and marginalized communities, from a traditional approach centered on specific diseases. Further to this in 2005, the WHO proposed to use a sharply focused term "neglected tropical diseases" in place of the vaguely defined term "other communicable diseases" following the second meeting of partners in Berlin. Dealing of NTDs with a new approach is a result of proper encapsulation of the paradigm shift. Many parties concerned with improving the health of the millions of people suffering from NTDs wanted to work in cohesion and so there was an urgent and important need to find a means of steering them. To meet this need in 2005, the WHO established the Department for Control of Neglected Tropical Diseases (WHO/NTD) at its headquarters in Geneva, Switzerland. The first meeting of Global Partners on NTDs, dedicated to contributing their efforts and resources to tackling these diseases, convened by the WHO in April 2007, was attended by more than 200 participants, including representatives from Member States, United Nations agencies, the World Bank, philanthropic foundations, universities, pharmaceutical companies, international NGOs, and other institutions.

A report on NTDs which included a range of diseases caused by individual pathogens, and groups of conditions caused by related microbial species, was published first of its kind by the WHO in 2010. As listed in **Box 1**, 17 conditions were considered as the main NTDs in this report.[6]

As per available data, 534,000 deaths annually (approximately) in the year 2004 were attributed to the NTDs.[5] As shown in **Figure 1**, they rank closely in terms of DALYs with the most important health problems in the developing world such as diarrheal diseases, ischemic heart disease, cerebrovascular diseases, malaria, and tuberculosis. Even the latest Global Burden of Disease Study (GBD) from 2017 provides very scary estimates, which is often underappreciated. NTDs and malaria together cause an estimated 720,100 deaths and 62 million

DALYs, which rank these conditions at par with our leading global health threats. Looking closely at the GBD 2017 numbers, especially at various age groups, highlight the fact that approximately one-half of those deaths and DALYs are in children under the age of 5 years, whereas approximately two-thirds of deaths and DALYs are in children and adolescents under the age of 20 years. This reiterates that what we know as the field of tropical medicine is in true sense the field of tropical pediatrics.

To address the NTDs of children worldwide over and above the workforce, there is an urgent need to apply new technologies. The major product development partnerships for these diseases prepared a consensus document in 2016,[6] but it needs to be updated recognizing that in the last few years, innovation in the area of global health has seen remarkable shifts. It is realized that major stress as well as focus should be on the needs of pediatric tropical medicine. Inventions of so many new basic science approaches in medicine, such as sci-RNA-seq (single-cell combinatorial indexing RNA sequencing), functional and comparative OMICs, gene editing, and systems biology, need to be applied in this field also. It was felt that we need new and alternative funding streams for such applications. For the support of new diagnostics, drugs, and vaccines, the world is seeing change in the governance also, some of which may be similar to the installation of new global health leaders. In the year 2017, the Global Health Task Force of the American Board of Pediatrics (ABP) emphasized on seven "guiding principles"—equity, sustainability, mutual benefit, humility, inclusivity, social justice, and prevention of adverse impact—and four "core practices" of communications, leadership, conflict resolution, and evaluation in the mechanisms for

---

Box 1: Main neglected tropical diseases.

The main neglected tropical diseases:
- Dengu
- Rabies
- Trachoma
- Buruli ulcer
- Endemic treponematoses (including yaws)
- Leprosy
- Chagas disease (American trypanosomiasis)
- Human African trypanosomiasis (sleeping sickness)
- Leishmaniasis
- Cysticercosis
- Dracunculiasis (Guinea-worm disease)
- Echinococcosis
- Foodborne trematode infections
- Lymphatic filariasis (elephantiasis)
- Onchocerciasis (river blindness)
- Schistosomiasis (bilharziasis)
- Soil-transmitted helminthiases (intestinal parasitic worms)

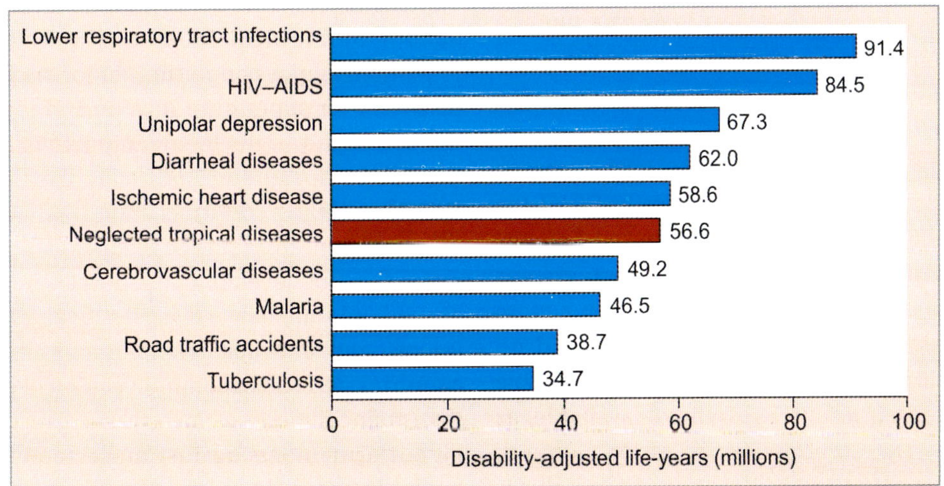

Fig. 1: Disability-adjusted life-years with the most important health problems in the developing world.

advancing global child health systems by partnerships.[6,7] An organized antiscience movement in the last few years has threatened these activities which include anti-vaccine initiative in the US, Europe, and now in Asian countries.

The vision of TDR is to give impetus to an effective global research effort on infectious diseases persisted due to poverty, in which disease-endemic countries have to play a pivotal role. It has a dual mission of developing new tools and strategies against these diseases and of developing the research and leadership capacity in the countries where the diseases occur. Some examples of work include helping to develop new treatments for diseases, such as ivermectin for onchocerciasis (river blindness), showing how packaging can improve use of artemisinin-combination treatment (ACT) for malaria, demonstrating the effectiveness of bed nets to prevent mosquito bites and malaria, and documenting how community-based and community-led programs increase distribution of multiple treatments. Using private sector approaches to attack R&D challenges and to develop products for developing countries is a big step forward by nonprofits that embrace industry practices and collaboration. This is known as the Product Development–Private-Public-Partnership (PD–PPP).[5] Vaccine development initiatives for leishmaniasis, hookworm, and infectious diarrheas, and drug development initiatives for leishmaniasis, African trypanosomiasis, and Chagas disease are examples of such new PPPs **(Box 2)**.[5] For the control or elimination of the seven most prevalent neglected tropical diseases—ascariasis, trichuriasis, hookworm infection, schistosomiasis, lymphatic filariasis, trachoma, and onchocerciasis—a blueprint developed by a group of private, public, and international organizations working together with pharmaceutical partners and national ministries of health is a very welcome step. The Bill and Melinda Gates Foundation's contribution in 1999 played a major role in giving big push in the funding PPPs (referred to as "push mechanisms") which worked as a major stimulus to establish such partnership. With updated guidelines for drug administration issued by the WHO, the newly established Global Network for Neglected Tropical Diseases has provided a platform to these partnerships for coordinating their activities in order to launch a more integrated assault on these conditions.[8] A scaled-up approach to simple interventions could lead to sustainable decreases in poverty if resources are made available, as recommended by the Commission for Africa. Some of the world's poorest countries may see new dawn if this is

> **Box 2:** Major public-private-partnerships committed to the neglected tropical diseases.
>
> - Drugs for Neglected Diseases initiative – DNDi (Geneva)
> - WHO partnership for parasite control – PPC (Geneva)
> - Institute for OneWorld Health (IOWH) (San Francisco, CA)
> - Diseases of the most impoverished - DOMI (Seoul, Korea)
> - Human Hookworm Vaccine Initiative – HHVI (Washington, DC)
> - International trachoma initiative (New York)
> - Infectious diseases research institute (Seattle, WA)
> - Global Alliance to Eliminate Lymphatic Filariasis (Liverpool, UK)
> - Schistosomiasis control initiative (London, UK and Boston, MA)
> - African Programme for Onchocerciasis Control (APOC)
> - Onchocerciasis Elimination Programme in the Americas (OEPA)

(WHO: World Health Organization)

realized and would represent a major success story for the United Nations Millennium Declaration.

Recent Ebola, Zika, Chikungunya, Nipah, and yellow fever outbreaks have warned the world including the developed countries that how the tropical diseases can reemerge or expand their ranges and cause havoc in a short span of time. Over and above these infectious diseases, many tropical countries are also witnessing increasing burden of chronic and degenerative diseases because of an epidemiological transition and other socioeconomic and health factors. It is realized by all the authorities that the tropical diseases can have great impact on tourists, business travelers, expatriate workers, migrants, and refugees in endemic regions, and in turn travel can also facilitate the spread of infectious diseases globally.

The vast variety of diseases prevalent in tropical countries provides research opportunities to doctors practicing in these areas and should take full advantage of the opportunities. "The malaria vaccine is the biggest need, but it gets virtually no funding, but male baldness does," philanthropic investor Bill Gates laments.[5] Sir Patrick Manson, one of the founder fathers of the London School of Tropical Medicine, stated, "The tropical practitioner enjoys opportunities for original research and discovery far superior in novelty and interest to those at the command of his fellow inquirer in the well-worked field of European and American research." Researchers from developing countries should take inspiration from this statement from one of the great scientists. If medical researchers of developing countries where these diseases are endemic and newer diseases are emerging will not take interest and show leadership, minor ailments of affluent countries and socioeconomic class will get more priority than major ailments of poverty. It is time to get started with all our armaments against neglected diseases affecting pediatric population of tropical countries.

■ REFERENCES

1. Banerjee A. The British Raj and rise and fall of tropical medicine. Medical Journal of Dr. D.Y. Patil Vidyapeeth. 2013;6(2):121-2.
2. Farrar J, Hotez P, Junghanss T, et al. History of Tropical Medicine, and Medicine in the Tropics. Manson's Tropical Diseases, 23rd edition. Edinburgh: Saunders Elsevier; 2013. pp. 1-8.
3. Hotez P, Ottesen E, Fenwick A, et al. The neglected tropical diseases: the ancient afflictions of stigma and poverty and the prospects for their control and elimination. In: Pollard AJ, Finn A (Eds). Hot Topics in Infection and Immunity in Children. New York: Springer; 2006.
4. Hotez PJ, Odom John AR, LaBeaud AD. Pediatric tropical medicine: The neglected diseases of children. PLoS Negl Trop Dis. 2019;13(5):e0007008.
5. Hotez PJ, Molyneux DH, Fenwick A, et al. Current concepts: control of neglected tropical diseases. N Engl J Med. 2007; 357:1018-27.
6. World Health Organization. Intensified Control of Neglected Diseases–Report of an International Workshop Berlin, 10–12 December 2003; 2004. [online] Available from: https://apps.who.int/iris/bitstream/handle/10665/68529/WHO_CDS_CPE_CEE_2004.45.pdf;jsessionid=0F5469D0335DDFA1499EBAF53D680D80? sequence=1. [Last accessed on November, 2019].
7. World Health Organization. Working to overcome the global impact of neglected diseases; First WHO report on Neglected Tropical diseases (2010). [online] Available from: https://apps.who.int/iris/bitstream/handle/10665/44440/9789241564090_eng.pdf?sequence=1. [Last accessed on November, 2019].
8. World Health Organization. Accelerating work to overcome the global impact of Neglected Tropical Diseases: A Roadmap for Implementation (2010). [online] Available from: https://apps.who.int/iris/bitstream/handle/10665/70809/WHO_HTM_NTD_2012.1_eng.pdf?sequence=1. [Last accessed on November, 2019].

Burden of Childhood Diseases in Tropics

Chabungbam Smilie, Piyush Gupta

WHAT ARE TROPICAL DISEASES?

Tropical diseases are a group of parasitic, bacterial, viral, and fungal infections that are uniquely more prevalent in the tropical and subtropical areas.[1] The term "tropics" refers to the geographical areas between the tropic of cancer and the tropic of capricorn; and the aterm "subtropics" covers the areas just outside the tropic zone latitudinally. These include sub-Saharan Africa, China, South Asia, and the Americas—Latin America and the Caribbean.[2] South Asia incorporates the nations of India, Afghanistan, Bangladesh, Bhutan, Nepal, Pakistan, Maldives, and Sri Lanka. These countries represent almost one-quarter of the global population, with India accounting for approximately 75% of the total population living in South Asia.[3] Diseases prevalent in these areas are typically infectious, although noninfectious diseases are also accelerating in the aforementioned areas. These diseases not only account for significant morbidities and mortality, but also affect certain subsets of the population disproportionately, especially children, and often impose a large share of economic burden. Later, they often cause disfigurement, social stigma, considerable morbidities and mortality.

PORTFOLIO OF TROPICAL DISEASES

Broadly, tropical diseases include the following:[1]
- Vaccine-preventable diseases, e.g. rabies, Japanese encephalitis
- Diseases responsible for major epidemics and those endemic in certain geographical areas, e.g. malaria, dengue, Chagas disease, human African trypanosomiasis
- Relatively neglected tropical diseases (NTDs), e.g. hookworm infestation, schistosomiasis, lymphatic filariasis, leishmaniasis, etc.

The NTD roadmap 2021–2030 of the World Health Organization (WHO) is mainly focused on 20 NTDs, which include Buruli ulcer, Chagas disease, chikungunya, cysticercosis, dengue fever and severe dengue, dracunculiasis, echinococcosis, human African trypanosomiasis, leishmaniasis (kala-azar), leprosy, lymphatic filariasis, onchocerciasis, rabies, schistosomiasis, soil-transmitted helminthiasis (ascariasis, hookworm infestation, trichuriasis), trachoma, foodborne trematodiasis (clonorchiasis, fascioliasis, opisthorchiasis, and paragonimiasis), and yaws and other vector-borne diseases.[4,5] Other vector-borne diseases include malaria, Rift Valley fever, yellow fever, Zika virus infection, Japanese encephalitis, West Nile fever, sandfly fever (phlebotomus fever), Crimean-Congo hemorrhagic fever, Lyme disease, rickettsial diseases (spotted fever and Q fever), tick-borne encephalitis, tularemia, plague, rickettsiosis, typhus, and louse-borne relapsing fever. The WHO included mycetoma, scabies and snake-bite in the list of NTDs at the 10th meeting of the Strategic and Technical Advisory Group for NTDs in 2017.[5] Today, these diseases are endemic in 149 countries, affecting 1 billion people, mostly infants and children, and are focused more in areas of urban and rural poverty. Major NTDs listed by WHO and Center for Disease Control and Prevention (CDC) are shown in **Table 1**.[5,6] Other diseases which are not included in the NTDs but are more prevalent in the tropics include pneumonia, diarrhea, malnutrition, iron deficiency anemia (IDA), vitamin A deficiency, iodine deficiency disorders, etc.

BURDEN OF TROPICAL DISEASES

Global Burden

The burden of tropical diseases differs significantly according to various geographical regions, which include

Table 1: Major neglected tropical diseases (NTDs) listed by the World Health Organization (WHO)[5] and Center for Disease Control and Prevention (CDC).[6]

Diseases	WHO	CDC
Buruli ulcer (*Mycobacterium ulcerans* infection)	+	+
Chagas disease	+	+
Chikungunya	+	
Cysticercosis	+	+
Dengue fever and severe dengue	+	+
Dracunculiasis (Guinea-worm disease)	+	+
Echinococcosis	+	+
Foodborne trematodiasis	+	
Human African trypanosomiasis (sleeping sickness)	+	+
Human rabies	+	+
Leishmaniasis (kala-azar)	+	+
Onchocerciasis (river blindness)	+	+
Schistosomiasis	+	+
Soil-transmitted helminthiasis (ascariasis, hookworm infestation, trichuriasis)	+	+
Trachoma	+	+
Yaws	+	+
Other vector borne diseases	+	+
Mycetoma	+	
Scabies	+	
Snakebite	+	

sub-Saharan Africa, China, South Asia, and the Americas—Latin America and the Caribbean. These diseases are more focused in areas of poverty, and affect specific subsets of the population, especially children. More than one billion people, or almost one-sixth of the world's population suffer from one or more of the major NTDs.[7] However, the burden of tropical diseases stratified by age is seldom available.

The disease burden is generally expressed in terms of disability-adjusted life years (DALYs). DALY is calculated as the summation of years of life lost (YLL) and years lived with disability (YLD). According to the WHO 2015 data on 14 out of 20 NTDs, the global burden attributed to the NTDs was estimated to be 25,135.59 thousand DALYs lost.[8] These diseases account for approximately 25% of the DALYs and 10% of the total mortality contributed by communicable diseases.[9] The diseases responsible for majority of the burden are soil-transmitted helminthiasis (ascariasis, hookworm infestation, and trichuriasis), schistosomiasis, dengue fever, lymphatic filariasis, human

rabies, leishmaniasis, onchocerciasis, and foodborne trematodiasis. However, data for YLL were not available for hookworm infestation, lymphatic filariasis, onchocerciasis, trachoma, and trichuriasis, so interpretation of the WHO 2015 data on DALYs should be done with caution. The global burden of major NTDs as estimates of DALYs according to the data published in WHO, Health Statistics and Information Systems (2015)[8] are compared with previous data reported by Bhutta et al. (published in 2014, using DALY estimates by WHO for 2010),[10] Hotez et al. [2014, using Global Burden of Disease (GBD) Study 2010][11] and Mathers et al.[12] (2007, using the WHO data 2002) in **Table 2**. According to the GBD 2010 study, the total burden of NTDs as estimated by DALYs was 26.06 million years, with maximum burden attributed to soil-transmitted helminthiasis, followed by leishmaniasis, schistosomiasis, lymphatic filariasis, and food-borne trematodiasis.

According to the GBD 2017 study, malaria and NTDs are ranked among the leading global health threats, with an estimated 720,100 deaths and 62 million DALYs.[13-15] Among these, it can be highlighted that one-half of the total deaths and DALYs affect children under 5 years of age; and two-third of deaths and DALYs affect children and adolescents less than 20 years of age.[16] The most ubiquitous tropical diseases found in children less than 5 years of age are malaria, followed by soil-transmitted helminthiasis (ascariasis, hookworm infestation, and trichuriasis), and dengue.[16] Similar pattern follows for children and adolescents under 20 years of age, although schistosomiasis is also common in this group of children and adolescents. Common childhood tropical diseases are ranked in terms of their prevalence and incidence in **Table 3**.

Tropical Diseases in South Asia and India

In 2018, South Asian nations represent a total population of 1.8 billion, or almost 25% of the world's population.[17] The region accounts for almost one-quarter of the global soil-transmitted helminth infections, one-half of the total burden of lymphatic filariasis, visceral leishmaniasis and leprosy, and more than one-third of the global deaths from rabies.[3] Major NTDs in India and Southeast Asia include the following—ascariasis, trichuriasis, hookworm infection, lymphatic filariasis, trachoma, visceral leishmaniasis, leprosy, and rabies.[3] Besides these, there is also an emerging burden of major arbovirus infections, namely Japanese encephalitis, dengue, and chikungunya.

Today, India is the second most populous country in the world, with a population of 1.35 billion which is almost 18% of the world's population and 75% of the population

Table 2: Comparison of global burden of major tropical diseases as estimates of disability-adjusted life years (DALYs) (in thousands) in last decade.

Disease	WHO 2015 Data[8]	Bhutta et al.[10] (WHO 2010)	Hotez et al.[11] (GBD 2010)	Mathers et al.[12] (WHO 2002)
Soil-transmitted helminthiasis	4,443.47	5,043	5,190	3,796
Ascariasis	1,094.67	1,254	1,320	1,817
Trichuriasis	542.80	630	640	1,006
Hookworm infestation	1,739.58	3,159	3,230	973
Schistosomiasis	3,513.85	3,971	3,310	1,702
Dengue fever	2,610.08	1,243	830	616
Lymphatic filariasis	2,070.85	2,740	2,780	5,777
Cysticercosis	1,856.36	503	500	–
Rabies	1,672.17	2,297	1,460	–
Leishmaniasis	1,356.46	3,754	3,320	2,090
Onchocerciasis	1,135.57	564	490	484
Foodborne trematodiasis	1,066.34	665	1,880	–
Echinococcosis	641.43	600	140	–
Leprosy	488.64	215	–	198
Human African trypanosomiasis	371.65	1,346	560	1,525
Trachoma	278.97	308	330	2,329
Chagas disease	252.70	499	550	667

(GBD: Global Burden of Disease; WHO: World Health Organization)

Table 3: Prevalence of most common tropical diseases in children and adolescents under 20 years of age.[16]

	Prevalence (million)		Percentage of global DALYs (%)	
Disease	Children under 5 years	Children and adolescents <20 years	Children under 5 years	Children and adolescents <20 years
Malaria*	77.0	155.3	69	82
Ascariasis	45.3	221.9	32	66
Dengue*	7.2	43.0	23	50
Hookworm infestation	16.7	93.3	7	41
Trichuriasis	13.4	109.1	3	38

*Data given as incidence (million).
(DALYs: disability-adjusted life years)

in South Asia.[17] The country accounts for the world's largest absolute burden of major NTDs—ascariasis, hookworm infestation, trichuriasis, dengue, lymphatic filariasis, trachoma, cysticercosis, echinococcosis, visceral leishmaniasis, and rabies **(Table 4)**.[15,18] According to the GBD 2016 study, India accounts for almost one-half of the global prevalence of visceral leishmaniasis, and nearly one-half of the world's total incidence of dengue and visual impairment due to trachoma.[15] Additionally, India also accounts for almost one-quarter of the global prevalent cases of ascariasis and hookworm infestation.[18]

EPIDEMIOLOGY OF MAJOR CHILDHOOD TROPICAL DISEASES

Brief descriptions of major tropical diseases are described as follows.

Dengue Fever and Severe Hemorrhagic Dengue

Dengue fever is a viral illness, caused by four serotypes of the Flaviviridae family (DEN-1, DEN-2, DEN-3, and DEN-4), which is transmitted by female mosquitoes of the species *Aedes aegypti* and *Aedes albopictus*. The disease is distributed throughout the tropics, mainly influenced

Table 4: Major neglected tropical diseases (NTDs) in India.[15,18]

| Disease | Number of cases | | % of cases in India | India's rank globally |
	Global	India		
Ascariasis	799.7 million	222.2 million	28	1
Hookworm infestation	450.7 million	102.4 million	23	1
Trichuriasis	435.1 million	67.8 million	16	1
Dengue	101.1 million	53.2 million	53	1
Lymphatic filariasis	29.4 million	8.7 million	29	
Trachoma (visual impairment)	3.3 million	1.8 million	53	1
Cysticercosis	2.7 million	0.82 million	31	1
Echinococcosis	973,662	119,320	12	1
Visceral leishmaniasis	30,067	13,530	45	1
Rabies	13,340	4,370	33	1

by heavy rainfall, hot and humid climate, and rapid urbanization. Approximately 3.9 billion people living in the tropics and subtropics are at risk, of which 390 million people acquire the infection each year and 96 million manifest clinically.[19,20] According to WHO, the number of cases reported has increased dramatically over the last few years, from 2.2 million in 2010 to 3.34 million in 2016, with the cases widely distributed over the Americas, Southeast Asia, and Western Pacific.[21] Among the total number of cases, approximately 500,000 people develop severe dengue per year, with a case-fatality rate of 2.5% annually. Since 2006, Delhi (India) recorded its worst outbreak in 2015 with more than 15,000 cases.

Dengue fever affects infants, young children, and adults. The infection causes fever and flu-like illness, and may potentially lead to lethal complications. Treatment is supportive with analgesics (acetaminophen), fluid replacement, and bed rest. Severe cases may require platelet transfusion or whole blood transfusion. Methods to control and prevent the disease include vector-control measures, removing artificial habitats for mosquitoes, improving community participation, and public health measures.

Soil-transmitted Helminthiasis

Soil-transmitted helminthiasis is a group of parasitic infections caused by intestinal nematodes, which are transmitted through soil contaminated with eggs present in human feces. Three main parasites that infect humans include roundworm (*Ascaris lumbricoides*), hookworms (*Necator americanus* and *Ancylostoma duodenale*), and whipworm (*Trichuris trichiura*). Almost 1.5 billion people, or one-quarter of the world's population, are infected with helminthiasis globally, with maximum

distribution in the tropical and subtropical regions of sub-Saharan Africa, East Asia, China, and the Americas.[22] Approximately 267 million preschool-age children and over 568 million school-age children are at risk of acquiring the infection.[22]

Children infected with these intestinal parasites lead to anemia, malnutrition, impaired growth and development, and cognitive delay. Prevention and control measures include health education on proper hygiene and encouraging healthy behaviors, e.g. proper handwashing technique and maintaining adequate sanitation. WHO recommends the drugs—albendazole (400 mg) and mebendazole (500 mg). Approximately 598 million children, which account to 69% of all children at risk received antihelminthic drugs in 2017.[22] Currently, the global target is elimination of morbidity due to helminthiases in children by 2020. This will be achieved by covering at least 75% of the children in endemic regions with antihelminthic drugs (at-risk population estimated was 836 million in 2016).

Schistosomiasis

Schistosomiasis is a parasitic disease caused by trematode worms (blood flukes) of the genus *Schistosoma*. The infection is acquired through contact with contaminated water, infested with the larval forms of the parasite which are released by freshwater snails. The disease is prevalent in the tropical and subtropical countries, especially in communities with unsafe drinking water and poor sanitation. School-age children are especially vulnerable to the infection because of improper hygiene and certain play habits, e.g. swimming and fishing in unsafe water infested with the parasite. In 2017, there were approximately 220.8 million people at risk for the disease of which 102.3 million people or 46% of the total at risk population were treated.[23] Almost 90% of those people requiring treatment live in Africa.

There are two main forms of the disease—*intestinal* and *urogenital*. Intestinal schistosomiasis causes abdominal pain, diarrhea, and blood in stools. Hepatomegaly, splenomegaly, and ascites may be present. Urogenital schistosomiasis is classically associated with hematuria. In advanced cases, there may be fibrosis of the bladder and ureters and kidney damage. The WHO-recommended drug is praziquantel. Control measures include large-scale treatment of at-risk population, health education on proper hygiene and adequate sanitation, access to clean and safe water, and snail control.

Malaria

Malaria is a febrile illness caused by *Plasmodium* parasites, which are transmitted by the bites of female *Anopheles* mosquitoes. *Plasmodium falciparum* and *Plasmodium vivax* are the two species that pose the greatest threat. In 2017, *P. falciparum* was responsible for a majority of the cases reported in the WHO African Region (99.7%), Southeast Asia (62.8%), the Eastern Mediterranean (69%) and the Western Pacific (71.9%), while *P. vivax* accounted for 74.1% of the malaria cases in the WHO region of the Americas.[24] There were 219 million cases of malaria reported in 2017 from 87 countries.[24] Five countries were responsible for almost half of the global burden of malaria: Nigeria (25%), the Democratic Republic of the Congo (11%), Mozambique (5%), India (4%) and Uganda (4%).[24] The most affected subset of the population are under-five children, with 266,000 deaths, accounting for 61% of the total malaria deaths in 2017.[24]

Symptoms include fever with chills, malaise, headache, and may progress to severe disease, particularly in children. Hypoglycemia, severe anemia, respiratory distress due to metabolic acidosis, and cerebral malaria are manifestations of severe malaria in children. Any child with suspected malaria should be confirmed with parasite-based diagnostic testing (microscopy or rapid diagnostic test) before treatment is initiated. Preventive measures include vector control, use of long-lasting insecticidal nets, etc.

Japanese Encephalitis

Japanese encephalitis is a viral disease caused by a *Flavivirus*, transmitted by infected mosquitoes of the species *Culex*. According to WHO, an estimated 68,000 cases occur each year, with a majority of cases occurring in the Southeast Asian and Western Pacific regions.[25] Approximately 13,600–20,400 Japanese encephalitis deaths occur every year worldwide.

In children, gastrointestinal symptoms including abdominal pain and vomiting may be the initial dominant symptoms. Severe disease is associated with high-grade fever, headache, neck rigidity, altered sensorium, seizures, and ultimately death. Case-fatality rate is as high as 30% and among those who survive, almost 20–30% have neurological sequelae, such as intellectual impairment, behavioral problems, epilepsy, paralysis, inability to speak, etc.

Chikungunya

Chikungunya is a mosquito-borne viral illness caused by a virus belonging to the family Togaviridae. It is transmitted by the bites of female mosquitoes of the species *Aedes aegypti* and *Aedes albopictus*. The disease is identified over 60 countries and mostly occurs in the regions of Indian subcontinent, Asia, and Africa.[26] Over 1.9 million cases have been reported from India, Indonesia, Maldives, Myanmar, and Thailand since 2005.

Chikungunya causes fever, severe debilitating joint pain and muscle pain, headache, nausea, vomiting, fatigue, and rash. There is no specific cure for the disease, and treatment is usually focused on symptomatic management. Preventive and control measures include vector control, spraying of insecticides to kill mosquitoes and treating water containers, using bed-nests, long-sleeved shirts, and mosquito repellants.

Leishmaniasis

Leishmaniasis is a vector-borne illness caused by the protozoan *Leishmania donovani* parasites which are transmitted by infected female sandflies (*Phlebotomus argentipes*). The disease affects the poorest people, with an estimation of 700,000 to 1 million new cases and 26,000–65,000 deaths each year, according to WHO data.[27] It is associated with malnutrition, migration of nonimmune people into endemic areas, and incursion into forests. More than 95% of the new cases reported to WHO in 2017 occur mainly in 10 nations—India, China, Nepal, Bangladesh, Kenya, Ethiopia, Somalia, Brazil, South Sudan, and Sudan.

There are three forms of the disease—(1) visceral leishmaniasis (also called kala-azar, most serious form), (2) cutaneous (most frequent), and (3) mucocutaneous. Visceral leishmaniasis or kala-azar is the main form of the disease in Southeast Asia region; however, the region is also endemic for cutaneous leishmaniasis. Approximately 5–10% of cases with kala-azar develop into post-kala-azar dermal leishmaniasis, and mainly occurs in East Africa and Indian subcontinent. Treatment depends on the type of the disease. All cases of visceral leishmaniasis require complete treatment, while cutaneous lesions may heal with local therapy, if large ulcers or lesions are present over face, joints, fingers, disfiguring lesions, and systemic therapy may be required. Drugs recommended include liposomal amphotericin B, pentavalent antimonials, combination regimens of miltefosine, and paromomycin for visceral leishmaniasis. Local therapy for cutaneous leishmaniasis include methylbenzethonium chloride, intralesional antimonials, thermotherapy, while systemic therapy for the same includes fluconazole, ketoconazole, pentavalent antimonials, and amphotericin B.

Foodborne Trematodiases

Foodborne trematodiases are caused by flukes (*Clonorchis sinensis, Opisthorchis viverrini, Fasciola hepatica,* and *Paragonimus spp.*). Infections are acquired through the consumption of raw or undercooked fish, crustaceans and vegetables that harbor the parasites. It is estimated that almost 200,000 infections and more than 7,000 deaths occur each year, leading to more than 2 million DALYs globally.[28] While clonorchiasis and opisthorchiasis are confined to Asia, paragonimiasis is distributed over the regions of Asia, Africa, and Latin America.

Symptoms include general malaise and abdominal pain. Clonorchiasis and opisthorchiasis may lead to cholangiocarcinoma while fascioliasis causes inflammation and fibrosis of large bile ducts and gall bladder, colic pain, jaundice, liver fibrosis, and anemia. Paragonimiasis causes chronic cough, associated with blood-stained sputum, dyspnea, and fever. Treatment includes administration of praziquantel and triclabendazole.

Rabies

Rabies is a fatal viral disease, which occurs in all continents, except Antarctica, across 150 nations, with more than 95% deaths in Asia and Africa.[5] The infection is transmitted to humans by rabid dogs in almost 99% of the cases. Children between 5 years and 15 years of age are the frequent victims. More than half of the global burden of the disease occurs in South-Asian countries, with India accounting for 17,000–20,000 of the total 55,000–70,000 deaths that occur globally per year.[29,30] The postexposure prophylaxis recommended by WHO includes immediate extensive local wound management and administration of a course of effective and potent rabies vaccine.[31] For high-risk exposures, rabies immunoglobulin should be given.

Yaws

Yaws is a chronic debilitating disease of childhood, caused by *Treponema pallidum* subspecies *pertenue*. The disease primarily affects the poorest people, living in the warm, humid and tropical forests of Asia, Africa, Latin America, and the Pacific. A majority of the affected population are children under 15 years of age, accounting for almost 75–80% of the total cases.[32] In 2018, a total of 80,472 suspected cases of yaws were reported to WHO, among which 888 cases were confirmed. India was declared to be free of yaws in May 2016.[32]

Lymphatic Filariasis

Lymphatic filariasis is a chronic disfiguring illness caused by nematodes of the family Filarioidea. *Wuchereria bancrofti* is responsible for a majority (>90%) of the cases worldwide, while *Brugia malayi* and *Brugia timori* can cause the disease in Asia.[33] The disease is transmitted by different types of mosquitoes, depending on the geographical area—*Anopheles* in Africa, *Culex quinquefasciatus* in America, *Aedes* and *Mansonia* in Asia, and the Pacific. Most of the infections are acquired during childhood, causing hidden damage to the lymphatic system and leading to elephantiasis and marked swelling in genitals (hydrocele, scrotal swelling). At present, it is estimated that 886 million people living in 52 countries are still at risk of infection and require preventive chemotherapy.[33]

Diethylcarbamazine citrate (DEC) is the drug of choice; however, DEC should not be given in patients coinfected with onchocerciasis as the same may aggravate the eye disease. WHO recommends mass drug administration (MDA) for prevention of lymphatic filariasis: albendazole (400 mg) twice per year in areas co-endemic with loiasis, ivermectin (200 mcg/kg) plus albendazole (400 mg) in regions with onchocerciasis, and ivermectin (200 mcg/kg) plus DEC (6 mg/kg), and albendazole (400 mg) in countries without onchocerciasis.[33]

Cysticercosis or Taeniasis

Taeniasis is an intestinal disease caused by tapeworms—*Taenia solium, Taenia saginata,* and *Taenia asiatica,* but major health problems are caused by *T. solium* only. The infection is acquired through the ingestion of infected undercooked pork meat (cysticerci or larval cysts), and thereby, passing eggs with the feces, which are infective for pigs as well as humans. Sometimes, *T. solium* eggs also infect humans via the fecal-oral route by ingesting contaminated food or water. The larvae or cysticerci may develop in the muscles, eyes, skin, and the central nervous system (neurocysticercosis). Symptoms of neurocysticercosis include severe headache, blindness, and epilepsy. It is responsible for 30% of the cases of epilepsy in endemic areas and is the most common preventable cause of epilepsy.[34] Currently, it is estimated that 2.56–8.30 million people are suffering from neurocysticercosis. *T. solium* was identified as the leading cause of deaths from foodborne diseases, according to the WHO Foodborne Disease Burden Epidemiology Reference Group, and is responsible for 2.8 million DALYs.[34]

Echinococcosis

Echinococcosis is a parasitic disease caused by tapeworms of the genus *Echinococcus*. It occurs in four forms—(1) cystic (*Echinococcus granulosus*), (2) alveolar (*Echinococcus multilocularis*), (3) polycystic (*Echinococcus vogeli*), and (4) unicystic (*Echinococcus oligarthrus*). Humans are accidental hosts and infection leads to the development of hydatid cysts in the liver and lungs. Symptoms include abdominal pain, nausea and vomiting in case of hydatids in the liver, while chronic cough, chest pain, and shortness of breath are the clinical manifestations when the lung is infected. Cystic echinococcosis is distributed worldwide, whereas the alveolar form is confined to the regions of Russia, Europe, North America, and China. The incidence of cystic echinococcosis in endemic regions is estimated to be 50 per 100,000 person-years, and the prevalence rate is 5–10%.[35] Treatment options include percutaneous treatment with the PAIR (puncture, aspiration, injection, and reaspiration) technique, surgery or anti-infective treatment with albendazole.

Chagas Disease (American Trypanosomiasis)

Chagas disease is a potentially life-threatening disease caused by *Trypanosoma cruzi*, which is mainly transmitted through contacts with feces or urine of infected triatomine bugs. Currently, 6–7 million people are infected with the disease, and is predominantly distributed in regions of Latin America; however, in the past few years, the disease has spread to other continents.[36] Benznidazole and nifurtimox are the drugs recommended for the disease, and are effective if given during the acute phase, including congenital transmissions. Chronic illness causes cardiac complications (cardiomyopathy) in 30% cases and gastrointestinal (megacolon, megaesophagus) or neurological alterations in 10% cases. Most effective method for prevention of the disease is vector control.

Dracunculiasis (Guinea-worm Disease)

Dracunculiasis is a parasitic disease caused by *Dracunculus medinensis*, transmitted through drinking contaminated water from open surface water sources, containing water fleas (tiny crustaceans or copepods) infected with the parasite. The disease was endemic in 20 countries in the mid-80s with an estimated 3.5 million cases. Since then, the Global Guinea Worm Eradication Program has made a tremendous progress and now, the disease is on the verge of eradication with only 28 human cases reported from three countries—Angola, Chad, and South Sudan in 2018.[37] Treatment includes extraction of the worm from the skin surface using a stick and winding few centimeters per day. There is no specific drug for the disease.

Buruli Ulcer

Buruli ulcer is a chronic debilitating illness caused by *Mycobacterium ulcerans*, mainly affecting the skin; but it may also affect the bone, leading to long-term disability and permanent disfigurement. The disease has been reported in 33 countries with tropical and subtropical climates, including Africa, South America, and Western Pacific. In 2018, there were 2,713 suspected cases reported from 14 countries.[38] Approximately 48% of cases in Africa are children under 15 years of age. It starts as a painless swelling or nodule that ulcerates within 4 weeks and later may involve the bone, resulting in deformities. The exact mode of transmission of the disease is still not known. WHO recommends a combination of rifampicin (10 mg/kg once daily) and clarithromycin (7.5 mg/kg twice daily) for a duration of 8 weeks for treatment of the disease.

Human African Trypanosomiasis

Human African trypanosomiasis or sleeping sickness is a vector-borne disease caused by the parasite *Trypanosoma brucei*, which is transmitted by tsetse fly (genus *Glossina*). The disease is endemic in 36 sub-Saharan African countries, with a total number of 1,446 cases reported in the year 2107, of which 77% cases occur in the Democratic Republic of Congo.[39]

In the first stage, sleeping sickness causes headache, fever, joint pain, and itching. Later in the second stage, the parasite can cross the blood-brain barrier and cause behavioral changes, confusion, poor coordination, and disturbances in sleep cycle. Pentamidine and suramin are recommended for first-stage treatment. Drugs used for treatment of second stage include melarsoprol, eflornithine and nifurtimox. A coordination network to ensure sustained control efforts was established in 2014 under the leadership of WHO and these efforts have led to a reduction in the number of cases.[39]

OTHER CHILDHOOD DISEASES IN THE TROPICS

Apart from the NTDs, there are diseases and nutritional deficiencies that are widespread all over the world but with maximum incidence, prevalence and mortality in the tropical and subtropical countries. Burden of some of these diseases are discussed as follows.

Tuberculosis

Tuberculosis (TB) is caused by *Mycobacterium tuberculosis*. Children can present with clinical manifestations of the disease at any age, but in endemic countries, they present most commonly between 1 year and 4 years.[40] The most common type of TB in children is pulmonary TB. In 2017, almost 1 million children aged <14 years were reported to have TB, of which 230,000 children died from the disease. TB occurs in almost every part of the world with the largest number of new TB cases (62%) in Southeast Asia and Western Pacific regions.[40] Two-thirds of new TB cases occurred in eight countries—India, Bangladesh, China, Indonesia, Nigeria, Philippines, Pakistan, and South Africa.

Human Immunodeficiency Virus

Human immunodeficiency virus (HIV) impairs the function of the immune system, thereby increasing susceptibility to various infections and some cancers. It continues to be a global health problem, affecting approximately 37.9 million people by the end of 2018.[41] In 2018, there were 1.7 million (1.3–2.2 million) children less than 15 years of age living with HIV globally, which accounts to 5% of all people living with HIV.[42] They also constitute 9% of new HIV infections and 13% of all acquired immunodeficiency syndrome (AIDS)-related deaths.[42] Infants less than 1 year of age are among the most vulnerable to the infection. Of the 1.7 million children living with HIV, only 54% were on antiretroviral therapy (ART) in 2018. The most affected region according to the 2018 data was the WHO African region, with 89% of the estimated 1.7 million children.

Malnutrition

Undernutrition (wasting/stunting/underweight) is mainly prevalent in low- and middle-income countries with poor socioeconomic status. According to the WHO 2016 data, 52 million under-five children are wasted, 17 million are severely wasted and 155 million are stunted.[43] In India, 21% under-five children are wasted, 7.5% severely wasted, 35.8% underweight and 38.4% stunted.[44] Almost 45% of deaths in under-five children are related to undernutrition. According to the GBD 2013 data, an estimated 225,906 deaths occurred globally due to protein energy malnutrition (PEM) in children under 5 years of age, of which India accounted for 19,483 (8.6%) PEM deaths.[45]

Vitamin A Deficiency

Vitamin A deficiency is a public health issue in more than half of all countries, mainly affecting preschool children. It is mainly prevalent in Africa and Southeast Asia. It is the leading cause of preventable blindness in children.[46] Currently, almost 250 million preschool children have vitamin A deficiency. Approximately 250,000–500,000 of these children become blind each year and 50% of them die within 1 year of losing their sight.[46] Children with vitamin A deficiency have severe visual impairment and blindness. The condition also increases the risk of severe infections and deaths from common childhood illnesses like measles and diarrhea.

Iron Deficiency Anemia

Iron deficiency anemia is the most common nutritional disorder worldwide, currently affecting 2 billion people or 30% of the world's population.[46] The high prevalence of IDA in the tropical and subtropical countries is attributed to the high prevalence of hookworm infestation, schistosomiasis, malaria, TB, HIV/AIDS and other infections in the region. It disproportionately affects the poorest people. Children and adolescents, especially girls, are the vulnerable age groups.

Diarrheal Diseases

Diarrhea is the second leading cause of death in children under 5 years of age and the leading cause of malnutrition in this group of children.[47] Each year, approximately 1.7 million cases of childhood diarrheal diseases occur globally, with almost 525,000 deaths annually.[47] It mainly affects the low-income countries with unsafe drinking water and poor sanitation. Children under 3 years of age in these countries experience on an average three episodes of diarrhea each year. According to GBD 2013 data, an estimated 519,666 global deaths were attributed to diarrheal diseases, of which 80,225 (15.4%) diarrheal deaths occurred in India.[45]

Pneumonia

Pneumonia can be caused by viruses, bacteria, or fungi. It can occur anywhere in the world, but most prevalent in

South Asia and sub-Saharan Africa.[48] It accounts for 15% of all deaths of under-five children, killing 808,694 children in 2017.

Measles

Measles is a highly contagious viral disease, which is most common in developing countries, especially in parts of Africa and Asia.[49] The disease resulted in 110,000 deaths globally in 2017, mostly under 5 years of age. Measles vaccination has led to 80% reduction in the measles death worldwide between 2000 and 2017.[49]

■ MORBIDITY AND MORTALITY CAUSED BY NEGLECTED TROPICAL DISEASES

Although information on health outcomes of tropical diseases among specific age groups of children and adolescents is scarce, it has been observed that a vast majority of tropical diseases (except onchocerciasis and leprosy) occurs disproportionately in children and adolescents.[2] The tropical diseases inflict morbidity and suffering by causing life-long disfigurement, disabilities, social stigma and poor economic productivity, rather than deaths. NTDs result in impaired growth and development, cognitive delay, malnutrition, reduced productive capacity, and ultimately, poverty.

Major tropical diseases have a disproportionate impact on children and adolescents. This subset of the population is not only prone to get infected more frequently with the tropical diseases, but also the infections are more severe. Some of the diseases are life threatening, and those which are not, may have profound permanent impacts on growth, cognitive development, disfigurements, and subsequently hampering socioeconomic development. For example, intestinal nematode infections which include hookworm infestation, ascariasis and trichuriasis cause moderate to severe anemia in school-age children (5–15 years of age), malnutrition, growth and cognitive delays. More than 50% of IDA in Africa and Asia is attributed to hookworm infestation.[50] Malaria is one of the major causes of death in children and when there is coinfection with hookworm infestation, which occurs frequently, it can lead to profound and incapacitating anemia.[51] Leishmaniasis can lead to social stigma caused by cutaneous and mucocutaneous disfigurement. Schistosomiasis is associated with hematuria, urogenital disease, intestinal and liver fibrosis, growth and cognitive delays. Two-third of the world's blindness cases are preventable and 90% of them occurs in the developing world.[50] Trachoma is one of the major causes of blindness and contributes almost 16%

of the same. Its prevalence is the highest in children aged 1–5 years. Tropical diseases also cause major afflictions in adolescents, particularly adolescent girls, in whom these diseases not only lead to anemia and malnutrition, but also cause genitourinary tract diseases which may promote the transmission of HIV and other sexually transmitted diseases.[52] Many of these diseases, including malaria and dengue, in women of reproductive age group, may have harmful effects on pregnancy and birth, leading to poor outcomes, and neonatal and early childhood mortality.[53-55] Similarly, diarrheal diseases and pneumonia have short-term mortality risks.[47,48] Diarrheal diseases also lead to long-term impacts on growth and development. The important clinical manifestations and associated disabilities are listed in **Table 5**.

Approximately 152,000 deaths were estimated to be caused by NTDs according to the GBD 2010 study. Among the NTDs for which deaths were estimated, majority of the deaths due to NTDs was accounted for leishmaniasis (primarily due to visceral leishmaniasis). Other killer NTDs included rabies, dengue, schistosomiasis, and African trypanosomiasis. The latest GBD data 2017 provides an estimated 720,100 deaths if malaria is included in the list along with the NTDs, and almost 50% of the total deaths occurred in children under 5 years of age.[13-16]

■ REASONS FOR THE HUGE DISEASE BURDEN

The tropical and subtropical regions have characteristic disease ecology that facilitates the transmission of tropical diseases. This includes hot climate, humidity, abundant rainfall, a large number of potential pathogens, potential vector breeding grounds, and a large number of potential insect vectors.[1] These diseases strike the poorest people living in remote rural areas and slum dwellings, thus, caught in a vicious cycle of diseases and poverty. They inflict morbidity by causing lifelong disfigurements and disabilities thereby resulting in deferral of help-seeking and interfere with the adherence to treatment due to social stigma.

Limited access to public health control measures and weaknesses of current approaches are partly responsible for the huge disease burden. The reasons for the ineffective control of tropical diseases include poor surveillance, lack of appropriate diagnostic tools, limited access to essential medicines and public health interventions, rapid reinfection, potential drug resistance and inadequate vector control measures.[2] The affordable and easily accessible diagnostic tools currently used to screen and measure tropical diseases in resource-limited settings are mostly inaccurate.[11]

Table 5: Major characteristics, clinical manifestations and associated disabilities of some major tropical diseases.[2]

Disease	Population at risk	Clinical characteristics and associated disabilities
Ascariasis	School-age children	Malnutrition, delay in growth and development, cognitive delay
Trichuriasis	School-age children	Inflammatory bowel disease, delay in growth and development, cognitive delay
Hookworm infestation	School-age children	Moderate-to-severe anemia, malnutrition, delay in growth and development, cognitive delay
Schistosomiasis	School-age children	Hematuria and urogenital disease, delay in growth and development, cognitive delay intestinal and liver fibrosis, malnutrition
Trachoma	Children	Trachomatous inflammation and folliculitis, severely visually impaired, blindness
Lymphatic filariasis	Adolescents	Lymphedema, hydrocele, genital and limb deformities, secondary bacterial infections
Leishmaniasis	Children	Cutaneous and mucocutaneous disfigurement, social stigma, death due to visceral leishmaniasis
Chagas disease	Children	Cardiomyopathy, megacolon, megaesophagus
Human African trypanosomiasis	All ages	Sleeping sickness
Buruli ulcer	Children	Disfigurement
Dracunculiasis	All ages	Disfigurement, secondary bacterial infections

Moreover, major NTDs do not receive enough international attention unlike the big three global threats—HIV/AIDS, malaria, and TB. NTDs technologies are not considered profitable by the pharmaceutical manufacturers of the developed countries as these diseases do not occur in the industrialized world.[56] The low- and middle-income countries in the tropics and subtropics continue to face a huge burden of these diseases.

■ CONCLUSIONS AND FUTURE DIRECTION

Some of the most important major tropical diseases are on the verge of effective control and elimination through the expanded use of MDA, targeted treatments and preventive chemotherapy.[2] WHO has classified NTDs into broadly two categories based on the methods required for effective control and elimination, for the programmatic point of view—preventive chemotherapy and transmission control (PCT) NTDs and innovative and intensified disease management (IDM) NTDs.[5] The former group includes soil-transmitted helminthiasis, lymphatic filariasis, schistosomiasis, trachoma, onchocerciasis, and foodborne trematodes. These diseases can be controlled through MDA of effective and safe drugs to entire at-risk population. On the other side, the IDM group of NTDs include those diseases which lack adequate tools for large-scale management, e.g. Buruli ulcer, leishmaniasis, Chagas disease, human African trypanosomiasis, etc.

Comprehensive programs on MDA, targeted treatments and preventive chemotherapy to effectively control and eliminate some of the most prevalent tropical diseases are underway in South Asia.[3] These include conducting national programs on MDA, under the Global Program to Eliminate Lymphatic Filariasis, with more emphasis in the areas of India, Bangladesh and Nepal; national programs on MDA to eliminate soil-transmitted helminthiasis (ascariasis, hookworm infestation, and trichuriasis); comprehensive vaccination for the elimination of Japanese encephalitis and rabies; preventive chemotherapy MDA for trachoma in addition to SAFE (surgery for trichiasis, antibiotics, facial cleanliness and environmental improvement) strategies. Recently, India has made considerable progress toward the control and elimination of major tropical diseases that include helminthiasis and lymphatic filariasis. According to WHO (2015), almost three-fourth of the total Indian children that require deworming for intestinal helminth infestation received mass treatment.[22] These national programs are integrated with improvements in sanitation, easy access to clean water and vector control measures including treatment of bed-nets with insecticides for the control of malaria, dengue, Japanese encephalitis and leishmaniasis. New emerging control tools which are under development including developing vaccines for dengue, malaria, leishmaniasis, and hookworm.[3]

However, there is a need to further strengthen and improve surveillance for better assessment and control of childhood diseases in the tropical countries. More policies on public health and research are required to find adequate diagnostic tools for large-scale use, effective and safe drugs, and vaccines. Public-private partnerships involving political leaders, pharmaceutical companies, charitable organizations, non-governmental organizations (NGOs), donor agencies and stakeholders are crucial to fight against childhood diseases in the tropics and subtropics as these regions mainly include the low- and middle-income countries. Continued progress to fight against tropical diseases depends on improved surveillance, strengthening public health policies and health systems, political support, and collaboration from all participants.

◼ REFERENCES

1. Bärnighausen, Bloom DE, Humair S. Global health-governance and tropical diseases. In: Farrar J, Hotez PJ, Junghanss T, Kang G, Lalloo D, White NJ (Eds). Manson's Tropical Diseases. Oxford: Saunders Ltd; 2013. pp. 16-22.
2. Hotez PJ, Molyneux DH, Fenwick A, et al. Control of neglected tropical diseases. N Engl J Med. 2007;357(10):1018-27.
3. Lobo DA, Velayudhan R, Chatterjee P, et al. The neglected tropical diseases of India and South Asia: review of their prevalence, distribution, and control or elimination. PLoS Negl Trop Dis. 2011;5(10):e1222.
4. World Health Organization (WHO). Neglected Tropical Diseases Roadmap Targets 2021-2030. [online] Available from: https://www.who.int/docs/default-source/ntds/ntd-roadmap-targets-2021-2030.pdf?sfvrsn=639f2b8a_2. [Last accessed on October, 2019].
5. World Health Organization (WHO). Tropical Diseases. [online] Available from: https://www.who.int/topics/tropical_diseases/en/. [Last accessed on October, 2019].
6. Centers for Disease Control and Prevention (CDC). Global Health - Neglected Tropical Diseases. [online] Available from: https://www.cdc.gov/globalhealth/ntd/index.html. [Last accessed on October, 2019].
7. Mitra AK, Mawson AR. Neglected tropical diseases: epidemiology and global burden. Trop Med Infect Dis. 2017;2(3):pii: E36.
8. WHO. Disease Burden and Mortality Estimates. [online] Available from: http://www.who.int/healthinfo/global_burden_disease/estimates/en/. [Last accessed on October, 2019].
9. Engels D, Savioli L. Reconsidering the underestimated burden caused by neglected tropical diseases. Trends Parasitol. 2006;22(8):363-6.
10. Bhutta ZA, Sommerfeld J, Lassi ZS, et al. Global burden, distribution, and interventions for infectious diseases of poverty. Infect Dis Poverty. 2014;3:21.
11. Hotez PJ, Alvarado M, Basáñez MG, et al. The global burden of disease study 2010: interpretation and implications for the neglected tropical diseases. PLoS Negl Trop Dis. 2014;8(7):e2865.
12. Mathers CD, Ezzati M, Lopez AD. Measuring the burden of neglected tropical diseases: the global burden of disease framework. PLoS Negl Trop Dis. 2007;1(2):e114.
13. GBD 2017 DALYs and HALE Collaborators. Global, regional, and national disability-adjusted life-years (DALYs) for 359 diseases and injuries and healthy life expectancy (HALE) for 195 countries and territories, 1990-2017: a systematic analysis for the Global Burden of Disease Study 2017. Lancet. 2018;392(10159):1859-922.
14. GBD 2017 Causes of Death Collaborators. Global, regional, and national age-sex-specific mortality for 282 causes of death in 195 countries and territories, 1980–2017: a systematic analysis for the Global Burden of Disease Study 2017. Lancet. 2018;392(10159):1736-88.
15. GBD 2016 Disease and Injury Incidence and Prevalence Collaborators. Global, regional, and national incidence, prevalence, and years lived with disability for 328 diseases and injuries for 195 countries, 1990–2016: a systematic analysis for the Global Burden of Disease Study 2016. Lancet. 2017;390(10100):1211-59.
16. Hotez PJ, Odom John AR, LaBeaud AD. Pediatric tropical medicine: The neglected diseases of children. PLoS Negl Trop Dis. 2019;13(5):e0007008.
17. The World Bank. Databank. [online] Available from: https://databank.worldbank.org/home.aspx. [Last accessed on October, 2019].
18. Hotez PJ, Damania A. India's neglected tropical diseases. PLoS Negl Trop Dis. 2018;12(3):e0006038.
19. Bhatt S, Gething PW, Brady OJ, et al. The global distribution and burden of dengue. Nature. 2013;496(7446):504-7.
20. Brady OJ, Gething PW, Bhatt S, et al. Refining the global spatial limits of dengue virus transmission by evidence-based consensus. PLoS Negl Trop Dis. 2012;6(8):e1760.
21. World Health Organization (WHO). Dengue and Severe Dengue. [online] Available from: https://www.who.int/news-room/fact-sheets/detail/dengue-and-severe-dengue. [Last accessed on October, 2019].
22. World Health Organization (WHO). Soil-transmitted Helminth Infections. [online] Available from: https://www.who.int/en/news-room/fact-sheets/detail/soil-transmitted-helminth-infections. [Last accessed on October, 2019].
23. World Health Organization (WHO). Schistosomiasis. [online] Available from: https://www.who.int/news-room/fact-sheets/detail/schistosomiasis. [Last accessed on October, 2019].
24. World Health Organization (WHO). Malaria. [online] Available from: https://www.who.int/news-room/fact-sheets/detail/malaria. [Last accessed on October, 2019].
25. World Health Organization (WHO). Japanese Encephalitis. [online] Available from: https://www.who.int/news-room/fact-sheets/detail/japanese-encephalitis. [Last accessed on October, 2019].
26. World Health Organization (WHO). Chikungunya. [online] Available from: https://www.who.int/news-room/fact-sheets/detail/chikungunya. [Last accessed on October, 2019].
27. World Health Organization (WHO). Leishmaniasis. [online] Available from: https://www.who.int/news-room/fact-sheets/detail/leishmaniasis. [Last accessed on October, 2019].
28. World Health Organization (WHO). Foodborne Trematodiases. [online] Available from: https://www.who.int/news-room/fact-sheets/detail/foodborne-trematodiases. [Last accessed on October, 2019].
29. Hampson K, Coudeville L, Lembo T, et al.; Global Alliance for Rabies Control Partners for Rabies Prevention. Estimating the global burden of endemic canine rabies. PLoS Negl Trop Dis. 2015;9(4):e0003709.
30. Kakkar M, Venkataramanan V, Krishnan S, et al.; Roadmap to Combat Zoonoses in India (RCZI) initiative. Moving from rabies research to rabies control: lessons from India. PLoS Negl Trop Dis. 2012;6(8):e1748.
31. World Health Organization (WHO). Rabies. [online] Available from: https://www.who.int/news-room/fact-sheets/detail/rabies. [Last accessed on October, 2019].

32. World Health Organization (WHO). Yaws. [online] Available from: https://www.who.int/news-room/fact-sheets/detail/yaws. [Last accessed on October, 2019].

33. World Health Organization (WHO). Lymphatic Filariasis. [online] Available from: https://www.who.int/news-room/fact-sheets/detail/lymphatic-filariasis. [Last accessed on October, 2019].

34. World Health Organization (WHO). Taeniasis/Cysticercosis. [online] Available from: https://www.who.int/news-room/fact-sheets/detail/taeniasis-cysticercosis. [Last accessed on October, 2019].

35. World Health Organization (WHO). Echinococcosis. [online] Available from: https://www.who.int/news-room/fact-sheets/detail/echinococcosis. [Last accessed on October, 2019].

36. World Health Organization (WHO). Chagas Disease. [online] Available from: https://www.who.int/news-room/fact-sheets/detail/chagas-disease-(american-trypanosomiasis). [Last accessed on October, 2019].

37. World Health Organization (WHO). Dracunculiasis (Guinea-worm Disease). [online] Available from: https://www.who.int/en/news-room/fact-sheets/detail/dracunculiasis-(guinea-worm-disease). [Last accessed on October, 2019].

38. World Health Organization (WHO). Buruli Ulcer. [online] Available from: https://www.who.int/news-room/fact-sheets/detail/buruli-ulcer-(mycobacterium-ulcerans-infection). [Last accessed on October, 2019].

39. World Health Organization (WHO). Trypanosomiasis, human African (Sleeping Sickness). [online] Available from: https://www.who.int/news-room/fact-sheets/detail/trypanosomiasis-human-african-(sleeping-sickness). [Last accessed on October, 2019].

40. World Health Organization (WHO). Tuberculosis (TB). [online] Available from: https://www.who.int/news-room/fact-sheets/detail/tuberculosis. [Last accessed on October, 2019].

41. World Health Organization (WHO). HIV/AIDS. [online] Available from: https://www.who.int/news-room/fact-sheets/detail/hiv-aids. [Last accessed October, 2019].

42. World Health Organization (WHO). Paediatric Care and Treatment. [online] Available from: https://data.unicef.org/topic/hivaids/paediatric-treatment-and-care/. [Last accessed on October, 2019].

43. World Health Organization (WHO). Malnutrition. [online] Available from: https://www.who.int/news-room/fact-sheets/detail/malnutrition. [Last accessed on October, 2019].

44. International Institute for Population Sciences (IIPS). National Family Health Survey-4. [online] Available from: http://rchiips.org/nfhs/factsheet_nfhs-4.shtml. [Last accessed on October, 2019].

45. Kyu HH, Pinho C, Wagner JA, et al. Global and national burden of diseases and injuries among children and adolescents between 1990 and 2013: findings from the global burden of Disease 2013 study. JAMA Pediatr. 2016;170(3):267-87.

46. World Health Organization (WHO). Micronutrient deficiencies. [online] Available from: https://www.who.int/nutrition/topics/vad/en/. [Last accessed on October, 2019].

47. World Health Organization (WHO). Diarrhoeal disease. [online] Available from: https://www.who.int/news-room/fact-sheets/detail/diarrhoeal-disease. [Last accessed on October, 2019].

48. World Health Organization (WHO). Pneumonia. [online] Available from: https://www.who.int/news-room/fact-sheets/detail/pneumonia. [Last accessed on October, 2019].

49. World Health Organization (WHO). Measles. [online] Available from: https://www.who.int/news-room/fact-sheets/detail/measles. [Last accessed on October, 2019].

50. Hotez PJ, Remme JH, Buss P, et al. Combating tropical infectious diseases: report of the disease control priorities in developing countries project. Clin Infect Dis. 2004;38(6):871-8.

51. Hotez PJ, Molyneux DH. Tropical anemia: one of Africa's great killers and a rationale for linking malaria and neglected tropical disease control to achieve a common goal. PLoS Negl Trop Dis. 2008;2(7):e270.

52. Downs JA, Dupnik KM, van Dam GJ, et al. Effects of schistosomiasis on susceptibility to HIV-1 infection and HIV-1 viral load at HIV-1 seroconversion: A nested case-control study. PLoS Negl Trop Dis. 2017;11(9):e0005968.

53. Rogerson SJ, Desai M, Mayor A, et al. Burden, pathology, and costs of malaria in pregnancy: new developments for an old problem. Lancet Infect Dis. 2018;18(4):e107-18.

54. Harrington WE, Kakuru A, Jagannathan P. Malaria in pregnancy shapes the development of foetal and infant immunity. Parasite Immunol. 2019;41(3):e12573.

55. Xiong YQ, Mo Y, Shi TL, et al. Dengue virus infection during pregnancy increased the risk of adverse fetal outcomes? An updated meta-analysis. J Clin Virol. 2017;94:42-9.

56. Hotez P, Ottesen E, Fenwick A, et al. The neglected tropical diseases: the ancient afflictions of stigma and poverty and the prospects for their control and elimination. Adv Exp Med Biol. 2006;582:23-33.

Child Health Services in the Tropics

Omar Irfan, Amira M Khan, Zulfiqar A Bhutta

INTRODUCTION

Nearly 80% of the world's population resides in low- and middle-income countries (LMICs) which bear the greatest burden of maternal, neonatal, and child mortality. The bulk of these deaths occur in the communities at homes.[1] Much of this mortality is attributable to preventable and treatable conditions through interventions that are affordable, feasible and delivered without complex technical resources. The challenge lies in reaching the most vulnerable communities, making it imperative that maternal, newborn, and child health (MNCH) interventions should focus on communities in tandem with facility-based strategies. This chapter primarily focuses on the different levels and components of child health services available in LMICs which are employed to effectively deliver health interventions through the continuum of care, starting from pregnancy to delivery and then to the newborn, infant, and the young child, to ensure an optimal health and nutrition status of children. Strengthening the health system and integrating facility and community-based interventions into packages of care at all levels will be key to increasing the coverage of health interventions and in further reducing child morbidity and mortality.

GLOBAL BURDEN OF NEWBORN AND CHILD MORBIDITY AND MORTALITY

Health status of children is defined by tracking their mortality, morbidity, nutrition, growth, and development. An overview of the current health situation of children in the developing countries is presented in this section.

Global Burden and Epidemiology of Mortality and Morbidity in Under-five Children

The under-five mortality rate (U5MR) has seen a remarkable reduction, decreasing from 93 per 1,000 live births in 1990 to 39 per 1,000 live births in 2017.[2] Despite this progress, an estimated 5.4 million children died in 2017; 2.5 million of those were neonates. It is concerning to note that the mortality in the neonatal period only saw a decrease of 41% as compared to a striking 60% reduction in the 1–59 month age group between 2000 and 2017.[2]

An estimated 80% of all the under-five deaths are clustered in parts of South Asia and the sub-Saharan Africa. The latter leads with the highest global U5MR of 76 deaths per 1,000 live births in 2017. About half of all under-five deaths are concentrated in just six nations: India, Pakistan, Ethiopia, Nigeria, Democratic Republic of Congo, and China.[2] The leading causes of under-five mortality are those occurring in the neonatal age group; premature birth complications (18%), intrapartum complications (12%), and neonatal infections including sepsis and meningitis (7%) **(Fig. 1)**. In 2014, an estimated 10.6% (14.84 million) of live births occurred before 37 weeks' gestation, of which 80% were in sub-Saharan Africa and South Asia.[3] Birth weight is a key indicator of maternal and fetal health during pregnancy, and in 2015, an estimated 14.6% (20.5 million) of newborns had low birth weight (LBW), defined as less than 2,500 g.[4]

The leading infectious causes of postneonatal under-five mortality include pneumonia (16%), diarrhea (8%), and malaria (5%).[2] Pneumonia is the leading cause of under-five deaths in sub-Saharan Africa with nearly 490,000 annual deaths. Malaria and neglected tropical diseases (NTDs) cause an estimated 720,100 deaths and 62 million disability-adjusted life years (DALYs), ranking these conditions among the leading global health threats. The 2017 Global Burden of Disease numbers highlight that approximately one-half of these deaths and DALYs affect children under-five, whereas approximately two-third affect children and adolescents under the age of 20 years.[5,6] Nearly 8% of the total under-five mortality is attributed to

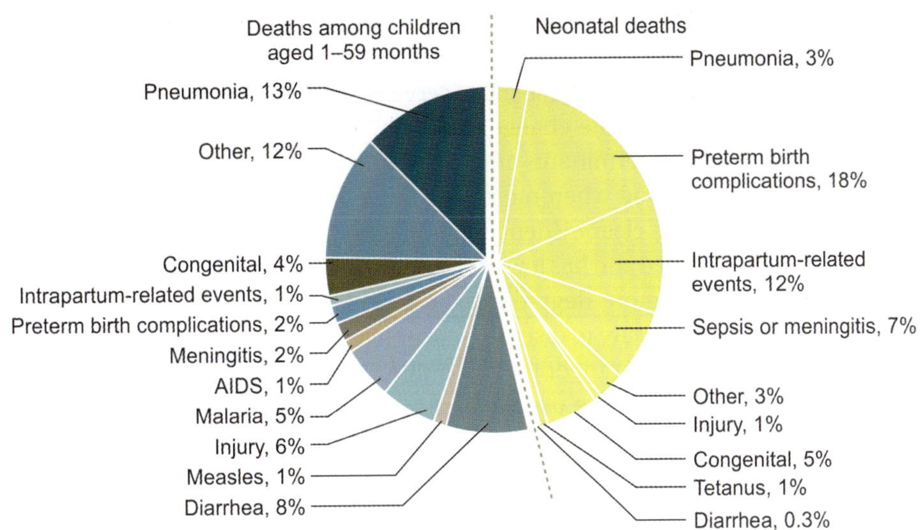

Fig. 1: Causes of the global distribution of deaths among children under-five, 2016.
Source: United Nations Inter-agency Group for Child Mortality Estimation (UNIGME). (2017). Levels and Trends in Child Mortality Report 2017. [online] Available from: https://www.unicef.org/publications/files/Child_Mortality_Report_2017.pdf. [Last accessed on October, 2019].

diarrheal disease and 90% of these diarrheal deaths are reported to occur in South Asia and sub-Saharan Africa. Incidence of both pneumonia and diarrhea are closely associated with poor home environments, undernutrition, and lack of access to health services. Malnutrition is an underlying determinant of nearly 45% of all under-five deaths. In many instances, overweight and obesity coexist with undernutrition, wasting and stunting, giving rise to the double burden of malnutrition.[5,6]

Global Burden and Epidemiology of Mortality and Morbidity in School-age Children

Between 1990 and 2016, the global mortality rate for children between 5 years and 10 years decreased from 10.3 deaths to 4.5 deaths per 1,000 children.[7] Despite this global trend, the mortality rate of older children remained high in 2016 in sub-Saharan Africa at 11.9 deaths per thousand. In 2016, an estimated 585,000 deaths were reported globally among children 5–9 years, with approximately 351,000 and 192,000 occurring in sub-Saharan Africa and South Asia, respectively.[7]

Mortality rates are substantially lower, and the breakdown of causes of mortality in children above-five is quite different from that of younger children, with noncommunicable diseases (NCDs) and injury-related causes are the leading causes. A high percentage of infection-related deaths, characteristic of early childhood, extends into later age for those countries with higher levels of under-five infectious morbidities. For example, in 2016, the nutritional and communicable disease-related death rate of children 5–14 years old in India was 32.6 and 26.2 per 100,000 for girls and boys, respectively, but the same rates for China were only 1.7 and 1.5.[8] NCDs and injuries in this age group were the principal causes of death in China, Brazil, and Mexico; however, India still experienced higher mortality rates due to infectious causes. This shows that, in some countries, the epidemiological transition has not yet occurred, resulting in a significant double burden of communicable and NCDs in older children.

The main causes of morbidity and mortality in children under-five, including respiratory infections, malaria, and diarrhea remain a significant burden for school-age children in the poorest LMICs. NCDs that have become increasingly prominent and cause significant morbidity and disability include asthma, rheumatic heart disease, hemoglobinopathies and neurological disorders. Additionally, school-age children experience a higher burden of injury-related causes including drowning, road traffic accidents, poisoning, burns, and maltreatment.

■ DETERMINANTS OF CHILD HEALTH

Despite seeing a declining trend in the under-five mortalities over the last two decades, there are still differences in the reduction of mortality and utilizing the maternal and child health indicators within and across countries. Such differences in health outcomes which are often seen as health inequities—are socially engraved, systematically distributed across the population, and are unjust.[9] In addition to the child's biological characteristics the factors which determine child health, growth and survival can be categorized into determinants related to the social and physical environment. Some important social determinants can include education, inequity, social security, poverty, lack of empowerment, climate change, and state of conflict and anarchy. These determinants are most critical in infancy and early childhood when most preventable child deaths happen. There is clear evidence that the population which is less empowered and has lower socioeconomic status, tend to live in a more degraded environment and in turn have a higher exposure to disease risk factors, as well as more physiologic derangements from chronic stress. Biological determinants are usually related to maternal risk factors (which influence a child's health in prebirth period), birth conditions if any, and the health and nutritional status of child with age. Unless this inequity is addressed, it is estimated that between 2016 and 2030, 69 million under-five children will die with nearly half of them in sub-Saharan Africa.[10]

Poverty has been a major underlying cause for many deaths, with nearly 99% of global maternal and newborn mortality occurring in LMIC.[11] In the tropical regions, the causes of most infectious diseases (especially TB, diarrhea, malaria, and the NTDs) are closely linked to poverty, poor sanitation, and food insecurity. NTDs are a group of tropical infections which are common in low-income populations in LMICs of Africa, Asia, and the Americas. As the 13 NTDs are all infectious (and largely vector-borne), they are more dependent on the external physical or biological conditions. Better socioeconomic status automatically reduces the probability of child illness by improving a child's nutritional status, uptake of child health interventions by the parents and guardians, and health-seeking behavior.[12,13] Healthcare has simply been unaffordable for many in the sub-Saharan Africa. User and informal healthcare fees, the cost of tests and medicines remain a major barrier to accessing health services, especially for the poor. Many African nations including South Africa, Ghana, and Uganda have all witnessed some success in user fee elimination for MNCH services.[14]

Low literacy in female, gender partiality, and lack of empowerment prevent women from seeking care, having the autonomy to make own decisions, and accessing the best possible services for themselves and their child's health, resulting in critical delays and deaths. Maternal factors can affect child health during preconception, pregnancy, childbirth, and the postnatal period. Family planning, pregnancy intervals, and early marriages are some of the decisions which can affect early child health. Studies from Ethiopia and Gambia indicate that child mortality may be between 3 times and 12 times higher, respectively, among mothers with limited autonomy.[15]

Changes in climate and the geographical disparities can contribute to inequitable access to food, health services, and education. Geography distribution dictates the physical environment in which children live, and their exposure to pathogens and pollutants. In addition to direct negative effects and increased risks of climate change associated disasters such as floods or drought, global climate change has been associated with major changes in risks of infectious diseases. The annual cases of dengue fever have doubled over the decades since 1990, with 58.4 million cases in 2013. Other infectious diseases, such as chikungunya, yellow fever and Zika viruses, are probably similarly responsive to climate change.[16] In 2011, Lloyd et al. developed a statistical model for moderate and severe stunting in children less than 5 years old at the national level in 44 countries under low and high climate change scenarios. Their numbers indicated that climate change-attributable stunting ranged from 570,000 in the best-case scenario to over 1 million under the high climate change scenario.[17] Around 160 million children live in extreme drought conditions, and an additional 500 million live in areas at extreme flood risk.[15]

Moreover, the total number of people affected by conflict and humanitarian emergencies has been on the rise. Children suffer a variety of physical and social deprivations, including lack of social security, loss of social and family structure, loss of food, and poor physical environments. Countries with the highest mortality rates in the sub-Saharan Africa have recently seen conflicts and complex emergency situations. One study in the Democratic Republic of the Congo reported that maternal deaths were more common in the conflict-stricken eastern provinces, compared to in the western region.[18] Complex emergencies, such as conflict and natural disasters, present difficulties to delivering MNCH services. These situations often suffer from poor referral systems, lack of equipment and supplies, loss of human workforce for health, and a deteriorating infrastructure.[19] Addressing the social determinants is a colossal task which will require higher level interdisciplinary policy making strategies and strong commitment by the stakeholders at all levels to implement and then assess the outcomes of the executed policies.

PROGRESS FROM MILLENNIUM DEVELOPMENT GOALS TO SUSTAINABLE DEVELOPMENT GOALS

In 2015, the Millennium Development Goals (MDGs) were succeeded by the Sustainable Development Goals (SDGs). Progress was slow on the education and health-related

MDGs. MDG 4 "Reduce child mortality" was the MDG most directly related to child health. MDGs related to infant, child and maternal mortality (MDGs 4a and 5a), and access to basic sanitation (MDG 7c) lagged behind in their progress by 2015. A report was compiled in 2015 under supervision of the United Nations to assess the periodic success of MDG which reported the global U5MR to decline substantially by 50% between 1990 and 2015.[20] Moreover, in the sub-Saharan Africa, the annual reduction in U5MR was over five times faster during the period of 2005–2013 as compared to 1990–1995.[20] Measles vaccination helped prevent nearly 15.6 million deaths between 2000 and 2013 with global measles cases declined by 67% for the same period.[20] MDGs are interrelated. Another MDG 5 which is linked to neonatal and child health is MDG 5 to improve maternal health. Since 1990, the maternal mortality ratio has declined by 45% globally. Between 1990 and 2013, the maternal mortality ratio declined by 64% and 49% in South Asia and sub-Saharan Africa, respectively. In North Africa, the proportion of pregnant women who received more than three antenatal visits increased from 50% to 89% between 1990 and 2014. Moreover, the contraceptive usage among women aged 15–49 years substantially increased.[20]

If the current child mortality figures persist, the SDG child mortality targets (reducing neonatal mortality to at least as low as 12 per 1,000 live births and under-five mortality to at least as low as 25 per 1,000 live births in all countries by 2030) will not be met in the 47 countries, 34 of which are in the sub-Saharan Africa. Reversing the current trends will require not only applying the lessons learned from MDGs but also addressing the determinants of child health and wellbeing. Indeed, evidence has shown that about half of the reduction in child mortality in LMICs between 1990 and 2010 was due to indirect influences beyond the scope of the health sector.[21] The focus on the health of children has to expand broadly to include healthy growth, development, and wellbeing, in addition to mortality.[22]

Poor health outcomes relate to complex issues such as lack of skilled birth attendants and qualified health workers, sociocultural restrictions, maternal empowerment, and care-seeking behaviors during pregnancy and childbirth.[23] It is crucial to reach the rural and urban poor settings through community health workers (CHWs) and volunteers to maximize the community outreach.

The global evidence for interventions for newborn care services in community settings has substantially improved through various healthcare providers, especially the CHWs, with a series of interventions that can be packaged for delivery at different times during pregnancy, childbirth, and after birth. CHWs have been effective previously in improving maternal and child health outcomes in a range of research settings.[1]

Studies assessing the women's groups, in support by community volunteers have shown consistent significant benefits on improving maternal and newborn outcomes.[24] The role of community-based interventions and platforms will become more significant along the road. These strategies will be instrumental in ensuring several of the key themes of the SDGs, such as reaching the marginalized populations and reducing inequities, are achieved within the said timeline.

INTERVENTIONS TO PREVENT AND MANAGE CHILD HEALTH MORBIDITIES AND MORTALITY

To optimize newborn health and survival, it is crucial to focus on the most effective evidence-based interventions with intentional investment and implementation. The interventions can be classified into two main types—first, preventive measures to reduce specific disease morbidities; second, case management interventions to treat disease, reduce illness severity, and improve the child health. Key interventions for each of the major causes of child mortality and morbidity are summarized in **Table 1**.

ORGANIZATION OF CHILD HEALTH SERVICES

The delivery of healthcare services in the LMICs does depend on groups of various trained professionals coming together as interdisciplinary teams. This can include professionals from medicine, physiotherapy, nursing, dentistry, midwifery, allied health, public health practitioners, and CHWs, who systematically provide individual and population-based preventive, curative, and rehabilitative care services. While there exist different definitions of the types of healthcare based on the different political, cultural, organizational and disciplinary perspectives, there appears to be some agreement that the primary healthcare (PHC) is the first element of the healthcare process and can also include the provision of secondary and tertiary levels as continuum of care.

Primary Healthcare

Primary healthcare is the first level of contact between a patient and the health system. Categorization of healthcare is usually based on the population served, hospital size (usually the number of beds), and the provision of clinical subspecialty and intensive care

Table 1: A summary of key interventions to address risk factors for the major causes of child mortality and morbidity.

Child conditions	Preventive interventions	Case management interventions
Newborn (<1 month)		
• Preterm birth • Neonatal sepsis • Perinatal asphyxia • Low birth weight • Congenital conditions	*Preconception:* • Maternal iron-folic acid or multiple micronutrient supplementation • Balanced protein-energy supplements for mothers at risk for undernutrition • Counseling for cessation of smoking, alcohol and other substances • Delaying age at first pregnancy, and promoting optimal inter-pregnancy intervals *Antenatal:* • Routine antenatal care visits • Maternal vaccination and prevention of rhesus disease • Intermittent preventive treatment of malaria in pregnancy (IPTp) • Screening and treatment of infectious diseases • Antenatal steroids for fetal lung maturation *Labor and childbirth:* • Skilled care and support during labor and birth • Care at the time of birth: Warmth, delayed cord clamping, hygienic cord care, and early initiation of breastfeeding *Postnatal:* Care during the first days and weeks after birth: Exclusive breastfeeding, warmth, kangaroo mother care, hygienic cord and skin care, vaccination, and prompt care-seeking for any illness	• Timely detection and management of hypertension, diabetes, and fetal growth restriction during pregnancy • Tocolytics and antenatal corticosteroids for preterm labor (in appropriate populations) • Antibiotics for preterm premature rupture of membranes • Timely detection and management of maternal GBS, helminthic, malaria, tuberculosis and HIV infections • Cesarean section or assisted vaginal delivery in case of fetal distress • Neonatal resuscitation if unable to breathe after birth • Diagnosis and treatment of neonatal sepsis and local infections
Infancy (<1 year) and early childhood (1–5 years)		
Pneumonia	• Immunization against pneumococcus, *Haemophilus influenzae*, pertussis, diphtheria, and measles • Exclusive breastfeeding up to 6 months; continued breastfeeding with appropriate complementary feeding at least up to 2 years • Reduction in environmental risk factors—e.g. indoor air pollution, overcrowding	• Treatment of pneumonia with amoxicillin • Treatment of severe pneumonia with parenteral antibiotics, oxygen, and other supportive treatment
Diarrhea and enteric infections	• Early and exclusive breastfeeding up to 6 months; continued breastfeeding with appropriate complementary feeding at least up to 2 years • Preventive vitamin A and zinc supplementation • Immunization against measles, rotavirus, cholera, and typhoid • Improved water and sanitation; hand washing with soap	• Oral rehydration therapy to prevent dehydration • Zinc treatment for 10–14 days during diarrhea • Antibiotics for dysentery and typhoid
Malaria	• Vector control • Use of long-lasting insecticide-treated bed nets • Intermittent preventive treatment in infants (IPTi)	Treatment of non-severe malaria with oral antimalarial drugs recommended for the area and treatment of severe malaria with parenteral antimalarial drugs
HIV/AIDS	• Primary prevention of HIV and of unintended pregnancies in HIV-infected women • Antiretroviral (ARV) treatment of pregnant women when indicated • Cotrimoxazole prophylaxis for HIV-exposed and HIV-infected children	Antiretroviral therapy (ART) for children when indicated
Malnutrition	• Early initiation of breastfeeding and exclusive breastfeeding up to 6 months of age • Continued breastfeeding with appropriate complementary foods for at least 2 years • Preventing vitamin A, iron, iodine, and zinc deficiencies • Community-based screening for severe acute malnutrition using mid-upper arm circumference (MUAC) measurements, and growth monitoring and promotion strategies	• Community-based management of children with severe malnutrition without complications • Hospital management of severely malnourished children with complications

Contd...

Contd...

Child conditions	Preventive interventions	Case management interventions
School age (5–10 years)		
Overweight and obesity	Education on healthy lifestyle measures	Anthropometric screening, management, and treatment of comorbidities
Non-communicable diseases • Sickle cell disease • Asthma • Epilepsy • Rheumatic heart disease	• Improving air quality • Early detection and treatment of streptococcal pharyngitis and rheumatic fever	• Treatment of sickle cell with hydroxyurea • Screening, ongoing treatment, and supportive care for congenital and chronic conditions
Communicable diseases	• Vaccination for HPV and tetanus • Vaccination for typhoid, cholera, dengue where indicated • Improved water and sanitation; hand washing with soap	Detection and case management of infections from early childhood described above
Unintentional injuries: • Drowning • Road injuries • Burns	• Swimming lessons • Helmet use • Improved cooking stoves and fire safety measures	Emergency basic life support and trauma management

(GBS: group B *Streptococcus*; HIV: human immunodeficiency virus; HPV: human papillomavirus; AIDS: acquired immunodeficiency syndrome)

services. The principles of PHC were first outlined in the declaration of Alma-Ata in 1978, a pioneering milestone in global health. According to the declaration of Alma-Ata, PHC "addresses the main health problems in the community, providing preventive, curative, and rehabilitative services accordingly...[it] relies, at local and referral levels, on health workers, including physicians, nurses, midwives, auxiliaries and community workers as applicable, as well as traditional practitioners as needed, suitably trained socially and technically to work as a health team and to respond to the expressed health needs of the community".[25] Forty years later, the declaration of Astana was ratified at the Global Conference on PHC in Astana, Kazakhstan in October 2018. PHC is widely recognized as the most cost-effective strategy for delivering essential health interventions, e.g. to reduce maternal and child mortality.[26] PHC encompasses care for mother and child, which can include services for family planning, immunization, prevention and treatment of injuries and common diseases, provision of essential facilities, health education, provision of food and nutrition and adequate supply of safe drinking water. Reducing maternal and child mortality are key public health targets, embodied in the SDGs. An important constraint in implementing them has been the shortage of human workforce, particularly among the PHC providers.

Given the emergence of maternal and newborn burden of disease in poor settings, we need strategies for promoting appropriate outreach through CHWs and volunteers. The global evidence for strategies and interventions in community settings has substantially improved, with a range of interventions that can be potentially packaged for delivery at different times during pregnancy, childbirth, and after birth, through various healthcare providers.[1] Progress has been made through adoption of the decentralization concept by countries, relocating the decision-making power to community and district levels with increased community participation through community-based committees and availability of various types of community-owned resource providers, such as CHWs, traditional birth attendants (TBAs), and community drug distributors to name a few.

Over time, countries have initiated evidence-based health practices that will impact the future of PHC outcomes. Through kangaroo mother care (KMC), Malawi was able to reduce mortality among preterm babies in hospitals by 51% when implemented in the first week of life as compared to late KMC or conventional care. Progress was made in reducing maternal and neonatal deaths in Eritrea by the introduction of community maternity homes for women living in remote areas.[27] South Africa has seen a widespread use of life-saving antiretroviral therapy (ART) than anywhere else in the world, estimated at 2.4 million people receiving ART. Majority of them have been treated in primary care settings (including clinics, community health centers, and district hospitals).[27]

Asia too has seen considerable progress in PHC-related services in child healthcare. In India, a group of accredited social health activists (ASHAs) were introduced in 2005 as part of a National Health Mission, with roles as community-level healthcare providers, especially for maternal and

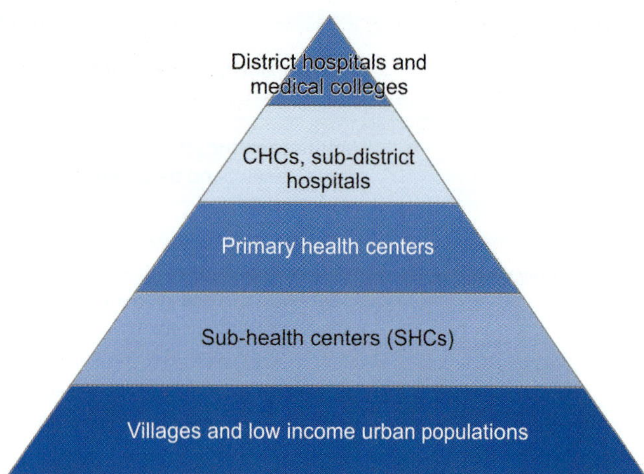

Fig. 2: Schematic diagram of the Indian Public Health System, showing the distribution of healthcare infrastructure in India. (CHCs: community health centers)

child health. Schematic diagram of the Indian Public Health System, showing the distribution of healthcare infrastructure is as shown in **Figure 2**.[28] Similarly in Nepal, female Community Health Volunteers were introduced in 1988, with a focus on maternal and child health, and have nationwide coverage. They are judged to have contributed significantly to improvements in maternal and child health outcomes.[29]

Research has shown that PHC can be largely beneficial in delivering quality maternal and child health interventions even without secondary-care.[30] Pakistan's PHC system comprises of a network of rural health centers (RHCs), basic health units (BHUs) and dispensaries spread in different parts of the country.[31] Over the last two decades, BHUs have been stressed upon as key sources for the PHC services delivery in the rural areas of country. The Ethiopian health system has been structured into three levels; primary, secondary and tertiary. PHC units comprise of a health center and satellite health posts. This primary system functions with aid of Health Extension Workers (HEWs) who can refer patients to health centers or the primary hospital for care, counseling, and basic primary care services like contraceptives, immunizations, and treatment for common childhood illnesses. The Health Extension Program uses "community ownership" and task shifting to provide basic health services at the grassroots. Since the implementation of the program, maternal and child health has improved.

Despite the progress made, several bottlenecks remain, including inequity in access, poor health infrastructure, lack of skilled health personnel, poor access to health services for people in remote areas, poor referral systems, inadequate focus on preventive services, and inefficient allocation of available resources. Strong PHC is the foundation of efficient, equitable, and sustainable health systems, and can address the majority of care needs for the locals, regardless of where they reside.

Secondary Healthcare

In LMICs, secondary healthcare is the second tier of health system, in which patients are referred to specialists in higher hospitals from PHC. Moreover, they also provide services on basic and emergency obstetric and newborn care services. Secondary care also includes skilled attendance during childbirth, intensive care, and medical imaging services. Some primary care services are delivered within hospitals.

Depending on the national policies, patients may be required to see a primary care provider for a referral before they can access secondary care. In countries like Tanzania and Ghana, patients often make secondary, regional and tertiary level health facilities their entry point into the health system and thus bypassing primary levels.[32] It has been observed that parents and guardians are willing to prioritize quality over quantity for childcare by traveling long distances to distant health centers. It can lead to congestion at higher-level health facilities and unnecessary costs for both the patients and the health system. The reasons for bypassing PHC facilities can include poor services (including lack of diagnostic services and medicines) and lack of trust in health workers at such facilities.[33] Improving the quality of care at PHC facilities could reduce delays in seeking the required care. Hence, in a situation of limited resources, strengthening the already existing PHC facilities to provide better services to rural populations should be prioritized before increasing the number of PHC facilities.

In India and Pakistan, the health centers for secondary healthcare include community health centers and district hospitals at block level. District hospitals are a hub of secondary care services in India, with one hospital present in each district. Cases requiring advanced care are referred from a PHC center to a community health center or a district hospital.[28] In India, district hospitals, subdivisional hospitals or community health centers can be declared a fully operational first referral unit (FRU) only if it is equipped to provide the three critical services—(1) emergency obstetric care including surgical interventions such as cesarean sections; (2) care for sick newborns; and (3) round-the-clock blood storage facility.[28]

Tertiary Healthcare

Tertiary healthcare is the third level of a health system, in which specialized care is provided usually after a referral from primary and secondary care. The tertiary level hospitals provide multispecialty clinical services and intensive care facilities to a wider population. Tertiary care hospitals also serve as teaching centers for education of various healthcare professionals on different levels. In India, like in many other LMICs, under the public health system, tertiary care service is provided by medical colleges and advanced medical research institutes. Examples of tertiary care services can include cancer management, specialized surgery services, management of severe burns, specialized neonatology services, palliative care, and other complex medical interventions.

In LMICs, healthcare services, including specialized and tertiary care, pose a significant financial burden on the people belonging to lower socioeconomic levels. Hence, provision of healthcare services by the public sector is a vital instrument in addressing the health morbidity and mortality burden for this population.[34] In countries such as Pakistan, families usually use public sector tertiary care hospitals affiliated with medical institutions as a relatively affordable source of quality specialized healthcare for their children. In lesser developed nations of Asia such as Nepal, in order to increase the access to healthcare services in tertiary level hospitals for poor and marginalized locals who have no ability to pay, the Ministry of Health and Population has defined six target groups for free healthcare services based on socioeconomic statuses; these groups are entitled to free services in tertiary-level hospitals.

■ SIGNIFICANCE OF COMMUNITY-BASED PRIMARY HEALTHCARE AND MATERNAL, NEWBORN AND CHILD HEALTH

Community Health Workers and Home Visitation

To succeed in achieving the health-related SDGs and universal health coverage (UHC), adequate numbers of health workers are required to provide services in an enabling environment.[35] For this reason, many LMICs have used CHWs to support the population living in resource-limited settings and ensure delivery of key healthcare and health promotion interventions. Similarly, there is an increasing task sharing with TBAs and midwives to deliver the MNCH services with documented beneficial effects of such programs.[36] The level of training CHWs receive and their affiliations, varies widely between and within countries. Generally, they work in coordination with health workers across the primary healthcare spectrum to provide health education, distribute intervention packages, diagnose and manage illness, and provide referrals to higher level centers.

Significant evidence exists that proves that community-based interventions are an important mode of improving healthcare delivery and outcomes.[1,37,38] CHWs are being "institutionalized" in the health workforce in Asia and Africa through incentives and enhanced training.[39] Recent studies from the poor communities in south Asia and Africa conclude that CHWs' home visiting during the antenatal and postnatal periods can improve both the antenatal care use, delivery, and reduce maternal and newborn mortality by at least 15–20%.[1] Moreover, home visiting is likely to improve the demand for and use of maternal and childcare services in conflict-affected and fragile states such as Afghanistan.[40] CHW programs have been effective in implementing maternal and child health interventions, such as breastfeeding and KMC.[41] Yuan et al. identified three studies from Bangladesh showing improved equity in immunization coverage between families with home visit intervention.[42] Childbirth and newborn care packages using home visits and community mobilization reduced neonatal mortality by 40%. Home visitation significantly reduced maternal morbidity as well.[1,43]

The Shasthya Shebika (SS) Program in Bangladesh, focuses on the need for female health workers to address the sociocultural barriers to healthcare services access. SSs provide health promotion sessions and educate families on safe delivery, nutrition, family planning, immunizations, and sanitation by making home visits. Over time, skilled delivery, healthy cord care practice, delayed bathing of the newborn and reduction of infant mortality has been reported after the introduction of the SS program.[44] The second most populous country, India, has three categories of CHWs—auxiliary nurse midwife (ANM), anganwadi worker (AWW), and ASHA. ASHA workers focus on promotion of maternal and child health, including immunizations and institutional-based deliveries. Agrawal et al. found that initiation of breastfeeding in the first hour of birth and hygienic cord care, were significantly higher among women visited by ANMs or AWWs with better knowledge.[45] Moving onto its neighbor, Pakistan, CHWs are an important part of the existing health system in the form of lady health workers (LHWs). In 2008, a group of researchers found that the villages where trained LHWs and TBAs provided newborn care and service delivery, had significant reduction in number of stillbirths and the neonatal mortality rate.[46]

Community Participation

The Alma-Ata declaration stressed upon community participation as pivotal to the planning, organizing, and implementation of primary healthcare.[25] In recent time, community participation has once again emerged as a prioritized commodity following the introduction of the SDGs. Integrated people-centered health services are central in achieving UHC and this requires participatory approaches as important tools.[47] Furthermore, with the increasing global prevalence of chronic disease, strategies encompassing community participation have been identified as key for implementing health promotion and the prevention and control of chronic diseases.[48]

There is little substantial evidence on the effectiveness of community involvement programs, particularly on intermediate and long-term health-related outcomes.[49] Much of the research done on community participation has focused only on LMICs despite evidence of its universal utility.[50] Community mobilization based packages have shown significant reduction in neonatal and perinatal mortality.[43] Community-based cares may improve breastfeeding behaviors and may increase referrals to higher health facilities for pregnancy related morbidities and other healthcare services during pregnancy.[51] The integration of community participation in the health service delivery will have positive effects on the sustainability, efficacy and longevity of community health systems, bringing all nearer to achieving the SDGs.

Integrated Community Case Management

The World Health Organization (WHO) and the United Nations International Children's Emergency Fund (UNICEF) collaborated with other development partners in the 2000s, to develop an approach—integrated community case management (ICCM) which aimed to bring treatment services "closer to home" and advocated for LMICs to implement it.[52,53] It is an extension of integrated management of childhood illness (IMCI) and it provides treatment services at community level; primarily executed in rural and hard-to-reach areas. ICCM is an approach to providing integrated case management services for two or more morbidities, including diarrhea, pneumonia, or malaria among children younger than 5 years of age at community level by lay health workers where there is limited access to health facility-based case management services.[54]

There are three main components of ICCM:
1. Training and deployment component—interventions with the motive of increasing access to ICCM services for children under 5 years of age by increasing the number of lay health workers trained on the WHO/UNICEF guidelines for integrated case management services.
2. Systems component—interventions with the motive of improving implementation of ICCM by strengthening health systems' organization and management.
3. Communication and community mobilization component—interventions with the motive of promoting good practices for health and nutrition and generating demand for case management services.[54]

With respect to pneumonia and diarrhea, ICCM has made remarkable progress. Studies have estimated ICCM to potentially reduce mortality in children under-five by 70%.[55] Management of diarrhea has substantially improved with an increase of 9% in care seeking for diarrhea, a remarkable 160% increase in the use of oral rehydration solution, and an 80% increase in the use of zinc supplements.[56] Amouzou et al. undertook a nonsystematic review of the effect of ICCM on child mortality in sub-Saharan Africa and found a greater decline in mortality among children aged 2–59 months in intervention areas compared to the comparison areas.[57] Moreover, community-based strategies have significantly decreased the prevalence and incidence of malaria.[58]

Despite significant reductions in under-five morbidity and mortality between 1990 and 2015, the overall impact of ICCM on childhood survival in LMICs is affected by a variety of factors. These include poor CHW adherence to guidelines, incomplete patient recording, inefficient monthly aggregation, and reporting of cases to higher health offices, as well as infrequent and irregular training and supervision.[59]

■ GAPS AND CHALLENGES

Despite the progress made in the maternal and child health indicators in the tropics, over the last few decades, there exists several gaps and challenges in the service delivery and the evidence generated for their effectiveness. Although most CHW programs are based in sub-Saharan Africa and South Asia, maximum studies have come out of Asia with paucity of research from LMICs in Africa.[60] There is a need for more high quality randomized study designs to identify gaps and limitations of interventions and to inform the future of PHC programs. There is also a lack of evidence on impact of integrated PHC programs with pure community-based implementation and the cost-effectiveness of community-based interventions. Studies are needed to evaluate the emerging innovative strategies of community-based PHC such as mobile health and their impact on service utilization and on maternal and child health outcomes.

The WHO has identified a global shortage of skilled health staff with an estimated deficit as high as 4.25 million in Asia and Africa alone. Severe shortage of qualified health workers and lack of political will to recruit and make them work according to their training is currently a serious concern. The challenges faced by the CHW programs are more or less similar in all the LMICs. These include the financial and administrative difficulties in supporting the CHW programs; the challenge of field supervision and effectively equipping CHWs to perform their duties; low community participation in the health sector and the strong influence of cultural beliefs and medicines. Conversely, many African nations such as Rwanda face a challenge of an increasing number of CHWs. Owing to insufficient resources the governments face a constant battle of providing CHWs with sufficient training and equipment. The Health Extension Program in Ethiopia has faced a number of challenges including delayed provision of health kits to workers, inadequate supervision, and deficient training.[14]

In India, lack of supervision and mentoring are major challenges within the ANM program, where ANMs are often left to manage the health centers on their own. Security is another primary concern to community workers. Iyer and Jesani report how incidents of ANMs being called out to homes on false pretenses and are sexually assaulted in their study areas.[61] Some of the challenges faced by the Pakistan's Lady Health Worker Program (LHWP) are insufficient funds, low coverage, low-quality training, inadequate supplies, and lack of timely payment of salary.[62] Moreover, LHWs and vaccinators face security threats and violence. CHWs' dissatisfaction with their work environment, lack of resources, inadequate linkages with the health system, and ignorance of government policies all impact PHC programs negatively.[63]

Regardless of the gaps and challenges in research and service delivery, several effective community-based PHC preventive and health promoting strategies have been proven to impact maternal, neonatal, and child health positively. It is necessary to ensure implementation of these strategies in LMICs on a large scale and in partnership with all stakeholders including the private and the public sector, the communities, and the donors to ensure political, financial, and social stability.

WAY FORWARD

The WHO assessed the main hurdles that prevent countries to achieve the MDGs. Looking at the gaps of the MDG era, WHO published a report in 2008 stressing on the lack of health services integration, identifying it as one of the major limitations to programs' efficacy in LMICs. Based on this assessment, WHO suggested a big change in the global health strategies to tackle this challenge, with the 2008 report entitled "primary healthcare: now more than ever". The new orientation toward "integrated primary healthcare" was adopted at the 62nd World Health Assembly the following year and was re-emphasized in the 2015 WHO Global Strategy on People-centered and Integrated Health Services. This represented a major undertaking—it was a call for a "fundamental paradigm shift in the way health services are funded, managed, and delivered".[64] It is imperative to note that attaining the SDGs is unlikely without coordinated efforts to improve maternal and child health outcomes through the spectrum of continued care. The target to achieve UHC is now one of the most prominent global health strategies.[65]

It is crucial to bring together the vertical and horizontal approaches of interventions, and fragmented and cohesive models of governance of health services in the form of an integrated model. For PHC to be integrated, the coordination of aid and health interventions in tandem with its implementation, is important.[66] Coordination is vital at all levels of implementation and should be the responsibility of the State. It is necessary to develop partnerships among the nongovernmental organizations (NGOs) and health authorities to better involve the stakeholders. There exist several coordination mechanisms, with some proven to be effective such as intersectoral approaches that bring the governments, stakeholders, and donors in close proximity within any sector to develop interventional policies.[67]

Another important measure for achieving integrated PHC is strengthening the existing public health systems. Integrating PHC requires capacity building of the health sector. It is important to realize that a multidisciplinary and multisectoral perspective is necessary for an integrated PHC.[68] This will involve stepping outside the mindset of sector-wide approaches and encouraging all the stakeholders from different sectors to participate in the decision-making process. Several multisectoral approaches have been tested as a framework for health interventions, including few recent UNICEF projects to improve water, sanitation, and hygiene (WASH) or to reduce malnutrition.[69] Strengthening also involves scaling up the health interventions in the form of expansion of interventions, whether on a population or a geographical basis, and sustaining their use. Strong stable political system along with mechanisms for monitoring political targets and commitments are essential components of large-scale implementations.

As emphasized by WHO, lack of trained healthcare workers is one of the most serious hindrances to scaling up UHC.[70] Informal providers with little or no medical training often deliver a below par service. Evidence suggests that intensive training sessions with these providers can help come near if not the same level of care that is provided by formal providers.[71] Training should be acceptable culturally as well as religiously. CHWs, especially in LMIC, may belong to lower socioeconomic groups and would benefit from regular salaries. CHWs would benefit from a full-time status which would help improve performance and encourage them to ensure delivery of quality care. Furthermore, nonfinancial incentives can help motivate the CHWs.[36] It is vital to maintain community worker's satisfaction in terms of work environment, safety, communication facilities, and monetary compensation.

In recent times, it has become important for health systems to have integration of innovative technologies including electronic medical records, telemedicine, digital medication technologies, and diagnostic tests. These can facilitate UHC by improving the reach, time management, efficiency, and public health monitoring. Moreover, they can help provide CHWs with information about healthcare protocols via text messaging.[72,73] A cluster randomized clinical trial (RCT) from Kenya conducted at rural health facilities showed that health workers who received mobile phone text messages for 6 months about malaria case management as reminders provided better management for malaria in children.[74]

Lastly, it is imperative to engage the community to make decisions about their health and becoming empowered producers of health services. Special attention should be given to engaging the marginalized populations to voice their own needs and so direct the way in which care is provided and funded. Such steps can serve as a platform for them to develop knowledge, skills and confidence. Integrating communities with the primary healthcare system can help both in effectively utilizing the available resources and infrastructure. Home visits, community mobilization, and community-based programs are critical to strengthen the PHC system. Once this link is established, the healthcare system can benefit significantly from the support and resources provided by national and local governments and the NGOs. As part of the SDGs, all United Nations States are targeting to achieve UHC by 2030. The role of primary healthcare in achieving UHC needs to be emphasized. Having a strong health system and a skilled workforce is pivotal in achieving the targeted health outcomes.

■ CONCLUSION

Despite substantial progress in reducing maternal and child mortality during the MDG era, a growing population, limited resources and political instability, pose serious challenges for existing health programs in LMICs, especially in their marginalized and rural areas.

Affordable and accessible PHC facilities, operating on the principles of community engagement and community mobilization are the need of the hour. Recognizing CHWs as a formal commodity and integrating community-based services in PHC will impact child health outcomes positively. Strengthening health systems, and integrating facility and community-based interventions into packages of care at all levels will be key to increasing the availability and coverage of health interventions and reduce child morbidity and mortality.

■ REFERENCES

1. Lassi ZS, Bhutta ZA. Community-based intervention packages for reducing maternal and neonatal morbidity and mortality and improving neonatal outcomes. Cochrane Database Syst Rev. 2015;(3):CD007754.
2. UNICEF, WHO, World Bank Group, United Nations. Levels and Trends in Child Mortality Report 2018. New York: UNICEF; 2018.
3. Chawanpaiboon S, Vogel JP, Moller AB, et al. Global, regional, and national estimates of levels of preterm birth in 2014: a systematic review and modeling analysis. Lancet Glob Health. 2019;7(1):e37-46.
4. Blencowe H, Krasevec J, de Onis M, et al. National, regional, and worldwide estimates of low birthweight in 2015, with trends from 2000: a systematic analysis. Lancet Glob Health. 2019;7(7):e849-60.
5. GBD 2017 DALYs and HALE Collaborators. Global, regional, and national disability-adjusted life-years (DALYs) for 359 diseases and injuries and healthy life expectancy (HALE) for 195 countries and territories, 1990-2017: a systematic analysis for the Global Burden of Disease Study 2017. Lancet. 2018;392 (10159):1859-922.
6. GBD 2017 DALYs and HALE Collaborators. Global, regional, and national age-sex-specific mortality for 282 causes of death in 195 countries and territories, 1980-2017: a systematic analysis for the Global Burden of Disease Study 2017. Lancet. 2018;392(10159):1736-88.
7. Masquelier B, Hug L, Sharrow D, et al. Global, regional, and national mortality trends in older children and young adolescents (5-14 years) from 1990 to 2016: an analysis of empirical data. Lancet Glob Health. 2018;6(10):e1087-99.
8. Fadel SA, Boschi-Pinto C, Yu S, et al. Trends in cause-specific mortality among children aged 5-14 years from 2005 to 2016 in India, China, Brazil, and Mexico: an analysis of nationally representative mortality studies. Lancet. 2019;393(10176): 1119-27.
9. Whitehead M, Dahlgren G. Concepts and principles for tackling social inequities in health: Levelling Up Part 1: Studies on Social and Economic Determinants of Population Health. World Health Organization; 2006.

10. United Nations Children's Fund. The State of the World's Children 2016: A Fair Chance for Every Child. New York: United Nations Children's Fund; 2016.

11. Lawn JE, Cousens S, Zupan J, et al. 4 million neonatal deaths: when? Where? Why? Lancet. 2005;365(9462):891-900.

12. Quansah E, Ohene LA, Norman L, et al. Social factors influencing child health in Ghana. PLoS One. 2016;11(1):e0145401.

13. Jacobs B, Ir P, Bigdeli M, et al. Addressing access barriers to health services: an analytical framework for selecting appropriate interventions in low-income Asian countries. Health Policy Plan. 2011;27(4):288-300.

14. Admassie A, Abebaw D, Woldemichael AD. Impact evaluation of the Ethiopian health services extension programme. J Dev Effect. 2009;1(4):430-49.

15. Rutherford ME, Mulholland K, Hill PC. How access to healthcare relates to under-five mortality in sub-Saharan Africa: systematic review. Trop Med Int Health. 2010;15(5):508-19.

16. Watts N, Amann M, Ayeb-Karlsson S, et al. The Lancet Countdown on health and climate change: from 25 years of inaction to a global transformation for public health. Lancet. 2018;391(10120):581-630.

17. Lloyd SJ, Kovats RS, Chalabi Z. Climate change, crop yields, and undernutrition: development of a model to quantify the impact of climate scenarios on child undernutrition. Environ Health Perspect. 2011;119(12):1817-23.

18. Deribe A, Tessema GA, Deribe K, et al. Trends, causes, and risk factors of mortality among children under 5 in Ethiopia, 1990-2013: findings from the Global Burden of Disease Study 2013. Popul Health Metr. 2016;14(1):42.

19. Shaw B, Amouzou A, Miller NP, et al. Access to integrated community case management of childhood illnesses services in rural Ethiopia: a qualitative study of the perspectives and experiences of caregivers. Health Policy Plan. 2015;31(5):656-66.

20. Way C. The Millennium Development Goals Report 2015. New York: United Nation (UN); 2015.

21. Temmerman M, Khosla R, Bhutta ZA, et al. Towards a new global strategy for women's, children's and adolescents' health. BMJ. 2015;351:h4414.

22. de Onis M, Branca F. Childhood stunting: a global perspective. Matern Child Nutr. 2016;12(Suppl 1):12-26.

23. Bhutta ZA, Black RE. Global maternal, newborn, and child health—so near and yet so far. N Engl J Med. 2013; 369(23):2226-35.

24. Prost A, Colbourn T, Seward N, et al. Women's groups practising participatory learning and action to improve maternal and newborn health in low-resource settings: a systematic review and meta-analysis. Lancet. 2013;381(9879): 1736-46.

25. Passmore R. The declaration of Alma-Ata and the future of primary care. Lancet. 1979;2(8150):1005-8.

26. Darmstadt GL, Lee AC, Cousens S, et al. 60 million non-facility births: who can deliver in community settings to reduce intrapartum-related deaths? Int J Gynaecol Obstet. 2009;107(Suppl 1):S89-112.

27. World Health Organization. The Africa Health Transformation Programme 2015-2020: A Vision for Universal Health Coverage. Geneva: World Health Organization; 2015.

28. Chokshi M, Patil B, Khanna R, et al. Health systems in India. J Perinatol. 2016;36(s3):S9-12.

29. Engel J, Glennie J, Adhikari SR, et al. Nepal's story: understanding improvements in maternal health. London: Overseas Development Institute; 2013.

30. Bhutta ZA, Ali S, Cousens S, et al. Alma-Ata: rebirth and revision interventions to address maternal, newborn, and child survival: what difference can integrated primary healthcare strategies make? Lancet. 2008;372(9642):972-89.

31. Khowaja K. Healthcare systems and care delivery in Pakistan. J Nurs Adm. 2009;39(6):263-5.

32. Nyonator F, Ofosu A, Segbafah M, et al. Monitoring and evaluating progress towards universal health coverage in Ghana. PLoS Med. 2014;11(9):e1001691.

33. Kahabuka C, Kvåle G, Moland KM, et al. Why caretakers bypass Primary Health Care facilities for child care—a case from rural Tanzania. BMC Health Serv Res. 2011;11:315.

34. Basu S, Andrews J, Kishore S, et al. Comparative performance of private and public healthcare systems in low- and middle-income countries: a systematic review. PLoS Med. 2012;9(6):e1001244.

35. World Health Organization. Global Strategy on Human Resources for Health: Health Workforce 2030. Geneva: World Health Organization; 2015-2016.

36. Bhutta ZA, Lassi ZS, Pariyo G, et al. Global experience of community health workers for delivery of health related millennium development goals: a systematic review, country case studies, and recommendations for integration into National Health Systems. Geneva: World Health Organization; 2010. p. 61.

37. Singh P, Sachs JD. 1 million community health workers in sub-Saharan Africa by 2015. Lancet. 2013;382(9889):363-5.

38. Lewin S, Munabi-Babigumira S, Glenton C, et al. Lay health workers in primary and community healthcare for maternal and child health and the management of infectious diseases. Cochrane Database Syst Rev. 2010;(3):CD004015.

39. Pfaffmann Zambruni J, Rasanathan K, Hipgrave D, et al. Community health systems: allowing community health workers to emerge from the shadows. Lancet Glob Health. 2017;5(9):e866-7.

40. Edmond KM, Yousufi K, Anwari Z, et al. Can community health worker home visiting improve care-seeking and maternal and newborn care practices in fragile states such as Afghanistan? A population-based intervention study. BMC Med. 2018;16(1):106.

41. Gilmore B, McAuliffe E. Effectiveness of community health workers delivering preventive interventions for maternal and child health in low- and middle-income countries: a systematic review. BMC Public Health. 2013;13:847.

42. Yuan B, Målqvist M, Trygg N, et al. What interventions are effective on reducing inequalities in maternal and child health in low- and middle-income settings? A systematic review. BMC Public Health. 2014;14:634.

43. Lassi ZS, Das JK, Salam RA, et al. Evidence from community level inputs to improve quality of care for maternal and newborn health: interventions and findings. Reprod Health. 2014;11(Suppl 2):S2.

44. Rahman M, Jhohura FT, Mistry SK, et al. Assessing community based improved maternal neonatal child survival (IMNCS) program in rural Bangladesh. PLoS One. 2015;10(9): e0136898.

45. Agrawal PK, Agrawal S, Ahmed S, et al. Effect of knowledge of community health workers on essential newborn healthcare: a study from rural India. Health Policy Plan. 2011;27(2):115-26.

46. Bhutta ZA, Memon ZA, Soofi S, et al. Implementing community-based perinatal care: results from a pilot study in rural Pakistan. Bull World Health Organ. 2008; 86(6):452-9.

47. Marston C, Hinton R, Kean S, et al. Community participation for transformative action on women's, children's and adolescents' health. Bull World Health Organ. 2016;94(5):376-82.

48. Narain JP. Integrating services for noncommunicable diseases prevention and control: use of primary healthcare approach. Indian J Community Med. 2011;36(Suppl 1):S67-71.

49. Rifkin SB. Examining the links between community participation and health outcomes: a review of the literature. Health Policy Plan. 2014;29(Suppl 2):ii98-106.

50. Milton B, Attree P, French B, et al. The impact of community engagement on health and social outcomes: a systematic review. Community Dev J. 2012;47(3):316-34.

51. Lassi ZS, Majeed A, Rashid S, et al. The interconnections between maternal and newborn health—evidence and implications for policy. J Matern Fetal Neonatal Med. 2013;26 (Suppl 1):3-53.

52. Bennett S, Dalglish SL, Juma PA, et al. Altogether now... understanding the role of international organizations in iCCM policy transfer. Health Policy Plan. 2015;30(Suppl 2):ii26-35.

53. Diaz T, Aboubaker S, Young M. Current scientific evidence for integrated community case management (iCCM) in Africa: findings from the iCCM Evidence Symposium. J Glob Health. 2014;4(2):020101.

54. World Health Organization, UNICEF. WHO/UNICEF Joint Statement Integrated Community Case Management: an equity-focused Strategy to Improve Access to Essential Treatment Services for Children. Geneva/New York: World Health Organization/UNICEF; 2012.

55. Theodoratou E, Al-Jilaihawi S, Woodward F, et al. The effect of case management on childhood pneumonia mortality in developing countries. Int J Epidemiol. 2010;39(Suppl 1):i155-71.

56. Das JK, Lassi ZS, Salam RA, et al. Effect of community based interventions on childhood diarrhea and pneumonia: uptake of treatment modalities and impact on mortality. BMC Public Health. 2013;13(Suppl 3):S29.

57. Amouzou A, Morris S, Moulton LH, et al. Assessing the impact of integrated community case management (iCCM) programs on child mortality: Review of early results and lessons learned in sub–Saharan Africa. J Glob Health. 2014;4(2):020411.

58. Salam RA, Das JK, Lassi ZS, et al. Impact of community-based interventions for the prevention and control of malaria on intervention coverage and health outcomes for the prevention and control of malaria. Infect Dis Poverty. 2014;3:25.

59. Nsona H, Mtimuni A, Daelmans B, et al. Scaling up integrated community case management of childhood illness: update from Malawi. Am J Trop Med Hyg. 2012;87(Suppl 5):54-60.

60. Lassi ZS, Middleton PF, Bhutta ZA, et al. Strategies for improving healthcare seeking for maternal and newborn illnesses in low- and middle-income countries: a systematic review and meta-analysis. Global Health Action. 2016;9:31408.

61. Iyer A, Jesani A. Barriers to the quality of care: the experience of auxiliary nurse-midwives in rural Maharashtra. In: Koenig M, Khan ME (Eds). Improving Quality of Care in India's Family Welfare Programme: The Challenge Ahead. New York: Population Council; 1999.

62. World Health Organization, Global Health Workforce Alliance. Country Case Study: Pakistan's Lady Health Worker Programme. Geneva: World Health Organization/Global Health Workforce Alliance; 2008.

63. Banchani E, Tenkorang EY. Implementation challenges of maternal healthcare in Ghana: the case of healthcare providers in the Tamale Metropolis. BMC Health Serv Res. 2014;14:7.

64. Bennett S, Fancourt N, Peters D, et al. WHO Global Strategy on People-Centred and Integrated Health Services: Interim report. Geneva: World Health Organization; 2015.

65. Rumbold B, Baker R, Ferraz O, et al. Universal health coverage, priority setting, and the human right to health. Lancet. 2017;390(10095):712-4.

66. Sundewall J, Jönsson K, Cheelo C, et al. Stakeholder perceptions of aid coordination implementation in the Zambian health sector. Health Policy. 2010;95(2-3):122-8.

67. Walford V. A review of health sector wide approaches in Africa. London: HLSP Institute; 2007. p. 30.

68. Link BG, Phelan JC. McKeown and the idea that social conditions are fundamental causes of disease. Am J Public Health. 2002;92(5):730-2.

69. Olu O, Usman A, Manga L, et al. Strengthening health disaster risk management in Africa: multi-sectoral and people-centred approaches are required in the post-Hyogo Framework of Action era. BMC Public Health. 2016;16:691.

70. Walley J, Lawn JE, Tinker A, et al. Primary healthcare: making Alma-Ata a reality. Lancet. 2008;372(9642):1001-7.

71. Frenk J. Reinventing primary healthcare: the need for systems integration. Lancet. 2009;374(9684):170-3.

72. Freifeld CC, Chunara R, Mekaru SR, et al. Participatory epidemiology: use of mobile phones for community-based health reporting. PLoS Med. 2010;7(12):e1000376.

73. Guy R, Hocking J, Wand H, et al. How effective are short message service reminders at increasing clinic attendance? A meta-analysis and systematic review. Health Serv Res. 2012;47(2):614-32.

74. Zurovac D, Sudoi RK, Akhwale WS, et al. The effect of mobile phone text-message reminders on Kenyan health workers' adherence to malaria treatment guidelines: a cluster randomised trial. Lancet. 2011;378(9793):795-803.

Nutritional Disorders in the Tropics

Piyush Gupta

Nutritional Considerations for Children in the Tropics

Aaradhana Singh, Piyush Gupta

INTRODUCTION

The nutritional status of children is a reflection of the developmental status of a country. Nutrition impacts not only the physical but also the mental health of children. Proper nutrition prevents communicable as well as noncommunicable diseases (NCDs). Malnutrition encompasses undernutrition (underweight, stunting, and wasting), overweight/obesity, and micronutrient deficiencies. With a change in lifestyle and easy availability of ultraprocessed food, there is continuous rise in the prevalence of overweight and obesity worldwide leading to a growing risk of NCDs including cardiovascular diseases, diabetes, chronic respiratory diseases, and cancers.

BURDEN OF UNDERNUTRITION AND OVERWEIGHT

Global Burden

As per UNICEF/WHO/World Bank Group Joint Child Malnutrition estimates 2019, 149 million (21.9%) children were stunted, 49 million (7.3 %) were wasted, and 40 million (4.9%) were overweight globally in the under-five age group.[1] Asia and Africa bear the greatest share of malnutrition. In 2018, more than half (55%) of all stunted under-five children lived in Asia and more than one third (39%) lived in Africa. More than two thirds (68%) of all wasted children in the under-five age group lived in Asia and more than one quarter (28%) lived in Africa. Almost half (47%) of all overweight under-five children lived in Asia and one quarter (24%) lived in Africa.[1] **Figures 1 and 2** show the prevalence of stunting and overweight, respectively, in UNICEF regions from 1990 to 2018. **Figure 3** shows the prevalence of wasting in UNICEF regions in 2018. Malnutrition rates continue to remain high. Stunting is declining very slowly while wasting still affects the lives of many young children. Prevalence of overweight/obesity is on the rise.

Burden in South Asia

South Asia has the highest burden of malnourished children. Two out of five stunted children in the world live in South Asia. South Asia is the only region with high wasting prevalence (10–15%). More than half of all wasted children in the world live in South Asia. **Table 1** shows the prevalence of childhood malnutrition in 10 countries of South Asia.[1]

Burden in India

As per the National Family Health Survey (NFHS-4) (2015–16), approximately 38% of under-five children in India were stunted, 21% were wasted, and 36% were underweight.[2] **Figure 4** depicts the trends of nutritional status as found in four NFHS surveys conducted between 1992 and 2016. The Ministry of Health conducted the Comprehensive National Nutrition Survey (CNNS) from 2016 to 2018 to collect data on the nutritional status of Indian children from 0 to 19 years of age. **Table 2** provides the prevalence of malnutrition as per NFHS-4 and CNNSs in India.[2,3] **Figures 5 to 7** show the prevalence of stunting, wasting, and underweight, respectively, in Indian states as per the CNNS.

Stunting prevalence was highest in Bihar, Madhya Pradesh, Rajasthan, and Uttar Pradesh (37–42%) and lowest in Goa and Jammu and Kashmir (16–21%). Madhya Pradesh, West Bengal, Tamil Nadu, and Jharkhand had high prevalence (≥20%) of wasting. The states with the lowest prevalence of under-five wasting were Manipur, Mizoram, and Uttarakhand (6% each). The states with the highest prevalence (≥39%) of underweight were Bihar,

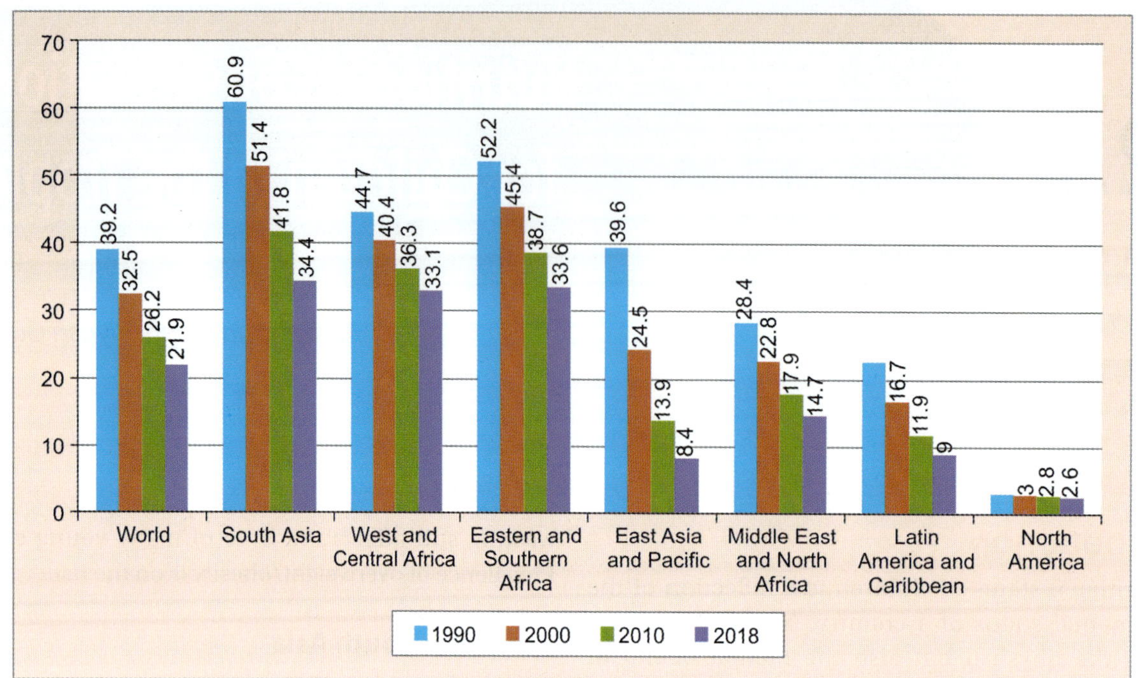

Fig. 1: Prevalence of stunting in under-five children by the UNICEF region, 1990–2019.
Source: Reproduced from UNICEF/WHO/World Bank Joint Malnutrition Estimates, 2018.[1]

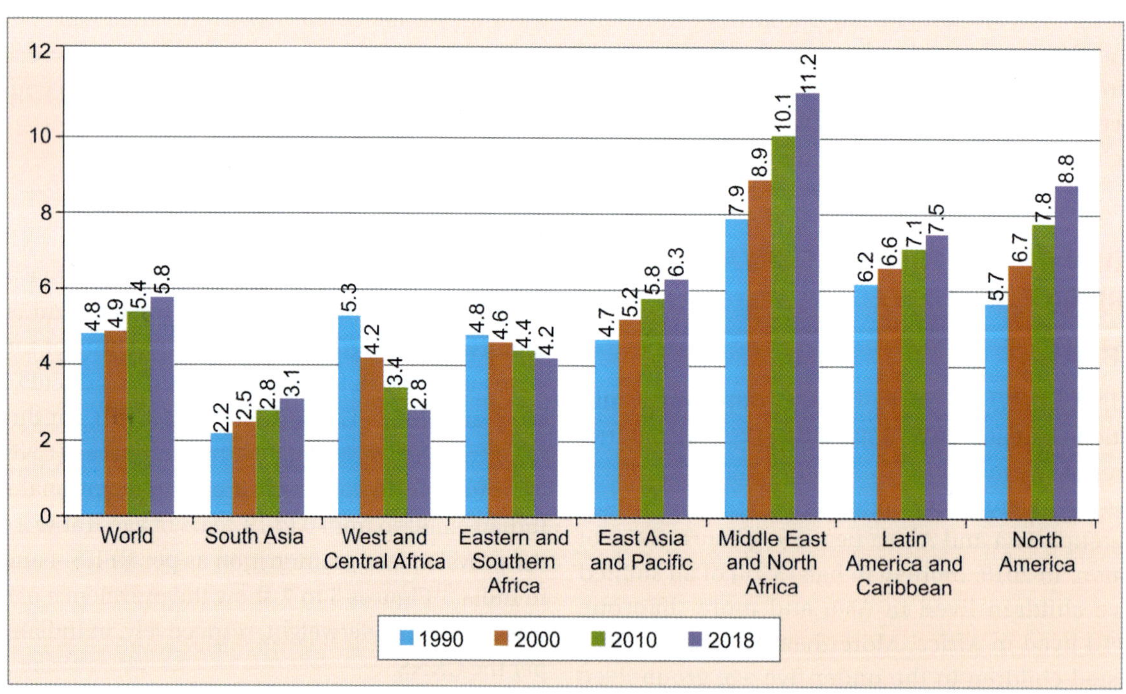

Fig. 2: Prevalence of overweight in under-five children by the UNICEF region from 1990 to 2018.
Source: Reproduced from UNICEF/WHO/World Bank Joint Malnutrition Estimates, 2018.[1]

Chhattisgarh, Madhya Pradesh, and Jharkhand. Mizoram, Sikkim, Manipur, Arunachal Pradesh, and Nagaland had the lowest prevalence (≤16%) of underweight.

The CNNS evaluated the anthropometric status of children as well as adolescents. **Figure 8** shows the prevalence of malnutrition in 0–4-year, 5–9-year, and 10–19-year age groups as per the CNNS.

Among adolescents, the prevalence of overweight and obesity were 5% and 1% respectively. The states with the highest prevalence (>12%) of overweight in adolescents

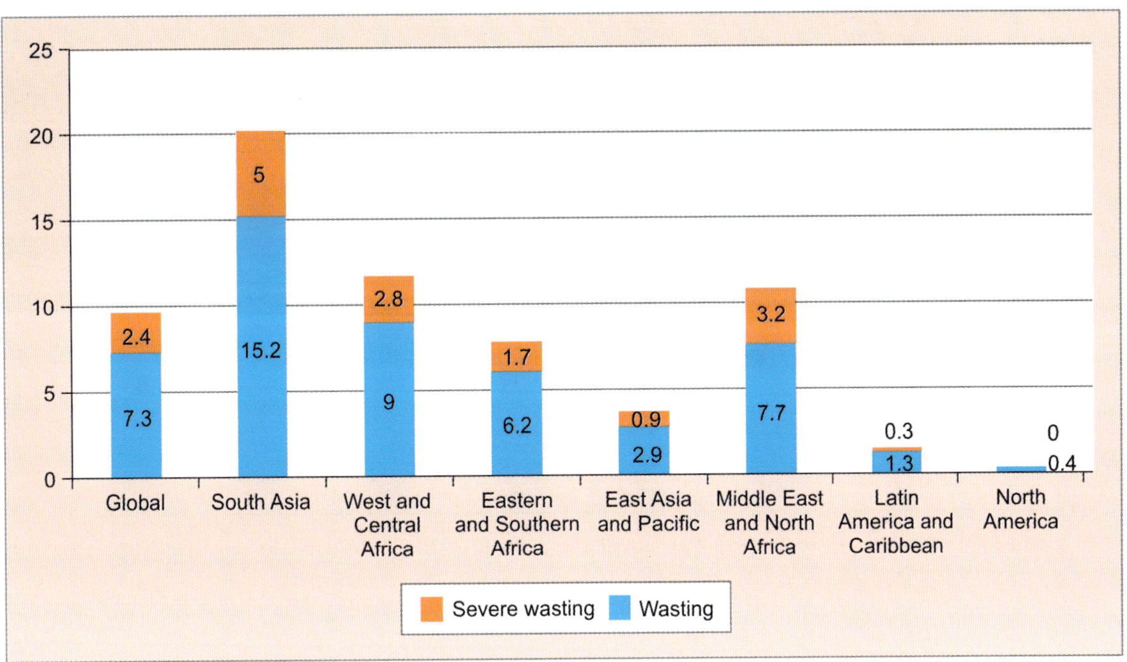

Fig. 3: Prevalence of under-five children with wasting by the UNICEF region, 2018.
Source: Reproduced from UNICEF/WHO/World Bank Joint Malnutrition Estimates, 2018.[1]

Table 1: Prevalence of malnutrition in under-five children in South Asia.						
Country	Survey year	Underweight (%)	Stunting (%)	Wasting (%)	Severe wasting (%)	Overweight (%)
Afghanistan	2013	25.0	40.9	9.5	4	5.4
Bangladesh	2014	32.8	36.2	14.4	3.2	1.6
Bhutan	2010	12.7	33.5	5.9	2.0	7.6
China	2013	2.4	8.1	1.9	–	9.1
India	2015–16	36.3	37.9	20.8	7.7	2.4
Maldives	2009	17.7	18.6	10.8	2.7	6.1
Myanmar	2015–16	18.5	29.4	6.6	1.3	1.5
Pakistan	2017–18	23.1	37.6	7.1	2.4	2.5
Sri Lanka	2016	20.5	17.3	15.1	3.0	2.0
Nepal	2014	30.1	37.5	11.3	3.2	2.1

Source: UNICEF/WHO/World Bank joint child malnutrition estimates (country level) 2009-18.[1]

were Delhi, Goa, and Tamil Nadu while the lowest prevalence (< 3%) of overweight was in Bihar, Madhya Pradesh, Uttar Pradesh, Jharkhand, and Rajasthan.[2]

Infant and Young Child Feeding practices: The CNNS 2018 has collected data not only on Infant and Young Child Feeding practices but also on diversity of food consumed by children and adolescents. **Table 3** depicts Infant and Young Child Feeding practices as per the CNNS 2018, NFHS-3, NFHS-4, and UNICEF 2018 (global data). More than 85% of children and adolescents consumed dark green leafy vegetables and pulses or beans at least once per week; one-third consumed eggs, fish, or chicken or meat at least once per week; and 60% consumed milk or curd at least once per week.[2]

■ MICRONUTRIENT DEFICIENCIES IN INDIA

The prevalence of anemia in the 6–35-month age group was 74%, 79%, and 59% in NFHS-2, NFHS-3, and NFHS-4 surveys, respectively. The CNNS was the largest survey for micronutrient deficiencies. **Table 4** shows the prevalence of anemia, vitamin A deficiency, vitamin D deficiency, vitamin B12 deficiency, and folate deficiency in 0–4-year, 5–9-year, and 10–19-year age groups as per the CNNS.

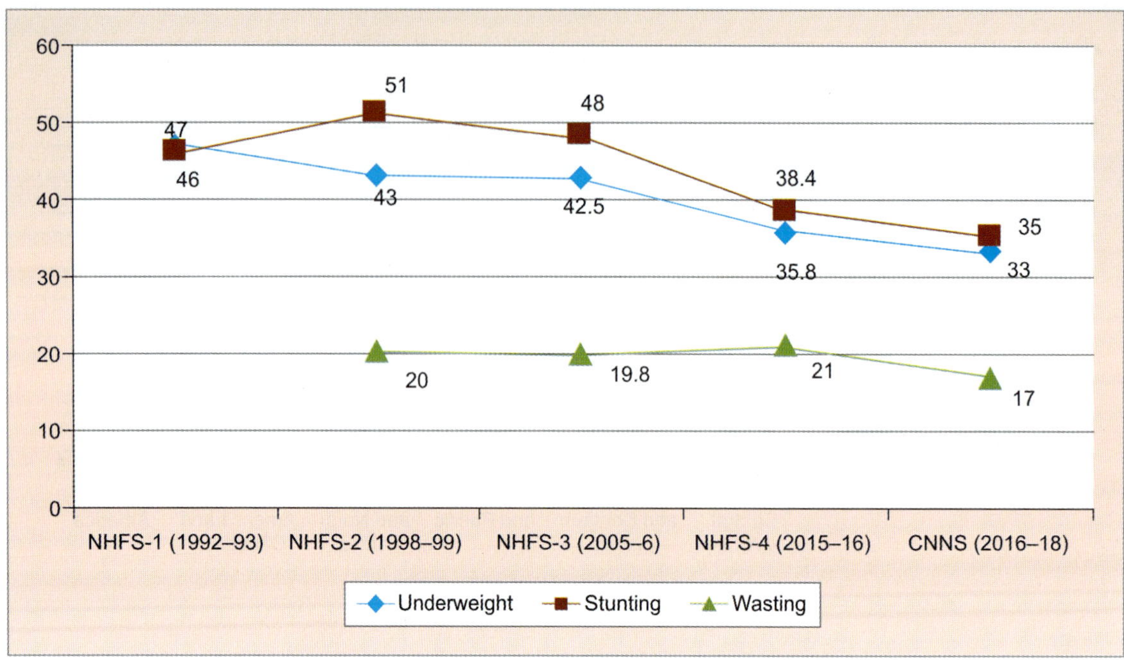

Fig. 4: Trends of malnutrition in under-five children, India.
(CNNS: Comprehensive National Nutrition Survey; NFHS-4: National Family Health Survey-4; UNICEF: United Nations Children's Fund)
Source: NFHS-3 (1998–99), NFHS-4 (2005–06), CNNS (2016–18), UNICEF Global (2018).

Table 2: Prevalence of malnutrition as per NFHS-4 and CNNS in India.			
	*NFHS-4 survey[3] (2015–16)**	*CNNS[2] (2016–18)**	*UNICEF Global[1] (2018)**
Children under 5 years who are stunted (height-for-age)	38.4	35.0	21.9
Children under 5 years who are wasted (weight-for-height	21.0	17.0	7.3
Children under 5 years who are severely wasted (weight-for-height)	7.4	NA	2.4
Children under 5 years who are underweight (weight-for-age)	35.8	33.0	15 (2014)

(CNNS: Comprehensive National Nutrition Survey; NFHS-4: National Family Health Survey-4; UNICEF: United Nations Children's Fund)
*All figures are in percentages.
Source: NFHS-3 (1998–99), NFHS-4 (2005–06), CNNS (2016–18), UNICEF Global (2018).

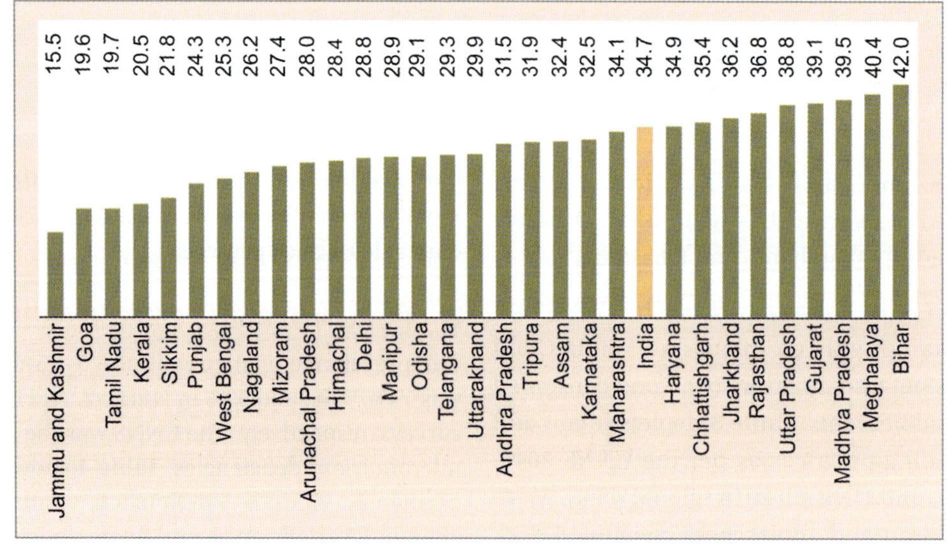

Fig. 5: Prevalence (%) of stunting among children aged 0–4 years by state, India.
Source: Reproduced from Comprehensive National Nutrition Survey, 2016–18.[2]

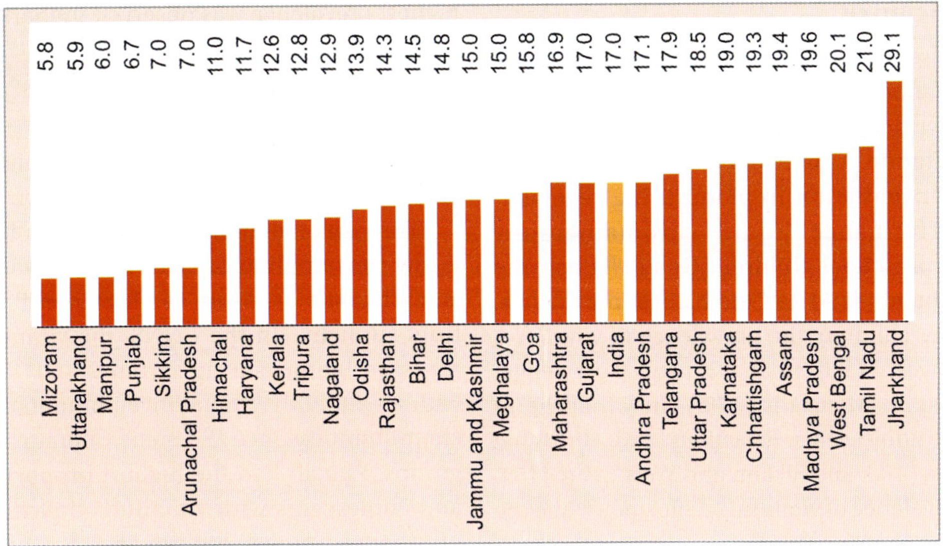

Fig. 6: Prevalence (%) of wasting among children aged 0–4 years by state, India.
Source: Reproduced from Comprehensive National Nutrition Survey, 2016–18.[2]

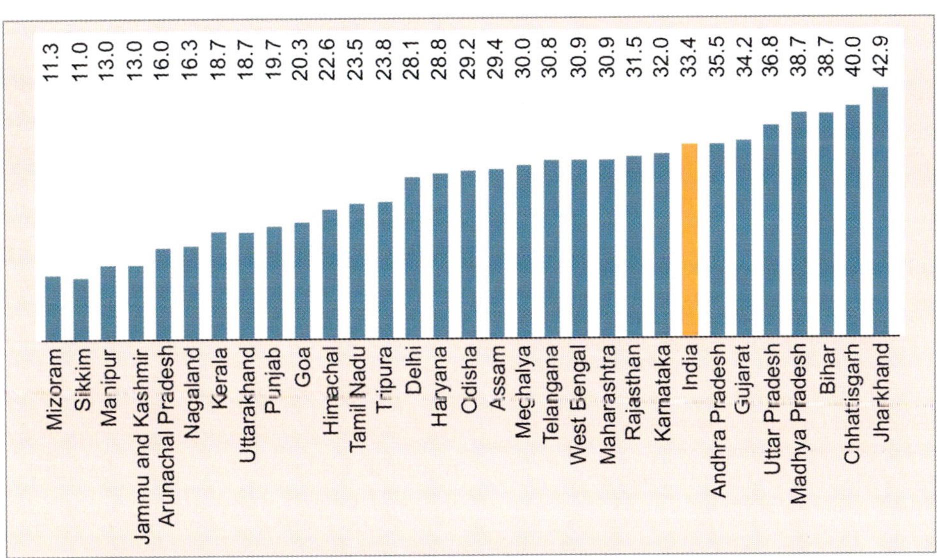

Fig. 7: Prevalence (%) of underweight among children aged 0–4 years by state, India.
Source: Reproduced from Comprehensive National Nutrition Survey, 2016–18.[2]

Nutritional Anemia

Anemia results from deficiency of iron, folate, vitamin B_{12}; malaria; helminthic infestations; genetic hemoglobinopathies such as thalassemia and sickle cell disease; chronic infection and inflammation; and chronic disease conditions such as renal failure.[4] In preschool children, the prevalence of anemia is highest in Madhya Pradesh (54%) and lowest in Nagaland (8%). Among school-age children, Tripura (41%) and Kerala (3%) had the highest and lowest prevalence, respectively. Among adolescents, West Bengal had the highest (46%) while Nagaland (8%) and Kerala had the lowest prevalence.[2]

Iron Deficiency

Iron deficiency is one of the most common nutritional deficiencies worldwide. In the CNNS, low serum ferritin among children and adolescents with normal C-reactive protein levels was considered as a biomarker for iron deficiency. In all three age groups, Punjab had the highest prevalence (67% among preschool children, 51% among school-age children, and 45% among adolescents) and Mizoram had the lowest prevalence of iron deficiency (4% among preschool children, 2% among school-age children, and 9% among adolescents).

Vitamin A Deficiency

Vitamin A is an essential micronutrient that is particularly important for immune function.

Vitamin A is critical during periods of rapid growth. In the CNNS, Vitamin A deficiency was measured by serum retinol concentration in blood using reversed-phase high-performance liquid chromatography (HPLC). Among preschool children, Goa (2%) had the lowest and Jharkhand (43%) had the highest prevalence. Among school-age children, the prevalence of vitamin A deficiency was lowest in Rajasthan (1%) and West Bengal (4%) and highest in Mizoram (47%) and Jharkhand (42%). Among the adolescents, Rajasthan (2%), Himachal Pradesh (3%), Goa (4%), and Sikkim and West Bengal (5% each) had low prevalence of vitamin A deficiency while the highest prevalence was observed in Jharkhand (30%) and Chhattisgarh (26%).[2]

Vitamin D Deficiency

Vitamin D is essential for bone metabolism and may also play a role in immune system regulation.

The risk of vitamin D deficiency is high where there is low consumption of foods rich in vitamin D and there is inadequate exposure to ultraviolet B (UVB) radiation from sunlight.[5] In the CNNS, the vitamin D status was assessed by measuring serum 25(OH)D concentration with an antibody-competitive immunoassay using direct chemiluminescence (Siemens Centaur). In all three age groups, Punjab had the highest proportions of children and adolescents with vitamin D deficiency, with a 52% prevalence among children aged 1–4 years, 76% among children aged 5–9 years, and 68% among adolescents aged 10–19 years.

Iodine Deficiency

Iodine is an essential nutrient required for the thyroid hormone synthesis. Its deficiency causes hypothyroidism in children. Worldwide, 88% of people consume iodized salt. The CNNS provided national- and state-level estimates of median urinary iodine concentrations (mUICs) among children and adolescents. In all states except Tamil Nadu where mUIC was >300 µg/L, children and adolescents had adequate urinary iodine status.[2]

Zinc Deficiency

Deficiency of zinc causes growth retardation, impaired immune function, hair loss, diarrhea, skin lesion, and delayed sexual maturation. Among children aged 1–4

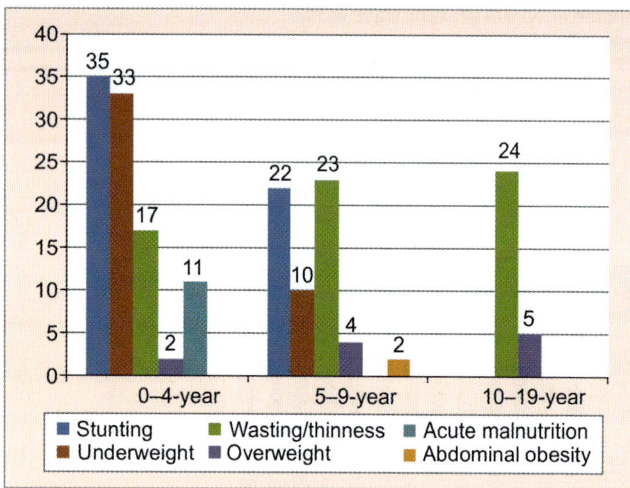

Fig. 8: Prevalence (%) of malnutrition in 0–4-year, 5–9-year, and 10–19-year age groups.
Source: Reproduced from Comprehensive National Nutrition Survey 2016–18.[2]

Table 3: Infant and Young Child Feeding practices in Indian children.

	NFHS-3 (1998–99)*	NFHS-4 (2005–06)*	CNNS (2016–18)*	UNICEF Global (2018)
Children breastfed within 1 hour after birth	23.5 (<3 years)	41.6 (<3 years)	56.6 (0–23 months)	44 (<3 years)
Children under age 6 months who are exclusively breastfed	46.4	54.9	58.0	42.0
Children 6–8 months receiving solid/semisolid food and breast milk	42.7	52.6	53.0	69.0
Minimum diet diversity in 6–23 months	NA	NA	21.0	29.0
Minimum meal frequency 6–23 months	NA	NA	42.0	53.0
Minimum acceptable diet	NA	NA	6.0	19.0
Continued breastfeeding aged 12–15 months at 1 year	NA	NA	83.0	65.0

(CNNS: Comprehensive National Nutrition Survey; NFHS-4: National Family Health Survey-4; UNICEF: United Nations Children's Fund)
*All figures are in percentages.
Source: NFHS-3 (1998–99), NFHS-4 (2005–06), CNNS (2016–18), UNICEF Global (2018).

Table 4: Prevalence of micronutrient deficiencies in children, India 2016–18.

	0–4 years	5–9 years	10–19 years
Anemia (%) 1–4 yr: Hb < 11.0 g/dL; 5–11 yr: Hb < 11.5 g/dL; 12–14 yr: Hb Girls: <12.0 g/dL, Boys: <13.0 g/dL	41.0	24.0	28.0
Iron deficiency (%) 1–4 yr: S. ferritin < 12 µg/L; ≥5 yr: S. ferritin < 15 µg/L	32.0	17.0	22.0
Vitamin A deficiency (%) 1–9 years: S. retinol concentration < 20 µg/dL 10–19 years S. retinol concentration < 20 µg/dL	18.0	22.0	16.0
Vitamin D deficiency (%) Serum 25(OH)D concentration < 12 ng/mL (30 nmol/L)	14.0	18.0	24.0
Zinc deficiency (%) <10 yr: <65 µg/dL >10 yr: Nonpregnant Females Males Morning fasting <70 µg/dL <74 µg/dL Morning nonfasting <66 µg/dL <70 µg/dL	19.0	17.0	32.0
Vitamin B_{12} deficiency (%) Serum vitamin B_{12} < 203 pg/mL	14.0	17.0	37.0
Folate deficiency (%) Serum erythrocyte folate < 151 ng/mL	23.0	28.0	37.0
Iodine (urinary iodine) status Adequate: >100 to ≤330 µg/L)	Adequate 213	Adequate 175	Adequate 173

(S. ferritin: serum ferritin; S. retinol: serum retinol)
Source: Comprehensive National Nutrition Survey, 2016–18.[2]

years, the highest prevalence was in Himachal Pradesh (41%) and lowest in Nagaland (1%). Among children aged 5–9 years, zinc deficiency ranged from 2% in Nagaland to 38% in Himachal Pradesh and among adolescents from 4% in Nagaland to 55% in Gujarat.[2]

Vitamin B12 and Folate Deficiency

Vitamin B12 and folate are necessary for the formation of healthy red blood cells, for the repair of body cells and tissues, and for the synthesis of DNA. Vitamin B12 is also important for maintaining normal nerve function. It is found primarily in foods of animal origin, and the risks for deficiency are therefore higher where access to these foods is limited.

In the CNNS, vitamin B12 and folate levels were assessed by estimating circulating levels of serum vitamin B12 and erythrocyte folate by a competitive immunoassay using direct chemiluminescence. Gujarat had the highest prevalence of vitamin B12 deficiency at 29% and West Bengal had the lowest prevalence at 2% among children aged 1–4 years. In the 5–9-year age group, prevalence ranged from 0% in Nagaland and 1% in Kerala to 31% in Uttar Pradesh and 32% in Punjab. A prevalence of 2% was reported in Kerala and Nagaland and 48% in Gujarat among adolescents aged 10–19 years.

◼ IMPACT OF MALNUTRITION

Around 45% of deaths among children under 5 years of age are linked to undernutrition.[6] Malnutrition increases susceptibility to infections and delays recovery from illness. Malnourished children have lower intelligence quotient. The degree of cognitive impairment is related to iron deficiency anemia and to the severity of stunting.

As per UNICEF, stunting in early life leads to loss of 0.7 grade in schooling, a delay of 7 months in starting school, and 22–54% reduction in lifetime earning.[7] Malnutrition has a negative impact on the economic growth of a country which is caused by the economic burden of high mortality and morbidity due to malnutrition and by decreasing the productivity of malnutrition-affected individuals. Adults undernourished as children earn 20% less than normally nourished.[8] Asia and Africa lose 80% of GNP (gross national product) every year.[8] An increase of 1 cm in height is associated with an increase of 4% and 6% in wages of men and women, respectively.[8] It is estimated that malnutrition may cost society up to US $3.5 trillion per year and overweight and obesity may cost up to US $500 billion per year. Health consequences of overweight contribute to 120 million of Disability Adjusted Life Years (DALYs) globally.[8]

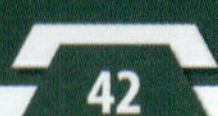

DETERMINANTS OF MALNUTRITION

Malnutrition is multifactorial caused not only by unavailability of adequate nutritious food but also by frequent illness and poor access to health services. Knowledge of determinants is essential to tackle this long-standing problem. **Figure 9** depicts the UNICEF conceptual framework of malnutrition.[9] The causes of malnutrition are classified as follows:

- *Immediate causes*: Inadequate dietary intake and diseases are the immediate causes.
- *Underlying causes*: These are household food insecurity (unavailability of food, poor access to food, or poor utilization of a diverse diet), improper feeding practices for children, unhealthy environments of household and surroundings, and poor access to adequate health care.
- *Basic causes*: These include social, economic, and political factors existing in a country which ultimately influence the nutritional status of children, adolescents, and pregnant women. Poverty limits the access of vulnerable populations to essential resources.

Stunting is a consequence of chronic undernutrition during pregnancy and during early childhood while wasting is an acute life-threatening condition resulting from poor feeding and diseases. Emergence of overweight and obesity is because of changing lifestyle resulting in poor physical activity and increased accessibility to processed food. Moreover, the causes of undernutrition and overweight, in many ways, are similar and interlinked. Stunting during early life has been linked to increased risk of overweight and NCDs in later life.

In Africa, Habyarimana et al.[10] found that the age and gender of the child, birth weight, mother's knowledge about nutrition, birth order, recent fever, multiple births, mother's education level, age of mother at child birth, body mass index, anemia prevalence, province, source of drinking water, and wealth quintiles were the key determinants of under-five malnutrition.

STRATEGIES TO COMBAT MALNUTRITION

It is well recognized now that nutrition is a life-long issue. The effect of poor nutrition starts in utero and infancy to persist in adulthood and perpetuates across generations.

Lifecycle Approach of UNICEF

The lifecycle approach of UNICEF highlights the need to target nutrition programs to different stages of life:

- Pregnancy through infancy (*first 1000 days*) is the most critical period of growth and development in a child's life. Inadequate nutrition during this critical period affects

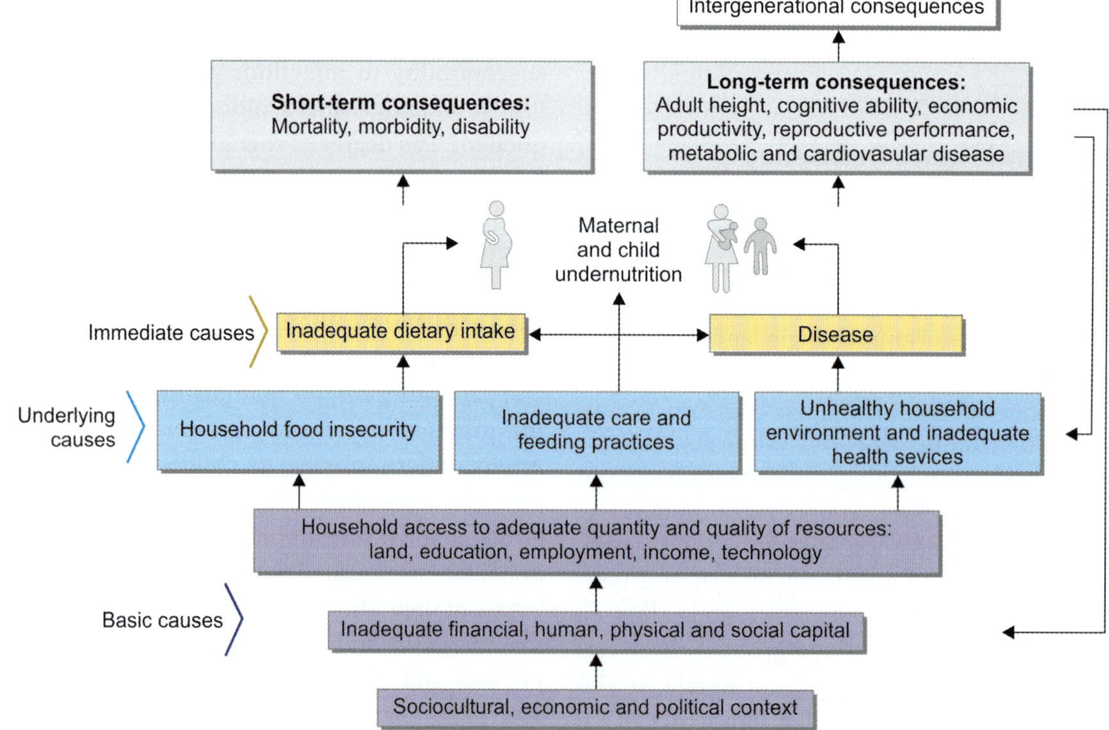

Fig. 9: Conceptual framework of determinants of malnutrition.
Source: Reproduced from United Nations Children's Fund. Strategy for improved nutrition of children and women in developing countries. New York: UNICEF, 1990.

the growth of child which lasts lifelong. Interventions targeted to this key period by improvement of maternal nutrition, exclusive breastfeeding for the first 6 months of life, and appropriate complementary feeding may reduce malnutrition prevalence.[11]

- Throughout childhood, good nutrition is important for the growth and health of children. Improving WASH (Water Access, Sanitation, and Hygiene) practices, nutritional support, vitamin A supplementation, immunization, and deworming in children are some targeted approaches. UNICEF provides ready-to-use therapeutic food (RUTF) in countries where children are suffering from acute malnutrition.
- From adolescence through pregnancy: Many adolescent girls and women have nutrient deficits. Micronutrient supplementation helps support healthy pregnancy and prevents low birth weight in babies.

Nutrition-Specific versus Nutrition-Sensitive Approaches

Nutrition-specific interventions target the factors which affect nutrition directly. These include promotion of exclusive breastfeeding up to 6 months of age, continued breastfeeding till 2 years of age, and appropriate complementary feed up to 2 years of age; food fortification; micronutrient supplementation; and treatment of severe acute malnutrition. Nutrition-sensitive interventions address the underlying determinants such as agriculture, clean water and sanitation, education, employment, healthcare, and women's empowerment.[12,13]

Global Nutrition Targets for 2025

In 2012 and 2013, the member states of WHO adopted nutrition targets to reduce the burden of malnutrition by 2025.[8]

- *Target 1*: Reduction in the number of children who are stunted by 40%
- *Target 2*: Reduction in anemia in women of reproductive age by 50%
- *Target 3*: Reduction in low birth weight by 3–30%
- *Target 4*: No increase in childhood obesity
- *Target 5*: At least 50% increase the rate of exclusive breastfeeding in the first 6 months
- *Target 6*: Reduce and maintain childhood wasting to less than 5%.

Of the 194 countries analyzed, 38 were found to be on track for overweight, 37 for wasting, 31 for exclusive breast-feeding, and 24 for stunting.[1]

Strategies in India

Poshan Abhiyaan

Poshan Abhiyaan (National Nutrition Mission) is a multiministerial convergence mission launched by Prime Minister Shri Narendra Modi in Rajasthan in March 2018.[14]

Mission Goals

It aims to improve the nutritional status in children (0–6-year age), adolescent girls, pregnant women, and lactating mothers through the life cycle concept. The Mission aims to achieve reduction in stunting from 38.4% (NFHS-4) to 25% by 2022 (*Mission 25 by 2022*). **Table 5** shows the objective and targets of the Mission. The objective of the *Abhiyaan* is to reduce the stunting in the identified districts with the highest burden by improving the quality of nutrition services. *Poshan Abhiyaan* is being implemented in 315 districts in the first year, 235 districts in the second year, and the remaining districts in the third year by the Ministry of Women and Child Development (MWCD).[15]

There are several nutrition programs in India. But there is lack of co-ordination among them. The *Abhiyaan* will monitor, fix targets, supervise, and guide the nutrition-related interventions through a robust convergence mechanism. The Mission will ensure convergence of various ongoing programs:

- Anganwadi Services
- Pradhan Mantri Matru Vandana Yojana
- Scheme for Adolescent Girls of MWCD
- Janani Suraksha Yojana (JSY)
- National Health Mission (NHM) of Ministry of Health and Family Welfare (MoH and FW)

Table 5: Objectives and targets of national nutrition mission.		
Sl. No	Objective	Target
1.	Prevent and reduce Stunting in children (0–6 years)	By 6% @ 2% p.a.
2.	Prevent and reduce undernutrition (underweight prevalence) in children (0–6 years)	By 6% @ 2% p.a.
3.	Reduce the prevalence of anemia among young children (6–59 months)	By 9% @ 3% p.a.
4.	Reduce the prevalence of anemia among women and adolescent girls in the age group of 15–49 years	By 9% @ 3% p.a.
5.	Reduce low birth weight (LBW)	By 6% @ 2% p.a.

Source: Poshan Abhiyaan Guidelines, Ministry of Women and Child Development, Government of India.[14]

- Swachh Bharat Mission of Ministry of Drinking Water and Sanitation (DW and S)
- Public Distribution System (PDS) of the Ministry of Consumer Affairs, Food and Public Distribution (CAF and PD)
- Mahatma Gandhi National Rural Employment Guarantee Scheme (MGNREGS) of the Ministry of Rural Development (MoRD)
- Drinking Water and Toilets with Ministry of Panchayati Raj and Urban Local Bodies through the Ministry of Urban Development.

Mission Components

- *Information and communication technology enabled real time monitoring (ICT-RTM) system*: ICDS-CAS (Common Application Software) preloaded mobiles will be made available to Anganwadi Workers (AWWs), tablets to lady supervisors, and desktops at block, district, state, and national levels for ICT-RTM monitoring.
- *Training and capacity building*: Incremental Learning Approach (ILA) will be adopted for training of personnel.
- *Community mobilization and Behavior Change Communication (BCC)*: The following activities will be included in this component:
  - *Community-based events*: Each Anganwadi Center (AWC) will organize one community-based traditional event every month to promote maternal and child health, and ₹250/- shall be reimbursed for the same. Information Education and Communication (IEC) to support nutrition behavior change. The IEC strategy aims to create awareness among general public regarding the various nutrition- and health-related government schemes. It guides the citizens on how to access them. The IEC activities mostly will be done through television, radio, print media, and social media.
  - *Jan Andolan*: Through the involvement of Panchayati Raj Institutions and Village Organizations, the Mission will ensure wide public participation by converting the nutrition-related issues into a *Jan Andolan*.
- *Innovations*: Any innovative idea that has the ability to significantly transform or enhance the Mission to achieve any of its stated outcomes may be developed into a pilot project and implemented later on.
- Incentives for AWWs for using the digital tools and for states/UTs based on their performance will be provided.

- *Grievance redressal and citizen engagement*: A Call Centre will be set up to effectively engage with the beneficiaries to provide grievance redressal and to monitor and follow-up on the nutritional indicators so that targeted action may be taken.
- *Nutrition surveillance system, social surveys, and audit monitoring*: Surveys will be conducted based on the data collected from the digitized systems and feedback will be provided for improvement in the programs.

The prevalence of malnutrition may be reduced by a multipronged approach which includes improving maternal nutrition before and during pregnancy and lactation; exclusive breastfeeding up to 6 months of age with continued breastfeeding till 2 years of life; adequate nutrition in early childhood; and access to basic health and WASH services. Many countries are on the right track.

Despite all the efforts done so far, the UNICEF, WHO, and World Bank global and regional child malnutrition estimates reveal that we are still far from a world without malnutrition. The joint estimates, published in March 2019, reveal insufficient progress to reach the World Health Assembly targets set for 2025 and the Sustainable Development Goals set for 2030.[1]

■ REFERENCES

1. United Nations Children's Fund (UNICEF), World Health Organization, International Bank for Reconstruction and Development/The World Bank. Levels and trends in child malnutrition: key findings of the 2019 Edition of the Joint Child Malnutrition Estimates. Geneva: World Health Organization; 2019.
2. Comprehensive National Nutrition Survey (CNNS): 2016-2018. Ministry of Health and Family Welfare (MoH and FW), Government of India, UNICEF and Population Council. New Delhi; 2019.
3. National Family Health Survey (NFHS-4), 2015-16: India. International Institute for Population Sciences (IIPS) and ICF. Mumbai: IIPS; 2017.
4. World Health Organization. Anemia. [online] Available from: https://www.who.int/topics/anaemia/en/. [Last accessed on November, 2019].
5. Roth DE, Abrams SA, Aloia J, et al. Global prevalence and disease burden of vitamin D deficiency: a roadmap for action in low- and middle-income countries. Ann N Y Acad Aci. 2018;1430(1):44-79.
6. The Lancet. The Lancet Series on Maternal and Child Undernutrition, Executive Summary. [online] Available from: http://www.thelancet.com/series/maternal-and-child-nutrition. [Last accessed on November, 2019].
7. UNICEF. Improving Nutrition Security in Africa, an EU-UNICEF Joint Action. [online] Available from: http://www.unicef.org/eu/files/EU-UNICEF_Africa.pdf. [Last accessed of November, 2019].

8. Global Nutrition Report. (2018). 2018 Global Nutrition Report, Executive Summary. [online] Available from: https://globalnutritionreport.org/reports/global-nutrition-report-2018/. [Last accessed on November, 2019].

9. United Nations Children's Fund. UNICEF's approach to scaling up nutrition for mothers and their children. Discussion paper. New York: Programme Division, UNICEF; 2015.

10. Habyarimana F, Zewotir T, Ramroop S. Key determinants of malnutrition of children under five years of age in Rwanda: Simultaneous measurement of three anthropometric indices. African Population Studies. 2016; 30(2):2328-40.

11. UNICEF. (2017). First 1000 days: The critical window to ensure that children survive and thrive. [online] Available from: https://www.unicef.org/southafrica/saf_brief_1000days.pdf. [Last accessed on November 2019].

12. Bhutta ZA, Das JK, Rizvi A, et al. Evidence-based interventions for improvement of maternal and child nutrition: what can be done and at what cost? Lancet. 2013;382:452-77.

13. Ruel M, Alderman T. Nutrition-sensitive interventions and programmes: how can they help to accelerate progress in improving maternal and child nutrition? Lancet. 2013;382: 536-51.

14. Ministry of Child Development and Government of India. Poshan Abhiyaan. [online] Available from: https://icds-wcd.nic.in/nnm/home.htm. [Last accessed on November, 2019].

15. National Nutrition Mission Administrative Guidelines. [online] Available from: https://icds-wcd.nic.in/nnm/NNM-Web-Contents/UPPER-MENU/AdministrativeApproval-Guidelines/Administrative_Guidelines_NNM-26022018.pdf [Last accessed on November, 2019].

Infant and Young Child Nutrition in Tropics

Satish Tiwari, Rupal Dalal

■ INTRODUCTION

In India, out of 1.2 million children aged 0–59 months who die, 58% of those deaths occur during the neonatal period.[1] Infant mortality rate is at present 41 and under-5 mortality rate is 50 per 1,000 live births as per National Family Health Survey (NFHS-4) data. Childhood undernutrition accounts for 45% of under-5 mortality alone and remains a key public health challenge in India. India is striving to reach an under-5 mortality rate of 25 deaths per 1,000 live births by 2030 as part of the Sustainable Development Goals set out by the UN.[2] To achieve good physical and mental development as well as long-term health, optimum nutrition starting in early stages of life is crucial.

■ INFANT AND YOUNG CHILD FEEDING STATISTICS IN INDIA

In India, breastfeeding is inadequate as only 55% babies are exclusively breastfed for 0–6 months and 41% are able to begin breastfeeding within an hour of birth.[3] For infants born by cesarean section, breastfeeding initiation can be delayed. Out of 92% institutional deliveries, 40% deliveries in Andhra Pradesh and 58% deliveries in Telangana are by cesarean section, but the early initiation of breastfeeding is only 40% and 37% in these respective states as per India's NFHS 2015.[4] According to a new study on the cost of not breastfeeding and an accompanying tool, annually, inadequate breastfeeding results in 100,000 preventable child deaths (mainly due to diarrhea and pneumonia), 34.7 million cases of diarrhea, 2.4 million cases of pneumonia, and 40,382 cases of obesity in India.[5] Only, 14.3% of nonbreastfeeding and 8.7% of breastfeeding children and thus mere 9.6% children aged 6–23 months receive an adequate diet as per NFHS-4 data.

Recommendations of Infant and Young Child Feeding

If every child from 0 month to 23 months was optimally breastfed, then we would have saved over 820,000 children under 5 years of age. Breastfeeding improves cognition, decreases school absence, and is associated with better income in adult life. Overweight and obesity is lower in babies who were breastfed as babies.[6] Optimum maternal, infant, and young child nutrition practices result in improvement in child development and they reduce health costs which results in economic gains for individual families as well as for the country.

World Health Organization (WHO) recommends:[7]
- Initiation of breastfeeding within 1 hour of birth
- First 6 months of exclusive breastfeeding
- Continued breastfeeding up to 2 years or beyond with introduction of nutritionally adequate and safe complementary foods on the completion of 6 months of age.

■ BREASTFEEDING

Antenatal Preparation

When a pregnant woman receives personal and professional guidance during pregnancy till she is discharged from the hospital postdelivery and beyond, her decision to initiate and maintain breastfeeding improves.[8] Breastfeeding counseling guides mother on proper positioning and latching techniques improving mother's confidence. It also prevents or resolves breastfeeding problems. Breastfeeding support in the community also results in increasing rates of initiation of breastfeeding as well as duration of exclusive breastfeeding.[9] Pregnant women should be informed about the benefits of exclusive breastfeeding up to 6 months and dangers of artificial feeding and bottle-feeding, breastfeeding techniques, expression of breast milk (press, compress, and release technique), and cup feeding technique. Women need to be encouraged to discuss their myths and doubts. They should be counseled to avoid prelacteal feeds.[10] Phone helplines for antenatal counseling and breastfeeding support after delivery for women from the urban areas showed remarkable improvement (95% adherences at all visits) in the exclusive breastfeeding rates in the intervention group as compared to control group that received only standard care.[11] Topics to be covered in Antenatal Education are given in **Table 1**.

Concept of "1,000 Days"

All parents share a common goal for their children to grow up to be happy and healthy who achieve their full potential. To that end, parents want to give their children the very best start. At no other time in life is there a greater opportunity to influence so many aspects of a child's development than during the "first 1,000 days" from pregnancy until 2 years of age. This period offers a unique period of opportunity to build healthier and more prosperous generations. Appropriate nutrition during 1,000 days influences a child's ability to thrive, learn, and have a lasting effect on a country's health and prosperity. Good nutrition during this period offers the essential infrastructure for brain development, growth, and immune system. The footings for lifelong health including predilections to obesity and certain chronic diseases are largely set during this 1,000-day period.[12] There are three crucial stages in the first 1,000 days: pregnancy, infancy, and early childhood. During pregnancy, if a mother's diet is not giving her the nutrients she needs to support a healthy pregnancy and her baby's development or if it is contributing to excessive weight gain or both, it can have serious, long-term consequences. There are some important nutrients which support neurodevelopment, these which includes protein; zinc; iron; choline; folate; iodine; vitamins A, D, B_6, and B_{12}; and long-chain polyunsaturated fatty acids (LCPUFAs) besides other nutrients. If the child is deprived of these key nutrients during this critical period of brain development, it may result in lifelong inadequacies in brain function despite subsequent nutrient repletion.[14]

Concept of Breast Crawl

Breast crawl is the movement of the newborns to move toward the nipple of the mother and attach to it for breastfeeding, all by themselves.[15] The newborn baby, when put on the mother's abdomen, starts moving 12–44 minutes after the birth, followed by spontaneous suck at 27–71 minutes after birth.[16] A Swedish nurse-midwife Ann-Marie Widstrom in early 70s began to observe a pattern in the behaviors of babies that were placed skin to skin with their mother's immediately after birth and allowed to quietly adjust to extrauterine life without interruptions. During these phases, the newborn moves in a focused manner but without being impatient or haste (*www.breastcrawl.org*). It is prerogative for those who are observing to relax, allow the baby and the mother to be alone and wonder at the marvelous drama unfolding as the baby discovers the breast, attaches, and suckles without any support or interference.[17] Advantages of early skin-to-skin care are given in following section.

Visit date	Topics
Table 1: Topics to be covered in antenatal education, model schedule.[13]	
Gest. Week:__ Visit # ___	1. The right to receive respectful maternity care, which refers to care organized for and provided to all women in a manner that maintains their dignity, privacy, and confidentiality, ensures freedom from harm and mistreatment, and enables informed choice and continuous support during labor and childbirth
Gest. Week:___ Visit #_____	2. Nonpharmacologic pain relief methods during labor and the influence of delivery methods on breastfeeding success
Gest. Week:___ Visit #_____	3. Global recommendations and importance of breastfeeding, the importance of exclusive breastfeeding for the first 6 months, the risks of giving breast milk substitutes, and the importance of continuing breastfeeding after 6 months with appropriate complementary foods, for the first 2 years or beyond
Gest. Week:___ Visit #_____	4. The importance of immediate and sustained skin-to-skin contact after birth
Gest. Week:___ Visit #_____	5. The importance of early initiation of breastfeeding and rooming-in on a 24-hour basis
Gest. Week:___ Visit #_____	6. The basics of milk supply and demand, to ensure the infant's adequate nourishment
Gest. Week:___ Visit #_____	7. The basics of good positioning and attachment and recognition of feeding cues
Gest. Week:___ Visit #_____	8. Management of most common initial challenges such as pain, cluster feeding, sleepy newborns, latching issues, engorgement, and practice of safe sleep

Concept of "Golden Hour"

The first hour after birth and the way it is handled may have short- and long-term consequences. Uterus is the "natural habitat" for the fetus. The intrauterine milieu have provided oxygen, nutrients, safety and security, as well as close and continual proximity to the mother's heart and voice. After birth, the mother's body and breasts take over these functions in providing warmth, protection, nutrition, and stabilization of newborn respiration; increasing glucose level (reducing hypoglycemia); reducing cortisol; maintaining BP; decreasing crying; and increasing quiet alert state and support for optimal oxygenation as well as close proximity to the mother's heart and voice.[18] Oxytocin, which facilitates relaxation, bonding, facial recognition, and maternal instincts, is increased during skin-to-skin contact whenever the newborn's hand massages mother's breasts.[19] Babies cried 10 times more, and the duration of crying was 40 times more when human infants separated from their mothers compared to those who were in skin to skin with their mothers.[20] The amygdala which is a part of limbic system matures in the first 2 months after birth and is involved in emotional learning, memory modulation, and activation of the sympathetic nervous system which is activated by skin-to-skin contact via prefrontal-orbital pathway, thus contributing to its maturation.[21] One-year-old infants who had spent the first 1–2 hours skin to skin with their mother were less easily irritated, were crying less, and were found to have better self-regulation during a structured play session.[22] Immediate skin-to-skin contact between mother and infant after birth helps to start early breastfeeding and increases the possibility of exclusive breastfeeding as well as the duration of breastfeeding.[23]

Responsive Feeding

Responsive feeding (RF) involves a mother understanding her baby's hunger cues and her own desire to feed her baby. Feeding time is not just for nutrition, but also for love, comfort, and reassurance between baby and mother. Many mothers know instinctively when to feed the baby but some are misinformed. Every baby and every mother have different requirements and many babies feed more frequently than the desired pattern recommends. This can leave the baby unsatisfied and irritable, which in turn demoralizes mother and the family's confidence in the adequacy of milk. Limiting feeds to fit into a regime can also threaten the mother's milk supply, and reduces the chance of successful on-going breastfeeding. Pediatricians, by learning about feeding cues at different phases of development, can guide in boosting parental feeding responsiveness. RF encourages a child to eat in a competent and responsible manner, being attentive to internal hunger and satiety cues, and cultivate the skills of optimal self-regulation and self-control of food intake. It also encourages the child's attention and interest in feeding, and the ability to communicate his or her needs by distinct and meaningful signals. In the long term, RF may ensure healthy eating habits, growth, as well as reduce child under- and overnutrition.[24,25] Responsiveness to Child Feeding Cues Scale (RCFCS) are given in **Table 2**. Strategies to promote RF are given in **Table 3**.

Adequacy of Milk

Human milk is unparalleled when it comes to providing perfect nutrition and protection against pathogens to the babies, while the neonatal immune system completes its development.[26] Time of lactation, length of gestation, maternal diseases, genotype, and diet, they all influence composition of milk.[27,28] Human lactation stage is divided into three major phases—colostrum, transitional milk, and mature milk. The first milk which is also called colostrum contains a high concentration of whey proteins, while the difficult to digest casein is almost undetectable, whereas the lactose and fat content is lower compared to that in mature milk.[29] The adequacy of milk can be approximately measured by frequency of urine output in 24 hours and the weight gain in an exclusively breastfed baby. The protein and sodium increased, whereas lactose, calcium, and zinc decreased when the milk volume falls below 300 mL/day.[30] A recent study compared many nutritional components of human milk between obese and lean lactating women. Human milk from obese mothers differs in fatty acid, vitamins, and carotenoid composition, contained lower docosahexaenoic acid (DHA), vitamin D, and lutein + zeaxanthin content than lean women.[31]

Composition of Milk

The mature human milk has protein content of 8–10 g/L[32] which is important for infants' healthy growth and has immune and antimicrobiological activity.[33] The high concentration of lactose in human milk, 6.7 g/100 mL, reflects the high nutritional requirements of human brain. Lipids contribute to the 44% of the total energy provided by human milk.[34] They provide essential nutrients such as polyunsaturated fatty acids (PUFAs), complex lipids, lipid-soluble vitamins, and bioactive compounds.[35] Predominant saturated fatty acids in the human milk are provided in the form of palmitic acid. The LCPUFAs, which are largely affected by mother's diet, exert several major

Table 2: Responsiveness to Child Feeding Cues Scale (RCFCS).[36]

Child feeding cues	Early	Active	Late
Hunger/receptiveness	Sucking	Rooting/nuzzling	Moving head frantically from side to side
	Opening/closing mouth repeatedly	Asking for food/excitatory or affirming vocalization	Crying
	Smacking/licking lips	Excitatory limb movement	Temper tantrums
	Increased alertness	Leaning/crawling/walking toward food	
		Bring or show bottle/spoon/cup/food to caregiver	
		Hitting caregiver on arm/chest	
		Motion to be placed in feeding location	
		Postural attention	
		Settling into feed/decrease in tension	
		Open mouth wide/latching on/feeding self	
		Fidgeting or squirming	
		Fussing or whining	
Fullness/disinterest	Hand-to-face	Pushes tray or feeding hand away	Crying
	Decreased muscle tone	Gives back food/utensils/bottle/cup	Sleeping
	Does not open mouth until spoon at lips	Pulls/turn away abruptly	Physically struggling/arching
	Takes interest in surroundings/looks away	Falling asleep	Vomiting
	Decreased activity level	Maximal lateral gaze aversion	
	Lip grimace/pout/frown	Refuse to open mouth	
	Slow or pauses	Takes off bib/attempts to leave feeding location	
	Gaze aversion	Biting spoon/nipple	
	Turning head in response to food	Detach from nipple	
		Saying "no" or shaking head "no"	
		Play with food items or surrounding items	
		Spitting or ejecting food from the mouth	
		Fussiness of whining	
		Physically agitated/squirming	

biological effects, particularly on membrane functions, including growth and immune response. In addition, it positively affects retinal and brain cortical functional development in infants.[37] A recorded increase in the omega-6/omega-3 ratio that underlines a suboptimal intake of omega-3 associated with a higher consumption of omega-6 which affects the level of omega-3 in human milk.[38] Minerals in human milk have major minerals such as calcium, magnesium, and phosphorus, which are tightly regulated in maternal serum. It has electrolytes such as sodium, chloride, and potassium, which in milk are determined by an electrical potential gradient in the secretory cell and trace elements such as iron, copper, and zinc may be influenced to a large extent by maternal diet.[39] Bioactive component of human milk is given in **Table 4**.

Breastfeeding and Associated Outcomes

Nutrient density and biological compounds in human milk contribute to the short- and long-term health benefits in infants as well as mothers.

Health Outcomes

- A 88% reduction of mortality in comparison to infants who are never been breastfed.[40]

Table 3: Strategies to promote responsive feeding.[41]

How to feed responsively	
Actively engage in: • Conversations and eye-to-eye contact with your child during feeding times • Clear communication regarding expectations • Responding to hunger and satiety cues • Feeding infants directly, or assisting older children to feed themselves	*Feeding progression*: • Slowly and patiently, while encouraging and motivating the child to eat • Never force-feed children
Modeling healthy behavior: Parents, caregivers, and family members should all make healthy food-based choices	*Required environment*: • Pleasant feeding environment • Child is seated in a relaxed and comfortable manner • Child is face to face with other family members • Distractions are minimized during meals • Routines are established as a result of organizing mealtimes, following a predictable schedule, and eating preferably at the same time and place
Offered food must be: Healthy, tasty, and developmentally appropriate	
To overcome food refusal, experiment with: • Different food combinations, tastes, and textures • Various methods of encouragement	
Additional responsive feeding strategies during special circumstances	
When the child is sick: • Feed slowly and patiently • Give mashed or soft food, especially if the child has difficulty swallowing • Give the child his or her favorite foods • Give small, frequent meals • Breastfeed more often and for longer at each feed, and increase fluid intake	*When the child is recovering from illness*: Be responsive to the child's increased hunger and escalate the amount of food by giving additional meals or snacks each day for 2 weeks, and offering more food per meal
When the child refuses to eat: • Give an alternative food • Make food more presentable to the child, e.g. in the shape of a character or a smiley face • Talk and/or sing to the child • Ensure that the child does not eat alone	*When the child has a reduced appetite*: • Feed slowly and patiently • Feed the child his or her favorite food • Breastfeed more often • Provide more feeding opportunities • Prepare smaller portion sizes, as opposed to three main meals

Table 4: Bioactive component in human milk.[42]

Anti-infective	Impact on intestinal microbiota	Immunomodulatory	Antioxidant	Tissue maturation/ development
Immune cells: lymphocytes, macrophages, neutrophils	Oligosaccharides— prebiotic	Soluble CD14	Inositol	Long-chain polyunsaturated fatty acid
Secretory immunoglobulin (IgA, IgG, and IgM)	Lactic acid bacteria— probiotic	Soluble toll-like receptor 2	Vitamin E	EGF, VEGF, G-CSF, and erythropoietin
Oligosaccharides		Transforming growth factor-β	Beta carotene	Stem cells
Lactoferrin		Platelet-activating factor acetylhydrolase	Lactoferrin	Osteopontin
Lysozyme		IL-10		
Haptocorrin		Osteopontin		
Transforming growth factor-β		Lactoferrin		
Human milk fat globule membrane proteins				

(Ig: immunoglobulin; EGF: epidermal growth factor; VEGF: vascular endothelial growth factor; G-CSF: granulocyte-colony stimulating factor; IL: interleukin)

- A 36% reduction of sudden infant death syndrome.
- A 72% reduction in diarrhea-associated hospitalization and relative risk of 0.69 of developing diarrhea within the first 5 years of age.[43]
- A 57% reduction in the respiratory infection-associated hospitalization.
- A 70% reduction in mortality from lower respiratory infections.

- A 68% reduction in risk of malocclusion.[44]
- A 35% reduction in the risk of developing diabetes type 2 with longer exposure to breastfeeding.[45]
- A 26% reduction in overweight/obesity.
- A 19% reduction in leukemia.[46]
- 3.4 points higher intelligent quotient.[47]
- Reduce complication including retinopathy of prematurity, necrotizing enterocolitis, late-onset sepsis, bronchopulmonary dysplasia, and late-onset sepsis.[48,49]

Maternal Health Outcome

- Each increase in 12 months duration in lifetime breastfeeding associated with a reduction of 4.3% in the incidence in breast cancer.[50]
- A 30% reduction in the incidence of ovarian cancer with longer periods of breastfeeding.[51]
- A 32% reduction in type 2 diabetes.[52]
- For every 6 months increase in the lifetime breast-feeding duration, Mean Body Mass Index 1% lower for every 6 months increase in the lifetime breastfeeding duration.[53]

Contraindications for Breastfeeding

There are very few contraindications of breastfeeding as mentioned in **Table 5**.

COMPLEMENTARY FEEDING

Complementary feeding (CF) as defined by WHO is the process which is started when breastmilk alone is insufficient to meet the nutritional requirements of infants. CF should be started at the completion of 6 months, even though breastfeeding should continue beyond 2 years.[54,55] Complementary foods are often of poor nutritional quality than breast milk. In addition, they are often given in inadequate amounts and, if offered too early or too frequently, they replace breast milk. Since the gastric capacity of a young child is small, it limits the amount of food consumed during each meal. Repeated infections decrease appetite and also infants and young children need a caring adult or other responsible person who not only selects and offers appropriate foods but assists and encourages them to consume these foods in sufficient quantity.

Amount of calories needed from complementary food is as follows:

- For 6–8 months—200 kcal/day
- For 9–11 months—300 kcal/day
- For 12–23 months—550 kcal/day.

Why Thick Consistency is Important?

Since the stomach capacity of young children in small, it is essential that they are offered food with thick consistency.

Table 5: Potential contraindications to breastfeeding.[13]	
Mother's condition	
Ebola virus	Suspected (until ruled out) or confirmed maternal Ebola virus
Herpes virus	Mothers with active herpetic lesions on the breast(s) should not breastfeed from the affected breast, but may breastfeed from the unaffected breast. Milk can be pumped from the affected breast, as there is no concern of hematologic transmission through the milk itself. However, milk can become contaminated via the breast pump, and thus should any part of the breast pump come in contact with herpetic lesions, that milk should be discarded. In this case, expression with discarding of milk should be encouraged to maintain milk supply until breastfeeding is resumed
HTLV I and II	Mothers with human T-cell lymphotropic virus type I or type II
Varicella	If there is onset of varicella within 5 days before or up to 48 hours after delivery, separation of mother and infant with feeding of expressed milk until mother is no longer contagious is recommended, with administration of varicella-zoster immune globulin to the infant as soon as possible. Avoid close contact with skin lesions. (For older infants, separation of the mother and infant is not recommended, as the mother was contagious prior to the appearance of skin lesions and thus the infant was already exposed.) Expert consultation is advised
Brucella	Untreated maternal brucellosis
Tuberculosis	Mothers with active, untreated pulmonary tuberculosis should not directly breastfeed but infant can be given mother's own expressed milk. While direct breastfeeding, the infant will receive prophylaxis with isoniazid. There might thus be no reason to separate them, if the infant is already being treated. Expert consultation is advised
Medication	Treatment with some medications such as chemotherapy, temporary or permanent cessation of breastfeeding may be advised. Check with LactMed, InfantRisk.com, or e-lactancia, Lactation Study or other local available accurate resources
Illicit drugs	Current use of illicit drugs (e.g. cocaine, heroin, phencyclidine) as determined on a case-by-case basis by the infant's healthcare provider
Infant's condition	
Inborn error of metabolism	Galactosemia (except for Duarte variant, in which partial breastfeeding is possible). Congenital lactase deficiency Some inborn errors of metabolism may require supplementation (phenylketonuria, maple syrup disease)

Watery food in the form of dal water and rice water which is given universally as first foods in India will cause growth faltering due to lack of nutrient density in such thin consistency foods. Start with pureed foods to begin with gradually increasing the food consistency and variety, as the infant gets older, adapting to the infant's requirements and abilities.

- For 6–8 months—pureed or pasty nutrient dense food
- For 9–11 months—mashed/soft chunky nutrient dense food, finger foods (snacks that can be eaten by children alone)
- By 12 months, most children can eat table foods which are the same types of foods as consumed by the rest of the family. Avoid foods that may cause choking (i.e. items that have a shape and/or consistency that may cause them to choke such as nuts, grapes, and raw carrots).

Information to Mothers about Consistency of Food

- The food should be prepared in such a way that its consistency is thick enough to stay on the spoon without running off when the spoon is tilted.
- Avoid using blender to prepare baby's foods, instead mash the food with hands or forks. When the blender is used, it may need extra fluids to work.
- Porridge, veggie, or meat stews that are so thin that they do not provide enough energy or nutrient.
- The consistency or thickness of foods makes a big difference to how well that food meets the child's energy needs and helps to fill the energy gap.

Why do Mothers do not Give Thick Consistency?

- Fear of choking
- Fear that thick food is difficult to swallow
- Fear of constipation
- Watery food is faster to give.

Meal Frequency (Table 6)

- The appropriate number of feedings depends on the energy density of the foods and the amounts consumed at each feeding.
- Feed 2–3 times per day at 6–8 months.
- Feed 3–4 times per day at 9–11 and 12–24 months of age.
- Additional nutritious snacks may be offered 1–2 times per day, as desired. Snacks are defined as foods eaten between meals, usually self-fed, convenient, and easy

Table 6: Meal frequency for complementary feeding as per WHO guideline.

Age in months	Frequency	Amount
7 months	2 meals a day	Start with 1 tbsp, go up to 4 tbsp
8 months	3 meals a day	1/2 cup a meal (125 mL)
9 months	3 meals a day + 1 snack	1/2 cup a meal
10 months	3 meals a day + 2 snack	1/2 cup a meal
11 months	3 meals a day + 2 snacks	1/2 cup a meal
12–23 months	3 meals a day + 2 snacks	1 cup a meal

to prepare. If energy density or amount of food per meal is low, or the child is no longer breastfed, frequent meals may be required.

BABY-LED WEANING[56]

Baby-led weaning (BLW) is an approach to introducing solid food that is based on the infant's developmental readiness to ingest foods other than breast milk. BLW is starting solid food instead of pureed food from day 1 of the CF. The baby herself takes the solid food, instead of spoon-feeding by parents. It allows the infant to control when to start eating other foods, what to eat, how quickly to eat, and how much to consume at a sitting. BLW is an alternative approach to the introduction of complementary foods in infancy. It is one way of RF.

Key Recommendations

- Exclusive breastfeeding from birth and introduction of complementary foods at the completion of 6 months of age.
- On-demand breastfeeding until 2 years of age or beyond.
- Responsive feeding, applying the principles of psychosocial care.
- Good hygiene and proper food handling by:
  - Wash caregivers' and children's hands before food preparation and eating
  - Store foods safely and serving foods immediately after preparation
  - Use clean utensils to prepare and serve food
  - Avoid the use of feeding bottles, which are difficult to keep clean.
- Gradually increase food consistency and variety, adapting to the infant's requirements and abilities.
- Increase the frequency that the child is fed as he/she gets older. The appropriate number of feedings

depends on the nutrient density of the foods and the usual quantity consumed at each feeding.

- Vegetarian diets may be unable to meet nutrient needs unless nutrient supplements or fortified products are used, especially iron, zinc, calcium, and vitamin B_{12}.
- Calorie density should be at least 0.8 kcal/g of complementary food.
- Provide diets with adequate fat from natural foods like ghee, butter, peanuts, sesame and other seeds, etc.
- Avoid giving low nutrient value drinks, such as tea, coffee and sugary drinks such as soda.
- Increase fluid intake as well as more frequent breastfeeding during illness and encourage eating soft, varied, appetizing, nutrient dense foods. After illness, increase the frequency of the food with lots of encouragement.

■ DIET DIVERSITY

To ensure healthy growth and organs formation, with strong immunity and neurological and cognitive development in early childhood, providing adequate nutrition is the key.[57] WHO[58] defines minimum dietary diversity percent as a proportion of children 6 months to 2 years of age who receive foods from four or more food groups making their diet diverse in quality. These food groups include grains, roots and tubers, legumes and nuts, dairy products (milk, yoghurt, and cheese), flesh foods (meat, fish, poultry, and liver/organ meats), eggs, vitamin A-rich fruits and vegetables, and other fruits and vegetables. Based on WHO recommendation of minimum acceptable diet (MAD), the NFHS-4 report[59] illustrates the need for dietary diversity. Without it, infants and young children are vulnerable to undernutrition, especially stunting and micronutrient deficiencies, and to increased morbidity and mortality. However, with increased globalization and easy access to processed and packaged foods, a higher consumption of sweets and fried food items is observed. These foods can be deficient in micronutrients, especially type 2 nutrients

(Table 7) which are important for growth and development of children.

Food Classification

Based on the nutrient requirement, **Table 8** explains the different food groups, which assist in obtaining the mentioned nutrients.

Food-to-food Fortification

Traditionally, we have always eaten varan bhath (pulse and rice), idlis, khichdis, dal dhokli, or even puran poli. This age-old combination took into considerations that cereals lack in amino acid lysine, whereas pulses lack in amino acid methionine. Addition of vegetables to cereal and pulse combination further enhances the availability of vitamins and minerals in the diet; hence go ahead and add dark green leafy vegetables, yellow, red, or orange vegetables such as carrot, yellow pumpkin, and a variety of gourds, to add taste and health value to the meal. This combination gives us better quality protein rich in vitamin and minerals than if we would have consumed them alone. This strategy is called food-to-food fortification.[61]

Ready-to-use Therapeutic Food[62,63]

Ready-to-use therapeutic food (RUTF) is energy-dense, micronutrient-enhanced pastes used in therapeutic feeding. Typical primary ingredients for RUTF include peanuts, oil, sugar, milk powder, and vitamin and mineral supplements. It provides all the nutrients required for recovery. It has a good shelf life, and does not spoil easily even after opening. Since RUTF is not water based, the risk of bacterial growth is very limited, and consequently, it is safe to use without refrigeration at household level. Finally, it can be used in combination with breastfeeding and other best practices for infant and young child feeding.

Ready-to-use therapeutic food should be used only:
- As therapeutic and not supplementary feeding
- Above 6 months of age

Table 7: Classification of nutrients.[60]	
Type 1 nutrients	*Type 2 nutrients*
The nutrients are required principally for specific metabolic functions in the body, rather than for metabolism in general. They are stored in the body	These are growth nutrients, the deficiency of which over a long period of time could result in growth failure
Minerals: Iron, iodine, copper, calcium, and selenium	Nitrogen and essential amino acids—histidine, isoleucine, leucine, lysine, methionine, cysteine, phenylalanine, threonine, tryptophan, and valine
B-complex vitamins: Thiamine, riboflavin, niacin, pyridoxine, folate, and cobalamin	*Minerals*: Potassium, magnesium, phosphorus, sulfur (sulfur-containing amino acids—methionine and cysteine), zinc, sodium, and chloride
Fat-soluble vitamins: A, D, E, and K	*Essential fatty acids*: Linoleic acid, alpha-linolenic acid, and arachidonic acid

Table 8: Classification of food groups.

Food groups	Common food names
Cereals/millets	Wheat flour, broken wheat, rava, bajra flour, jowar flour, rice flour, corn flour ragi flour. Rice products like poha, kurmura, etc.
Pulses	Whole dals and flours of toovar, moong, massoor, mutki, all types of channa chick peas, urad, kulith, all types of vatana. Soya bean and its products like soya chunks, granules, tofu, and all types of rajma, etc.
Green leafy and stem vegetable	Palak, methi, cabbage, colocasia leaves, spring onions, coriander leaves. Mint leaves, suva bhaji, mayalu, amaranth leaves, radish leaves, curry leaves, drumstick leaves cauliflower greens, lettuce, celery, parsley, garlic greens asparagus, lotus stem leek, etc.
Roots and tubers	Potato, sweet potato, turnip, cassava, yam, ginger, carrot, radish beetroot, arbi, onions, and garlic. Bamboo shoots, artichoke, water chestnuts, parsnip, etc.
Other vegetables	Tendli, brinjal, carrots, chavli, capsicum, bhendi, tindola, yellow pumpkin, french beans, karela, lauki, cauliflower, ash gourd, snake gourd, cucumber, green tomatoes, broccoli, green peas, walor, mushrooms sweet corn, all varieties of green chillies, zucchini, etc.
Milk and milk products	Milk, paneer, cheese, buttermilk, lassi, curd, skimmed milk, butter, ghee, etc.
Non-vegetarian	Chicken, mutton, egg, fish, etc.
Fats and oils	Butter, ghee, vegetable and seed oils, nut oils, etc.
Fruits	Banana, apple, chickoo, mango, guava, papaya, orange, sweet lime, watermelon, grapes, etc.
Nuts and dried fruits	Groundnuts, almond, walnuts, dates, figs, raisins, etc.
Oilseeds	Flax seeds, sunflower seeds, pumpkin seeds, sesame seeds, etc.

Table 9: The difference between homemade and home available foods.[64]

Homemade	Home available or commercial infant foods
Homemade infant foods are generally prepared in households by parents/caretakers, using fresh ingredients	Commercially prepared infant foods also known as "readymade" infant foods, are typically mass produced and purchased in a preprepared format requiring minimal, if any, cooking or heating before consumption
Homemade infant foods contains average (as per the taste of family) amounts of sugar, salt, and some amount of fat	These foods have high sugar, sodium levels and fat levels as compared to homemade foods
• Homemade infant foods have more use of vegetables in daily diet of the infant as compared to commercial preparations • Feeding fruits and vegetables in infancy is associated with increased uptake of fruits and vegetables in later years as well	Commercial foods have more quantity of fruits in the preparation as compared to vegetables

■ For a limited time period (4–8 weeks) until the child recovers from severe acute malnutrition (SAM), which should be defined in explicit treatment protocols.

Homemade versus Home Available Food

The benefits of homemade food are very well known. Still in the present era of consumerism and globalization, the consumption of artificial, packaged, and tinned food is increasing by leaps and bounds at the cost of child nutrition. The differences between homemade and home available food are given in **Table 9**.

■ CHILD NUTRITION IN DISEASES

The nutrition of the child in some of the metabolic and other disorders is discussed in **Table 10**. Dietary modifications may be required in different types of disorders.

Allergies and Disorders and Child Nutrition

A food allergy is an adverse reaction to food involving an immunological mechanism. The clinical symptoms of food allergies range from mild discomfort to severe or life-threatening reactions, which require immediate medical intervention. The prevalence of food allergies has been estimated to be around 1–3% in adults and 4–6% in children.[65] The foods which cause the most severe reactions and most cases of food allergies are as follows:

■ Cereals containing gluten
■ Crustacean
■ Eggs
■ Fish
■ Peanuts
■ Soybeans
■ Milk
■ Tree nuts.

Table 10: Disorders and child nutrition.[67]

Disorder type	Description
Carbohydrate malabsorption	• Carbohydrate malabsorption occurs when the main dietary carbohydrates, sugars, and starches are not absorbed from the gastrointestinal (GI) tract • Carbohydrate malabsorption is detected by testing a child's stool and finding a pH less than 5.5, which is caused by carbohydrate fermentation from malabsorption. It is also detected by testing the stool for glucose or other sugars such as sucrose and starches. This type of malabsorption can lead to watery diarrhea with dehydration and acidosis
Disorders of amino acid absorption/ protein digestion	Amino acids are the building blocks of proteins. Disorders of amino acid absorption occur when there are defects in these transporters in gut lining. Disorders of protein digestion can occur when any of the digestion process is altered or abnormal
Disorders of fat digestion	Fat digestion begins in the stomach. Some of the by-products of fat digestion can be directly absorbed in the stomach. When the fat enters the small intestine, the gallbladder and pancreas secrete substances to further break down the fat. Small bowel syndrome, liver disorders, as well as cystic fibrosis may increase the risk of fat digestion disorders and lead to fat malabsorption
Disorders of metal absorption	Deficiency of the metals due to defect in the metabolism process are noted. Commonly known metal deficiencies are zinc, copper, selenium, chromium, and iodine
Disorders of vitamin absorption	Deficiency of the vitamins due to defect in the metabolism process are observed. Commonly known vitamin deficiencies are biotin, vitamin B_{12}, folate, niacin, vitamin A, D, E, and K
Growth problems	The cause of a growth problem depends on the type of growth disorder in question. Some growth problems are genetic, while others may be caused by hormonal disorders or poor absorption of food leading to undernutrition
Malnutrition	Malnutrition is an imbalance between nutrient requirements and intake. Children who are undernourished can lack energy, protein, or micronutrients and the condition may negatively affect growth, development, and other outcomes. Overnutrition is caused by excessive nutrient intake. Being overnourished can lead to various health problems, noncommunicable diseases, and obesity

Food Faddism and Nutrition Quackery

Based on findings from researches related to the myths and beliefs surrounding CF are mentioned below:[66]

- Most mothers avoided pulses because it was considered difficult to digest and produce gas in the child's stomach.
- Jaggery, spicy food, papaya, eggs, mangoes, etc., were considered "hot" for the child. Chicken, mutton, fish, papaya, beet root, and brinjal were also considered "hot."
- Spicy and fried foods, eggs, tea/coffee, non-vegetarian foods were considered as "harmful."
- Banana, curd/butter milk, ice creams, and fruits such as guava were considered "cold." Banana, curd, and rice cause cold and cough. Lemon juice and other citrus fruits were also considered to be "cold."
- Ghee is heavy to digest and causes cough.
- Only liquid foods such as dal and rice water are good to start with. Solid/thick consistency food cannot be given.
- Wheat/daliya/moti suji is heavy.
- Maggi/biscuits/marketed foods help in weight gain.
- Milk is whole and complete food till 1 year of age.
- Vegetables choke in food pipe.

■ INNOVATIONS IN CHILD NUTRITION

Antinutrients[68]

They are compounds which reduce the nutrient utilization and/or food intake of plants, or plant products used as human food. There are several compounds in the foods we eat classified as antinutrients. Many traditional methods of food preparation such as fermentation, germinating, cooking, and malting increase the nutritive quality of plant foods through reducing certain antinutritional factors (ANFs) as given in **Table 11**.

Cooking Techniques to Improve Nutrient Availability

To improve the contents of certain B vitamins (thiamine, riboflavin, and niacin), fermentation of cereals has been found to be potent process. Studies have shown that malting enhances the ascorbic acid and B-vitamins content and increases iron, zinc, and phosphorus absorption and bioavailability. Soaking legumes and grains in water (up to 24 hours) will allow germinating or sprouting. The grains are then dried, dehusked, and milled. In this malting process, some of the starch in the grains is degraded into sugars, protein quality and digestibility are improved, the contents of riboflavin, niacin, and vitamin C are increased, and the contents of antinutrients are reduced. Malting produces amylase, this converts starch into sugars and thereby makes the porridge or gruel less thick. This is of special importance for children with moderate malnutrition, as it allows more cereal or legume to be added, thereby increasing the energy and nutrient density. Several studies have shown that the energy and nutrient intake can be improved if germinated amylase-rich flour

Table 11: Antinutritional factors, sources in foods, the effect on nutrients, and cooking techniques to decrease it.

Name	Present in foods	Effect on absorption of	Cooking techniques used to decrease ANFs
Glucosinolates	Cruciferous vegetables (broccoli, brussels sprouts, and cabbage)	Iodine	Boiling, stir-frying, stir-frying followed by boiling
Lectins and protease inhibitors	Legumes (beans, peanuts, and soybeans), whole grains	Calcium, iron, phosphorus, and zinc	Leaching in water
Oxalates	Green leafy vegetables and tea	Calcium	Leaching in water
Phytates (phytic acid)	Whole grains, seeds, legumes, some nuts	Iron, zinc, magnesium, and calcium	Soaking, germination, fermentation, malting, dehulling, sprouting, roasting, etc.
Saponins	Legumes, whole grains	Can interfere with normal nutrient absorption such as zinc and by inhibiting metabolic and digestive enzymes	Soaking and blanching
Tannins	Tea, coffee, and legumes	Iron	De-hulling, soaking, and germination

is used as porridge or if some of this flour is added to other porridges. A combination of soaking, sprouting, and dehulling beans followed by heating generally increased nutrient digestibility and bioavailability. Soaking reduces phytates by ~50% but when the water in which the pulses are soaked is discarded, the phytates reduce to ~60%. Hence, the water in which the pulses are soaked should be discarded prior to germination or fermentation or cooking.[69] Soaking of split dals may also wash out soluble vitamins and minerals into the soaking water. Hence, the product must incorporate good sources of vitamins and minerals.

Recipe Ideas

- *Hot milk booster*: Make a powder of almonds, walnuts, and elaichi and keep in an air tight jar. When you come home wet and hungry, heat the milk, add the masala, add honey or sugar as desired and drink. Alternatively chop up dates or anjeer and add while heating the milk. Milk and cereal-based preparation are better than only milk.
- All kinds of vegetables either alone or in combination and be boiled like tomato–onion garlic, spinach–onion–tomato, beetroot–tomato–white pumpkin, corn–French beans–carrots, with or without pieces of chicken. One can have the preparation pureed or just leave the vegetables pieces in the preparations. We can add more flavors by making a thin white sauce by sautéing wheat flour in a little butter and add milk and water mix.
- *Vegi-paneer chapati wraps*: Take leftover chapatis, add sliced onions, tomatoes, green chilies, coriander leaves, garam masala or masala of your choice and grate paneer roll, add salt. Wrap and press over a tava

with or without butter, serve with a tomato chutney or green chutney.

- *Chapati pizzas*: Cut leftover chapatis to desired shape and size. Place on top cream styled corn or boiled corn, add your choice of finely chopped veggies such as capsicum, French beans, green chilies, carrots, green peas or alternatively add pizza sauce and veggies, boiled chicken or even boiled rajma. Add cheese on top and bake in an oven or put on tava and cover heat till the base is crispy.
- *Sweet pancakes*: Make a batter with wheat flour mixed with egg and milk, add cinnamon powder for extra flavor. Take a nonstick pan, make just like thick or thin uttappas. Before removing from pan, you can add chopped bananas, apple, or even dates. Fold and drizzle with honey or just add a little butter.
- *Savory desi pancakes*: Make a batter of mixed attas of besan, wheat-flour, rice, ragi, and soya. Add grated vegetables of your choice such as carrots, cabbage, onions, ginger, spinach, and methi. Add salt, haldi, and garam masala. Pour the batter on nonstick and make small omelettes. Serve hot with chutneys or pickles.
- *Steamed dumplings*: Make rice atta dough with warm water. Roll out small puris stuff with veggies, boiled pulses, chicken of your choice, make into modak, karanji or packet shaped. Steam and serve with chutneys.
- *Veggie idlis*: If little lazy, just bring idli batter. Grate variety of veggies into the batter. Eat fresh or sauté. Alternatively make them into dhoklas and season with rai, jeera, curry leaves, green chilies, and haldi.

■ BARKER'S HYPOTHESIS

The Barker's hypothesis proposed that noncommunicable diseases including metabolic syndrome were associated with malnutrition or some other cause of growth restriction during early development, if there was later exposure to a high-energy diet.[70] It could be the result of more complex multifactorial contributors including the relationship between nutrition during pregnancy, maternal metabolic status, and the socioeconomic and even psychosocial status of the mother and child.[71] There was an inverse correlation between birth weight and the severity of several measures of the metabolic syndrome. Fetuses survived malnutrition by irreversible adoption of a thrifty phenotype, which they called the fetal programing or thrifty phenotype hypothesis and later broadened to developmental origins of health and disease.[72] By limiting the growth or function of some organs such as the kidneys, liver, and pancreas that were essential to immediate survival and adopting a state of insulin resistance, crucial glucose or other limited energy supplies would be diverted to the heart and brain which were crucial for survival, so the fetus survived the period of malnutrition. The irreversible reduction of hepatic, pancreatic, and renal size and/or function was assumed to be chosen by the fetus as a protective mechanism in response to malnutrition. This would improve the survival of fetuses or older children programed this way as long as they were exposed to malnutrition.[73,74] On the other hand, it would mean they would be poorly suited to any subsequent period of high-energy consumption as the permanent reduction of hepatic, renal, and pancreatic capacity and peripheral insulin resistance would result in the metabolic syndrome.

LEGISLATIONS AND CHILD NUTRITION

To get a good start in life is the birth right of each and every individual. Proper nutrition is the mother's and child's right. Since there were violations of these rights by various stakeholders, many national and international agencies have come up with various declarations from time to time. These include *Innocenti Declaration*, *The Conventions of the Right of the Child*, International Code, *Codex Alimentarius*, ILO Conventions 2000, IMS Act, etc.[75,76]

The Infant Milk Substitutes (IMS) Act was passed by the Government of India in 1992 and amended in 2003. The Act regulates and prohibits the production, promotion, supply, and distribution of infant milk substitutes, feeding bottles, and infant food for the baby under 2 years of age.[77] The detailed provisions of the Act and the consequences of violations of these provisions are beyond the scope of this article for the constraint of the space.

There are many International recommendations and World Health Assembly Resolutions that there should be Government legislations and laws to regulate the activities of multinationals companies to prevent commerciogenic malnutrition and improve the health of future generation of our nation.

Ethical Issues in Infant and Young Child Feeding

The ethical issue in child nutrition includes the misguided propaganda, unscientific and biased information, and publicity by the multinationals. Projecting any food with exaggerated health claims or as "Magic food" is the part of such propaganda. There is need to regulate these unethical acts by strong regulatory acts and legislations.[78]

Role of Government

The Government of India has enacted many laws such as IMS Act, Food Safety and Standards Act 2006, Cable Television Network Regulation Act 2000, which regulates the unscientific promotion, biased advertisements, false and exaggerated claims regarding baby foods, junk foods, infant milk substitutes and feeding bottles, etc. The need of the hour is that all of us must now see that these legislations do not become a mere "teethless paper tigers."[79]

Role of Academic Organizations

The various academic organizations of Neonatologist, Pediatricians, Obstetricians, Community Medicine graduates, Nutritionist, Lactation Consultants, and other stake-holders must now be proactive in implementing the provisions of various acts and the legislations enacted by the government. It has been observed that there are no significant improvements in most of the health parameters related to maternal and child nutrition in spite of so many laws. One of the reasons for this is that we have badly failed in monitoring the violations of these legislations.[80] No matter how long we have traveled in wrong direction, we can always turn around in the right direction.

KEY MESSAGES

- Do not fry foods instead bake, boil, poach, or sauté in a cast iron pan.
- Use just enough water for cooking vegetables.
- Limit the use of processed foods such as ketchup, mustard, and salad dressing—they are high in salt and can be high in sugar, too.
- Limit your salt intake in food (sodium content).
- Choose fresh foods over canned and processed. Read labels carefully. Soy sauce, brine and monosodium glutamate (MSG), e.g. contain a lot of sodium.

- Do not select ready-to-eat and junk food items available to you and do not skip meals.
- Increase fiber intake in the form of raw fruits, vegetables, whole cereals, etc.
- Avoid using soda-bicarb while cooking vegetables and pulses, it destroys vitamins.
- When you make paneer use the whey, it contains good proteins in making curries or for binding dough.
- Dry the curry leaves they are good source of vitamin A, crush them, and sprinkle while seasoning vegetables, dals, etc.
- Include vitamin C-rich source in every meal. It could be a fresh fruit; seasonal ones are cheap and add variety to meals.
- Whenever eating boiled egg have it with cut slices of tomato, lettuce, onion, cabbage or any raw vegetables with a dash of lime juice. Best is make the masala omelet or bhurji (savory scrambled eggs) with finely chopped onions, tomatoes, green chilies, and coriander leaves, turmeric powder, salt, and pepper.
- When the weather is hot, besides sufficient water, juicy fruits such as watermelon, oranges, and sweet limes or buttermilk, lemon juice, coconut water, and sugarcane juice must be eaten along with the meals.
- Add rock salt, (pink) instead of white table salt in your buttermilk, this will increase our mineral content of the dish. Use of spices like ajwain, jeera, red chilies, even seeds such as aliv, alsi, sauf, ground nuts, black and white til, rai ka khura, can make your juices and salads high in antioxidants.
- The meal must be a combination of various food groups such as cereal–pulse, cereal–nonveg, cereal–green leafy vegetable, cereal–root vegetable, cereal–other vegetables or cereal–milk, this increases the nutritional quality and gives variety to the diet.
- Wash vegetables and then cut them and do not wash again as nutrients will be lost in the water.
- Cook vegetables just before eating, avoid reheating, and always cook in a covered pan to save nutrients and gas.

ACKNOWLEDGMENT

Nutrition Team from Research Centre, College of Home Science, Nirmala Niketan:

Dr Ratnaraje Thar, PhD Biological Sciences, PG Dip. Education Management
BSc. MSc, MPhil in Foods Nutrition and Dietetics,
Research Director
Hon. Nutritionist, Police Hospital, Nagpada, Mumbai, Maharashtra, India

Ms Aarti Jain, BSc, MSc in Nutrition and Dietetics
Research Associate
Corporate Nutritionist at Connect and Heal Primary Pvt. Ltd. and Wellness Associates Fitness Solutions and Management Pvt. Ltd.

Ms Rima Ved, BSc, MSc in Dietetics and Food Service Management
Field Nutrition and Research Assistant for Community Projects.

REFERENCES

1. United Nations Children's Fund (UNICEF); World Bank Group (WBG); World Health Organization (WHO); United Nations (UN) for the UN Inter-agency Group for Child Mortality Estimation. Levels and trends in child mortality. New York: UNICEF; 2015.
2. Research and Information System for Developing Countries. (2016). India and Sustainable Development Goals: The Way Forward. Available from: http://ris.org.in/sdg/india-and-sustainable-development-goals-way-forward#. [Last accessed on November, 2019].
3. International Institute of Population Sciences (IIPS). (2019). National Family Health Survey, India: Key Findings from NFHS-4. Available from: http://rchiips.org/NFHS/ factsheet_NFHS-4.shtml. [Last accessed on November, 2019].
4. Aguayo VM, Gupta G, Singh G, et al. Early initiation of breast feeding on the rise in India. BMJ Glob Health. 2016;1(2):e000043.
5. Walters DD, Phan LTH, Mathisen R. The cost of not breast-feeding: global results from a new tool. Health Policy and Planning. 2019;34(6).
6. Victora CG. Breastfeeding in the 21st century: epidemiology, mechanisms, and lifelong effect. Lancet. 2016;387(10017):475-90.
7. WHO. The optimal duration of exclusive breastfeeding. Report of the expert consultation. Geneva: WHO; 2001. Available from: http://apps.who.int/iris/bitstream/ 10665/67219/1/WHO_NHD_01.09.pdf?ua=1. [Last accessed on November, 2019].
8. Brand E, Kothari C, Stark MA. Factors related to breastfeeding discontinuation between hospital discharge and 2 weeks postpartum. J Perinat Educ. 2011;20:36-44.
9. Leite AJ, Puccini RF, Atalah AN, et al. Effectiveness of home-based peer counselling to promote breastfeeding in the northeast of Brazil: a randomized clinical trial. Acta Paediatr. 2005;94(6):741-6.
10. Gupta A, Dadhich JP, Ali SM, et al. Skilled Counseling in Enhancing Early and Exclusive Breastfeeding Rates: An Experimental Study in an Urban Population in India. Indian Pediatr. 2019;56(2):114-8.
11. Patel A, Kuhite P, Puranik A, et al. Effectiveness of weekly cell phone counseling calls and daily text messages to improve breastfeeding indicators. BMC Pediatr. 2018;18:337.
12. https://fhop.ucsf.edu/sites/fhop.ucsf.edu/files/custom_download/1000Days-NourishingAmericasFuture-Report-Final-Webversion-Singles_0.pdf. Accessed on 18th Aug 2019.
13. Hernández-Aguilar MT, Bartick M, Schreck P, et al. ABM Clinical Protocol #7: Model Maternity Policy Supportive of Breastfeeding. Breastfeed Med. 2018;13(9):559-74.

14. Schwarzenberg SJ, Georgieff MK.; Committee On Nutrition. Advocacy for Improving Nutrition in the First 1000 Days To Support Childhood Development and Adult Health. Pediatrics. 2018;141(2):e20173716.

15. Marchlewska-Koj A, Lepri JJ, Müller-Schwarze D. Chemical Signals in Vertebrate 9. Switzerland: Springer Science and Business Media; 2012. p. 419.

16. Desai SN, Daftary SV. Selected Topics in Obstetrics and Gynaecology-4: For Postgraudate and Practitioners. New Delhi: BI Publications Pvt Ltd.; 2008. p. 281.

17. Phillips R. The Sacred Hour: Uninterrupted Skin to Skin Contact Immediately After Birth. Newborn and Infant Nursing Reviews. 2013;13(2):67-72.

18. Moore ER, Anderson GC, Bergman N, et al. Early skin-to-skin contact for mothers and their healthy newborn infants. Cochrane Database Syst Rev. 2012;5:CD003519.

19. Matthiesen AS, Ransjö-Arvidson AB, Nissen E, et al. Postpartum maternal oxytocin release by newborns: effects of infant hand massage and sucking. Birth. 2001;28(1):13-9.

20. Christensson K, Cabrera T, Christensson E, et al. Separation distress call in the human neonate in the absence of maternal body contact. Acta Paediatr. 1995;84(5):468-73.

21. Schore AN. Effects of a secure attachment relationship on right brain development, affect regulation, and infant mental health. Infant Mental Health J. 2001;22:7-66.

22. Bystrova K, Ivanova V, Edhborg M, et al. Early contact versus separation: effects on mother–infant interaction one year later. Birth. 2009;36:97-109.

23. Balogun OO, O'Sullivan EJ, McFadden A, et al. Interventions for promoting the initiation of breastfeeding. Cochrane Database Syst Rev. 2016;(11):CD001688.

24. DiSantis KI, Hodges EA, Johnson SL, et al. The role of responsive feeding in overweight during infancy and toddlerhood: a systematic review. Int J Obesity. 2011;35(4):480-92.

25. Black MM, Aboud FE. Responsive feeding is embedded in a theoretical framework of responsive parenting. J Nutr. 2011;141(3):490-4.

26. Sharp JA, Modepalli V, Enjapoori AK, et al. Bioactive functions of milk proteins: a comparative genomics approach. J Mammary Gland Biol Neoplasia. 2014;19:289-302.

27. Andreas NJ, Kampmann B, Mehring Le-Doare K. Human breast milk: a review on its composition and bioactivity. Early Hum Dev. 2015;91:629-35.

28. Gidrewicz DA, Fenton TR. A systematic review and meta-analysis of the nutrient content of preterm and term breast milk. BMC Pediatr. 2014;14:216.

29. Institute of Medicine. Milk volume. In: Nutrition during lactation. Washington, DC: National Academies Press, 1991. pp. 80-112.

30. Dewey KG, Finley DA, Lönnerdra B. Breast milk volume and composition during late lactation (7-20 months). J Pediatr Gastroenterol Nutr. 1984;3(5):713-20.

31. Panagos PG, Vishwanathan R, Penfield-Cyr A, et al. Breastmilk from obese mothers has pro-inflammatory properties and decreased neuroprotective factors. J Perinato. 2016;36(4):284-90.

32. Butte N, Lopez-Alarcon M, Garza C. Nutrient adequacy of exclusive breastfeeding for the term infant during the first 6 months of life. Geneva: WHO; 2001.

33. Haschke F, Haiden N, Thakkar SK. Nutritive and Bioactive Proteins in Breastmilk. Ann Nutr Metab. 2016;69(Suppl 2): 17-26.

34. Grote V, Verduci E, Scaglioni S, et al. Breast milk composition and infant nutrient intakes during the first 12 months of life. Eur J Clin Nutr. 2016;70:250-6.

35. Koletzko B. Human Milk Lipids. Ann Nutr Metab. 2016;69 (Suppl 2):28-40.

36. Hodges EA, Johnson SL, Hughes SO, et al. Development of the responsiveness to child feeding cues scale. Appetite. 2013;65:210-9.

37. Del Prado M, Villalpando S, Elizondo A. Contribution of structural and functional role. Proc Nutr Soc. 2000;59:3-15.

38. Ballard O, Morrow AL. Human milk composition: nutrients and bioactive factors. Pediatr Clin North Am. 2013;60:49-74.

39. Institute of Medicine (US) Committee on Nutritional Status during Pregnancy and Lactation. Milk composition. In: Nutrition during lactation. Washington, DC: National Academies Press; 1991. pp. 113-52.

40. Sankar MJ, Sinha B, Chowdhury R, et al. Optimal breastfeeding practices and infant and child mortality. A systematic review and meta-analysis. Acta Paediatr. 2015;104:3-13.

41. Janetta H, Sharmilah B, Baheya N, et al. Responsive feeding: establishing healthy eating behaviour early on in life. South African Journal of Clinical Nutrition. 2013;26(3):S141-9.

42. Patel AL, Kim JH. Human milk and necrotizing enterocolitis. Semin Pediatr Surg. 2018;27:34-8.

43. Horta BL, Victora CG. Short-term effects of breastfeeding: a systematic review of the benefits of breastfeeding on diarrhoea and pneumonia mortality. Geneva: World Health Organization; 2013.

44. Peres KG, Cascaes AM, Nascimento GG, et al. Effect of breastfeeding on malocclusions: a systematic review and meta-analysis. Acta Paediatr. 2015;104(467):54-61.

45. Horta BL, Loret de Mota C, Victoria CG. Long-term consequences of breastfeeding on cholesterol, obesity, systolic blood pressure, and type 2 diabetes: a systematic review and meta-analysis. Acta Paediatr. 2015;104(467):30-7.

46. Amitay EL, Keinan-Boker L. Breastfeeding and Childhood Leukemia Incidence: A Meta-analysis and Systematic Review. JAMA Pediatr. 2015;169(6):e151025.

47. Horta BL, Loret de Mota C, Victora CG. Breastfeeding and intelligence: a systematic review and meta-analysis. Acta Paediatr. 2015;104(467):14-9.

48. Menon G, Williams TC. Human milk for preterm infants: why, what, when and how? Arch Dis Child Fetal Neonatal Ed. 2013;98:F559-62.

49. Radmacher PG, Adamkin DH. Fortification of human milk for preterm infants. Semin Fetal Neonatal Med. 2017;22:30-5.

50. Collaborative Group on Hormonal Factors in Breast Cancer. Breast cancer and breastfeeding: collaborative reanalysis of individual data from 47 epidemiological studies in 30 countries, including 50302 women with breast cancer and 96973 women without the disease. Lancet. 2002;360(9328):187-95.

51. Chowdhury R, Sinha B, Sankar MJ. Breastfeeding and maternal health outcomes: a systematic review and meta-analysis. Acta Paediatr. 2015;104(467):96-113.

52. Aune D, Norat T, Romundstad P, et al. Breastfeeding and the maternal risk of type 2 diabetes: a systematic review and dose-response meta-analysis of cohort studies. Nutr Metab Cardiovasc Dis. 2014;24:107-15.

53. Bobrow KL, Quigley MA, Green J, et al. Persistent effects of women's parity and breastfeeding patterns on their body mass index: results from the Million Women Study. Int J Obes (Lond). 2013;37:712-7.

54. World Health Organization. (2019). Nutrition: Complementary feeding. [online] Available from: https://www.who.int/nutrition/topics/complementary_feeding/en/. [Last accessed on November, 2019].

55. Appendix V, Guiding Principles for Complementary Feeding of the Breastfed Child (2003). Guidelines for an Integrated Approach to the Nutritional Care of HIV-Infected Children (6 Months-14 Years). Geneva: World Health Organization; 2009.

56. D'Auria E, Bergamini M, Staiano A, et al. Baby-led weaning: what a systematic review of the literature adds on. Ital J Pediatr. 2018;44(1):49.

57. de Onis M, Brown D, Blössner MB, et al. Levels and trends in child malnutrition. UNICEF-WHO-The World Bank joint child malnutrition estimates. 2012.

58. World Health Organization. Nutrition: Data sources and inclusion criteria. [online] Available from: https://www.who.int/nutrition/databases/infantfeeding/data_source_inclusion_criteria/en/. [Last accessed on November, 2019].

59. International Institute for Population Sciences (IIPS) and ICF. National Family Health Survey (NFHS-4), 2015-16.

60. Golden MHN. Specific deficiencies versus growth failure: Type I and Type II nutrients. J Nutri Environ Med. 1996;6:301-8.

61. World Health Organization. Guidelines on food fortification with micronutrients. Allen L, de Benoist B, Dary O, Hurrell R (Eds). World Health Organization; 2006.

62. Caron O. RUTF product specifications. In: UNICEF SD, RUTF pre-bid conference, MSF/UNICEF. 2012.

63. UNICEF. Ready-to-use therapeutic food for children with severe acute malnutrition. (2013). Position Paper, 1.

64. Maslin K, Venter C. Nutritional aspects of commercially prepared infant foods in developed countries: a narrative review. Nutr Res Rev. 2017;30(1):138-48.

65. Chop.edu. (2019). Breastfeeding a Baby with Food Allergies. Children's Hospital of Philadelphia. [online] Available from: https://www.chop.edu/pages/breastfeeding-baby-food-allergies. [Last accessed on November, 2019].

66. Sabharwal V. Myths and beliefs surrounding complementary feeding practices of infants in India. Journal of Community Nutrition and Health. 2014;3(1):34.

67. Chop.edu. (2019). Nutritional Disorders. Children's Hospital of Philadelphia. [online] Available from: https://www.chop.edu/conditions-diseases/nutritional-disorders. [Last accessed on November, 2019].

68. Mihrete Y. Review on Anti Nutritional Factors and their Effect on Mineral Absorption. Acta Scientific Nutritional Health. 2019;3(2):84-9.

69. Helbig E, de Oliveira AC, Queiroz Kda S, et al. Effect of soaking prior to cooking on the levels of phytate and tannin of the common bean (Phaseolus vulgaris, L.) and the protein value. J Nutr Sci Vitaminol (Tokyo). 2003;49(2):81-6.

70. Hales CN, Barker DJ. Type 2 (non-insulin-dependent) diabetes mellitus: the thrifty phenotype hypothesis. Diabetologia. 1992;35(7):595-601.

71. Barker DJ. Fetal programing of coronary heart disease. Trends Endocrinol Metab. 2002;13(9):364-8.

72. Gillman MW. Developmental origins of health and disease. N Engl J Med. 2005;353(17):1848-50.

73. Stanner SA, Yudkin JS. Fetal programing and the Leningrad Siege study. Twin Res. 2001;4(5):287-92.

74. Victora CG, Adair L, Fall C, et al.; Maternal and Child Undernutrition Study. Maternal and child undernutrition: consequences for adult health and human capital. Lancet. 2008;371(9609):340-57.

75. Gupta A, Singh CU, George J. In: Under attack: an Indian law to protect breastfeeding. BPNI. New Delhi: D K Fine Arts Press, 1998. pp. 10-11.

76. UNICEF. National Implementation of the International Code of marketing of breast-milk substitutes. Nutrition section. New York; 2003.

77. Tiwari S, Chaturvedi P. The IMS Act 1992: need for more amendments and publicity. Indian Pediatr. 2003;40:743-6.

78. Bang A, Tiwari S, Agarwal RK. Legal and ethical issues in infant growth. In: Preedy VR (Ed). Handbook of Growth and Growth Monitoring in Health and Disease, Volume 1. New York: Springer Science + Business Media, LLC; 2012. pp. 115-29.

79. Tiwari S. Legislations and infant feeding. In; Gupte S. (Ed) Text Book of Nutrition. New Delhi: Peepee Brothers; 2006. pp. 126-34.

80. Doctors must shun baby food seminars - IAP. Times of India. Available from: http://articles.timesofindia.indiatimes.com/2011-04-18/india/29442996_1_ims-act-seminars-infant-milk-substitutes-act. [Last accessed on November, 2019].

Severe Acute Malnutrition

Akash Bang, Payal Meshram

■ SEVERE ACUTE MALNUTRITION

World Health Organization (WHO) defines the term *malnutrition* as a state of deficiency, excess or improper intake of energy and/or nutrients, that can lead to undernutrition, deficiency of vitamins and minerals, overweight, obesity, and chance of development of noncommunicable diseases.[1] However, in common usage, the term is generally used to denote undernutrition traditionally. Malnutrition can be broadly classified as acute and chronic. Anthropometric parameters play an important role in this differentiation. *Chronic* malnutrition is characterized by stunting (decrease in linear growth) and undernutrition (poor weight gain over a long time) with loss of body fat (adipose tissue), whereas *acute* malnutrition is characterized by wasting [decrease in weight for height, body mass index (BMI) and mid-upper arm circumference (MUAC)]. Acute malnutrition is usually associated with one of the two clinical scenarios called marasmus (wasting syndrome) and kwashiorkor (edematous malnutrition) or combination of these two (marasmic kwashiorkor).

Acute malnutrition is further graded as moderate or severe acute malnutrition (SAM) based on the following WHO diagnostic criteria based on anthropometric parameters—wasting, MUAC, and presence or absence of edema. *Wasting* is low weight for height Z score (based on WHO standard growth charts); the lower the Z score, higher is the risk of mortality. *MUAC* is a very sensitive indicator for determining the severity due to its single cutoff value. It is especially important at resource-limited setups like drought or refugee camps with a scarcity of trained personnel. The peripheral health workers can also easily measure MUAC ensuring early detection and management even in remote areas.[2] The presence of *edema* heightens the sensitivity of the above diagnostic parameters and

increases mortality risk. Hence, it has been given special importance in the diagnostic criteria. The WHO diagnostic criteria for children from 6 months through 59 months for SAM and moderate acute malnutrition (MAM) are summarized in **Box 1**.

For children younger than 6 months of age, no specific criteria are available and generally weight for length and bilateral edema these two parameters are used. For children older than 5 years of age, BMI is used to determine malnutrition, ($\leq$2 SD for moderate and $\leq$3 SD for severe).[3]

The Burden

Malnutrition is one of the most important causes of morbidity and mortality worldwide accounting directly or indirectly for about 45% mortality globally. WHO reports on the recent global trends show that the children under 5 years of age from developing countries are the worst affected with nearly 52 million children suffering from wasting and 17 million from SAM.[1] As per National Family Health Survey (NFHS)-4 data (2015–16), the under-five mortality rate in India is 50/1,000 live births which are less than the NFHS-3 data (75/1,000 live births). In spite of this, India is performing poorly as far as nutrition is concerned. Decline in percentage of stunted and underweight children in these years indicates an improvement in chronic malnutrition, but the percentage of wasted and

Box 1: Diagnostic criteria for SAM and MAM for children aged 6–59 months.

Severe acute malnutrition	*Moderate acute malnutrition*
• MUAC < 115 mm, *or* • Weight-for-length Z-score ≤ –3, *or* • Bilateral pitting edema	• MUAC 115 to 124 mm, *or* • Weight-for-length Z-score –2 to –3

(MAM: moderate acute malnutrition; MUAC: mid-upper arm circumference; SAM: severe acute malnutrition)

severely wasted children has increased from 19.8% to 21% and 6.4% to 7.5%, respectively, as per NFHS-4 data, thus clearly proving that SAM is still a burning problem in India. State-wise prevalence of wasting is highest in Jharkhand (29.0%) and above the national average in eight other states (Haryana, Goa, Rajasthan, Chhattisgarh, Maharashtra, Madhya Pradesh, Karnataka, and Gujarat) and three union territories (Puducherry, Daman and Diu, and Dadra and Nagar Haveli).[4]

Risk Factors

Infections like diarrhea or pneumonia precipitate malnutrition but vice versa is also true, as malnourished children are more susceptible to infection due to their impaired immune system. The malnutrition–infection–malnutrition is thus a vicious cycle. *Poor nutritional and educational status of the mother, low birth weight, inadequate breastfeeding, suboptimal infant and young child feeding (IYCF) practices, poor hygiene and chronic illnesses like human immunodeficiency virus (HIV) and tuberculosis* are the underlying causes which precipitate this vicious cycle. Socioeconomic and sociopolitical factors like *poverty, socioeconomic disparities, illiteracy, political disputes, inadequate housing, food, and water facilities, lack of easy access to healthcare* play a crucial role too. Many of these causes of malnutrition are correctable and preventable. So the recent understanding is that optimal emphasis should be given on *"1,000 days nutrition concept"* which includes 9 months conception period (270 days) plus an additional 24 months (730 days). By 2 years of age, the child attains 20% of adult weight, 50% of adult height, and 80% of the total brain development, and thus is a very crucial period for growth and development of the child.

Pathophysiology

Due to the inadequacy of carbohydrates and energy in the diet, the body starts utilizing the fat stores followed by protein sources to meet the energy needs. To preserve the limited resources of energy, malnourished child curtails its activity to a minimum—this is called *reductive adaptation*. This, in turn, affects the physiology of major regulating organs of the body as follows:

Cardiovascular System

Impairment of cardiac function in the form of decreased cardiac output is seen in malnourishment. Increase in body fluids may further worsen the condition leading to cardiac failure and death. Proper titration of fluid is important during the management of malnutrition.

Hepatobiliary System

Accumulation of fats in the liver impairs its process of gluconeogenesis, albumin synthesis, and removal of toxic proteins and metabolites from the body. Impaired gluconeogenesis and glycogen reserves make the child prone to frequent hypoglycemia episodes.

Renal System

Retention of sodium and fluids in the body occurs due to decreased glomerular filtration rate (GFR) leading to fluid overload and edema.

Gastrointestinal System

The small intestinal villi get atrophied during malnourishment which reduces the absorption of nutrients and decreases the synthesis of digestive enzymes and transportation membrane proteins. Gut motility decreases leading to bacteremia and sepsis. This *malnutrition enteropathy* is characterized with villous atrophy, mucosal thinning, increased intestinal permeability, loss of tight junction proteins (leading to loss of gut barrier function), and lymphocytic infiltration. This leads to diarrhea and loss of essential nutrients further worsening the malnutrition.

Immune System

Immune dysfunction occurs due to atrophy of lymph glands, thymus, tonsils and decreased levels of complements, immunoglobulin, and cell-mediated immunity. Due to an impaired immune system, these children are more susceptible to infections but at the same time, may not show classic manifestation of infections or inflammation.

Metabolic System

Due to impaired heat generation and loss mechanism, these children are more susceptible to hypothermia as well as hyperthermia. The basal metabolic rate also gets reduced by 30% during this period. Loss of subcutaneous fat causes loose skin folds; so in these cases, it is difficult to determine the level of dehydration. A decrease in sodium pump activity and increased membrane permeability allows intracellular transport of sodium and decrease in the level of potassium and chloride, rendering them more prone to dyselectrolytemias, particularly hypernatremia and hypokalemia.

Endocrine System

Malnutrition also affects the endocrine organs like pancreas, leading to a decrease in insulin and insulin-like growth factor levels and an increase in growth hormone and cortisol levels.

Clinical Triage

Often children with malnutrition come to notice when they seek treatment for some acute illnesses. Very few children need hospital-based management. Based on triage, SAM patients are classified as either uncomplicated or complicated SAM. *Triage* parameters include *the Appetite Test* **(Box 2 and Table 1)**, *presence or absence of medical complications, and access for follow-up.* The indications for inpatient management are—failed appetite test, child with acute illness needing treatment, poor response to outpatient management, and any chronic illness like tuberculosis, HIV, etc. **(Box 3)**. For infants below 6 months of age, hospitalization is a better option, as the mother needs counseling and assistance for initiating breastfeeding. The complicated cases need facility-based care in a healthcare facility or nutritional rehabilitation center (NRC) or malnutrition training center (MTC). The uncomplicated cases, i.e. those with a good appetite, no medical illness and edema can be managed at home.

Bilateral edema is one of the diagnostic parameters of SAM. *Edema* is classified as *mild* (+) if involving both feet/ankles, *moderate* (++) if in both feet plus lower legs, hands or lower arms, *severe* (+++) if generalized including both feet, legs, hands, arms, and face. Presence of edema worsens the clinical outcome; so special criteria are recommended for hospitalization in cases of only edema **(Box 4)**.

- Every child of SAM who presents with bilateral severe (+++) edema even if the child has a good appetite and no medical complications
- Mild-to-moderate edema with medical complications and poor appetite
- Every child <6 months with edema.

Children above 6 months of age with mild-to-moderate edema, no medical complications and good appetite can be managed on an outpatient basis.

■ FACILITY-BASED MANAGEMENT OF COMPLICATED CASES OF SEVERE ACUTE MALNUTRITION[5-7]

Initial Assessment

During hospitalization, first look for the *danger signs* like severe dehydration, shock, convulsion, unconsciousness, or respiratory distress. Immediately initiate the management for the emergency issues. Meanwhile, an attempt should be made to find out the *underlying illness* that worsened the child's health, e.g. diarrhea, pneumonia, any other infections, etc. for which detailed history and physical examination is very crucial. *History* should include the details of current illness like duration and frequency to determine the severity, birth history, dietary history (initiation of breastfeeding, breastfeeding practices, complementary feeding history, premorbid diet assessment), history of immunization, family history (to find out the socioeconomic status), and any chronic illness in the family. *Examine* the child with specific focus on vital signs; signs of acute illnesses to determine the severity; anthropometry to categorize the child in SAM; head-to-toe examination for signs of malnutrition, micronutrient deficiencies and for systemic illness; and systemic examination for determining the pathological impact on the vital systems of the body. The *laboratory tests* should

---

Box 2: Appetite test.

- Appetite test should be carried out in quiet, comfortable environment
- Mother/caregiver should wash his/her hands first
- Allow the child to sit comfortably on lap and offer RTUF
- Encourage the child to finish the food
- If child is able to finish the amount as recommended for weight, child can be shifted to outpatient management

(RTUF: ready-to-use food)

Table 1: Criteria for passing Appetite Test.

Body weight (kg)	Minimum amount needed to be consumed to pass the Appetite Test
<4	15 mL
4–6.9	25 mL
7–9.9	35 mL
10–14.9	50 mL

Box 3: Indications for hospitalization.

- Child who fails the appetite test
- Child with acute illness needing treatment
- No or poor response to outpatient management
- Any chronic illness like tuberculosis, HIV, etc.
- Prefer hospitalization in infants below 6 months

(HIV: human immunodeficiency virus)

Box 4: Criteria for hospitalization in severe acute malnutrition (SAM) cases with only edema.

- Severe bilateral edema (+++)
- Mild-to-moderate edema with medical complications and poor appetite
- Infants <6 months with edema

include biochemistry—blood sugar level, electrolytes; hematological—complete blood count, anemia workup if relevant; workup for identification of infection—leukocyte count and differentials, blood culture, urine culture, stool examination; radiological including chest radiographs; investigations to rule out chronic illnesses like tuberculin test, erythrocyte sedimentation rate (ESR), sputum analysis and HIV testing; and special tests, e.g. tests for celiac disease **(Table 2)**.

The hospital-based management of SAM includes three overlapping phases as follows:

1. *Initial stabilization*: Initially more emphasis is given on early recognition and prompt treatment of acute life-threatening conditions like hypoglycemia, hypothermia, dehydration, and infection. During this phase, the child's caretaker is also trained to cut short the inpatient stay of the next phase.

2. *Rehabilitation phase*: As the clinical condition improves, the child is started on ready-to-use food (RTUF). The child is mostly discharged within a week once a steady weight gain and/or decreased edema is observed to complete rehabilitation on outpatient follow-up basis.

3. *Follow-up*: Mental, emotional and physical growth of child is monitored.

World Health Organization recommended 10 steps of management of SAM which fulfill the abovementioned phases are as follows **(Table 3)**:

*Step 1: Treat and prevent hypoglycemia **(Fig. 1)**:* Children with SAM are more prone to hypoglycemia due to impaired

Table 2: Management of severe acute malnutrition.

History	• Details of current illness • Birth history • Detailed dietary history • History of immunization • Family history • Any chronic illness in the family
Examination	• Signs of acute illness • Anthropometry to categorize • Head to toe examination for signs of malnutrition and micronutrient deficiencies • Detailed systemic examination
Laboratory investigations	• Blood sugar level and electrolytes • Complete blood count • Anemia workup • Workup for acute infections • Investigations to rule out chronic illnesses

Table 3: World Health Organization's 10 steps of management of severe acute malnutrition.

Step no.	Steps of management
1.	Treat and prevent hypoglycemia **(Fig. 1)**
2.	Treat or prevent hypothermia
3.	Give antibiotics
4.	Treat and prevent dehydration **(Fig. 2)**
5.	Correct electrolyte imbalance
6.	Give micronutrients
7.	Initiate feeding
8.	Catch up growth
9.	Sensory stimulation
10.	Discharge and follow-up

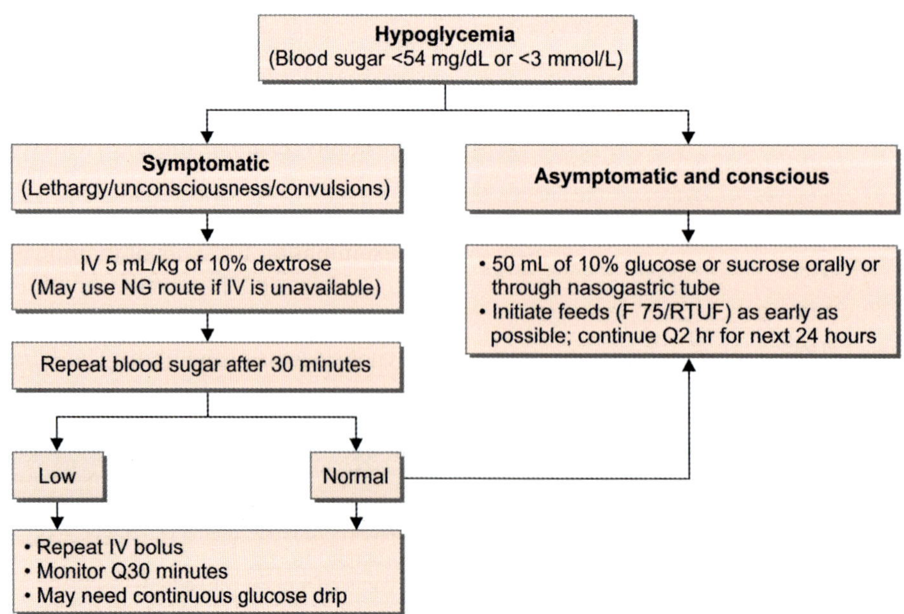

Fig. 1: Management of hypoglycemia in SAM.
(RTUF: ready-to-use food; SAM: severe acute malnutrition; IV: intravenous; NG: nasogastric)

gluconeogenesis, as explained earlier. Monitoring the child for hypoglycemia (blood sugar level <54 mg/dL or <3 mmol/L) is very necessary. Hypoglycemia and hypothermia may occur together and can be further precipitated by any underlying infection. Hence, management or prevention of all the three complications is crucial in SAM.

If the child is *asymptomatic and conscious,* administer 50 mL of 10% glucose or sucrose (one rounded teaspoon of sugar in three tablespoons of water) orally or by nasogastric (NG) tube followed by first feed. Initiate feeding with F-75 (Formula 75) or RTUF as early as possible and then continue every 2 hourly for 24 hours.

If the child is *symptomatic* (has lethargy, convulsions) or *unconscious,* administer 5 mL/kg of 10% dextrose intravenously (IV). If IV is not established, give the same with a NG tube. If both routes are not available, put one teaspoon of sugar moistened with 1–2 drops of water sublingually and repeat every 20 minutes while taking precaution to avoid aspiration. Monitor blood glucose level after 30 minutes; if sugar is still low repeat the bolus and monitor every 30 minutes after starting continuous glucose drip at 6 mg/kg/min. If the child responds to initial treatment, try to start feeding with F-75.

Step 2: Treat or prevent hypothermia: SAM children are more prone for hypothermia due to their poor heat regulatory mechanism. Hypothermia is diagnosed when the *axillary temperature is <35°C or rectal temperature is <35.5°C* in these children. As soon as it is documented, rewarm the child under a radiant warmer or cover them in warm blankets. If these options are not available, have the mother hold the baby in skin-to-skin contact and cover both of them. Avoid direct and vigorous warming to prevent burns. Start feeding immediately and continue every 2 hourly. As mentioned earlier, see for hypoglycemia and sepsis if hypothermia is documented and start with IV/IM antibiotics, if needed. Monitor the child every 2 hourly for hypothermia or every half-hourly if the heater is being used. *Prevent* further hypothermia by keeping the child covered especially head mainly during night time, continuing skin-to-skin contact [kangaroo mother care (KMC)] to infants, keeping the child dry by changing nappies, clothes, bedsheets and by feeding every 2 hourly.

Step 3: Give antibiotics: Due to impaired immunity, majority of SAM children do not manifest the classic signs of infection; hence it is better to keep a high index of suspicion and start antibiotics empirically. Oral amoxicillin can be prescribed in uncomplicated cases on outpatient basis. Complicated cases like septic shock, hypoglycemia, and infections of respiratory tract, urinary tract and skin should be started on IV broad-spectrum antibiotics like a combination of cephalosporin or penicillin group, e.g. benzylpenicillin [50,000 U/kg intramuscular (IM) or IV every 6 hours] or ampicillin (50 mg/ kg IM or IV every 6 hours) for 2 days, then oral amoxicillin (25–40 mg/kg every 8 hours for 5 days) combined with an aminoglycoside like gentamicin (7.5 mg/kg IM or IV) once a day for 7 days. These regimens should be adapted to local resistance patterns.

Start appropriate antibiotics if any specific infection is present like pneumonia, meningitis, skin infections, dysentery, etc. Antimalarials can be started if peripheral blood smear is positive for malarial parasite. Initiate the treatment for chronic infections like tuberculosis or HIV, if diagnosed.

Step 4: Treat and prevent dehydration (Fig. 2): Most of the SAM children present with acute or persistent diarrhea due to malabsorption of nutrients or chronic infections. Due to pre-existing loose skin fold, apathetic look, sunken eyes, etc., assessment of dehydration is difficult in these children. In such cases detailed history and examination findings like vital signs, feeling for the moistness of buccal mucosa and tongue, recent eye changes and urine output should help. Similarly, differentiation between dehydration and shock is also difficult and they can coexist. An apathetic or lethargic child with low volume pulse, cold extremities, and decreased urine output could be present in case of shock as well as dehydration. For this, history from the mother like the history of diarrhea, recent change in child's thirst pattern, and eyes may be of help.

The WHO recommended that full strength standard low osmolarity oral rehydration solution (ORS) should not be used in these children because its sodium (75 mmol/L) content is high. Due to the defect in sodium pump and transcellular membrane in children with SAM, there is an intracellular shift of sodium and extracellular shift of potassium. Rehydrating the children with the standard low osmolarity ORS will increase the body sodium which may worsen again with the normalization of membrane function. So, WHO recommends a special rehydration solution for malnourished children called *ReSoMal (Rehydration Solution for Malnourished children).* This solution has low sodium content and increased potassium, zinc, magnesium, and copper content which helps in overcoming hypernatremia, hypokalemia and other electrolyte derangements. For composition of ReSoMal, see **Table 4**. ReSoMal can be prepared from ready to dilute sachets or by adding one packet of standard ORS into 2 liters of water (half strength ORS) with 50 g of sugar and 40 mL of mineral mix solution. If the mineral mix is

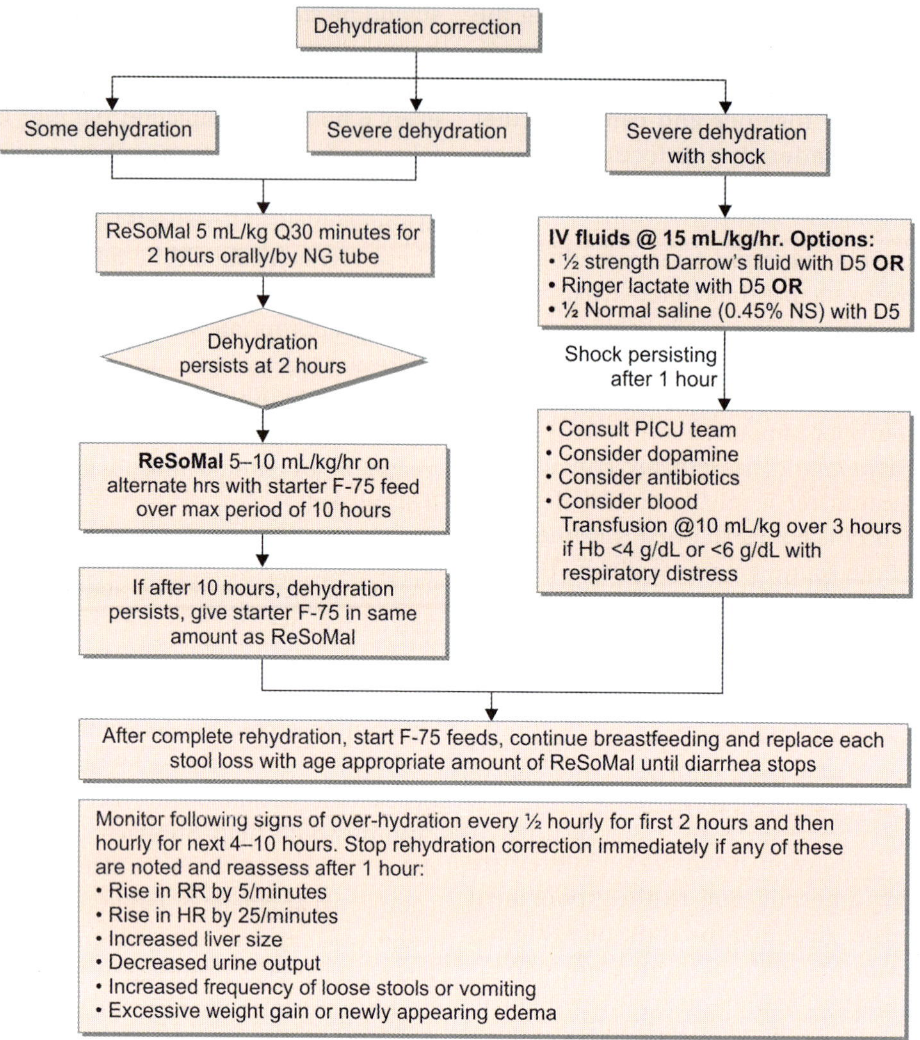

Fig. 2: Management of dehydration in SAM.
(D5: 5% dextrose; Hb: hemoglobin; HR: heart rate; IV: intravenous; NG: nasogastric; NS: normal saline; RR: respiratory rate; PICU: pediatric intensive care unit; SAM: severe acute malnutrition)

Table 4: Composition of ReSoMal (rehydration solution for malnourished).

Components	Concentration mmol/L
Glucose	125
Sodium	45
Potassium	40
Chloride	70
Citrate	7
Magnesium	3
Zinc	0.3
Copper	0.045
Osmolarity	300

not available then add 40 mEq of IV potassium chloride solution (either 40 mL of 10% potassium chloride, or 50 mL of 7.5% potassium chloride).

In children with *SAM with some or severe dehydration with no signs of shock*, rehydration can be done slowly with ReSoMal either orally or by NG tube at 5–10 mL/kg/hr over up to 12 hours to avoid sudden stress on the heart. A child should receive ReSoMal 5 mL/kg every 30 minutes for 2 hours. Even after that if dehydration persists, then give 5–10 mL/kg/hr ReSoMal on alternate hours over a maximum period of 10 hours with F-75 feeds. If the child needs dehydration correction after 10 hours, then give starter F-75 in the same amount of that of ReSoMal. *The full-strength WHO standard ORS is recommended only in cases of cholera or profuse watery diarrhea with SAM.*

Children with *SAM and severe dehydration with signs of shock* should be started on IV fluids like half-strength Darrow's fluid with 5% dextrose or ringer lactate with 5% dextrose or, if neither is available, on half normal saline with 5% dextrose. IV infusion for rehydration is only recommended in cases of circulatory collapse and should begin immediately @*15 mL/kg/hr* with above-recommended fluid. If shock persists even after 1 hour of IV fluid, then give blood transfusion at 10 mL/kg slowly over 3 hours if hemoglobin is <4 g/dL or <6 g/dL with respiratory distress. If there is no anemia, vasoactive drugs like dopamine should be considered in consultation with pediatric intensive care unit (PICU) team. Also, consider infections and start antibiotics within first hour, if indicated (*see* Step 3).

Monitoring: Monitor the child during rehydration to assess the progress in form of fall in heart rate and respiratory rate, improvement in urine output, return of tears, less sunken eyes/fontanelle, moistening of mouth with improvement in skin turgor. Monitoring should be done every half-hourly for the first 2 hours, then hourly for next 4–10 hours. The signs of improvement will not be very obvious in these children because of the underlying pathology. But, the threat of *overhydration* is also very high in these children so monitoring for the same is equally important. While monitoring, check for *rise in respiratory rate by 5 breaths/ min, pulse rate by 25 beats/min, excessive weight gain, palpable liver, urine output and frequency of loose stool and vomiting. Stop rehydration correction immediately if you get any of the abovementioned signs of overhydration and assess after 1 hour.* After complete rehydration, to prevent further dehydration, start F-75 feeds; continue breastfeeding if child breastfeeds; and replace each stool loss with ReSoMal. For less than 2 years, 50–100 mL and for more than 2 years, 100–200 mL of ReSoMal can be given for each stool loss. This therapy is continued until diarrhea stops.

Zinc supplementation (10–20 mg/day) for total 10–14 days is recommended in all these children after reduction in stool frequency. For children >6 months, a dose of 20 mg/day is given for 14 days. As WHO recommended therapeutic food contains zinc in adequate amounts, additional supplementation is not recommended.

Step 5: Correct electrolyte imbalances: As potassium and magnesium are deficient in children with SAM, extra potassium (3–4 mEq/kg/day) and extra magnesium (0.3 mL/kg of 50% magnesium sulfate IM once) must be started and continued up to 2 weeks. On day 1, 2 mL of magnesium solution, and then 0.2–0.3 mL/kg/day is recommended orally. Magnesium facilitates the intracellular shift of potassium and thus helps to correct the electrolyte imbalance and edema. Premixed sachet or combined mineral electrolyte solution is added in the feeds of children to provide this extra potassium and magnesium (20 mL of the solution is added in 1 liter of feed).

Step 6: Give micronutrients: According to 2013 WHO guidelines, vitamin A should be started in a dose of 5,000 IU/day in a therapeutic diet or as multivitamin supplements. For treating signs suggestive of vitamin A deficiency like night-blindness, xerophthalmia, corneal ulcerations, etc. high dose of vitamin A is given as per age recommendations (50,000 IU below 6 months, 1 lac IU for 6–12 months and 2 lacs IU above 12 months) on days 1, 2 and 14. Therapeutic feeds like F-75, F-100, and RTUF already contain multivitamins like vitamin A, folic acid, zinc, and copper. Additional supplementation of these is not needed in children taking these feeds. If abovementioned feeds are not available, then vitamins should be supplemented in a dose of twice their recommended daily allowance (RDA), e.g. *folic acid 5 mg on day 1 followed by 1 mg/ day, elemental zinc 2 mg/kg/day, copper 0.3 mg/kg/day daily for 2 weeks.* Start iron supplementation at 3 mg/kg/day only after initiation of F-100 feed in the rehabilitation phase when the child develops a good appetite and start gaining weight. Iron started early in the stabilization phase can worsen the infection, may induce gastric intolerance, and may not be utilized well due to hypoproteinemia.

Step 7: Initiate feeding: Feeding is initiated after the child gets hemodynamically stable. The starter feed F-75, which is a milk-based formula, is generally started in all children who fail the appetite test. The F-75 contains 75 kcal/100 mL of feed and 1–1.5 g proteins. The composition of starter F-75 is given in **Table 5**. F-75 is given in a dose of 80–100 kcal/kg (approximately 100–135 mL/kg) in a day in small frequent feeds, i.e. every 2–3 hours. Frequent small doses are given initially due to decreased gastric acid production and gut motility in these children. As a child's appetite improves, may be within a week, the child is able to take large and less frequent feeds. Initiate feeding with cup or bowl, but if there is any difficulty like an oral ulcer or the child cannot take enough amount (not able to finish

Table 5: Composition of formula 75 (F-75) feeds.		
Components	*Starter F-75*	*Starter F-75 cereal based*
Dried skimmed milk	25 g	25 g
Sugar	100 g	70 g
Cereal flour	–	35 g
Vegetable oil	27 g	27 g
Mineral mix	20 mL	20 mL
Vitamin mix	140 mg	140 mg
Boiled water to make	1000 mL	1000 mL
Energy	75 kcal/100 mL	75 kcal/100 mL
Protein	0.9 g/100 mL	1.1 g/100 mL
Lactose	1.3 g/100 mL	1.3 g/100 mL

80% of the feed offered for 2–3 consecutive days) then go for NG tube feeding. Monitor and record the daily weight gain, amount consumed and leftover, vomiting episodes, stool frequency, and consistency. Breastfeeding should be continued over and above the starter feed.

Step 8: Catch up growth: This step is undertaken once the child makes a transition from stabilization to rehabilitation phase **(Box 5)**. The criteria that indicate this transition include regression or disappearance of edema, return of good appetite and metabolic stability (no hypoglycemia or dyselectrolytemia). The child can be started on F-100 or RTUF feeds in this phase. F-100 is a therapeutic feed with more calories and protein. Each 100 mL of feed contains 100 kcal of energy and 2.9 g of proteins. The composition of F-100 is given in **Table 6**. The composition of milk-based preparations of F-75 and F-100 is given in **Table 7**.

The transition from F-75 to F-100 or RTUF feed should be gradual. If started on F-100, give F-100 feed in the same amount that of F-75 every 2 hourly for at least 2 days and then increase 10 mL in each feed every 2 hourly till the child tolerates well. The goal is to achieve a calorie intake of 150–220 kcal/kg/day and protein 4–6 g/kg/day. The child with complicated SAM gaining weight on F-100 feeds should be shifted on RTUF feeds and observed for the acceptance or tolerance of diet before shifting them to outpatient or community-based centers.

If the child is directly started on RTUF then give small regular meals initially, i.e. initially 8 and later 5–6 meals per day. Increase the amount gradually to reach the prescribed requirement. If the child is not able to finish the amount of RTUF, then top it up with F-75 during the transition phase. Stop RTUF and switch to F-75 if the child is not able to finish more than 50% of the prescribed amount in 12 hours. Try to restart RTUF after 1–2 days. Give plenty of fluids when the child on RTUF because it does not contain fluids. Breastfeeding should be continued if the child is on breastfeeding. The child should be monitored for weight and loss of edema to determine the progress of therapy. Weight gain is evaluated after every 3 days and categorized according to the weight gain criteria **(Table 8)**. In cases with only moderate weight gain (5–10 g/kg/day), check whether the calorie intake criteria are met and search for infections. Cases with poor weight gain (<5 g/kg/day) must undergo full assessment for the reason for poor weight gain. In cases of edema, this transition from stabilization to the rehabilitation phase must be done only when there is a regression of edema and return of appetite.

Step 9: Sensory stimulation: These children need mental, emotional and behavioral support along with nutrition,

Box 5: Transition from initial stabilization and rehabilitation phase.

Criteria for transition from F-75 to F-100 / RTUF (stabilization to rehabilitation phase)
- Disappearance of edema
- Return of appetite
- Metabolic stability (no hypoglycemia or dyselectrolytemia)

If started on F-100 food
- Start in same amount that of F-75 every 2 hourly for at least 2 days
- Later increase 10 mL in each feed every 2 hourly till the child tolerates well
- Goal is ensuring calorie intake of 150–220 kcal/kg/day and protein 4–6 g/kg/day

If started on RTUF
- Initially 8 meals per day and later upto 5–6 meals per day
- Gradually increase the amount of RTUF
- Top up with F-75 during the transition phase (if not able to finish RTUF)
- Give plenty of fluids and continue breastfeeding

Stop RTUF and switch to F-75 if not able to finish more than 50% of the prescribed amount in 12 hours. Try to restart RTUF after 1–2 days

(RTUF: ready-to-use food)

Table 6: Composition of formula 100 (F-100) feeds.

Components	Catch up F-100 feed
Dried skimmed milk	80 g
Sugar	50 g
Cereal flour	–
Vegetable oil	60 g
Mineral mix	20 mL
Vitamin mix	140 mg
Boiled water to make	1,000 mL
Energy	100 kcal/100 mL
Protein	2.9 g/100 mL
Lactose	4.2 g/100 mL

Table 7: Whole milk-based formula 75 (F-75) and formula 100 (F-100) feeds.

Components	Starter F-75	Catch up F-100
Boiled whole milk	150 mL	440 mL
Sugar	50 g	40 g
Vegetable oil	10 mL	10 mL
Electrolyte solution	10 mL	10 mL
Boiled water to make	500 mL	500 mL

Table 8: Weight gain criteria.

Weight gain	g/kg/day
Good	>10
Moderate	5–10
Poor	<5

<table>
<tr><td>

Box 6: Criteria for shifting from health facility to outpatient care.

Medical
- Completion of parenteral antibiotics
- Clinically well and alert
- Medical complications resolved fully
- Return of normal appetite
- Regression or disappearance of edema

Socioeconomical
- Preparedness of caregiver—their availability for child care and appropriate knowledge and skills related to child feeding practices
- Availability of resources to feed the child

</td><td>

Box 7: Criteria for discharge from treatment.

- Improvement in the anthropometric parameter used initially to diagnose SAM
  - If MUAC was used initially, then MUAC ≥125 mm *and* no edema for at least 2 weeks
  - If weight for height/length was used initially, then Z-scores ≥−2 *and* no edema for at least 2 weeks
- No acute illness
- Good appetite and gaining weight
- Fully immunized
- Community support for child health
- Mother willing and able to take care of the child
- Knows how to prepare the food of child
- Gives assurance for regular follow-up

</td></tr>
</table>

(MUAC: mid-upper arm circumference; SAM: severe acute malnutrition)

so physical and play activities are encouraged during the rehabilitation phase. The child should play for at least 15–30 minutes a day with its parents apart from other informal plays. Mother is advised to play with their children using simple toys in a loving, relaxed, and playful environment.

Step 10: Shifting from health facility and further follow-up: The child with complicated SAM can be shifted to outpatient care during the rehabilitation phase. The criteria for discharge are summarized in **Box 6** and include:

- Completion of parenteral antibiotics
- Clinically well and alert
- Medical complications resolved fully
- Return of normal appetite
- Regression or disappearance of edema.

The anthropometric parameters used for diagnosing SAM are not used for shifting the child to outpatient care because an improvement in these parameters takes time. Even though the child fulfills the above criteria, various other social factors such as loss of earnings for the mother, poverty, and care of the other siblings should be taken into account. Therefore, community support should be carefully assessed before shifting. This includes availability of mother/caregiver for child care, resources to feed the child, and appropriate knowledge on child feeding practices. This preparation of parents for outpatient treatment is important because a child will require continuing care as an outpatient to complete its rehabilitation phase and for prevention of relapse. To achieve this, the caregivers are instructed to bring the child weekly for therapeutic food, vaccination if any, and routine vitamin A supplementations.

CRITERIA FOR DISCHARGING THE PATIENT FROM TREATMENT (BOX 7)

A SAM child should be discharged from treatment only when he/she shows improvement in the anthropometric indicator originally used for confirmation of SAM. Children who got diagnosed on account of bilateral pitting edema should be discharged based on either MUAC or weight for height/length parameter—whichever is used in that particular region as diagnostic or discharge parameter.

At the time of discharge, advice mother to give appropriate meals at least five times a day, high-calorie snacks in between, help and encourage a child to complete feeds, give food separately to quantify child's intake, and continue breastfeeding.

Follow-up

A child with SAM should be periodically monitored to prevent relapse after shifting for outpatient treatment. Follow-up plan of weekly weight measurement should be made with the community rehabilitation center under which the child is enrolled. If the child fails to gain weight after 2 weeks or edema reappears or loss of appetite is noted, then shift the child again to the hospital for reassessment.

TREATMENT OF ASSOCIATED CONDITIONS[5]

Worm Infestation

If there is evidence of any worm infestation, deworming should be done after the stabilization phase with albendazole single dose (400 mg above 2 years of age, 200 mg for age 1–2 years) or mebendazole 100 mg orally twice a day for 3 days. If worm infestation is very prevalent in the geographical area, mebendazole can also be given empirically after 7 days of admission.

Eye Problems

Start oral vitamin A supplementation as discussed earlier. For corneal ulcers or clouding, topical eyedrops of antibiotics chloramphenicol or tetracycline four times a day for 7–10 days, atropine drops one drop three times a day for 3–5 days, covering with saline-soaked pads and bandaging is recommended.

Skin Lesions

Skin lesions due to kwashiorkor or zinc deficiency improve after oral zinc supplementation but the care of the affected area is also important. Soak or bathe the affected areas for 10 minutes in 0.01% potassium permanganate solution, apply zinc barrier creams on raw areas and gentian violet on skin sores.

Diarrhea

If diarrhea continues, stool examination must be undertaken for diagnosing giardiasis and lactose intolerance. In case of giardiasis, give metronidazole (7.5 mg/kg every 8 hours for 7 days). In cases of lactose intolerance, stop milk-based feeds and switch to F-75 cereal-based feeds. Improvement in stool frequency and consistency after stopping milk-based feeds indicates the existence of lactose intolerance in a child.

Severe Anemia

Blood transfusion is indicated if hemoglobin is less than 4 g/dL or less than 6 g/dL with respiratory distress. A child should be transfused with whole blood 10 mL/kg slowly over 3 hours, with IV furosemide 1 mg/kg at the start of transfusion. Packed cells @10 mL/kg should be transfused if a child is in heart failure. In cases of edema, due to redistribution of fluids, apparent fall in hemoglobin may be noted and needs no transfusion. Transfusion in cases of malnutrition should be given slowly and of small volumes to avoid stress on the heart. Monitor pulse, respiratory rate, palpate liver, listen to lung fields, and check jugular venous pressure every 15 minutes during transfusion.

Chronic Infections

Human immunodeficiency virus and tuberculosis are important chronic infections of consideration.

In cases of a child with *HIV*, start antiretroviral therapy (ART) after treating acute infection and metabolic complications. A child is monitored for metabolic complications and opportunistic infections after initiation of treatment for about 6–8 weeks. Doses of ART are the same as recommended in a normal child. High dose vitamin A supplementation and zinc supplementation should be started for diarrhea. Co-trimoxazole prophylaxis should be given in these children to prevent opportunistic infections.

If *tuberculosis* is suspected, get a tuberculin (Mantoux) test and a chest X-ray done. Tuberculin test may turn out to be false negative due to impaired immunity in a SAM child with tuberculosis. If the test is positive or tuberculosis is strongly suspected, begin antitubercular therapy.

■ MANAGEMENT OF MALNUTRITION IN UNCOMPLICATED CASES[8]

Children, older than 6 months of age, who have no acute infection or medical complication and have passed the appetite test, are treated on outpatient basis. Outpatient management is provided through the community-based management of acute malnutrition (CMAM). CMAM program is a decentralized, low-cost model of care beneficial not only for children but also to the caregivers. It protects the child from nosocomial infections, provides modalities for early identification of relapse and also reduces the caregivers' financial burden. The beneficiaries are provided with high energy, micronutrient RTUF.

Ready-to-use Therapeutic Food

It is a peanut-based formulation available commercially as soft, semisolid paste containing peanuts, sugar, oil, powdered milk, and vitamins and minerals mix. RTUF can also be prepared locally by replacing peanuts (protein) with sesames or grains (rice, barley, jawar, maize, and wheat) and adding it into milk powder and mineral-vitamin mix. *Advantages* of RTUF are—high energy dense food compared to F-100, that can be readily consumed by >6 months old children in small quantities at frequent intervals, can be kept unrefrigerated for almost 2 years because of low water content. It provides all the macro- and micronutrients needed for nutritional rehabilitation. Easy transportation, less spoilage and no need of cooking make RTUF the cornerstone of outpatient management of SAM. One foil sachet of RTUF contains 500 kcal. The child is started on 175 kcal/kg/day. Caregiver is advised on maintenance of hygiene, proper hand washing, and provision of clean drinking water.

Child should be empirically started on antibiotics like amoxicillin 40 mg/kg/day twice a day for 7 days on outpatient basis.

Follow-up

Child is followed up weekly or two weekly by community health workers for monitoring of weight gain, counseling for avoidance of relapse and to refill the food. If the child is not gaining weight, it is hospitalized and evaluated to find

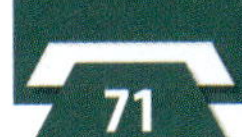

out the underlying pathology. The criteria to discharge the child from the treatment are the same as above (*see* **Box 7**).

Severe Acute Malnutrition Management in Children Less than 6 Months[5-7]

Severe acute malnutrition is less common in children below 6 months of age. Diagnostic criteria of SAM in children below 6 months include weight-for-length less than –3 Z-score *or* presence of bilateral pitting edema.

A child should be hospitalized if there is no adequate weight gain or failure to thrive, presence of medical complications, bilateral pitting edema, ineffective breastfeeding, and any social or medical issue (like disability or depression of caregiver) requiring detailed assessment and management. An *admitted child* should be started on parenteral antibiotics just like an older child with SAM. Infections like tuberculosis, HIV, pneumonia, meningitis, etc. should be treated similarly. Oral amoxicillin should be started in outpatient cases. Establishment or reestablishment of breastfeeding is very important. When the infant is hospitalized, mother is encouraged for feeding. If the infant is not feeding well, the mother is supported to re-lactate. Supplementary feeds like infant formula feeds F-75 and diluted F100 are also prescribed along with breastfeeding. Supplementary suckling approaches are also prioritized. Clean and safe preparations of the supplementary feed are recommended.

Criteria for shifting child from inpatient care to outpatient care are absence of medical complications, regression of edema, clinically alert child with good appetite, weight gain (above the median as per WHO growth velocity charts or >5 g/kg/day for 3 consecutive days), appropriate immunization and linkage to community-based center for follow-up.

Criteria for complete discharge of the child include adequate breastfeeding or supplementary feeding, adequate weight gain, and weight for height > –2 Z score. Infants whose caregiver declines admission or who do not need inpatient care can be managed on outpatient basis by monitoring weight gain weekly, by counseling and supporting the mother for reestablishment of feeding, by assessing the physical and mental health of mother. If the infant does not show any improvement, hospitalization is recommended for evaluation and management.

■ REFERENCES

1. World Health Organization. Joint Child Malnutrition Estimates—Levels and Trends (2017 edition). New York/Geneva: UNICEF/WHO/The World Bank Group; 2018.
2. Walters T, Sibson V, McGrath M. Mid Upper Arm Circumference and Weight-for-Height Z-score as Indicators of Severe Acute Malnutrition. Oxford: Emergency Nutrition Network; 2012.
3. World Health Organization, UNICEF. WHO Child Growth Standards and the Identification of Severe Acute Malnutrition in Infants and Children. Geneva/New York: WHO/UNICEF; 2018.
4. National Family Health Survey (NFHS-4) 2015-16 India. [online] Available from: http://www.rchiips.org/nfhs. [Last accessed on October, 2019].
5. World Health Organization. Pocket Book of Hospital Care for Children: Guidelines for the management of common childhood illnesses, 2nd edition. Geneva: WHO; 2013.
6. Dalwai S, Choudhury P, Bavdekar SB, et al. Consensus statement of the Indian Academy of Pediatrics on integrated management of severe acute malnutrition. Indian Pediatr. 2013;50(4):399-404.
7. World Health Organization. (2013). Guideline Updates on the Management of Severe Acute Malnutrition in Infants and Children. [online] Available from: https://apps.who.int/iris/bitstream/handle/10665/95584/9789241506328_eng.pdf?ua=1. [Last accessed on October, 2019].
8. WHO, UNICEF. Community-Based Management of Severe Acute Malnutrition. Geneva/New York: WHO/ UNICEF; 2004.

Vitamin Deficiencies in Tropics

Upendra Kinjawadekar

INTRODUCTION

Vitamin deficiencies have always been a major consideration in pediatrics. Although the classic forms of many of the vitamin deficiencies are memorized in undergraduate medical education days, the deficiencies in otherwise asymptomatic normally growing children are often overlooked. These deficiencies are very common in tropics and can have a significant impact on the overall health of a child. In this chapter we shall briefly overview the common water- and fat-soluble vitamin deficiencies seen in tropics.

WATER-SOLUBLE VITAMIN DEFICIENCIES

Vitamin B1 (Thiamine)

Carbohydrate containing foods are the main sources of energy and thiamine is essential for the conversion of food into energy. Brain, heart, and nerve cells also require B1 to remain healthy. Beriberi, Wernicke–Korsakoff syndrome, and Leigh syndrome are associated with thiamine deficiency. Good dietary sources of B1 are pork, beef, liver, seeds, peas, whole grain products, oatmeal, etc. Consuming polished white rice has become a status symbol and just to increase its shelf-life lipid rich outer bran is removed. Therefore even though rice makes up to 60% of the daily dietary energy, vast majority of population is thiamine deficient. Even cooking, baking, and canning can destroy thiamine. Thiamine deficiency can also occur as a complication of total parenteral nutrition (TPN) if adequate thiamine supplements are not provided.

It takes about 8–12 weeks for the symptoms to appear after deficient intake of thiamine containing food. Clinical picture is usually divided into a dry (neuritic) type and a wet (cardiac) type. The cardiac and renal dysfunction resulting in fluid accumulation, ultimately leads to wet beriberi.

Dry beriberi has peripheral neuropathy as predominant feature. A cyanotic and dyspneic infant occasionally may present with tachycardia and cardiomegaly with a loud piercing cry. Wernicke encephalopathy presents with ophthalmoplegia, nystagmus, ataxia, intracranial hemorrhage, and confusion. Korsakoff psychosis results in short-term memory loss and confabulation with normal cognition.

Infancy and toddlerhood is the period of very fast growth and development compared to the body size, for which high B1 dose is usually required. Although developed nations do not see thiamine deficiency commonly, it is not uncommon to see in tropics, a typical 5–7-year-old child with poor cognitive and neurological development once in a while due to marginal B1 status.

On a background of compatible symptoms and related clinical setting the diagnosis can be suspected. A high index of suspicion in children presenting with unexplained cardiac failure may sometimes be lifesaving.

Prevention

Thiamine can be retained in rice by parboiling, a process of steaming the rice in the husk before milling. During complementary feeding special care needs to be taken to include meat, whole grain cereals, etc.

There are no easily available biochemical markers to suggest thiamine deficiency nor do we have information on its exact prevalence.

Treatment

Oral thiamine administration is sufficient in most cases. In central nervous system (CNS)/cardiac manifestations, 10 mg thiamine intramuscular/intravenous (IM/IV) daily for a week followed by 3–5 mg/day PO for 6–12 weeks. The

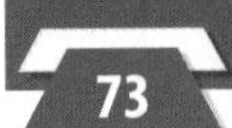

response is dramatic in those with cardiovascular system (CVS) manifestations compared to those with neurologic manifestations where the response could be slow and often incomplete.

Riboflavin (Vitamin B2)

Apart from playing a key role in energy metabolism, riboflavin is essential not only for the formation of red blood cells (RBCs) but also for healthy skin and vision. A dry scaly skin coupled with cracks on lips and/or at the corners of moth is suggestive of riboflavin deficiency. Eyes can have hypersensitivity to light. The main cause of riboflavin deficiency is lack of consumption of vitamin B2. Malnutrition or malabsorption can precipitate the deficiency. The side chain of this vitamin is photochemically destroyed during phototherapy for neonatal jaundice. Studies have shown a higher prevalence in adolescent females and those of a low socioeconomic status.

Prevention

Adequate consumption of milk, milk products and eggs, legumes, and mushrooms prevents riboflavin deficiency.

Treatment

Oral administration of 3–10 mg of riboflavin as a part of B complex vitamin.

Niacin (Vitamin B3)

Another vitamin which is also involved in energy metabolism. Digestive system, nerves, and skin also need niacin to maintain healthy status. Recently large doses of niacin are also being used for lowering cholesterol which should strictly be done under medical supervision. Dietary niacin deficiency is known as pellagra which is characterized by the three Ds: diarrhea, dementia, and dermatitis. The dermatitis looks like a sunburn on the photosensitive areas of the skin.

Causes of Niacin Deficiency

Malnutrition and tryptophan-deficient corn diets are the main causes of niacin deficiency. However, pellagra can occur in association with anorexia nervosa, prolonged isoniazid therapy, and malabsorptive diseases. Primary deficiency secondary to poor dietary intake is rare as niacin is widely distributed in plant and animal foods with the exception of cereal corn or sorghum. Pellagra has not been documented in normally growing children. A severe dietary imbalance, such as in anorexia nervosa and in war or famine conditions, also can cause pellagra.

Diagnosis

There is no good functional test to evaluate niacin status so the diagnosis is usually made from the physical signs of symmetric dermatitis, glossitis, and gastrointestinal (GI) symptoms.

Treatment

Usually 50–300 mg of dietary niacin is sufficient. In severe cases or with in poor intestinal absorption, 100 mg can be given IV along with other B complex vitamins.

Pyridoxine (Vitamin B6)

All chemical reactions involving proteins and amino acids need pyridoxine. For the formation of insulin, antibodies, and RBCs, pyridoxine is important. The Revised National Tuberculosis Control Program (RNTCP) 2019 guidelines have recommended routine pyridoxine supplementation for those taking isoniazid (INH) containing antitubercular treatment (ATT) for treatment or prevention.

The clinical features of deficiency are irritability, vomiting, listlessness, seizures, and failure to thrive. Whenever any young infant presents with seizure, vitamin B6 deficiency or dependency should be suspected. Once more common causes are eliminated 100 mg pyridoxine should be injected IM.

Biotin and pantothenic acid are both essential for energy metabolism, there is not a set recommended dietary allowance (RDA) for either one. They are both found in a wide variety of animal and plant foods therefore deficiency is very rare. Although presenting with protein calorie malnutrition, reports of patients consuming diets high in raw eggs, in which avidin binds to biotin and affects absorption, have produced biotin deficiency. Patients treated with valproic acid can also have biotin deficiency.

Pantothenic acid was discovered as a growth factor for yeast and certain bacteria. It also plays a role in the formation of certain hormones and neurotransmitters.

Vitamin B12 (Cobalamin)

Out of the total body stores of 2–5 mg of B12, roughly around 50% is stored in liver. The recommended daily intake (RDI) of B12 in children is 0.7 µg/day B12 and 2 µg/day in adults. As only microorganisms synthesize B12, it is found only in foods of animal origin. Foods like meats, seafood, egg yolk, and poultry are rich sources of B12. The children belonging to strict vegetarian families have low intake of foods of animal origin and therefore will have B12 deficiency. Furthermore, this unique vitamin needs the help of intrinsic factor for absorption. Because intrinsic factor is made by the lining of the stomach any malabsorption disorder like chronic atrophic gastritis can also result in its deficiency. The dietary sources are expensive and not a part of staple diet in tropical countries. Exclusively breastfed baby whose mother is B12 deficient can develop B12 deficiency and the problem can remain uncorrected with faulty complementary feeding. B12 deficiency impairs the normal hematological, neurological and GI function. The hematological features of megaloblastic anemia are indistinguishable from those of folate deficiency. The neurological symptoms can vary from tingling, numbness sensation in extremities, cognitive changes to irreversible paralysis in extreme cases. Foods and supplements of B12 causing adverse effects are not reported. Mexico, The Indian subcontinent, selected areas in Africa, Central and South America are the places where B12 deficiency is more common than the rest of the world.

Vitamin B12 deficiency amongst Kenyan school children was 70% and amongst preschool children of India was 80%. A study conducted by Kapil U et al., deficiency of folate, vitamin B12 was high amongst children between 5 years and 18 years of age.

The first manifestation of folate deficiency is a decline in serum folate levels usually seen 14 days after consumption of folate deficient diet; gradually leading to megaloblastic anemia and elevated homocysteine concentration. It is generally believed that folate deficiency does not induce neurological complications.

Adequate folate status early in pregnancy greatly reduces the risk of neural tube defects. Infants fed on goat's milk can have folate deficiency. The good dietary sources of folate are found naturally mainly in fruits such as orange and papaya, leafy vegetables, beans, etc. Fortified foods and supplements contain folic acid.

Folate deficiency is usually caused by dietary folate deficiency. Though medications such as methotrexate, phenytoin, and pyrimethamine can cause folate deficiency; it is usually caused by faulty diet which is deficient in folate containing foods.

Treatment

Folic acid given in the dose of 0.5–1 mg/day for 3–4 weeks or until a definite hematologic response is established. Vitamin B12 deficiency responds promptly to parental administration of 250–1,000 µg of B12. Children with only hematologic presentation recover fully within 2–3 months whereas up to 6 month therapy may be required for those with neurology disease. Wheat flour fortification is a simple, inexpensive, and effective food-based strategy to improve the micronutrient status of populations in tropics. Fortification refers to the practice of restoring the nutrients lost during the milling process while adding other vitamins and minerals, as needed, in order to improve the nutritional quality of the food supply. The World Health Organization (WHO) recommends this approach as part of a multipronged strategy to control iron and other micronutrient deficiencies in the general population. India produces an average 75 million tons of wheat annually. The majority of this production is transformed into flour and widely consumed by all socioeconomic categories in the form of flat bread, or *chapatti*. Therefore, wheat flour fortification has the potential to effectively improve the micronutrient status of a large segment of the Indian population. Strict vegans should ensure regular consumption of vitamin B12.

Vitamin C (Ascorbic Acid)

Dietary sources high in vitamin C include fresh, uncooked fruits, and vegetables. The best sources are citrus fruits and fruit juices, melons, guava, tomatoes, green leafy vegetable (GLV), cauliflower, etc. If these sources are not ingested in adequate amounts, humans of any age can develop scurvy.

Infantile scurvy results from lack of intake of vitamin C rich foods such as fresh fruits and vegetables. Affected infants present with irritability, failure to thrive, swollen and painful extremities with restriction of movements (pseudoparalysis), frog posture, gum bleeding, and scorbutic rosary. Characteristic radiological findings and rapid response to treatment with vitamin C confirms the diagnosis. Costochondral beading may suggest the diagnosis of rickets but rachitic rosary is round and nontender, while rosary in scurvy is sharp and tender. All these conditions can generally be distinguished by the presence of associated clinical features such as fever, rash, or trauma. Ancillary investigations and radiography help in confirming the diagnosis. Some of the specific signs are the Frankel sign (zone of calcification at the margin of growth plate), Wimberger sign (calcification around the epiphysis), and scurvy line (lucency adjacent to metaphyseal sclerotic line) rarefaction.

The true prevalence of scurvy in tropical pediatric population is unknown. Humans and other primates cannot synthesize their own vitamin C due to mutation in the gene coding for L-gulonolactone oxidase. This is the enzyme required for the biosynthesis of vitamin C; a water-soluble essential micronutrient involved in many biologic and biochemical functions. It is a potent antioxidant and a cofactor for several enzymes which are involved in the biosynthesis of collagen, carnitine, and neurotransmitters.

The symptoms of scurvy are due to decreased synthesis of collagen which leads to weakening of skeleton and vasculature.

Some of the musculoskeletal manifestations of scurvy are myalgia, arthralgia, limb weakness, extremity swelling, subperiosteal hemorrhage, hemarthrosis, IM hematoma, and osteopenia/osteoporosis. In a retrospective study of 28 children with scurvy in Thailand, the most common presenting complaints were inability to walk (96%) and tenderness of lower limbs (86%).

Limited intake of fresh fruits and vegetables is the chief cause of scurvy; the RDI of vitamin C in children varies with age: 0–6 months—40 mg/dL; 6–12 months—50 mg/dL; 1–3 years—15 mg/dL; 4–8 years—25 mg/dl; 9–13 years—45 mg/dL; 14–18 years—65–75 mg/dL.

In children, groups reported to be at risk include those with oral aversions or inadequate nutritional intake due to various causes including developmental delay, cerebral palsy, and pervasive developmental disorders. Infants who are fed evaporated or super boiled milk are also at risk of developing scurvy. Ratanachu-Ek et al. found that 89% of the cases were supplemented with ultra-heat temperature milk.

On a background history of poor dietary intake the classic clinical features along with X-ray can help to diagnose scurvy. The practical and best confirmatory method for diagnosis of scurvy is the resolution of the manifestations with vitamin C supplementation. Plasma vitamin C level can be used, although it does not always reflect tissue levels of vitamin C. This is because a recent intake in vitamin C-containing food can give normal blood levels. The diagnosis of vitamin C deficiency is usually considered when the plasma concentration is <0.19 mg/dL.

The treatment of scurvy is vitamin C supplementation and to correct the condition that led to the deficiency. There is no established regimen for vitamin C supplementation in scurvy. Regimens of 1 g/day for 2 weeks or 100–200 mg/day for up to 3 months have achieved complete recovery.

VITAMIN A

Malnourished children from tropical countries have increased risk of death from various infectious and noninfectious causes, but vitamin A deficiency is a significant comorbid condition in most of them. Unfortunately, blindness due to vitamin A deficiency which is completely preventable is still prevalent in many tropical countries. Any Green, Yellow, Orange (GYO) vegetable or fruit, e.g. green, yellow, red vegetable/fruits like amaranth, papaya, mangoes, pumpkin, carrots, dairy products like milk, fish, egg yolk, and red palm oil are excellent sources of vitamin A from diet. Unless the mother/caretaker is aware of dangers of vitamin A deficiency and importance of its inclusion in diet the child will not get adequate amount from the routine staple diet. Hence, vitamin A deficiency along with many other micronutrients (MNs) becomes a part of hidden hunger syndrome wherein the body does not give any specific hunger clues for it. Even a subclinical vitamin A deficiency can have serious consequences in the growing child.

Apart from the eye manifestations like xerophthalmia or nyctalopia, the bacterial binding to mucus membrane is increased resulting in negative health consequences. Low serum retinol and staining of the eyes with 1% rose Bengal are helpful in diagnosis though not routinely recommended. The dietary sources never result in hypervitaminosis which is very much possible by accidental over ingestion of vitamin A capsules/syrup. Plasma and skin will have yellowish orange discoloration due to hypercarotenemia. Whenever the prevalence of vitamin A deficiency is more than 0.55% it is advised to give pulse doses at 6 monthly intervals.

All the health monitoring bodies including United Nations International Children's Emergency Fund (UNICEF)/WHO have stated that vitamin A deficiency is an important public health issue, especially in children from 6–59 months; with South Asia (44%) and Sub-Saharan Africa (48%) amongst the most affected regions.

The Government of India launched the National Prophylaxis Programme against nutritional blindness due to vitamin A deficiency in 1970 targeting children aged 1–6 year with the specific aim of preventing nutritional blindness due to keratomalacia. The program was modified in 1994, under the National Child Survival and Safe Motherhood Programme where the target group was restricted to 9–36 months children. The age of the target group was later modified as 6–59 months in 2006. It is gratifying to note that the percentage of children aged 9–59 months who received a vitamin A dose in the past

6 months has gone up to 60.2% in 2015–2016 as compared to 16.5% in 2005–2006.

The metacentric study carried out by Indian Council of Medical Research (ICMR) in 16 districts covering 1.64 lakh preschool children revealed the prevalence of vitamin A deficiency (Bitot's spots) as 0.83%. Another survey carried out by National Nutrition Monitoring Bureau (NNMB) (ICMR) during 2002–2005 in eight states (Andhra Pradesh, Karnataka, Kerala, Madhya Pradesh, Maharashtra, Odisha, Tamil Nadu, and West Bengal) reported similar prevalence of Bitot's spots (0.8%) among 71,591 rural preschool children. Repeat surveys carried out by NNMB in seven states of the country covering rural preschool children have indicated reduction in the prevalence of vitamin A deficiency (Bitot's spots) from 0.7 (1996–1997) to 0.2% (2011–2012). The Central India Children Eye Study carried out among 11,829 schoolchildren of government schools in Nagpur and Maharashtra reported the prevalence of Bitot's spots as 0.1%. The prevalence of Bitot's spots was also reported as 0.19% among children 0–5 years in Meghalaya.

The prevalence of subclinical vitamin A deficiency (serum retinol <20 µg/dL) among preschool children was reported to be around 62% as revealed by NNMB survey carried out during 2002–2005. A recent study carried out in Phek District of Nagaland covering 661 preschool children aged less than 5 years reported the prevalence of subclinical vitamin A deficiency as 32.6%. The prevalence of subclinical vitamin A deficiency (serum retinol <20 µg/dL) was reported as 4% among tribal rural women of reproductive age in Central India.

The main preventive measures against vitamin A deficiency are the following:

High-dose vitamin A supplementation: based on the principle that vitamin A is a fat-soluble vitamin which is stored in liver. So large doses, if given every 6 months, should be sufficient to overcome dietary deficiency. There is growing evidence which is questioning the effectiveness of routine vitamin A supplementation in reducing mortality even with subclinical deficiency. Hence, this program should ideally be reserved in areas with high incidence of Bitot spots (>0.5%).

Fortification of foods particular of those children belonging to vulnerable groups like street children/under institutional care/poor socioeconomic class, etc.

The local governing bodies should encourage not only the consumption but also the local production and marketing of vitamin A containing fruits and vegetables.

Effective and mass measles immunization should be monitored.

Simple measure like encouragement of breastfeeding and its continuation even during illnesses like diarrhea/lower respiratory infection (LRI).

Biofortification, wherein the B-carotene content of the food is improved with through plant breeding. Feeding programs needs to be researched for the feasibility, acceptability, and cost-effectiveness like impact of golden rice rich in provitamin A, ultra rice rich in iron and other MN and red palm oil.

Treatment for Deficiency

Xerophthalmia is treated by giving 1,500 µg/kg vitamin A orally for 5 days followed by IM 7,500 µg of vitamin A in oil until recovery. Vitamin A is also used in preterm infants to improve respiratory function and prevent development of chronic lung disease.

Vitamin—Rich Cures

Nutrition history is full of fascinating stories of nutrient deficiency diseases that confounded doctors of the past.

- The scourge of scurvy, which plagued seafarers several hundred years ago, was finally cured by stocking ships with lemons, oranges, and limes; hence, British sailors were called "limeys". Scurvy is caused by a deficiency of vitamin C, a nutrient that citrus fruits provide in abundance.
- Night blindness, often caused by a deficiency of vitamin A, was known in ancient Egypt. The recommended cure of the day: eating ox or rooster livers. Today it is well known that liver contains more vitamin A than many other foods.
- Giving children cod liver oil to prevent rickets was practiced in the 19th century. But not until 1922, when vitamin D was discovered, did scientists know what substance in cod liver oil gave protection.
- Beriberi, a deficiency of thiamine, was noted in Asia as polished, or white, rice became more popular than unrefined, or brown, rice. The cure was discovered accidentally when chickens with symptoms of beriberi ate the part of rice that was discarded after polishing. It contained the vitamin-rich germ. Today the process of enrichment adds thiamine and other B vitamins back to polished rice; today rice is fortified with folic acid, too.

■ VITAMIN D

What it does?

- Helps almost every part of the body.
- Promotes absorption of calcium and phosphorus; regulates how much calcium remains in the body.
- Helps deposit these minerals in bone and teeth, helps keeping them strong and so reduces fracture risk.
- Helps cell growth regulation.

Immunomodulator Role

Low bone mass, weakness of muscles, and increased risk of fracture are definitely associated with vitamin D deficiency. Although studies are exploring the links to vitamin D's potential role in preventing cancer, diabetes, autoimmune disorders, cardiovascular disease, among other health conditions, the evidence is not sufficient to offer guidance.

Vitamin D (calciferol), which consists of a group of fat-soluble sterols. The age, gender, race, and geographical differences do not have any bias on the prevalence of vitamin D deficiency. The RDA for vitamin D assumes little or no sunlight exposure. The recommendation also allows for margin of safety that recognizes differences in season, latitude, skin pigment, and genetic factors among other factors and considers risks for skin cancer with more sun exposure. In recent years there has been confusion about identifying a vitamin D deficiency because laboratory tests do not have standardized cutoffs to define a deficiency.

Since vitamin D is stored in the body, too much of it can be toxic possibly leading to confusion, dysrhythmias, renal calculi or damage, hypercalcemia, hypercalciuria, and clouding of corneas. Dietary supplements or injectable route can cause an overdose. Aluminum hydroxide is useful for the treatment.

Because the body limits its own vitamin D production, excessive sun exposure will not result in vitamin D toxicity.

Where it is Mostly Found?

Some oily fish like salmon/tuna as well as fortified foods like milk, yogurt, cheese, and juices have good amount of vitamin D. Some mushrooms that are new in the market are exposed to ultraviolet light to boost their vitamin D content. Summer milk produced by cows grazing on green plants is found rich in vitamin A and D.

Fortified foods and dietary supplements supply vitamin D in two different forms. D2 ergocalciferol and D3, i.e. cholecalciferol. Both are equally good for bone health.

Based on the findings from some Indian studies, a high prevalence of hypovitaminosis D was observed among different age groups. Hypovitaminosis D ranged from 84.9% to 100% among school-going children, 42% to 74% among pregnant women, 44.3% to 66.7% among infants, 70% to 81.1% among lactating mothers, and 30% to 91.2% among adults.

Management of Hypovitaminosis D

Children with nutritional vitamin D deficiency should receive vitamin D and should ensure adequate intake of calcium (minimum of 500 mg/day) and phosphorous. Dose of vitamin D is 2,000 IU/day for a minimum of 3 months. It should be followed by daily intake of vitamin D 400 IU/day for <1 year old and 600 IU/day for >1 year old.

■ VITAMIN E

The main role of vitamin E, a fat-soluble vitamin, appears to be an antioxidant. It may help prevent the oxidation of low-density lipoprotein (LDL) (bad) cholesterol, which contributes to plaque buildup in the arteries. For prevention and treatment of retinopathy of prematurity, hemolytic anemia of prematurity neuromuscular diseases, and bronchopulmonary dysplasia, vitamin E has a proven role.

Amongst alpha, beta, gamma, and delta-tocopherols which have vitamin E activity, alpha compounds are most bio-potent.

In vegetable oils, nuts, and seeds, vitamin E protects their unsaturated fats from oxidation. Typically foods high in unsaturated fats are also good sources of vitamin E.

A "Garden" of Antioxidants?

An eating style with plenty of fruits and vegetables is undisputed as the wisest approach to good health. Eating plenty of whole grain foods as well as nuts containing vitamin E provides them too. Too much of vitamin E (only when taken as supplement) may increase the risk of bleeding, may impair vitamin K action, and can increase the action of anticoagulant medication. In newborn, excess of vitamin E can lead to necrotizing enterocolitis.

By reducing the proinflammatory cytokines vitamin E also has an additional positive effect on autoimmune disease. While treating children with cholestasis it should be remembered that about 50–70% of them could be vitamin E deficient.

■ VITAMIN K

Vitamin K makes proteins which are essential for blood clotting. Apart from regulating calcium metabolism, it also plays important in cellular signaling and proliferation.

Vitamin K is present in many foods. It is found in highest concentrations in green vegetables such as cabbage, spinach, and lettuce and broccoli. Additionally, (like vitamin D) vitamin K can be synthesized by human body via bacteria in the large intestine. The exact amount of vitamin K synthesized by bacteria that is actually absorbed in the lower intestine is not known, but likely contributes less than 10% of the recommended intake. Newborns have low vitamin K stores and it takes time for the sterile newborn gut to acquire the good bacteria it needs to produce vitamin K. So, it has become a routine practice to inject newborns with a single IM dose of vitamin K. This practice has significantly reduced vitamin K-dependent bleeding disorders in babies.

Daily requirement is not characterized. Deficiency leads to increased prothrombin time and bleeding tendency. Breast milk has lower concentration (15 µg/mL) as compared to cow's milk (60 µg/mL). Apart from routine supplementation in newborns, vitamin K may also need to be given in liver disease, persistent diarrhea, and malabsorption. It is used both orally and parenterally.

CONCLUSION

Vitamin deficiencies occur at all age groups and are especially more prevalent in tropical countries. Children due to their rapid growth; pregnant and lactating women due to their physiological demands have serious consequences when faced with a challenge of water or fat soluble vitamin deficiencies. Co-existence of many vitamin deficiencies is also a common finding. Early diagnosis and immediate interventions to treat deficiencies as well as education of population on inclusion of specific food groups in their diet and participation in Government programs such as food fortification or supplementation are important steps to tackle the problem of vitamin deficiencies in tropics.

SUGGESTED READING

1. Bailey RL, West KP Jr, Black RE. The Epidemiology of Global Micronutrient Deficiencies. Ann Nutr Metab. 2015;66(Suppl 2):22-33.
2. Bemeur C, Butterworth RF. Thiamin. In: Ross AC, Caballero B, Cousins RJ, Tucker KL, Ziegler TR (Eds). Modern Nutrition in Health and Disease, 11th edition, Lippincott Williams and Wilkins, Philadelphia; 2014. p. 317.
3. Clinicalgate. (2015). Vitamin B Complex Deficiency and Excess. [online] Available from: https://clinicalgate.com/vitamin-b-complex-deficiency-and-excess/ [Last accessed on November, 2019].
4. Coverage at a crossroads: New Directions for Vitamin A Supplementation Programmes. UNICEF, May 2018.
5. Duggan C, Watkins JB, Koletzko B, et al. Nutrition in Pediatrics Basic Science, Clinical Applications, 5th edition.
6. Elizabeth KE. Vitamins, minerals and micronutrients. In: Elizabeth KE (Ed). Nutrition and Child Development, 5th edition. Hyderabad: Paras Medical Publisher; 2015. pp. 98-120.
7. Gathwaia G, Yadav S, Lal OG. Vitamin E level in normal Indian children. Indian J Clin Practice. 2013;24(3).
8. Gonmei Z, Toteja GS. Micronutrient status of Indian population. Indian J Med Res. 2018;148(5):511-21.
9. Gwirtz JA, Garcia-Casal MN. Processing maize flour and corn meal food products.Ann NY Acad Sci. 2014;1312:66.
10. Kamboj P, Dwivedi S, Toteja GS. Prevalence of hypovitaminosis D in India & way forward. Indian J Med Res. 2018;148(5):548-56.
11. Kaur S, Goraya JS. Infantile scurvy. Indian Pediatr. 2017;54(8): 699.
12. Kliegman R, Geme ST. Nelson Textbook of Pediatrics, 21st edition. Amsterdam, Netherlands: Elsevier; 2019.
13. Kupka R, Villamor E, Fawzi WW, et al. Vitamins. In: Duggan C, Watkins J, Walker WA (Eds). Nutrition in pediatrics: basic science, clinical applications. 4th edition. Hamilton: BC Decker; 2009. pp. 99-114.
14. LibreText. (2019). Fat-Soluble Vitamins. [online] Available from: https://med.libretexts.org/Bookshelves/Nutrition/Book:_Human_Nutrition_(University_of_Hawaii)/9:_Vitamins/9.2:_Fat-Soluble_Vitamins [Last accessed on November, 2019].
15. Mimouni-Bloch A, Goldberg-Stern H, Strausberg R, et al. Thiamine deficiency in infancy: long-term follow-up. Pediatr Neurol. 2014;51:311.
16. Misra M. Vitamin D Deficiency and Insufficiency in Children and Adolscents, uptodate.com accessed on 15th July 2019.
17. Rao SN, Chandak GR. Cardiac beriberi: often a missed diagnosis. J Trop Pediatr. 2010;56:284.
18. Sasidharan PK. B12 deficiency in India archives of medicine and health sciences. 2017;5(2):261-8.

Iodine Deficiency Disorders

Aakriti Gupta, Umesh Kapil

■ INTRODUCTION

Iodine deficiency is the leading cause of preventable mental impairment and brain damage in the world.[1,2] Iodine deficiency disorders (IDDs) refers to all adverse health consequences of iodine deficiency in a population. IDDs may originate before birth, jeopardize children's mental health and often their very survival. IDD with its causal association with brain development, cognition, and learning disabilities impairs the economic productivity of adults and progress of the country.[1-6] Even mild iodine deficiency increases the risk of stillbirth, spontaneous abortion, and congenital abnormalities, such as cretinism, a serious irreversible form of mental retardation amongst pregnant women living in iodine-deficient areas.[1-3]

Iodine is an essential element for the synthesis of thyroid hormones by the thyroid gland. Thyroid hormones, i.e. triiodothyronine (T3) and thyroxine (T4) are iodinated molecules of the essential amino acid tyrosine which regulates cellular oxidation. They affect calorigenesis, thermoregulation, intermediary metabolism, protein synthesis, and promote nitrogen retention, glycogenolysis, lipolysis, glucose and galactose absorption in intestine and their uptake by adipocytes.[3,7,8] These hormones are crucial to the metabolism of tissues and development of the central nervous system in the fetus and children.[8,9]

Thyroid gland and physiology: Iodide (I⁻) absorption in the stomach and small intestine is mediated by the sodium-iodide symporter (NIS), which also mediates the uptake of iodide from the bloodstream into the thyroid follicular cell.[3,8-10] Iodide is incorporated into thyroglobulin (Tg), a process referred to as organification. Iodide is oxidized to iodine (I₂) which immediately reacts with tyrosine in Tg protein to form monoiodotyrosine or diiodotyrosine.[3,8-10] These reactions are catalyzed by thyroid peroxidase. The iodinated compounds, in turn, couple to form T3 and T4, which are then secreted from the thyroid into the circulation.[3,8-10]

Thyroid-stimulating hormone (TSH), secreted from the anterior lobe of the pituitary gland, is regulated by the "feedback" mechanism regulated by the level of thyroid hormones (T3 and T4) in the blood. TSH stimulates the transport of iodide from the blood into thyroid cells, oxidation of iodide to iodine, and its binding to tyrosine.[3,8-10]

Both deficient and excessive iodine intakes have been reported to impair thyroid function and lead to thyroid disorders in populations.[3] Deficient iodine intake triggers secretion of TSH and increases the expression of the NIS to maximize the uptake of iodine into thyroid cells and clearance of circulating iodine.[11] The thyroid accumulates an increased proportion of ingested iodine, reuses the iodine from the degradation of thyroid hormones efficiently, thus reducing the renal clearance of iodine.[11] Even small increases in iodine intake in previously iodine-deficient populations are sufficient to reset the thyroid system at different serum TSH levels and change the pattern of thyroid diseases.[12]

In a population living in regions of mild-to-moderate iodine deficiency have been reported to have increased serum Tg concentrations and thyroid size, whereas serum TSH, T3, and T4 are in the normal range.[13-15] Subclinical hypothyroidism with increased serum TSH concentration and normal T4 is observed in a population with moderate-to-severe iodine deficiency.[16,17] As iodine deficiency becomes more severe, TSH might rise further along with stimulation of the trapping mechanism of iodide by the thyroid and intrathyroidal metabolism of iodine. Hence, T3 increases slightly or remains unchanged and T4 decreases because of preferential secretion of T3 by the thyroid.[18]

ETIOLOGY OF IODINE DEFICIENCY DISORDERS

Development of IDD is mainly due to the following reasons:

Environmental Iodine Deficiency

The iodine content of crops, fruits, and vegetables is dependent on the soil in which they are grown. Iodine concentration of plant foods grown in deficient soils may be significantly lower (10 µg/kg dry weight) than plants grown in iodine-sufficient soils (≈1 mg/kg).[19] Iodine deficient soils are most common in inland regions, mountainous areas, and areas of frequent flooding. Rapid changes in environmental conditions leads to melting of glaciers, change of river beds, leaching effects of snow, water and heavy rainfall, and loss of forest cover, which removes iodine from the soil.[9] The erosion of soils in riverine areas due to overgrazing of fields by livestock and deforestation results in continued increase in the loss of iodine from the soil. Groundwater in these areas also lacks iodine. The resultant low iodine content of soil leads to low iodine in livestock and vegetation and also in humans consuming these iodine deficient foods. New areas, which were relatively free of this problem, are now being identified as iodine-deficient possibly because of the intensive agricultural technologies and multiple cropping.

Addition of iodine to foods (e.g. iodization of salt) becomes necessary to combat iodine deficiency in populations residing in iodine deficient areas.[20]

About 90% of the iodine requirements are met through the diet.[21] It is estimated that iodine in foods is lost in varying amounts (20–70%) during the cooking process.[21] Use of iodized salt is therefore advocated to meet the daily requirements, in addition to the iodine present in foods.

Iodine content of common foods is given below in **Table 1**.[22]

Recommended Daily Intake of Iodine

- 90 µg for preschool children (0–59 months);
- 120 µg for school children (6–12 years);
- 150 µg for adolescents (above 12 years) and adults;
- 250 µg for pregnant and lactating women.

Goitrogens in Food

Presence of certain substances called goitrogens adversely influences the utilization of iodine in staple foods.[23] Goitrogens may directly or indirectly affect the thyroid gland. Depending on the level of interference with iron metabolism, direct goitrogens may be classified in three

Table 1: Iodine content of common foods.

Food	Iodine content (µg per 100 g)
Bread (made with iodized salt)	46
Bread (without iodized salt)	3
Eggs	22
Regular milk	13
Beef, pork, and lamb	<1.5
Tap water (varies depending on site)	0.5–20.0
Apples, oranges, grapes, and bananas	<0.5

classes: (1) Class I goitrogens inhibit the entry of iodide into the thyroid glands (thiocyanate, isothiocyanate, and cyanogenic glycosides) and interfere with TSH; (2) Class II goitrogens inhibit intrathyroidal oxidation, organic binding process of iodide and/or the coupling reaction in the process of thyroxine synthesis [thiourea, thionamides, flavonoids, phenolic compounds, and some phthalate derivatives (disulfides and goitrin)]; and (3) Class III goitrogens interfere with proteolysis (necessary step for utilization of thyroxine), dehalogenation, and hormone release (iodide and lithium).[20] Indirect goitrogens increase the rate of thyroid hormone metabolism (2,4-dinitrophenol and biphenyls).

Goitrogens are usually active only if iodine supply is limited and/or if goitrogen containing foods are consumed for a long duration in the diet. A variety of naturally occurring agents have been identified that might be goitrogenic in man. Some of these substances are found in abundance in certain tubers and vegetables, like tapioca, cabbage, and cauliflower **(Table 2)**.

These compounds belong to the following chemical groups:

- Sulfurated organics (thiocyanate, isothiocyanate, goitrin, and disulfides)
- Flavonoids (polyphenols)
- Polyhydroxyphenols and phenol derivatives
- Pyridines, phthalate esters, and metabolites
- Polychlorinated and polybrominated biphenyls
- Organochlorines [Like dichlorodiphenyltrichloro-ethane (DDT)]
- Polycyclic aromatic hydrocarbons
- Inorganic iodine (in excess)
- Lithium (used in the treatment of some neurological disorders).

Intrinsic Factors

Some of the intrinsic factors such as failure to synthesize thyroid hormones due to inherited or congenital defects

Table 2: Dietary goitrogens.

Goitrogen	Mechanism
Foods	
Dietary fat	Dietary fat composition may influence TSH secretion and thyroid peroxidase activity
Cassava, linseed, bamboo shoot, sorghum, sweet potato	Contain cyanogenic glucosides; they are metabolized to thiocyanates that compete with iodine for thyroidal uptake
Cruciferous vegetables: Cabbage, kale, cauliflower, broccoli, turnips, rapeseed	Contains glucosinolates; metabolites compete with iodine for thyroidal uptake and impair thyroid peroxidase activity
Mustard, turnip, and radish	Thiocyanate impair thyroid peroxidase activity
Millet	Flavonoids impair thyroid peroxidase activity

(TSH: thyroid-stimulating hormone)

and peripheral resistance to thyroid hormones can cause IDD.[24]

CURRENT MAGNITUDE OF IODINE DEFICIENCY DISORDER

Iodine deficiency is defined by the World Health Organization (WHO) in terms of median urinary iodine concentration (UIC) of the population. Globally, 1.88 billion people and 241 million children (~30%) are at risk of iodine deficiency due to insufficient dietary intake of iodine.[25] In 1990, 11.2 million children had overt cretinism, and 43 million people suffered with some degree of intellectual impairment.[26] Based primarily on surveys of UIC in school-age children, an estimated 9 countries have excessive iodine intake, 105 countries have adequate iodine nutrition, and 14 countries remain iodine deficient.[27] Over half the children with insufficient iodine intake live in Southeast Asia (76 million) and Africa (58 million).[25] Unlike other micronutrient deficiencies, which is concentrated in the developing world, iodine deficiency is a problem in both developed and developing countries **(Fig. 1)**.[27]

In India, more than 200 million people were estimated to be at risk of IDDs (prevalence of IDD is >10%) and 71 million persons were suffering from goiter and other IDDs.[28]

Iodine deficiency disorder surveys conducted all across the country found that of the 414 districts surveyed till the year 2015–2016, 337 districts were found to be endemic for IDD with total goiter rate (TGR) >5%.[29] Majority of the IDD surveys conducted in the country have also reported TGR of more than 5% (range: 2–42%).[30-42] A study carried out in high altitude region of Himachal Pradesh, reported total goiter rate of more than 15% among schoolchildren aged 6–12 years. However, these children had adequate iodine intake as indicated by median UIC.[31] High TSH of more than 5 mUI/L was reported amongst more than 60% of the neonates in Himachal Pradesh.[43,44] Studies have reported insufficient iodine intake among pregnant women with median UIC of <150 µg/L.[30,32,33,45,46]

HEALTH CONSEQUENCES OF IODINE DEFICIENCY

Iodine deficiency affects all the stages of human development starting from the fetal life **(Table 3)**. Maternal iodine deficiency is recognized as the greatest cause of preventable mental impairment in the world. In developing countries, 38 million newborns each year are at risk of iodine deficiency.[25] Iodine deficiency in pregnancy causes disturbances in thyroid hormones in both mothers and fetuses. Lack of thyroid hormones supply to the developing brain may cause adverse cognitive impairments and even brain damage in fetus. As thyroid hormones function to ensure normal growth and development, consequences of their disturbances are noticeable on the proportion of cell differentiation and gene expression.[47] Mild-to-moderate iodine deficiency in a population increases thyroid volume and the overall risk of goiter in all the population. Severe iodine deficiency is associated with an array of adverse effects, including goiter, cretinism, neonatal hypothyroidism, and growth retardation. Severe iodine deficiency during pregnancy increases risk of stillbirths, abortions, congenital abnormalities, and infant mortality.

Brain Development and Cognition

If the diet of a pregnant woman lacks iodine, the fetus is also deprived of adequate iodine and, hence, cannot produce enough thyroxin. Maternal thyroxine crosses the placenta before onset of fetal thyroid function at 10–12 weeks.[48] Iodine required for the synthesis of thyroid hormones, exerts an action through binding of T3 to nuclear receptors. Nuclear T3 receptors and the amount of T3 bound to these receptors increases six- to ten fold

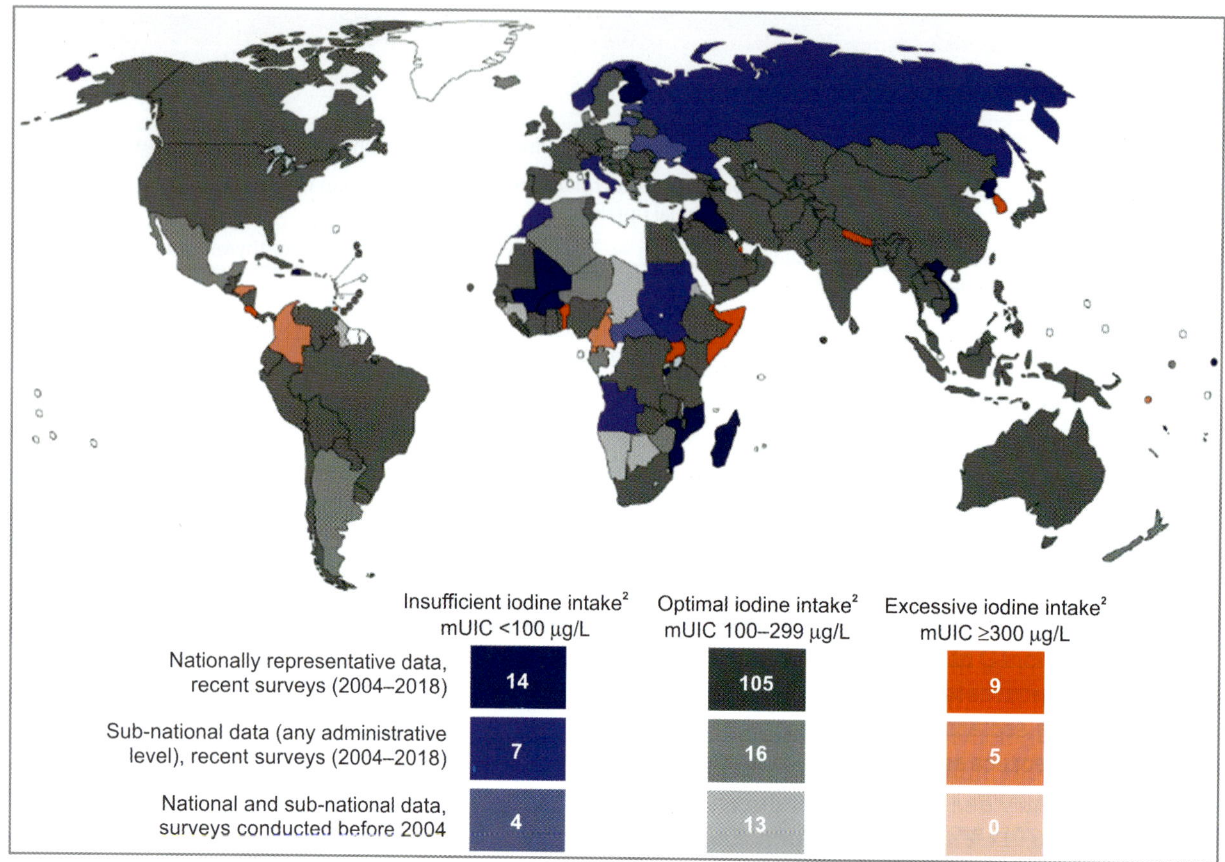

Fig. 1: Global scorecard of iodine nutrition in 2019 in the general population based on median urinary iodine concentration (mUIC) in school-age children (SAC).
Source: The Iodine Global Network. Global scorecard of iodine nutrition in 2019 based on median urinary iodine concentration (mUIC) in school-age children (SAC). Zurich, Switzerland: Iodine Global Network; 2019.[27]

Table 3: The spectrum of iodine deficiency disorders.	
Fetus	Miscarriage Stillbirths Congenital anomalies Increased perinatal morbidity and mortality Neurological cretinism Myxedematous cretinism Psychomotor defects
Neonate	Neonatal goiter Neonatal hypothyroidism Endemic neurocognitive impairment Increased susceptibility of the thyroid gland to nuclear radiation
Child and adolescent	Goiter Juvenile hypothyroidism (subclinical) Impaired mental function Retarded physical development Increased susceptibility of the thyroid gland to nuclear radiation
Adult	Goiter with its complications Hypothyroidism Impaired mental function Spontaneous hyperthyroidism in the elderly Iodine-induced hyperthyroidism Increased susceptibility of the thyroid gland to nuclear radiation

between 10 weeks and 16 weeks. The critical period for maximal brain growth and maturation comprises of the third to fifth month of gestation. T4 is critical during this period for many aspects of brain development including neurogenesis, neuronal migration, organization, axon and dendrite formation, myelination, synaptogenesis, and neurotransmitter regulation. The other period of brain development occurs from third trimester onwards up to the second and third years postnatally. It corresponds to glial cell multiplication, migration, and myelinization.[49]

Substantial amounts of T4 are transferred from mother to fetus during late gestation. These nuclear receptors regulate the expression of specific sites in different brain regions following a precise developmental schedule. Thyroid hormones affect ribonucleic acid (RNA) polymerase II in assembling messenger RNA and in influencing transfer RNA (tRNA) sulfurtransferase. This confers the release of polypeptide chains from ribosomes which plays an important role in the timing, rate, and quantity of brain cell proliferation.[50] The growth and differentiation of the central nervous system is closely related to iodine and thyroid hormones. Impairment of cerebral functions in the fetus is directly related to maternal thyroxinemia. This may lead to fetal growth retardation **(Fig. 2)**.

Combined maternal and fetal hypothyroidism occurs mostly in regions with dietary iodine deficiency. Fetuses with hypothyroidism often do not survive in the womb, and many infants die within few weeks of birth.[51] Iodine induced hypothyroidism during the fetal period also leads to a decrease in the proportion and density of radial glial cells fibers of the hippocampal formation of the brain.[52] Experimental studies conducted amongst thyroidectomized animals to demonstrate effect of severe iodine deficiency on the brain of neonates showed a decrease in axodendritic connections primarily in the neuropil, small size and abnormally densely-packed perikarya and reduced number of axons and dendrites in the interperikaryonal space.[53] Several other research studies have also documented the harmful effect of thyroid hormone deficiency during the development.[54,55]

Mild maternal iodine deficiency during pregnancy is associated with either lower child intelligence quotient (IQ) or educational assessment scores. Children born with hypothyroidism have global developmental delay and remain intellectually subnormal with low IQ. They are often incapable of completing school. In areas with prevalence of mild-to-moderate iodine deficiency, the schoolchildren are 9–13.5 points of IQ below those living in iodine-sufficient areas.[1,9,56,57]

Thyroid hormone deficiency, whether produced by removal or absence of the thyroid due to disease or congenital defects is associated with severe retardation of growth and maturation of almost all organ systems. The most critical period for the brain in human life cycle is from the second trimester of pregnancy to the first year after birth. Impairment in brain development is observed in areas of iodine deficiency, where thyroid hormone levels are low. In its most extreme form, this results in cretinism, but of much greater public health importance are the more subtle degrees of brain damage and reduced cognitive capacity which affects the entire population.[58-60]

Goiter

The healthy human body contains 15–20 mg of iodine, of which about 70–80% is present in the thyroid gland. The thyroid gland which weighs only 15–20 g possesses a remarkable concentrating power for iodine.

Less availability of iodine to thyroid gland impairs its ability to synthesize T3 and T4. This results in the hyperactivity of the thyroid gland to increase the secretion of TSH and produce the requisite amounts of T3 and T4 thereby enlarging itself by hyperplasia.[9] Tg accumulates in the thyroid gland follicles, increasing their deposits of colloid in the thyroid gland. The accumulation of colloid increases the overall size of the thyroid gland, a condition called a goiter **(Fig. 3)**. Simple goiter is due to a lack of iodine in diet due to iodine deficiency in soil, ingestion of a goitrogen, or a demonstrable defect in a hormone biosynthetic pathway, leading to impaired thyroid hormone synthesis.[11] It could also be due to when one or more factors impair the capacity of the thyroid to secrete active hormones sufficient to meet the needs of the peripheral tissues.

When the underlying disorder is severe, compensatory responses, including hypersecretion of TSH, are inadequate to overcome the impairment. This results in

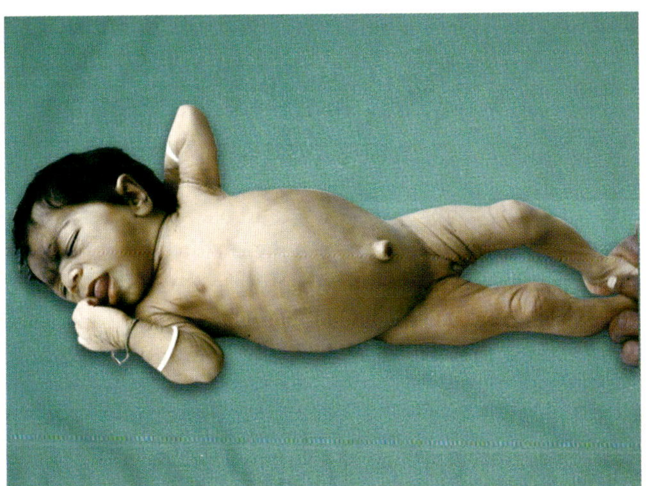

Fig. 2: A 3-month-old infant with hypothyroidism. Note abdominal distension, large tongue, umbilical hernia, and dry skin.
Source: Dr PSN Menon, Dr Anurag Bajpai.

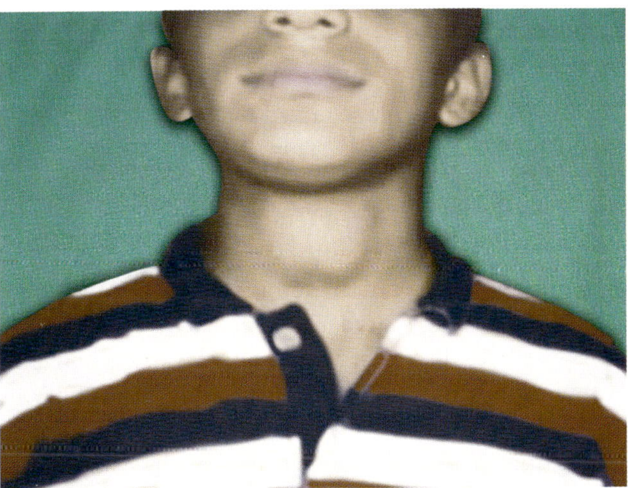

Fig. 3: Goiter in a school-age child.
Source: Dr Umesh Kapil.

the patient to become both goitrous and hypothyroid. Thus, simple goiter cannot be clearly separated in the pathogenetic sense from goitrous hypothyroidism. Initially, goiter is characterized by diffused homogenous enlargement, but over time nodules often develop.

Cretinism

Cretinism or neonatal hypothyroidism is caused by low blood levels of thyroid hormones. It is characterized by severe cognitive deficits, short stature, and may cause deafness and muteness in children and adults born to mothers who were iodine-deficient during pregnancy.

Clinically two forms of cretinism are known which are as following:

- *Neurological cretinism*: The three characteristic features of neurological endemic cretinism in its fully developed form are: (1) extremely severe mental retardation; (2) squint and deaf mutism; and (3) spastic diplegia—motor spasticity affecting the arms and lower limbs leading to characteristic gait and brisk reflexes.[61-63] The patients usually have a goiter.
- *Myxedematous cretinism*: The typical myxedematous cretinism has a less severe degree of mental retardation than the neurological cretinism.[64,65] However, they exhibit all the features of extremely severe hypothyroidism such as severe growth retardation, incomplete maturation of the facial features including the naso-orbital configuration, atrophy of the mandibles, short stature, puffy features, myxedematous, swollen tongue, thickened and dry skin, dry and decreased hair, eyelashes and eyebrows and markedly delayed bone, and sexual maturation. The patients usually had a thyroid normal in size and position, and were seldom deaf.

Hypothyroidism

Hypothyroidism is characterized by low serum T4 levels and elevated TSH levels. This condition is generally encountered in adults.[3,54,66] It leads to coarse and dry skin, husky voice, delayed tendon reflexes, epiphyseal dysgenesis, low metabolic rate, weight gain, cold extremities, constipation, reduced libido, menstrual irregularities, and reduced mental activity.

Hyperthyroidism—an abnormally elevated blood level of thyroid hormones—is often caused by a pituitary or thyroid tumor.[3,67] In Graves' disease, the hyperthyroid state results from an autoimmune reaction in which antibodies overstimulate the follicle cells of the thyroid gland. Hyperthyroidism can lead to an increased metabolic rate

and heart rate, excessive body heat, weight loss, sweating, diarrhea, and tremors.

ASSESSMENT OF IODINE STATUS IN POPULATIONS

Four methods are generally recommended for assessment of iodine nutrition in populations: (1) UIC, (2) the goiter rate, (3) serum TSH, and (4) serum Tg **(Table 4)**.

The UIC is a sensitive indicator of recent iodine intake (days), Tg shows an intermediate response (weeks to months), whereas changes in the goiter rate reflect long-term iodine nutrition (months to years).

Total Goiter Rate

Clinically, presence of goiter is considered a marker of iodine deficiency. WHO staging of goiter is listed in **Table 5**.[68] Two methods are available for measuring goiter: (1) palpation of thyroid gland and (2) thyroid ultrasonography. A thyroid is considered goitrous when each lateral lobe has a volume greater than the terminal phalanx of the thumbs of the subject being examined by palpation.[69] Palpation of goiter in areas of mild iodine deficiency has poor sensitivity and specificity. Measurement of thyroid volume by ultrasound is preferable,[70] but operationally not feasible in all areas. Thyroid ultrasound is noninvasive, quick (2–3 minutes per subject), and feasible even in remote areas using portable equipment.

The size of the thyroid gland inversely changes in response to alterations in iodine intake. It depends on various factors such as severity and duration of iodine deficiency, the type and effectiveness of iodine supplementation, age, sex, and possible additional goitrogenic factors.[71,72]

According to WHO, TGR (goiter grades 1 and 2) of 5% or more, in 6–12 years school children is characterized as endemic goiter and indicates a severe public health problem. The cutoff of 5% allows some margin of inaccuracy of goiter assessment and also for goiter which may occur in iodine-replete population due to other causes such as goitrogens and autoimmune thyroid diseases. TGR of 5–19.9, 20–29.9, and 30% and more indicate mild, moderate, and severe endemicity of iodine deficiency; respectively.[68,69]

Urinary Iodine

Urinary iodine (UI) is an excellent indicator of recent iodine intake as >90% of ingested iodine is excreted in

Table 4: Indicators of iodine status at population level.

Indicator (units)	Age group	Advantages	Disadvantages	Application
Median urinary iodine concentration (µg/L)	School-age children, adults, and pregnant women	• Spot urine samples are easy to obtain • Relatively low cost • External quality control program in place	• Not useful for individual assessment • Assesses iodine intake only over the past few days • Meticulous laboratory practice needed to avoid contamination • Sufficiently large number of samples needed to allow for varying degrees of subject hydration	See Table 6
Goiter rate by palpation (%)	School-age children	• Simple and rapid screening test • Requires no specialized equipment	• Specificity and sensitivity are low due to a high inter-observer variation • Responds only slowly to changes in iodine intake	Degree of IDD by goiter rate: • 0–4.9%—none • 5–19.9%—mild • 20–29.9%—moderate • ≥30%—severe
Goiter rate by ultrasound (%)	School-age children	• More precise than palpation • Reference values established as a function of age, sex, and body surface area	• Requires expensive equipment and electricity • Operator needs special training • Responds only slowly to changes in iodine intake	
Thyroid stimulating hormone (mIU/L)	Newborns	• Measures thyroid function at a particularly vulnerable age • Minimal costs if a congenital hypothyroidism screening program is already in place • Collection by heel stick and storage on filter paper is simple	• Not useful if iodine antiseptics used during delivery • Requires a standardized, sensitive assay • Should be taken by heel prick at least 48 hours after birth to avoid physiological newborn surge	A <3% frequency of TSH values >5 mIU/L indicates iodine sufficiency in a population
Serum or whole blood thyroglobulin (µg/L)	School-age children and adults	• Collection by finger stick and storage on filter paper is simple • International reference range available • Measures improving thyroid function within several months after iodine repletion	• Expensive immunoassay • Standard reference material is available, but needs validation	Reference interval in iodine-sufficient children is 4–40 µg/L

(IDD: iodine deficiency disorder; TSH: thyroid-stimulating hormone)

Table 5: Simplified classification of goiter* by palpation.

Grade 0	No palpable or visible goiter
Grade 1	A goiter that is palpable but not visible when the neck is in the normal position (i.e. the thyroid is not visibly enlarged). Thyroid nodules in a thyroid, which is otherwise not enlarged, fall into this category
Grade 2	A swelling in the neck that is clearly visible when the neck is in a normal position and is consistent with an enlarged thyroid when the neck is palpated

*A thyroid gland will be considered goitrous when each lateral lobe has a volume greater than the terminal phalanx of the thumbs of the subject being examined.

the urine. Spot UI concentration is the most widely used biochemical measurement for assessing and monitoring the iodine status at the population level. According to WHO criteria, the recommended median iodine concentrations should be greater than 100 µg/L and less than 20% of the population should have UICs <50 µg/L. Median UI less than 20, 20–49, 50–99 µg/L indicate severe, moderate or mild iodine deficiency in a given population.[69] In community-based surveys, UICs in casual or spot urine samples provides the iodine status of the population.

Thyroid-stimulating Hormone

Serum TSH concentration reflects the iodine intake of the individual and is determined by the level of circulating thyroid hormone in the body. TSH can therefore be used as an indicator of iodine nutrition **(Table 6)**. Iodine deficiency in older children and adults may slightly increase the serum TSH; however, the values often remain within the normal range. Hence, TSH is not a sensitive indicator of iodine nutrition in adults.

Table 6: Epidemiological criteria for assessing iodine nutrition in a population based on median and/or range of urinary iodine concentrations.

Median urinary iodine (µg/L)	Iodine intake	Iodine nutrition
School-aged children		
<20	Insufficient	Severe iodine deficiency
20–49	Insufficient	Moderate iodine deficiency
50–99	Insufficient	Mild iodine deficiency
100–199	Adequate	Optimal
200–299	More than adequate	Risk of iodine-induced hyperthyroidism in susceptible groups
>300	Excessive	Risk of adverse health consequences (iodine-induced hyperthyroidism, autoimmune thyroid disease and hypothyroidism)
Pregnant women		
<150	Insufficient	
150–249	Adequate	
250–499	More than adequate	
≥500	Excessive[a]	
Lactating women[b]		
<100	Insufficient	
≥100	Adequate	
Children less than 2 years old		
<100	Insufficient	
≥100	Adequate	

[a] The term "excessive" means in excess of the amount required to prevent and control iodine deficiency.
[b] In lactating women, the figures for median urinary iodine are lower than the iodine requirements because of the iodine excreted in breast milk.

Thyroid-stimulating hormone in neonates is a valuable indicator for assessing iodine deficiency because it reflects iodine status during a period when the developing brain is sensitive to iodine deficiency.[72,73] The neonatal thyroid has a low iodine content compared to that of the adult, and hence, iodine turnover is much higher. This high turnover leads to increased stimulation by TSH due to iodine deficiency. TSH levels are therefore elevated in iodine-deficient newborns in the first few weeks of life. The prevalence of neonates with elevated TSH levels serves as a valuable indicator to assess the severity of iodine deficiency in a population.

Concentration of TSH is determined either using dried whole blood spots on filter paper or from serum. These methods are well established and widely available.

The increase in the number of neonates with moderately elevated TSH concentrations (above 5 mLU/L whole blood) is proportional to the degree of iodine deficiency during pregnancy. It may be higher than 40% in severe endemic areas. When a sensitive TSH assay is used on samples collected three to four days after birth, a <3% frequency of TSH values >5 mLU/L indicates iodine sufficiency in a population.[72,73]

Thyroglobulin

Thyroglobulin is a protein, which is synthesized only in the thyroid gland. Serum Tg is secreted in small amounts into the circulation and is normally <10 µg/L when iodine is sufficient in the body.[74] In endemic goiter areas, serum Tg increases due to greater thyroid cell mass and TSH stimulation. Mild-to-moderate iodine deficiency may be associated with elevated serum Tg concentrations in adults and children. Serum Tg measurement correlates with the severity of iodine deficiency as measured by UI.[75] Intervention studies reported that Tg falls rapidly after iodine repletion with iodized oil and potassium iodide. Hence, Tg is a more sensitive indicator of iodine repletion than TSH or T4.[76,77]

■ PREVENTION OF IODINE DEFICIENCY DISORDERS

There are several modes of iodine supplementation used for prevention of IDD. These are: (1) iodized salt, (2) iodized oil, (3) iodized capsules, (4) iodized bread, and (5) iodized water. Out of these, the most cost-effective and operationally feasible method is iodized salt.

Iodized Salt

Iodized salt is considered the most appropriate measure for iodine fortification[1] as it is used by all sections of a community, irrespective of social and economic status. Its production is often confined to a few centers so that fortification can occur on a large scale and with better controlled conditions, making it an economical method of supplying iodine.

The WHO recommends that all food-grade salt, used in household and food processing should be fortified with iodine as a safe and effective strategy for the prevention and control of IDDs in populations living in stable and emergency settings.[2]

Salt iodization was first used as an intervention strategy to present goiter in the United States of America and Switzerland in 1920s.[78] The National Goitre Control Programme was launched by the Government of India in 1962, which was later renamed as National Iodine Deficiency Disorders Control Programme (NIDDCP) in 1992 focusing on Universal Salt Iodization (USI).

At present, sale of noniodized salt for direct human consumption is banned under the Food Safety and Standards Act, 2006.[79] The NIDDCP has the following goals: (1) To bring the prevalence of IDD to below 5% in the country, (2) To ensure 100% consumption of adequately iodated salt (15 ppm) at the household level.[80] Fortification concentration was calculated based on the mean recommended nutrient intake of 150 µg iodine/day + 30% losses from production to household level before consumption, and a 92% iodine bioavailability.[69,81,82] Minimum standard of 30 ppm iodine is mandated at production level and 15 ppm at the retail level.[80]

The initiatives taken by the government has resulted in an increase in percentage of households National Family Health Survey-2 (NFHS-2) using iodized salt, i.e. from 71.6% during 1998–1999[83] to 93.1% during 2015–2016.[84] The National Iodine and Salt Intake Survey (2014–2015) reported that 78% of the households were consuming adequate iodized salt.[85] However, still significant percentage of the population continues to consume inadequately iodized salt (14%) or nil iodine salt (8%). The use of iodized salt varied dramatically from one state to another. The use of iodized salt was high (90% and more) in the northeastern parts of India where salt is transported by railways. This was possibly due to mandatory monitoring of iodized salt before and during rail transport, unlike road transport. However, all the states in the southern region had low levels of use of adequately iodized salt, ranging from only 21% in Tamil Nadu to 43% in Karnataka. There is a need to reach the unreached population and cover the "last mile" of USI success story of India.[86]

Salt iodine content at the production and packaging site, wholesale and retail levels and in households are indicators for monitoring and evaluating IDD control programmes.[1]

A systematic review reported that iodized salt has a large effect on reducing the risk of goiter, cretinism, low cognitive function, and iodine deficiency.[55] Robust monitoring of salt iodization may help in ensuring safe and effective levels of iodine consumption.

Double Fortified Salt

The National Institute of Nutrition, Hyderabad, has developed technology for iron-fortified iodized salt [double fortified salt (DFS)] and has transferred the technology to the industry.[87] Food Safety and Standards Authority of India (FSSAI) has approved two technologies for manufacture of DFS. DFS formulations are intended to provide 100% of daily dietary iodine requirement, and approximately 30–40% of daily dietary iron requirement.[88] In 2009, the Ministry of Health and Family Welfare has endorsed the addition of iron in double fortified salt at 0.8–1.1 ppm (mg/g of salt).[89] The use of DFS has been made mandatory in hot cooked meals under the Mid-Day Meal (MDM) and Integrated Child Development Service (ICDS) programmes.[90] Some states are currently providing DFS through the Public Distribution System (PDS) in selected districts.

The use of DFS in the daily diet increases iron intake by 10 mg/day; consistent use of DFS has been shown to improve the hemoglobin level by 0.5 g/year.[91,92] The pace of increase in hemoglobin by use of DFS is slow. Hence, more rapid improvement in hemoglobin is needed in vulnerable groups such as pre-school and school children.

Iodized Oil

Salt iodization is the best method for supplying iodine to the deficient populations. In some cases iodized salt is unable to meet the requirement of women during pregnancy, exposing the progeny to potential developmental risks. Hence, iodized oil can be regarded as an emergency measure for the control of severe IDD until an effective iodized salt program can be introduced.

Iodized oil may be provided to both pregnant women and children less than 2 years of age as a single oral dose of iodized oil every 6–12 months. Single oral dose of Lipiodol containing 240 mg iodine for 6 months coverage or 480 mg for 12 months is recommended. Evidence has reported effectiveness of a single iodized oil injection (4 mL) in correcting iodine deficiency for a period of up to 4.5 years,[93] prevention of endemic cretinism and a reduction in fetal and neonatal deaths.[94] In regions of moderate-to-severe iodine deficiency without effective salt iodization, lactating women who receive single iodized oil soon after delivery can provide adequate iodine to their infants through breast milk for at least 6 months, enabling the infants to achieve euthyroidism.[95]

Recommendations from WHO-United Nations Children's Fund (UNICEF)-International Council for Control of Iodine Deficiency Disorders (ICCIDD) for oral iodized oil supplementation of women and children are shown in **Table 7**.

Recent evidence on the effect of iodine fortification of foods, beverages, condiments, or seasonings other than salt on reducing goiter, improving physical development measures, and any adverse effects are uncertain.[96]

Table 7: WHO-recommended dosages of daily and annual iodine supplementation.

Population group	Daily dose of iodine supplement (µg/day)	Single annual dose of iodized oil supplement (mg/year)
Pregnant women	250	400
Lactating women	250	400
Women of reproductive age (15–49 years)	150	400
Children <2years[a,b]	90	200

[a] For children 0–6 months of age, iodine supplementation should be given through breast milk. This implies that the child is exclusively breastfed and that the lactating mother received iodine supplementation as indicated above.

[b] These figures for iodine supplements are given in situations where complementary food fortified with iodine is not available, in which case iodine supplementation is required for children of 7–24 months of age.

RISKS OF EXCESS IODINE INTAKE

Excessive iodine intake can cause alterations in thyroid function by decreasing the release of thyroid hormone and serum levels of thyroid hormone and increasing the serum level of TSH to the upper limit of the normal range. In normal individuals, high iodine exposure can cause transient inhibition of thyroid hormone synthesis by a mechanism known as the acute Wolff-Chaikoff effect.[97-99] Wolff and Chaikoff leads to the generation of several inhibitory substances (such as intrathyroidal iodolactones, iodoaldehydes, and/or iodolipids) on thyroid peroxidase activity, resulting in decreased synthesis of thyroid hormones.

Wolff-Chaikoff effect disappears within a few days through downregulation of the iodide transporter in thyroid cells, and normal thyroid hormone synthesis resumes.[100-102] However, lack of the normal adaptation of the thyroid to iodide excess amongst subjects with endemic iodine deficiency goiter can result in thyrotoxicosis. This response, termed iodide-induced hyperthyroidism or the Jod-Basedow effect, occurs in only a small fraction of individuals at risk.[100] This is seen most frequently in those with mild, autoimmune thyroid disease, such as Hashimoto thyroiditis during several weeks after the exposure.[101] By contrast, iodine-induced hyperthyroidism represents a failure of the acute Wolff-Chaikoff effect. Iodine-induced hyperthyroidism might be transient or permanent, and risk factors include nontoxic or diffuse nodular goiter, latent Graves' disease, and long-standing iodine deficiency.[103] In addition, iodine-induced hyperthyroidism in euthyroid patients with nodular goiter in iodine-sufficient areas has also been reported when iodine supplementation is excessive.[104] The Wolff-Chaikoff effect does not mature until 36–40 weeks gestation; therefore, preterm infants are vulnerable to the effects of iodine overload.[105-107]

High iodine intake is associated with autoimmune thyroid disease.[108] A sudden increase in iodine intake in an iodine-deficient population may induce thyroid autoimmunity.[109] People with antithyroid antibodies have a higher risk of developing thyroid dysfunction when the iodine intake is high.[110] The overall incidence of thyroid carcinoma in populations does not appear to be influenced by iodine intake.[111]

CONCLUSION

Impressive progress has been achieved in the control of iodine deficiency in India and globally. Successful adoption and scaling up of universal iodised salt has resulted in adequate iodine status in pre-school children (UIC: 213 µg/L), school-age children (UIC: 175 µg/L) and adolescents (UIC: 173 µg/L) in India as documented in recent Comprehensive National Nutrition Survey (2016-2018).[112] However, still significant percentage of the population continues to consume inadequately iodized salt or nil iodine salt. Achieving sustainable elimination of the IDD would require accelerated and coordinated effort and development of new strategies to achieve and maintain sustainable IDD elimination.

REFERENCES

1. World Health Organization. (2007). Assessment of iodine deficiency disorders and monitoring their elimination: a guide for programme managers. [online] Available from: https://apps.who.int/iris/handle/10665/43781 [Last accessed on November, 2019].
2. World Health Organization. (2013). Micronutrient deficiencies. [online] Available from: https://www.who.int/nutrition/topics/idd/en/ [Last accessed on November, 2019].
3. Zimmermann MB, Boelaert K. Iodine deficiency and thyroid disorders. Lancet Diabetes Endocrinol. 2015;3:286-95.
4. Gordon RC, Rose MC, Skeaff SA, et al. Iodine supplementation improves cognition in mildly iodine-deficient children. Am J Clin Nutr. 2009;90:1264-71.
5. Zimmermann MB. The adverse effects of mild-to-moderate iodine deficiency during pregnancy and childhood: a review. Thyroid. 2007;17:829-35.
6. Bath SC, Steer CD, Golding J, et al. Effect of inadequate iodine status in UK pregnant women on cognitive outcomes in their children: results from the Avon Longitudinal Study of Parents and Children (ALSPAC). Lancet (London, England). 2013;382:331-7.
7. Mullur R, Liu Y-Y, Brent GA. Thyroid hormone regulation of metabolism. Physiol Rev. 2014;94:355-82.
8. Leung A, Pearce EN, Braverman LE. Role of iodine in thyroid physiology. Expert Rev Endocrinol Metab. 2010;5:593-602.

9. Zimmermann MB, Jooste PL, Pandav CS. Iodine-deficiency disorders. Lancet. 2008;372:1251-62.

10. Gibney MJ, Lanham-New SA, Cassidy A, et al. Introduction to Human Nutrition. 2nd edition. United States: Wiley-Blackwell; 2009.

11. Zimmermann MB. Iodine Deficiency. Endocr Rev. 2009;30: 376-408.

12. Laurberg P, Jørgensen T, Perrild H, et al. The Danish investigation on iodine intake and thyroid disease, DanThyr: status and perspectives. Eur J Endocrinol. 2006;155:219-28.

13. Rasmussen LB, Ovesen L, Bülow I, et al. Relations between various measures of iodine intake and thyroid volume, thyroid nodularity, and serum thyroglobulin. Am J Clin Nutr. 2002;76:1069-76.

14. Thomson C, Woodruffe S, Colls A, et al. Urinary iodine and thyroid status of New Zealand residents. Eur J Clin Nutr. 2001; 55:387-92.

15. Vejbjerg P, Knudsen N, Perrild H, et al. Thyroglobulin as a marker of iodine nutrition status in the general population. Eur J Endocrinol. 2009;161:475-81.

16. Chopra IJ, Hershman JM, Hornabrook RW. Serum thyroid hormone and thyrotropin levels in subjects from endemic goiter regions of New Guinea. J Clin Endocrinol Metab. 1975; 40:326-33.

17. Delange F, Hershman JM, Ermans AM. Relationship between the serum thyrotropin level, the prevalence of goiter and the pattern of iodine metabolism in Idjwi Island. J Clin Endocrinol Metab. 1971;33:261-8.

18. Delange F, Camus M, Ermans AM. Circulating thyroid hormones in endemic goiter. J Clin Endocrinol Metab. 1972; 34:891-5.

19. Assey VD, Greiner T, Mzee RK, et al. Iodine Deficiency Persists in the Zanzibar Islands of Tanzania. Food Nutr Bull. 2006; 27:292-9.

20. Eastman CJ, Zimmermann MB. The Iodine Deficiency Disorders. Endotext; 2018.

21. National Institute of Nutrition. Nutrient Requirements and Recommended Dietary Allowances for Indians; 2010.

22. Nutrition Australia. Iodine Facts. [online] Available from: http://www.nutritionaustralia.org/national/resource/iodine-facts [Last accessed on November. 2019].

23. Vanderpas J. Nutritional Epidemiology and Thyroid Hormone Metabolism. Annu Rev Nutr. 2006;26:293-322.

24. Bamji M, Krishnaswamy K, Brahmam G. Textbook of human nutrition, 3rd edition. New Delhi: Oxford and IBH Publishing Co. Pvt. Ltd; 2009.

25. UNICEF. Sustainable Elimination of Iodine Deficiency; 2008.

26. World Health Organisation. Indicators for assessing iodine deficiency disorders and their control through salt iodization; 2001.

27. The Iodine Global Network (IGN). Global scorecard of iodine nutrition in 2019 based on median urinary iodine concentration (mUIC) in school-age children (SAC). Zurich, Switzerland: Iodine Global Network; 2019.

28. Tiwari B, Ray I, Malhotra R. Policy guidelines on national iodine deficiency disorders control programme-nutrition and IDD cell. Directorate of Health Services, Ministry of Health and Family Welfare. New Delhi: Government of India; 2006 pp. 1-22.

29. National Health Mission. National Iodine Deficiency Disorders Control Programme (NIDDCP). [online] Available from: https://www.nhm.gov.in/nrhmcomponents/national-disease-control-programmes-ndcps/iodinedeficiency-disorders.html [Last accessed on November; 2019].

30. Sareen N, Kapil U, Nambiar V, et al. Iodine nutritional status in Uttarakhand State, India. Indian J Endocrinol Metab. 2016; 20:171-6.

31. Kapil U, Pandey RM, Kabra M, et al. Status of iodine deficiency in district Kangra, Himachal Pradesh after 60 years of salt iodization. Eur J Clin Nutr. 2013;67:827-8.

32. Kapil U, Sareen N, Nambiar V, et al. Status of iodine nutrition among pregnant mothers in selected districts of Uttarakhand, India. Indian J Endocrinol Metab. 2015;19:106-9.

33. Kapil U, Prakash S, Sareen N, et al. Status of iodine deficiency among pregnant mothers in Himachal Pradesh, India. Public Health Nutr. 2014;17:1971-4.

34. Shetty A, Rao CR, Kamath A, et al. Goiter Prevalence and Interrelated Components from Coastal Karnataka. Indian J Pediatr. 2019;86:159-64.

35. Ahmed M, Khan M, Nagarajarao V, et al. Iodine deficiency in children: A comparative study in two districts of south-interior Karnataka, India. J Fam Community Med. 2014;21:48-52.

36. Manjunath B, Suman G, Hemanth T, et al. Prevalence and Factors Associated with Goitre among 6–12-year-old Children in a Rural Area of Karnataka in South India. Biol Trace Elem Res. 2016;169:22-6.

37. Gupta R, Langer B, Raina S, et al. Goiter prevalence in school-going children: a cross-sectional study in two border districts of sub-Himalayan Jammu and Kashmir. J Fam Med Prim Care. 2016;5:825-8.

38. Bali S, Singh AR, Nayak PK. Iodine Deficiency and Toxicity Among School Children in Damoh District, Madhya Pradesh, India. Indian Pediatr. 2018;55:579-81.

39. Sridhar PV, Kamala CS. Iodine status and prevalence of Goitre in school going children in rural area. J Clin Diagn Res. 2014;8(8):PC15-PC17.

40. Chaudhary C, Pathak R, Ahluwalia SK, et al. Iodine deficiency disorder in children aged 6-12 years of Ambala, Haryana. Indian Pediatr. 2013;50:587-9.

41. Das D, Chakraborty I, Biswas A, et al. Goiter prevalence, urinary iodine, and salt iodization level in sub-Himalayan Darjeeling district of West Bengal, India. Indian J Public Health. 2014;58:129-33.

42. Zama SY, Ahmed M. Prevalence of Goitre in School Children of Chamarajanagar District, Karnataka, India. J Clin Diagnostic Res. 2013;7:2807-9.

43. Kapil U, Kabra M, Sareen N, et al. Iodine nutrition status amongst neonates in Kangra district, Himachal Pradesh. J Trace Elem Med Biol. 2014;28:351-3.

44. Kapil U, Kabra M, Prakash S, et al. Iodine Nutritional Status Among Neonates in the Solan District, Himachal Pradesh, India. J Community Health. 2014;39:987-9.

45. Kant S, Haldar P, Lohiya A, et al. Status of iodine nutrition among pregnant women attending antenatal clinic of a secondary care hospital: a cross-sectional study from Northern India. Indian J Community Med. 2017;42:226-9.

46. Rao S, Toteja G, Bhatia N, et al. Iodine status of pregnant women residing in urban slums of Delhi. Asian J Pharm Clin Res. 2018;11:506-8.

47. Hetzel BS, Chavadej J, Potter BJ. The brain in iodine deficiency. Neuropathol Appl Neurobiol. 1988;14:93-104.

48. Sack J. Thyroid function in pregnancy—maternal-fetal relationship in health and disease. Pediatr Endocrinol Rev. 2003;1 Suppl 2:170-6.

49. DeLong R. Neurological involvement in iodine deficiency disorders. Amsterdam: Elsevier; 1987.

50. Koibuchi N, Chin WW. Thyroid Hormone Action and Brain Development. Trends Endocrinol Metab. 2000;11:123-8.

51. Menon KC, Skeaff SA, Thomson CD, et al. The effect of maternal iodine status on infant outcomes in an iodine-deficient Indian population. Thyroid. 2011;21:1373-80.

52. Martínez-Galán JR, Pedraza P, Santacana M, et al. Early effects of iodine deficiency on radial glial cells of the hippocampus of the rat fetus. A model of neurological cretinism. J Clin Invest. 1997;99:2701-9.

53. Eayrs JT. Endocrine influence on cerebral development. Arch Biol (Liege). 1964;75:529-65.

54. Ahmed RG. Hypothyroidism and brain developmental players. Thyroid Res. 2015;8:2.

55. Aburto NJ, Abudou M, Candeias V, et al. Effect and safety of salt iodization to prevent iodine deficiency disorders: a systematic review with meta-analyses. World Health Organization; 2014.

56. Bleichrodt N. A metaanalysis of research on iodine and its relationship to cognitive development. United States: Cognizant Communication Corporation; 1996. pp. 195-200.

57. Parag K, Kumar D, Sinha RR, et al. Iodized Salt Consumption and its Association with Intelligence Quotient (IQ) Among 6–12 years Age Group Children in Bihar. Indian J Pediatr. 2019;86: 256-62.

58. Delange F. Iodine requirements during pregnancy, lactation and the neonatal period and indicators of optimal iodine nutrition. Public Health Nutr. 2007;10:1571-80.

59. Stanbury JB, Delange F, Ermans A, et al. The varied manifestations of endemic cretinism. Trans Am Clin Climatol Assoc. 1974;85:6-17.

60. Delange F. The role of iodine in brain development. Proc Nutr Soc. 2000;59:75-9.

61. McCarrison R. Observations on Endemic Cretinism in the Chitral and Gilgit Valleys. Ind Med Gaz. 1908;43:441-9.

62. DeLong GR, Stanbury JB, Fierro-Benitez R. Neurological signs in congenital iodine-deficiency disorder (endemic cretinism). Dev Med Child Neurol. 2008;27:317-24.

63. Boyages SC, Halpern JP, Maberly GF, et al. A comparative study of neurological and myxedematous endemic cretinism in western China. J Clin Endocrinol Metab. 1988;67:1262-71.

64. Dumont JE, Ermans AM, Bastenie PA. Thyroidal Function in a Goiter Endemic IV. Hypothyroidism and Endemic Cretinism. J Clin Endocrinol Metab. 1963;23:325-35.

65. Delange F, Ermans AM, Vis HL, et al. Endemic cretinism in Idjwi Island (Kivu Lake, Republic of Congo). J Clin Endocrinol Metab. 1972;34:1059-66.

66. Sullivan SA. Hypothyroidism in Pregnancy. Clin Obstet Gynecol. 2019;62:308-19.

67. Michalska J, Milczek T, Olszewski J, et al. Hyperthyroidism and pregnancy. Ginekol Pol. 1998;69:1016-9.

68. World Health Organization. Goitre as a determinant of the prevalence and severity of iodine deficiency disorders in populations; 2014.

69. World Health Organisation, United Nations Children's Fun and the IC for the C of IDD. Assessment of the iodine deficiency disorders and monitoring their elimination. A guide for programme managers. Geneva: WHO; 2007. pp. 1-107.

70. Zimmermann M, Saad A, Hess S, et al. Thyroid ultrasound compared with World Health Organization 1960 and 1994 palpation criteria for determination of goiter prevalence in regions of mild and severe iodine deficiency. Eur J Endocrinol. 2000;143:727-31.

71. Aghini-Lombardi F, Antonangeli L, Pinchera A, et al. Effect of Iodized Salt on Thyroid Volume of Children Living in an Area Previously Characterized by Moderate Iodine Deficiency. J Clin Endocrinol Metab. 1997;82:1136-9.

72. Zimmermann MB, Hess SY, Adou P, et al. Thyroid size and goiter prevalence after introduction of iodized salt: a 5-y prospective study in schoolchildren in Côte d'Ivoire. Am J Clin Nutr. 2003;77:663-7.

73. Li M, Eastman CJ. Neonatal TSH screening: is it a sensitive and reliable tool for monitoring iodine status in populations? Best Pract Res Clin Endocrinol Metab. 2010;24:63-75.

74. Spencer CA, Wang CC. Thyroglobulin measurement. Techniques, clinical benefits, and pitfalls. Endocrinol Metab Clin North Am. 1995;24:841-63.

75. Knudsen N, Bülow I, Jørgensen T, et al. Serum Tg—A Sensitive Marker of Thyroid Abnormalities and Iodine Deficiency in Epidemiological Studies. J Clin Endocrinol Metab. 2001;86: 3599-603.

76. Benmiloud M, Chaouki ML, Gutekunst R, et al. Oral iodized oil for correcting iodine deficiency: optimal dosing and outcome indicator selection. J Clin Endocrinol Metab. 1994;79:20-4.

77. Missler U, Gutekunst R, Wood WG. Thyroglobulin is a more sensitive indicator of iodine deficiency than thyrotropin: development and evaluation of dry blood spot assays for thyrotropin and thyroglobulin in iodine-deficient geographical areas. Eur J Clin Chem Clin Biochem. 1994;32:137-43.

78. Kimball OP. History of the prevention of endemic goitre. Bull World Health Organ. 1953;9:241-8.

79. Pandav C. Evolution of iodine deficiency disorders control program in India: A journey of 5,000 years. Indian J Public Health. 2013;57:126-32.

80. Ministry of Health and Family Welfare. Revised policy guidelines on National Iodine Deficiency Disorders Control Programme; 2006.

81. World Health Organization. Recommended iodine levels in salt and guidelines for monitoring their adequacy and effectiveness. World Health Organization; 1997.

82. World Health Organization. Iodine and health. Eliminating iodine deficiency disorders safely through salt iodization: a statement by the World Health Organization; 1994.

83. Indian Institute of Population Science. National Family Health Survey (NFHS-II) 1998-99 Report. India: IIPS; 2000.

84. International Institute for Population Sciences (IIPS) and Macro International. National Family Health Survey (NFHS-4), 2015–16. India: IIPS; 2016.

85. IDD Newsletter. Across India, women are iodine sufficient. Indai: IDD; 2015.

86. International Institute for Population Sciences (IIPS) and Macro International. National Family Health Survey (NFHS-3), 2005–06. India: IIPS; 2007.

87. Narasinga Rao BS, Prasad S, Apte SV. Iron Absorption in Indians Studied, by Whole Body Counting: a Comparison of Iron Compounds Used in Salt Fortification. Br J Haematol. 1972;22:281-6.

88. Venkatesh Mannar MG, Raman JK. Double Fortified Salt in India: Coverage, Efficacy and Way Forward. Indian J Community Heal. 2018;30:63-71.

89. Food Safety and Standards Authority of India. (2019). Double Fortified Salt. [online] Available from: https://ffrc.fssai.gov.in/commodity?commodity=double-fortified-salt [Last accessed on November, 2019].

90. Ministry of Health and Family Welfare. (2018) Anemia Mukt Bharat: Intensified National Iron Plus Initiative (I-NIPI). [online] Available from: https://anemiamuktbharat.info/portal/wp-content/uploads/2018/09/Anemia-Mukt-Bharat-Brochure_English.pdf [Last accessed on November, 2019].

91. Sivakumar B, Brahmam GN, Nair KM, et al. Prospects of fortification of salt with iron and iodine. Br J Nutr. 2001;85:S167.

92. Sivakumar B, Nair KM. Double fortified salt at crossroads. Indian J Pediatr. 2002;69:617-23.

93. Buttfield IH, Hetzel BS. Endemic goitre in eastern New Guinea, with special reference to the use of iodized oil in prophylaxis and treatment. Bull World Health Organ. 1967;36:243-62.

94. Pharoah PO, Buttfield IH, Hetzel BS. Neurological damage to the fetus resulting from severe iodine deficiency during pregnancy. Lancet (London, England). 1971;1:308-10.

95. Bouhouch RR, Bouhouch S, Cherkaoui M, et al. Direct iodine supplementation of infants versus supplementation of their breastfeeding mothers: a double-blind, randomised, placebo-controlled trial. Lancet Diabetes Endocrinol. 2014;2:197-209.

96. Santos JAR, Christoforou A, Trieu K, et al. Iodine fortification of foods and condiments, other than salt, for preventing iodine deficiency disorders. Cochrane database Syst Rev. 2019;2:CD010734.

97. Wolff J, Chaikoff IL. Plasma inorganic iodide as a homeostatic regulator of thyroid function. J Biol Chem. 1948;174:555-64.

98. Morton M, Chaikoff I, Rosenfeld S. Inhibiting effect of inorganic iodide on the formation in vitro of thyroxine and diiodotyrosine by surviving thyroid tissue. J Biol Chem. 1944;154:381-7.

99. De la Vieja A, Dohan O, Levy O, et al. Molecular analysis of the sodium/iodide symporter: impact on thyroid and extrathyroid pathophysiology. Physiol Rev. 2000;80:1083-105.

100. Melmed S, Polonsky K, Larsen P, et al. Williams textbook of endocrinology. 13th edition. Amsterdam, Netherlands: Elsevier; 2015.

101. Markou K, Georgopoulos N, Kyriazopoulou V, et al. Iodine-induced hypothyroidism. Thyroid. 2001;11:501-10.

102. Eng PH, Cardona GR, Fang SL, et al. Escape from the acute Wolff-Chaikoff effect is associated with a decrease in thyroid sodium/iodide symporter messenger ribonucleic acid and protein. Endocrinology. 1999;140:3404-10.

103. Pramyothin P, Leung AM, Pearce EN, et al. Clinical problem-solving: a hidden solution. N Eng J Med. 2011;365:2123-7.

104. Lazarus J, Brown RS, Daumerie C, et al. 2014 European thyroid association guidelines for the management of subclinical hypothyroidism in pregnancy and in children. Eur Thyroid J. 2014;3:76-94.

105. Brook C, Clayton P, Brown R. Brook's clinical pediatric endocrinology, 6th edition. United States: Wiley-Blackwell; 2009.

106. Parravicini E, Fontana C, Paterlini GL, et al. Iodine, thyroid function, and very low birth weight infants. Pediatrics. 1996;98:730-4.

107. Chung HR, Shin CH, Yang SW, et al. Subclinical Hypothyroidism in Korean Preterm Infants Associated with High Levels of Iodine in Breast Milk. J Clin Endocrinol Metab. 2009;94:4444-7.

108. Laurberg P, Cerqueira C, Ovesen L, et al. Iodine intake as a determinant of thyroid disorders in populations. Best Pract Res Clin Endocrinol Metab. 2010;24:13-27.

109. Kahaly GJ, Dienes HP, Beyer J, et al. Iodide induces thyroid autoimmunity in patients with endemic goitre: a randomised, double-blind, placebo-controlled trial. Eur J Endocrinol. 1998;139:290-7.

110. Li Y, Teng D, Shan Z, et al. Antithyroperoxidase and Anti-thyroglobulin Antibodies in a Five-Year Follow-Up Survey of Populations with Different Iodine Intakes. J Clin Endocrinol Metab. 2008;93:1751-7.

111. Feldt-Rasmussen U. Iodine and Cancer. Thyroid. 2001;11:483-6.

112. Ministry of Health and Family Welfare (MoHFW), Government of India, UNICEF and Population Council, 2019. Comprehensive National Nutrition Survey (CNNS) National Report. New Delhi.

Micronutrient Disorders in Tropics

Elizabeth KE, Gibby Koshy

■ INTRODUCTION

Micronutrient malnutrition is a spectrum of nutritional disorders, a subset of malnutrition, which cuts across all ages. Overt micronutrient deficiency disorders (MDDs) are major public health issues in middle- and low-income tropical countries. Deficiency is often subclinical and is referred to as the "hidden hunger". It can be rarely a toxicity like hypervitaminosis or heavy metal excess. These often get magnified due to factors like infections, poor dietary intake with respect to quantity and quality and reduced bioavailability. Even though the major micronutrient disorders are related to iron, iodine and various vitamin deficiencies, malnutrition resulting from major elements like calcium, potassium, sodium, magnesium, sulfur, and phosphorous and various other microminerals is a great challenge.

Vitamins are classified as *fat soluble*: A, D, E, and K and *water soluble*: B complex and C. Minerals are classified as:

- *Essential trace elements*—iron, iodine, zinc, selenium, copper, chromium, molybdenum
- *Elements which are probably essential*—manganese, silicon, nickel, boron, vanadium
- *Potentially toxic elements*—fluorine, lead, cadmium, mercury, arsenic, tin, aluminum, lithium.

More awareness about the importance of micronutrients and knowledge about their biochemical functions and antioxidant properties have recently enhanced growing interest in their role in treatment and prevention of micronutrient-related disorders. This chapter summarizes the disorders related to micronutrients among children from tropical areas including functions of micronutrients, interventions, prevention, and future implications. Detailed information on iodine deficiency disorders (IDDs) and vitamin deficiency disorders (VDDs) is discussed in separate sections.

■ WHY IN CHILDREN AND WHY IN TROPICS?

Micronutrients play a very significant role in child growth and development, and in treatment and prevention of childhood diseases. Children especially under the age of 5 years are more vulnerable to the long-term consequences and effects of micronutrient deficit, either directly or indirectly. These occur through interactions, which could have untoward effects on childhood growth and mental development, leading to impaired cognitive development, decreased immunity, and stunted growth.[1] Multiple micronutrient deficiencies are more prevalent in infants and schoolchildren, especially in the tropics, among low-to-middle income countries.[2] Tropical diseases like malaria, tuberculosis, soil transmitted helminthiasis, etc. pose added impact on micronutrient requirement and metabolism. Micronutrient deficiency affects school performance and, moreover, results in increased childhood morbidity and mortality. Early identification and correction of micronutrient deficiencies in early childhood is essential for reducing morbidity and mortality. Excess or deficiency of micronutrients could influence the mental and physical functioning and can also affect child health and quality of survival later in life with adverse outcomes. Young children are more vulnerable to micronutrient deficiencies because of the relatively greater need for vitamins and minerals, reduced intake of a variety of food groups and as they are more susceptible to the harmful consequences of micronutrient deficiencies in later childhood. Children are in the growth and development phase and have nutritional requirements that change with stages of growth, when compared to adults. They also require micronutrients based on changing requirements, increased loss during infections and inadequate dietary intake.

In developing countries and tropical countries, school-aged children are found vulnerable to micronutrient deficiencies due to inadequate consumption of nutrient-rich foods, lack of access to adequate healthcare, cultural and dietary taboos, inefficient utilization of essential and available micronutrients related to infections and parasitic infestations in children. Some of the major causes for micronutrient disorders include poor diet, infections, helminthic infestations, and poor health caring practices and could lead to increased child and maternal morbidity and mortality and intellectual capacity. In tropics, the micronutrient status and the impact of micronutrient interventions in children also depend on the presence of underlying infections, socioeconomic factors, interactions between medical treatment and the micronutrient supplementations and on the interactions between single and multiple micronutrients as part of the supplementation.

■ MICRONUTRIENT MALNUTRITION

Micronutrients are essential as these cannot be synthesized by the body. Micronutrient deficiency, known as the "hidden hunger", occurs when the absorption or intake of essential vitamins and minerals falls below the levels needed for growth and development in children and for maintenance of physical and cognitive function. This also means that these are not visible like protein energy malnutrition and can have severe health consequences especially during the growing-up phase. Micronutrients play a major role in maintaining the body homeostasis and serve as cofactors for metabolic enzymes and helps in body's defensive mechanism against oxidative stress.

Micronutrients and Breastfeeding

Breastfeeding meets the needs of infants and the concentrations of most micronutrients like calcium, copper, and magnesium are regulated by the maternal homeostatic mechanisms independent of the maternal nutritional status and diet, and provide protection against micronutrient deficiency or excess. The concentrations of essential elements like iron and zinc in breast milk are also regulated by the mammary gland in order to protect the newborn infant against the deficiency and excess. But, beyond 6 months, breast milk alone cannot meet the needs for zinc and iron and needs to be supplemented as supplements or by diverse complementary foods.[3]

■ MICRONUTRIENTS AND THEIR FUNCTIONS

Micronutrients are essential vitamins and minerals that are needed only in small amounts and they play a significant role in the production of enzymes and hormones and help to regulate the cognitive development, functioning and growth and immune activity. The sources, functions, deficiencies, clinical features, requirements, and toxicity of the various micronutrients are summarized in **Tables 1 and 2.**

Micronutrient Excess versus Deficiency

Micronutrients are often considered to be the "magic bullets" and may turn dangerous, if consumed in excess. A paradoxical situation of increasing overeating has also been reported among children struggling with micronutrient deficiency in many of the countries located in the tropical areas.

Micronutrients with Public Health Importance

Iron

Iron deficiency is the most common micronutrient disorder and the main cause of anemia worldwide, especially in children in tropics.[4] Iron is essential for the transportation of oxygen and for generating energy and vital for normal neurological development. Any change in iron storage and metabolism could contribute to adverse outcome in neonatal disorders such as retinopathy of prematurity (ROP), necrotizing enterocolitis (NEC), and hypoxic ischemic encephalopathy (HIE).[5] Even though, zinc protoporphyrin/heme ratio has been useful as a better sensitive marker of iron deficiency and correlates with other iron biomarkers such as ferritin or transferrin, it varies with age and does not measure the functional iron status. In tropical countries, the most common cause of iron deficiency among children includes poor dietary intake, malnutrition, infections and helminthic infestations especially hookworm and trichuriasis. Iron deficiency and iron deficiency anemia is more prevalent during the second 6 months of life due to poor intake, rapid growth and development, depletion of prenatal iron stores, and increased demands. In India, the National Iron Plus Initiative (NIPI) program recommends universal daily iron supplementation during pregnancy and first 6 months of lactation, followed by biweekly during 6–59 months of age, weekly during 5–15 years of age in all children and also till 49 years to women in the reproductive age group (WRA). This is of utmost importance as iron deficiency is the rule in tropical countries like India. The role of iron in physical stamina, cognition, myelination, learning ability, preventing frequent breath holding spell, febrile convulsion, and hyper-cyanotic blue spell in cyanotic congenital heart disease is also now in highlight.

Table 1: Sources, functions, and requirements of various micronutrients.

Micronutrient TE	Sources	Functions	Requirements
Iron	• Heme—7–35% and nonheme—2–20% • Fish, meat, liver, 3 Gs: grams, grains, greens • Jaggery/molasses, asafetida, turmeric, dates, watermelon • Cooking in iron vessels	• Constituent of myoglobin and enzymes, role in oxygen transport. For physical stamina, learning ability and myelination • Also known as the "energy mineral"	• *Prophylaxis*: 2–3 mg/kg/day, children 10–20 mg/day, pregnancy and lactation 30–40 mg/day • *Treatment oral*: 4–6 mg/kg/day for 3–4 months Inj: Weight in kg × deficit in g/dL × 2.5 + 25%, iron sucrose IV/IM • *Packed red cell transfusion*: 5–10 mL/kg. Always treat the cause
Iodine	Seafoods, drinking water (two-thirds requirement), iodized salts	Constituent of thyroxine, for metabolic control, modulation of estrogen and fetal health	50–150 µg/day
Copper	Liver, fish, meat, oyster, legumes, competes with Zn and Mo for absorption	• Constituents of enzymes, ceruloplasmin, and hormone function, role in hemopoiesis, essential for Zn, iron and vitamin C function, bone • Also called twin mineral of iron	1–2 mg/day
Zinc	Liver, beef, oyster, cereals, nuts, grapes	Constituents of enzymes, role in protein and nucleic acid synthesis, epithelial repair, fluid electrolyte transport, taste function, immunity	• 5–15 mg/day • *Treatment*: Diarrhea; Zn : 2–6 m 10 mg/day and >6 m 20 mg/day • Dose 1–2 mg/kg/day up to 150 mg elemental zinc
Chromium	Yeast, liver cereals, nuts, cocoa, pepper	Facilitates insulin action and weight loss, helps to prevent diabetes	10 µg/day *Treatment*: Single dose 180 µg in hyperglycemia
Fluorine	Drinking water, seafoods, tea, cheese	Constituent of bone and teeth	1–5 mg/day drinking water up to 1 ppm
Selenium	Meat groups, green, garlic	Antioxidant, cofactor of enzyme function, maintains liver integrity	100 µg/day
Manganese	Cereals, legumes, greens, tea	Component of superoxide dismutase, role in oxidative phosphorylation	1–5 mg/day
Nickel	Chocolate	Component of urease and nickel plasmin, stabilizes membranes	Not known
Silicon		Cross-linkage of collagen. Helps in bone formation	Not known
Vanadium	Protein rich food	Regulation of enzyme Na+/K = ATPase, adenylate cyclase, and protein kinase	Not known
Molybdenum	Legumes and green leafy vegetables, liver	Molybdenum containing enzymes in humans are xanthine oxidase/dehydrogenase, aldehyde oxidase and sulfite oxidase	2–3 µg/kg/day

(TE: trace element; ORS: oral rehydration solution; IV: intravenous; IM: intramuscular)

Zinc

Zinc is essential for maintaining the body homeostasis and regulating gene expression, and deficiency of zinc could result in recurrent infections, poor appetite and growth retardation, impaired immune function, diarrhea, alopecia, and poor wound healing. There is increased risk of zinc deficiency associated with low birth weight, NEC, and severe pneumonia. In tropical countries, deficiency of zinc increases the incidence, morbidity and mortality from diarrhea, acute respiratory infections, and malaria. In the absence of systemic inflammation, a good indicator of zinc intake would be measurement of the plasma zinc; however, it does not indicate the total zinc status, and serum alkaline phosphatase may be used as a surrogate marker of zinc status. Zinc supplementation in children with stunting has been found to be beneficial. It is also used in babies with stunted growth and intrauterine growth restriction (IUGR). Even though zinc supplementation has been found to be beneficial in shortening the duration of severe pneumonia, recent evidences do not support the use of

Table 2: Deficiencies, clinical features and toxicity of the various micronutrients.

Micronutrient TE	Deficiencies	Clinical features	Remarks and toxicity
Iron	LBW, excess cow's milk, blood loss, hookworm, whipworm, malabsorption, poor intake, increased demand	• Pallor, dyspnea, CCF, irritability, lack of concentration, pica, koilonychia • *Investigation*: S. iron (50–150 μg/dL), iron-binding capacity (100–400 μg/dL) S. ferritin (50–250 ng/mL), transferrin saturation <15%, blood smear hypochromic microcytic anemia, MCV, MCH, MCHC reduced and RDW increased	• Oxalate, phytates, Zn, coffee/tea inhibit absorption. Vitamin C, cobalt, lime juice and acid medium increase absorption • *Toxicity*: Chronic-hemosiderosis, hemochromatosis • *Acute*: GI upset, stages of quiescent phase, metabolic derangement, hepatic failure and strictures. Gastric lavage (GL) with soda bicarbonate and desferrioxamine • IV desferal 50 mg/kg followed by 10 mg/kg/hr × 24 hrs • S. iron >1,800 μg/dL is fatal
Iodine	Low content in water, especially mountainous areas, excessive intake of brassica species; cabbage, cauliflower	• Endemic goiter, hypothyroidism, stillbirth, CNS defect • *Investigation*: Urinary iodine, PBI, T3, T4, TSH, iodine uptake study	Iodized salt to contain 15 μg/g (15 ppm); up to 30 ppm added to tackle loss. Excess can cause iodism, reversible dermatitis and cobalt deficiency/excess, iron deficiency, manganese excess and fluorine excess may aggravate goiter
Copper	LBW, preterm TPN, PEM, nephrotic syndrome, Menkes kinky hair syndrome is an X-linked metabolic disturbance of copper metabolism characterized by mental retardation, abnormal hair texture, hypocupremia (<65 μg/dL) and low circulating ceruloplasmin (<20 mg/dL)	• Hypochromic anemia, neutropenia, hypopigmented hair, bony defects • *Investigation*: S. Cu 75–150 μg/dL S. ceruloplasmin 10–50 μg/dL	*Toxicity*: Indian childhood cirrhosis, hepatitis, cirrhosis, Coombs negative hemolytic anemia, Zn deficiency, Cu deposition occurs in Wilson's disease
Zinc	PEM, TPN, hepatitis, nephrotic syndrome, acrodermatitis enteropathica, especially as a genetic defect	• Growth retardation, anorexia, gonadal atrophy, alopecia, dermatitis, diarrhea, reduced taste sensation. • *Investigation*: S. Zn 60–150 μg/dL, Zn in hair	• Phytates reduce absorption, excess reduces iron and copper levels. Used as adjuvant in Wilson's disease • *Toxicity*: GI upset, Cu deficiency
Chromium	PEM, TPN	• Hyperglycemia, encephalopathy • *Investigation*: S. Cr 0.02 μg/dL	*Toxicity*: Renal failure, dermatitis
Fluorine	Poor water content	Dental caries	*Excess*: Dental and skeletal fluorosis, genu valgus with excess in drinking water and increased sorghum intake, >2–3 ppm in drinking water needs defluoridation by alum and/or by reverse osmosis
Selenium	PEM, TPN, poor soil content	• Keshan cardiomyopathy, arthritis, myalgia, growth retardation, liver necrosis, risk of liver cancer • Kashin–Beck disease (Endemic osteoarthropathy) • *Investigation*: S. Se 13 μg/dL	Dental caries, alopecia, garlic odor in breath
Manganese	TPN	• Growth retardation, reddening of hair, increased prothrombin time • *Investigation*: S. Mn 0.06 μg/dL	• Iron decreases Mn absorption • *Toxicity*: Encephalitis, goiter, cardiomyopathy, cholestasis
Nickel	TPN	*Investigation*: S. nickel 0.02 μg/dL	*Excess*: Dermatitis, liver necrosis, nasal and lung cancers

Contd...

Contd...

Micronutrient TE	Deficiencies	Clinical features	Remarks and toxicity
Silicon	TPN	Growth retardation, defective bone growth	*Excess*: Granuloma and fibrosis of lung Silicosis, urolithiasis
Vanadium	PEM	Deficiency associated with nutritional edema	
Molybdenum	—	• Molybdenum deficiency coexisting with selenium deficiency may be obligatory for the development of Keshan disease • Tachycardia, central scotoma, irritability, coma and probably increased incidence of mouth and esophageal cancers	Excess may unmask hyperuricemia, gout and genu valgus. Abnormally high levels lead to copper deficiency

(CCF: congestive cardiac failure; CNS: central nervous system; IM: intramuscular; IV: intravenous; LBW: low birth weight; MCH: mean corpuscular hemoglobin; MCHC: mean corpuscular hemoglobin concentration; MCV: mean corpuscular volume; PBI: protein-bound iodide; PEM: protein energy malnutrition; RDW: red cell distribution width; TE: trace element; TPN: total parenteral nutrition; TSH: thyroid-stimulating hormone)

zinc as supportive treatment in lower respiratory infections in children. Zinc needs to be supplemented through dietary intake as there is no long-term storage of zinc when compared to iron. Studies have shown that the prevalence of deficiencies of zinc and iron were significantly lower in children who received multiple micronutrient supplements along with anthelminthic treatment. Currently, there is a targeted zinc supplementation program during episodes of diarrhea starting beyond the newborn period, 10 mg/day below 6 months of age and 20 mg/day above 6 months for 14 days. This has several benefits including mucosal repair and prevention of further episodes of diarrhea. Acrodermatitis enteropathica is a rare genetic disorder with diarrhea, periorificial and acral symmetric skin lesions, and alopecia that responds to zinc supplements. Zinc supplementation has been useful in improving the outcome of malaria, pneumonia, and diarrheal infections among children from lower socioeconomic areas in low-income developing countries. Clinical trials on zinc supplementation have clearly demonstrated the positive benefits of improved zinc status in children and their role in reducing the incidence of various infectious diseases. Zinc supplementation is essential for optimal immune function and has been found to be effective in reducing the diarrheal morbidity in malnourished children with HIV compared to children without HIV infection.

Selenium

Selenium plays a key role in the regulation of the endocrine, immune, cardiovascular, and neurological functions and acts as a cofactor for enzymes responsible for protection against oxidative damage such as glutathione peroxidase (GPx). This may be assessed for the sufficiency of selenium levels. Measurement of the serum levels of selenium associated with selenoprotein P, glutathione peroxidase (GSHpx), and albumin reflects the short-term storage and hair, nail, and erythrocyte levels of selenium are indicative of the long-term selenium exposure. The direct impact of selenium on clinical outcomes is unknown. Selenium supplementation is more suitable for selenium-depleted, very low birth weight babies and preventing severe infection in these babies. Keshan cardiomyopathy has been attributed to selenium deficiency.

Copper

Copper is essential for the neurotransmitter biosynthesis, transportation of iron, and protection against oxidative injuries, and deficiency could result in hematological and neurological disorders. It could also present as psychomotor retardation, iron-resistant sideroblastic anemia, and neutropenia among infants. Copper is essential for the normal functioning of various organs and metabolic process including hemoglobin synthesis, iron oxidation, cellular respiration and connective tissue formation and plays a significant role as cofactor for important enzymatic pathways. Assessment of copper includes the measurement of serum copper and ceruloplasmin and measuring the activity of copper-zinc superoxide dismutase, a sensitive indicator of the functional status of copper. Copper is one of the essential components of the antioxidant enzymes that provide protection against the free radicals especially in cardiovascular diseases and hypercholesterolemia, and oxidative stress disorders might be triggered by imbalance in the copper metabolism. Copper supplementation is recommended for children with severe malnutrition and refractory anemia.

OTHER MICRONUTRIENTS OF CLINICAL RELEVANCE

The functional role and significance of chromium in the control of glucose and lipid metabolism has been well documented. Manganese is an essential nutrient involved in bone formation, carbohydrate, amino acid and cholesterol metabolism and important cofactor for arginase, pyruvate decarboxylase and superoxide dismutase enzymes. Excess amounts can have neurotoxic effects and can lead to psychological disturbances. Deficiency is reported to be associated with epilepsy, Perthes disease and phenylketonuria. Molybdenum is essential for many vital body functions and helps in prevention of buildup of toxins and acts as cofactor for enzymes sulfite oxidase, aldehyde oxidase, and xanthine oxidase.

MACROMINERALS OR MAJOR ELEMENTS

These are needed in larger amounts when compared to trace minerals in order to perform their specific function in body. Calcium is necessary for the proper structure and functioning of bones and teeth, and assists in the muscle function and required for vascular contraction and dilatation and hormonal secretion. Only <1% of total body calcium is needed for supporting critical metabolic functions. The body uses bone tissue as a reservoir for and source of calcium in order to maintain constant calcium concentrations in blood, muscle, and intercellular fluids. Serum calcium concentration is a poor indicator of calcium status because of the complex mechanism regulating the calcium homeostasis. Phosphorous is a major structural component of the bone in the form of calcium phosphate salt, and phospholipids forms major structural components of cell membranes with all energy production and storage depending on phosphorylated compounds. It also helps in the normal acid-base balance and acts as a cofactor for several enzymes, hormones and cell signaling molecules. Sodium is essential for maintaining blood pressure and fluid-electrolyte balance. Chloride helps with maintaining the fluid-electrolyte balance and digestive juice. Potassium is helpful with nerve transmission and muscle function and maintaining fluid balance. Sulfur-containing amino acids helps in the maintenance and integrity of cellular systems by influencing the cellular redox state and the capacity of the cells in detoxification of the toxic compounds, free radicals and reactive oxygen species.

MICRONUTRIENT DEFICIENCY RELATED DISORDERS

Micronutrients and Immunity

It has been well documented that infectious diseases with substantial morbidity and mortality in children occur as consequences of under nutrition including deficiency of micronutrients. Micronutrient deficiencies coexist along with infectious diseases and complex interactions often lead to the vicious cycle of infections and malnutrition especially among preschool children from lower socioeconomic areas living in tropical countries. Children from developing countries and from lower socioeconomic backgrounds with subclinical deficiencies of micronutrients are more at increased risk of infections due to impaired immune function. Accurate assessment of the micronutrient status is difficult especially in disease related to immune dysfunction. The effects of human immunodeficiency virus (HIV) disease among children from lower socioeconomic background in tropical countries are compounded by the widespread presence of micronutrient deficiencies. Multiple micronutrient supplementation may be effective and safe in reducing the burden of tuberculosis and HIV disease.

Micronutrients Deficiency and Infestations

Helminthic infestations could result in reduction of serum levels of multiple micronutrients including iron, copper, selenium, cobalt, and zinc, and there is some evidence that these effects can be reversed by periodic deworming along with micronutrient supplementation like iron and vitamin A, added to complement deworming efforts. Even though the helminth infestation with micronutrient deficiency could be just a mere association, linking the micronutrient supplementation with the deworming program can be justified as the poor children from lower socioeconomic area in tropics are more likely to benefit from both the interventions. A systematic review reported that moderate to heavy hookworm infestations among school-age children were associated with lower hemoglobin levels and iron deficiency anemia. There is need for more research on the helminth species-specific effects related to micro-nutrients and better understanding of the interactions between helminthic infections and micronutrients in order to plan integrated and sustainable strategies in affected children in tropics. Systematic reviews and meta-analysis have reported that iron supplementation did not have any effect on helminth infection and reinfection and no protective effect on infectious illness. Gaining more insight into the interrelations between helminthic infections and micronutrients is essential for designing of adequate public health interventions to improve the health and development of children. Improvement in all anthropometric measurements in children has been reported after anthelminthic treatment in high endemic areas.

Micronutrients Deficiency and Chronic Diseases and Malignancies

A randomized study trial on micronutrient deficiencies in neutropenic children with cancer reported that there was no correlation between the dietary intake and the micronutrient deficiency status and emphasized the need for more research into the prevalence and etiology of micronutrient deficiencies among children with cancer. Selenium levels measured by plasma mass spectroscopy using hair, serum and urine samples reported that the serum and hair levels of selenium were significantly lower among pediatric cancer patients with lymphomas, leukemias and solid tumors when compared to the healthy control group of children, whereas the urine levels of selenium were quite higher. The study concluded that selenium deficiency might be associated with development of pediatric cancer, and that there is need for further additional future studies for determining the role of selenium in cancer pathogenesis. Assessment of growth and nutritional status in cerebral palsy children aged 1–16 years reported that majority of the children had multiple micronutrient deficiencies and recommended correction of these deficiencies especially vitamin D deficiency and anemia along with physical and emotional support for wellbeing of affected children.

Antioxidant Properties and Free Radical Related Disorders

Of special significance is the role of trace elements and other micronutrients in antioxidant defense in various free radical related disorders. Zinc and copper are essential for cytoplasmic superoxide dismutase, manganese for the mitochondrial enzyme, and selenium is part of the prosthetic group of GPx. The micronutrients play a significant role in the antioxidant mechanisms and are essential part of the different enzymatic systems for disposal of the products of oxidation. For example, zinc and copper are essential for cytoplasmic superoxide dismutase, selenium for GPx and manganese for the mitochondrial enzyme activity.

Micronutrients Deficiency in Overweight and Obesity

Two major public health nutritional problems—undernutrition and obesity—among children are arising in tropical countries due to micronutrient deficiencies with cultural factors, shift in socioeconomic status, dietary practices, lifestyle preferences, genetic and environmental factors contributing to this double burden of nutritional transition. The other end of the spectrum of malnutrition includes adverse effects resulting from the excessive intake of micronutrients which carries significant implications for micronutrient intervention programs. Infants and young children are vulnerable and ingestion of micronutrients in excess amounts in a short period or higher intakes over a longer term above the upper limits are more likely to result in increased likelihood of adverse health effects, even though tolerance may develop if the micronutrient intake are at or near to the upper limit. The assessment of total intake of micronutrients needs to consider all the sources of micronutrients such as food and water, fortified and biofortified food and micronutrient supplements.[6] Majority of overweight and obese children are anemic and are deficient in vitamin D, zinc, and so on. Studies have reported reduction in the serum zinc concentrations on obese children and the underlying mechanism could be explained by the role of zinc in metabolism of the hormones involved in the pathophysiology of obesity. Zinc concentration is directly associated with serum leptin concentration, an obesity related hormone associated with satiety through zinc alpha 2 glycoprotein (ZAG). There might be greater risk of developing micronutrient imbalance in obese children especially significantly lower levels of serum zinc, selenium and iron levels, and higher levels of copper, which may play a significant role in the pathogenesis of obesity and related metabolic risk factors.

ASSESSMENT OF MICRONUTRIENT STATUS

Micronutrient status assessment remains a challenge among children when compared to adults due to many complicating factors such a changing metabolic demand, immature organ functions and varied feeding patterns affecting the food intake and depends on a combination of biomarkers. Even though measurement of serum or plasma levels of micronutrients are helpful to some extent, these do not measure the total body storage adequately. It warrants atomic absorption spectrophotometry, which may not be feasible in the tropical countries. Measuring the micronutrient-related enzyme activities could be helpful to some extent for evaluation of the true status of micronutrients in children especially during systemic illnesses. Associated protein deficiency can be a confounding factor in this context.

Identification and early diagnosis and treatment of single micronutrient deficiencies are much easier when compared to that of multiple micronutrient deficiencies. Physiological or biochemical consequences and impaired metabolism can result from progressive depletion of one or more micronutrients and could have detrimental effects. Milder form of micronutrient deficiencies is much more common and quite difficult to recognize and quantify.

MONITORING FOR MICRONUTRIENT DEFICIENCY AND INTERVENTIONS

The health of young children needs to be monitored along with the existing micronutrient programs in order to ensure that they are protected from micronutrient deficiencies as well as from excess amounts and using the indicators set aside by World Health Organization (WHO). Micronutrient supplementation and interventional programs needs to be monitored to assess the impact of these measures on micronutrient disorders in children, which could be helpful for planning regional initiatives and for planning diversification of diets as per local needs at affordable rates and for proposing recommendations. Even though, there is still no clear consensus on the most effective method of improving micronutrient status in children including dietary diversity, fortification and supplementation or on micronutrient intervention in treatment of underlying infections, micronutrient interventions still remain the most cost-effective method to improve global health in tropical countries, especially the low- and middle-income countries.

INTERVENTIONS/MICRONUTRIENT SUPPLEMENTATION

Even though food fortification is one of the best methods of meeting the recommended daily intake of micronutrients and for preventing from getting worse among affected children; foods fortified with micronutrients may not fully meet the needs among nutritionally vulnerable young children nor reach the needy. Micronutrient interventions in the form of supplementation or fortification have been reported to be useful in the improvement of both immediate and long-term health effects of deficiency of micronutrients including reduced prevalence of low birth weight, increased child survival and improved cognitive development. In India, there are national programs or national consensus for three vitamins and three minerals including vitamin A, folate, vitamin D, iron, iodine and zinc. For better understanding of the impact of the micronutrient interventions, there is a need to periodically assess the baseline micronutrient deficiency in children.

PREVENTION OF MICRONUTRIENT RELATED DISORDERS

A national consultative meeting convened by the Infant and Young Child Feeding (IYCF) chapter of the Indian Academy of Pediatrics (IAP) concluded that proper maternal and infant-young child feeding strategies were essential for prevention of micronutrient deficiencies.[7] It was also suggested to follow measures such as encouraging delayed cord clamping for 1 minute, use of germinated foods and dietary diversification and scaling up of micronutrient supplementation in high-risk group of children. One of the best approaches for reducing micronutrient deficiency would be increasing the simultaneous intake of many nutrients, which could be helpful in improving the diet quality. In a systematic review on intervention strategies aiming at improving micronutrient status in children under 5 years of age from lower- or middle-income countries, 4,235 reviews were included and it was concluded that there was a positive effect on single or multiple micronutrient deficiencies in preschool children after supplementation with single or multiple micronutrients.[1] It was also reported that there was increased serum ferritin and hemoglobin levels and also height gain following anthelminthic treatment, reduced risk of anemia with delayed cord clamping in infants up to 6 months of life and improved ferritin with antimalarial treatment in malaria endemic areas. WHO has recommended the use of multiple micronutrient powders (MMPs) containing at least iron, vitamin A and zinc for home fortification of foods as one of the options in order to improve the iron status and also to reduce anemia in infants and children between the age of 6 months and 23 months and also implementing iron provision in conjunction with adequate measures taken for prevention, diagnosis and treatment of malaria. These are single dose packets of powder containing these micronutrients which could be sprinkled onto any semisolid food anywhere in order to increase the content of the essential micronutrients in the diet. Measures such as school health program, nutrition education and micronutrient intervention methods like supplementation and fortification of essential micronutrients are found to be effective along with dietary diversification, improving economic growth and eradicating poverty. A coordinated multi-micronutrient program in order to deal with the coexisting micronutrient deficiencies in children is expected to improve the micronutrient status, rather than a pill for each. A well-balanced diet is also essential to get the added benefits.

ADDRESSING MULTIPLE MICRONUTRIENT DEFICIENCIES

Studies have shown that the coexistence of multiple micronutrient deficiencies were more common than single micronutrient deficiency occurring in isolation in tropical countries emphasizing the need for focusing on several micronutrients and their interactions as part of the screening and treatment process for MDDs in children.[8] In tropical countries, the higher prevalence of concurrent micronutrient deficiencies along with macronutrient deficiencies could also be related to several circumstances, which might lead to multiple micronutrient deficiency, which could be different factors including the dietary diversity and lower socioeconomic status.[9] The density of micronutrients in diets consumed by families, especially children from predominantly rural areas of low-income countries are comparatively low when compared to families from urban areas, where there is access to high quality fortified foods and micronutrient supplements.[10]

CHALLENGES IN MICRONUTRIENT SUPPLEMENTATION IN THE TROPICAL COUNTRIES

Higher prevalence of infectious diseases, malnutrition and helminthic infections among children from lower socioeconomic backgrounds and from tropical and developing countries poses a complex challenge, when targeting micronutrient disorders. Other factors include purchasing power, availability of nutrient rich food, family practices, dietary practices and cultural and traditional practices. There is a need to identify and understand the critical gaps in the knowledge in order to evaluate or test possible affordable interventions and to provide evidence to the decision or policymakers and stake holders and to address this public health problem. Improving the nutritional status of children and ensuring dietary diversity along with micronutrient supplementation through fortification can have a positive impact on the economic growth and development.

CHALLENGES IN TREATMENT OF MICRONUTRIENT MALNUTRITION

Micronutrients deficiencies are difficult to be diagnosed clinically especially in children because of the subclinical nature and existence of multiple micronutrient deficiencies and as they are progressive and cannot be identified until they are in their later stages. The prevalence of micronutrient disorders is quite common in tropical countries, and children under 5 years of age are vulnerable. The coexistence of multiple micronutrient deficiency along with protein and/or energy malnutrition makes it more challenging for early identification and treatment. For example, in malaria-endemic areas, iron supplementation combined with antimalarial treatment is more effective than iron supplementation alone in children with iron deficiency. Similarly, anthelminthic treatment needs to be considered along with micronutrient supplementation for effective and complete treatment. It has also been reported that irrespective of iron supplementation with or without simultaneous zinc supplementation, there was significant decrease in the levels of serum zinc. Zinc is considered as an opponent of iron and copper. Even though, the risk of anemia was significantly reduced, with iron supplementation in exclusively breastfed infants, there was no significant increase in the serum ferritin levels. *Helicobacter pylori* infection is yet another factor for less effectiveness of iron supplementation in the tropics. The presence of antinutrients and phytates are yet other factors, similar to caffeine in coffee and tannin in tea that hinder iron absorption. Polyphenols present in amla (Indian gooseberry) is now identified to be an antinutrient to iron, despite the presence of lot of vitamin C that is thought to be beneficial in iron absorption.

Even though, it is possible to reverse MDDs, some deficiency disorders could result in irreversible and long-term consequences, which in turn might be influenced by the severity and extent of the deficiency. Mild-to-moderate iron deficiency anemia is identified to put a negative signature on the cognitive abilities of a growing young child. Diagnosis and assessment of micronutrient deficiency and excess in children poses a challenge due to diverse dietary practices and feeding methods, changes influenced by systemic infections or inflammation, varying grades of deficiency and nonavailability of accessible standardized tools for assessment.

FUTURE STRATEGIES AND POLICIES

There seems to be no clear consensus on the most effective methods of improving micronutrient status, even though micronutrient deficiency remains a major public health problem among children in tropical countries. There is need for further research and data on micronutrient deficiencies and related disorders in tropical countries. Future research needs to consider further development of improved biomarkers and their application in early identification of micronutrient disorders. This could be helpful for guidance toward intervention programs in tropical countries. Interventions for micronutrient deficiencies and anemia in school-aged children need to consider the local needs for effective micronutrient supplementation and fortification programs. Multiple micronutrient disorders, that are preventable, are much more common than the single micronutrient deficiency and the consequences in longer term have deleterious impacts on the economic development and human capital at the country level.

There needs to be more investment into the technical expertise for assessment of micronutrient status among children in tropical countries as part of the prevention and treatment programs and biomarkers for micronutrient status specific for metabolic and antioxidant activities and single or combined micronutrient intervention strategies for supplementation, fortification, public health nutritional interventions, and dietary strategies. It is essential to understand the epidemiology in order to plan the intervention strategies for prevention and treatment of micronutrient disorders. The extent of global burden of micronutrient disorders could only be assessed by understanding more about the influence of inflammation and infections on biomarkers of nutritional status and interpretation of clinical, functional and biochemical indicators.

More research is needed in future on genetic and epigenetic mechanisms underlying micronutrient status in malnutrition and infectious diseases among children from tropical areas. Assessment of micronutrient intervention programs and using information from systematic reviews and meta-analysis on micronutrient intervention programs and recommendations based on evidence could be useful for implementation of effective micronutrient intervention programs which in turn would be helpful in achieving the goal of prevention of micronutrient malnutrition globally. Evidence-based approaches are essential for prevention at global level taking into consideration the epidemiology for planning intervention strategies under different conditions.

CONCLUSION

Micronutrient malnutrition and multiple deficiencies of varying grades are major public health problems in the tropics. However, there are no uniform standardized tools for assessment or optimum strategies for effective prevention and treatment. The extent and complexity of the problem in relation to tropical infections, infestations, and diseases pose further challenges. Further research into prevalence, long-term consequences of micronutrient deficiencies in children and their underlying mechanisms in relation to childhood disorders is essential and critical knowledge gaps need to be considered when formulating recommendations on micronutrient supplementation in children. Modified and affordable interventions along with evidence-based measures need to be reported to decision and policy makers for addressing this key public health problem among children in tropical countries. Micronutrient supplementation programs needs to be modified and targeted based on local needs and treating the underlying causes as well. The higher prevalence of malnutrition and infectious diseases among children in tropical countries poses a complex challenge in targeting specific treatment for specific and multiple micronutrient deficiencies. However, behavioral change communication with respect to dietary diversity, micronutrient supplementation, and food fortification are helpful.

REFERENCES

1. Campos Ponce M, Polman K, Roos N. What approaches are most effective at addressing micronutrient deficiency in children 0–5 years? A review of systematic reviews. Matern Child Health J. 2018;23(Suppl 1):4-17.
2. Bailey RL, West KP Jr, Black RE. The epidemiology of global micronutrient deficiencies. Ann Nutr Metab. 2015;66(Suppl 2):22-33.
3. Bellows AL, Smith ER, Muhihi A, et al. Micronutrient Deficiencies among Breastfeeding infants in Tanzania. Nutrients. 2017;9(11). pii: E1258.
4. Camaschella C. New insights into iron deficiency and iron deficiency anemia. Blood Rev. 2017;31(4):225-33.
5. Dao DT, Anez-Bustillos L, Cho BS, et al. Assessment of micronutrient status in critically ill children: challenges and opportunities. Nutrients. 2017;9(11). pii: E1185.
6. Pike V, Zlotkin S. Excess micronutrient intake: defining toxic effects and upper limits in vulnerable populations. Ann N Y Acad Sci. 2019;1446 (1):21-43.
7. Bharadva K, Mishra S, Tiwari S, et al. Prevention of Micronutrient Deficiencies in Young Children: Consensus Statement from Infant and Young Child Feeding Chapter of Indian Academy of Pediatrics. Indian Pediatr. 2019;56(7):577-86.
8. Abeywickrama IIM, Koyama Y, Uchiyama M, et al. Micronutrient Status in Sri Lanka: A Review. Nutrients. 2018; 10(11). pii: E1583.
9. Chowdhury MH, Shill LC, Purba NH, et al. Adverse Effect of micronutrient deficiencies on children's development: The Wasting Syndrome. Food Nutr Current Res. 2019;2(1):136-47.
10. Biesalski HK, Jana T. Micronutrients in the life cycle: Requirements and sufficient supply. NFSJ. 2018;11:1-11.

Obesity in the Tropics

M Singaravelu, AR Karthick

INTRODUCTION

Overweight and obesity are defined as abnormal or excessive fat accumulation that presents a risk to health. Obesity has been labeled as childhood epidemic. The problem has risen to alarming levels with one in 10 children being overweight and India has the second highest number of obese children in the world after China.[1] According to the World Health Organization (WHO) estimate, the number of overweight children under age of 5 years is around 41 million and nearly half of them are in Asia. If this trend continues, globally there will be 70 million overweight or obese infants and young children by 2025.[2] Obesity is now linked with more deaths than underweight. Comorbidities associated with obesity has increased over the years and it is imperative that healthcare providers identify them and provide treatment at the earliest in order to prevent both medical and psychological complications of obesity. Therefore, there should be high priority set for preventing childhood obesity.

DEFINITIONS

The term "obesity" refers to an excess of fat. It is difficult to measure body fat directly in daily practice. The relationship between weight and height gives a good estimate of body fat which is now advocated for clinical purposes. Body mass index (BMI) gives a good correlation between weight and height defined as weight (in kilograms) divided by height (in meters) squared. This estimate holds good for children more than 2 years of age. Other measures of childhood obesity include weight for height (for children less than 2 years) and regional fat estimate (waist circumference, waist-to-hip ratio). Level of body fat changes during childhood with infants having higher adipose tissue which gradually decreases till about 5–6 years. This period is called "adiposity rebound" when body fat is typically at its lowest level.[3] Fat tissues then gradually increase until early adulthood. Child is said to be overweight when the BMI is between 85th percentiles and 95th percentiles and obese when BMI is ≥95th percentile. The WHO recommends using WHO growth charts for identifying children with overweight and obesity. It is prudent to use WHO growth charts for children less than 5 years of age and the Indian Academy of Pediatrics (IAP) growth chart after the age of 5 years.

ETIOLOGY AND PATHOGENESIS

Obesity results from imbalance between energy intake and expenditure. Inappropriate dietary preferences and sedentary lifestyle promote positive energy balance resulting in obesity. Individual's genetic background is also an important determinant of obesity. The first 2 years of age is increasingly recognized as modifiable period related to risk for childhood obesity.[4] High gestational weight gain, higher birth weight, and maternal smoking are associated with increased risk. Breastfeeding is protective and children who are breastfed for longer durations have significantly lower risk of becoming obese. Many factors like appetite, nutritional intake, physical activity, energy expenditure and genetically predisposed body habitus determine individual's risk for becoming obese. According to the Avon Longitudinal study, the odds of children aged 7 years becoming obese if father, mother or both had obesity were 2.93, 4.66, and 11.75, respectively.[5] This clearly shows that parental obesity has a dominant influence over childhood obesity.

Neuroendocrinology of Energy Metabolism

Complex neuroendocrine interactions exist which influence individual's food intake and energy expenditure. The major hormone in this mechanism is leptin, an exclusive product of adipose tissue which acts centrally in hypothalamus. During fasting and weight loss states, leptin and insulin are found in low concentrations. This promotes increase in food intake and decrease in energy expenditure by stimulating neuropeptide Y synthesis and by inhibiting sympathetic activity and other catabolic pathways. After feeding and during weight gain, increased levels of leptin and insulin decreases food intake and increases energy expenditure through melanocortin and corticotropin-releasing hormones. Orexins A and B from hypothalamus and ghrelin from stomach are other major peptides that stimulate feeding.[1,3]

Numerous social and environmental factors influence food habits and physical activity which are the key determinants of childhood obesity. India is sailing the same boat when it comes to fast food consumption. Recent decade witnessed impressive economic growth and resulted in steadily increasing income. Emerging fast food culture with ease of access, ready availability, taste and marketing strategies, makes children consume larger portion sizes and increased snacking between meals. Reduced sleep time has significantly contributed to development of obesity. Children have started sleeping less due to increased time in watching television, studying and in general due to faster pace of life. Studies have found out that decreased sleep is associated with decreased leptin levels and increased ghrelin levels with tendency for increased appetite.[1,5]

Lack of Physical Activity

Many factors have played their role in making our kids lack physical activity. Overindulgence in indoor leisure activities and entertainment like television and computer games with increasing pressure to perform in academics and lack of open spaces and playgrounds in communities have contributed much to childhood obesity. Fear of child predators and nonavailability of safe walking routes is forcing parents to use vehicles for transportation instead of using bicycle and walking as modes of transportation.[6]

Excess Caloric Intake

Increased intake of energy-dense, high calorie foods/snacks that are high in fat and sugar but low in proteins, vitamins and minerals has largely contributed to the obesity epidemic. Overweight is also prevalent among adolescents who regularly eat out and among those who replaced snacks for meals. Nutrient-poor sugar-sweetened beverages are often consumed along salty and high-fat food choices. Past decade has witnessed increase in portion size and consumption of large portions with frequent snacking has contributed to energy imbalance resulting in weight gain and obesity.[7]

Lifestyle-related Factors

Daily allowance to purchase lunch, easy availability of maids to take care of household chores, use of bus or car for commuting instead of walking or bicycling and aggressive advertising campaigns by fast-food chains and beverages have all contributed to obesity in children.[5,6]

Sociocultural Factors and Urbanization

False traditional beliefs about health and nutrition, forced feeding by parents and lack of knowledge about nutrition also contributed to obesity. Using food as a reward, as a part of socializing, and as a means to control others have encouraged the development of unhealthy relationship with food. Due to population expansion and illegal settlements, open grounds and parks have dwindled.[5,6]

Genetics

Body mass index is 25–40% heritable. However, genetic factors account for less than 5% of cases of childhood obesity. Some children tend to have melanocortin-4 receptor (MC4R) mutations which results in food-seeking behavior and early onset obesity. There is some evidence that appetite traits are heritable and some genes modulating appetite also relate to weight. Fat mass and obesity-associated (FTO) gene polymorphism results in dysregulation of orexigenic hormone, ghrelin, and results in poor postprandial appetite suppression. There are also recent studies in Indian children indicating association of *AMD1* gene variant with obesity and plasma leptin levels.[8] Leptin deficiency and mutations in leptin receptors have also been identified to cause human obesity.

Syndromes and Obesity

In an obese child with dysmorphic features, presence of characteristic syndromes like Down syndrome, Prader–Willi syndrome, Bardet–Biedl syndrome, etc. must be looked for and evaluated. These children tend to be short and obese in contrast to children with exogenous obesity who are either with normal or tall stature. Adipose tissue functions as an active endocrine organ and it metabolizes sex steroids, which in turn plays a role in fat distribution. Hence hypogonadal states like Turner, Klinefelter syndromes cause increased fat deposits.

Drugs and Medical Causes

Rapid weight gain can occur in children taking glucocorticoids, valproate, carbamazepine and certain antipsychotics. This may need dose modification or discontinuation of the drug. If the child has poor linear growth and rapidly gaining weight, an underlying medical cause should be ruled out.

OBESITY ASSOCIATED COMORBIDITIES

There is growing evidence of many comorbidities associated with pediatric obesity **(Fig. 1)** and these persist into adulthood. Results from Harvard Growth Study reveal that overweight adolescence boys were twice likely to die from cardiovascular disease compared to their peers with normal weight. Though such studies are lacking from Indian population, considerable risk also exists for Indian children. As fatty tissue increases, insulin resistance increases and affects both cardiovascular health and lipid metabolism. Nonalcoholic fatty liver disease is common in asymptomatic obese Indian children and can present with nonalcoholic steatohepatitis or advanced fibrosis.[9] Obesity also negatively affects school performance creating low self-esteem. Some of the major comorbidities associated with obesity are tabulated in **Table 1**. Adiponectin is a peptide with anti-inflammatory property and it is reduced in obese children. Adipocytes secrete proinflammatory peptides like interleukin 6 (IL-6) and tumor necrosis factor α (TNF α) and in turn cause subclinical inflammation leading to cardiovascular diseases.[3]

CLINICAL EVALUATION

Clinical evaluation begins with identification of children with obesity and overweight during routine checkups and during immunization visits. The following are performed step-by-step while evaluating a child with overweight and obesity **(Fig. 2)**.

- Examination of growth chart for weight, height, and BMI trajectories
- Detailed analysis of nutritional, family eating and activity patterns
- Complete pediatric history to look for associated comorbidities
- Family history of obesity and obesity-associated disorders
- Physical examination and laboratory diagnosis to identify comorbidities.

Table 1: Comorbidities associated with obesity.

Disease	Symptoms/clinical data
Cardiovascular	
Dyslipidemia	HDL <40, LDL >130, total cholesterol >200 mg/dL
Hypertension	Systolic BP >95% for sex, age, height
Endocrine	
Type 2 diabetes mellitus	Polyuria, polydipsia, acanthosis nigricans
Metabolic syndrome	Central adiposity, insulin resistance, dyslipidemia, hypertension, glucose intolerance
Polycystic ovary syndrome	Acne, hirsutism, irregular menstrual period, insulin resistance
Gastrointestinal	
Nonalcoholic fatty liver disease	Hepatomegaly, increased transaminases
Gallbladder disease	Abdominal pain, vomiting, jaundice
Orthopedic	
Blount disease (tibia vara)	Severe bowing of tibia, knee pain, limp
Slipped capital femoral epiphysis	Hip pain, knee pain, limp
Neurological and psychological problems	
Migraines	Headaches, hemicrania
Behavioral complications	Low self-esteem, anxiety, depression
Pulmonary	
Asthma	Wheezing and shortness of breath
Obstructive sleep apnea	Snoring, apnea, restless sleep

(HDL: high-density lipoprotein; LDL: low-density lipoprotein)

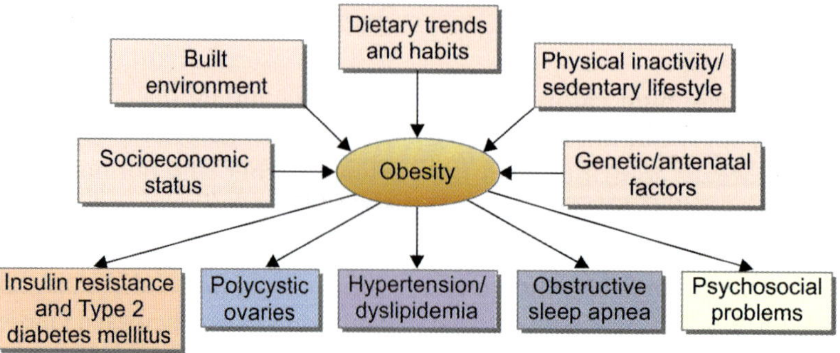

Fig. 1: Causes and consequences of obesity in children.

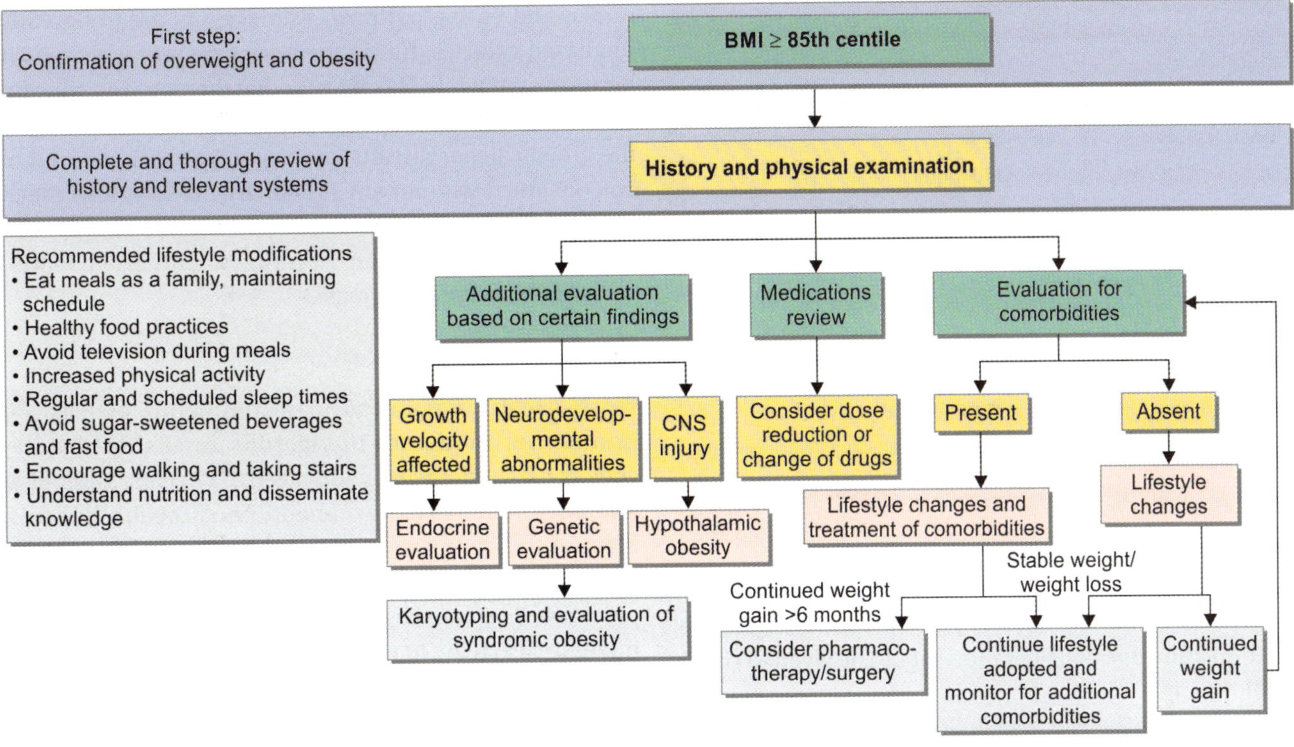

Fig. 2: Approach to obesity in children.
(BMI: body mass index; CNS: central nervous system)

It is prudent to maintain growth charts during periodic health visits so that timely identification of overweight and obesity can be made. Growth charts help in identifying the timing of onset, duration, and severity of obesity. Children with BMI ≥99th percentile are more likely to have comorbidities and they must be examined carefully. There exists "sensitive periods" during childhood wherein there is increased risk of developing obesity.[3] Careful monitoring of growth is mandatory during infancy, adiposity rebound, and adolescent period. A child consuming excess of calories will exhibit higher weight and height centile. However, at some point, weight centile exceeds height centile and child's BMI comes in overweight or obese range. Tracing of height trajectory is helpful in identifying children with endocrine problems. These children exhibit slowing of linear growth with increasing weight centiles. Growth hormone deficiency, hypothyroidism and Cushing's syndrome are some of the endocrine causes of childhood obesity. Genetic disorders must be suspected in children with hyperphagia, facial dysmorphism, cognitive impairment, vision and hearing abnormalities. Children taking antipsychotic medication or antiepileptics like sodium valproate can have excessive appetite leading to overweight and obesity.

Assessment of calorie intake can be done using 24-hour dietary recall method with special attention to intake of water, fruits, vegetables, and consumption of fast foods and sugar-sweetened beverages. This initial information will be useful to make changes in eating behavior during intervention. Assessment of physical and recreational activities including screen time helps getting an insight into family's activity pattern and the necessary changes can be planned during treatment.[10] Comorbidities associated with obesity should be looked for during physical examination and complete review of all bodily systems should be done.

LABORATORY EVALUATION

It is recommended to evaluate fasting plasma glucose, triglycerides, low-density lipoprotein (LDL), high-density lipoprotein (HDL), cholesterol, and liver functions during initial evaluation of children with obesity. Overweight children with family history of diabetes or with signs of insulin resistance should have fasting plasma glucose evaluated. Reference of normal values can be seen in **Table 2**.

MANAGEMENT

Treatment of overweight and obese children requires multidisciplinary approach with a holistic outlook.

Table 2: Normal laboratory values for recommended tests.

Laboratory test	Normal value
Glucose	<110 mg/dL
HbA1C	<5.7%
LDL	<110 mg/dL
HDL	>45 mg/dL
Total cholesterol	<170 mg/dL
Triglycerides	<75 mg/dL (0–9 years group) <90 mg/dL (10–19 years group)
AST	<58 U/L (2–8 years) <46 U/L (9–15 years) <35 U/L (15–18 years)
ALT	<35 U/L

(ALT: alanine transaminase; AST: aspartate transaminase; HbA1C: glycosylated hemoglobin; HDL: high-density lipoprotein; LDL: low-density lipoprotein)

Family-based interventions have produced most successful outcomes and due consideration should be given to child's developmental age. The immediate goal in management is to reduce rate of weight gain, followed by period of weight maintenance and finally achieving weight reduction to improve BMI percentile. In long-term, the intention is to improve quality of life and to reduce morbidity as well as mortality associated with complications of obesity.

Targets for Obesity Treatment

There are no clear targets defined for treating children less than 2 years who have overweight or obesity. Weight maintenance is all that is required in 2–5 years age group children with overweight and obesity. In 6–11 years age group, weight maintenance is adequate for overweight children whereas for obese children in the same age group, weight maintenance or minimal weight loss of 0.5 kg/month may be attempted. However, if the child's BMI is more than 99th percentile, weight loss up to 1 kg/ week may be allowed. Weight maintenance is sufficient for overweight adolescent in age group of 12–18 years. For obese adolescents of the same age group, weight loss up to 1 kg/week may be attempted.[11,12]

Diet Therapy

Availability of and repeated exposure to healthy food forms the ultimate background for developing preferences and can overcome dislike of foods. The practice of family meals should be encouraged and structured mealtimes promote consumption of healthy foods. Unless family members involve in planning diet change, it will be difficult for a child to make any changes in nutritional intake and eating patterns. Adolescents require greatly increased calories during their growth spurt which must be addressed while planning for diet therapy. The concept of "traffic light" diet groups is popular wherein those in the green category (fruits and vegetables) are allowed to be consumed without any limitations, yellow (lean meat, dairy, starches, and grains) in moderation and red (fatty meats, sugar-sweetened beverages, and fried foods) reserved for infrequent treats.[13]

Physical Activity

World Health Organization recommends at least 60 minutes of moderate-to-vigorous intensity physical activity for children and youth aged 5–17 years. Additional amounts of activity provide additional health benefits. Most of the daily activities should be aerobic. Vigorous intensity activities should be incorporated at least 3 times per week. For inactive children and youth, a progressive increase in activity to eventually achieve the target shown above is recommended. It is appropriate to start with smaller amounts of physical activity and gradually increase duration, frequency and intensity over time. It should also be noted that if children are currently doing no physical activity, doing amounts below the recommended levels will bring more benefits than doing none at all.[13]

Behavior Modification and Social Support

Television viewing is often associated with eating and many fast-food products are marketed directly to children. Families should be assisted to develop goals to change nutritional intake and physical activity. They should be provided with necessary information and counseled about gradual rate of BMI percentiles and not to expect immediate lowering of BMI centiles on initiating behavioral changes. Behavioral changes linked with improving BMI percentiles include consumption of high-quality diets, increasing exercise, avoidance of sugar-sweetened beverages, decreased screen time, and weight monitoring.

Treatment of Comorbidities

Children may have associated problems like hypertension, impaired glucose tolerance, polycystic ovarian syndrome, skin problems, and sleep apnea which need to be addressed while planning for intervention.

Medications

Drugs for promoting weight loss in children are understudied and only sparse data is available. They have a role only as an add-on after initial management with diet, exercise, and behavioral changes have failed. The efficacy of medications even with combined behavioral interventions has resulted in modest weight loss. They are used only in severely obese adolescents. Orlistat is a lipase inhibitor and it decreases absorption of fat up to 30%, resulting in modest weight loss. It is approved for use in adolescents ≥12 years. However, it produces abdominal cramps, oily stools, flatulence, spotting, and deficiency of fat-soluble vitamins like A and D.[12]

Surgery

Bariatric surgery can be considered only in adolescents with complete or near-complete skeletal maturity and very severe obesity (BMI of ≥40) with medical complication from obesity, after having no results with 6 months of multidisciplinary weight management program. Roux-en-Y and adjustable gastric bands are the preferred surgical approaches. Nutritional complications like malabsorption, vitamin and mineral deficiencies must be taken care of after surgical intervention.[12]

■ PREVENTION

In 2016, WHO has developed a set of recommendations to successfully tackle childhood obesity which is brought forward as commission on ending childhood obesity.[13]

Promote Intake of Healthy Food

Simple nutrient labeling such as traffic light labels or health star ratings is not sufficient. Health and nutrition literacy should be included in the educational program. It is also necessary to have context-specific food-based dietary guidelines for both children and adults. Such information should reach all segments of the society so that healthier choices can be made. Taxation influences purchasing behavior and it is recommended to implement an effective tax on sugar-sweetened beverages and other unhealthy foods and it requires development of nutrient profiles. Implementing restrictions on marketing of foods and beverages helps reduce exposure of children and adolescents to the power of marketing of unhealthy foods.[14]

Promote Physical Activity

Nearly 81% of adolescents do not achieve the recommended 60 minutes of physical activity each day.[15] Children and adolescents, their parents, caregivers, teachers, and health professionals must be encouraged on knowing what constitutes healthy body size, physical activity, sleep behaviors, and appropriate use of screen-based entertainment. Schools and public spaces must be equipped with adequate facilities for physical activity during recreational time.

Preconception and Pregnancy Care

Maternal overweight or obesity and excess pregnancy weight gain increases the likelihood of obesity during infancy and childhood. The care that a woman receives before, during and after pregnancy has profound implications for later health and development of her child. Evidence indicates that health of fathers at the time of conception can also influence the risk of obesity in their children. So, healthy lifestyle guidance is necessary for both would-be fathers and mothers. Hyperglycemia and gestational hypertension should be screened for and managed appropriately. Young people are often uninformed of what constitutes a healthy diet. There is a need to develop clear guidance and support with additional focus on appropriate nutrition for the promotion of healthy diets and physical activity for the prospective mothers and fathers before conception and during pregnancy.

Early Childhood Diet and Physical Activity

Six months of exclusive breastfeeding followed by introduction of appropriate complementary foods significantly reduce the risk of obesity. Government should ensure all maternal facilities practice 10 steps to successful breastfeeding. Family's belief and perceptions of eating and ideal body weight are significant impetus to follow certain complementary feeding practices. Providing them with clear guidance and support encourages the consumption of wide variety of healthy foods and avoidance of specific categories of foods (sugar-sweetened milk, fruit juices or energy-dense nutrient poor foods) during initiation of complementary feeding. Physical inactivity is a leading contributor to overweight and obesity and WHO has recently published guidelines on physical activity, sedentary behavior, and sleep for children under 5 years of age.[16] It is summarized below:

Infants should:
- Be physically active several times a day through interactive floor-based play and includes at least 30 minutes in prone position
- Not be restrained for more than 1 hour at a time (e.g. prams and strollers)
- Screen time is not recommended
- Have 14–17 hours (0–3 months of age) or 12–16 hours (4–11 months of age) of good quality sleep including naps

Children 1–2 years of age should:

- Spend at least 180 minutes in variety of physical activities, including moderate-to-vigorous physical activity throughout the day.
- Not be restrained for more than 1 hour at a time. Screen time is not recommended for 1-year-olds. For children more than 2 years, sedentary screen time should be no more than an hour. Children should be engaged in reading and storytelling by caregiver when sedentary.
- Have 11–14 hours of good quality sleep including naps with regular sleep and wake-up times.

Children 3–4 years of age should:

- Spend at least 180 minutes in variety of physical activities, including moderate-to-vigorous physical activity throughout the day, more being better.
- Not be restrained for more than 1 hour at a time. Sedentary screen time should be no more than 1 hour; less is better.
- Have 10–13 hours of good quality sleep including naps with regular sleep and wake-up times.

Metabolic equivalent of task (MET) is a physiological measure used for connoting energy cost of physical activities. One MET is the energy equivalent spent by an individual while seated at rest. Moderate physical activity is equivalent to 4–7 METs or 4–7 times the energy expenditure at rest for that child and vigorous physical activity is equivalent to more than 7 METs.

Health, Nutrition and Physical Activity for School-age Children

Programs to improve nutrition and physical activities in children can be successful by integration of activities into a health promoting school initiative. The interventions need to be integrated into the school day and curriculum. It is an absurdity to encourage and educate children on healthy behaviors while allowing sale of inappropriate foods and beverages in school environment. It is prudent to eliminate provision of unhealthy foods and establish standards for meals provided in schools that meet healthy nutrition guidelines. Schools and sports facilities must also ensure access to potable water. Inclusion of nutrition and health education within core curriculum in schools improves the nutritional literacy. Schools can make food preparation classes available to children, their parents and caregivers. Regular participation in quality physical education improves child's attention span, enhances their cognitive control and processing, reduces symptoms of depression and improves psychosocial outcomes. Schools should include it in their curriculum and provide adequate staffing and facilities to support this.

Weight Management

Regular growth monitoring at school or primary healthcare facility gives an opportunity to identify children at risk of overweight and obesity. As a part of universal health coverage, government should develop and support appropriate weight management services for children and adolescents who are overweight or obese. It must be family-based, multicomponent (including nutrition, physical activity, and psychosocial support) and delivered by multi-professional teams with appropriate training and resources.

India should also formulate a national policy and partner with the private sector to end the childhood obesity epidemic. It is necessary to create a database for childhood obesity and initiate community-based research to document the burden of obesity at state and national level.

■ SUMMARY

There is an urgent need for the society to focus on the causes of childhood obesity and the methods to tackle them. In developing countries like India, we need to have practical and cost-effective community-based strategies with strong policy changes in order to curb the escalating epidemic of childhood obesity. Improving physical activity, reducing sedentary time, and ensuring quality sleep in young children will improve their physical health, mental health and wellbeing, and help prevent childhood obesity and associated diseases later in life.

■ REFERENCES

1. Ranjani H, Pradeepa R, Mehreen TS, et al. Determinants, consequences and prevention of childhood overweight and obesity: an Indian context. Indian J Endocrinol Metab. 2014;18(Suppl 1):S17-25.
2. WHO | Facts and figures on childhood obesity [Internet]. WHO. [cited 2019 Jul 31]. Available from: http://www.who.int/end-childhood-obesity/facts/en/
3. Kliegman RM, Geme J St. Nelson Textbook of Pediatrics, 21st edition. Vol. 2. Elsevier; 2019.
4. Ranjani H, Mehreen TS, Pradeepa R, et al. Epidemiology of childhood overweight and obesity in India: a systematic review. Indian J Med Res. 2016;143(2):160-74.
5. Parthasarthy LS, Phadke N, Chiplonkar S, et al. Association of fat mass and obesity-associated gene variant with lifestyle factors and body fat in Indian children. Indian J Endocrinol Metab. 2017;21(2):297.

6. Sahoo K, Sahoo B, Choudhury AK, et al. Childhood obesity: causes and consequences. J Family Med Prim Care. 2015;4(2):187-92.

7. Keshari P, Mishra CP. Growing menace of fast food consumption in India: time to act. Int J Community Med Public Health. 2017;3(6):1355-62.

8. Tabassum R, Jaiswal A, Chauhan G, et al. Genetic Variant of AMD1 is Associated with Obesity in Urban Indian Children. PLoS One [Internet]. 2012 Apr 9 [cited 2019 Aug 4];7(4). Available from: https://www.ncbi.nlm.nih.gov/pmc/articles/PMC3322123/

9. Pawar SV, Zanwar VG, Choksey AS, et al. Most overweight and obese Indian children have nonalcoholic fatty liver disease. Ann Hepatol. 2016;15(6):853-61.

10. Spear BA, Barlow SE, Ervin C, et al. Recommendations for treatment of child and adolescent overweight and obesity. Pediatrics. 2007;120(Suppl 4):S254-88.

11. Styne DM, Arslanian SA, Connor EL, et al. Pediatric Obesity—Assessment, Treatment, and Prevention: An Endocrine Society Clinical Practice Guideline. None. 2017;102(3):709-57.

12. August GP, Caprio S, Fennoy I, et al. Prevention and Treatment of Pediatric Obesity: An Endocrine Society Clinical Practice Guideline Based on Expert Opinion. J Clin Endocrinol Metab. 2008;93(12):4576-99.

13. WHO. Commission on Ending Childhood Obesity [Internet]. WHO. [cited 2019 Aug 3]. Available from: http://www.who.int/end-childhood-obesity/en/

14. Kar SS, Kar SS. Prevention of childhood obesity in India: way forward. J Nat Sci Biol Med. 2015;6(1):12-7.

15. Raj M. Obesity and cardiovascular risk in children and adolescents. Indian J Endocrinol Metab. 2012;16(1):13.

16. NCDs. Information sheet: global recommendations on physical activity for health 5-17 years old [Internet]. WHO. [cited 2019 Jul 31]. Available from: http://www.who.int/ncds/prevention/physical-activity/recommendations5_17years/en/

Neonatal Mortality and Morbidity in Tropics

Shashi Kant Dhir

INTRODUCTION

The first 28 days of life starting from the birth are referred to as neonatal period. It is further divided into early neonatal period including less than 7 days and late neonatal period between 7 days of life and 28 days of life. The age distribution of the mortality of children shows that the highest risk of death is during the neonatal period. Various indicators are used in describing the mortality parameters in children **(Table 1)**.

Despite the substantial progress in neonatal care over last quarter century, in 2018, 6,850 neonates died daily, majority of them occurring in low-income and low and middle income countries (LMICs). The ratio of the neonates to children dying postneonatal age to less than 5 years is 0.89:1, which is a matter of huge concern.[1] The importance of strategies to decrease neonatal deaths was recognized by global agencies and "A Promise Renewed"[2] and "Every Newborn Action Plan" initiatives were launched by the United Nations and the World Health Organization, respectively.[3] The targets of decreasing neonatal mortality rate (NMR) to 12 by 2030, set by these initiatives to decrease the neonatal and under-five mortality by working on preventable causes of death, were embedded in the Sustainable Development Goals (SDGs).[4] This chapter delineates the magnitude, trend, and causes leading to neonatal deaths along with description of common neonatal morbidities at global and national levels and way forward to address them.

MAGNITUDE OF NEONATAL MORTALITY

Global Estimates

The United Nations Inter-agency Group for Child Mortality Estimation (UN IGME) is an agency for estimating the NMR globally by reconciling the differences across data sources, for taking into account the systematic biases associated with the various types of data for 195 countries since 2011, and for producing trend estimates from 1990 to 2018. As per the 2018 estimates from UN IGME, globally 5.3 million under-5 children died accounting for 85% of all children deaths; out of these, 2.5 million (47%) were less

Table 1: Mortality parameters in children.	
Indicator	**Definition**
Neonatal mortality rate (NMR)	Number of deaths among all live births during the first 28 days of life expressed per 1,000 live births
Early neonatal mortality rate (ENMR)	Number of neonatal deaths <7 days of life expressed per 1,000 live births
Late neonatal mortality rate (LNMR)	Number of neonatal deaths between 7 days and 28 days of life expressed per 1,000 live births
Infant mortality rate	Number of infant deaths between birth and 1 year of age expressed per 1,000 live births
Under-five child mortality rate	Number of infant deaths between birth and 5 years of age expressed per 1,000 live births
Stillbirth	Death of a fetus weighing at least 500 g (or if birth weight unavailable, after 22 completed weeks of gestation or crown heel length of 25 cm or more) before the complete expulsion from its mother
Perinatal mortality rate (PMR)	Number of deaths of fetuses weighing at least 500 g (or if birth weight unavailable, after 22 completed weeks of gestation or crown heel length of 25 cm or more) plus the number of early neonatal deaths per 1,000 total births

than 1 month of age.[1] **Figure 1** depicts global mortality rates and number of deaths by age categories over the years 1990–2018.

Estimates from Tropical Countries

The tropical countries contribute substantially to the global burden of neonatal mortality because of high birth rate, socioeconomic and demographic factors. India, Pakistan, and Nigeria are top three among tropical countries in neonatal mortality rates. Sub-Saharan Africa had the highest neonatal mortality rate in 2018 at 28 deaths per 1,000 live births, followed by Central and Southern Asia with 25 deaths per 1,000 live births. The NMR in 1990 and 2018 of few of the tropical countries are depicted in **Table 2**. The complete list can be viewed at UN IGME website.[5]

Estimates from India

As per the estimates from 2018, India had the maximum absolute number of neonatal deaths in the world. Although there has been a trend of decrease in the neonatal deaths from 1.58 million in 1990 to 0.55 million in 2018, a reduction of 60%; yet there is a long way to match the global NMR. As per the sample registration survey report 2017, the neonatal mortality rate in India is 23, ranging from 5 in Kerala to 33 in Madhya Pradesh.[6] The various indicators related to perinatal and neonatal mortality are being shown in **Table 3**. The percentage of neonatal deaths to total infant deaths is 70.7% at the national level. The state-wise neonatal mortality status and the ratio of neonatal death to infant death in 2017 are depicted in **Figure 2**.

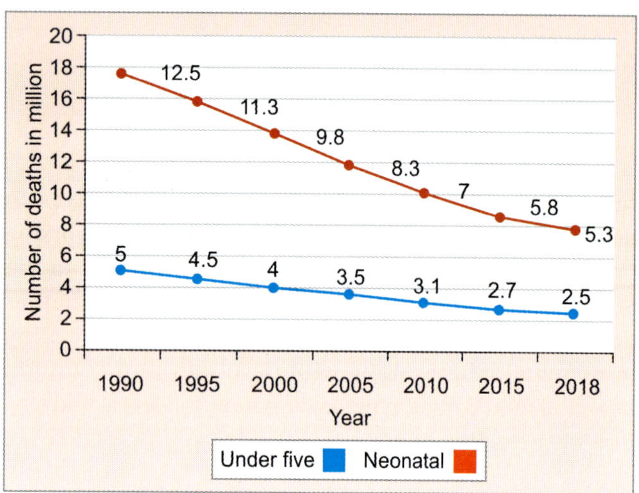

Fig. 1: Global number of deaths in children over 1990–2018. *Source:* United Nations Inter-agency Group for Child Mortality Estimation. (2019). Levels and trends of child mortality Report 2019. [online] Available from: https://www.unicef.org/media/60561/file/UN-IGME-child-mortality-report-2019.pdf. [Last accessed on December, 2019].

◼ CAUSES OF NEONATAL MORTALITY

Global

According to a recent global estimate of causes of neonatal deaths, prematurity-related complications (32%),

Table 2: Neonatal mortality estimates in tropical countries.*

Country	NMR 1990	NMR 2018	Percentage decline	Country	NMR 1990	NMR 2018	Percentage decline	Country	NMR 1990	NMR 2018	Percentage decline
Angola	54	28	48	Djibouti	50	32	36	Madagascar	39	21	46
Benin	46	31	33	Equatorial Guinea	48	30	38	Malawi	50	22	56
Brazil	25	8	68	Ethiopia	59	28	53	Mauritania	46	33	28
Burkina Faso	46	25	46	Gambia	49	26	47	Niger	54	25	54
Burundi	40	22	45	Guinea	62	31	50	Nigeria	50	36	28
Cameroon	40	27	33	Guinea-Bissau	64	37	42	Pakistan	65	42	35
Central African Republic	52	41	21	Haiti	39	26	33	Sierra Leone	53	33	38
Chad	52	34	35	India	57	23	60	Somalia	45	38	16
Comoros	50	32	36	Kenya	28	20	29	Sudan	43	29	33
Côte d'Ivoire	49	34	31	Liberia	59	24	59	Togo	43	25	42

(NMR: neonatal mortality rate)

*The list is not complete. Please refer to UN IGME website for latest complete and updated list.[5]

Source: United Nations Inter-agency Group for Child Mortality Estimation. (2019). Levels and trends of child mortality Report 2019. [online] Available from https://www.unicef.org/media/60561/file/UN-IGME-child-mortality-report-2019.pdf. [Last accessed on December, 2019].

intrapartum-related events (birth asphyxia; 22%), and sepsis/pneumonia (20%) accounted for most neonatal deaths.[1] Previous large global estimates have also depicted that major causes have remained same over many decades.

India and Tropical Countries

In LMICs, preterm-related sepsis and intrapartum events constitute the most common cause of mortality, whereas in high-income countries, preterm birth and congenital malformations are the most common causes of neonatal mortality. In a study done on around 7 lakh neonatal deaths in India, the leading causes were preterm birth complications (44.0%), intrapartum-related events (19.1%), and neonatal sepsis or meningitis (13.7%).[7] The Million Death Study showing trends of neonatal mortality causes over 16 years recently reported that in India, neonatal deaths from prematurity have been showing an increasing trend over the last 16 years, whereas deaths due to sepsis and birth asphyxia are decreasing in India.[8] **Figures 3 and 4** show the breakup of causes of neonatal mortality in world and India, respectively.

Perinatal Mortality and Stillbirth Rate

The perinatal mortality rate in India has been estimated to be 23 and ranges from 26 in rural areas to 15 in urban areas. The estimate of stillbirth rate for the year 2017, at the National level, was 5. The highest level of stillbirth rate was in Chhattisgarh (13 per 1,000 live births) and the lowest in Jammu & Kashmir, Jharkhand, and Telangana (1 per 1,000 live births).[6] The reporting of perinatal rate and stillbirth does have issues of underreporting as most of these may occur at home also and never get reported, and this may be the cause of gross difference between the Indian and the global estimates. Stillbirths are extremely difficult to capture and there is a big scope for better capturing of the data.

Table 3: Neonatal and perinatal mortality in India.

Indicators (per 1,000 live birth)	Total	Rural	Urban
Neonatal mortality rate	23	27	14
• Early neonatal mortality rate	18	21	10
• Late neonatal mortality rate	5	6	3
Stillbirth rate	5	5	4
Perinatal mortality rate (per 1,000 total birth)	23	26	15

Source: SRS 2017[6]

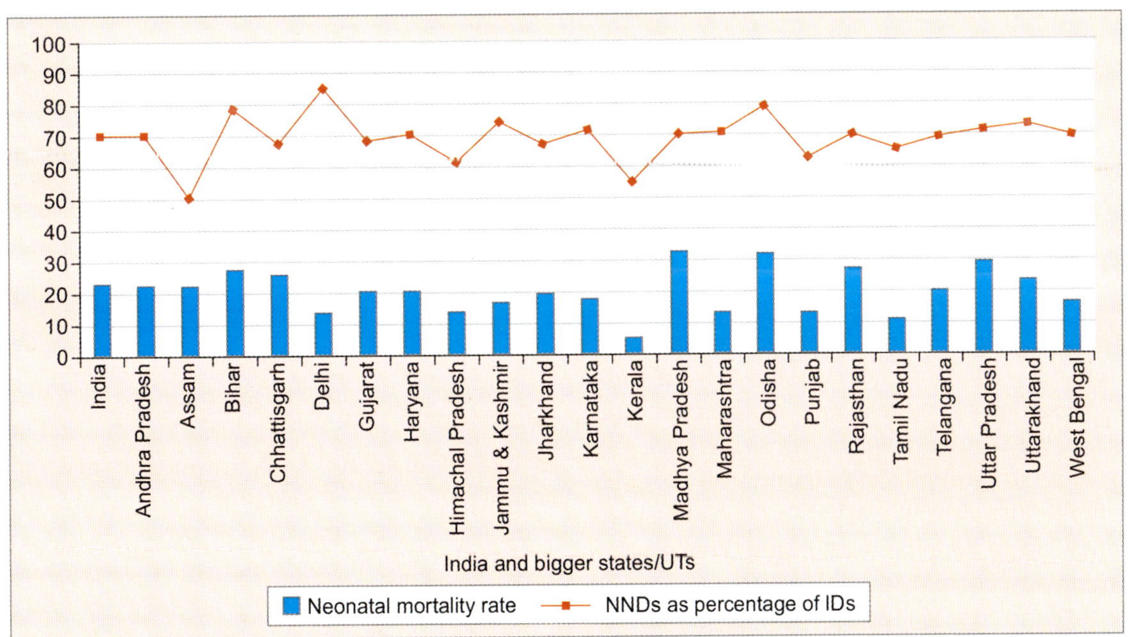

Fig. 2: Neonatal mortality rate and percentage share of neonatal deaths to infant deaths, in India and bigger states, 2017. (NND: neonatal death; ID: infant death)

Source: Ministry of Home Affairs, Government of India. Census of India: SRS Statistical Report 2017. [online] Available from: http://www.censusindia.gov.in/vital_statistics/SRS_Reports_2017.html. [Last accessed on December, 2019].

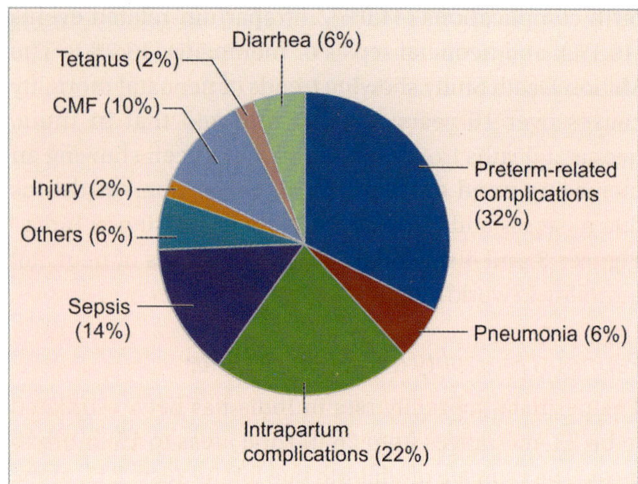

Fig. 3: Causes of neonatal deaths in world.
(CMF: congenital malformations)
Source: Population Division, Department of Economic and Social Affairs, United Nations Levels and Trends in Child Mortality Report 2018. [online] Available from: https://www.un.org/en/development/desa/population/publications/mortality/child-mortality-report-2018.asp. [Last accessed on December, 2019].

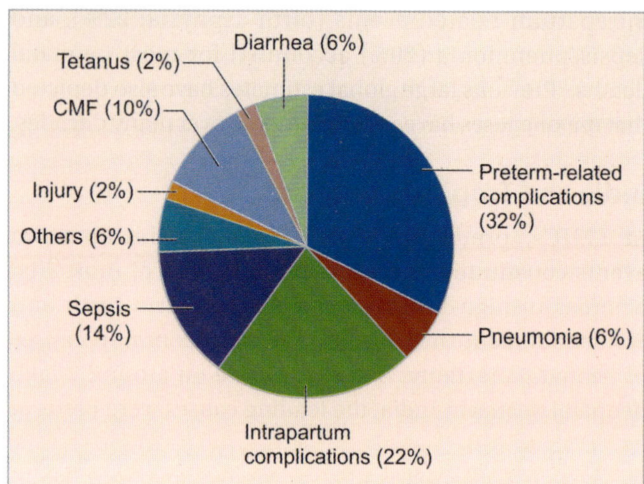

Fig. 4: Causes of neonatal deaths in India.
(CMF: congenital malformations)
Source: Ministry of Home Affairs, Government of India. Census of India: SRS Statistical Report 2017. [online] Available from: http://www.censusindia.gov.in/vital_statistics/SRS_Reports_2017.html. [Last accessed on December, 2019].

Timing of Neonatal Deaths

Seventy five percent of all neonatal mortality occurs in the early neonatal period. The first 72 hours are most crucial and roughly half of the neonates die during this period. The birth asphyxia-related deaths usually occur within the first 3 days and prematurity-related deaths occur within the 1st week. Sepsis is an important cause of mortality at all ages and is the most common cause of death in late neonatal period.[9]

Neonatal Morbidities

Neonatal morbidities do affect the long-term outcomes for the children and morbidity-free condition determines the intact survival of the children. They vary from region to region across the globe as they depend not only upon the weight and gestation of the neonate but also upon other factors such as socioeconomic status of the country, family education and background, and quantum of available care. The morbidities also differ in babies depending upon whether they are in hospital or at home. Prematurity-related morbidities, low birth weight (LBW), and infections are among the most commonly seen neonatal morbidities. **Table 4** shows the common morbidities seen in the neonatal period.

Low Birth Weight

Low birth weight is defined as birth weight less than 2,500 g at birth and is a composite measure of fetal growth and

Table 4: Morbidities commonly seen in neonates.

Healthcare facility based	*Community based*
Preterm birth	Preterm birth
Low birth weight	Breastfeeding issues
Birth asphyxia	Low birth weight
Neonatal jaundice	Hypothermia
Sepsis	Birth asphyxia
Hypoxic-ischemic encephalopathy	Neonatal jaundice
Respiratory distress syndrome	Sepsis
Seizures	Congenital malformations
Hypoglycemia	Conjunctivitis
Cardiac malformations	Diarrhea

gestational length. It is an important predictor of adverse short-term as well as long-term health outcomes. LBW includes both appropriately grown preterm neonates (<37 completed weeks of gestation), and term and preterm growth-restricted neonates (<10th centile of weight for gestational age and sex) and can be used as a surrogate marker in settings where accurate gestational age assessment is not possible. About 60% of LBW neonates are born at term after fetal growth restriction while rest are born due to prematurity. LBW babies born because of preterm delivery also have complications leading to death and long-term morbidities in children younger than 5 years of age. According to Born Too Soon: The Global Action Report on Preterm Birth, 80% preterm were born in south

Asia and sub-Saharan Africa with India at the top of the list of 10 nations contributing 60% of the world's premature deliveries.[10] A recent systematic analysis of estimate of LBW revealed some progress in reducing LBW between 2000 and 2015 (17.5% vs 14.6%); still majority (91%) of the whole LBW prevalence is from LMICs, mainly southern Asia (48%) and sub-Saharan Africa (24%). Hence, the average annual reduction rate (AARR) of 2.74% required between 2012 and 2025 to achieve SDG will require more than doubling the existing progress, more in LMICs.[11]

Community-based studies indicate that the short-term outcomes in LBW infants include 11–13 times increased risk of dying, higher risk of asphyxia, sepsis, and hypothermia. LBW newborns have a higher risk of morbidity at a later age like stunting in childhood, lower intelligent quotient, long-term neurodevelopmental disability, and physical ill health. There are more chances of adult-onset chronic conditions such as cardiovascular disease, obesity, and diabetes mellitus due to epigenetic modifications.[9]

Neonatal Sepsis and Other Infections

Neonatal sepsis may manifest as septicemia alone or in form of pneumonia, meningitis, or osteomyelitis. The incidence ranges from 30 to 170 versus 1 to 3 per 1,000 live births in developing versus developed countries of the world. South Asia and sub-Saharan Africa have the highest burden of neonatal sepsis in the world.[9] The pooled incidence of culture-positive sepsis in hospital-based reports from South Asia is 15.8 per 1,000 live births,[12] and about 50–70% of the common Gram-negative isolates are now multidrug resistant.[12] The high incidence of sepsis may be due to poor hand hygiene and suboptimal infection control practices. In India, DeNIS study, a multicenter prospective cohort study from LMICs, was conducted with 13,500 enrolled neonates with high degree of methodological rigor in contrast to passive surveillance in previous studies. In this study, the incidence of total sepsis was 14.3% and of culture-positive sepsis, two-third isolates were Gram-negative bacteria such as *Acinetobacter* spp, *Klebsiella* spp, and *Escherichia coli*. Nearly two thirds of the total episodes occurred in ≤72 hours of life which was a sharp contrast to high-income countries where late-onset sepsis is predominant. The pathogens in early-onset sepsis did not differ from that of late-onset sepsis, and high rates of multidrug resistance were observed in most of the isolates.[13] The presence of sepsis in the neonates predisposes them to other comorbid conditions leading to increased hospital admissions, neurodevelopmental disabilities, financial implications for the family as well as community, and even late neonatal mortality.

Birth Asphyxia

Impaired blood flow and gas exchange *in utero* can trigger a cascade of neuronal injury, leading to neonatal encephalopathy and resultant long-term damage. Majority of infants recover quickly and have completely normal survival; a subset may be affected with evolving clinical encephalopathy termed hypoxic-ischemic encephalopathy. The outcome in children with perinatal asphyxia without clinical encephalopathy may not be completely normal and it may be associated with abnormal motor, sensory, cognitive, and behavioral outcomes in the child.

Hypoglycemia

Hypoglycemia is a preventable cause of developmental delay and is a common morbidity present in neonates. It leads to typical topographical distribution of brain injury at posterior limb of internal capsule, occipital lobe, basal ganglia, thalamus leading to significant long-term neurodevelopmental disorders. The number of days with moderate hypoglycemia has been found to be strongly related to lesser mental and motor developmental scores at a corrected age of 18 months, even after statistical adjustments for a wide range of factors known to influence development. It is found to be associated with a dose-dependent increased risk of poor executive function and visual motor function, even if asymptomatic, and may thus influence later learning.

Neonatal Jaundice

As many as 60% of otherwise healthy, newborns develop some degree of elevated bilirubin levels yet most of them do not have any sequelae. Acute bilirubin encephalopathy sometimes may be transient and reversible, but chronic bilirubin encephalopathy with resultant permanent neuronal damage is known to occur in neonates having high bilirubin levels, especially if other risk factors such as sepsis, acidosis, or blood group incompatibility are coexistent.

Hypothermia

Hypothermia defined as body temperature <36.5°C is associated with increased rates of preventable morbidity, including increased risk of neonatal infections, coagulation defects, acidosis, delayed fetal-to-newborn circulatory adjustment, hyaline membrane disease, and brain hemorrhage. Hypothermia can be prevented by simple

Table 5: Predicted scenario-based global NMR (per 1,000 live births).

Scenario	Global NMR in 2017	Predicted NMR in 2030
No change from NMR in 2017	18	19.0
Continuing annual rate of reduction in NMRs between 2000 and 2017	18	13.2
NMR same as country in that region showing best trend over 2000–2017	18	10.0
All countries achieving SDG target	18	8.8

(NMR: neonatal mortality rate; SDG: sustainable developmental goal)
Adapted from: Hug L, Alexander M, You D, et al. National, regional, and global levels and trends in neonatal mortality between 1990 and 2017, with scenario-based projections to 2030: a systematic analysis. Lancet Glob Health. 2019;7(6):e710-20.

Table 6: Highly effective Interventions having potentials to decrease neonatal mortality rate.

Preconceptional	Antenatal	Intrapartum	Postnatal
Folic acid supplementation	• Tetanus toxoid immunization • Syphilis screening and treatment • Pre-eclampsia and eclampsia: Prevention (calcium supplementation) • Intermittent presumptive treatment for malaria • Detection and treatment of asymptomatic bacteriuria	• Antibiotics for preterm premature rupture of membranes • Corticosteroids for preterm • Detection and management of breech (cesarean section) • Labor surveillance (including partograph) for early diagnosis of complications • Clean delivery practices	• Resuscitation of newborn baby • Breastfeeding • Prevention and management of hypothermia • Kangaroo mother care • Community-based pneumonia case management

Adapted from: Darmstadt GL, Bhutta ZA, Cousens S, et al. Evidence-based, cost-effective interventions: how many newborn babies can we save? Lancet Lond Engl. 2005;365(9463):977-88.

measures such as ensuring a warm environment during delivery; early breastfeeding and skin-to-skin contact with the mother; proper bathing, drying, and swaddling; and prompt identification and rewarming of hypothermic neonates.

CONCLUSION

The neonatal mortality continues to be very high and despite the formulation of SDGs, the progression to decrease it has been very slow. Hug et al. on basis of the systematic analysis of the global trends of all the countries have predicted the likely NMR based upon various scenarios **(Table 5)**.[14] It would be virtually impossible to attain the SDGs, if the causes of neonatal mortality and ways to prevent them are not looked into with newer and efficacious insights. The majority of the deaths occurs in the early neonatal period; therefore, cost-effective, easy, culturally acceptable, and efficacious interventions within these first 7 days of birth must be researched as they have the potential to significantly decrease the total number of deaths.

The 16 interventions suggested by Lancet Neonatal Survival Series two decades ago **(Table 6)** having potential to reduce perinatal or neonatal mortality and providing intact survival, especially in low-income and middle-income countries, still hold true and a universal coverage of these interventions could avert a significant number of preventable neonatal deaths worldwide, a way forward to achieve SDGs for the developing countries.[15] Strengthening and utilization of the existing healthcare services with special focus on community, communication, transportation, and identification of obstacles at the facility level would probably help further in curbing the neonatal mortality.

REFERENCES

1. United Nations Inter-agency Group for Child Mortality Estimation. (2019). Levels and trends of child mortality Report 2019. [online] Available from: https://www.unicef.org/media/60561/file/UN-IGME-child-mortality-report-2019.pdf. [Last accessed on December, 2019].
2. Ki-moon B. Global strategy for women's and children's health; 2010. [online] Available from: https://www.who.int/pmnch/knowledge/publications/fulldocument_globalstrategy/en/. [Last accessed on December, 2019].
3. World Health Organization. Every Newborn Action Plan; 2014. [online] Available from: https://www.healthynewbornnetwork.org/hnn-content/uploads/Every_Newborn_Action_Plan-ENGLISH_updated_July2014.pdf. [Last accessed on December, 2019].
4. Sustainable Development Knowledge Platform. Sustainable Development Goals. [online] Available from: https://sustainabledevelopment.un.org/?menu=1300. [Last accessed on December, 2019].

5. Population Division, Department of Economic and Social Affairs, United Nations. Levels and Trends in Child Mortality Report 2018. [online] Available from: https://www.un.org/en/development/desa/population/publications/mortality/child-mortality-report-2018.asp. [Last accessed on December, 2019].

6. Ministry of Home Affairs, Government of India. Census of India: SRS Statistical Report 2017. [online] Available from: http://www.censusindia.gov.in/vital_statistics/SRS_Reports_2017.html. [Last accessed on December, 2019].

7. Liu L, Oza S, Hogan D, et al. Global, regional, and national causes of under-5 mortality in 2000-15: an updated systematic analysis with implications for the Sustainable Development Goals. Lancet Lond Engl. 2016;388(10063):3027-35.

8. Million Death Study Collaborators. Changes in cause-specific neonatal and 1-59-month child mortality in India from 2000 to 2015: a nationally representative survey. Lancet Lond Engl. 2017;390(10106):1972-80.

9. Sankar MJ, Neogi SB, Sharma J, et al. State of newborn health in India. J Perinatol. 2016;36(Suppl 3):S3-8.

10. World Health Organization. Born Too Soon: The Global Action Report on Preterm Birth; 2012. [online] Available from: https://www.who.int/pmnch/media/news/2012/201204_borntoosoon-report.pdf. [Last accessed on December, 2019].

11. Blencowe H, Krasevec J, Onis M de, et al. National, regional, and worldwide estimates of low birthweight in 2015, with trends from 2000: a systematic analysis. Lancet Glob Health. 2019;7(7):e849-60.

12. Chaurasia S, Sivanandan S, Agarwal R, et al. Neonatal sepsis in South Asia: huge burden and spiralling antimicrobial resistance. BMJ. 2019;364:k5314.

13. Investigators of the Delhi Neonatal Infection Study (DeNIS) collaboration. Characterisation and antimicrobial resistance of sepsis pathogens in neonates born in tertiary care centres in Delhi, India: a cohort study. Lancet Glob Health. 2016;4(10):e752-60.

14. Hug L, Alexander M, You D, et al. National, regional, and global levels and trends in neonatal mortality between 1990 and 2017, with scenario-based projections to 2030: a systematic analysis. Lancet Glob Health. 2019;7(6):e710-20.

15. Darmstadt GL, Bhutta ZA, Cousens S, et al. Evidence-based, cost-effective interventions: how many newborn babies can we save? Lancet Lond Engl. 2005;365(9463):977-88.

Essential Issues in Neonatal Care in Tropics

Rahul Kadam, BD Bhatia

INTRODUCTION

Tropics are the region of the earth surrounding equator which usually has hot and humid conditions and two seasons, namely dry and wet season. Sub-Saharan Africa and Southern Asia are the major tropics. India is one of the tropical countries. There are many health-related issues which are classical of tropical region both in adults and in pediatric population.

Neonate is defined as an infant less than 4 weeks old. Tropics account for 52% of all live births worldwide and whooping 78% of all neonatal deaths worldwide, with almost 50% of these deaths happening at home. About 50% of the neonatal mortality is in the first 24 hours of life whereas only 25% of the neonatal deaths happen after the first week of life.[1,2] Globally, severe infections (36%) are the major cause of neonatal deaths followed by prematurity related issues (29%) and birth asphyxia (23%).[3] Many issues are encountered while taking care of these vulnerable groups; few of them such as hypothermia, birth asphyxia, sepsis, hyperbilirubinemia, hypernatremia, neonatal transport, and intrauterine growth restriction (IUGR) are essential particularly in tropical countries.

NEONATAL HYPOTHERMIA

Neonatal hypothermia is progressive reduction in body temperature below 36.5°C. The mechanisms of heat loss in a newly born include conduction, convection, evaporation, and radiation.[4] World Health Organization (WHO) has categorized hypothermia into three stages: (1) mild hypothermia (36.0–36.4°C), (2) moderate hypothermia (32.0–35.9°C), and (3) severe hypothermia (<32.0°C).

In tropics, hypothermia is still a major concern and has so far been a neglected challenge.[4,5] In many communities still, the practices leading to heat loss in the newborn are prevalent and are difficult to change.[6,7] Hypothermia prevention technologies are at a developmental stage.[8] The healthcare providers and parents lack the awareness of the problem. They either do not or insufficiently practice the simple interventions which protect a newborn from hypothermia. Hypothermia and its adverse consequences contribute to the neonatal morbidity and mortality.

Maintenance of a normal body temperature is critical for newborn survival and is performed by hypothalamus through shivering and nonshivering thermogenesis.[9] However, in neonates, these mechanisms are compromised leading to metabolic derangements and mortality either directly because of hypothermia or indirectly from associated morbidities such as sepsis,[10] hypoglycemia, or hemorrhage.

Immature thermal regulation, low birth weight (LBW), prematurity, IUGR, and birth asphyxia are significantly associated with hypothermia.[11,12] Hypoglycemia also contributes to hypothermia. Early bathing is a common practice in tropics[13] and can lead to significant heat loss and hypothermia.[14] The infants born to a mother from low socioeconomic strata, young and inexperienced mother, or a multipara mother can have low body temperature.[11]

In any setting, an important therapeutic principle during and after resuscitation is prevention or treatment of hypothermia.[15,16] The delivery room temperature should be set at 26°C and above.[17] At birth, baby should be received in a warm towel, dried, and covered with a prewarmed towel/blanket. The emphasis should be on skin-to-skin contact [kangaroo mother care (KMC)] and baby should be kept with the mother (bedding in). Bath should not be given for first 6 hours of life, and possibly should be postponed longer, till the discharge from the hospital.

In preterm infants, the combination of strategies such as warm delivery room, radiant warmer, thermal mattress,[18] warmed humidified respiratory gases,[19] plastic/polythene wrap, and a cap should be used to maintain normal temperature during transition.

Treatment of hypothermia is rewarming. However, current evidence is insufficient to support either rapid ($\geq$0.5°C/hr) or slow rewarming (<0.5°C/hr). Either approach is reasonable. Once euthermia is achieved, all further resuscitation procedures should be carried out with temperature-controlling interventions in place. The goal should be to achieve and maintain normothermia and avoid iatrogenic hyperthermia.

Breastfeeding is therapeutic in hypothermia. It replenishes newborn's glucose levels, thus provides energy for thermogenesis. It also provides warmth through the contact with mother.

■ NEONATAL SEPSIS

In tropics, neonatal sepsis is a major contributor of neonatal mortality.[3] In tropics, the impact of neonatal infections on neonatal deaths may be even higher as most of the cases are not even registered and they die at home due to lack of a surveillance system.[20]

The factors responsible for higher prevalence of neonatal sepsis in tropics are high rates of home births, poverty, shortages of medical personnel, and poor environmental conditions.[21]

The organisms causing neonatal sepsis are acquired either before or during delivery from the mother's blood, skin or vaginal tract,[21] whereas the nosocomial and environmental pathogens can lead to neonatal infections, after the delivery.

In tropics, the classification of sepsis as an early and late onset based upon the causative organisms is difficult. Unclean delivery practices can lead to early nosocomial sepsis (within 72 hours of birth) in hospital settings,[22] whereas community-acquired pathogens can lead to late-onset sepsis in neonates who are born at the household.[23] Predominant organisms in both community and hospital settings are Gram-negative; the most common pathogens are *Klebsiella* and *Escherichia coli.*[24,25]

Often clinical picture of sepsis is similar to other common neonatal problems and neonatal mortality due to sepsis can be significantly reduced by training community healthcare workers to recognize and promptly refer to the hospital the neonates with any of the following clinical signs:[26,27] axillary temperature >37.5°C or <35.5°C, poor feeding, abnormal movements or movement only when stimulated, fast breathing (respiratory rate >60/min) or severe chest indrawing.

The access to laboratory tests for diagnosis of sepsis is limited in developing countries.[28] Complete blood-cell count (CBC) varies at different gestations and even with day of life.[29] Despite its association with infection, CBC findings have low sensitivities.[30,31] The gold standard for the diagnosis of neonatal sepsis is blood culture. However, the yield depends upon the amount of blood inoculated, the degree of bacteremia, and previous use of antibiotics.[29] The newer molecular diagnosis methods for the identification of pathogens such as real-time polymerase chain reaction are promising.[32] However, they are not freely available at most of the health facilities in tropics.

The utility of lumbar puncture is controversial and the practice guidelines vary between centers.[33] Lumbar puncture should be deferred in asymptomatic newborn evaluated for early-onset sepsis. It should be performed for every symptomatic newborn and all neonates with bacteremia.

Antibiotic therapy should be started empirically in neonates with risk factors for early-onset sepsis or clinical features suggestive of sepsis.[34] The combination of ampicillin and aminoglycoside should be the initial choice as the reported antibiotic resistance to them has remained at less than 10% in the past decade.[35,36]

The empiric antifungal therapy[37] should be initiated for those with risk factors for candida sepsis such as exposure to broad-spectrum antibiotics, thrombocytopenia, and extreme prematurity.

It is safe to stop antibiotics by 48 hours for stable neonates with negative blood culture.[34] A 7–10-day antibiotic course is enough in neonates with culture-positive sepsis, who are >32 weeks gestational age, >1,500 g birth weight, and have non-*Staphylococcus aureus* infection.[34] Neonates with culture-positive sepsis, who are <32 weeks of gestation, less than 1,500 g birth weight, and have *S. aureus* bacteremia, should receive a 14-day antibiotic course.

For early-onset meningitis, ampicillin in combination with either cefotaxime or an aminoglycoside should be used,[38] whereas in late-onset meningitis, combination of third-generation cephalosporin and vancomycin is recommended.[34] The recommended duration of antimicrobial therapy for Gram-positive meningitis is 14 days and for Gram-negative meningitis is 21 days.[38] Newborns with *Listeria monocytogenes* meningitis and complicated meningitis warrant prolonged course of antimicrobial therapy.[34,38] Neuroimaging is mandatory in all cases of meningitis, to rule out complications.

In tropics, few parents refuse hospitalization or beds might be unavailable in hospitals.[39] In such cases, mortality can be significantly reduced by administration of antibiotics at home.[26,27] The broad-spectrum antibiotics which can be easily administered once a day include gentamicin, procaine penicillin, and ceftriaxone.[40]

In developing countries, there has been a significant increase in antibiotic resistance to both community- and hospital-acquired infections.[22,41] Due to inappropriate use of higher antibiotics, many neonatal units harbor resistant pathogens.[42] Prolonged use of antibiotics increases the risk of necrotizing enterocolitis, late-onset sepsis, fungal sepsis, and death.[43,44]

Neonatal sepsis can be reduced significantly by following clean practices during and after delivery.[45] The application of substances such as clove oil and surma[46] and mustard seed oil[47] and cow dung on umbilical stump is still a prevalent practice in the tropics which can lead to serious infections such as tetanus and other infections. Cutting the umbilical cord by bamboo piece or crushing it with stone is a traditional practice in some tropics. The 6 Cs advocated by WHO should be practiced at every birth, namely clean hands of the birth attendant, clean delivery surface, clean perineum, clean blade to cut the cord, clean cord tie, and clean clothes to wrap the baby and mother. Chlorhexidine has been effective in reducing the neonatal sepsis in tropics when used for vaginal washes during delivery, for cleaning umbilical stump, or for skin antisepsis.[48]

Exclusive breastfeeding reduces neonatal infections[49] by virtue of anti-inflammatory, anti-infective, and immunoregulatory factors transmitted to the baby through milk.

Hand washing is the single most effective measure to reduce cross infections and has shown to reduce bacteremia in very low birth weight (VLBW) babies by 60%.[50,51] After hand wash, one should not touch any fomites till the necessary task is over.

The other effective strategies to reduce neonatal sepsis include, avoiding overcrowding in neonatal intensive care units (NICUs), adequate number of nurses, use of plenty of disposables, minimal handling policy, strict asepsis during procedures and while handling intravenous lines, antibiotic stewardship program, and regular microbiological surveillance in the unit.

◼ NEONATAL TRANSPORT

In the first week of life, 1 in 10 babies requires admission to a neonatal unit.[52] Although in utero transport is the "gold standard", it is sometimes unavoidable for neonates to be born in facilities that may be incapable of adequately supporting them. As a result, ex utero transfer remains a reality.

Neonatal transport is a challenge in tropics because of several reasons which include scarce and inaccessible facilities, lack of organized transport systems, road networks are poor or nonexistent, long distance road transports, communication systems are not developed, ill-equipped healthcare facilities, families have inadequate financial or other resources, and virtually no healthcare provider accompanying the neonate en route. Most neonates are transported without any stabilization. Any available vehicle is used, and the receiving hospital is not defined and contacted prior to transport.

Many smaller centers with inadequate facilities attempt to provide level III care which leads to deficiencies in the quality or consistency of care. Often, these neonates are transferred by less experienced staff from one center to another[53] and the risk of adverse events on these transports is significantly higher compared to the transport with trained and well-equipped staff.[54] The babies transported with inadequate facilities en route are often received at the tertiary centers cold, blue, and hypoglycemic, with cardiorespiratory compromise, and close to 75% of them have serious clinical implications in ultimate outcome. One of the iatrogenic factors contributing to the neonatal mortality is poor transportation.

A specialized retrieval team can deliver intensive care to neonates who are critically ill and transport them to a NICU with minimal morbidity and mortality related to the transfer. A capable neonatal transport system rapidly delivers an advanced neonatal intensive care at the patient's bedside at the referring hospital and is capable of maintaining the almost level of care en route to the receiving hospital.

The key components of a neonatal transport system are human resources, modes of transportation, appropriate equipment, communication, and family support.

The success of transport system depends upon the selection and training of the team members. Team member should have the necessary medical skills and should be able to deal sensitively with colleagues, parents, and personnel at the referring and receiving hospital. This pool includes fellows/registrars trained in level III care, respiratory therapists, nurses, and emergency medical technicians. For neonates with complex problems, a neonatologist should be a team leader.

A family member or a paramedic can be the accompanying person, in resource-limited settings or for community transports. They should be trained in identification of danger signs and their immediate possible treatment, and also in routine care during transport.

The neonatal transport ambulance should at least fulfill the requirements for a basic life support ambulance.

The principles of neonatal transport include[55] assessment, pretransport stabilization, and care en route. At the referring hospital, assess the baby and check for temperature, airway, breathing, circulation, and sugar.

The temperature of the infant on arrival at the accepting institution is a measure of the effectiveness of thermal support and medical care before and during transport. Ideally, use a transport incubator. In case of unavailability of the transport incubator, as in resource-limited settings, KMC is a good method of maintaining a neonate's temperature.[56] Thermocol boxes have been used for neonatal transport in resource poor settings and are found effective. Plastic/polythene wraps or transwarmer mattresses reduce hypothermia by keeping newborns warmer.[57]

If airway is unstable, the neonate should be intubated before commencing transport. The aim should be to avoid or prevent hypoxemia as well as hyperoxemia. If a baby requires a minimal oxygen, then supplement it through the nasal prongs with a flow rate of less than 2 L/min. However, if there is moderate to severe respiratory distress with increasing oxygen requirements, continuous positive airway pressure (CPAP) or mechanical ventilation may be considered. Assess perfusion at regular intervals by capillary refill time (CRFT). Continue maintenance intravenous fluids as per protocol. Initiate and titrate inotropes as per need. Hypoglycemia if any should be corrected.

Inform the referral unit to arrange the bassinet ahead of arrival, and to keep the overhead radiant warmer on and to arrange mode of respiratory support necessary for the baby. The newborn's condition prior to the transport, vitals monitoring en route, and the details of treatment provided before and during transport should be meticulously documented and handed over to the treating team.

The parents of the sick newborn are usually under tremendous stress. The transport team leader should counsel them emphatically about baby's general condition, provisional diagnosis, treatment options, approximate hospitalization duration, overall prognosis, and the finances involved.

■ BIRTH ASPHYXIA

Birth asphyxia is defined by WHO as "failure to initiate or sustain breathing at birth," which accounts for approximately one quarter of the neonatal deaths globally. Amongst survivors, it can lead to cognitive impairment, cerebral palsy, and seizures in later life.[1] India contributes to 27% of global neonatal deaths[58] and birth asphyxia accounts for 26.8% neonatal deaths in India.

In tropics, still a lot of births occur at home and are conducted by untrained birth attendants. At birth, neonatal resuscitation is often not initiated, or inadequate or wrong methods are used. To prevent asphyxia, high-risk cases should be transferred in utero to a higher center where facilities and expertise for adequate neonatal resuscitation are available. Neonatal resuscitation is a simple, inexpensive, and cost-effective key skill which will significantly reduce the deaths related to birth asphyxia. At birth, around 10% of the newborns need some assistance for transition, and 1% of them require some extensive resuscitation measures making neonatal resuscitation a frequently performed medical intervention.[59]

Every birth is a potential emergency and at least one person should attend it, whose only responsibility should be to take care of the newborn. He/she should be capable of performing the initial steps of resuscitation and can administer at least positive pressure ventilation, if required.

The presence of perinatal risk factors enhances the need for resuscitation, wherein additional personnel who is capable of performing endotracheal intubation, chest compressions, and umbilical vein catheter insertion should be immediately available.

The major organs such as brain, kidneys, lungs, gut, and liver suffer a hypoxic ischemic injury as a consequence of perinatal asphyxia. Hypoxic ischemic encephalopathy (HIE) refers to the clinical manifestations of brain injury and the survivors may have long-term neuromotor sequelae. Birth asphyxia is the earliest multiorgan dysfunction syndrome in the life and can lead to a spectrum of clinical manifestations ranging from seizures, encephalopathy, shock, persistent pulmonary hypertension (PPHN), respiratory distress, pulmonary hemorrhage, acute kidney injury, feed intolerance, disseminated intravascular coagulation, and metabolic derangements.

A baby who requires a resuscitation at birth should be transferred to a facility where close monitoring for a hypoxic injury and anticipatory treatment is possible. The crux of the treatment after asphyxia is the prevention of ongoing brain injury through a supportive care in the first 48 hours. Constant monitoring and the reassessment at periodic intervals are the key for better outcome. Oxygenation and perfusion should be assessed and supported accordingly.

All our attempts are to attenuate, prevent, and treat the effects of the secondary neuronal injury which sets in within 6 hours of birth. The neonates with features of stage II–III HIE should reach higher center with the facility of therapeutic hypothermia within 6 hours of birth. Therapeutic hypothermia reduces risk of death and morbidity in stage II and stage III HIE by 32% and 18%, respectively.

■ HYPERNATREMIC DEHYDRATION

Hypernatremia, defined as a serum sodium level of more than 145 mEq/L, is a frequently encountered electrolyte disorder. Severe hypernatremia refers to serum sodium level of >160 mEq/L. Hypernatremic dehydration depicts a deficit in body water in relation to total body sodium.[60]

One should suspect a hypernatremic dehydration in a neonate if there are clinical signs suggestive of dehydration or if there is more than 10% of weight loss in the first week of life.[61,62] Neonatal hypernatremic dehydration can lead to serious central nervous system consequences such as intracranial hemorrhage, thrombosis, or even a death.[63] With early diagnosis and timely management of this condition, devastating consequences can be avoided.

Neonates are worst affected due to immaturity of their kidney which hinders the excretion of excess sodium. They are dependent on caretakers for provision of appropriate and adequate fluids and feeds as they cannot express the thirst and cannot feed themselves.[64] The etiology of hypernatremic dehydration is multifactorial such as pure water loss as in diabetes insipidus, loss of hypotonic fluid as in vomiting or diarrhea, or an excess sodium consumption through improperly prepared hypertonic infant formula. At birth, breast milk sodium content is higher and it rapidly declines over subsequent days. Inadequate mother–infant bonding leads to decline in human milk production, as a consequence of which the physiologic fall in sodium content of human milk does not occur.

Hypernatremic dehydration usually manifests clinically between 3 days and 3 weeks. Symptoms and signs are usually nonspecific and include poor feeding, fever, lethargy or irritability, tachycardia, and poor perfusion. Few patients may present with jaundice, convulsions, or excessive weight loss.[63] There can be an intense thirst,[64] mucous membranes are dry, and skin may have doughy feel and is thick.

Complications include subarachnoid or intracranial hemorrhage or thrombosis, extensive pontine, and extrapontine myelinolysis. Other recognized complications of hypernatremia include hyperglycemia, hypocalcemia,

renal tubular injury, and renal vein thrombosis. In acute severe hypernatremia, the mortality is around 45%.[64]

The treatment of hypernatremic dehydration in a newborn is rehydration at very slow pace. The first emergency phase is restoration of vascular volume with 10–20 mL/kg of normal saline. The next phase is a rehydration phase, in which the sum of maintenance fluid and free water deficit is administered evenly over 48 hours. The choice of fluid during rehydration phase is 5% dextrose in 0.45% normal saline.[60] Edema in brain, seizures, and death can occur if hypernatremia is corrected too rapidly. The rate of fall of serum sodium level should not exceed 15 mEq/L per day. If serum sodium level is >200 mEq/L, peritoneal dialysis should be considered.[65]

Prevention of hypernatremic dehydration:

- Injudicious use of sodium bicarbonate in neonate should be prohibited.
- Physician should alert himself regarding possibility of hypernatremic dehydration in breastfed newborn infant. Follow-up visit of mother and newborn infant is to be practiced to reinforce the signs of successful breastfeeding as well as to detect any problem of baby at earlier.[66]
- If weight loss is more than 10%, the weight of a neonate should be checked on a daily basis till the growth velocity returns to the normal.

■ NEONATAL JAUNDICE

Neonatal jaundice is a global clinical problem. However, the incidence is the highest in Asian and Southeast Asian regions because of high prevalence of late preterm births, poor exclusive breastfeeding rates, glucose 6 phosphate dehydrogenase (G6PD) deficiency, and poor prevention of Rh isoimmunization.

Delayed referral, improper phototherapy, and high prevalence of comorbid conditions such as asphyxia, IUGR, and sepsis contribute to increased incidence of bilirubin encephalopathy in developing countries.

Jaundice is visible manifestation of yellowness of the skin and sclera due to elevated serum bilirubin levels above 5–7 mg/dL. It can be either physiologic or pathologic. Around 80% of the preterm infants and 50–60% of term infants suffer from jaundice. In most of the neonates, jaundice is physiologic. However, recent evidence suggests that severe neonatal jaundice (SNJ) can lead to significant morbidity and mortality.[67] SNJ has been recognized to cause deafness, learning difficulties, cerebral palsy, auditory neuropathy, and cognitive impairment. Nearly 65–75% of VLBW require treatment for neonatal jaundice.

In neonates discharged home after birth, jaundice is the most common cause of readmission.

Physiologic jaundice is almost a universal phenomenon in every newborn due to their immaturity to handle increased bilirubin production and is usually appearant by 2–3 days of life. The peak level of total serum bilirubin (TSB) level in term neonates is 12–15 mg/dL and in preterm neonates can rise above 15 mg/dL.

Any jaundice which does not fit to the time frame of physiologic jaundice is designated as pathological jaundice. Grossly, in term neonates, TSB of more than 5 mg/dL on day 1, of more than 10 mg/dL on day 2, and of 12–13 mg/dL thereafter is considered as pathologic.[68] Any TSB value of more than or equal to 17 mg/dL anytime should be considered pathologic.

The characteristic features of pathologic jaundice include the following:
- Clinically appearant jaundice in first 24 hours of life
- Rise in serum bilirubin at the rate of more than 0.2 mg/dL/hr or more than 5 mg/dL in 24 hours
- Based on the age-specific nomogram, if TSB level is above 95th percentile
- Direct bilirubin of greater than 1.5 mg/dL anytime
- Jaundice persisting beyond 2 weeks in a term baby and 3 weeks in a preterm baby
- If there are signs of acute bilirubin encephalopathy.

The major risk of SNJ is bilirubin induced neuronal injury. The more the duration of SNJ, the more the chances of neuronal damage. There are three clinical phases of acute bilirubin encephalopathy with increasing severity.

Initial phase: Initially baby will be lethargic, stuporous, hypotonic, and has poor sucking, high-pitched cry, and decreased movements. Early recognition of these signs is essential so that prompt therapeutic intervention is planned to prevent progression/reversal.

Intermediate phase: Within 2–3 days, baby develops moderate stupor, irritability, fever, and hypertonia predominately in extensor group of muscles (opisthotonos and retrocollis). These infants would progress to the advanced phase, if untreated.

Advanced phase: Over the next several days, if untreated baby develops deep stupor or coma, consistently elevated tone, inability to feed, and shrill cry. There can be spontaneous retrocollis and opisthotonos or can be easily elicited by stimulation. They may also have dysconjugate eye movements, paresis of upward gaze, eyelid retraction, or facial dystonia.

The main clinical features of chronic encephalopathy include extrapyramidal movement abnormalities, disturbances of gaze, hearing deficits, and dental dysplasia. Investigations are required for:
- Assessing the severity of jaundice
- Differentiating conjugated from unconjugated jaundice
- Identifying the etiology
- Predicting the risk of bilirubin encephalopathy. (1) As a routine, in all babies with severe jaundice a TSB with direct and indirect fractions, packed cell volume, reticulocyte count, direct Coombs test (DCT), peripheral smear, serum albumin, and G6PD screening are advised. (2) When sepsis is suspected, a sepsis screen along with blood and urine cultures is recommended. (3) In Rh isoimmunized mothers, cord blood should be screened for TSB, hematocrit, blood grouping, and DCT. (4) If there is a direct hyperbilirubinemia persisting beyond 2 weeks, a thyroid profile, urine culture, and galactosemia screen should be performed as first line investigations.

Principles of management of neonatal hyperbilirubinemia include prevention, early detection, phototherapy, and exchange transfusion.

Predischarge universal screening of neonates, use of phototherapy if required, and timely follow-up after the hospital discharge are among the most important steps to prevent severe neonatal hyperbilirubinemia. In majority of the neonates, jaundice is benign and parents should be reassured about it and at the same time, they should be educated about how to clinically assess the jaundice in natural sunlight and to seek a medical help if baby appears too yellow. One of the common causes for exaggerated jaundice during initial few days include inadequate breastfeeding. The common breastfeeding related issues include faulty positioning, poor attachment, cracked or sore nipple, engorged breasts, and inadequate production of milk. They should be addressed during hospital stay and subsequent visits.

Other important aspects of prevention include screening of mothers for isoimmunization and maternal use of anti-Rh immunoglobulin in Rh-negative pregnancy.

Important aspects of surveillance and early detection are identifying infants at risk of severe jaundice which include:
- Infants with predischarge TSB in high-risk zone
- Jaundice within 24 hours of life
- Cephalohematoma or significant bruising
- Significant weight loss
- Feeding not established before discharge
- G6PD deficiency
- Late preterm neonates
- Previous sibling having SNJ.

Visual assessment should be performed in these at risk neonates every 12–24 hours during initial 3–5 days of life. Visual assessment should be supplemented with transcutaneous or total bilirubin estimation. Serum bilirubin levels should be plotted on the hour-specific nomograms.

The requirement of treatment either in the form of phototherapy or exchange transfusion is determined based on the criteria of American Academy of Pediatrics (AAP).[69] AAP provides different age-specific nomograms for phototherapy and exchange transfusion.

Indications of exchange transfusion include the following:

- Isoimmune hemolytic disease with any of the following:
  - Hydrops
  - Cord TSB >5 mg/dL and cord Hb <11 g/dL
  - TSB value rises at the rate of >1 mg/dL/hr despite phototherapy
  - TSB value rises at the rate of >0.5 mg/dL despite phototherapy with corresponding Hb value of 11–13 g/dL
- Any baby having features of acute bilirubin encephalopathy
- TSB level in exchange range in accordance to age-specific nomograms.

Other suggested therapies include high-dose intravenous immunoglobulin, metalloporphyrins, phenobarbitone, and probiotics. However, there is insufficient evidence to support their use.

■ INTRAUTERINE GROWTH RESTRICTION

Intrauterine growth restriction is another commonly encountered problem in tropics, which is defined as a fetal growth less than the normal growth potential for a specific neonate. Globally, IUGR is seen in around one quarter of the newborns. The significant burden of IUGR is contributed by tropical countries. Asia, Africa, and Latin America account for nearly 75%, 20%, and 5% cases of IUGR, respectively. The maternal, placental, or fetal factors usually lead to IUGR. Maternal undernutrition, poor socioeconomic status, neglected girl child, and medical and obstetric disorders complicating pregnancy contribute a large number of cases of IUGR in developing countries. The various conditions[70-73] cause mismatch between nutritional or respiratory demands of the fetus and the supply from placenta which in turn lead to impaired fetal growth. The fetal growth restriction occurs in any trimester which results in either symmetric or asymmetric IUGR.

Severely affected IUGR infants are prone to mortality and morbidities in immediate newborn period such as birth asphyxia, meconium aspiration syndrome, PPHN, or pulmonary hemorrhage. Other neonatal complications include hypothermia, polycythemia, jaundice, hypoglycemia, hyperglycemia, hypocalcemia, feed intolerance, necrotizing enterocolitis, and late-onset sepsis. The long-term sequelae include growth failure, abnormal neurodevelopment, poor scholastic performance, and behavioral issues.[74,75]

Prevention of IUGR births is extremely important as they contribute significantly to the neonatal mortality and are burden to health infrastructure of the country. The essential factors which determine the fetal growth in tropics which need improvement are nutrition of adolescent girls, prepregnancy weight, poverty, and interpregnancy spacing. The interventions to improve maternal nutrition and reduce fetal growth restriction in developing countries[76] are balanced energy protein supplementation, calcium supplementation, micronutrient supplementation, and antimalarial drug prophylaxis for pregnant women in malaria-endemic areas.

In mothers diagnosed to have IUGR babies, certain interventions can be tried which include bed rest, parenteral nutrition, oxygen therapy, and pharmacological therapy such as antibiotics, aspirin, beta-adrenergic agonist, or atrial natriuretic peptide.

Intrauterine growth restriction still remains a major challenge for the neonatologists and obstetricians in tropics.

■ BREASTFEEDING PRACTICES

In tropics, there are several prevalent newborn feeding traditions, especially the first feed. In many Indian communities, breastfeeding is not even initiated till the third day of life, the reason being some ceremony need to be completed before initiation of breastfeeding such as breast washing by mother-in-law or an elder sister. Few women wait for night fall to happen and for some it is a family custom. Many women do not even attempt breastfeeding with the assumption that they will not have any milk at this stage. Few women perceive the early milk "unclean" as it appears "different." Few communities discard the colostrum as they think that it is harmful and newborn may find it difficult to digest.[77]

Many inaugural or prelacteal feeds such as glucose, sugar, honey, ghuttis, jaggery, and animal milk are offered to a newborn during this interim period. With prelacteal feeds, there is a risk of contamination, aspiration, and adverse toxic effects such as botulism.

Mothers should be motivated to initiate breastfeeding as soon as possible, ideally within half an hour of vaginal delivery and within 4 hours of cesarean section, preferably within an hour. They should be informed about the benefits of breastfeeding to the baby, mother, and society as well. The colostrum is the first vaccination of the baby, meet the baby's nutritional requirements in first few days, and has certain constituents which a baby should not miss. Delayed initiation of breastfeeding predisposes to breast engorgement which in turn inhibits further milk production. The rate of exclusive breastfeeding is unlikely to improve with a mere counseling and actual physical support by lactation expert (any healthcare worker) is essential. Every healthcare facility should adopt baby friendly hospital initiative (BFHI) policy.

In tropics, over a past decade, neonatal health has gained a lot of importance. It is possible to prevent majority of the neonatal deaths by implementing simple, cost-effective solutions which are readily available. Simple perinatal interventions have reduced preterm morbidity and mortality: KMC, antenatal steroids, delivery room CPAP, and delayed cord clamping have proved to be game changers. SpO_2 monitoring has reduced retinopathy of prematurity (ROP) significantly. Major challenge remains the implementation of these interventions. Currently, in tropics, these interventions are not reaching the most vulnerable newborns at community level. The pressing priority is to identify the approaches to overcome existing barriers in care-seeking which are either physical, economic, or cultural. This can be achieved by developing close partnership between the research and health policy community. There is a need of strong local and national leadership and adequate funding. Quality initiatives are equally important. Intense counseling on few essential practices such as institutional delivery, early initiation of breastfeeding, maintaining good thermal care, KMC, and asepsis should go long way in the tropics to tackle the essential issues in neonatal care.

■ REFERENCES

1. Lawn JE, Cousens S, Zupan J. 4 million neonatal deaths: when? Where? Why? Lancet. 2005;365:891-900.
2. Zupan J, Aahman E. Perinatal Mortality for the Year 2000. Estimates Developed by WHO Geneva. Switzerland: World Health Organization; 2005.
3. Black RE, Cousens S, Johnson HL, et al. Global, regional, and national causes of child mortality in 2008: a systematic analysis. Lancet. 2010;375:1969-87.
4. Kumar V, Shearer JC, Kumar A, et al. Neonatal hypothermia in low resource settings: a review. J Perinatol. 2009;29:401-12.
5. Mullany LC. Neonatal hypothermia in low-resource settings. Semin Perinatol. 2010;34:426-33.
6. Thairu L, Pelto G. Newborn care practices in Pemba Island (Tanzania) and their implications for newborn health and survival. Matern Child Nutr. 2008;4:194-208.
7. Hill Z, Tawiah-Agyemang C, Manu A, et al. Keeping newborns warm: beliefs, practices and potential for behaviour change in rural Ghana. Trop Med Int Health. 2010;15:1118-24.
8. Lunze K, Yeboah-Antwi K, Marsh DR, et al. Prevention and management of neonatal hypothermia in rural Zambia. PLoS One. 2014;9(4):e92006.
9. Knobel R, Holditch-Davis D. Thermoregulation and heat loss prevention after birth and during neonatal intensive-care unit stabilization of extremely low-birthweight infants. J Obstet Gynecol Neonatal Nurs. 2007;36:280-7.
10. Lunze K, Hamer DH. Thermal protection of the newborn in resource-limited environments. J Perinatol. 2012;32:317-24.
11. Zayeri F, Kazemnejad A, Ganjali M, et al. Incidence and risk factors of neonatal hypothermia at referral hospitals in Tehran, Islamic Republic of Iran. East Mediterr Health J. 2007;13:1308-18.
12. Mance MJ. Keeping infants warm: challenges of hypothermia. Adv Neonatal Care. 2008;8:6-12.
13. Sreeramareddy CT, Joshi HS, Sreekumaran BV, et al. Home delivery and newborn care practices among urban women in western Nepal: a questionnaire survey. BMC Pregnancy Childbirth. 2006;6:27.
14. Bergström A, Byaruhanga R, Okong P. The impact of newborn bathing on the prevalence of neonatal hypothermia in Uganda: a randomized, controlled trial. Acta Paediatr. 2005;94:1462-7.
15. The American Academy of Pediatrics. Textbook of Neonatal Resuscitation, 6th edition. Elk Grove, IL: American Academy of Pediatrics; 2011.
16. Singhal N, Niermeyer S. Neonatal resuscitation where resources are limited. Clin Perinatol. 2006;33:219-28, x-xi.
17. DeMauro SB, Douglas E, Karp K, et al. Improving delivery room management for very preterm infants. Pediatrics. 2013;132: e1018-25.
18. McCarthy LK, Molloy EJ, Twomey AR, et al. A randomized trial of exothermic mattresses for preterm newborns in polyethylene bags. Pediatrics. 2013;132:e135-41.
19. te Pas AB, Lopriore E, Dito I, et al. Humidified and heated air during stabilization at birth improves temperature in preterm infants. Pediatrics. 2010;125:e1427-32.
20. Thaver D, Zaidi AK. Burden of neonatal infections in developing countries: a review of evidence from community-based studies. Pediatr Infect Dis J. 2009;28(Suppl 1):S3-9.
21. Edmond K, Zaidi A. New approaches to preventing, diagnosing, and treating neonatal sepsis. PLoS Med. 2010;7:e1000213.
22. Zaidi AK, Huskins WC, Thaver D, et al. Hospital-acquired neonatal infections in developing countries. Lancet. 2005;365: 1175-88.
23. Ganatra HA, Zaidi AK. Neonatal infections in the developing world. Semin Perinatol. 2010;34:416-25.
24. Zaidi AK, Thaver D, Ali SA, et al. Pathogens associated with sepsis in newborns and young infants in developing countries. Pediatr Infect Dis J. 2009;28(Suppl 1):S10-8.
25. Downie L, Armiento R, Subhi R, et al. Community acquired neonatal and infant sepsis in developing countries: efficacy of WHO's currently recommended antibiotics–systematic review and meta-analysis. Arch Dis Child. 2013;98:146-54.
26. Young Infants Clinical Signs Study Group. Clinical signs that predict severe illness in children under age 2 months: a multicentre study. Lancet. 2008;371:135-42.

27. Baqui AH, El-Arifeen S, Darmstadt GL, et al. Effect of community-based newborn-care intervention package implemented through two service-delivery strategies in Sylhet district, Bangladesh: a cluster-randomised controlled trial. Lancet. 2008;371:1936-44.

28. Shane AL, Stoll BJ. Neonatal sepsis: progress towards improved outcomes. J Infect. 2014;68:S24-32.

29. Camacho-Gonzalez A, Spearman PW, Stoll BJ. Neonatal infectious diseases: evaluation of neonatal sepsis. Pediatr Clin North Am. 2013;60:367-89.

30. Hornik CP, Benjamin DK, Becker KC, et al. Use of the complete blood cell count in early-onset neonatal sepsis. Pediatr Infect Dis J. 2012;31:799-802.

31. Hornik CP, Benjamin DK, Becker KC, et al. Use of the complete blood cell count in late-onset neonatal sepsis. Pediatr Infect Dis J. 2012;31:803-7.

32. Yager P, Edwards T, Fu E, et al. Microfluidic diagnostic technologies for global public health. Nature. 2006;442: 412-8.

33. Patrick SW, Schumacher RE, Davis MM. Variation in lumbar punctures for early onset neonatal sepsis: a nationally representative serial cross-sectional analysis, 2003-2009. BMC Pediatr. 2012;12:134.

34. Sivanandan S, Soraisham AS, Swarnam K. Choice and duration of antimicrobial therapy for neonatal sepsis and meningitis. Int J Pediatr. 2011;2011:712150.

35. Stoll BJ, Hansen NI, Sanchez PJ, et al. Early onset neonatal sepsis: the burden of group B Streptococcal and E. coli disease continues. Pediatrics. 2011;127:817-26.

36. Muller-Pebody B, Johnson AP, Heath PT, et al. Empirical treatment of neonatal sepsis: are the current guidelines adequate? Arch Dis Child Fetal Neonatal Ed. 2011;96:F4-8.

37. Hsieh E, Smith PB, Jacqz-Aigrain E, et al. Neonatal fungal infections: when to treat? Early Hum Dev. 2012;88(Suppl 2): S6-10.

38. Tunkel AR, Hartman BJ, Kaplan SL, et al. Practice guidelines for the management of bacterial meningitis. Clin Infect Dis. 2004;39:1267-84.

39. Darmstadt GL, Batra M, Zaidi AK. Oral antibiotics in the management of serious neonatal bacterial infections in developing country communities. Pediatr Infect Dis J. 2009;28(Suppl 1):S31-6.

40. Darmstadt GL, Batra M, Zaidi AK. Parenteral antibiotics for the treatment of serious neonatal bacterial infections in developing country settings. Pediatr Infect Dis J. 2009;28(Suppl 1):S37-42.

41. Thaver D, Ali SA, Zaidi AK. Antimicrobial resistance among neonatal pathogens in developing countries. Pediatr Infect Dis J. 2009;28(Suppl 1):S19-21.

42. Tzialla C, Borghesi A, Perotti GF, et al. Use and misuse of antibiotics in the neonatal intensive care unit. J Matern Fetal Neonatal Med. 2012;25(Suppl 4):35-7.

43. Kuppala VS, Meinzen-Derr J, Morrow AL, et al. Prolonged initial empirical antibiotic treatment is associated with adverse outcomes in premature infants. J Pediatr. 2011;159:720-5.

44. Cotten CM, Taylor S, Stoll B, et al. Prolonged duration of initial empirical antibiotic treatment is associated with increased rates of necrotizing enterocolitis and death for extremely low birth weight infants. Pediatrics. 2009;123:58-66.

45. Rhee V, Mullany LC, Khatry SK, et al. Maternal and birth attendant hand washing and neonatal mortality in southern Nepal. Arch Pediatr Adolesc Med. 2008;162:603-8.

46. Ayaz A, Saleem S. Neonatal Mortality and Prevalence of Practices for Newborn Care in a Squatter Settlement of Karachi, Pakistan: A cross-sectional study. Plos One. 2010;5: e13783.

47. Thatte N, Mullany LC, Khatry SK, et al. Traditional birth attendants in rural Nepal: knowledge, attitude, and practices about maternal and new born health. Glob Public Health. 2009; 4:600-17.

48. Mullany LC, Darmstadt GL, Tielsch JM. Safety and impact of chlorhexidine antisepsis interventions for improving neonatal health in developing countries. Pediatr Infect Dis J. 2006;25:665-75.

49. Vohr BR, Poindexter BB, Dusick AM, et al. Persistent beneficial effects of breast milk ingested in the neonatal intensive care unit on outcomes of extremely low birth weight infants at 30 months of age. Pediatrics. 2007;120:e953-9.

50. Borghesi A, Stronati M. Strategies for the prevention of hospital acquired infections in the NICU. J Hosp Infect. 2008;68: 293-300.

51. Pessoa-Silva CL, Hugonnet S, Pfister R, et al. Reduction in health care associated infection risk in neonates by successful hand hygiene promotion. Pediatrics. 2007;120:e382-90.

52. Chalmers S, Mears M. Neonatal pre-transport stabilisation-caring for infants the STABLE way. Infant. 2005;1:34-7.

53. Mathur NB. Comprehensive neonatal care in India: Experiences in planning and implementation. J Neonatol. 2006;20:204-5.

54. Cornette L. Contemporary neonatal transport: problems and solutions. Arch Dis Child Fetal Neonatal Ed. 2004;89: F212-4.

55. Neonatal transfer and transportation: NNF Training module. Saluja S, Mathur NB (Eds). National Neonatology Forum: New Delhi; 2005.

56. Conde-Agudelo A, Belizán JM, Diaz-Rossello J. Kangaroo mother care to reduce morbidity and mortality in low birth-weight infants. Cochrane Database Syst Rev. 2011:CD002771.

57. McCall EM, Alderdice F, Halliday HL, et al. Interventions to prevent hypothermia at birth in preterm and/or low birth weight infants. Cochrane Database Syst Rev. 2008:CD004210.

58. Liu L, Johnson HL, Cousens S, et al. Global, regional, and national causes of child mortality: an updated systematic analysis for 2010 with time trends since 2000. Lancet. 2012; 379(9832):2151-61.

59. Kattwinkel J, Perlman JM, Aziz K, et al. Part 15: neonatal resuscitation: 2010 American Heart Association Guidelines for Cardiopulmonary Resuscitation and Emergency Cardiovascular Care. Circulation. 2010;122(18 Suppl 3): S909-19.

60. Schwaderer AL, Schwartz GJ. Treating hypernatremic dehydration. Pediatrics in Review. 2005;26(4):148-51.

61. Konetzny G, Bucher HU, Arlettaz R. Prevention of hypernatremic dehydration in breastfed newborn infants by daily weighing. Eur J Pediatr. 2009;168:815-8.

62. Cohn A. A simple method for assessing if weight loss is greater or less than 10%. Arch Dis Child. 2005;90(1):88.

63. Boskabadi H, Maamouri G, Ebrahimi M, et al. Neonatal hypernatremia and dehydration in infants receiving inadequate breastfeeding. Asia Pac J Clin Nutr. 2010;19:301-7.

64. Elamin A, Nair P. Case reports: hypernatremic dehydration in infancy. Sudan J Paediatr. 2007;8:161-70.

65. Bolat F, Oflaz MB, Güven AS, et al. What is the safe approach for neonatal hypernatremic dehydration? A retrospective

study from neonatal intensive care unit. Pediatr Emer Care. 2013;29:808-13.

66. Oh YJ, Lee JE, An SH, et al. Severe hypernatremic dehydration in a breast-fed neonate. Korean Journal of Pediatrics. 2007;50(1): 85-8.

67. Bhutani VK, Zipursky A, Blencowe H, et al. Neonatal hyperbilirubinemia and Rhesus disease of the newborn: incidence and impairment estimates for 2010 at regional and global levels. Pediatr Res. 2013;74(Suppl 1):86-100.

68. Madan A, MacMohan JR, Stevenson DK. Neonatal Hyper-bilirubinemia. In: Teush HW, Ballard RA, Gleason CA (Eds). Avery's Diseases of the Newborn, 8th edition. WB Saunders: Philadelphia; 2005. pp. 1226-56.

69. American Academy of Pediatrics Subcommittee on Hyperbilirubinemia. Management of hyperbilirubinemia in the newborn infant 35 or more weeks of gestation. Pediatrics. 2004;114(1):297-316.

70. Ananth CV, Peltier MR, Chavez MR, et al. Recurrence of ischemic placental disease. Obstet Gynecol. 2007;110:128-33.

71. Redline RW. Placental pathology: a systematic approach with clinical correlations. Placenta. 2008;29(Suppl A):S86-91.

72. Wilkins-Haug L, Quade B, Morton CC. Confined placental mosaicism as a risk factor among newborns with fetal growth restriction. Prenat Diagn. 2006;26:428-32.

73. Boog G. Chronic villitis of unknown etiology. Eur J Obstet Gynecol Reprod Biol. 2008;136(1):9-15.

74. De Jesus LC, Pappas A, Shankaran S, et al. Outcomes of small for gestational age infants born at <27 weeks' gestation. J Pediatr. 2013;163:55-60.

75. Guellec I, Lapillonne A, Renolleau S, et al. Neurologic outcomes at school age in very preterm infants born with severe or mild growth restriction. Pediatrics. 2011;127:e883-91.

76. Bhutta ZA, Das JK, Rizvi A, et al. Evidence-based interventions for improvement of maternal and child nutrition: what can be done and at what cost? Lancet. 2013;382:452-77.

77. Bandyopadhyay M. Impact of ritual pollution on lactation and breastfeeding practices in rural West Bengal, India. Int Breastfeed J. 2009;4:2.

Ketan Bharadva, Hitesh Patel

INTRODUCTION

Good neonatal nutrition is essential for survival, physical growth, mental development, performance, productivity, health, and well-being across the entire life span. Mortality and morbidities as fall out of malnutrition and overnutrition are well known. Similarly roots of adult onset diseases in fetal and infant nutrition are enfolding more. Large number of populations belongs to surviving cohort of premature babies with improvement in antenatal management of high-risk pregnancy and advanced neonatal care of extremely low birth weight (ELBW) babies. So, ignorance or improper nutritional care of these babies will result into a large number of nutritionally deprived populations. Developing world like sub-Saharan Africa and South Asian countries contributes 80% of total preterm births in world.[1]

Neonatal nutrition, especially low birth weight (LBW) babies, pose a special challenge in nutrition. About 97% of all very low birth weight (VLBW) infants and 99% of infants <1,000 g at birth weighed <10th percentile at 36 weeks' postmenstrual age.[2]

Evidence-based nutritional intervention at the time of birth and in early infancy such as exclusive breastfeeding and use of breast milk and fortification in a LBW infants has proven outcomes respiratory and gastrointestinal infections, in cognitive development in preterm and term babies, and long-term morbidity like obesity, type 2 diabetes, and hypertension.[3]

Improving nutritional status of neonates and infants needs multisector interventions which include government as well as nongovernment health sector which can cover vast majority of populations in a community by various community-based interventions. Various evidence-based nutritional intervention targeting adolescent girl and female in child bearing age in a preconception period, apart from nutritional care of pregnant and lactating mother and newborn babies immediately after birth and then up to early childhood has a potential role to improve overall maternal and children health statistics.[4]

NUTRITIONAL REQUIREMENTS

Table 1 shows nutritional requirements of neonates in different weight categories.

NUTRIENT SOURCES

Breast milk is the gold standard nutrition for growth, development, immune maturation, and behavior and healthy microbial colonization. When mother's own milk (MoM) is not available, next choice is pasteurized donor human milk (DHM), and then comes commercial infant milk formulae and lastly animal milk.

Breast Milk and Breastfeeding

Detailed description of breastfeeding is out of scope of this article. Below are few salient features to be noted.

Exclusive breastfeeding is nutritionally adequate for first 6 months of life in *term healthy* newborns. "Exclusive breastfeeding" is defined as no other food or drink, not even water, except breast milk (including expressed milk or from a wet nurse) or oral rehydration salts (ORS), vitamins, minerals, and medicines. Exclusive breastfeeding from birth is possible except for a few medical conditions **(Annexure 1)**,[5] and unrestricted exclusive breastfeeding results in optimal milk production.[6-8]

Apart from nutritional constituents human milk acts as medium of transfer of defense and other components to the offspring, which has lifelong impact also, through its bioactive factors like cells, anti-inflammatory, antioxidative and anti-infective agents, growth factors, and

Table 1: Enteral nutrient requirements.[9]

Nutrient	ELBW (<1,000 g)	VLBW (>1,000 g)	DRI/AI (0–6 months)
Fluid	150–200 mL/kg	135–190 mL/kg	0.7 L/day
Energy	110–120 kcal/kg	110–130 kcal/kg	555 kcal/day
Carbohydrate	9–20 g/kg	7–17 g/kg	60 g/day
Protein	3.8–4.4 g/kg	3.4–4.2 g/kg	9.1 g/day
Fat	6.2–8.4 g/kg	5.3–7.2 g/kg	31 g/day
DHA	>21 mg/kg	>18 mg/kg	
ARA	>28 mg/kg	>24 mg/kg	
Minerals			
Calcium	100–220 mg/kg		210 mg/day
Phosphorus	60–140 mg/kg		100 mg/day
Magnesium	7.9–15 mg/kg		30 mg/day
Sodium	69–115 mg/kg (3–5 mEq/kg)		120 mg/day
Potassium	78–117 mg/kg (2–3 mEq/kg)		400 mg/day
Chloride	107–249 mEq/kg		180 mg/day
Trace elements			
Zinc	1,000–3,000 µg/kg		2 mg/day
Iron	2–4 mg/kg		0.27 mg/day
Iodine	10–60 µg/kg		110 µg/day
Vitamins			
Vitamin A	700–1,500 IU/kg		400 µg/day
Vitamin D	150–400 IU/kg		5 µg/day
Vitamin E	6–12 IU/kg		4 mg/day
Vitamin K	8–10 µg/kg		2 µg/day
Vitamin C	12–24 mg/kg		40 mg/day
Vitamin B12	0.3 µg/kg		0.4 µg/day
Folic Acid	25–50 µg/kg		65 µg/day
Pyridoxine	150–210 µg/kg		0.1 mg/day
Thiamin	180–240 µg/kg		0.2 mg/day
Riboflavin	250–360 µg/kg		0.3 mg/day
Niacin	3.6–4.8 mg/kg		2 mg/day

(AI: adequate intake; ARA: arachidonic acid; DHA: docosahexaenoic acid; DRI: dietary reference intakes; ELBW: extremely low birth weight; VLBW: very low birth weight)

prebiotics. Thus, it is not just nutrition, but an overall driver of survival and health of newborn, the content of which is not just produced in mammary cells but also transferred from maternal serum and may be coming from as far as maternal gut!! It has a direct major role in development of gastrointestinal, immune, and central nervous system development. Extensive studies have shown it to be protective against infectious diseases like diarrhea, pneumonia, urinary tract infection (UTI), meningitis, otitis, etc. It also influences infant programming of late metabolic diseases, protecting against obesity, and type 2 diabetes. Breastfed children have better cognition by 4–7 intelligence quotient (IQ) points. It obviates risks with artificial feeding like atopy, inflammatory bowel diseases, cardiovascular diseases, and hyperlipidemia.[10]

The first 4–6 weeks are full of dynamic changes that convert colostrum of lactogenesis I stage through transitional milk of lactogenesis II from 3 days to 15 days phase to mature milk. They suffice for the different needs of the actively changing metabolic milieu of the newborns.

Colostrum

- It is the key support to insulin predominated fetal metabolism (dependent on continuous transplacental glucose supply) to a glucagon predominated newborn metabolism (dependent on variable fat based fuel economy).[11,12] It is through its contents of gluconeogenic amino acid precursors (alanine); long-chain fatty acids in initiation of transcription of carnitine palmitoyltransferase enzyme for ketogenesis; and through lactose which minimizes insulin secretion. Hence, feeding glucose water is discouraged as it increases insulin secretion; decreases glucagon; and delays initiation of natural metabolic changes to maintain basal sugar levels.

- Colostrum has loads of immune and trophic factors. It is found to be beneficial in protecting against late-onset sepsis (LOS) and necrotizing enterocolitis (NEC) by virtue of immune and trophic factors leading to inhibition of proinflammatory cytokines and has increased breastfeeding success rates. Oropharyngeal feeding or smearing application of mothers' own colostrum is a simple, novel and low-cost intervention in ELBW or extreme premature newborns.[13-15]

*Baby-friendly Hospital Initiative (BFHI) 2018 revision, gives excellent evidence-based recommendations to successful breastfeeding (**Box 1**).*

Early initiation of breastfeeding within first hour of birth has a potential to reduce neonatal mortality by 22%. It can be done for all stable newborns including postcesarean births.

Key to successful breastfeeding and answer to most common problems is proper comfortable positioning of mother and infant with good latching and frequent feeding; and counseling with active listening and confidence building of all mothers. Trained lactation counselors have a big role to play but all staff taking care of mother-infant dyad including neonatologists should be *trained* to support.

Conditions like hypotonic infants, cleft lip or palate, ankyloglossia, twins/triplets, etc. need specific technique assistance by trained lactation counselor and vigorous steps to maintain breastfeeding and mother's confidence. Similarly maternal conditions like diabetes, breast problems, surgery, medications, low milk output, etc. demands specific extra care. It is recommended to refer to specific guidelines for them.

Low Milk Transfer and Milk Output

- Perceived low milk output in presence of optimal weight gain is the most common scenario.

- Premature neonates, sick neonates, and neonates with congenital anomalies like cleft palate, severe ankyloglossia, cardiac or renal problems may not be able to suck properly can lead to poor milk transfer and breast stimulation.

- Presence of maternal endocrine problems (pituitary failure after severe hemorrhage and retained piece of placenta), hypoplastic breast development, hormone-containing contraceptive pills, pregnancy, severe malnutrition, smoking and alcohol consumption, diabetes, pregnancy-induced hypertension, and chorioamnionitis should alert the doctors to anticipate possible low milk production.

- There are more chances of inadequacy of breast milk transfer to neonate in unsupported mothers, primiparas, and unmonitored cases.

Box 1: Ten steps to successful breastfeeding (BFHI-2018).

Critical management procedures:
1a. Comply fully with the *International Code of Marketing of Breast-milk Substitutes* and relevant World Health Assembly resolutions.
1b. Have a written infant feeding policy that is routinely communicated to staff and parents.
1c. Establish ongoing monitoring and data-management systems.
2. Ensure that staffs have sufficient knowledge, competence, and skills to support breastfeeding.

Key clinical practices:
3. Discuss the importance and management of breastfeeding with pregnant women and their families.
4. Facilitate immediate and uninterrupted skin-to-skin contact and support mothers to initiate breastfeeding as soon as possible after birth.
5. Support mothers to initiate and maintain breastfeeding and manage common difficulties.
6. Do not provide breastfed newborns any food or fluids other than breast milk, unless medically indicated.
7. Enable mothers and their infants to remain together and to practice *rooming-in 24 hours* a day.
8. Support mothers to recognize and respond to their infants' cues for feeding.
9. Counsel mothers on the use and risks of feeding bottles, teats, and pacifiers.
10. Coordinate discharge so that parents and their infants have timely access to ongoing support and care.

(BFHI: Baby-friendly Hospital Initiative)

Note: For details of proper skin-to-skin contact, early initiation of breastfeeding, breastfeeding methods, maintenance and augmentation, hunger cues, detailed assessment, and counseling techniques refer to appropriate literature.

Signs of Inadequate Milk Transfer

- Most sensitive sign is weight loss at beyond 3 days of life of more than 10% [7% for the smaller and/or intrauterine growth restriction (IUGR) infant] or weight loss continuing beyond 5 days of life, or more than 3% per day. It demands a thorough evaluation and support to breastfeeding before prescribing supplemental feeds. Loss beyond 12.5% may need supplementation.
- Delayed transition to yellow stools (continued meconium passage) beyond 5 days.
- Clinical or laboratory evidence of dehydration (high Na, lethargy, poor feeding, low urine output, etc.) not improving despite skilled management of breastfeeding may need supplemental feeds.
- Simply crying baby without above signs is not indicative of inadequacy.

Indications of Supplemental Feeds

Healthcare providers should know proper monitoring for adequacy and indications for supplementations to prevent secondary hypernatremic dehydration and hypoglycemia and at the same time prevent abuse of it. Some guides to supplemental feeding for term healthy neonates.[16] First choice of supplemental feeds is DHM.

- Asymptomatic hypoglycemia unresponsive to appropriate frequent breastfeeding may need supplementation. If intravenous (IV) glucose therapy is indicated for hypoglycemia, breastfeeding should be continued with it.
- Temporary cessation of breastfeeding (e.g. maternal chemotherapy or critical illness, etc.) may need supplement feeding.
- Weight loss beyond 12.5% or dehydration may need supplementation after thorough evaluation and when skilled steps to support breastfeeding fail.
- When supplementation is done all steps should be taken to maintain breastfeeding, e.g. restricting the supplement amount to suffice normal newborn physiology, avoiding bottle feeding, frequent hand expression or pumping (at least eight times in 24 hours) to completely drain the breasts and prevent engorgement, and infant continues to practice at the breast—supplement given after breastfeeding attempt.
- Use of supplemental nursing systems (or simpler ways by using dropper or syringe or feeding tube attached to breast) is recommended. It helps to stimulate breasts to produce more milk, encourages skin-to-skin contact and infant sucking at breasts, provides breastfeeding experience to mother.

- Clear psychological message should be passed to parents that supplemental feeding is purely temporary and not a permanent inclusion of artificial feedings.
- Interruption of breastfeeding is not indicated for breast milk jaundice in an otherwise thriving well infant. Thorough evaluation takes first priority.
- Policies should be in implemented strongly by hospitals to mandate doctor's orders for medically indicated supplemental feeding and when to terminate it, and informed consent of mother.

Breastfeeding Late Preterms[17]

- Implementation of the Ten Steps to Successful Breastfeeding of the BFHI gives better chances of success in term neonates, but these steps may not be able to meet certain nutritional issues in late preterms and occasional sleepy early term infants. Late preterms (between 34 0/7 and 36 6/7 weeks of gestation) are often having morbidity and mortality related to inadequate breast milk transfer, especially when there is lack of proactive support to mothers. They have higher rehospitalization rates related to poor breastfeeding.
- Late preterms may have low alertness and are often more sleepy, less vigorous and agile, and may have frequent difficulties with positioning and latching, sucking and swallowing in comparison with full-term neonates. It may be misdiagnosed as sepsis or other medical illness, and thus unwarranted mother-child separation, investigation and treatment, as well as poor nutrition.
- Some large agile late preterms cannot achieve effective suckling to transfer enough breast milk on test weighing immediately in first few days despite seemingly proper latching and sucking. They may miss to get due attention. So all late preterms should be monitored vigorously to make sure adequacy and maintenance of breast milk supply and transfer.
- It may be necessary to wake up the sleepy neonate 3 hours after previous feed if it does not show hunger cues.
- It is observed that late preterm newborns lend up with more use of breastfeeding supports like nipple shields, formula supplementation, milk expression, and breast compressions.
- All mothers should start expressing colostrum 3 hourly starting from first hour of birth. Hand expression seems better than pumps.
- Stable and healthy neonates should not be separated from mother for IV antibiotics or phototherapy.

- Test weighing should be considered to check adequacy of milk transfer.
- Problems of more premature neonates have been discussed later in this article.

Expressed Breast Milk

- Expression of breast milk is indicated for better initiation and maintenance of breastfeeding; or for conditions when optimal direct breastfeeding is not possible (e.g. sick or preterm neonate); or when there is separation of mother and neonate (e.g. neonate and mother in different hospitals).
- All mothers should be trained in expression of milk. Manual expression is preferable for short-term needs. Pumps may give better yields but are difficult in hygiene maintenance. (For details please refer relevant literature.)
- Expression under hygienic condition and then immediate storage under very clean conditions is a must to ensure safety (**Annexure 2**). Do not add fresh milk to a frozen container. Human milk should not be stored in hospital grade plastic containers used for collection of specimen, but instead food grade plastic containers be used. Pyrex containers are the best bet amongst others like steel, polypropylene, polyethylene, glass or bisphenol containing containers. Containers or collection kits of pumps do not need sterilization but need thorough cleaning with hot soapy/boiling water and then drying completely. Do not use chemical disinfection. Frozen or cold milk should be allowed to come to room temperature before feeding by thawing slowly. Do not use microwave. It should not be refrozen.[17] Colostrum can be stored up to 24 hours, and mature milk up to 6 hours at room temperature. Beyond that, it should be stored at 3–4°C before use. If not used for more than 5 days, it should be frozen.

Maternal Supplementation and Breast Milk

Maternal intake of nutrients directly influencing its content in breast milk is variable for different nutrients. Amongst macronutrients no much influence is seen except for mild increase in fats by increasing fat content of maternal diet. Amongst micronutrients; iron, zinc, copper, vitamin D, folic acid, and calcium supplementation of lactating mothers do not have influence on its breast milk content. Water-soluble vitamins (thiamine, pyridoxine, riboflavin, and cobalamin), vitamin A, iodine, and selenium supplementation of lactating mother may improve its content in breast milk.[18]

Galactogogues are indicated when there is proven poor breast milk production despite of proper actions to improve the status.

Donor Human Milk

The concept of human milk banking was established way back in 1909 in Vienna, Austria but with emergence of human immunodeficiency virus (HIV) and other safety issues it went almost obsolete then. Later with advent of Holder method of pasteurization rendering killing of HIV and other pathogens the concept again has picked up. With consensus and guidelines coming up in international pediatric, neonatal, and other health bodies there is increasing interest in establishing human milk banks and use of human milk.[3,19-22] WHO has recommended it as Category 1 Intervention for LBW infants and is supported by Essential Nutrition Actions targeting the first 1,000 days of life.

Worldwide there is increasing acceptance of DHM as an alternative to feed newborn in cases of nonavailability or insufficient MoM. It is most recommended for its effect on intestinal disorders, especially due to significant reduction in possibility of dreaded NEC and late onset sepsis, more so in newborns with birth weights less than 1,500 g, even though it has slower growth rates as compared to formula.[23] This effect may be due to immunoprotective factors for immature mucosa; and also due to the absence of deleterious antigens of animal milk. In addition it has trophic value in gut with early achievement of full enteral feedings. There are potential neurocognitive, cardiovascular, and other long-term advantages like fresh human milk.

Donor human milk is safe when appropriate methods of screening donors, collection, pasteurization, storage, and disbursement are taken through a human milk bank. Nonpasteurized donor milk, informal sharing, and human milk procured from sources other than a scientific milk banks are strongly discouraged due to risks of microbial contamination, infectious diseases, drugs, herbs or toxins passage from donor, spoiling in other ways, etc.[24]

A complete human milk-based diet (mother's milk fortified with DHM-based fortifiers) may result in substantial financial savings on medical care resources by preventing NEC.[25,26]

A lot of expectations are kept with use DHM as compared to formula milk, but still the evidences have not built up in literature. Cochrane review with limitations like studies funded by infant formula manufacturers and other methodological flaws shows moderately strong evidence that for preterm and LBW neonates, partial or complete formula feeding when compared with donor breast milk, results in higher rates of weight gain, linear growth, and head growth but also higher risk of developing NEC. The trial data did not show an effect on all-cause mortality, or on long-term growth or neurodevelopment. Further research is needed in this area.[27,28]

Even though Holder's heat treatment reduces effects of by destruction of many enzymes, cellular and other bioactive immune components (like immunoglobulins and white cells, lipase, and certain growth factors), and by damage to unsaturated fatty acids and milk fat globule membrane, but it still retains oligosaccharides, long-chain polyunsaturated fatty acid (LCPUFA), gangliosides, vitamin A, D, E, B12, folic acid, lactose, some cytokines and growth factors; and also renders significant anti-infective, protective, and nutrient properties to benefit recipient.[29] Newer methods of heat treatment which preserves more functions are under research [like high-temperature–short-time (HTST) pasteurization: 72°C for 5–15 seconds). But the skepticism of slower growth and loss of biologic components should not be reason for denial of DHM.[24,29,30]

Donor human milk should be fortified to meet early nutrient requirements and achieve better short-term growth. Individualized fortification is advised.[29]

Indications for Use

Donor pasteurized human milk is usually used for variety of indications like premature infants, especially <1,500 g, infants with gastrointestinal surgery leading to short bowel syndrome (SBS), when the mother is ill or hospitalized and temporarily unable to feed her infant; weaning from parenteral nutrition; metabolic disorders especially amino acid disorders, and before the MoM comes in initial days after birth.

Otherwise it is occasionally used for older children with severe allergic disorders, failure to thrive on formula feeds, feeding intolerance, chronic rotaviral enteritis, cancer chemotherapy, and absence of biological mother due to various reasons. It is being tried in variety of adult disorders like cancers and immunoglobulin A (IgA) deficiency etc. as a therapeutic tool.

Commercial Infant Formula

Commercial infant formula is intended as an effective substitute to breast milk and is formulated to mimic the nutritional composition of breast milk. But all are far inferior to breast milk as they lack the non-nutritional, bioactive components of human milk (protective and trophic factors), and the quality of their proteins and lipids

(amino acid and fatty acid profiles) may not be optimal for the needs of the baby.

Compositional guidelines for commercial infant formulas have been agreed in the Codex Alimentarius, and these are defined according to the energy density of feeds, that is the energy per 100 mL using products with 65 kcal/100 mL as typical (**Annexure 3**).

Infant formulas are available in three forms: (1) Powder: The least expensive form of infant formula that must be mixed with water before feeding; (2) Liquid: Concentrated liquid that must be mixed with an equal amount of water; and (3) Ready-to-feed: The most expensive form of infant formula that requires no mixing.

The instructions on the tin or carton for preparing the formula should be followed exactly to ensure that it is not too concentrated or diluted. Overconcentration can overload the infant with salts and protein, which can be dangerous, and overdilution can lead to malnutrition.

To prevent its abuse and protect breastfeeding, production, distribution and sale of infant milk formulas, bottles and teats is regulated by Infant Milk Substitutes (IMS) Act in India.

Bovine milk is the basis for most infant formula. Milk formulas from different animals (goat, ewe, mare, donkey, or camel), or formulas based on lamb or chicken, have been widely marketed as substitutes for cow milk in the management of cow milk allergy.

Soy-based formulas are effective options for infants with galactosemia or congenital lactase deficiency. Soy products should not be used in infants under 6 months of age with food allergy.

Hypoallergenic formulas: Protein hydrolysate formulas are meant for infants who are unable to tolerate cow milk or soy-based formulas.

Amino acid formulas are another option for infants who have severe cow milk allergy with reactions to or refusal to ingest appropriate amounts of extensively hydrolyzed formula. They provide protein in the form of free amino acids with no peptides.

Animal Milk

Whole cow's milk contains greater amounts of protein and minerals (calcium, sodium, phosphorus, chloride, magnesium, and potassium) and less carbohydrate, essential fatty acids (linoleic and α-linolenic acids) and long-chain polyunsaturated fatty acids, iron, zinc, vitamin C, and niacin (**Annexure 4**). Not only does cow's milk have a higher concentration of total protein, but its quality differs from human milk and its proteins are potentially allergenic to the human infant. It is not advisable to use whole unmodified animal milk due to its excess solute load with tendency to cause hypernatremic dehydration under conditions of water stress and gastrointestinal bleeding, and possibility of sensitization from intact proteins.

Parenteral Nutrition

It is described later in this article.

Fortification of Breast Milk

Breast milk alone does not meet the high nutrient requirements of preterm newborns when fed at usual feeding volumes, so as to fulfill optimal growth and development in early few months of life. This may lead to extra uterine growth retardation (EUGR) if there is lack of early aggressive nutrition during the first few days of life. Early postnatal growth failure that continues after discharge results in growth below the 10th percentile. It places the infant at risk of impaired neurodevelopment. Protein and mineral (especially calcium, phosphorus, and sodium) contents of breast milk is suboptimal which makes a VLBW babies susceptible to develop growth faltering, hyponatremia, and poor bone mineralization. Also protein content of breast milk progressively reduces in initial months after delivery. Fortification of a human milk aids weight gain, head growth, bone mineralization, and accretion of lean body mass. Hence, fortification of breast milk is suggested for preterm infants.[31] Evidence showed that protein supplementation of human milk fed to preterm infants as early aggressive nutrition plan that includes early parenteral nutrition administration with 3–4 g/kg/day of protein, minimal enteral feedings, and increased short-term growth.[2] Human milk fortifiers (HMF) can provide extra 10% of nutrients. The calorie requirement of a preterm infant is usually met with the addition of HMF, which provides about 4 g/kg/day of protein and 3.5–4 g/kg/day of fats. Though fortification will increase an osmolarity of milk, it did not increase an incidence of NEC.[32]

In clinical practice, 1 g of HMF sachet is added to 25 mL of expressed breast milk (EBM) or pasteurized DHM depending up on the product guideline. All preterm infants <1,500 g, or ≤34 weeks gestation, or >1,500 g (who receives >2 weeks parenteral nutrition and fails to achieve standard growth), should be fed fortified human milk. Fortification of human breast milk is continued till 40 weeks of postmenstrual age.[33]

There are two types of fortification: standard or individualized. Human milk fortification can be started safely with multinutrient fortifiers when the milk volume reaches 50–80 mL/kg/day. Routinely, standard fortification is used and if proper growth is not achieved switch to individualized fortification is done using single nutrient products of protein, lipids, or carbohydrates. Individualized fortification can be targeted fortification (based on milk analysis) or adjustable fortification [based on blood urea nitrogen (BUN) measurements]. Neonatal intensive care unit (NICU) facilities and experiences decides the type of individualized fortification.[34] There is no strong evidence to support the use of hydrolyzed protein source in fortifiers. Postdischarge fortification shows some benefits and no reduction of breastfeeding rates, but there is no consensus on it.[31]

Usually HMF is manufactured from bovine milk and is supplied as powder or liquid. Liquid fortifiers are made to prevent *Enterobacter sakazakii* like infections associated with powder milks, but they are very less studied so far.

Human milk fortifiers increase growth rates of preterm infants during initial hospital stay, but do not provide consistent longer term growth or development.[32,35] The human milk based fortifier use is significantly associated with lower incidence of overall and surgical NEC than the bovine milk based fortification. They further enhance the antibacterial activity of human milk.[36] They are very expensive currently. Recent research is on providing more and more bioactive factors in HMF to improve the outcomes.

Supplements

Calcium, phosphorous, iron, zinc, vitamin A, vitamin D, and multivitamin liquids are used to supplement LBW neonates. They are described later in this chapter.

NUTRITIONAL STRATEGIES IN LOW BIRTH WEIGHT/PRETERM NEWBORNS

Exact goal for nutrition for prematures is still not fully defined, but postnatal growth should be like the intrauterine growth of a normal fetus with the same postconceptual age. Intrauterine nutrient accretion rates are considered to be the gold standard for neonatal nutrition. In practice it is seen that amino acids are restricted due to fear of intolerance, glucose is often the only energy source given at high rates resulting in hyperglycemia, and fat, as intralipids, is usually withheld due to hyperglycemia and fear of lung injury or kernicterus. The drastic change from a nutrient enriched environment as seen in utero to the nutrient sparse extrauterine environment puts additional stress on an already vulnerable sick premature infant.[37]

Nutritional deficiencies in early life lead to permanent growth and development failure.

Clinical practices amongst NICUs across the world differ despite the evidences to support a comprehensive nutritional plan to attain reasonably optimal postnatal growth in small premature infants. This variation is due to a lack of knowledge, systematic planning, practice implementation, healthcare provider habit, unit history, and a lack of evidence-based guidelines to standardize practice. After implementation of the standardized nutrition plan, EUGR decreased from 57% to 28%. Chronic lung disease (CLD), days of parenteral nutrition, and central line use also significantly decreased.[38]

Often the MoM is not adequate to provide optimal nutrition for a very preterm baby, non-nutrient content of breast milk confers many benefits to a growing preterm baby like immunological boost, easy tolerance due to low renal solute load, reduced risk of NEC, and a significant higher intelligent quotient at later age. There are challenges of feed tolerance, maturity of suck-swallow also.

Enteral feeding is the preferred physiologic method provided maturity, size, and condition of neonate permits. If it is not possible to meet nutrition enterally or enteral nutrition can be hazardous, parenteral nutrition can meet nutritional demands of premature neonate, critically ill neonate, neonates with gastrointestinal immaturity, malformations or major gastrointestinal tract (GIT) surgery or with protracted diarrhea.

Evidence-based Enteral Feeding

Minimal Enteral Feeding/Nutrition

- Delaying progression of feedings beyond 4 days of life delays establishment of full enteral feedings by a few days. Delaying enteral feedings in small premature infants does not prevent NEC.[39]
- Enteral starvation is known to lead to loss of gastrointestinal structure and function like blunting of villi, loss of mucosal deoxyribonucleic acid (DNA), protein content, and enzymatic activity. It occurs with parenteral nutrition even if there is maintenance of anabolic status. To prevent these changes trophic

subnutritive feeds are used which are known as minimal enteral feeding, gastrointestinal priming, gut priming, or early hypocaloric feeding.
- Typically, starting within 24 hours of life or soon as the critically sick neonate stabilize, 10–20 mL/kg per milk day is given at the same rate for at least 5 days. Milk tolerance, reaching full feeds, liver function, metabolic bone disease, days to hospital discharge, and weight gain are improved after trophic feeding.[38] Trophic feeds are contraindicated in intestinal obstruction or ileus. It is not contraindicated in a patient of perinatal asphyxia, respiratory distress syndrome, hypotension, mechanical ventilation, glucose disturbance, umbilical lines, and sepsis.[40]

Choice of Milk

- Infant's MoM is the first choice. Every mother of a preterm baby should be encouraged to express breast milk immediately after delivery to provide breast milk as early as possible for an enteral feeding.
- Those who cannot be fed MoM should be fed DHM; preterm donor's milk is more preferred.
- When neither is available then till 6 months of age infants should be fed standard formula milk and VLBW be given preterm formula milk when do not gain weight on proper feeding with standard formula milk.[19]

Feeding Methods

- Method for enteral feeding depends on the gestational maturity **(Table 2)**. Preterm babies less than 34 weeks of gestational age (GA) should be allowed for non-nutritive sucking (NNS), which helps them to achieve breastfeeding skill rapidly and also improves milk secretion in their mothers.[33]
- In preterm babies orogastric tube feeding is preferred method for enteral nutrition compared to nasogastric tube feeding. Nasogastric tube feeding increases air way resistance by 30–50% and work of breathing in preterm babies and has higher incidence of periodic breathing and central apnea.[40]
- Unlike continuous feeding intermittent bolus feeding is more physiological way of feeding as it induces

Table 2: Oral feeding skills maturation and initial feeding method.[33]

Gestation	Feeding skills	Initial feeding method
<28 weeks	No proper sucking efforts or propulsive motility in the gut	Intravenous fluids
28–31 weeks	Sucking bursts develops. No coordination of suck-swallow and breathing	Oro/Nasogastric tube feeding
32–34 weeks	Slightly mature sucking pattern. Coordination between swallowing-breathing begins	Spoon/Palladai feeding
>34 weeks	Mature sucking pattern with coordination between swallowing and breathing	Breastfeeding

gastrointestinal hormonal surges such as secretion of gastrin, gastrointestinal inhibitory peptides, and enteroglucagon suitable for GIT development, better feeding tolerance and growth. With continuous feeding there is loss of nutrients like fat and calcium due to with tube.

- Intermittent bolus feeding may increase pulmonary resistance and fluctuation of cerebral blood flow. So some author recommends use of continuous feeding method in an unstable preterm and a babies with less than 1,250 g.[40]
- Gavage feeding is given via an indwelling nasogastric tube during mechanical ventilation. An indwelling orogastric tube is used after endotracheal extubation.
- Continuous transpyloric feeding can be tried in selected preterm infants with extremely poor gastric emptying and symptomatic gastroesophageal reflux (GER).

Initiation of Feedings

- Clinically stable LBW infants with ability to breastfeed should be started breastfeeding as soon as possible after birth.
- Very low birth weight infants should receive 10 mL/kg/day of enteral feeds, preferably EBM from the first day of life, and remaining fluid requirement be given as IV fluids.[19]

Progression of Feeds

- Advancing enteral feed volumes at daily increments less than 24 mL/kg/day do not reduce the feeding intolerance, risk of NEC or death in very preterm or VLBW infants, extremely preterm or ELBW infants, small for gestational age (SGA) or growth-restricted infants, or infants with antenatal vascular flow problems. Advancing the volume of enteral feeds at faster rates (daily increase of 30–40 mL/kg as compared to slow increment 10–15 mL/kg/day) reduces the time taken to regain birth weight and establish full enteral feeds by many days, and may reduce the risk of late-onset invasive infection.[38]
- Low birth weight infants fed partially or completely by an alternative oral feeding method should be fed based on infants hunger cues (demand feeding) with maximal interval of 3 hours of sleep once full feeds are established.
- Non-nutritive sucking is beneficial without side effects.

Assessment of Feeding

- Routine Ryle's tube (RT) aspiration is not recommended to assess feeding. When baby reaches to minimum

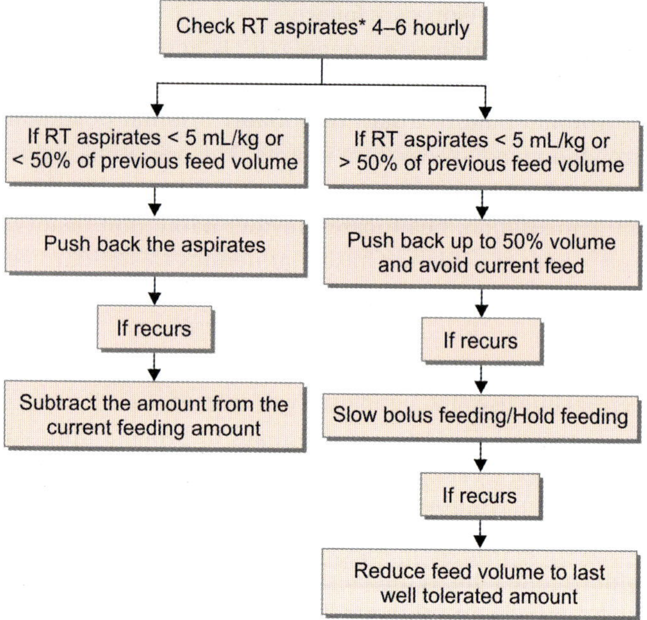

Flowchart 1: Feeding tolerance and progression.

(RT: Ryle's tube)
* Brown colored, green color aspirates are always pathological which requires further evaluation.

RT feeding volume of 2 mL for <0.5 kg, 3 mL for 0.5–0.75 kg, 4 mL for 0.75–1 kg, 5 mL for >1 kg newborns, RT aspiration should be checked. Abdominal girth monitoring is very much observer dependent and is not reliable indicator to assess feed tolerance. Further assessment for the feed tolerance can be done as shown in **Flowchart 1**.

Fortification

- Very low birth weight infants on MoM or DHM should not routinely be given bovine milk-based HMF. Those who fail to gain weight despite adequate breast milk feeding should be given human-milk fortifiers, preferably which are human milk based.[19]
- Human milk fortifier is indicated in preterm infants <31 weeks and/or <1,800 g.

Supplements

- Very low birth weight infants should receive 400–1,000 IU/day vitamin D supplements till 12 months age. Those fed on MoM or DHM should receive 120–140 mg/kg/day calcium and 60–90 mg/kg/day phosphorus supplementation during the first months of life daily till 4 kg weight is achieved; and 2–4 mg/kg/day iron supplementation from 2 weeks to 12 months of age.
- Current evidences do not suggest daily oral vitamin A or zinc supplements in LBW newborns on MoM or DHM.

- Multivitamin supplement is started when the infant has established full enteral feeds.
- Medium-chain triglycerides (MCTs) can be used as an energy supplement for preterm infants who fail to thrive.

Optimal duration of Exclusive Breastfeeding

Low birth weight infants should be exclusively breastfed until 6 months of age.

Parenteral Nutrition

Early parenteral nutrition prevents catabolic state, induces anabolism, and establishes protein accretion rate similar to that of in utero to promote linear growth. Total parenteral nutrition (TPN) therapy consists of providing sufficient fluids according to maturity and environmental condition of a patient and to provide sufficient calorie in form of 60% from carbohydrate, 30% from lipid and 10–15% from protein. Total kilocalories in 10% dextrose is 0.34 kcal/mL, while 10% lipid solution contains 0.9 kcal/mL **(Annexure 5)**.[41] Neonate on a prolong parenteral nutrition must be monitored two to three times a week by clinical examination, anthropometry, laboratory workup for assessment of growth, and complications related to prolong parenteral nutrition.

Carbohydrate: Glucose is only carbohydrate recommended for parenteral nutrition because it is readily available to brain compared to other nonglucose carbohydrate. In preterm and term neonate IV glucose is started with 6 g/kg/day (4–5 mg/kg/minute) on first day after birth and can be increased gradually up to 18 g/kg/day (12–13 mg/kg/minute) if tolerated well. Baby should be monitored carefully to avoid hypoglycemia as well as hyperglycemia for a better long-term neurodevelopmental outcome.

Lipid is provided as emulsions in parenteral nutrition supplies. In VLBW babies lipid is started on first day at 2 g/kg/day and increased by 0.5–1 g/kg/day up to 3–4 g/kg/day. Commercial lipid emulsions based on soya-bean oil or SMOF-mixtures of soy-bean oil, MCTs, olive oil and fish oil are considered safe for prolonged parenteral nutrition therapy. Monitor for a risk of hypertriglyceridemia and cholestasis.

Protein is provided as amino-acid infusion containing nine essential amino acids and semi-essential amino acids like tyrosine, taurine, cysteine, and arginine. Goal is to prevent catabolism, maintain protein stores, and provide sufficient energy and protein for growth. Starting on first day at 2 g/kg/day and it is increased to 3–4 g/kg/day.

In prolonged cases monitor BUN and metabolic acidosis.

Vitamin and minerals should be provided in a sufficient amount to meet its in utero accretion rate. Calcium and phosphorus should be provided in a dose of 75–90 mg/kg/day and 60–70 mg/kg/day respectively to prevent osteopenia of prematurity.[42] Fat- and water-soluble vitamins should be added in form of commercially available multivitamin at a dose of 1 mL/kg/day.

Early Aggressive Nutrition Approach

It is aimed at preventing the catabolic state of initial days of life in small premature infant includes the giving TPN with 3–4 g/kg/day amino acids beginning within hours of birth, 0.5–1 g/kg/day intralipids with advancement to 3 g/kg/day beginning in the first 24 hours of life and minimal enteral feedings at 10–20 mL/kg/day started within the first 1–2 days of life.[37] Aggressive intake of amino acids and intralipids can be tolerated immediately after birth by VLBW infants. Aggressive early TPN significantly increased positive nitrogen balance and caloric intake, without increasing the risk of metabolic acidosis, hypercholesterolemia, or hypertriglyceridemia.[43,44]

■ NUTRITION IN SPECIAL CIRCUMSTANCES

Critically Sick Neonates in NICU

Enteral feeding is sometime very challenging in critically sick babies such as extreme preterm babies with patent ductus arteriosus (PDA), NEC, with abnormal antenatal Doppler, septicemia, shock requiring vasopressors and inotropes, with medication like steroids, ibuprofen, indomethacin, etc. There is no clear cut feeding guideline in all these babies. But research has shown to adopt a slow advancement of enteral feeding in first 10 days in an extreme premature babies with <29 weeks of GA and those babies with 29–34 weeks with abnormal antenatal Doppler to avoid NEC. Also aggressive nutritional strategy in first week of life in form of TPN in a critically sick baby will improve the long-term neurodevelopmental outcome.

Chronic Lung Disease

Neonates with CLD have higher metabolic needs due to more work of breathing and oxygen dependency. They require fluid restriction to improve pulmonary mechanics. So calorie dense feeding is recommended to optimize the growth. Parenteral nutrition is an option for a patient poorly tolerating enteral feeding.

Cholestatic Liver Disease

Nutritional problems in a cholestatic liver disease are due to increase in energy expenditure and poor nutritional uptake due to intestinal malabsorption of fat and fat-soluble vitamins. Cholestasis associated with prolonged use of parenteral nutrition can be managed by restricting the lipid infusion of 1–2 g/kg/day. It can be prevented by using mixed lipid emulsion composed of soybean oil, medium chain triglyceride, olive oil, and fish oil (SMOF-LE) instead of using soybean oil based lipid emulsion. Diet with sodium restriction is advised in a baby with chronic cholestasis associated edema and ascites. Additional vitamin and mineral supplementation are recommended **(Annexure 6).**[45]

Short Bowel Syndrome

Anatomical shortening of a bowel after surgery makes baby vulnerable for nutritional deficit due to loss of the surface area for the intestinal function and because of physiological dysfunction of an intestine. Prognosis depends on the site and length of a resection. To compensate fluid loss from ostomy site or high stool output, an ultimate goal for fluid and calorie intake should be 150–200 mL/kg/day and 100–140 kcal/kg/day. Enteral feeding should be started as early as possible to improve small bowel adaptation. Establishment of oral feed has an additional benefit of release of salivary epidermal growth factor. So, breastfeeding is preferably given. If not possible, then breast milk via tube feeding is given. Infant formula containing hydrolyzed protein is preferred in selected group of the patient with SBS as it is lactose free and contains MCTs which is easy to digest. Current evidence does not support use of amino-acid based formula. Zinc supplements are often used empirically. Additionally vitamin B12 and fat-soluble vitamins are required in SBS with ileal resection.

Gastroesophageal Reflux and Gastroesophageal Reflux Disease

Frequent regurgitation (GER) with normal weight gain is physiological and common before 2 months age. Gastroesophageal reflux disease (GERD) diagnosis is for significant clinical presentation (frequent nonbilious vomiting episodes with nontender/nondistended abdomen, poor weight gain, and arching of neck or respiratory symptoms). Frequent and small feeding, supervised prone or left lateral positioning, thickening milk feed can help to reduce an episodes of regurgitation. Commercial thickened infant formula in preterms has

risk of NEC. Cow's milk protein allergy can mimic GERD. For a baby with exclusive breastfeeding, mother should be advised to restrict milk and milk products in her own diet and for infant formula consuming baby, hydrolyzed protein formula be tried for 2–4 weeks. On failure of such approaches H2 receptor blockers, proton pump inhibitors, and prokinetics can be tried.[46]

Inborn Errors of Metabolism

Goal is avoidance or controlled intake of dietary precursors of toxic metabolites. Special diet along with macronutrient and micronutrient as per the recommended dietary allowance (RDA) is essential for long-term management of patient with inborn errors of metabolism (IEM). Breastfeeding is contraindicated in a classic galactosemia while breastfeeding along with special protein free diet is recommended in other metabolic disorders. Few IEM like fatty acid oxidation disorder requires avoiding prolonged fasting and a regular glucose supply is needed in glycogen storage disorder. Special diet with low phenylalanine for phenylketonuria (PKU) and low in branched chain amino acids for maple syrup urine disease (MSUD) are commercially available. Protein restricted diet is needed in organic acidemia and urea cycle disorder.

Human Immunodeficiency Virus and Newborn Feeding

The presence of HIV in breast milk and transmission is the main concern surrounding breastfeeding in HIV positive mothers. There is high probability of infant succumbing to infectious diseases and malnutrition in absence of breastfeeding in developing countries. With increasing evidences of significant reduction of transmission by antiretroviral therapy (ART) to mother and child, there is confidence built in continuing breastfeeding by HIV positive mother.

Summary of Recommendations in Neonate by WHO and National AIDS Control Organization[47,48]

- Human immunodeficiency virus-infected mothers or whose status is unknown and whose infants are HIV uninfected or of unknown HIV status or when the infant is living with HIV, exclusive breastfeeding infants for the first 6 months is recommended, then introduce appropriate complementary foods, and continue breastfeeding. Mothers whose status is unknown should be offered HIV testing.

- Human immunodeficiency virus positive mothers with HIV should breastfeed for at least 12 months, and even up to more than 2 years but should be properly supported to ART compliance [lifelong ART is recommended now instead of antiretroviral (ARV) drug prophylaxis]. Although exclusive breastfeeding is recommended, practicing mixed feeding is not a reason to stop breastfeeding in the presence of ARV drugs. When ARV drugs are not immediately available (like in emergencies), breastfeeding may still provide infants born to mothers living with HIV a greater chance of HIV-free survival.
- When the infant is living with HIV, mothers are strongly encouraged to exclusively breastfeed for the first 6 months and continue breastfeeding up to 2 years or beyond. For infant diagnosed HIV positive, ART should be started.
- Duration of breastfeeding should not be restricted where there is provision and adherence support for lifetime ART and support in breastfeeding. Mothers living with HIV and healthcare workers can be reassured that even shorter duration of breastfeeding of less than 12 months is better than never initiating breastfeeding at all.
- Breastfeeding can be stopped gradually over a month once a nutritionally adequate and safe diet without breast milk is provided. Stopping breastfeeding abruptly is not advisable.
- When mothers known to be living with HIV decide to stop breastfeeding at any time (only in situations where breastfeeding cannot be done or on individual parents' informed decision), infants should be provided with safe and adequate replacement feeds to enable normal growth and development. For infants less than 6 months of age alternatives to include (1) infant milk formula if AFASS (acceptable, feasible, affordable, sustainable, and safe) criteria are met but it is expensive and (2) heat-treated expressed breast milk. Home-modified animal milk is not recommended as a replacement food in the first 6 months of life. Heat-treated EBM be considered by mothers known to be living with HIV as an interim feeding strategy in special circumstances, like LBW or ill neonate is unable to breastfeed; the mother is unwell or temporarily unable to breastfeed; to assist mothers in stopping breastfeeding; or if ARV drugs are temporarily not available.
- Bottle-feeding should be strongly discouraged and not practiced at all.
- Do not use leftover milk at the end of a feeding session to refeed the infant.

- Regularly monitor for early detection of nutritional deficiencies, growth faltering, and infection among the infants.
- Avoid non-nutritive or comfort suckling.
- In National AIDS Control Organization (NACO) guidelines there is a mention of advices when wet nursing is pursued, but WHO guidelines do not have it. Neither of these guidelines have mentioned about DHM.

MONITORING OF NUTRITIONAL STATUS

Monitoring of growth of infants should be comprehensive, as recommended for term infants, and include assessments of length, head circumference, weight/length ratio, and, if possible, fat and fat-free mass.

The WHO Multicentre Growth Reference Study Group gives growth velocity tables from birth onwards for newborns 2 kg or more. Preterm postnatal growth standards are available to assess preterm infants until 64 weeks postmenstrual age (6 months corrected age). Beyond that time there is no need for any adjustment with the World Health Organization Child Growth Standards for term newborns. Ninety percent moderate to late preterm infants can be monitored by using the International Fetal and Newborn Growth Consortium for the 21st Century Preterm Postnatal Growth Standards from birth until life at home. The late preterm infants should be monitored for weight every week till 40 weeks postconceptual age or until it is gaining weight regularly adequately.

Average weight gain should average 20–30 g/day, and length and head circumference should increase by an average of 0.5 cm/week. Protein markers of nutritional status (albumin, prealbumin, transferrin, and retinol-binding protein (RBP), hormonal markers (somatomedin C, visfatin, and ghrelin), dual energy X-ray absorptiometry (DEXA) scan, etc. may be used as per need and availability.

There should be proper discharge and follow-up policies.

HUMAN MILK BANKING

Human milk bank is the scientific safe system of counseling and screening donors, collection, pasteurization, storage, and disbursement of human milk. It should include ethical promotion of breastfeeding and human milk without any direct or indirect commercial interests; and follow international code of protection of breastfeeding and law of the land in spirit and action. They are now integral part of Comprehensive Lactation Management Centres (CLMC) in India in public health facilities as a step to make human milk available universally. Presence of human milk bank in NICU improves breastfeeding rates postdischarge and reduces use of formula milks.[29]

Procedures in Human Milk Bank

For detailed description of the processing please refer the standard guidelines.[21,22,24,49] Its basic principles are given below.

- *Counseling*: Donor mothers are generally driven by altruistic motivation and have good family support. Donation is completely voluntary, noncommercial—without any pecuniary or compensatory benefits. A counselor explains potential donors about the use of donated milk, principles of voluntary donation, and the process of donation and processing of milk at the bank. Donors do not have any claim on their donated milk. Necessary consent forms are filled and signed by donors. Usually donors are counseled from well-baby clinics, postnatal wards, and in community. Lactating mothers 3–10 months postdelivery are best donors with maximal outputs. A single donor can contribute over a long period of time by regular visit to bank or transporting breast milk from home to the bank under cold chain. Alternatively, many donors can gather at one place and donate a large amount over a few hours' time in form of a camp by the bank.
- *Screening donor*: Donor and her infant both should be in good health. By filling a checklist of risk factors donors are screened for infective illness, high risk behaviors, medications, drugs of abuse, toxins (e.g. pesticides, mercury, and herbs), etc. Eligible donors are then screened for HIV, hepatitis B virus surface antigen (HBsAg), and venereal disease research laboratory (VDRL) by serologic testing.
- *Collection of milk*: Under supervision and assistance from bank staff hygienic expression of breast milk is done either by pump or manually. Double pumping with hospital grade electric pumps gives better results, but risk of contamination is least with manual expression. Often milk of preterm delivered donors is segregated and used for preterm recipients. Donated milk is kept in earmarked prepasteurization refrigerator till serologic reports are clear. If any donor is found to be positive in serologic testing her donation is discarded, and she is counseled and directed to necessary medical care.
- *Bacterial cultures*: Milk may undergo bacterial cultures before pasteurization and if it does not meet standards it is discarded. For low resource settings this may be avoided as most often the commensals are grown which do not cause any problems. Most of pathogens

are taken care of by pasteurization. Postpasteurization cultures are mandatory and it should be sterile, if any bacterial growth is found then the whole batch is discarded.

- *Pasteurization*: Pasteurization with Holder's method is done at 62.5°C for 30 minutes followed by quick cooling to below 5°C. Milk from multiple donors may be pooled in larger containers before pasteurization. It helps reducing variations in composition from different donors.
- Storage by freezing at below –20°C is done immediately in the same container that was pasteurized. It can be stored up to 6 months.
- Disbursal on prescription of doctor after counseling and consent from recipient infant's parents, on first-in, first-out basis is done. Before use it is thawed hygienically as per protocol.
- Labeling and record keeping meticulously of the whole process is mandatory to ensure safety of the milk and tracing of the donors if needed.

◼ CONCLUSION

Neonatal macro and micro nutrition is crucial for lifelong outcomes. It often demands lots of expertise especially in preterms, growth retarded and critically ill children. Human (Mother's own) milk is undoubtably the first choice. All the health staff including neonatologists should be thoroughly trained in science, practice, promotion and protection of breastfeeding. Also important is nutrition of pregnant and lactating mothers.

◼ REFERENCES

1. Chawanpaiboon S, Vogel JP, Moller AB, et al. Global, regional, and national estimates of levels of preterm birth in 2014: a systematic review and modelling analysis. Lancet Glob Heal. 2019;7(1):e37-46.
2. Fenton TR, Premji SS, Al-Wassia H, et al. Higher versus lower protein intake in formula-fed low birth weight infants. Cochrane Database Syst Rev. 2014;(4):CD003959.
3. Breastfeeding and the Use of Human Milk. Pediatrics. 2012; 129(3):e827-41.
4. WHO. Essential Nutrition Actions: improving maternal, newborn, infant and young child health and nutrition. Geneva, Switzeland: World Health Organization (WHO); 2013.
5. WHO. Acceptable Medical Reasons for Use of Breast-Milk Substitutes. Geneva: World Health Organization; 2009.
6. Butte NF, Lopez-Alarcon MG, Garza C. Nutrient adequacy of exclusive breastfeeding for the term infant during the first six months of life. Geneva: World Health Organization; 2002.
7. Nielsen SB, Reilly JJ, Fewtrell MS, et al. Adequacy of Milk Intake During Exclusive Breastfeeding: A Longitudinal Study. Pediatrics. 2011;128:e907-14.

8. Kramer MS, Kakuma R. Optimal duration of exclusive breast-feeding. Cochrane Database Syst Rev. 2012;8(4):CD003517.

9. Groh-wargo S, Sapsford A. Enteral nutrition support of the preterm infant in the neonatal intensive care unit. Nutr Clin Pract. 2009;24(3):363-76.

10. WHO. SESSION 1, The importance of infant and young child feeding and recommended practices. Infant and Young Child Feeding: Model Chapter for Textbooks for Medical Students and Allied Health Professionals. Geneva: World Health Organization; 2009.

11. Morton SU, Brodsky D. Fetal Physiology and the Transition to Extrauterine Life. Clin Perinatol. 2016;43(3):395-407.

12. de Rooy L, Hawdon J. Nutritional factors that affect the postnatal metabolic adaptation of full-term small- and large-for-gestational-age infants. Pediatrics. 2002;109(3):E42.

13. Nasuf AW, Ojha S, Dorling J. Oropharyngeal colostrum in preventing mortality and morbidity in preterm infants. Cochrane Database Syst Rev. 2018;9:CD011921.

14. Snyder R, Herdt A, Mejias-Cepeda N, et al. Early provision of oropharyngeal colostrum leads to sustained breast milk feedings in preterm infants. Pediatr Neonatol. 2017;58(6): 534-40.

15. Lee J, Kim H-S, Jung YH, et al. Oropharyngeal colostrum administration in extremely premature infants: an RCT. Pediatrics. 2015;135(2):e357-66.

16. Kellams A, Harrel C, Omage S, et al. ABM Clinical Protocol #3: Supplementary Feedings in the Healthy Term Breastfed Neonate, Revised 2017. Breastfeed Med. 2017;12:188-98.

17. Boies EG, Vaucher YE. ABM Clinical Protocol #10: Breastfeeding the Late Preterm (34-36 6/7 Weeks of Gestation) and Early Term Infants (37-38 6/7 Weeks of Gestation), Second Revision 2016. Breastfeed Med. 2016;11:494-500.

18. WHO. Effects of maternal nutrient intake and status on breastmilk composition. Complementary Feeding of Young Children in Developing Countries. Geneva: World Health Organization; 2014. p. 85.

19. World Health Organization. Guidelines on optimal feeding of low birth-weight infants in low-and middle-income countries. Geneva: WHO; 2011.

20. Moro GE, Arslanoglu S, Bertino E, et al. XII. Human Milk in Feeding Premature Infants: Consensus Statement. J Pediatr Gastroenterol Nutr. 2015;61:S16-19.

21. Balmer SE, Williams AF. Guidelines for the establishment and operation of human milk banks in the UK. J Hosp Infect. 1995;31:155-6.

22. Bharadva K, Tiwari S, Mishra S, et al. Human milk banking guidelines. Indian Pediatr. 2014;51(6):469-74.

23. Schanler RJ, Shulman RJ, Lau C. Feeding strategies for premature infants: Beneficial outcomes of feeding fortified human milk versus preterm formula. Pediatrics. 1999;103(6 I):1150-7.

24. Abrams SA, Landers S, Noble LM, et al. Donor human milk for the high- risk infant: Preparation, safety, and usage options in the United States. Pediatrics. 2017;139(1):e20163440.

25. Ganapathy V, Hay JW, Kim JH. Costs of Necrotizing Enterocolitis and Cost-Effectiveness of Exclusively Human Milk-Based Products in Feeding Extremely Premature Infants. Breastfeed Med. 2011;7(1):29-37.

26. Trang S, Zupancic JAF, Unger S, et al. Cost-ffectiveness of supplemental donor milk versus formula for very low birth weight infants. Pediatrics. 2018;141(3):e20170737.

27. Quigley M, Embleton ND, McGuire W. Formula versus donor breast milk for feeding preterm or low birth weight infants. Cochrane database Syst Rev. 2018;6(6):CD002971.

28. Boyd CA, Quigley MA, Brocklehurst P. Donor breast milk versus infant formula for preterm infants: systematic review and meta-analysis. Arch Dis Child Fetal Neonatal Ed. 2007;92(3):F169-75.

29. Arslanoglu S, Corpeleijn W, Moro G, et al. Donor human milk for preterm infants: Current evidence and research directions. J Pediatr Gastroenterol Nutr. 2013;57(4):535-42.

30. Arslanoglu S, Ziegler EE, Moro GE. Donor human milk in preterm infant feeding: Evidence and recommendations. J Perinat Med. 2010;38(4):347-51.

31. Arslanoglu S, Boquien C-Y, King C, et al. Fortification of Human Milk for Preterm Infants: Update and Recommendations of the European Milk Bank Association (EMBA) Working Group on Human Milk Fortification. Front Pediatr. 2019;7:76.

32. Brown JV, Embleton ND, Harding JE, et al. Multi-nutrient fortification of human milk for preterm infants. Cochrane Database Syst Rev. 2016;(5):CD000343.

33. Naidu S. Feeding of low birth weight neonates. J Neonatol. 2008;22(2):123-5.

34. Agostoni C, Buonocore G, Carnielli V, et al. Enteral Nutrient Supply for Preterm Infants: Commentary From the European Society of Paediatric Gastroenterology, Hepatology and Nutrition Committee on Nutrition. J Pediatr Gastroenterol Nutr. 2010;50(1):85-91.

35. Amissah EA, Brown J, Harding JE. Protein supplementation of human milk for promoting growth in preterm infants. Cochrane Database Syst Rev. 2018;(6):CD000433.

36. Sullivan S, Schanler RJ, Kim JH, et al. An exclusively human milk-based diet is associated with a lower rate of necrotizing enterocolitis than a diet of human milk and bovine milk-based products. J Pediatr. 2010;156(4):562-567.e1.

37. Lunde D. Extrauterine Growth Restriction: What Is the Evidence for Better Nutritional Practices in the Neonatal Intensive Care Unit? Newborn Infant Nurs Rev Medscape Pediatr. 2014;14(3):92-8.

38. Oddie SJ, Young L, McGuire W. Slow advancement of enteral feed volumes to prevent necrotising enterocolitis in very low birth weight infants. Cochrane Database Syst Rev. 2017;(8):CD001241.

39. Morgan J, Young L, McGuire W. Delayed introduction of progressive enteral feeds to prevent necrotising enterocolitis in very low birth weight infants. Cochrane Database Syst Rev. 2014;(12):CD001970.

40. Dutta S, Singh B, Chessell L, et al. Guidelines for feeding very low birthweight infants. Nutrients. 2015;7(1):423-42.

41. Ayede A. Achieving optimal feeds for preterm babies, recommendations and realities in practice: Nigerian perspective. Ann Ibadan Postgrad Med. 2011;9(1):1-7.

42. De Curtis M, Rigo J. The nutrition of preterm infants. Early Hum Dev. 2012;88(Suppl 1):S5-7.

43. Wilson DC, Cairns P, Halliday HL, et al. Randomised controlled trial of an aggressive nutritional regimen in sick very low birthweight infants. Arch Dis Child Fetal Neonatal Ed. 1997;77(1):F4-11.

44. Ibrahim HM, Jeroudi MA, Baier RJ, et al. Aggressive early total parental nutrition in low-birth-weight infants. J Perinatol. 2004;24(8):482-6.

45. Koletzko B. Nutritional management in cholestatic liver disease. In: Koletzko B, Bhatia J, Bhutta ZA, Cooper P, Makrides

M, Uauy R, Wang W (Eds). Pediatric Nutrition in Practice, 2nd edition. Basel: Karger Publishers; 2015. pp. 178-81.

46. Denne SC. Neonatal nutrition infant nutrition breastfeeding infant formula gastroesophageal reflux. Pediatr Clin North Am. 2015;62(2):427-38.

47. World Health Organization, UNICEF. Updates on HIV and infant feeding : the duration of breastfeeding, and support from health services to improve feeding practices among mothers living with HIV. Geneva: WHO; 2016. p. 58.

48. NACO. Nutrition Guidelines for HIV-Exposed and Infected Children (0-14 years of age). Ministry of Health & Family Welfare. Goverment of India; 2013. pp. 4-11.

49. Weaver G, Bertino E, Gebauer C, et al. Recommendations for the Establishment and Operation of Human Milk Banks in Europe: A Consensus Statement From the European Milk Bank Association (EMBA). Front Pediatr. 2019;7:53.

50. Eglash A, Simon L, Brodribb W, et al. ABM Clinical Protocol #8: Human Milk Storage Information for Home Use for Full-Term Infants, Revised 2017. Breastfeed Med. 2017;12(7): 390-95.

51. Michaelsen KF. Breastfeeding. In: Koletzko B, Bhatia J, Bhutta ZA, Cooper P, Makrides M, Uauy R, Wang W (Eds). Pediatric Nutrition in Practice, 2nd edition. Basel: Karger Publishers; 2015. pp. 92-6.

52. Kolaček S. Parenteral Nutritional Support. In: Koletzko B, Bhatia J, Bhutta ZA, Cooper P, Makrides M, Uauy R, Wang W (Eds). Pediatric Nutrition in Practice, 2nd edition. Basel: Karger Publishers; 2015. pp. 158-62.

53. Ramirez-Mayans J, Neto UF, Cleghorn G, et al. Global Standard for the Composition of Infant Formula: Recommendations of an ESPGHAN Coordinated International Expert Group. J Pediatr Gastroenterol Nutr. 2005;41(5):584-99.

Annexure 1: Acceptable medical reasons for use of breast milk substitutes.[5]

Infants who should not receive breast milk or any other milk except specialized formula: Infants with classic galactosemia, MSUD, or PKU

Infants for whom breast milk remains the best feeding option but who may need other food in addition to breast milk for a limited period
- VLBW infants <1,500 g or preterm infants <32 weeks of gestation
- Newborn at risk of hypoglycemia if their blood sugar fails to respond to optimal breastfeeding or breast milk feeding. (e.g. preterm, SGA, severe intrapartum hypoxic/ischemic stress, sick, and newborns of diabetic mothers)

Maternal conditions that may justify permanent avoidance of breastfeeding: HIV infection if replacement feeding meets AFASS criteria.

Maternal conditions that may justify temporary avoidance of breastfeeding:
- Severe illness that prevents a mother from caring for her infant.
- HSV-1: Direct contact between lesions on the mother's breasts and the infant's mouth should be avoided until all active lesions have resolved.

Maternal medication:
- Sedating psychotherapeutic drugs, antiepileptic drugs and opioids and their combinations may cause side effects such as drowsiness and respiratory depression and are better avoided if a safer alternative is available;
- Radioactive iodine-131 is better avoided given that safer alternatives are available—a mother can resume breastfeeding about two months after receiving this substance;
- Excessive use of topical iodine or iodophors (e.g. povidone-iodine), especially on open wounds or mucous membranes, can result in thyroid suppression or electrolyte abnormalities in the breastfed infant and should be avoided;
- Cytotoxic chemotherapy requires that a mother stops breastfeeding during therapy.

Maternal conditions during which breastfeeding can still continue, although health problems may be of concern:
- *Breast abscess*: Breastfeeding should continue on the unaffected breast; feeding from the affected breast can resume once treatment has started.
- *Hepatitis B*: Infants should be given hepatitis B vaccine, within the first 48 hours or as soon as possible thereafter.
- Hepatitis C.
- *Mastitis*: If breastfeeding is very painful, milk must be removed by expression to prevent progression of the condition.
- *Tuberculosis*: Mother and baby should be managed according to national tuberculosis guidelines.
- *Substance use*:
    - Maternal use of nicotine, alcohol, ecstasy, amphetamines, cocaine, and related stimulants has been demonstrated to have harmful effects on breastfed babies;
    - Alcohol, opioids, benzodiazepines, and cannabis can cause sedation in both the mother and the baby.

(AFASS: acceptable, feasible, affordable, sustainable, and safe; HIV: human immunodeficiency virus; HSV: herpes simplex virus; MSUD: maple syrup urine disease; PKU: phenylketonuria; SGA: small for gestational age; VLBW: very low birth weight)

Annexure 2: Milk storage guidelines.[50]

Storage location temperature	Maximum recommended storage duration
Room temperature 16–29°C (60–85°F)	4 hours optimal 6–8 hours (under very clean conditions)
Ice packs 15°C (59°F)	24 hours (under very clean conditions)
Refrigerator ~4°C (39.2°F)	4 days optimal 5–8 days (under very clean conditions)
Freezer < −4°C (24.8°F)	6 months optimal 12 months acceptable

Annexure 3: Compositional requirements of infant formula proposed by the ESPGHAN.[53]

Component/unit	Minimum	Maximum
Energy, kcal/100 mL	60	70
Proteins, g/100 kcal		
Cow's milk protein	1.8	3
Soy protein isolates	2.25	3
Hydrolyzed cow's milk protein	1.8	3
Lipid g/100 kcal	4.4	6
Carbohydrates, mg/100 kcal	9	14
Vitamins		
Vitamin A, µg RE/100 kcal	60	180

Contd...

Contd...

Component/unit	Minimum	Maximum
Vitamin D3, µg/100 kcal	1	2.5
Vitamin E, mg/100 kcal	0.5	5
Vitamin K, µg/100 kcal	4	25
Vitamin B12, µg/100 kcal	0.1	0.5
Folic acid, µg/100 kcal	10	50
Thiamin, µg/100 kcal	60	300
Minerals and trace elements		
Iron (formula based on cow's milk protein and protein hydrolysates) mg/100 kcal	0.3	1.3
Iron (formula based on soya protein isolates) mg/100 kcal	0.45	2.0
Calcium, mg/100 kcal	50	140
Phosphorus (formula based on cow's milk protein and protein hydrolysates) mg/100 kcal	25	90
Phosphorus (formula based on soya protein isolates) mg/100 kcal	30	100
Ratio calcium/phosphorus	1:1	2:1
Sodium, mg/100 kcal	20	60
Potassium, mg/100 kcal	60	160
Chloride, mg/100 kcal	50	160
Iodine, µg/100 kcal	10	50
Zinc, mg/100 kcal	0.5	1.5

(ESPGHAN: European Society for Pediatric Gastroenterology Hepatology and Nutrition)

Annexure 4: Human milk versus cow's milk contents (per 100 g)[51]

Components	Mature human milk	Cow's milk
Protein	1.0 g (40% casein)	3.4 g (80% casein)
Fat	3.8 g	3.7 g
Lactose	7.0 g	4.6 g
Minerals	0.2 g	0.8 g
Energy	66 kcal	65 kcal

Annexure 5: Recommended dosages of parenteral nutrition substrate for stable patient.[52]

Category	Total fluid	Energy (kcal/kg)	Amino-acids (g/kg)	Glucose (g/kg)	Lipids (g/kg)	Sodium (mmol/kg)	Potassium (mmol/kg)
Preterm	140–160	110–120	1.5–4	18	Up to 3–4	3–5	2–5
Neonate (1st month)	140–160	90–100	1.5–3	18	Up to 3–4	2–3	1.5–3

Annexure 6: Vitamin and mineral supplementation for infant with cholestasis.[45]

Fat-soluble vitamin	
Vitamin A	10,000–15,000 IU/day as Aquasol A
Vitamin D	5,000–8,000 IU/day as D2
Vitamin E	50–400 IU/day as α-tocopherol aqueous
Vitamin K	2.5–5 mg every other day as Vitamin K1
Water soluble vitamins	2 times the recommended dietary allowance (RDA)
Minerals and trace elements	
Calcium	20–100 mg/kg/day
Phosphorus	25–50 mg/kg/day
Magnesium	1–2 mEq/kg/day
Zinc	1 mg/kg/day

Neonatal Infections in the Tropics

Arvind Shenoi, Uthaya Kumaran

INTRODUCTION

Globally, 2.6 million neonatal deaths are reported per annum in 2016 and not only 99% of these deaths are attributed by developing countries but also three-fourths of them occurring in the initial 7 days of life.[1] Worldwide neonatal sepsis (21%) is one of the major causes of neonatal deaths, the other two being prematurity (34%) and birth asphyxia (24%).[2] Neonatal mortality rate (NMR) in these countries varies widely from 8 to 45 per 1,000 live births with the risk of a child dying within a month is nine times higher in sub-Saharan Africa and South-East Asia than in high income countries. Infections are an important cause of neonatal mortality and this chapter will review bacterial, mycobacterial, viral, and fungal infections in the tropical countries.

DEFINITION OF NEONATAL SEPSIS[3]

Neonatal sepsis literature is rife with various terminologies and in order to have clarity we have adopted the definitions given in **Box 1**.

EPIDEMIOLOGY

Globally, the incidence of neonatal sepsis ranges from 1 to 5 cases per 1,000 live births. It is estimated that 3 million newborns and 1.2 million children suffer from sepsis globally every year. Three out of every 10 deaths due to neonatal sepsis are thought to be caused by resistant pathogens.[4] Clinically diagnosed sepsis is present in 49–170 per 1,000 live births, culture-proven sepsis in 16 per 1,000 live births and neonatal meningitis in 0.8–6.1 per 1,000 live births. Even though case definitions are clear-cut, we do not have exact incidence of probable sepsis, confirmed sepsis, systemic inflammatory response syndrome (SIRS), and septic shock. It is reasonable to conclude that neonates who have succumbed have done so from septic shock. Neonatal sepsis accounts for 21% of neonatal deaths, as confirmed by the Delhi Neonatal Infection Study (DeNIS) study. Data from the DeNIS study suggests that 14.5% of neonates develop sepsis of which 6.2% [95% confidence interval (CI) 5.8–6.6] were culture positive. The risk of mortality in the culture negative sepsis was 8.6%, and in culture positive sepsis was 15.7%.[5]

Mother-to-child transmission of infections is more common with viral than bacterial infections. Vertical transmission of viruses like *Cytomegalovirus* (CMV), rubella, and herpes is well known. Recently Zika virus has shown to cause microcephaly in babies of affected mothers. Human immunodeficiency virus (HIV) infection can spread through placenta, delivery process or breast milk to a neonate.

Maternal colonization with bacteria during delivery, especially genital infections, urinary tract infection (UTI) or any other bacteremia can cause early-onset sepsis (EOS) in neonates. Neonates in developing countries are at an even greater risk for developing EOS because of higher rates of prematurity, intrauterine growth restriction, birth asphyxia, lack of antenatal care, and unhygienic birth practices. Social factors include poverty, illiteracy, harmful traditional practices, lack of sanitation and clean water, and lack of access to medical facilities. Hospital settings in the developing world are a significant source of infections for neonates because healthcare workers in these settings receive inadequate infection control training and often lack the knowledge to identify and treat maternal or neonatal risk factors for nosocomial infection. The incidence, risk factors, and pathogens causing EOS and late-onset sepsis (LOS) in developing versus the developed world have been described in **Table 1**.

> **Box 1:** Definition of SIRS, infection, sepsis, severe sepsis, septic shock, and organ dysfunction.[3]
>
> *SIRS (systemic inflammatory response syndrome)*
> The presence of at least two of the following four criteria, one of which must be abnormal temperature or leukocyte count:
> 1. Core temperature of >38.0°C or <36°C
> 2. Tachycardia, defined as a mean heart rate >2 SD above normal for age in the absence of external stimulus, chronic rugs, or painful stimuli; or otherwise unexplained persistent elevation over a 0.5- to 4-hour time period OR bradycardia, defined as a mean heart rate <10th percentile for age in the absence of β-blocker drugs or congenital heart disease; or otherwise unexplained persistent bradycardia
> 3. Mean respiratory rate >2 SD above normal for age or mechanical ventilation for an acute process not related to underlying neuromuscular disease or the receipt of general anesthesia
> 4. Leukocyte count elevated or depressed for age or >20% immature to total neutrophil ratio or C-reactive protein >10 mg/dL.
>
> *Infection*: A suspected or proven (by positive culture, tissue stain, or polymerase chain reaction test) infection caused by any pathogen OR a clinical syndrome associated with a high probability of infection. Evidence of infection includes positive findings on clinical examination, imaging, or laboratory tests (e.g. white blood cells in a normally sterile body fluid, perforated viscus, chest radiograph consistent with pneumonia, petechial or purpuric rash, or purpura fulminans).
>
> *Sepsis*: Systemic inflammatory response syndrome in the presence of or as a result of suspected or proven infection.
>
> *Severe sepsis*: Sepsis plus one of the following: Cardiovascular organ dysfunction OR acute respiratory distress syndrome OR two or more other organ dysfunctions.
>
> *Septic shock*: Sepsis and cardiovascular organ dysfunction.
>
> *Cardiovascular organ dysfunction*: Despite administration of isotonic intravenous fluid bolus >40 mL/kg in 1 hour (>10 mL/kg in infants less than 32 weeks):
> - Decrease in BP (hypotension) <5th percentile for age or systolic BP >2 SD below normal for age or MAP <30 mm Hg with poor capillary refill time (>4 seconds) OR
> - Need for vasoactive drug to maintain BP in normal range (dopamine >5 mcg/kg/min or dobutamine, or epinephrine at any dose) OR
> - Two of the following:
>   - Unexplained metabolic acidosis: base deficit >5.0 mEq/L
>   - Increased arterial lactate >2 times upper limit of normal
>   - *Oliguria*: Urine output <0.5 mL/kg/hr
>   - *Prolonged capillary refill*: >4 seconds
>   - Core to peripheral temperature gap >3°C.
>
> *Pulmonary dysfunction*:
> - PaO_2/FiO_2 <300 in absence of cyanotic heart disease or pre-existing lung disease (excessive oxygen should be limited to avoid complications including retinopathy of prematurity) OR
> - $PaCO_2$ >65 torr or 20 mm Hg over baseline $PaCO_2$ OR
> - Proven need for >50% FiO_2 to maintain saturation >92% (88% for <32 weeks) OR
> - Need for nonelective invasive or noninvasive mechanical ventilation.
>
> *Neurological dysfunction*: Acute change in mental status.
>
> *Hematological dysfunction*:
> - Platelet count <80,000/mm³ or a decline of 50% in platelet count from highest value recorded over the past 3 days OR
> - International normalized ratio (INR) >2.
>
> *Renal dysfunction*: Serum creatinine >2 times upper limit of normal for age or twofold increase in baseline creatinine.
>
> *Hepatic dysfunction*: Alanine transaminase two times upper limit of normal for age or 50% increase over patient's baseline.
>
> *Probable sepsis*: A small subset of neonates has sterile blood cultures yet has a clinical course consistent with sepsis. In these infants, a clinical diagnosis of probable sepsis can be made based upon clinical assessment; subsequent laboratory tests show positive results, and the clinical course. A complete course of antibiotic therapy is generally warranted in neonates with probable sepsis diagnosis unless an alternative diagnosis is established that explains the findings.

(BP: blood pressure; MAP: mean arterial pressure)

■ ETIOLOGY AND CLINICAL FEATURES

Neonatal Bacterial Infections

Localized infections[6]

Localized infections can arise in any site of traumatized skin. These infections can become systemic when the organism colonizing the infected area enter the bloodstream and can cause septicemia. For well-appearing term-infant, local application of antimicrobials is sufficient while in sick infants or in preterm infants, treatment consists of a full sepsis evaluation and empiric intravenous (IV) antimicrobial therapy. Therapy is guided by the organism identified.

Table 1: Incidence, organisms, and risk factors involved in early-onset sepsis and late-onset sepsis in resource rich and limited countries.[5]

Factors		Early-onset sepsis	Late-onset sepsis
Time of onset		<72 hours of age	>72 hours of age
Incidence	Resource rich countries	• 1/1,000 live births in term infants • 4.4/1,000 live births in preterm	• 1–2/1,000 live births in term infants • *Preterm infants*: – <25 weeks—41% – 25–28 weeks—21% – >29 weeks—10%
	Resource limited countries	Two-thirds of total sepsis	One-third of total sepsis
Causative organisms in resource rich settings		• Group B *Streptococcus* • *Escherichia coli* • Coagulase-negative staphylococci	• Coagulase-negative staphylococci (48%) • *Staphylococcus aureus, Enterococcus* (22%) • Gram negative: *E. coli, Klebsiella, Pseudomonas* (18%) • Fungi (12%)
Causative organisms in resource limited settings		• *Acinetobacter* (22%) • *Klebsiella* (17%) • Coagulase-negative staphylococci (15%) • *E. coli* (12%)	• *Klebsiella* • *E. coli* • *Staphylococcus* species • Fungi
Risk factors		• Febrile illness in the mother with evidence of bacterial infection within 2 weeks prior to delivery • Prolonged rupture of membranes (PROM) >18 hours • Prematurity or low birth weight • Preterm (<37 weeks) premature rupture of membranes (pPROM) • Foul smelling liquor and/or meconium stained liquor • Perinatal asphyxia (Apgar score <4 at 1 minute) • Low birth weight (<2,500 g) or prematurity • Single unclean or >3 sterile vaginal examination(s) during labor • Prolonged labor (sum of 1st and 2nd stage of labor >24 hours)	• Low birth weight • Babies admitted to NICU and undergoing invasive procedures • Prolonged ventilation • Parenteral nutrition through central catheters • Not feeding orally • Admission to inadequately staffed units, poor compliance to unit policy on prevention of infections

(NICU: neonatal intensive care unit)

- *Cellulitis*: It usually occurs at traumatized skin sites: in the scalp at lesions caused by intrapartum fetal monitors, scalp blood gas samples, tissues in penile area due to circumcision, in the extremities at sites of venipuncture or cannulation, and in the umbilical stump. *Staphylococcus aureus* and Gram-negative organisms are commonly implicated.
- *Pustulosis*: Infectious pustulosis usually caused by *S. aureus* is common in the axillae, groin, and periumbilical area, and must be distinguished from the benign neonatal rash erythema toxicum and transient pustular melanosis, all of which have a more generalized distribution. Gram stain of infectious pustules will reveal neutrophils and Gram-positive cocci.
- *Omphalitis*: Omphalitis is characterized by erythema and/or induration of the periumbilical area with purulent discharge from the umbilical stump. Responsible organisms include both Gram-positive and Gram-negative species. Colonization of the umbilical stump by *Clostridium tetani* under conditions of poor hygiene can result in neonatal tetanus (NT) in the infant of an unimmunized mother.
- *Conjunctivitis*: Ophthalmia neonatorum refers to inflammation of the conjunctiva within the first month of life. Causative agents include bacteria *Staphylococci*, *Streptococci*, and Gram-negative organisms; *Neisseria gonorrhoeae*; *Chlamydia trachomatis*; and herpes simplex virus (HSV). Treatment usually involves topical application of antimicrobial for bacterial infections. Gonococcal conjunctivitis is prevented by instilling silver nitrate drops in the conjunctivae of both eyes soon after birth in areas of high prevalence of maternal gonococcal infections. Fortunately, it is not a common illness in our country and routine prophylaxis with silver nitrate drops is not recommended.

EARLY-ONSET SEPSIS

Common pathogens implicated in EOS can be acquired from the maternal genital tract, or horizontal transmission from delivery room or neonatal nursery, or through unhygienic obstetrical procedures carried out in community settings. EOS usually manifests as respiratory distress and pneumonia. Clinical manifestations can range from subtle symptoms to profound septic shock. Signs and symptoms of sepsis are nonspecific and include temperature instability, irritability, lethargy, respiratory distress, poor feeding, tachycardia, poor perfusion, and hypotension. Hence, it is important to identify neonates with risk factors for sepsis and to have a high index of suspicion for sepsis. Multivariate predictive models for risk of EOS have been developed and validated in clinical use, including the EOS calculator which is based on risk factors [e.g. newborn clinical condition, highest intrapartum maternal temperature, maternal group B *Streptococcus* (GBS) status, the administration of maternal intrapartum antibiotic prophylaxis administered at least >4 hours before delivery, gestational age, and duration of rupture of membranes]. The estimated risk of sepsis can be used to help guide decision-making regarding diagnostic evaluation and empiric antibiotic treatment. EOS risk calculators are not valid for preterm infants (<34 weeks gestation), and they do not apply to LOS.[7] In asymptomatic preterm infants with risk factors for EOS, limited evaluation consisting of a blood culture followed by the administration of empiric antibiotic therapy is necessary. A full diagnostic evaluation for EOS includes complete blood count (CBC) with peripheral smear to look for immature neutrophils, toxic granules, immature/total neutrophil ratio (I/T ratio), C-reactive protein (CRP), procalcitonin, blood culture, and lumbar puncture.

C-reactive Protein

C-reactive protein is an acute phase reactant synthesized in the liver that increases in inflammatory conditions, including sepsis. Although an elevated CRP greater than 1 mg/dL is 90% sensitive in detecting neonatal sepsis, its poor specificity makes it a poor predictor for neonatal sepsis, as it is elevated in other noninfectious inflammatory conditions (e.g. maternal fever and fetal distress). CRP levels do not seem to be affected by gestational age, and serial CRPs have been found to be useful to follow resolution of infection and guide antibiotic therapy even in extreme preterm infants.[8]

■ LATE-ONSET SEPSIS

Late-onset sepsis typically presents as septicemia and meningitis. Neonates can present with nonspecific symptoms as mentioned in EOS or a growing preterm can present with feed intolerance, poor weight gain, increase in

ventilator/oxygen requirements, and metabolic acidosis in blood gas. Evaluation involves CBC with peripheral smear, blood culture, lumbar puncture, urine culture, and culture from local sites like tracheal aspirate, purulent discharge from eye or pustules. Treatment is supportive by correction of shock by fluid boluses, inotropes, providing respiratory support, correction of anemia, thrombocytopenia by transfusion of blood products, and initiation of empiric antibiotic therapy.

■ NEONATAL TETANUS (NT)

It is caused by toxin of the bacteria *C. tetani* and is predominantly a disease of poorer developing countries where lack of maternal tetanus immunization, unhygienic birth practices, and poor neonatal care continue to contribute to high rates of disease. World Health Organization (WHO) reported that in 2017, 30,848 newborns died from NT, 85% reduction from the situation in 2000. Currently, 13 countries still have not eliminated maternal and NT. In 2012, NT constituted almost 2% of neonatal death worldwide.[9] Treatment is complicated with intensive care, antitetanus immunoglobulin (Ig), and penicillin therapy. Mortality is extremely high with case fatality rate of 85%. Clean cord care and antenatal tetanus toxoid vaccination have gone a long way in eliminating this disease.

■ NEONATAL TUBERCULOSIS

Neonatal tuberculosis caused by *Mycobacterium tuberculosis* can be either congenital or postnatally acquired. Cantwell diagnostic criteria are described in **Box 2**.[10]

Perinatal transmission of tuberculosis is through endometrial tuberculosis or disseminated disease in mother, hematogenous spread, amniotic fluid aspiration or ingestion of infected secretions. The definitive lesion of congenital tuberculosis is primary complex of liver with caseating granuloma from which the organism spreads to other organs. Uncommonly, primary foci can involve lungs or gastrointestinal (GI) tract from the rupture of placental lesion into the amniotic fluid. Neonatal tuberculosis can involve any organ systems of the body with features of septicemia, persistent or recurrent pneumonia, meningitis,

Box 2: Cantwell diagnostic criteria for congenital tuberculosis.[10]

Proven tuberculosis lesions plus one of the following:
- Tuberculous lesion in a newborn baby in the first week of life
- Primary liver complex or caseating hepatic granulomas
- Maternal genital tract or placental tuberculosis
- Exclusion of postnatal transmission by a thorough investigation of contacts

lymphadenopathy, jaundice, ascites, disseminated intravascular coagulation, otitis media, osteomyelitis or paravertebral abscess.

Culture of tuberculous bacilli from placenta or endometrial curettage along with HIV testing of mother should be done for suspected congenital tuberculosis. In neonates, confirmation of tuberculosis infection is done by testing of acid-fast bacilli smear and cultures from body fluids. Ultrasonography of the liver and the probe-guided biopsy of liver should be considered in case of diagnostic dilemma. Conventional Ziehl–Neelson stain light microscopy techniques, X-ray of chest to look for infiltrates, Mantoux test is routinely done in developing countries. Utility of Mantoux test in neonates is poor due to low reactogenicity and poor helper T-cell responses, a negative Mantoux test does not rule out the disease. Newer methods such as GeneXpert, light-emitting diode (LED) fluorescence microscopy, and Mycobacteria Growth Indicator Tube (MGIT) are effective but are expensive and not easily available in most tropical countries.

Antituberculous treatment (ATT) should be initiated promptly once culture is obtained in a neonate with suspected congenital tuberculosis **(Table 2)**.[11] Mothers who have completed ATT or have received 2 weeks of ATT before delivery are less likely to transmit the disease to their newborn. Infants receiving isoniazid (INH) prophylaxis should receive pyridoxine supplementation. Revised National Tuberculosis Control Program (RNTCP) and Indian Academy of Pediatrics (IAP) recommend Bacillus Calmette–Guérin (BCG) vaccination at birth even for those receiving INH prophylaxis after excluding active tuberculosis infection.

NEONATAL VIRAL INFECTIONS

Fever, rash, or flu-like symptoms during pregnancy in the mother can transmit viral infections vertically, and sometimes horizontally during neonatal period from healthcare workers and family members. Viral infections often present in syndromic manner such as encephalitis, hepatosplenomegaly, and respiratory distress. Viral infections are usually diagnosed by clinical features and serology as viral culture is not widely available. Polymerase chain reaction (PCR)-based detection of viral deoxyribonucleic acid (DNA) or ribonucleic acid (RNA) is a better option to culture, but these tests are expensive.

RUBELLA

Toxic fetal embryopathy, called congenital rubella syndrome **(Box 3)**,[12] abortion or fetal death are the results of maternal rubella infection in pregnancy. The risk of congenital defects, if the rubella affects a pregnant mother, is 85% in the first trimester, 50% if it occurs in 13–16 weeks, and 25% if it occurs in 17–24 weeks. Many of these children on follow-up manifest neurological problems like sensorineural hearing loss (SNHL), autism, and mental retardation. Sentinel surveillance from our country has confirmed the widespread presence of congenital rubella syndrome making a strong case for universal rubella vaccination in India.

Diagnosis depends upon the clinical spectrum and a positive rubella-specific IgM antibody. The virus can be cultured from a throat or nasal swab, or alternatively rubella virus RNA can be detected by PCR. The treatment is essentially symptomatic. The baby must be isolated from other neonates, children, and pregnant women as virus shedding has been documented till 1 year of age.

CYTOMEGALOVIRUS

Cytomegalovirus infections in the newborn can be both congenital and acquired. Only 10% of neonates with congenital CMV manifest features of intrauterine growth restriction, hepatosplenomegaly, conjugated

Table 2: Management of an exposed neonate in perinatal tuberculosis (TB).[11]

Condition	Mother and baby both active TB	Mother—active TB Baby—no disease/skin test positive	Mother—active TB Baby—no disease/no latent infection
Treatment	• Mother—ATT • Baby—ATT • Intensive phase—isoniazid (INH)/ rifampicin (RIF)/pyrazinamide (PZA)/ and either ethambutol (EMB) or amikacin for 2 months • Continuation phase—INH + RIF for 7–10 months	• Mother—ATT • Baby—INH prophylaxis for 9 months	• Mother—ATT • Baby—INH for 3–4 months followed by MTX test. If MTX is negative, stop INH by 3 months. If MTX is positive, search for disease. If the disease is positive then treat as congenital TB, and if no disease, give INH for 9 months
Isolation	Separation avoided; advised if MDR-TB, noncompliant to therapy, the mother has contagious TB before starting ATT		
Barrier method	Face mask		

(ATT: antituberculous treatment; MTX: Mantoux; MDR-TB: multidrug-resistant tuberculosis)

> **Box 3:** Case definitions for congenital rubella syndrome (CRS) surveillance.[12]
>
> *Suspected CRS*: The presence of any of the following conditions in an infant:
> - Structural heart defect [excluding patent ductus arteriosus (PDA)[*] or patent foramen ovale (PFO)[*]] in infants <37 weeks gestational age
> - Hearing impairment[§]
> - *One or more of the following eye signs*: Cataract, microphthalmos, microcornea, congenital glaucoma, and pigmentary retinopathy
> - Maternal history of suspected or confirmed rubella infection during pregnancy
> - Strong clinical suspicion.
>
> *Clinically confirmed CRS*: The detection by a physician of two clinical signs from group A or one from group A and one from group B in an infant:
> - *Group A*: Cataract(s), congenital glaucoma, pigmentary retinopathy, congenital heart defect, or hearing loss
> - *Group B*: Microcephaly, developmental delay, meningoencephalitis, splenomegaly, purpura, radiolucent bone disease, or jaundice with onset within 24 hours after birth.
>
> *Laboratory-confirmed CRS*: The presence in an infant of one condition from group A (above) and one of the following laboratory criteria:
> - Detection of rubella immunoglobulin M (IgM) antibody
> - Sustained detectable rubella immunoglobulin G (IgG) antibody level, as determined on at least two occasions at age 6–12 months, in the absence of receipt of rubella vaccine.
>
> *Congenital rubella infection*: Absence of any clinical signs from group A in an infant with a positive rubella-specific IgM test.
>
> *Clinically compatible case*: Signs or symptoms of CRS in a patient from whom a blood specimen could not be collected.
>
> *Excluded noncase*: A negative serologic result for rubella, irrespective of clinical signs present in an infant.

[*]Confirmed by echocardiography.
[§]Confirmed by auditory brainstem response or auditory steady-state response audiometry.

jaundice, thrombocytopenia, microcephaly, intracranial periventricular calcifications, and retinitis, while others remain asymptomatic. The most common sequelae of congenital CMV is SNHL with 50% of the symptomatic neonates and 15% of asymptomatic neonates developing this on follow-up. Blood transfusion, or infected breast milk ingestion has been described to cause acquired CMV in preterm neonates. Detection of viral DNA by PCR in blood spot confirms congenital CMV, but absence does not rule out the disease. A strongly positive IgM antibody titer in a newborn 14 days of age associated with chorioretinitis or intracranial calcifications is a diagnostic of CMV.

Asymptomatic congenital CMV does not require antiviral treatment currently whereas it is indicated for neonates with symptomatic CMV disease. Oral valganciclovir 16 mg/kg/dose or IV ganciclovir 6 mg/kg/dose given twice daily for 6 months has been shown to improve auditory and neurodevelopmental outcome at 2 years in neonates if started within 1 month of life.[13] Prevention of transmission of CMV by blood transfusion can be done by filtering the blood with leukocyte filters and irradiation. Freezing red cells in glycerol and removal of the buffy coat are the other methods described. Donor human milk can be pasteurized or frozen to decrease the risk of transmitting CMV.

HERPES SIMPLEX VIRUS

The two types of HSV viruses, HSV-1 and HSV-2, are enveloped double-stranded DNA viruses. Modes of transmission include transmission through the maternal genital tract at birth or through ascending infection with intact or ruptured amniotic membranes. The risk of transmission of virus to the fetus is 25–60% when the primary infection occurs in the mother around the time of delivery, while it is only about 2% if there is reactivation of infection acquired during the first two trimesters or earlier.

Clinical features include: (1) disseminated herpes infection—present with involvement of liver, lungs, and brain in about 25% of the cases; (2) localized meningoencephalitis—can occur with or without skin involvement in about 30% of cases; (3) skin, eyes, and mouth (SEM) disease can occur in 45% of cases and about 20% cases of SEM disease may have involvement of eyes or oral mucosa without any skin lesions. Diagnosis is done by PCR of the viral DNA in the cerebrospinal fluid (CSF), blood or from the vesicular fluid. The enzyme-linked immunosorbent assay (ELISA) test for HSV IgM or IgG is not useful as the median time for seroconversion is 21 days.

Treatment of HSV infection is with IV acyclovir 20 mg/kg/dose thrice a day for 14 days for SEM disease or 21 days in case of central nervous system (CNS) or disseminated disease. It is recommended that the CSF PCR be repeated at the end of 21 days of therapy and if positive the parenteral acyclovir therapy continued for 7 more days. Thereafter, oral suppressive therapy for 6 months of acyclovir at 300 mg/m^2/dose administered thrice a day is given to improve the neurodevelopmental outcome and to prevent skin recurrences. Topical 1% trifluridine, 0.1% iododeoxyuridine, or 0.15% ganciclovir, along with parenteral therapy as above should be used for eye disease. Treatment of a baby born to a woman with suspected or proven genital herpes requires the baby to be observed closely for clinical signs. Cultures from the surfaces of conjunctiva, mouth, nasopharynx, and rectum along with blood should be sent for PCR. If these are negative, the baby is discharged home after educating the family about the signs and symptoms of neonatal HSV infection. If the blood or surface PCR is positive, the baby is started on IV acyclovir therapy after collecting blood sample or CSF for HSV PCR and liver function tests. Neonatal HSV disease can be prevented by conducting cesarean section within 4 hours of rupture of membranes.

VARICELLA VIRUS (CHICKENPOX)

Varicella infection in pregnancy can cause severe illness in the mother, fetus (congenital varicella syndrome) or neonate. Mothers who have developed chickenpox in pregnancy need counseling and regular follow-up. The features of this syndrome are microcephaly, cortical atrophy, scarring of skin, microphthalmia, chorioretinitis, and hypoplasia of limbs. The diagnosis is essentially clinical. There is a recommendation to give VZIG (varicella-zoster immune globulin) to exposed pregnant women to prevent congenital varicella syndrome.

Varicella infection acquired in the peripartum period can also affect the neonate. If the mother develops varicella within 5 days prior to 2 days after the delivery, morbidity will be higher as no antibodies will be transferred to the baby. Dose of VZIG advised for these neonates is 62.5 units for those weighing less than 2 kg and 125 units for weight 2 kg or more. If the neonate develops chickenpox in spite of receiving VZIG or if VZIG was not available, IV acyclovir therapy 20 mg/kg/dose 8 hourly for 7–10 days is recommended.[14]

DENGUE VIRUS[15]

Dengue is caused by one of the four related RNA viruses of the genus *Flavivirus*. The incubation period in humans is 3–14 days. Careful evaluation for dengue illness should be done in a neonate with severe sepsis like illness, whose mother has dengue illness around the time of delivery, even if the initial screening came negative. Low viremia at birth can result in false negative result. Neonates can present with shock, thrombocytopenia, pleural effusion, and ascites with the characteristics of hemodynamic instability and capillary leak. Diagnosis is done by detection of the dengue nonstructural protein antigen (NS1) in the baby. Dengue IgM and IgG antibodies can take weeks or months

to develop. Management includes aggressive fluid and vasopressor therapy, with supportive intensive care.

CHIKUNGUNYA

Neonatal infection with chikungunya virus is reported from our country and Reunion Island. The disease is usually vertically transmitted if the mother has viremia around the time of delivery and can present with apnea, fever, and erythematous maculopapular generalized rash which leaves a diffuse perioral hyperpigmentation that may last for a few weeks. Rarely, neonatal encephalitis and white matter injury are also reported in neonatal chikungunya infection. Treatment is mainly supportive as no antivirals are effective.

HEPATITIS B VIRUS

Infection with hepatitis B virus (HBV) occurs mostly during labor and delivery, while, transmission to the fetus in utero is only 2%. If the mother is HBsAg and HBeAg positive, about 90% of the neonates develop chronic hepatitis without immunization. Whereas only 5–20% of newborns will develop chronic infection if she is HBsAg positive and HBeAg negative. The symptoms of perinatal HBV infection are usually mild, though rarely can present as fulminant hepatic failure. The diagnosis is made by detecting elevated levels of HBsAg, HBeAg, and HBV DNA. The treatment is supportive and follow-up is essential to detect chronic carrier state and reactivation of HBV disease. Prevention of HBV vertical transmission by immunization forms the rationale behind disease control (**Table 3**).

ENTEROVIRUS INFECTION

Polioviruses, Coxsackie, *Parechoviruses,* Echoviruses, and *Enterovirus* 71 are the viruses that belong to *Enterovirus* group. Enteroviral infection acquired through horizontal transmission tends to be milder while vertical transmission can be life-threatening. Clinically, an affected neonate can present either asymptomatically or with life-threatening myocarditis (Coxsackie B), hepatitis (Echovirus), encephalitis and white matter injury (*Parechovirus*, Herpesvirus, CMV, rubella, and chikungunya), meningitis or sepsis-like picture (any *Enterovirus*). Generally, the mother can have a viral illness around the time of delivery. Diagnosis is by PCR but the cost of the test is expensive. Treatment is with supportive care.

PARVOVIRUS B19

Parvovirus B19 infection during pregnancy causes hydrops fetalis and spontaneous abortion. Fetal myocarditis due

Table 3: Prevention of hepatitis B vaccine (HBV) infection in a neonate.

Status	HBsAg negative mother	HBsAg positive mother*
Neonates >2 kg	HBV at birth followed by 2nd and 3rd dose at 1–2 months and 6 months	HBV Hepatitis B immunoglobulin (HBIg) both should be given at birth preferably within 12 hours HBV 2nd and 3rd dose at 1–2 months and 6 months
Neonates <2 kg	HBV at birth followed by 3 additional doses at 1, 2–3 months, and 6 months	HBV HBIg both should be given at birth preferably within 12 hours HBV additional doses at 1, 2–3 months, and 6 months

*Anti-HBs and HBsAg titer should be rechecked in infants at 9–18 months.

to maternal parvovirus infection has also been reported. Intrauterine transfusion has been tried for the treatment of hydrops. Prognosis is guarded as in other causes of neonatal nonimmune hydrops.

RESPIRATORY SYNCYTIAL VIRUS, RHINOVIRUS, AND INFLUENZA VIRUS

Respiratory group of viruses includes respiratory syncytial virus (RSV), rhinovirus or influenza infections which may be transmitted to the neonate postnatally. The affected neonates present with apnea, tachypnea, increased oxygen or ventilator requirement, and feeding difficulties for which the treatment is essentially supportive. Nebulized ribavirin and monoclonal antibody palivizumab are mentioned as effective against RSV infection, currently its value and cost-effectiveness are questioned. Neonatal influenza infection has been described during the pandemics of classical as well as the H1N1 viruses. Oseltamivir is used in the treatment of H1N1 infection at a dose of 1 mg/kg × 12 hourly for 5 days. Maternal and staff immunization usually prevents influenza infection in newborn intensive care unit (NICU). Currently, no vaccine is available for other respiratory viruses.

ZIKA VIRUS

Zika virus is *Aedes* mosquito-borne *Flavivirus* and infection with Zika virus causes milder symptoms such as fever, arthralgia, maculopapular rashes, and rarely neurological manifestations in children or adult population. But when a pregnant woman gets infected in any trimester, fetus will be affected resulting in congenital Zika syndrome (CZS). First case of Zika virus related microcephaly was reported in US in 2016.[16] Zika virus is a neurotropic virus that particularly targets neural progenitor cells. The principal clinical features of CZS include severe microcephaly with partially collapsed skull, facial disproportion, marked early hypertonia, hyperreflexia, seizures, irritability, arthrogryposis, thin cerebral cortices with subcortical calcifications, macular scarring and focal pigmentary retinal mottling, and SNHL. Neonates born to mother with Zika virus infection during pregnancy and neonates with clinical features consistent with CZS should be evaluated with viral RNA reverse transcriptase polymerase chain reaction (RT-PCR) in serum, urine or CSF and serum Zika virus IgM ELISA. If both the tests are negative, Zika virus infection is unlikely. Neuroimaging is required for evaluation of brain damage. There is no specific treatment for Zika virus infection and management is supportive.

HUMAN IMMUNODEFICIENCY VIRUS INFECTION

Human immunodeficiency virus infection in the newborn is asymptomatic mostly. Prevention of mother-to-child transmission begins with screening of pregnant women, counseling of safe living, early initiation of antiretroviral therapy if found positive, birth planning, and infant feeding options; postpartum therapy for the mother and baby, followed by early infant diagnosis as per the National AIDS Control Organization (NACO) guidelines **(Flowchart 1)**.[17]

FUNGAL INFECTIONS

Neonatal fungal infections may be surface colonization or invasive fungal infections. Fungal isolation from the blood, CSF, bones, or tissues suggests invasive disease. Risk factors for invasive infections include prolonged antibiotic therapy, especially third generation cephalosporins, prolonged parenteral nutrition, presence of central venous catheter, prolonged ventilation, use of H2 receptor blockers, and abdominal surgery. Bottle feeding and maternal candida infection of the nipple are risk factors for oral thrush in the newborn.

Candida Infections

Infection with candida species occurs either at birth or soon after delivery. Clinical features can be a dermal infection,

Flowchart 1: Components of PPTCT program.[17]

Offer of HIV counseling and testing services to all pregnant women

HIV negative pregnant women
- Safe sex counseling
- Couple counseling
- Linkages to family planning services
- Free condoms
- Behavior change communication for high risk women and partner
- Repeat HIV testing, considering window period if spouse is positive or she have high risk behavior
- Infant feeding and nutrition counseling

HIV infected pregnant women
- Antenatal care (ensure at least four visits)
- Counseling on choices of continuation or medical termination of pregnancy—to undertake within the first 3 months of pregnancy only
- Screening for tuberculosis and other opportunistic infections
- Screening and treatment for sexually transmitted infections
- WHO clinical staging and CD4 testing
- Counseling on positive living, safe delivery, birth planning and infant feeding options
- Couple and safe sex counseling and HIV testing of spouse and other living children
- Linkage to antiretroviral therapy (ART) services
- Provide ART regardless of clinical stage and CD4 count
- Nutrition counseling and linkages to government/other nutrition programs
- Family planning services
- Exclusive breastfeeding reinforcement/infant feeding support through home visits
- Psychosocial support through follow-up counseling, home visits and support groups

HIV exposed infant (HEI)
- Exclusive breastfeeds up to 6 months and continued breastfeeds in addition to complementary feeds after 6 months up to 1 year for early infant diagnosis (EID) negative babies and up to 2 years for EID positive babies who receive pediatric ART
- Postpartum ARV prophylaxis for infant for minimum 6 weeks
- Early infant diagnosis at 6 weeks of age; repeat testing at 6 months, 12 months, and 6 weeks after cessation of breastfeeds
- Cotrimoxazole prophylaxis from 6 weeks of age
- HIV care and pediatric ART for infants and children diagnosed as HIV positive through EID
- Growth and nutrition monitoring
- Immunizations and routine infant care
- Gradual weaning after 6 months and introduction of complementary feeds from 6 months onwards along with continuation of breastfeeding for at least 1 year for adequate growth and development of the child
- Confirmation of HIV status of all babies at 18 months using all three antibody (rapid) tests

(PPTCT: Prevention of Parent-to-Child transmission; HIV: human immunodeficiency virus; WHO: World Health Organization; ARV: antiretroviral)

often present as diaper rash in term neonates or systemic candidiasis, respiratory distress, hepatosplenomegaly, and a fulminant disease with 40% mortality in extremely low birth weight (ELBW) infants. Systemic fungal infection with candida can be congenital or nosocomial. Clinical features include all the signs of sepsis with severe infections presenting with shock, circulatory failure, disseminated abscesses, and multiorgan involvement. All neonates with candidemia should undergo an eye examination, cranial scan, echocardiography, and renal scanning. Renal involvement could present as UTIs, parenchymal candidiasis or fungal ball in the pelvis. Endophthalmitis occurs in 3% of neonates with candidemia. Spontaneous intestinal perforation, which usually mimics necrotizing enterocolitis (NEC), is a complication of intestinal candidiasis and is amenable to treatment with systemic antifungals. CNS involvement includes meningitis and brain abscess which occur in 10–15% and 4% of candidemic patients, respectively. Candida endocarditis is diagnosed in 5% of infants with candidemia. Definitive diagnosis is growth of the fungus in blood and CSF. Molecular methods like PCR, though expensive, are now available in our country which give the diagnosis within 24 hours.

Treatment of candida infections depends on whether the infection is systemic or local **(Table 4)**. Invasive fungal infections are treated with systemic antifungal medications and the removal of indwelling catheters—urinary or intravascular. In case of a urinary fungal ball or fungal endocarditis, surgical resection may be required, if systemic fungal therapy fails. Oral and mucocutaneous candidiasis can be treated with either miconazole gel or oral fluconazole 3 mg/kg for 7 days. Prophylactic antifungal therapy with fluconazole or oral nystatin or miconazole gel reduces the incidence of colonization and invasive fungal infection in very low birth weight (VLBW) infants but no reduction in mortality.[18]

Table 4: Systemic antifungal and preventive measures to reduce invasive fungal infections.

Antifungals	Dose	Spectrum	Drawbacks
Polyenes: • Amphotericin B • Liposomal Amphotericin B (less toxicity)	1–1.5 mg/kg/day OD 5–7 mg/kg/day OD	• All candida except • Candida lusitaniae • Aspergillus • Zygomycetes	• Nephrotoxicity • Hypomagnesemia • Bone marrow depression • Elevated liver enzymes
Triazoles: Fluconazole	Treatment: • 12 mg/kg/day OD • Prophylaxis—3–6 mg/kg/dose twice weekly in high risk • VLBW infants	All candida	Resistance against Candida krusei, Candida glabrata, Candida parapsilosis
Nucleoside analogs: Flucytosine	25–100 mg/kg/day OD	• All candida except • C. krusei	Emergence of resistance if given as monotherapy

Preventive measures to reduce fungal infections in VLBW infants:
• Cesarean section delivery for high risk infants
• Reducing the duration of invasive ventilation
• Appropriate duration of antibiotics
• Less usage of central catheters
• Restricting parenteral nutrition for short duration
• Avoidance of H2 blockers and postnatal corticosteroids

(VLBW: very low birth weight)

■ PARASITIC INFECTIONS

Congenital toxoplasma infection and malaria can present in the neonatal period as the two organisms have been shown to be transmitted vertically.

Toxoplasmosis

Toxoplasma gondii (*T. gondii*) is a coccidian parasite in cats. Humans become infected with *T. gondii* by ingesting food or water contaminated with cat feces or occurs by eating undercooked meat of animals harboring tissue cysts. Vertical transmission of maternal infection with the parasite causes fetal infection which is lowest in the first trimester (14%), increasing to 29% and 59% in the second and third trimesters, respectively. Nevertheless, the severity of the disease falls with increasing gestation. The classic triad of congenital toxoplasmosis includes chorioretinitis, punctate intracranial calcification, and hydrocephalus. Other clinical findings are skin rash, hepatosplenomegaly, and conjugated jaundice. Diagnosis is done by detection of nucleic acid in CSF by PCR techniques and serology with *T. gondii*-specific IgM and IgA. Total duration of treatment is for 1 year **(Box 4)**.

Malaria[19]

Transmission of malaria to a neonate can occur transplacentally, or through blood transfusion, or mosquito bite postnatally. Congenital malaria is often defined as demonstration of the parasite on peripheral smear within 7 days of birth. Clinical features are fever, anemia, jaundice, hepatosplenomegaly, and thrombocytopenia. Treatment of the affected newborn is mainly with chloroquine base 25 mg/kg total dose over 3 days; reports mention use of parenteral quinine, mefloquine, and artesunate in individual cases. Prevention of malaria in pregnancy with antimalarials or insecticide-treated bed nets has been shown to reduce the incidence of severe antenatal anemia, antenatal parasitemia, and perinatal mortality.

■ COMPLICATIONS AND OUTCOMES OF NEONATAL SEPSIS

Neonatal sepsis is associated with increased chances of morbidity and mortality in the affected neonates. Mortality rate was 26% in septic neonates and 48% in case of culture positive sepsis as reported by DeNIS group. Case fatality rate was highest in pseudomonas sepsis (78%) followed by *Escherichia coli* (61%), *Acinetobacter* (59%), *Enterococcus* (59%), and coagulase-negative staphylococci (CoNS) (27%). There was not much difference between EOS and LOS in relation to mortality in contrast to that of developed countries where EOS constitutes 25% and LOS 18%. Multidrug-resistant (MDR) pathogen, defined as resistant to extended spectrum cephalosporins and carbapenems, has become a global issue. In the DeNIS multicenter study, *Acinetobacter* (82%), *Klebsiella* (54%), and *E. coli* (38%) showed an evidence of MDR. Methicillin resistance was detected in CoNS (61%) and *S. aureus* (38%). Death rates

Box 4: Treatment of congenital toxoplasmosis.

Pyrimethamine: 1 mg/kg/dose twice daily for 2 days followed by
1 mg/kg/day once daily from 3 days to 6 months of age, then 1 mg/kg/day thrice weekly till 1 year along with
Sulfadiazine: 50 mg/kg 12 hourly for 1 year
Folinic acid: 10 mg thrice weekly for 1 year
Prednisone therapy: 0.5 mg/kg twice daily is used for high CSF protein or severe chorioretinitis

(CSF: cerebrospinal fluid)

among MDR pathogens were slightly higher than that of sensitive pathogens.[5]

Morbidity associated with neonatal sepsis is also high. Risk factors for increased morbidity include VLBW, Gram-negative or fungal pathogen, need for intubation or vasopressor therapy, renal and cardiac dysfunction, metabolic acidosis, neutropenia, and bleeding. Short-term complications associated with sepsis in preterm includes increased risk of patent ductus arteriosus (PDA), prolonged ventilation, prolonged need for intravascular access, bronchopulmonary dysplasia, NEC, increased duration of hospital stay, and higher health costs. There is a greater risk of neurodevelopmental impairments, either by direct infection of CNS or indirectly through inflammation, including hearing and visual deficits, cerebral palsy, and impaired psychomotor and mental development in ELBW infants.[20]

PNEUMONIA[6]

Incidence of neonatal pneumonia ranges from 0.4 to 12.6 per 1,000 live births in developing countries. EOS often presents as congenital pneumonia, but it is difficult to distinguish from primary respiratory function disorders like transient tachypnea of newborn or respiratory distress syndrome at birth. A careful evaluation including sepsis screen, X-ray of chest, and blood culture will help in arriving at a diagnosis. Ventilator-associated pneumonia (VAP) in neonates who are ventilated for chronic lung disease is challenging to diagnose. Tracheal secretions culture along with the clinical status of the newborn, as well as laboratory and radiographic features is essential for the diagnosis of VAP. Treatment involves supportive care and empirical antibiotic therapy based on the antibiogram of prevailing organisms in the NICU.

URINARY TRACT INFECTION

Bacteremia may cause UTI or it can occur due to primary infection of the urinary tract in neonates with congenital anomalies of the kidney or urinary tract. In industrialized countries, incidence of UTI in febrile infants <3 months is around 7–15%. Term infants develop UTI in second and third week of life and the incidence is <1%, whereas in preterm infants, it is 8% which increased to 13% in ELBW neonates because of their relatively immunocompromised status and invasive devices. In developing countries, 6% of neonatal sepsis is UTI. *E. coli* is the predominant pathogen implicated in term infants diagnosed with UTI in community-acquired settings. In preterm infants with prolonged hospital stay, CoNS and *Klebsiella* are the most common organisms while candida UTI is peculiar to ELBW neonates. Symptoms include fever, poor weight gain, jaundice, vomiting, loose stools, poor feeding, and lethargy. Diagnosis is by suprapubic or catheterized urine routine microscopy and culture. Neonates diagnosed with UTI should undergo complete evaluation including sepsis screening, blood culture, CSF analysis, and renal ultrasonography. After the infection is treated, micturating cystourethrogram (MCU) and renal scintigraphy scanning with Technitium-99 dimercaptosuccinic acetate (DMSA) need to be done. Treatment involves appropriate antibiotic therapy and supportive care. Acute pyelonephritis may result in renal parenchymal scarring, chronic kidney disease, and high risk for hypertension. Antibiotic prophylaxis is advised for infants with renal tract anomalies and severe grades of vesicoureteric reflux.[21]

NECROTIZING ENTEROCOLITIS[22]

Necrotizing enterocolitis is a common GI emergency in neonates and is characterized by ischemic necrosis of the intestinal mucosa. Globally, the incidence of NEC reported among preterm infants <32 weeks is around 2–7% which decreases as the gestation increases. The prevalence of NEC varies geographically and temporally, sometimes occurring in clusters or epidemics with mortality varies between 15% and 30%. Prematurity, PDA, prolonged duration of antibiotic therapy, usage of H2 receptor blocker, and formula feeding increase the risk while orally administered probiotics and early introduction of breast milk feeding protects against the development of NEC. Diagnosis is based on laboratory, radiography, and clinical parameters using Bell's staging criteria. Treatment is supportive, appropriate antibiotic therapy, temporary cessation of feeding, and surgical management, if required.

MENINGITIS

The proportion of meningitis among septic neonates as reported by the DeNIS collaborative group is around 10.3% with the case fatality rate being around 51%.[5] The incidence of neonatal meningitis among studies published from developing countries ranged from 0.8 to 6.1 per 1,000 live births.[23] Neonatal meningitis presents as temperature instability, irritability, hypotonia, poor feeding, seizures, apnea, respiratory distress, and vomiting. Organisms commonly causing meningitis in our country are bacterial—*Acinetobacter*, *Klebsiella*, and CoNS; viral—*Enterovirus*, Herpesvirus, and Arbovirus; Fungal—Candida species and *Aspergillus*. Diagnosis is done by CSF analysis, Gram-staining and culture. Antibacterial therapy for 2–3 weeks is recommended for meningitis caused by bacteria depending on the sensitivity pattern. Antifungal therapy should be continued for 3 weeks after clearance of the fungus from CSF. Neurological complications of neonatal meningitis are cerebral edema (vasogenic and cytotoxic), increased intracranial pressure, ventriculitis, cerebritis, hydrocephalus, brain abscess, cerebral infarction, cerebral venous thrombosis, arterial stroke, and subdural effusion or empyema which may necessitate neurosurgical drainage and prolonged duration of antimicrobial therapy.[6] Neonates with meningitis should be screened weekly for complications and MRI of brain with or without angiography may be required for detailed evaluation of these complications **(Box 5)**.[24]

BONE AND JOINT INFECTIONS

Neonates with sepsis can progress to develop septic arthritis or osteomyelitis. Septic arthritis is infection of joints by bacteria, fungi, or viruses and osteomyelitis involves bone. Risk factors include umbilical vessel catheterization, central venous catheters, femoral vessel blood sampling, prematurity, skin infections or complicated delivery, and UTI. Pathogenesis involves entry of bacteria by hematogenous spread, direct inoculation, or extension of a contiguous focus of infection and the subsequent inflammatory response. Clues to joint/bone involvement include lack of use of the involved extremity, aversion to or discomfort on being handled, positional preferences, and unilateral swelling of the extremity, buttocks, or genitalia. Typical presentation in neonates is that of septicemia, cellulitis, or fever without a focus of infection. Bacterial arthritis usually affects the lower extremity and up to 10% of cases involve more than one joint. Delay in initiation of treatment is associated with long-term damage to bones and joints, particularly when the hip or shoulder joint is involved. *S. aureus* is the most common cause of bacterial arthritis in all age groups. Tubular bones are more frequently involved (femur and tibia constitutes 80%) in osteomyelitis and diagnosis is supported by a combination of clinical features suggestive of bone infection, an imaging study with abnormalities characteristic of osteomyelitis, a positive microbiologic specimen. Effective antimicrobial therapy for 4–6 weeks is recommended for bone and joint infections. In infants <1 month of age, the entire course of antimicrobial therapy should be given parenterally. Surgical intervention involves drainage of joint fluid in arthritis and drainage of subperiosteal and soft tissue abscesses and intramedullary purulence, debridement of contiguous foci of infection, and excision of sequestra in osteomyelitis. Complications of bacterial osteoarticular infections include sepsis, septic shock, deep vein thrombosis, septic pulmonary emboli, avascular necrosis, joint laxity, limited range of motion of the joint, limb-length discrepancy, pathologic fractures, and premature osteoarthritis.

NEONATAL INFECTION CONTROL STRATEGIES IN DEVELOPING COUNTRIES

Clinical features of sepsis in neonates are subtle and nonspecific and difficult to detect in community settings. The young infants clinical signs study group has identified seven clinical signs that has high sensitivity and specificity for detecting serious illness in neonates in primary care settings **(Box 6)**.[25] Recognizing these signs and initiating treatment with oral antibiotics is feasible by a community healthcare worker which reduces the neonatal mortality by 20%. Various intervention measures to reduce the neonatal mortality due to sepsis include antenatal care to the mothers, intrapartum, and postnatal measures **(Box 7)**.[26]

Golden hour breastfeeding within an hour and skin-to-skin contact by Kangaroo care helps to reduce the neonatal infection drastically. Promotion of early enteral feeding with breast milk reduces the need for or length of use of central venous lines and total parenteral nutrition. Essential components of the WHO and United Nations Children's Fund (UNICEF) nIMCI (neonatal integrated management of childhood illness) training program for primary healthcare workers in low resource settings[27] are given in **Box 8**.

Various measures to reduce hospital-acquired infection include hand hygiene, nutrition, and care bundles for prevention of catheter-associated bloodstream infections,

Box 5: Complications of meningitis.[24]

Ventriculitis:
- Inflammation of the ventricular fluid and the ependymal lining of the ventricles
- 20% of neonatal meningitis progress to ventriculitis
- Suspected when a neonate with meningitis not responding to effective antibiotic therapy
- Cranial imaging shows intraventricular strands, echogenic ependymal, and dilated ventricles
- Ventricular tap under neurosurgical guidance helps in relieving the CSF obstruction
- Treatment involves parenteral antimicrobial therapy for 6–8 weeks and can involve direct instillation of antibiotics into ventricles.

Hydrocephalous:
- Occurs in 25% of infants with neonatal meningitis and more common with Gram-negative organisms
- *Clinical findings*: Signs of increased intracranial pressure (ICP) (bradycardia, hypertension, and respiratory depression) and accelerated head growth
- Treatment is by prolonged duration of antibiotics and neurosurgical intervention including CSF diversion procedures.

Brain abscess:
- Occurs in 10% of neonatal meningitis and in 11–19% of patients with Gram-negative bacterial meningitis
- Risk is increased in neonates with meningitis caused by *Citrobacter koseri*, *Serratia marcescens*, *Proteus mirabilis*, and *Cronobacter sakazakii*
- New-onset seizures, prominent focal cerebral signs, or poor clinical response to antibiotic therapy
- CSF pleocytosis with predominance of mononuclear cells and elevated protein
- *Characteristic image findings*: Variably circumscribed region of decreased attenuation and contrast enhancement of the rim
- *Treatment*:
    - Pediatric neurosurgeon consultation for needle aspiration or excision
    - Serial brain imaging at regular intervals to monitor the evolution of the lesion
    - Duration of antibiotic therapy 6–8 weeks depending on the clinical and radiographic response.

Cerebral infarction:
- Neonatal stroke or cerebral infarction includes arterial ischemic stroke and cerebral sinovenous thrombosis
- Occurs in 30–50% of neonatal meningitis
- Tends to occur early within the first week after the diagnosis of meningitis
- Clinical manifestations may include focal seizures and hemiparesis
- Evaluation includes MRI of brain with angiography (MRA) and coagulation studies and echocardiogram
- *Management*: Supportive including adequate oxygenation and ventilation, control seizures, correct dehydration and anemia, and monitor and correct metabolic disturbances and electrolyte disorders
- If infection is suspected, antibiotic treatment should be started until culture results are available.

Subdural effusion:
- Occurs in 11% of neonates with bacterial meningitis and 7–13% of those with Gram-negative meningitis
- Clinical findings subtle include bulging fontanelle, accelerated head growth, or signs of increased ICP
- Most resolve spontaneously
- *Indications for aspiration*: Subdural empyema, imminent development of craniocerebral disproportion, focal neurologic findings, and/or evidence of increased ICP if the findings appear to be related to the effusion.

Chronic complications of meningitis:
- Hydrocephalus, multicystic encephalomalacia, porencephaly and cerebral cortical, and white matter atrophy
- 20–50% of neonates tend to have developmental delay
- Late-onset seizures in approximately 10–20%
- Cerebral palsy in approximately 15–20%
- Hearing loss in approximately 5–10%.

(CSF: cerebrospinal fluid; MRI: magnetic resonance imaging)

Box 6: The young infant clinical signs study group.[25]

- History of difficulty in feeding
- History of convulsions
- Movement only when stimulated
- Respiratory rate R60 breaths per minute
- Severe chest indrawing
- Axillary temperature >37.5°C
- Axillary temperature <35.5°C

antibiotic stewardship, quality improvement projects, and probiotics **(Box 9)**.[28]

■ CONCLUSION

Neonates are an immunocompromised group at risk for infections by a wide variety of microorganisms. These infections are a major cause of neonatal morbidity and mortality in the tropics. Early diagnosis and aggressive therapy is key to reducing mortality. Many complications can occur as nearly all organs can be involved in sepsis. Simple preventive strategies include early and exclusive breastfeeding, kangaroo mother care, and rooming in. Specific infections like hepatitis B and HIV have detailed

Box 7: Interventions to reduce mortality due to neonatal infections in developing countries.[26]

Antenatal care:
- Adequate antenatal care with at least four antenatal visits to a skilled health professional
- Maternal tetanus toxoid vaccination
- Screening and treatment of sexually transmitted diseases (STDs) with treatment of asymptomatic bacteriuria and urinary tract infection
- Educating mothers about importance of clean birth practices
- Improved nutrition.

Intrapartum care:
- Delivery by a skilled birth attendant
- Clean birth practices
- Appropriate management and referral for any complications arising out of delivery
- Clean cord cutting with sterile instruments
- Risk-based administration of intrapartum antibiotics.

Postnatal care:
- Encouragement of early and exclusive breastfeeding
- Hygienic skin and cord care
- Use of chlorhexidine to decrease skin colonization
- Kangaroo mother care, especially for low birth-weight babies
- Training of community healthcare workers to take healthcare to the home.

Box 8: Essential components of the WHO/UNICEF nIMCI training program for primary healthcare workers in low resource settings.[27]

Assessment of child:
- Examining the child and assessing for danger signs
- Checking for feeding problems and low birth weight
- Checking vaccination status.

Classification of illness:
Color-coded triage system used to classify illness according to the need for:
- Urgent referral
- Specific medical treatment and advice
- Simple advice and home-based care.

Identification of specific therapy:
- Algorithm-based identification of specific therapy based on classification of illness
- Essential treatment (e.g. intramuscular antibiotic injections) given before transfer for serious urgent conditions
- First dose of oral antibiotic therapy given in clinic for children requiring therapy at home
- Vaccinations provided according to immunization status.

Counseling:
- Counseling mother about exclusive breastfeeding and any feeding problems with child
- Counseling mother about her own health
- Counseling mother on techniques to keep low-weight infants warm at home
- Teaching caretaker to recognize danger signs and importance of seeking timely care
- Teaching caretaker to give oral drugs and general care for child
- Asking caretaker to return for follow-up at appropriate time.

Follow-up care: Reassess child for any new problems.

(WHO: World Health Organization; UNICEF: United Nations Children's Fund; nIMCI: neonatal integrated management of childhood illness)

Box 9: Preventive measures to reduce hospital-acquired infections.[28]

Hand hygiene—WHO recommendations:
- Wash visibly soiled hands (dirt, blood, or other body fluids) with soap and water
- For all clinical settings in which the hands are not visibly soiled, use an alcohol-based hand rub
- Adherence to hand hygiene before and after direct patient contact
- Jewelry and watches are removed before hand washing and remain off until after contact
- Sleeves of clothing should remain above the elbows during hand hygiene and while caring for patients
- Each patient should have a dedicated stethoscope that is cleaned with alcohol before and after each use
- Use of gloves does not replace the need for hand hygiene
- Do not wear artificial nails, and natural nails should be kept short
- Promote education and feedback from the staff regarding hand hygiene programs
- Monitor healthcare workers hand hygiene adherence and provide feedback on their performance.

Contd...

Contd...

Nutrition:
- Early and exclusive breastfeeding and ensuring proper collection and storage of human milk
- No alteration of hyperalimentation solutions after preparation
- Reduced exposure to intravenous lipids and hyperalimentation
- Kangaroo mother care.

Central line-associated bloodstream infections (CLABSI) care bundles:
- Setting and adhering to institutional guidelines for the insertion and care of indwelling lines
- Use of sterile technique and antiseptic agents at the site during line placement
- Daily monitoring of catheter sites, and redressing and cleaning the site on a weekly basis
- Scrub the hub for 15 seconds while handling any central lines and wait for 30 seconds to 1 minute before any infusion
- Tubing used to infuse dextrose and amino acids should be replaced every 4–7 days
- Catheters should be removed promptly when they are no longer essential because the risk of infection generally increases with time. Optimally, umbilical artery catheters should not be left in place for more than 5 days, umbilical venous catheters should be removed as soon as possible when no longer needed but can be used up to 14 days, if managed aseptically
- Remove and do not replace umbilical artery or venous catheters if any signs of central line-associated bloodstream infection, vascular insufficiency in the lower extremities, or thrombosis are present
- Do not use topical antibiotic ointment or creams on catheter insertion sites because of the potential to promote fungal infections and antimicrobial resistance
- Add low doses of heparin (0.25–1.0 U/mL) to the fluid infused through umbilical arterial catheter.

Antibiotic stewardship:
- *Judicious use of antibiotics in the NICU*:
    – Limiting use to only those situations in which a bacterial infection is likely
    – Discontinuing empirical treatment when a bacterial infection has not been identified
    – Changing the antibiotic agents administered to those with the narrowest spectrum on the basis of susceptibility testing
    – Treating for the appropriate duration.
- Curtailing the use of third-generation cephalosporins and using other antibiotic agents, such as aminoglycosides for empirical therapy, has been associated with less antibiotic resistance, including ESBL-producing organisms
- Good infection-control practices also play a significant role in reducing horizontal transmission of antibiotic-resistant bacteria
- Auditing antimicrobial use of practitioners and providing feedback
- Formulary restriction and preauthorization requirements for selected antimicrobial agents
- Education of prescribers and nurses concerning the role of antimicrobial use and the development of resistance
- Development of clinical guidelines/pathways for selected conditions
- Antimicrobial order forms
- Specific plans for streamlining (broad- to narrow-spectrum antibiotic agents) or deescalating (elimination of redundant or unnecessary) antimicrobial agents
- Dose optimization on the basis of individual characteristics (e.g. weight, renal status, and drug-drug interactions)
- Switching from parenteral to oral antibiotic agents when appropriate and feasible.

Quality improvement: Continued quality improvement focused on increasing healthcare staff awareness and education, establishing common improvement goals, training, environmental care, and setting guidelines for patient care.

Probiotics:[29]
- Probiotics are defined as live nonpathogenic microbial preparations that colonize the intestine
- A 2016 meta-analysis showed probiotics were associated with a small, but statistically significant, reduction in the risk of LOS compared with placebo or no treatment (13.9% vs. 16.3%; RR 0.86, 95% CI 0.78–0.94)
- Concerns and uncertainties regarding appropriate dosing, strain selection, safety, and regulation of these products
- Hence cannot be recommended routinely.

(WHO: World Health Organization; NICU: neonatal intensive care unit; ESBL: extended-spectrum beta-lactamase; LOS: late-onset sepsis; RR: relative risk; CI: confidence interval)

protocols for preventing maternal-to-infant transmission of infections. Viral and fungal infections also occur in neonates and care givers need to be aware of the dangers they pose, be able to diagnose them, and treat as needed.

■ REFERENCES

1. UNICEF. United Nations Inter-agency Group for Child Mortality Estimation (UN IGME); 2019. [online] Available from: https://data.unicef.org/topic/child-survival/neonatal-mortality. [Last accessed on November, 2019].
2. Bang A. Neonatal Resuscitation Capacity Building and Research on its Impact: Need of the Hour. Indian Pediatr. 2019; 56:365-7.
3. Wynn JL, Wong HR. Pathophysiology and Treatment of Septic Shock in Neonates. Clinics in Perinatology. 2010;37(2):439-79.
4. Fleischmann-Struzek C, Goldfarb DM, Schlattmann P, et al. The global burden of paediatric and neonatal sepsis: a systematic review. Lancet Respir Med. 2018;6(3):223-30.

5. Investigators of the Delhi Neonatal Infection Study (DeNIS) collaboration. Characterisation and antimicrobial resistance of sepsis pathogens in neonates born in tertiary care centres in Delhi, India: a cohort study. Lancet Glob Health. 2016;4:e752-60.

6. Puopolo KM. Bacterial and Fungal Infections. In: Eichenwald EC, Hansen AR, Martin C, Stark AR (Eds). Cloherty and Stark's manual of neonatal care, 8th edition. Philadelphia: Wolters Kluwer; 2016. pp. 714-6.

7. Puopolo KM, Draper D, Wi S, et al. Estimating the probability of neonatal early-onset infection on the basis of maternal risk factors. Pediatrics. 2011;128(5):e1155-63.

8. Isayama T. The clinical management and outcomes of extremely preterm infants in Japan: past, present, and future. Transl Pediatr. 2019;8(3):199-211.

9. Lawn JE, Blencowe H, Oza S, et al. Every Newborn: progress, priorities, and potential beyond survival. Lancet. 2014;384(9938):189-205.

10. Cantwell MF, Shehab ZM, Costello AM, et al. Brief report: congenital tuberculosis. N Engl J Med. 1994;330(15):1051-4.

11. Shenoi A, Kavitha HR. Perinatal Tuberculosis. Pediatr Inf Dis. 2019;1(1):30-3.

12. Murhekar M, Bavdekar A, Benakappa A, et al. Sentinel Surveillance for Congenital Rubella Syndrome – India, 2016-2017. MMWR Morb Mortal Wkly Rep. 2018;67:1012-6.

13. Manicklal S, Emery VC, Lazzarotto T, et al. The "silent"; global burden of congenital cytomegalovirus. Clin Microbiol Rev. 2013;26:86-102.

14. Shrim A, Koren G, Yudin MH, et al.; Maternal Fetal Medicine Committee. Management of varicella infection (chickenpox) in pregnancy. J Obstet Gynaecol Can. 2012;34:287-92.

15. Thomas J, Thomas P, George CR. Neonatal dengue. Int J Contemp Pediatr. 2017;4: 2234-6.

16. Moore CA, Staples JE, Dobyns WB, et al. Characterizing the Pattern of Anomalies in Congenital Zika Syndrome for Pediatric Clinicians. JAMA Pediatr. 2017;171(3):288-95.

17. National AIDS control organization. Updated Guidelines for prevention of parent to child transmission (PPTCT) of HIV using multi drug anti-retroviral regimen in India. New Delhi: National AIDS control organization; 2013. [online] Available from: http://www.naco.gov.in/sites/default/files/National_Guidelines_for_PPTCT_0.pdf. [Last accessed on November, 2019].

18. Cleminson J, Austin N, McGuire W. Prophylactic systemic antifungal agents to prevent mortality and morbidity in very low birth weight infants. Cochrane Database Syst Rev. 2015;24(10):CD003850.

19. Singh J, Soni D, Mishra D, et al. Placental and neonatal outcome in maternal malaria. Indian Pediatr. 2014;51:285-8.

20. Bakhuizen SE, de Haan TR, Teune MJ, et al. Meta-analysis shows that infants who have suffered neonatal sepsis face an increased risk of mortality and severe complications. Acta Paediatrica. 2014;103(12):1211-8.

21. Samayam P, Ravi Chander B. Study of urinary tract infection and bacteriuria in neonatal sepsis. Indian J Pediatr. 2012; 79(8): 1033-6.

22. Weitkamp JH, Premkumar MH, Martin CR. Necrotising enterocolitis. In: Eichenwald EC, Hansen AR, Martin C, Stark AR (Eds). Cloherty and Stark's manual of neonatal care, 8th edition. Philadelphia: Wolters Kluwer; 2016. pp. 355-66.

23. Ouchenir L, Renaud C, Khan S, et al. The Epidemiology, Management, and Outcomes of Bacterial Meningitis in Infants. Pediatrics. 2017;140(1):e20170476.

24. Edwards MS, Baker CJ. Bacterial meningitis in the neonate: neurological complications; 2018. [online] Available from: https://www.uptodate.com/contents/bacterial-meningitis-in-the-neonateneurologiccomplications?search=neonatal%20meningitis&source=search_result&selectedTitle=3~32&usage_type=default&display_rank=3#H4. [Last accessed on November, 2019].

25. Young Infants Clinical Signs Study Group. Clinical signs that predict severe illness in children under age 2 months: a multicentre study. Lancet. 2008;371:135-42.

26. Ganatra HA, Stoll BJ, Zaidi AK. International perspective on early-onset neonatal sepsis. Clin Perinatol. 2010;37(2):501-23.

27. WHO. Integrated management of childhood illnesses chart booklet; 2008. [online] Available from: http://whqlibdoc.who.int/publications/2008/9789241597289_eng.pdf. [Last accessed on November, 2019].

28. Polin RA, Denson S, Brady MT; Committee on Fetus and Newborn; Committee on Infectious Diseases. Strategies for prevention of health care-associated infections in the NICU. Pediatrics. 2012;129(4):e1085-93.

29. Rao SC, Athalye-Jape GK, Deshpande GC, et al. Probiotic Supplementation and Late-Onset Sepsis in Preterm Infants: A Meta-analysis. Pediatrics. 2016;137(3):e20153684.

Neonatal Transport

VP Goswami, Ravi Sachan

INDICATIONS FOR NEONATAL TRANSFER

- Refusal to feeds
- Lethargy
- Bleeding
- Hypothermia
- Prematurity
- Low birth weight neonate with feeding difficulty
- Respiratory distress needing respiratory support
- Inborn errors of metabolism
- Congenital anomalies requiring surgical intervention
- Birth asphyxia with hypoxic-ischemic encephalopathy (HIE)
- Hyperbilirubinemia needing exchange transfusion
- Refractory shock, seizures, and hypoglycemia
- Procedures unavailable at referring hospital.

Early identification of a sick neonate, prereferral stabilization, and care during transport are the key to success of neonatal transportation.[1-3]

TYPES OF NEONATAL TRANSFERS

- *Interhospital transfer*: From community to hospital/hospital to other hospital
- *Intrahospital transfer*: Transport within hospital
- Transport for specialized care
- Reverse transport after treatment
- *In utero transfer*: If delivery of a high-risk baby is expected and adequate facility is not available at the primary center, it is always better to transfer in utero.

PREPARATION BEFORE TRANSPORTATION

- *Assessment and stabilization*: Make complete assessment of the baby and make sure that there is a genuine reason for referral. While waiting for the transport team to arrive, the neonatologist responsible should be with the referring hospital staff. Stabilize with respect to temperature, oxygenation, perfusion, and blood sugar (*TOPS*).[4-6] First dose of injection ampicillin and gentamycin should be given before transport.
- *Obtain consent for the transport:* Explain the general condition of the baby, prognosis, and the reasons for transfer of the baby. Take consent for the referral.
- *Write a referral note*: Make a precise note regarding baby's clinical condition, reasons for referral, and treatment given to the baby. All copies of monitoring charts, consents, and radiographs should be given. A sample referral note is given at the end of the chapter **(Annexure 1)**.
- *Encourage mother to accompany*: Mother should be encouraged to accompany the baby for breastfeeding and for providing supportive care to the baby while on the way and in the hospital. If mother is not available, any other relatives should accompany the baby and the transport team.[7] *"Do not forget to take 5 mL of mother's blood sample in a plain vial, if mother is not able to accompany the new born."*
- *Arrange a healthcare provider to accompany*: A doctor, nurse or health worker [Auxiliary nurse midwife/accredited social health activist (ANM/ASHA)] should accompany the baby for en route care and to facilitate transfer.
- *Communication and counseling to the family*: It is one of the most difficult aspect of the neonatal transport. Hospitalization and the need for transport of a newborn can be a crisis for the entire family. All possible efforts should be made for providing emotional support and measure to reduce anxiety of the parents or family. Allow the parents to see and touch their child prior to transport. It should be clearly explained to the parents

where to go and whom to contact. If possible, inform the referral facility beforehand.

- *Vehicle*: The ambulance used for neonatal transport should be equipped with power backup, oxygen supply, etc. It should have proper place for fixation of the transport incubator and secure fastening of the other equipment such as infusion pump and monitoring devices.[7,8]
- *Equipment and drugs*: All the equipment needed for maintaining TABC (thermoneutral environment and to ensure airway, breathing, and circulation) and vital monitoring facility. A glucometer is required to check blood sugar. T-piece resuscitator/continuous positive airway pressure (CPAP)/mechanical ventilator should be available and functional. All the essential emergency drugs including surfactant should be ensured. Prepare all medications and intravenous fluids that may be needed during the transport in advance **(Annexure 2)**.

In order to improve the quality of neonatal transport and outcome, use the following checklist before transport:

- Introduction of transport team to parents
- Communication and counseling of parent (Give the reason for referral and possible complication during transport. Discuss the plan for transport.)
- Maternal history, if available, and maternal blood sample
- Neonatal identification band
- *Documents*: Referral letter and parent's consent for transport
- Neonatal case records, nursing monitoring sheet, etc.
- Secured [endotracheal (ET) tube if intubated] and maintained airway
- Pulse oximeter probe attached to baby for monitoring of oxygenation
- Maintain adequate blood glucose concentration
- Secure IV (intravenous) line for IVF (intravenous fluid) administration, umbilical venous, and arterial access
- Put an orogastric (OG) tube to decompress the stomach (if abdomen is distended)
- First doses of antibiotics and sample of blood cultures bottle, if available
- All the relevant laboratory investigation report, radiograph, etc.
- Address and contact details of parents, referring unit, and referral unit.

ORGANIZATION OF TRANSPORT SERVICES

India has a National Ambulance System (NAS) with dialing facility of 108 under the Janani Shishu Suraksha Karyakaram (JSSK) to transfer both mother and newborn from community to referring unit and back to community after delivery or treatment of the mother and neonate. All the hospitals with maternal and neonatal healthcare services should have facility for neonatal transport. Transport team should have a medical officer/neonatologists who should monitor and facilitate the transport.

- *Transport teams*: A multidisciplinary team is comprised of a neonatologist, neonatal nurse, respiratory therapists, and other supporting team members. Team members should introduce themselves to the staff of the referring hospital and family members. Photo identification should be worn by every team members. The team should coordinate with the referring hospital staff. Allow one parent to travel with the patient as long as all team members agree that the family member will not interfere with medical care.[8,9]
- *Modes of transport*: Every country has their own protocol and guideline regarding neonatal transport services depending upon availability of infrastructure, resources and geographical distances. It mainly includes surface and air transport.[8]
- *Equipment*: The team should be self-sufficient in terms of equipment, medications, and other supplies. The list of the essential equipment is given at the end of the chapter **(Annexure 1)**.
- *Legal issues*: The transport process may raise medicolegal issues, which may vary from country to country. All the protocol and procedures should be strictly followed to avoid any medicolegal issue.

PRINCIPLES OF MANAGEMENT DURING TRANSPORT (EN ROUTE CARE)

- *Stabilization during transport*: Elective intubation is preferable before transport in neonate with respiratory distress, recurrent apnea and abnormal sensorium. If a neonatal transport ventilator is not available, T-piece resuscitator can be used. However, if T-piece resuscitator is also not available, bag and tube ventilation can be provided.
- *Airway, breathing, circulation, and oxygenation*: Maintenance the head in slightly extended position. Clear the mouth and nose if there are any secretions. If the baby develops apnea, give gentle tactile stimulation by flicking the sole or CPAP can be provided.[9] Maintain adequate perfusion by giving judicious use of IVF and ionotropic support if required to maintain the perfusion. Oxygen can be administered to the baby via short binasal prong or via face mask to maintain oxygen saturation (SpO_2) between 90% and 94%. Heated,

humidified and blended gas should be administered to the neonate if the facility is available.

- *Maintain warm chain*: The baby should not be in cold stress. Provide skin-to-skin contact with the mother, if she is accompanying. If not any other family member can provide skin-to-skin care. This is the cost-effective and convenient method to keep the baby warm while on transport.[7] This method is applicable to all the hemodynamically stable neonate. Ensure warm transport by covering the baby with clothes including cap, gloves, and stockings. If the baby passes urine or stool, dry him promptly.
- *Transport incubator*: This is the ideal mode of transport but is often not available. Heating blankets or phase-changing material (PCM) devices can be used as an alternative method for keeping the neonate warm during transport.
- *Provide feeds*: If baby is active, breastfeed should be encouraged if mother is accompanying the baby. Frequent breastfeeding also helps the infant to maintain the body temperature. If the baby is able to feed, but the mother is unable to accompany, alternative feeding method must be used.
- Teams should use mobile phones to maintain contact with the NICU (neonatal intensive care unit) and seek advice for unexpected events.

NEONATE WITH SPECIAL CONDITIONS

- Respiratory distress syndrome (RDS) may require surfactant administration during transport. It is advisable to give surfactant before leaving the facility; however, the transport team should consult the neonatologist before surfactant administration and it should be documented.[10,11]
- A neonate with worsening respiratory distress, CPAP therapy during transport may be considered if the transport team has sufficient clinical experience to CPAP therapy. However, if the neonate is not maintaining oxygen saturation, intubation may be considered to provide mechanical ventilation or PPV.[10]
- Neonate with birth asphyxia needing therapeutic hypothermia: If criteria for therapeutic hypothermia are met, cooling should be started during transport while monitoring the process. Referring unit should have protocol for the same.
- Neonate with pneumothorax may worsen during transport. Therefore, it is suggested to drain the pneumothorax and keep a chest tube in place before departure.

- Infants with congenital diaphragmatic hernia (CDH) require immediate intubation and mechanical ventilation. Placement of a nasogastric tube prevents gaseous distention of herniated viscera during respiratory support.[9]
- *Cyanotic congenital heart disease (CCHD)*: In duct-dependent cyanotic heart disease, prostaglandin E1 (PGE1) should be initiated at the referring hospital and administered through a central venous catheter such as an umbilical venous catheter. ET intubation for transport of an infant requiring PGE1 infusion is warranted because of risk of apnea.[9]
- *Abdominal wall defects*: Both gastroschisis and omphalocele are treated by placing a nasogastric tube and immediately wrapping exposed abdominal contents with warm, sterile, saline-soaked (noncling) gauze. Wrapping with a plastic bag or plastic wrap decreases heat and insensible water losses.
- Tracheoesophageal fistula and esophageal atresia. Tube should be placed gently in the esophageal pouch to minimize the risk of aspiration. Positive-pressure ventilation (PPV) should be avoided in order to avoid over distention of the stomach.
- *Neural tube defects*: Should be wrapped in warm, sterile, saline-soaked noncling gauze and plastic wrap for protection and to minimize heat and fluid loss, as well as to prevent contamination with stool.
- *Neonate on inhaled nitric oxide (iNO)*: Treatment should be continued if transfer to an extracorporeal membrane oxygenation (ECMO) center is required. iNO decreases the need for ECMO in neonate with persistent pulmonary hypertension of the newborn (PPHN) and hypoxemic respiratory failure (HRF). In some cases, it may be appropriate to begin iNO treatment on transport.[9]

REVERSE TRANSPORT AFTER TREATMENT

Neonates who are stable after initial treatment but need further continuation of care, e.g. IV antibiotics or low birth care, can be referred back to the referring facility. A detailed case summary and plan of the treatment should be prepared. Prior information need to be communicated before referring back to the referred facility.

CONCLUSION

Early and safe transport of a neonate has shown improvement in neonatal outcome. The field of transport medicine has grown substantially in the past several decades and will continue to grow and changing.

Development of standards and guidelines will enable to assess the impact of neonatal transport. The role of developing technologies, such as telemedicine, will likely have an increasing presence in referral hospitals as well as for use by transport teams. In addition, there will likely be increasing attention paid to cost and value, especially of high-cost air transport that may lead to stricter criteria and a greater push toward national transport guidelines. Therefore as systems move forward, it is imperative to ensure the highest level of skill and competence both in the transport team and in the facilities that refer and receive these patients be it through team specialization, regionalization of high-level neonatal critical care, or support of telemedicine and outreach initiatives.

■ REFERENCES

1. Saluja S, Mathur NB. Neonatal transferal and transportation: NNF Training module. National Neonatology Forum, New Delhi; 2005.
2. Zodpey S, Paul VK, PHFI, et al. (2014). State of India's Newborn (SOIN) 2014 - A report New Delhi, India: Public Foundation of India, All India of Medical Sciences & Save the Children 2014. [online] Available from: https://www.newbornwhocc. org/SOIN_PRINTED%2014-9-2014.pdf. [Last accessed on December, 2019].
3. Sehgal A, Roy MS, Dubey NK, et al. Factors contributing to outcome in newborn delivered out of hospital and referred to a teaching institution. Indian Pediatr. 2001;38(11):1289-94.
4. Mathur NB, Arora D. Role of TOPS (a simplified assessment of neonatal acute physiology) in predicting mortality in transported neonates. Acta Paediatrica. 2007;96(2):172-5.
5. Daga SR, Daga AS, Dighole RV, et al. Rural neonatal care: Dahanu experience. Indian Pediatrics. 1992;29(2):189-93.
6. Mathur NB. Comprehensive neonatal care in India: Experiences in planning and implementation. Journal of Neonatology. 2006;20:204-5.
7. McCall EM, Alderdice FA, Halliday HL, et al. Interventions to prevent hypothermia at birth in preterm and/or low birthweight infants. Cochrane Database of Syst Rev. 2008;(1):CD004210.
8. Roy MP, Gupta R, Sehgal R. Neonatal transport in India: from public health perspective. Med J DY Patil Vidyapeeth. 2016;9(6:)566-9.
9. Orr RA, Felmet KA, Han Y, et al. Pediatric specialized transport teams are associated with improved outcomes. Pediatrics. 2009;124(1):40-8.
10. Bomont RK, Cheema IU. Use of nasal continuous positive airway pressure during neonatal transfers. Arch Dis Child Fetal Neonatal Ed. 2006;91(12):F85-9.
11. Mildenhall LF, Pavuluri NN, Bowman ED. Safety of synthetic surfactant use before preterm newborn transport. J Paediatr Child Health. 1999;35(6):530-5.

Annexure 1: A common sample referral note.

Date _______________ Time _______________

Address with phone no.: ____

Name _____________________ Mother's name__________________________ Father's name _______________________

Address of the parents with phone no.: ___________________________________

Date of birth: _____________________ Time of birth: _____________________

Sex: _____________________ Mother's blood group (MBG): _____________________

Clinical diagnosis: ____

Birth details:

Mode of delivery: _____________________

Place of delivery: ____

Time of 1st cry: ___________ APGAR 1 min: ___________ 5 min: ___________ 10 min: ___________

Resuscitation details:

 APGAR score: Details of CPAP if required:

Duration of O_2: _____________, Birth weight: ___________ grams

Clinical course:

Feeding well: Yes/No, Breastfeeds: Yes/No, Spoon feeds: Yes/No

Type of feeds: Mother's milk/formula milk/any other milk diluted milk: Yes/No

Passage of Urine: Yes/No Stool: Yes/No

Reason for transfer: Respiratory distress/Not feeding well/Convulsions/Jaundice/Malformation, etc.

Examination findings:

Jaundice Yes/No: ____

Any congenital malformations: ____

Temperature: _________ °C

HR: _________ /min, RR: _________ /min Chest retractions: Yes/No

Central cyanosis: Yes/No CFT < 3 sec/> 3 sec

Receiving oxygen: Yes/No with nasal cannula/Face mask/Oxyhood

SaO_2: _________% Blood sugar: _________ mg%

Time of last feed given:

Investigations with date: ____

Treatment given (Dosages and duration):

____

Place to which being referred: ____

Mode of transport: _____________________ Name of the accompanying person: _____________________

Details of the referral hospital with phone no.: _____________________

Signatures with name of referring doctor Signature of parents/Relatives

Date and Time (Relation with baby)

Phone no. Phone no.

Annexure 2: Equipment required during neonatal transport.

Thermal support equipment and supplies:
- Transport incubator
- Thermometer and/or temperature monitor and probes
- Plastic wrap, insulating blankets, and heat shield

Respiratory support equipment:
- Oxygen cylinders with indicators of line pressure and gas content
- Flow meters, oxygen tubing, and adapters
- Oxygen hood, neonatal size masks, and cannula
- Oxygen analyzer and pulse oximeter
- Neonatal positive-pressure bags
- CPAP machine with appropriate nasal prongs
- Mechanical ventilator with backup circuit
- *Endotracheal (ET) tubes*: 2.5, 3.0, 3.5, and 4.0 mm
- Laryngoscope with size 00, 0 and 1 blades, and extra batteries
- Tape to secure ET tube

Suction equipment:
- Mucus suction trap and suction catheters (5, 6, 8, 10, 12 F)
- Regulated suction with gauge limiting < 100 mm Hg
- Feeding tube (8 Fr) for orogastric decompression
- Sterile gloves and sterile water for irrigation

Monitoring equipment:
- Stethoscope, cardiac monitor, and pulse oximeter
- Glucometer for blood sugar monitoring

Parenteral infusion equipment:
- Intravenous catheters (24 and 26 guaze)
- Syringes (2, 5, 10, 20, and 50 mL)
- Splint and transparent dressings or micropore
- Three way stopcocks
- Intravenous (IV) chamber sets and micro drip sets
- Intravenous administration tubing compatible with infusion pump

Medications:
- Calcium gluconate 10%
- Epinephrine (1:10,000) prefilled syringes, sodium bicarbonate
- Dopamine, dobutamine, morphine, and midazolam
- Normal saline, phenobarbitone, and surfactant

Intrauterine Growth Retardation

Rhishikesh Thakre

DEFINITION

Intrauterine growth retardation (IUGR) is defined as a fetus that fails to reach its intrauterine potential for growth due to a pathologic cause. IUGR is also termed as fetal growth restriction (FGR). Small for gestational age (SGA) is a term used to describe infants whose weight and/or height is less than 10th percentile for gestational age, using gender-specific reference population charts. All IUGR infants are not SGAs and not all SGAs are IUGR. IUGR infants pose a significant burden in low income countries and are vulnerable to sudden fetal demise, neonatal morbidity, mortality, and adult-onset metabolic disorders.

ETIOPATHOGENESIS

Intrauterine growth retardation affects 5–10% of pregnancies. It is the most common cause of premature births and intrapartum asphyxia and second leading cause of perinatal mortality. It is responsible for up to 30% of stillborn infants. The incidence of IUGR varies among countries, populations, and races and increases with decreasing gestational age (up to 50% of very preterm babies are IUGR). Up to 26% neonates born in South Asia are low birth weight (LBW, weight less than 2.5 kg) and 44.5% are SGA, both figures being highest for any region in the world.[1-3]

Fetal growth is a complex process, influenced by multiple factors which are interdependent. Two-thirds of fetal growth occurs in third trimester. Disruption in anabolic hormones—placental, pancreatic, thyroid, adrenal, and pituitary—and gene polymorphism contribute to FGR. For ease of understanding, the causative factors (**Table 1**) are categorized as placental and nonplacental (fetal and maternal). The most common cause of IUGR is placental insufficiency. IUGR is classified based on etiology, severity, and timing of onset (**Box 1**).

The importance of classifying IUGR helps identify distinct phenotypes in terms of placental function and effects on the brain (**Table 2**). Type III IUGR is unique as it is early in onset with superadded placental insufficiency

---

Box 1: Classifying intrauterine growth retardation.

- *Timing on insult*: Early gestation (<32 weeks) and late gestation (>32 weeks)
- *Severity*: Symmetric (type I), asymmetric (type II), and mixed (type III)
- *Etiology*: Placental and nonplacental (materno-fetal)
- *Nutrition*: Stunted (proportionate) and wasted (disproportionate)

Table 1: Etiology of IUGR.

Fetal factors	Uteroplacental factors	Maternal factors
- Chromosomal abnormalities - Genetic syndromes - IU infections - Multiple gestation - Skeletal anomalies - IEM	- Maternal vascular disease - *Abnormal placentation*: Bilobed placenta, low-insertion placenta, chorioangioma, velamentous insertion of the umbilical cord, and presence of a single umbilical artery	- Malnutrition - *Diseases*: Eclampsia, diabetes, chronic disorders, immune mediated disorders, and severe anemia - *Abuse*: Smoking, heroin, alcohol, and cocaine - *Drugs*: Warfarin, antiepileptics, folic acid antagonist, and antineoplastic - *Miscellaneous*: High altitude, stress, depression, and ethnicity

(IUGR: intrauterine growth retardation; IU: intrauterine; IEM: inborn errors of metabolism)

Table 2: Classification of IUGR.

	Type 1 IUGR	Type 2 IUGR	Type 3 IUGR
Incidence	20–30%	70–80%	Variable
Timing	Early (<32 weeks)	Late (>32 weeks)	Variable
Anthropometry	Head, weight, and length decreased	Head spared. Weight and height near normal	Mixed
Pathology	Decrease in cell number	Cell number unaffected Decrease in cell size	Mixed
Fetal hypoxia in utero	+++	+	Variable
Tolerance to hypoxia	High High CVS adaptation	Low Low CVS adaptation	Variable
Prenatal US Doppler	• Estimated fetal weight and/or AC < the 10th percentile • Pulsatility index (PI) of the uterine artery > the 95th percentile • PI of the umbilical artery > the 95th percentile (two out of three)	Estimated fetal weight and/or AC < the 3rd percentile	Variable
Ponderal index	Normal (more than 2)	Low (less than 2)	
Appearance	Weight, HC and length less than 10th percentile, signs of malnutrition less pronounced	Weight less than 10th percentile and HC and length as per gestation age, malnutrition signs predominate	Mixed
HC:CC in term	<3 cm	>3 cm	
Cause	Genetic, chromosomal, and infection	Uteroplacental insufficiency	Mixed
Perinatal mortality	High	Low	Variable
Implication	• Difficult diagnosis • Difficult management • Low risk for asphyxia and hypoglycemia • Poor outcome	• Difficult diagnosis • High risk for asphyxia and hypoglycemia • Guarded outcome	Mixed

(IUGR: intrauterine growth retardation; CVS: cardiovascular system; AC: abdominal circumference; HC: head circumference; CC: chest circumference)

during third trimester. Pathophysiologic processes lead to preterm labor and preterm delivery in severe IUGR.

The key issue in IUGR is in utero hypoxia and diminished nutrition. The insult may be insidious, acute, chronic, acute on chronic, partial, total, or subtotal leading to hypoxemia, ischemia, acidosis, and growth retardation. The degree and severity of insult causes redistribution of blood supply to brain and heart at the cost of other organs. This leads to structural and functional "programing" of all developing organs which defines the clinical spectrum not only during neonatal period but also in adulthood.

CLINICAL ASSESSMENT

Many of the FGR fetuses are not LBW. Hence, relying on weight alone for diagnosis is error prone. Anthropometry (weight, height, and head circumference) is plotted on growth charts to identify growth status. In symmetric SGA infants, weight and height are below the 10th percentile and in asymmetric SGA, weight is less than 10th percentile but height is above the 10th percentile. Majority of SGA infants are asymptomatic. A structured and focused evaluation, anticipation of problems is required for care of these vulnerable infants **(Table 3)**. One of the most overlooked factors is placental examination, both gross and microscopic, which provides clue to cause of IUGR. Over half of those who are SGA have appropriate fetal growth and are constitutionally small.[4]

The spectrum of manifestations of IUGR are time specific **(Table 4)**.

INVESTIGATIONS

There is no gold standard test for diagnosis of IUGR. Prenatal diagnosis is difficult and relies on combination of clinical, ultrasound, and Doppler findings **(Table 5)**. Less than 50% of IUGR infants are diagnosed prenatally.[4]

Table 3: Focused examination.

Gestation and anthropometry	Gestational assessment using Dubowitz chart, plotting weight, and height and head circumference on growth charts which are gestation, gender, and population specific
Appearance	Generalized loss of subcutaneous fat, no buccal fat, large head with thin trunk and limbs, scaphoid abdomen, loose skin folds, long nails, peeling of skin, alert, jittery, large anterior fontanel, meconium staining, and poor breast bud
Growth indices	• Ponderal index (PI) = [Weight (in gram) × 100]/[length (in cm)^3] PI <10th percentile suggests type 1 IUGR and >10th percentile as type 2 IUGR • Midarm/head circumference (MAC/HC) <0.27 in term infant
Dysmorphism	With congenital anomalies suggestive of genetic or chromosomal defect
Parent weight/height	For identifying constitutional small infants
Stigmata of intrauterine infection	Microcephaly, cataract, murmur, hepatosplenomegaly, petechiae, purpura, and chorioretinitis
Thermal instability	Documenting and periodic assessment of temperature. Due to less brown fat and large body surface area
Polycythemia	Plethoric appearance and screening for hematocrit Due to chronic intrauterine hypoxia and increased erythropoiesis stimulated by erythropoietin
Hypoglycemia	Screening at 2 hours of age for glucose and periodically till first 48 hours of age

(IUGR: intrauterine growth retardation)

Table 4: Spectrum of manifestation of IUGR.

Perinatal	At birth	Neonatal period
• Cord prolapse • Placental abruption/infarct • Fetal distress • Meconium aspiration • Stillbirth • Cesarean section	• Hypothermia • Asphyxia • Meconium aspiration • Congenital anomalies	• Hypothermia • Hypoglycemia • Hypocalcemia • Polycythemia • Jaundice • Feed intolerance • Nosocomial sepsis • Congenital malformation • PPHN • ROP • Slow growth

(PPHN: persistent pulmonary hypertension of the newborn; ROP: retinopathy of prematurity; IUGR: intrauterine growth retardation)

Table 5: Identifying IUGR.

Prenatal	Postnatal

• LMP and fundal height
• USG study
  – First trimester (crown rump length)
  – Second/third trimester (weight, height, biparietal diameter, head/abdominal circumference, and femur length)
• Biophysical profile
• Doppler study
	• Gestation and anthropometry
	• Ponderal index
	• Body mass index
	• Midarm circumference/head circumference ratio
	• Clinical assessment of nutrition score

(IUGR: intrauterine growth retardation; LMP: last menstrual period; USG: ultrasonography)

Doppler abnormalities precede biophysical deterioration and are used for determining the frequency of monitoring. Deterioration in Doppler and biophysical profile is an indication for delivery.

Investigations are indicated based on clinical status. All IUGR infants are "at risk" and need to be observed and supervised during first 48 hours of life. Screening for temperature, sugar (2 hours of age and 4–6 hourly till 48 hours of age), and hematocrit (6–12 and 24 hours of age) is indicated in all. Based on clinical manifestations specific investigations are carried out.

■ TREATMENT

There is no specific treatment for IUGR. Care is essentially supportive. The priorities in neonatal care are outlined in **Table 6**. Treatment of common problems is depicted in **Table 7**.

Table 6: Management priorities.

Delivery room	• Resuscitation team • Anticipate asphyxia and meconium aspiration • Ensure thermal care • Search for congenital anomalies
First day	• Use growth charts for plotting weight, height and head circumference, and assess gestation. Determine SGA status using growth charts • Search for congenital anomalies • Anticipate and manage asphyxia, seizures, respiratory distress, thermal instability, and hypoglycemia • Ensure early feeding
NICU stay	Anticipate feed intolerance, jaundice, polycythemia, seizures, respiratory distress, seizures, and sepsis Ensure adequate proteins and calories. Monitor growth
At discharge	Growth pattern, ROP screen, and long-term follow-up plan

(SGA: small for gestational age; NICU: newborn intensive care unit; ROP: retinopathy of prematurity)

Table 7: Management of IUGR problems.

Problem	Diagnosis	Care
Hypothermia	Axillary temperature <36.5°C	Ensure warmth, periodically check temperature, and provide additional heat source
Hypoglycemia	B sugar <45 mg%	Early and supervised feeding, serial glucostix screening, if symptomatic hypoglycemia give a bolus of 2 cc/kg of 10% D, if asymptomatic provide 6–8 mg/kg/min of glucose infusion rate
Hypocalcemia	Serum calcium <9 mg%	Screen for serum calcium by 24 hours of age, calcium gluconate
Polycythemia	Venous hematocrit >65%	Increase fluid intake, ensure hydration, if Hct >70% partial exchange transfusion
Feed intolerance	Gastric residue >20%	Use mother's own milk, standardized feeding regimen, trophic feeds, cautious feed increase, monitor abdominal girth, use of probiotics, and rule out obstruction
Jaundice	Icterus and serum bilirubin (total)	Ensure adequate feeding, hour specific bilirubin estimation, phototherapy, and search for cause
Asphyxia	Low Apgar score at 5 minutes or need for resuscitation at birth	Anticipate, support and maintain temperature, airway, breathing, and circulation. Consider anticonvulsants. Monitor vital parameters, SpO_2, urine output, and perfusion
Respiratory distress	RR >60/min, chest indrawing or grunt	Oxygen, monitor vital parameters, consider CPAP, if unable to maintain SpO_2 consider ventilation, treat the underlying cause
Growth delay	Weight <15 g/kg/day	Monitor growth, adequate calories, proteins, and rule out occult infection
PPHN	Varying SpO_2, refractory hypoxia, upper-lower limb SpO_2 >10%	Sedation, minimal handling, maintain acid–base balance, correct electrolyte imbalance, perfusion and blood pressure. Consider ventilation, sildenafil, and nitric oxide support

(IUGR: intrauterine growth retardation; CPAP: continuous positive airway pressure; PPHN: persistent pulmonary hypertension of the newborn; Hct: hematocrit; RR: relative risk)

■ PREVENTION

At present, there is no specific preventive strategy for IUGR. Several interventions have been identified but few are clinically proven **(Tables 8 and 9)**.

■ FOLLOW-UP

Intrauterine growth retardation infants need long-term follow-up extending to adult life. They are at increased risk for growth and development disorders which emerge during the life span **(Box 2)**. The risk is more with preterm IUGR compared to term IUGR. Excessive weight gain, postnatal head growth, and head size at infancy are predictors for long-term neurodevelopmental outcome. Growth hormone therapy is indicated for growth failure at 2 years of age.

Table 8: Best prenatal practices for prevention of IUGR.

Intervention	Evidence
Balanced energy protein supplementation[5]	Mean birth weight was significantly increased (random-effects MD + 40.96 g, 95% CI 4.66–77.26, Tau = 1744, I^2 = 44%, 11 trials, 5,385 women, moderate-quality evidence); significant reduction in the risk of small for gestational age (RR 0.79, 95% CI 0.69–0.90, I^2 = 16%, seven trials, 4,408 women, moderate-quality evidence).
Intermittent preventive treatment of malaria in pregnancy	Decreased neonatal mortality [RR 0.68 (95% CI: 0.49–0.95)] and LBW [RR 0.71 (95% CI: 0.57–0.89)]
Multiple micronutrient supplementation[6]	Decrease in the number of newborn infants identified as LBW (RR 0.88, 95% CI 0.85–0.91; high-quality evidence) or small-for-gestational age (RR 0.90, 95% CI 0.83–0.97; moderate-quality evidence).
Insecticide-treated nets	Higher mean birthweight (kg) 0.06 (0.02–0.09)
Anti-platelets for preeclampsia[7,8]	About 10% reduction in small for gestational age babies (36 trials, 23,638 women, RR 0.90, 95% CI 0.83–0.98)
Smoking cessation[9]	Increase in mean birth weight by 53.91 g (95% CI 10.44 g to 95.38 g)

(IUGR: intrauterine growth retardation; CI: confidence interval; RR: relative risk; LBW: low birth weight; MD: mean difference)

Table 9: Interventions in practice but with variable benefit for IUGR.

- Bed rest to mother
- Parenteral nutrition to mother
- Calcium supplementation
- Calcium supplementation for hypertension
- Nutritional supplementation to fetus
- Antihypertensive for mild-to-moderate hypertension
- Oxygen therapy
- Prophylactic antibiotic therapy to mother
- Pharmacological therapy to mother including aspirin, beta adrenergic agonist, and atrial natriuretic peptide
- Nitric oxide donor
- Intermittent abdominal compression

(IUGR: intrauterine growth retardation)

Box 2: Follow-up and outcomes of intrauterine growth retardation.[10]

- Plot growth monthly for first 6 months, 2 monthly till 2 years
- Assess development, vision, and hearing at 3, 6, 9, 12, 18, and 24 months
- Assess for behavior and minor developmental issues during school age
- Yearly blood pressure and growth pattern till 5–6th decade

Infancy	Adolescent	Adult
• Short stature • Slow weight gain • Motor delay • Cognitive impairment • Scholastic backwardness • Low IQ • Behavior problems • (ADHD and ASD) • Speech delay • Auditory—visual delay	• Early or delayed puberty • PCOS	• Coronary artery disease • Diabetes/insulin resistance • Dyslipidemia • Obesity • Hypertension • Renal insufficiency • Subfertility • Osteoporosis

(PCOS: polycystic ovary syndrome; IQ: intelligence quotient; ADHD: attention deficit hyperactivity disorder; ASD: autism spectrum disorder)

■ REFERENCES

1. Lee AC, Katz J, Blencowe H, et al. National and regional estimates of term and preterm babies born small for gestational age in 138 low income and middle-income countries in 2010. Lancet Glob Health. 2013;1:e26-36.
2. Lee AC, Kozuki N, Cousens S, et al. Estimates of burden and consequences of infants born small for gestational age in low and middle income countries with INTERGROWTH-21st standard: analysis of CHERG datasets. BMJ. 2017;358:j3677.
3. Kesavan K, Devaskar SU. Intrauterine growth restriction postnatal monitoring and outcomes. Pediatr Clin North Am. 2019;66(2):403-23.
4. Nardozza LM, Caetano AC, Zamarian AC, et al. Fetal growth restriction: current knowledge. Arch Gynecol Obstet. 2017;295:1061-77.
5. Ota E, Hori H, Mori R, et al. Antenatal dietary education and supplementation to increase energy and protein intake. Cochrane Database Syst Rev. 2015;6:CD000032.
6. Haider BA, Bhutta ZA. Multiple-micronutrient supplementation for women during pregnancy. Cochrane Database Syst Rev. 2015;11:CD004905.
7. Jabeen M, Yakoob MY, Imdad A, et al. Impact of interventions to prevent and manage preeclampsia and eclampsia on stillbirths. BMC Public Health. 2011;11(Suppl 3):S6.
8. Duley L, Henderson-Smart DJ, Meher S, et al. Antiplatelet agents for preventing pre-eclampsia and its complications. Cochrane Database Syst Rev. 2007;(2):CD004659.
9. Lumley J, Chamberlain C, Dowswell T, et al. Interventions for promoting smoking cessation during pregnancy. Cochrane Database Syst Rev. 2009;(3):CD001055.
10. Hay WW, Thureen PJ, Anderson MS. Intrauterine growth restriction. NeoReviews June 2001;2(6):e129-38.

Neonatal Critical Care in Resource-Constrained Tropics

Varun K Sharma, Jaikrishan Mittal

INTRODUCTION

India contributes to 20% of global live births. However, due to high neonatal mortality rate (NMR), 25% of world neonatal deaths take place in India. The neonatal age group is the most vulnerable phase of a child's life and the risk of mortality is multiple times higher. In 2016, worldwide 2.6 million babies died during the first 28 days of life while in India this estimate was 0.75 million in 2013.[1] The current NMR in India is 24/1,000 live births as per World Health Organization (WHO) recent data. Other tropical countries also have a higher mortality rate when compared to developed countries. However, countries such as Sri Lanka, Malaysia, and Thailand despite being in tropics have lower NMR. There are striking global inequalities in survival rates for infants born preterm. In low-income settings, mortality for infants born at 32 weeks is about 50%; almost all of these babies survive in high-income countries. These stark disparities are due to a lack of basic and essential care, such as warmth, breastfeeding support, antibiotics, and supplemental oxygen. In low-income countries, more than 90% of extremely preterm babies (<28 weeks) die in the first few days of life.[2]

There has been a lot of focus on neonatal health in the last two decades in order to achieve the Millennium Development Goal of reducing child mortality by 66%. India could reduce child mortality by 62% by various health programs. Now, the new Sustainable Development Goals for the year 2035 targets to reduce NMR to 10/1,000 live births.[3] This is challenging for a resource-limited country like India. The common causes of neonatal mortality in India are prematurity and its related complications, asphyxia, sepsis, and congenital abnormalities. Most of the deaths in the neonatal period occur during the first 7 days of life (75%) of which the first 24 hours is more critical.[4] Neonatal care is a continuum of care, which involves multiple facets of healthcare programs. This will be incomplete if it does not come as a universal package.[1]

The outcome of newborn period depends upon multiple determinants such as adolescent girls' health, reproductive health facilities, maternal health in preconception period, provision of quality antenatal care, obstetric care during intrapartum phase, facilities of neonatal resuscitation at birth, provision of essential newborn care, availability of special care for high-risk babies and sick neonates, referral system for critically ill neonates, and intensive care facilities. Each determinant in this chain is important and healthcare package should focus on every aspect. Every newborn will need the basic newborn essential care but a significant proportion will also need special care or intensive care. In order to reduce NMR below 10/1,000 live births, the healthcare system must provide critical care along with essential newborn care.[5]

NEONATAL CRITICAL CARE IN INDIA

Neonatal critical care is available in both public and private healthcare settings. In a public hospital, the neonatal intensive care unit (NICU) facility is available mostly in medical colleges and attached hospitals. Such NICUs are few in any state; hence, they cannot cater to the entire population. These NICUs face problems such as limited resources, overcrowding, and lack of equipment, consumables, and medicines. With the development of special care neonatal unit (SCNU) in district hospital, some of the sick neonates are being managed in Level II neonatal care.[6] These units have the potential to decrease the burden on Level III neonatal units. There is a need to develop a good referral pathway between these units along with adequate transport services. Many of the neonates are also cared in private NICUs, which lead to out-of-pocket expenditure for the family. These units aim to provide standardized neonatal care. Trained neonatologists along with pediatricians usually provide services in these units. However, some of the units lack expertise, resources, and accreditation.

ROLE OF OBSTETRIC CARE IN IMPROVING NEONATAL OUTCOMES

The two important causes of mortality in neonates are prematurity and birth asphyxia (intrapartum events). The role of obstetrics is very crucial in the management of these conditions. Emergency obstetric facility along with availability of the anesthetist is required in the management of these babies. Studies have shown that neonatal mortality can be decreased if these services are available.[7] Prevention of premature delivery can decrease the burden on healthcare services. Use of antenatal steroids (ANSs) in pregnant mothers for threatened preterm delivery (<35 weeks) is beneficial in reducing mortality, respiratory distress syndrome, intraventricular hemorrhage (IVH), and necrotizing enterocolitis (NEC).[8] Both dexamethasone and betamethasone are easy to administer at minimal cost. Mothers with preterm onset of labor need adequate rest, tocolytics, ANS and timely referral to a center where preterm baby care is available. In an Indian health setting, where most of the deliveries take place in a Primary Health Center (PHC) and Community Health Center (CHC), there should be a facility to transport the baby in utero to district hospitals. For babies less than 30 weeks, Level III NICU with obstetric care facility will be ideal. Referral pathways need to be developed for assistance of health personnel to make prompt decisions in such situations. Ambulance services have been found to be helpful in transfer of high-risk pregnant females but need more community awareness for wide-scale use.[9] Public–private partnership has also played an important role in providing these services with efficacy and cost-effectiveness.[10]

In case a preterm delivery takes place in PHC or CHC, resuscitation or stabilization should be provided by trained staff. Equipment such as Ambu bag, face mask, and oxygen cylinder come at minimal cost and should be provided at all levels of healthcare where birthing facilities are available. Nurses can be trained to provide stimulation, warmth (use of cap, skin-to-skin contact with mother, or plastic bags), and free-flow oxygen. Facilities should be provided to transfer preterm babies to nearby special newborn care units (SNCUs). Maintaining normothermia is crucial in maintaining good outcomes for preterm babies. A neonatal transport incubator is ideal but in cost-constrained settings, Embrace Nest™ can be very useful.

In case the mother is stable, both mother and baby can be transferred together by providing skin-to-skin [kangaroo mother care (KMC)] contact enroute.[11]

Perinatal asphyxia (intrapartum events, poor perinatal adaptation) is the second most common cause of mortality. Birth asphyxia can be prevented by providing good monitoring during the process of labor.[12] Timely detection of fetal distress can help in early referral to a distant hospital where specialized obstetric care is available and prevent hypoxic-ischemic encephalopathy (HIE). Provision of emergency lower segment cesarean section instrumental delivery, and blood bank facility (antepartum hemorrhage) is needed at a district hospital to tackle such a condition. As per literature, only 10% of the babies need neonatal resuscitation. Ninety percent of these cases will respond to either stimulation or positive-pressure ventilation.[13] Nursing staff should be trained as per Neonatal Resuscitation Programs (NRPs) and basic equipment should be provided to prevent asphyxia. These interventions have the potential to decrease complications associated with birth asphyxia.[14] The concept of Newborn Corner has been emphasized in the current concept of newborn care. This is a place where the baby can receive warmth and resuscitation if needed. A trained auxiliary nurse midwife should be present at all deliveries.[15] She should be trained to identify babies who will need further postresuscitation care and referral to SNCU.

Improving Level II Neonatal Critical Care

In India, Level II neonatal care mainly comprises management of babies 1,200–1,800 g, 30–34 weeks gestation, sick neonates ≥1,800 g with birth asphyxia, meconium aspiration syndrome, jaundice, sepsis and need of tube feeding for nutrition and growth.[15] This is being made available in a district hospital or private NICU managed by the pediatrician (private health professional). In order to set up SCNU, adequate investment and resources are required. This has been appropriately highlighted in an article by Prinja et al.[16] The overall cost of SCNU care would be 20.4 billion rupees which amounts to 0.8% of Indian healthcare spending. Looking into the possible impact on improvement in neonatal care by these facilities, this amount is worth investing. However, the resources need judicious utilization for babies who actually need it.

Neonatal critical care can be improved by providing good-quality Level II neonatal care. Emphasis should be given on the development of teaching aids and protocol formulation for appropriate management of sick babies.[17]

Recently, there has been emphasis on delivery room management of preterm babies. Babies born more than 30 weeks of gestation can be easily stabilized in SCNU if appropriate care is provided right from birth.[18] Continuous positive airway pressure (CPAP) has become standard of care in the respiratory support of preterm babies. If adequate positive end expiratory pressure (PEEP) is provided right from birth, requirement of invasive ventilation and surfactant administration can be easily reduced even in cases of extreme preterm babies. Standard delivery room practice includes delayed cord clamping for 60 seconds, use of plastic bag and head cap, adequate PEEP by face mask and Neopuff™-like equipment, monitoring of SpO_2 by pulse oximeter, and temperature maintenance by radiant warmer.[19] All these interventions are of less cost when compared to providing invasive ventilation and surfactant therapy. This will improve good outcomes in preterm babies. SCNU can manage these babies at their own unit, hence decreasing the referral to tertiary care centers. Additional cost of transport (on both ambulance and staff) can be saved.

Once preterm babies are stabilized and admitted in SCNU, focus should be on prevention of infection and providing nutritional support. Babies >30 weeks of gestation or >1,200 g can be easily managed on expressed breast milk (EBM) via tube feeding. The duration of intravenous fluids can be decreased by having standard feeding regimens as per weight of the babies. Formula feed should be avoided as far as possible. Storage of EBM needs a dedicated refrigerator. Nursing staff should be educated on the importance of EBM. Lactation support to mother can be provided by a nurse or dietician. This will help in prevention of NEC in babies and hospital-acquired infection in preterm babies.[20]

Infection Control in Neonatal Critical Care

The most common cause of death and complication in preterm neonates is infection/sepsis. Units should practice evidence-based intervention for reduction of healthcare-associated infections (HAIs). Most common HAIs are bloodstream-related infections, ventilator-associated pneumonia, and sepsis.[21] Emphasis should be given on hygiene (handwash and hand rub), environmental cleaning, contact precaution, judicious use of antibiotics (antibiotics stewardship program), and safe injection practices.[22] Neonatal sepsis leads to increased usage of intravenous antibiotics, prolonged hospitalization, and increased comorbidities. This puts extra burden on health resources. Hence, adequate investment and importance should be given to prevention of infection. Handwashing

facility should be available at the entrance of NICU. An adequate-sized sink and elbow-operated tap are needed. A nonmedicated liquid soap dispenser should be fixed on the wall besides the sink and supply should be maintained. All health professionals and visitors should compulsorily wash their hands before entry in NICU. Display of poster (WHO) of handwashing steps along with regular monitoring and motivation of the staff can help in improvement of hand hygiene compliance. Before handwash, sleeves should be rolled and any ornaments (rings/bangles) should be removed. Cultural factors should be taken into consideration. Education can play a vital role in implementation of proper hand hygiene practices.[23] Cap, mask, and gown are not proven to decrease infection in NICU and hence undue emphasis on this can reduce hand hygiene rates. Visitors or staff with upper respiratory infections should not be allowed in NICU. Environmental cleaning is the responsibility of both nursing staff and housekeeping staff. Nursing staff should clean the warmer, monitor, and immediate surroundings of the baby with soap and water in each shift. Housekeeping staff should focus on cleaning floors, wall, sinks, and doors twice or thrice a day by wet mopping. An adequate checklist should be maintained to improve compliance. Neonates with sepsis can spread infections to other babies. Gram-negative infections usually occur by contaminated hands of health staff. Cross-contamination can be reduced by contact precaution (clean gloves and gown), nurse allocation (one nurse can see only the infected babies), isolation of infected neonates, disinfection of personal equipment of the baby, and proper disposal of biomedical waste.[22]

Temperature Maintenance in a Neonatal Intensive Care Unit

Hypothermia in newborns is associated with increased morbidity and mortality, especially in premature babies. As compared to term babies, premature babies have less subcutaneous fat, lack nonshivering thermogenesis, poor vasomotor control, larger skin surface area, and immature skin with minimal stratum corneum, which predisposes them to the risk of hypothermia.

As per the WHO, hypothermia in newborns is defined as axillary temperature <36.5°C. Temperature between 36.0°C and 36.5°C is cold stress (mild hypothermia), 32.0°C and –36.0°C is moderate hypothermia, and <32.0°C is severe hypothermia. Moderate and severe hypothermia are associated with increased risk of IVH, worsening respiratory distress, hypoglycemia, metabolic acidosis, NEC, late-onset sepsis, and mortality.[24]

The WHO recognizes newborn thermal care as a critical and essential component of essential newborn care. Various methods have shown to be efficacious in preventing neonatal hypothermia. For this purpose, 10 interlinked steps in the form of warm chain have been introduced, which can be easily practiced in resource-limited settings and carried out from birth and later to prevent hypothermia. These include maintaining delivery room temperature at 25°C at least (as recommended by the WHO),[25] drying the baby immediately after birth and wrapping in warm linen, providing skin-to-skin care contact, and initiating early breastfeeding. There should be warm transportation from the delivery room to NICU by using a transport incubator or in case it is unavailable we can use plastic wrap or Ziploc bags immediately after birth before drying.[26] The latest NRP guidelines also suggest the potential use of polyethylene bags or a portable warming pad on maintaining temperature in preterm infants.[27] Training and awareness of staff involved in newborn care about euthermia and its maintenance is also one of the most cost-effective and crucial approaches for hypothermia prevention. Babies in NICU can be kept warm by keeping them under a radiant warmer or inside an incubator or by providing KMC. In case the radiant warmer or incubator is not available, the nursery can be kept warm.

Safe Oxygen Therapy in Neonates

Oxygen is one of the commonly used therapies in neonates as they are prone to respiratory compromise either during or after birth. The aim of oxygen therapy is to achieve adequate tissue oxygenation, but one must monitor the oxygen delivery to prevent oxygen toxicity and oxidative stress. Pulse oximetry provides a safe, accurate, and noninvasive adjunct to the assessment of tissue oxygenation. Oxygen saturation is determined by infrared spectrometry, utilizing two electrodes and a small cuff that can be placed around a hand, foot, or toe without requiring heating or calibration. There is controversy regarding the acceptable level of SpO_2. Many studies have looked into this issue of targeting "low" oxygen saturation range of 85–89% versus "high" range of 91–95% in preterm infants.[28] Evidence available from some of these trials showed that targeting oxygen saturation range of 91–95%, compared to 85–89%, reduces the risk of mortality but increases the risk of severe retinopathy of prematurity (ROP).[29,30] Hence, in preterm neonates SpO_2 should be targeted in between 90% and 95% while in term neonates, it should be above 95%. Pulse oximeter should be made available of newborn care for safe delivery of oxygen despite the cost being involved in purchase and maintenance of this equipment. Reusable SpO_2 probe should be used to decrease the ongoing cost. Care should be taken in using the probe and teaching aids should be used to decrease its maintenance cost.

Safe Administration of Intravenous Fluids

Intravenous fluids are most commonly administered through intravenous cannulae inserted by trained medical or nursing staff. They require careful monitoring of the insertion site for signs of extravasation, safe injection practices for prevention of bloodstream infections as well as meticulous monitoring of fluid intake and output.[31] Sick neonates usually need monitoring of electrolytes and urine output along with daily weight. Fluid overload can increase the risk of NEC, bronchopulmonary dysplasia, and respiratory or cardiac overload. Newborns are at particularly high risk for extravasation because of their immature and fragile skin as well as the small diameter of their peripheral veins. Therefore, inadvertent continuous infusion increases the risk for extravasation. Along with lengthy hospitalizations and multiple medical treatments, NICU patients are highly susceptible to complications from therapy, and otherwise minor injuries can lead to severe morbidities when experienced by the NICU population.[32] The Association of Women's Health, Obstetric and Neonatal Nurses published an evidence-based clinical practice guideline for neonatal skin care in 2001.[33] The guidelines included some of the interventions such as use of IV cannula plastic/silicone catheters instead of steel needles, avoiding areas difficult to immobilize, especially near areas of flexion; securing IV devices with transparent adhesive dressing so that the insertion site is clearly visible; appropriate documentation, at least hourly inspection; and stopping the infusion immediately if any signs of extravasation.

Nasogastric Tube Feeding

Developmental immaturity of the preterm newborn (especially those born before 34 weeks gestation), or severe illness in a more mature neonate, may limit their ability to coordinate sucking and swallowing required for successful exclusive breastfeeding. In these instances, intragastric feeding is a commonly used low-tech intervention to deliver nutrition, using EBM where possible.[17] Enteral nutrition can reduce the need of intravenous fluids and the risk of infection and cannula extravasation. Nurses should be trained to identify feed intolerance in baby on tube feeding. The usual signs are vomiting, pre-feed gastric aspirates, abdominal distension, altered gastric aspirates, or blood in stools.[34]

Kangaroo Mother Care

Kangaroo mother care is an evidence-based, cost-effective approach for reducing mortality and morbidity in preterm infants. Overall, it is estimated that 15–20% of all births worldwide are low birth weight (LBW), representing more than 20 million births a year, the great majority of them being reported in low- and middle-income countries (WHO 2014).[35] As per WHO recommendation, "Newborns weighing 2,000 g or less at birth should be provided as close to continuous Kangaroo mother care as possible and intermittent KMC if continuous Kangaroo mother care is not possible."[36]

Kangaroo mother care is care of preterm infants carried skin to skin with the mother or care giver. It includes early, continuous, and prolonged skin-to-skin contact between the mother and the baby along with exclusive breastfeeding (ideally). KMC can be given to all LBW babies who are hemodynamically stable. KMC can be given by any member of family including mother, father, and other members. It can easily be practiced in hospital and at home with family support to mother and maintaining good hygiene. KMC is provided by mothers using front-open gown and by placing the baby between the mother's breasts in an upright position with the cap and nappy put on. Turn the head to the side, in a slightly extended position. This is to keep the airway open. It also allows eye-to-eye contact between mother and baby. Secure the baby with a binder or wrap. The top of the binder should be at the baby's ear. There are many benefits of KMC to baby which include better growth potentials, better growth of head circumferences, less chances of severe infection, and less mortality rates.[37] The baby who receives KMC has better weight gain, greater breastfeeding rates, lesser hypothermia, lower apnea, and higher oxygen saturations.[38] Mothers are less stressed during kangaroo care as compared with a baby kept in an incubator. They report a stronger bonding with the baby, increased confidence, and a deep satisfaction that they were able to do something special for their babies. Many studies have shown easy acceptability and feasibility of KMC in resource-limited settings. KMC is associated with significant cost savings as well as better outcomes, less dependence on incubators, less nursing staff necessary, and shorter hospital stay.[39]

Human Resources in Neonatal Intensive Care Unit

Another area of concern in managing Level II SCNU is availability of trained nursing staff and pediatrician.[40] Indian Academy of Pediatrics (IAP) and National Neonatology Forum (NNF) have started training of nurses in some accredited neonatal centers. These courses have to be planned to address the needs of sick neonates. Learning tools to meet the desired training need to be developed. Trained nurses have the potential to provide good neonatal care. They can also manage transport services for moderately sick babies on CPAP or ventilator. As the number of trained neonatologists (DM Neonatology, and IAP and NNF Neonatal Fellowship and International Fellowship), these doctors can be appointed in providing quality care in district hospitals' SCNU. Salaries of both nurses and doctors are the major expense in any NICU.[16] Support of the government along with nongovernmental organizations (NGOs) can be useful in smooth functioning and maintenance of SCNU.[4]

Role of Private Level II Care at District Level

Sixty percent of the inpatient care is still provided in a private healthcare setting. It is important that these SCNUs should be incorporated in the newborn care program to provide easy access to a broader section of the population. These units should be accredited and audited at a regular interval to maintain necessary standards and quality care. They should adhere to the protocols and guidelines set up by the expert committee for the management of sick neonates. For weaker socioeconomic families, financial support can be provided by various central or state government funded health schemes or private insurance companies. Appropriate remuneration can help in functioning of these private NICUs and provision of standard neonatal care to all sections of society.

Neonatal Critical Care at Tertiary Care Units (Level III Neonatal Care)

The emergence of the subspecialty of neonatology and the availability of dedicated NICUs with advanced technology designed for the newborn have improved the survival and outcomes of infants born prematurely or with serious medical or surgical problems. In high-income, high-resource countries, an entire workforce has evolved with expertise in the unique developmental physiology and congenital and acquired diseases of the newborn. This convergence of expertise and resources describes most modern-day NICUs in the United States (US), Canada, and high-income countries in Europe, UK, and across the globe. Multidisciplinary care has become the norm, and families are increasingly being integrated into the healthcare team. The infrastructure, resources, and workforce realities are quite different in developing countries, particularly not only in Africa and Southeast Asia but also in developing nations of North and South America.[41] The government in these countries should give greater emphasis to SCNU as these can decrease neonatal mortality by 70%.[16] This will also decrease the burden on tertiary neonatal units. Having said that, there is an important role of Level III neonatal care. Appropriate care at these centers is needed to decrease the mortality rate by another 20%. These units usually focus on extreme preterm babies (<30 weeks or 1,200 g) and critically sick neonates. These units should practice the same concept of providing essential newborn care for normal or high-risk delivery, SCNU care along with specialized intensive care. Such units should be developed in all medical colleges and major hospitals.

There are well-equipped private neonatal units in many cities of India where critical care is provided. These units also provide education for neonatology (DM Neonatology, fellowship programs under IAP and NNF). Some units are also training nurses under the guidance of training program designed by NNF. In developed countries such as UK and US, the capacity to care for high-risk newborns was expanded with the introduction of neonatal nurse practitioners (NNPs) into the workforce and formalized with certification beginning in the early 1980s. NNPs are registered nurses who have completed a master's degree and advanced clinical training, and they perform many complex activities. A policy statement of the American Academy of Pediatrics Committee of Fetus and Newborn recommended that care provided by NNPs be given in collaboration with or under the supervision of a physician, usually a neonatologist.[42] Similar courses can be designed by the NNF and they can be involved in providing quality neonatal care and procedures.

Tertiary neonatal units should be able to provide all forms of ventilation [high-frequency oscillatory ventilation (HFOV), conventional ventilation], management of extreme preterm neonates (24–30 weeks gestation), total parenteral nutrition (TPN), inotropic support, invasive monitoring via arterial lines, blood gas analysis, in-house radiology and laboratory investigation round the clock, blood products' availability, surfactant therapy, and emergency medications. These interventions are expensive and need highly trained doctors and nurses for prompt decision regarding treatment and appropriate execution. But tertiary care can be provided in resource-limited countries. The care provider should understand that resources need to be spent in a judicious manner. There are ethical dilemmas in dealing with extreme preterm neonates and severely asphyxiated babies with HIE and congenital abnormalities. Despite the best treatment, the outcomes in these groups of babies are not favorable and hence providing medically futile care can lead to prolongation of suffering and increase burden to a nation that already has few resources. Guidelines exist for withdrawal of intensive care in developed countries.[43] Such pathways should be medically legalized in India, so that a sound decision can be taken by the healthcare provider and the family of the neonate. Even for patients with good prognosis, the financial burden of an ICU care is often too great for families from a primarily lower socioeconomic background. To ensure availability of universal neonatal care, the cost of tertiary care needs to be included in the government health schemes. Adequate remuneration can support private tertiary neonatal units in providing these services.[16]

Concept of Regionalization in Providing Tertiary Neonatal Care

Perinatal care regionalization is an organized system of care in a geographic area in which infants are born at or transferred to hospitals that are able to provide the most appropriate care for each infant's needs. Hospitals within the region are designated by their capability of providing basic or more highly specialized care. The highest level facilities have the most specialized providers and advanced technology and equipment appropriate to care for the smallest, most critically ill, or most complex infants in order to ensure the best outcomes. The intent of providing risk-appropriate care to the population within a region is to achieve the best outcomes in the most cost-effective manner.[41]

However, many factors may affect the outcomes of preterm infants that may or may not be related to the site of delivery. These include characteristics of obstetric care (e.g. prenatal steroid use), experience of nursing staff, nurse-to-patient ratios, or other issues of practice, including an approach to resuscitation at the border of viability. Similar to three levels of newborn care in developed countries,[44] the Indian system has evolved in three levels of care.

Challenges in Providing Tertiary Neonatal Critical Care

Intensive monitoring and basic lifesaving intervention are essential in NICU. Multiple equipment are required to support sick neonates. When selecting equipment, due consideration needs to be given to the cost–benefit ratio, easy to use, availability of annual maintenance, and biomedical support. Local vendors should be given priority during purchase so that technical support can be made easily available. Multipara monitors, neonatal ventilators, CPAP delivery systems, humidifiers, infusion pumps, incubators, radiant warmers, phototherapy units, therapeutic cooling devices, blood gas analyzers, laminar flow units, and refrigerator are must in any tertiary unit. Additional bedside point-of-care facilities such as cranial ultrasonography, echocardiography, and amplitude electroencephalogram (EEG) can optimize management in some very sick neonates. Incubators should be used for babies of less than 30 weeks or weight less than 1,200 g. The number of incubators can be procured as per the local needs of the unit.

Mechanical ventilators for neonates are expensive, especially if they provide HFOV or volume-targeted ventilation. Adequate display of graphics and parameters is essential to guide optimal ventilation, weaning, and early extubation to CPAP. Volume guarantee ventilation has the potential to decrease hypocarbia, ventilator-induced lung injury, and intraventricular hemorrhage. The need of invasive ventilation can be decreased by providing adequate PEEP and standardized delivery room practices. There are multiple studies which have supported noninvasive support for extreme preterm babies.[30,45] This can reduce the need of intubation, ventilation, and surfactant therapy. This can immensely reduce the cost of providing respiratory support to preterm babies. Bubble CPAP can be provided at a significantly less cost compared to CPAP delivered by ventilators. Consumables used for CPAP interface are nasal mask/prongs, nasal tubing, and caps. These products if locally manufactured can reduce the cost immensely. Reusable circuits can be used for multiple patients with adequate disinfection and sterilization in between patients. Surfactant therapy has improved the respiratory outcomes in neonates with respiratory distress syndrome. Early and selective use of surfactant can help to provide judicious use of this costly product.[46]

Nutritional Support in Extreme Preterm Neonates

Total parenteral nutrition is needed to maintain adequate growth and development in neonates born below 30 weeks of gestation or babies less than 1,200 g. This will provide adequate nutritional support till the baby is on significant enteral feeds. TPN is also needed in babies with a surgical condition. Good nutrition is important at all stages of life. Babies are born at a time of rapid growth and formation of body tissues and organs. Optimal nutrition is required for achieving the adequate intake to maintain targeted growth. TPN is usually administered by an umbilical venous catheter or peripherally inserted central line (PIC line). TPN should be prepared in vertical laminar flow units to maintain asepsis. EBM should be started to promote enteral feeds and should be increased in a standardized manner.[47]

ROLE OF PEDIATRIC SUBSPECIALITIES

Pediatric surgery is an important division of neonatal services. Many congenital abnormalities such as tracheaesophageal fistula, congenital diaphragmatic hernia, and intestinal atresia need surgical correction. NEC is common in premature neonates and many times needs surgical evaluation and intervention. Pediatric ophthalmologist services are needed to perform ophthalmic evaluation for ROP in preterm neonates. ROP screening should be done as per guidelines and follow-up should be maintained. Pediatric cardiologist support is needed in management of congenital heart disease, echocardiography, and medical management. Referral to a cardiac center is needed for surgical intervention once the baby is stabilized medically. A high-risk newborn clinic should be run where neurodevelopment follow-up and assessment can be done appropriately. Some neonates may need the support of a pediatric neurologist.

CONCLUSION

India is witnessing a significant improvement in care of newborn. Several initiatives over the last few decades have contributed to decreasing NMR. There should be focus on neonatal critical care to improve the outcomes in sick neonates. Countries should improve emergency obstetrics services, training of neonatal nurses, transport of sick neonates, and sustained investment in neonatal health programs. High-quality, accessible, and family centered inpatient care should be provided at all levels of newborn care. Education of health professionals with evidence-based guidelines using standardized tools, development of skills, and formalized training program will have impact on providing Level III neonatal critical care. Universal health package and every newborn action plan along with focus on all levels of newborn care can help us achieve to reduce the NMR below 10/1,000 live births.

REFERENCES

1. Sankar MJ, Neogi SB, Sharma J, et al. State of newborn health in India. J Perinatol. 2016;36(s3):S3-8.
2. March of Dimes, PMNCH, Save the Children, WHO. Born too soon: The global action report on preterm birth. In: Howson CP, Kinney MV, Lawn JE (Eds). Geneva, Switzerland: World Health Organization; 2012.

3. World Health Organization. Every Newborn: an action plan to end preventable deaths. (2014). [online] Available from: https://www.who.int/maternal_child_adolescent/documents/every-newborn-action-plan/en/. [Last accessed on October, 2019].

4. Million Death Study Collaborators. Changes in cause-specific neonatal and 1–59-month child mortality in India from 2000 to 2015: a nationally representative survey. Lancet. 2017;390(10106):1972-80.

5. Basnet S, Adhikari N, Koirala J. Challenges in setting up pediatric and neonatal intensive care units in a resource-limited country. Pediatrics. 2011;128(4):e986-92.

6. Shantharam Baliga B, Raghuveera K, Vivekananda Prabhu B, et al. Scaling up of facility-based neonatal care: a district health system experience. J Trop Pediatr. 2007;53(2):107-12.

7. Rammohan A, Iqbal K, Awofeso N. Reducing neonatal mortality in India: critical role of access to emergency obstetric care. PLoS One. 2013;8(3):e57244.

8. Manktelow BN, Lal MK, Field DJ, et al. Antenatal corticosteroids and neonatal outcomes according to gestational age: a cohort study. Arch Dis Child Fetal Neonatal Ed. 2010;95(2):F95-8.

9. Singh S, Doyle P, Campbell OM, et al. Transport of pregnant women and obstetric emergencies in India: an analysis of the "108" ambulance service system data. BMC Pregnancy Childbirth. 2016;16(1):318.

10. Kumutha J, Rao GV, Sridhar BN, et al. The GVK EMRI maternal and neonatal transport system in India: a mega plan for a mammoth problem. Semin Fetal Neonatal Med. 2015;20(5):326-34.

11. Daga S. Reinforcing kangaroo mother care uptake in resource limited settings. Matern Health Neonatol Perinatol. 2018;4:26.

12. Phelan JP. Perinatal risk management: obstetric methods to prevent birth asphyxia. Clin Perinatol. 2005;32(1):1-17, v.

13. Kattwinkel J, Perlman JM, Aziz K, et al. Part 15: neonatal resuscitation: 2010 American Heart Association Guidelines for Cardiopulmonary Resuscitation and Emergency Cardiovascular Care. Circulation. 2010;122(18 Suppl 3):S909-19.

14. Barber CA, Wyckoff MH. Use and efficacy of endotracheal versus intravenous epinephrine during neonatal cardiopulmonary resuscitation in the delivery room. Pediatrics. 2006;118(3):1028-34.

15. Keene CM, Aluvaala J, Murphy GAV, et al. Developing recommendations for neonatal inpatient care service categories: reflections from the research, policy and practice interface in Kenya. BMJ Glob Health. 2019;4(2):e001195.

16. Prinja S, Manchanda N, Mohan P, et al. Cost of neonatal intensive care delivered through district level public hospitals in India. Indian Pediatr. 2013;50(9):839-46.

17. Moxon SG, Lawn JE, Dickson KE, et al. Inpatient care of small and sick newborns: a multi-country analysis of health system bottlenecks and potential solutions. BMC Pregnancy Childbirth. 2015;15(Suppl 2):S7.

18. Saugstad OD. Delivery room management of term and preterm newly born infants. Neonatology. 2015;107(4):365-71.

19. Lapcharoensap W, Bennett MV, Powers RJ, et al. Effects of delivery room quality improvement on premature infant outcomes. J Perinatol. 2017;37(4):349-54.

20. Kim JH, Unger S. Canadian Paediatric Society, Nutrition and Gastroenterology Committee. Human milk banking. Paediatr Child Health. 2010;15(9):595-8.

21. Yusef D, Shalakhti T, Awad S, et al. Clinical characteristics and epidemiology of sepsis in the neonatal intensive care unit in the era of multi-drug resistant organisms: a retrospective review. Pediatr Neonatol. 2018;59(1):35-41.

22. Tacconelli E, Cataldo MA, Dancer SJ, et al. European Society of Clinical Microbiology. ESCMID guidelines for the management of the infection control measures to reduce transmission of multidrug-resistant Gram-negative bacteria in hospitalized patients. Clin Microbiol Infect. 2014;20(Suppl 1):1-55.

23. Pittet D, Allegranzi B, Boyce J. World Health Organization World Alliance for Patient Safety First Global Patient Safety Challenge Core Group of Experts. The World Health Organization guidelines on hand hygiene in health care and their consensus recommendations. Infect Control Hosp Epidemiol. 2009;30(7):611-22.

24. Lunze K, Bloom DE, Jamison DT, et al. The global burden of neonatal hypothermia: systematic review of a major challenge for newborn survival. BMC Med. 2013;11:24.

25. World Health Organization. Thermal protection of the newborn: a practical guide; 1997. [online] Available from: https://www.who.int/maternal_child_adolescent/documents/ws42097th/en/. [Last accessed on October, 2019].

26. McCall EM, Alderdice FA, Halliday HL, et al. Interventions to prevent hypothermia at birth in preterm and/or low birth weight infants. Cochrane Database Syst Rev. 2008;(1):CD004210.

27. America Academy of Pediatrics. In: Kattwinkel J, Jerry S (Eds). Textbook of Neonatal Resuscitation, 5th edition. Illinois: American Academy of Pediatrics; 2006.

28. Askie LM, Henderson-Smart DJ, Irwig L, et al. Oxygen-saturation targets and outcomes in extremely preterm infants. N Engl J Med. 2003;349(10):959-67.

29. STOP-ROP Investigators. Supplemental therapeutic oxygen for prethreshold retinopathy of prematurity (STOP-ROP), a randomized, controlled trial. I: primary outcomes. Pediatrics. 2000;105(2):295-310.

30. Carlo WA, Finer NN, Walsh MC, et al. SUPPORT Study Group of the Eunice Kennedy Shriver NICHD Neonatal Research Network. Target ranges of oxygen saturation in extremely preterm infants. N Engl J Med. 2010;362(21):1959-69.

31. Atay S, Sen S, Cukurlu D. Incidence of infiltration/extravasation in newborns using peripheral venous catheter and affecting factors. Rev Esc Enferm USP. 2018;52:e03360.

32. Thigpen JL. Peripheral intravenous extravasation: nursing procedure for initial treatment. Neonatal Netw. 2007;26(6):379-84.

33. Lund CH, Osborne JW, Kuller J, et al. Neonatal skin care: clinical outcomes of the AWHONN/NANN evidence-based clinical practice guideline. Association of Women's Health, Obstetric and Neonatal Nurses and the National Association of Neonatal Nurses. J Obstet Gynecol Neonatal Nurs. 2001;30(1):41-51.

34. Dutta S, Singh B, Chessell L, et al. Guidelines for feeding very low birth weight infants. Nutrients. 2015;7(1):423-42.

35. World Health Organization. Global Nutrition Targets 2025: Low birth weight policy brief (WHO/NMH/NHD/14.5). Geneva: World Health Organization; 2014.

36. World Health Organization. WHO recommendations on interventions to improve preterm birth outcomes. Geneva: World Health Organization; 2015. p. 42.

37. Charpak N, Ruiz-Peláez JG, Figueroa de Calume Z. Current knowledge of Kangaroo Mother Intervention. Curr Opin Pediatr. 1996;8(2):108-12.

38. Conde-Agudelo A, Díaz-Rossello JL. Kangaroo mother care to reduce morbidity and mortality in low birth weight infants. Cochrane Database Syst Rev. 2016;(8):CD002771.

39. Broughton EI, Gomez I, Sanchez N, et al. The cost-savings of implementing kangaroo mother care in Nicaragua. Rev Panam Salud Publica. 2013;34(3):176-82.

40. Neogi SB, Malhotra S, Zodpey S, et al. Challenges in scaling up of special care newborn units—lessons from India. Indian Pediatr. 2011;48(12):931-5.

41. Avery GB, MacDonald MG, Seshia MMK. The scope and organization of neonatology: North American and global comparisons. Avery's Neonatology: Pathophysiology and Management of the Newborn. 7th edition. Philadelphia: Wolters Kluwer; 2016.

42. Wallman C, Committee on Fetus and Newborn. Advanced practice in neonatal nursing. Pediatrics. 2009;123:1606-7.

43. Withholding and Withdrawing Life Sustaining Treatment in Children: A Framework for Practice. 2nd edition. London, United Kingdom: Royal College of Paediatrics and Child Health; 2004.

44. American Academy of Pediatrics Committee on Fetus and Newborn. Levels of neonatal care. Pediatrics. 2012;130(3): 587-97.

45. Morley CJ, Davis PG, Doyle LW, et al. COIN Trial Investigators. Nasal CPAP or intubation at birth for very preterm infants. N Engl J Med. 2008;358(7):700-8.

46. Sandri F, Plavka R, Simeoni U; CURPAP Advisory Board. The CURPAP study: an international randomized controlled trial to evaluate the efficacy of combining prophylactic surfactant and early nasal continuous positive airway pressure in very preterm infants. Neonatology. 2008;94(1):60-2.

47. El Hassan NO, Kaiser JR. Parenteral nutrition in the Neonatal Intensive Care Unit. NeoReviews. 2011;12(3):e130-40.

Lalan Kumar Bharti, Kumar Ankur

Facility-based Newborn Care in Tropics

3.8 CHAPTER

INTRODUCTION

The Facility-based newborn care (FBNC) Program was launched by the Ministry of Health and Family Welfare, Government of India (MoHFW, GOI), to improve the outcome of newborn. Newborn Care Corners (NBCCs), newborn stabilization units (NBSUs), and special newborn care units (SNCUs) were established at different levels of facilities. The aim was to establish a continuum of care with the launch of home-based and FBNC components ensuring that every newborn receives essential care right from the time of birth at the health facility and then at home during the first 42 days of life. To implement this, the MoHFW has developed FBNC Operational Guideline to facilitate the states in planning, establishment, and monitoring of care of newborns[1] where round-the-clock services are being provided by skilled workers.[2,3]

During the late 90s, the government, under a national program, implemented a package of interventions for Essential Newborn Care (breastfeeding, warmth, and hygiene) at different levels of the health system.[4] This package was again expanded in subsequent national programs by adding essential components of neonatal health.[5] With the help of the National Neonatology Forum (NNF) accreditation committee, FBNC became functional in 26 districts with strengthening of district and subdistrict health facilities mainly through provision of equipment and trainings.[6] The first successfully operating district level unit was established in the Purulia district of West Bengal in the year 2003.[7] The results showed reduced neonatal mortality rate (NMR) by 14% in the 1st year and by 21% in the 2nd year among the admitted neonates after the SNCU became functional. It led to a 10% reduction in NMR at the district level within a span of 2 years.[8] With these initial initiatives, the present concept of FBNC was born.

NEED OF FACILITY-BASED NEONATAL CARE

Over the years, under-five mortality rate has shown a decline; however, there is minimal reduction in neonatal mortality as two-thirds of the infant mortality are contributed to by newborn deaths. Around 45% of the neonatal deaths occur within the first 48 hours of life and tackling this is a major challenge.[9] In 2016, out of 2.6 million deaths, 46% were of under-five deaths, and this translates to 7,000 neonatal deaths every day. The majority of them die on the 1st day and close to one million die within the next 6 days. That is why, reducing neonatal mortality is immensely important not only because the proportions of under-five deaths that occur during the neonatal period are increasing, but also because the interventions needed to address the major causes of neonatal deaths generally differ from those needed to address other under-five deaths. If current trends follow, then it is highly likely that more than 60 countries would miss the sustainable development goal of reducing NMR to at least as low as 12 deaths per 1,000 live births by 2030. The major causes of neonatal mortality are asphyxia, sepsis, and issues related to low birth weight (LBW) and prematurity which need skilled care in a facility. In these situations, the baby needs to be safely transferred to a health facility in a timely manner for early initiation of treatment. That is why, the facilities need to be developed in terms of appropriate infrastructure and resources. Optimum healthcare staff (physicians, nursing personnel, and support staff) needs to be positioned at such facilities, who have been adequately trained in neonatal care skills. These facilities ideally need to be in the close vicinity of the communities so that they would be able to access them in times of need for reasonably good outcomes.

STRUCTURE AND IMPLEMENTATION OF DELIVERY OF FACILITY-BASED NEWBORN CARE

Facility-based newborn care guidelines provide detailed information regarding civil design, infrastructure, manpower, and data management and provide protocols for case management.[1,10] It has two components, i.e. essential newborn care for all and care of sick newborns. Providing these services, three levels of newborn care were defined.[1] The cost of establishing a 12-bedded level-II unit (SNCU) in a district hospital is around 4,100,000 INR. However, the running cost comes around 1,000,000 INR per year. This is much less compared to what is incurred in developed world. Over the years, the need for FBNC has increased further, since the introduction of Janani Suraksha Yojana (JSY), where a cash incentive scheme for promoting institutional deliveries is being promoted. The aim is to reduce the overall maternal and infant mortality rates and to ensure 100% institutional deliveries among the underprivileged society. The program focuses on poor pregnant women, with special attention for states having low institutional delivery rates and high burden of maternal and neonatal mortalities. The scheme launched in 2010 on a pilot basis in 52 selected districts of the country, which provides a cash incentive of INR 4,000 directly to women aged above 19 years for the first two live births, subject to the woman fulfilling specific conditions relating to maternal child health and nutrition.[1,10]

ESTABLISHING FACILITY-BASED NEWBORN CARE

As per FBNC guideline, any facility having delivery load more than 3,000 per year should have a SNCU with a minimum of 12 beds, while facilities having less delivery load should have a NBSU with 4–6 beds. However, if the delivery load is more than 3,000 per year, then 4 beds should be added for every 1,000 additional deliveries. It is important to understand that if the number of beds is below 12, then the SNCU intervention does not remain cost-effective.[1] With the success of the JSY, more number of sick newborns are being referred from the community. That is why, the NNF suggested that there should be a link between the primary healthcare and the tertiary care centers, which led to establishing FBNC.[11] At the primary health centers (PHCs), a NBCC was planned where skilled

neonatal resuscitation can be provided at large, whereas at a community health center, a neonatal stabilization unit (NSU) was planned which would be a 4–6-bedded unit, where along with resuscitation, temperature management, feeding-related issues, oxygen therapy, treatment for jaundice, and intravenous (IV) therapy can be provided. At this unit, after stabilizing a sick neonate, he/she can be referred to the SCNU, in case the neonate requires longer stay. However, if the neonate does not require more specialized care, the same can be done at the NSU. At the SCNU, which is a 12–20-bedded unit, not only management related to resuscitation, temperature, feeding, oxygen, or IV drug infusion should be provided but also there should be a facility to do blood administration and exchange transfusion.[1,10,12] So, actually SCNU should be an advanced facility center in a multilayered health service structure that is geared to save lives of each and every sick newborn even in remotest part. The level-II care offered at SCNU is suitable for caring for sick and low-weight neonates born at the hospital or in other facilities.[13] The NNF has helped in capacity building of district and subdistrict level neonatal care staff and is also conducting a well-structured 4-day onsite exhaustive workshop to train the nursing staff and medical officers.[13]

Provision for Facility-based Newborn Care in All Districts

Each district should have newborn care facilities established as a three-tiered level system. **Table 1** gives the number of FBNC units required in an average district assuming that the district has one district and one subdistrict hospital with more than 3,000 deliveries per year, five first referral units (FRUs), and 20 24 × 7 PHCs. The facilities would be needed for newborn care in one such district is explained in **Table 1**.

Thus, this district will have approximately 34–35 NBCCs, 5 NBSUs, and at least 2 SNCUs and preferably a mother and newborn care unit (MNCU). The aim is to provide each district at least with one functional SNCU, NBCC at all levels, and functional NBSUs at the FRU level, especially those FRUs located at a distance from the District Hospital/Medical College.

Monitoring Facility-based Newborn Cares: Record Keeping and Reporting

To improve the status of FBNC, effective mechanisms have to be created to collect data, analyze, and utilize it for programmatic improvement. Uniform guidelines have been disseminated to the states, to improve the reporting

Table 1: Facilities required for newborn care in one district.

Newborn services	Level of facility	Number of units	Total number of units
Newborn care corner	SC, PHC, CHC (designated as 24*7 services)	20	34
	First referral unit-Labor room	5	
		5	
	District hospital, subdistrict hospital (with >3,000 deliveries/year)–Labor room	2	
	OT	2	
Newborn stabilization units	First referral unit	5	5
SNCU (MNCU)	District hospital, subdistrict hospital (with >3,000 deliveries/year)	2	2

(CHC: Community Health Center; MNCU: mother newborn care units; PHC: primary health center; SC: subcenter; SNCU: special newborn care units; OT: operation theater)

system. SNCU online monitoring system has been scaled up to ensure uniformity in data collection and getting real-time data for efficient monitoring and timely feedback. For this, State Programme Management Unit (PMU in FBNC cell) or child health nodal person will be supported by the state level SNCU Data Manager and the Clinical Care Coordinator for monitoring quality and completeness of clinical data entry and identifying areas for correcting actions including periodic reviews.[14] All units will have a computerized data entry system. Each unit will record information in the standard case-recording sheet for every newborn admitted. Standard case definitions would be used for recording the clinical diagnosis to ensure that the data is valid, reliable, and comparable across the units. Medical colleges have also been identified as National and Regional Collaborating Centers for capacity building, mentoring, and supervision of SNCUs.[1] The UNICEF (United Nations Children's Fund) supported National Health Mission (NHM) to develop a real-time online monitoring system, first piloted in Madhya Pradesh and is being scaled up across the country under the India Newborn Action Plan (INAP). This system actually monitors performance of SNCUs and tracks follow-up of baby till 1 year of age. As of now, 11 states and more than 300 SNCUs are reporting online.[15] The results from a pilot study conducted in 2010 over a 6-month period at a district level birth subcenter in Karnataka have shown that these checklists can help in markedly improving delivery of healthcare practices.[16]

Current Status of Facility-based Newborn Care in India

About 70% of the delivery in rural areas and 30% of urban delivery still happen at home in the hands of unskilled birth attendants, and neonatal care is provided to only 36.4% of live births.[3] As on June 2011, 253 SNCUs (40.1%) were reported to be operational out of the 631 units proposed by the states/UTs. The proportion of SNCUs reported operational was highest in the high-focus non-NE states (44.8%) followed by the non-high-focus states/UTs (39.8%), while the proportion was much less for the high-focus NE states (18%). Currently, there are 602 SNCUs, 2,228 NBSUs, and 16,968 NBCCs established across the country.

Details of the new units are as under:[17]

S. No.	Year	SNCU	NBSU	NBCC
1.	Existing in 2013–14	525	1,761	14,099
2.	Added in 2014–15	40	143	64
3.	Added in 2015 till date	37	324	2,805

However currently, FBNC has seen massive scale-up with more than 82% of the districts having a functional SNCU and almost 96% saturation of delivery points with NBCC. More than 90% of functional SNCUs now report the utilization data and patient-specific data online. Several states such as Andhra Pradesh, Telangana, Rajasthan, and Uttar Pradesh have established State Resource Centers to enhance capacity within the state to support the FBNC program *(Facility-based Newborn Care Operational Guideline, 2019)*. Under the NHM, states submit their annual plans and GOI helps them in either establishing new units or renovating and expanding of existing units. The support is also extended for recruiting human resources of all cadres and capacity building of medical officers and staff nurses. The procurement and maintenance support for equipment are also included in the annual budgets. The Kangaroo mother care units for care of small babies were also established at the district level with the support from GOI.[17] In 2015–2016, Gujarat has operationalized 40 SNCUs by saturating each district with at least one SNCU. The study found near proportion of inborn (53%) and outborn (47%) admissions and 44% admission of females. Out of 69,662 admissions, 67% were discharged, 16% died, 10% left against medical advice, and 7% were referred to higher centers. The most common reasons for admission in SCNU were respiratory distress syndrome (RDS) (22%) and sepsis (21%) and the common causes of mortality were RDS (23%) and infection (21%). However, the proportion of deaths in outborn was high compared to inborn.[18] Overall, 6–10% of all babies born are likely to need inpatient care as per population estimates and hence it is mandatory to plan and provide level-II care setups at district and subdistrict levels.

CONCLUSION

The FBNC program was launched for capacity building of the SNCU staff in the year 2009 by NNF and UNICEF and subsequently revised and launched in the year 2014 by the MoHFW. The feedback received from the states and facilitators over the last 5 years has been very encouraging and it is to note that many health personnel working in the SNCUs have been successfully trained and are continuing to be trained. An operational guideline was disseminated in 2011 to assist the Program Manager to plan newborn care facilities at the district and subdistrict levels. The total number of SNCUs, NBSUs, and NBCCs has increased with rapid pace; however, the quality of care is quite variable. The guidelines elaborated on the layout, infrastructure, equipment, and human resource and created dedicated budget lines for both establishment and recurring costs. However, linkages of SNCUs with NBSUs and NBCCs are weak, thus hampering the continuum of newborn care. NBSUs, in particular, have not received the required attention and have remained a weak link in most districts.

Recently, a revised package has been developed and edited with electronic inputs from the experts which have been prepared by MoHFW, with support from the WHO (World Health Organization), by incorporating the suggestions of the experts in the "FBNC Package "comprising the Participant's Manual with supplement/electronic book, the NRP (Neonatal Resuscitation Program) Module, and Program Manager's handbook with special emphasis on improving the core competencies, QI initiative projects, better harmonization of newborn training packages, and addition of CPAP (continuous positive airway pressure) and DSC (developmental supportive care) programs.

REFERENCES

1. Ministry of Health and Family Welfare, Government of India. Facility Based Newborn Care Operational Guide; 2011. [online] Available from: http://164.100.130.11:8091/rch/FNBC_Operational_Guideline.pdf. [Last accessed on December, 2019].
2. Darmstadt GL, Bhutta ZA, Cousens S, et al. Evidence-based, cost-effective interventions: how many newborn babies can we save? Lancet. 2005;365(9463):977-88.
3. Neogi SB, Malhotra S, Zodpey S, et al. Does facility-based newborn care improve neonatal outcomes? A review of evidence. Indian Pediatr. 2012;49(8):651-8.
4. A strategic approach to reproductive, maternal, newborn, child and adolescent health (RMNCH+A) in India. Ministry of Health & Family Welfare. Government of India; 2013. [online] Available from: https://www.nhm.gov.in/images/pdf/programmes/rmncha-strategy.pdf.
5. Ramji S, Modi M, Gupta N. 50 years of neonatology in India: progress and future. Indian Pediatr. 2013;50(1):104-6.
6. JHPIEGO. Shaping policy for maternal and newborn health: a compendium of case studies; 2013. [online] Available from: http://reprolineplus.org/system/files/resources/policy_compendium.pdf. [Last accessed on December, 2019].
7. Sen A, Mahalanabis D, Singh AK, et al. Development and effects of a neonatal care unit in rural India. Lancet. 2005;366(9479):27-8.
8. Sen A, Mahalanabis D, Singh AK, et al. Impact of a district level sick newborn care unit on neonatal mortality rate: 2-year follow-up. J Perinatol. 2008;29(2):150-5.
9. Registrar General and Census Commissioner, India. Projected Population. [online] Available from: http://censusindia.gov.in/Census_Data_2001/Projected_Population/Projected_population.aspx. [Last accessed on December, 2019].
10. UNICEF. Toolkit for setting up special care newborn units, stabilisation units and newborn care corners. [online] Available from: https://www.healthynewbornnetwork.org/hnn-content/uploads/UNICEF_Toolkit-for-Setting-Up-Special-Care-Newborn-Units-Stabilisation-Units-and-Newborn-Care-Corners.pdf. [Last accessed on December, 2019].
11. Ministry of Health and Family Welfare, Government of India. Annual Report. for the year 2013-14. [online] Available from: https://nhm.gov.in/images/pdf/media/publication/Annual_Report-Mohfw.pdf. [Last accessed on December, 2019].
12. State of India's Newborn (SOIN) report; 2014. Available from: https://www.newbornwhocc.org/SOIN_PRINTED%2014-9-2014.pdf.
13. Indian public health standards. [online] Available from: http://nrhm.gov.in/about-nrhm/guidelines/indian-public-health-standards.html (Last accessed on February 2013).
14. Report of the Working Group on National Rural Health Mission (NRHM) for the Twelfth Five Year Plan (2012-2017). Available from: http://planningcommission.nic.in/aboutus/committee/wrkgrp12/health/WG_1NRHM.pdf.
15. Child Health Division, Ministry of Health and Family Welfare, Government of India. State-wise progress under NRHM (as on March 2015). [online] Available from: http://nrhm.gov.in/nrhm-components/rmnch-a/child-health-immunization.html. [Last accessed on December, 2019].
16. Spector JM, Agrawal P, Kodkany B, et al. Improving quality of care for maternal and newborn health: prospective pilot study of the WHO safe childbirth checklist programme. PLoS One. 2012;7(5):e35151.
17. Press Information Bureau. Government of India. Ministry of Health and Family Welfare. 602 Special Newborn Care Units (SNCUs) operational in the country; 2015. Available from: (Release ID: 133548). https://pib.gov.in/newsite/pmreleases.aspx?mincode=31.
18. Shah HD, Shah B, Dave PV, et al. A step toward healthy newborn: an assessment of 2 years' admission pattern and treatment outcomes of neonates admitted in special newborn care units of Gujarat. Indian J Community Med. 2018;43(1):14-8.

INTRODUCTION

As mentioned in the chapters on mortality and morbidity statistics of newborns in India or globally, prematurity, asphyxia, and sepsis remain the major causes of deaths in newborns. These account for almost 70% of infant mortality rate and around 40% of under-5 child deaths. Neonatal death in the 1st week accounts for 70% of Neonatal Mortality Rate (NMR) and almost 50% of Infant mortality rate (IMR).[1,2] Hence, interventions aimed at this period were targeted in a landmark study done by Drs Rani and Abhay Bang in the tribal district of Gadchiroli in Maharashtra during 1993–2003. They trained village health workers (VHWs) who were selected from local villages and paid remunerations marginally more than the daily labor wages (to avoid more wealthy local villagers to vie for these jobs). The VHWs were provided 36 hours of training spread over a year making it merely 3 hours a month. Work efficiency of VHWs was strictly supervised by facilitator. As 90% of deliveries were happening at home in that period, VHWs were trained to resuscitate, start early breastfeeding, care of low birth weight (LBW) babies, early case diagnosis of sepsis, institution of antibiotics as oral cotrimoxazole and injectable gentamicin, etc. **(Fig. 1)**.

The NMR of the intervention area fell from 62 to 25 in the study period from 1993 to 2003, which was an impressive 70% reduction compared to control area. Case-specific fatality rates decreased by 72% in LBW sepsis, by 90% in sepsis-specific NMR, by 60% in mild asphyxia, 47.5% in severe asphyxia, and 90% in asphyxia-specific NMR[3,4] **(Figs. 2 and 3)**.

This study was then upscaled in different districts of Maharashtra as *Ankur Project* and in Lucknow, Patna,

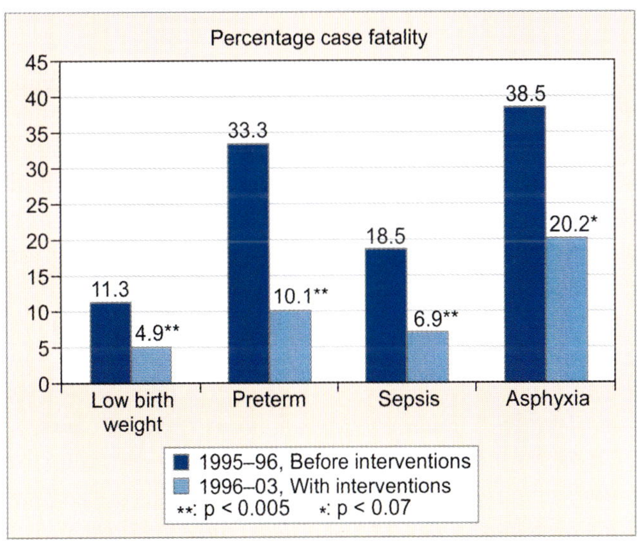

Fig. 2: Effect of home-based newborn care on case fatality in life-threatening morbidities (1995 to 1996 vs 2001 to 2003).

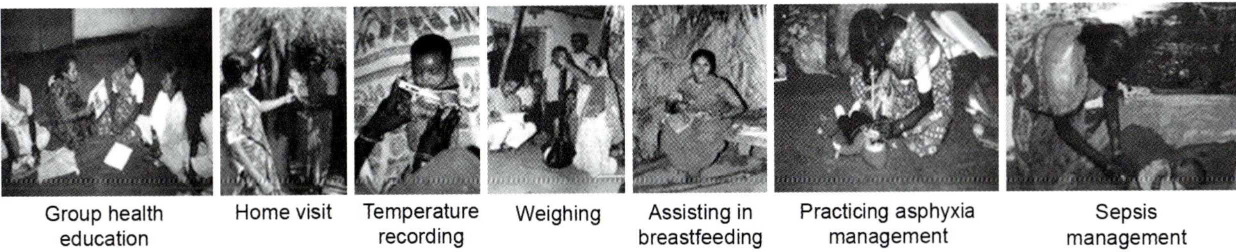

Fig. 1: Village health workers (VHWs) in Society for Education, Action and Research in Community Health, (SEARCH) study in Gadchiroli near Nagpur, Maharashtra.

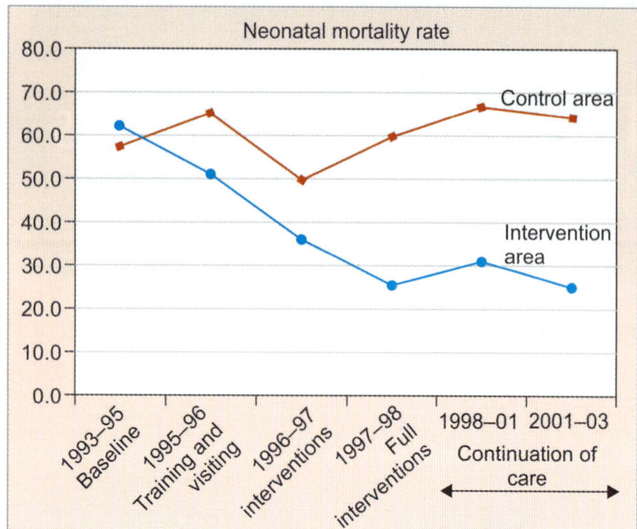

Fig. 3: Neonatal mortality rate (NMR) in the intervention and control area—1993 to 2003.

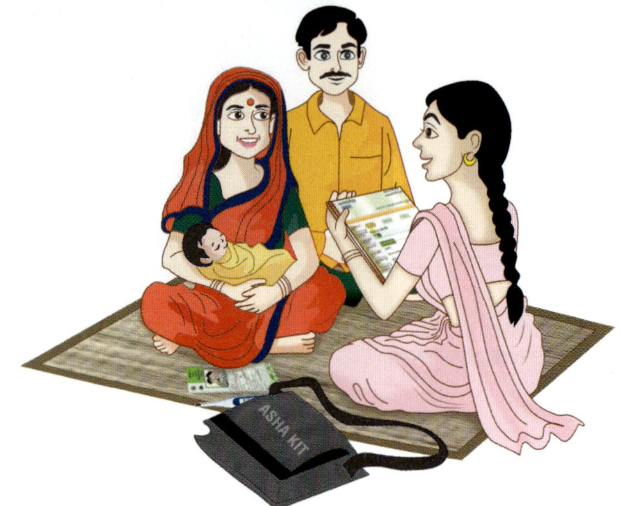

Fig. 4: ASHA using communication skills during home visits. (ASHA: Accredited Social Health Activist)

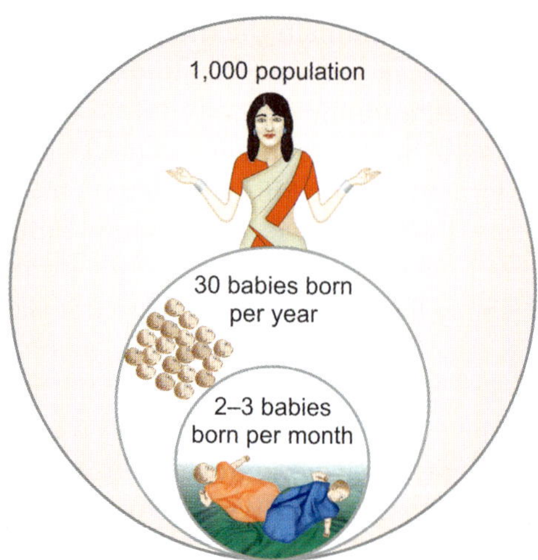

Fig. 5: Estimate of children under care of an ASHA.

Udaipur, and Cuttack in different states under the *ICMR (Indian Council of Medical Research) replication study*. The Ankur project involved replicating the effort in seven NGOs (nongovernmental organizations) throughout different parts of Maharashtra, and the NGOs selected included those working in tribal, rural, and urban slum areas. Community health workers (CHWs) were observing mothers in pregnancy and newborns up to 28 days of life. A 35-page booklet was needed to be filled in 8–13 weeks which had boxes mainly to be ticked or values to be put; very little writing was required. A CHW kit consisted of this booklet, spring weighing scale, AMBU bag for resuscitation, disposable syringes, needles, medicines, and drugs. The total score for seven coverage indicators [*(1) mothers who received one health education (HE) in pregnancy and one HE in postpartum, (2) home deliveries attended, (3) home-delivered newborns examined within 24 hours after birth, (4) newborns started on exclusive breastfeeding within 24 hours, (5) those who received four visits in neonatal period, (6) at least one supervisory visit in neonatal period, and (7) sepsis-diagnosed babies either treated or referred*] by the 3rd year of intervention, i.e. by 2005, was *84.6%*. This project demonstrated a decline of *50%* in NMR with *44%* in early NMR and *72%* in late NMR in around 80,000 population in those seven tribal areas or urban slums.[5]

ACCREDITED SOCIAL HEALTH ACTIVIST

The National Rural Health Mission (NRHM) was launched on April 12, 2005, which introduced ASHA (Accredited Social Health Activist).[6] Under this program, ASHA is selected as one woman per village (approximately 1 per 1,000 population) who would receive an initial training of 23 days on basic health topics; five rounds of trainings spread over 1 year followed by 2 days of refresher trainings every alternate month. ASHA is selected from local village/area who is well known to its residents, does not get any fixed remuneration, gets task-based incentives, and carries out following tasks **(Figs. 4 and 5)**:

- Linkage between auxiliary nurse midwife (ANM), trained birth attendant (TBA), anganwadi worker (AWW), and multipurpose worker (MPW)
- Escorting patients to hospital
- Primary medical care to needy people
- Acts as depot holder for oral rehydration salts (ORS) packets, zinc tablets, iron-folic acid (IFA) tablets,

chloroquine tablets, disposable delivery kit (DDK), oral pills, condoms, etc.

- Keeps records of ASHA register, diaries, their experiences, difficulties, AWW register, and registrations of births and deaths.

HOME-BASED NEWBORN CARE (REVISED GUIDELINES 2014)[1] (FIGS. 6 TO 10)

Institutional births have phenomenally increased over the last decade and more. This has put an extra deal of burden on already overworked and infrastructurally weak public health hospitals. The Government of India has timely targeted this anomaly by building special care newborn unit (SCNU) in almost all districts of the country, sometimes more than two or so. Facility-based newborn care (FBNC) remains the mainstay of guidelines on which these SNCU babies are managed.

Even these centers get overfull and not all mother–baby dyads can be kept in a hospital for more than 48 hours. The immediate neonatal care for the early 1st week and extended to first 42 days and later to 1–2 years requires a dedicated healthcare worker emerging from the community itself as proved in the Gadchiroli experiment. Hence, ASHA envisaged in NRHM acts as a vehicle for delivery of optimum care to all newborns and postpartum mothers. This completes the continuum of neonatal care from institutions to home and later till 2 years of optimum nutrition, growth, and development.

Home-based newborn care (HBNC) is well articulated in government policy aimed at improving newborn survival. The key policy documents that articulate this are the XIth plan document (2007–2012) and the Minutes of Meeting from the Mission Steering Group (MSG), dated June 21, 2011. In the XIth Plan document, the role and

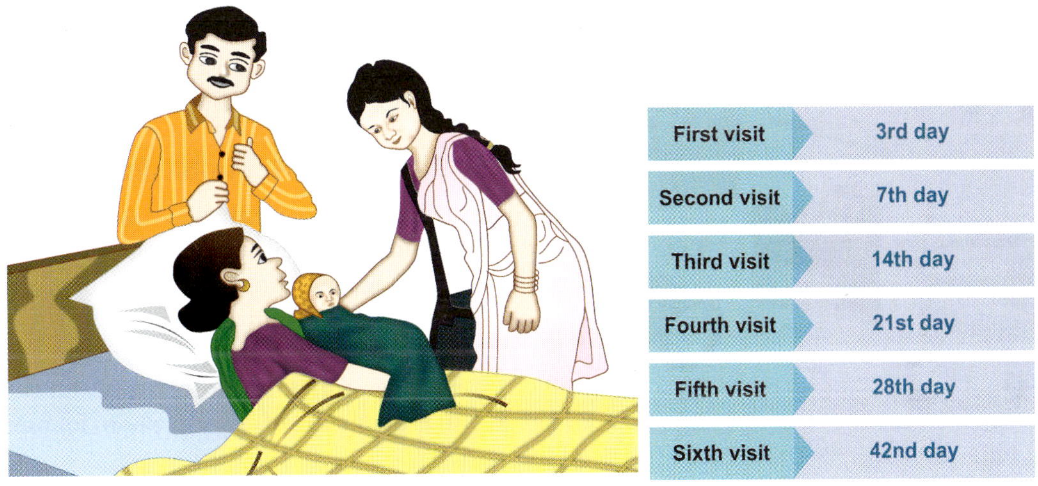

Fig. 6: ASHA counseling family during HBNC home visits in first month of life.

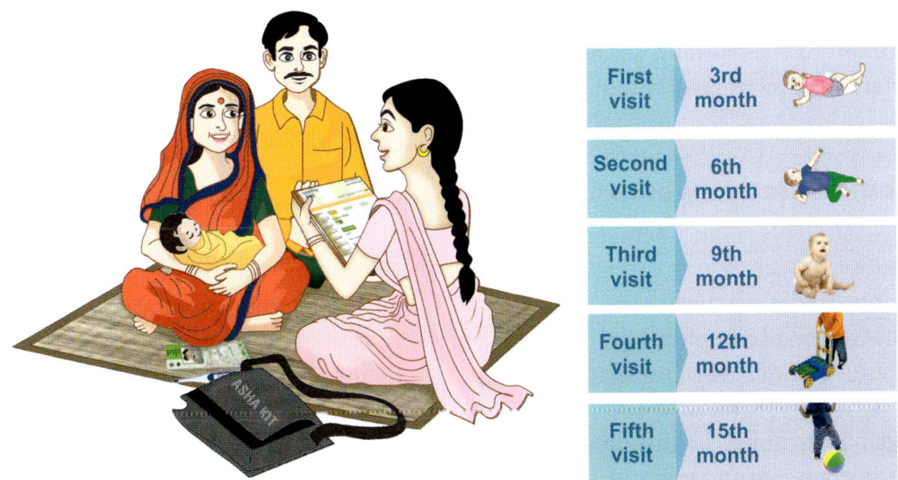

Fig. 7: ASHA counseling family during HBYC home visits in first year of life.

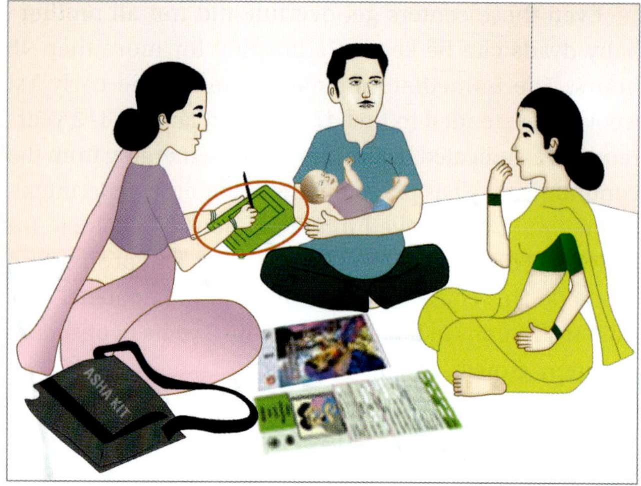

Fig. 8: ASHA filling diary during home visits.

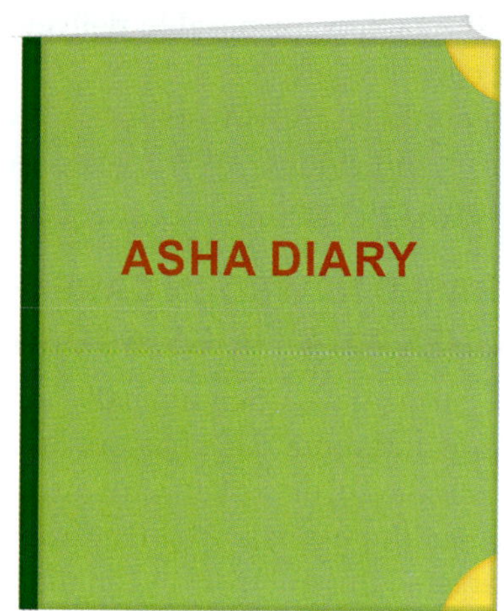

Fig. 10: ASHA diary.

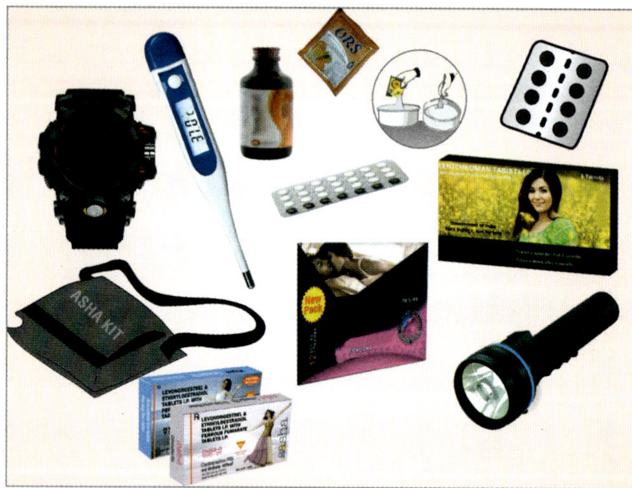

Fig. 9: ASHA kit for HBNC and HBYC.
(HBNC: Home-based newborn care;
HBYC: Home-based care for young child)

incentives of ASHA in HBNC were defined. The MSG fixed up an incentive amount of ₹ 250/- for a set of six home visits to assess newborn as well as postpartum care of the newborn.[1]

Objectives of Home-based Newborn Care

The major objective of HBNC is to decrease neonatal mortality and morbidity through:

- The provision of essential newborn care to all new-borns and the prevention of complications
- Early detection and special care of preterm and LBW newborns
- Early identification of illness in the newborn and provision of appropriate care and referral

- Support the family for adoption of healthy practices and build confidence and skills of the mother to safeguard her health and that of the newborn ASHA is also entrusted with postpartum care of mothers apart from her other many different tasks.

Key Services of Home-based Newborn Care

The key services under HBNC constitute the provision of:

- Care for every newborn through a series of home visits by an ASHA in the first 6 weeks of life. In most state contexts, this health worker is the ASHA
- Information and skills to the mother and family of every newborn to ensure better health outcomes
- An examination of every newborn for prematurity and LBW
- Extra home visits for preterm and LBW babies by the ASHA or ANM, and referred for appropriate care as defined in the protocols
- Early identification of illness in the newborn and provision of appropriate care at home or referral as defined in the protocols
- Follow-up for sick newborns after they are discharged from facilities
- Counseling the mother on postpartum care, recognition of postpartum complications, and enabling referral
- Counseling the mother for adoption of an appropriate family planning method
- In case of those deliveries that occur on the way to the health institutions or at home out of choice, despite motivation for institutional delivery, the ASHA must be equipped with the skills and competencies required to provide appropriate newborn care.

Skills as Provisioned for ASHA in HBNC

- Mobilize all pregnant mothers and ensure that they receive the full package of antenatal care.
- Undertake birth planning and birth preparedness with the mother and family to ensure access to safe delivery.
- Provide newborn care through a series of home visits which include the skills for:
  - Weighing the newborn
  - Measuring newborn temperature
  - Ensuring warmth
  - Supporting exclusive breastfeeding through teaching the mother proper positioning and attachment for initiating and maintaining breastfeeding
  - Diagnosing and counseling in cases of problems with breastfeeding
  - Promoting hand washing
  - Providing skin, cord, and eye care
  - Health promotion and counseling mothers and families on key messages on newborn care which include discouraging unhealthy practices such as early bathing and bottle feeding
  - Ensuring identification and prompt referral of sepsis or other illnesses.
- Assessing if the baby is high risk (preterm or LBW) through:
  - The use of protocols and managing such LBW or preterm babies through increasing the number of home visits
  - Monitoring weight gain
  - Supporting and counseling the mother and the family to keep the baby warm and enabling frequent and exclusive breastfeeding
  - Teaching the mother to express breast milk and feed baby using cup and spoon or paladai, if required.
- Detecting signs and symptoms of sepsis, providing first-level care and referring the baby to an appropriate center, after counseling the mother to keep the baby warm. If the family is unable to go, the ASHA should ensure that the ANM visits the sick newborn on a priority basis.
- Recognizing postpartum complications in the mother and referring appropriately.
- Counseling the couple to choose an appropriate family planning method.
- Using the checklist for the first Visit to the Newborn (Annexure 1b) and Home visit form (Annexure 1c) to remind her to ask the key questions and ensuring that she follows the steps of examination and counseling the mother.
- Providing immediate newborn care, in case of those deliveries that do not occur in institutions (home deliveries or those deliveries occurring on the way to the institution).

Capacity Building of Accredited Social Health Activist

The ASHA is required to acquire these skills by training in Modules 6 and 7 using ASHA trainers' manual. This entails four rounds of 5 days' training spanned over a year. No training rounds can be done within an interval of 10–12 weeks during which she is expected to practice the skills taught till then. The HBNC kit will be provided in the beginning itself so that the ASHA is well acquainted with it during the training rounds and interval periods. She will be evaluated after each round for knowledge and skills. On-site mentoring will be done by facilitators using supervisory checklists to assess correct application of skills.

Support to the ASHA to Ensure Positive Newborn Health Outcomes

Payments

The ASHA after training in Modules 6 and 7 are required to apply skills such as use of handwashing, taking temperature in newborns, managing hypothermia, taking weight correctly, assessing feeds, and looking out for sepsis. For this she is entitled:

- *For institutional deliveries*: ₹ 250/- for *six* visits (Days 3, 7, 14, 21, 28, and 42)
- *For home deliveries*: ₹ 250/- for *seven* visits (Days 1, 3, 7, 14, 21, 28, and 42)
- *For cesarean deliveries, where discharge takes place after 5–6 days*: ₹ 250/- for completing remaining *five* visits (Days 7, 14, 21, 28, and 42)
- *In case baby discharged from SNCU*: ₹ 250/- for the remaining visits and ₹ 50/- per monthly visit for arranging follow-up in SNCU for a period of 1 year
- *In case of LBW babies*: ₹ 50/- per monthly visit for arranging follow-up in SNCU for a period of 2 years
- *For deliveries taking place at maternal place and then moving back to her house*: ₹ 250/- is divided as ₹ 125/- between ASHAs of both places if each ASHA has made three visits. The ANM/AWW visiting the mother would verify this fact. If two or less visits are made by any ASHA, only the other ASHA completing five or more visits will get full payment of ₹ 250/-.

In order to reimburse the payments, ASHA is expected to fill two forms: Examination of newborn and Home visit form. The HBNC card can be used as a voucher for payment purposes and verification by facilitator/ANM/AWW.

The amount to be paid is based on the completed home visit form and first examination of the newborn form, validated by the ASHA facilitator/ANM. The payments to the ASHA should be made on time and with dignity. The payments are made on the *45th* day [using the state mechanism for JSY (Janani Suraksha Yojana) payment] subject to the following:

- Enabling that birth weight is recorded in the Maternal and Child Protection (MCP) Card
- Ensuring that the newborn is immunized with BCG, first doses of OPV, and DPT/Pentavalent*, and entering into the MCP card
- Enabling Birth Registration
- Both mother and newborn are safe until the 42nd day of delivery.

Ensuring Field Support

The ASHA facilitator must visit ASHA at least twice a month for on-job mentoring. The ANM must visit jointly with ASHA at least in 10% of newborns in her subcenter area to supervise the skills of ASHA using supervisory checklists. This would help in timely payment of ASHA. The Village Health and Nutrition (VHN) day will be utilized by ANM to check the coverage and review of quality of services rendered. VHN activity will be supervised by Medical Officers (MOs). Monthly meetings at the PHC (primary health center) level by MOs would also supervise ASHA's visits and referral supports and build linkages. Refresher trainings will be conducted once in 3 months. ASHA's kit is to be refurbished and replenished as per the checklist regularly.

Enabling Health Promotion by ASHA

The ASHA is expected to use her interpersonal communication to educate mothers and family about health promotion and care of newborns and postpartum mothers; to cover these aspects, she has a communication package.

Other Forms of Support

ASHA must be appreciated by the ANM and medical officers for her work especially during Village Health and Sanitation committee meetings. Her achievements like

---

*means wherever pentavalent is available and applicable.

no newborn deaths, etc., may be awarded. Support for grievance redressal should be provided.

Monitoring of Home-based Newborn Care Program

The Ministry of Health and Family Welfare (MoHFW), in each quarter of year, regularly monitors the progress of HBNC in each state by means of various indicators, namely *Process, Output, and Outcomes*. These indicators are shown in **Table 1**.

Steps of Monitoring

- ASHA's home visit form, which she fills during visit to each household, can be used to oversee the number and content of visits.
- During the monthly meetings with ASHA, ANM or ASHA facilitator will verify and sign the home visits form.
- ASHA facilitator/ANM then issues and submits a token/slip to the PHC staff (clerk/accountant).
- Payments to ASHA are then made after approval of Medical Officer in PHC who reviews the HBNC implementation monthly.
- At district level, nodal officer will monitor HBNC program. CMOs (Chief Medical Officers) of the district should also review in this monthly meetings. State NRHM Director would also review these meetings.
- At the national level, NHSRC, under guidance of Child Health Division, MoHFW, monitors the progress.

■ HOME-BASED CARE OF THE YOUNG[7]

Background (Fig. 11)

To provide support for nutrition and early childhood development, the Home-based care for young child (HBYC) has been launched as part of the National Health Mission and POSHAN Abhiyaan of the Ministry of Women and Child Development.

It is observed that:

- About half of the children under 6 months of age are exclusively breastfed.
- About four children out of 10 children under 3 years are breastfed within 1 hour of birth.
- One child out of 10 breastfeeding children aged 6–23 months receive an adequate diet (adequate diet means feeding several times a day as per the age recommendation and giving a diverse variety of foods to meet the requirement for optimal growth and development).

Table 1: Process and output indicators and outcomes.

Process indicators	Output indicators	Outcomes
• Percentage of ASHA trained in Round 1 of Modules 6 and 7 • Percentage of ASHA trained in Round 2 of Module 6 and 7 • Percentage of ASHA trained in Round 3 of Modules 6 and 7 • Percentage of ASHA trained in Round 4 of Module 6 and 7 • Percentage of ASHA with complete HBNC kit	• Percentage of newborns who were visited in the first 2 days of birth at home • Percentage of newborns who received full schedule of HBNC visits • Percentage of newborns who were weighed at birth • Percentage of low birth weight recorded • Percentage of sick newborns referred • Percentage of SNCU discharged babies visited as per schedule	• Percentage of newborn received home visit for HBNC by ASHA against total estimated live births • Percentage of newborns who were breastfeed in the 1st hour • Percentage of low birth weight • Preterm (high risk) babies reported • Percentage of sick newborns admitted at referral sites (SNCUs) • Number of newborns deaths

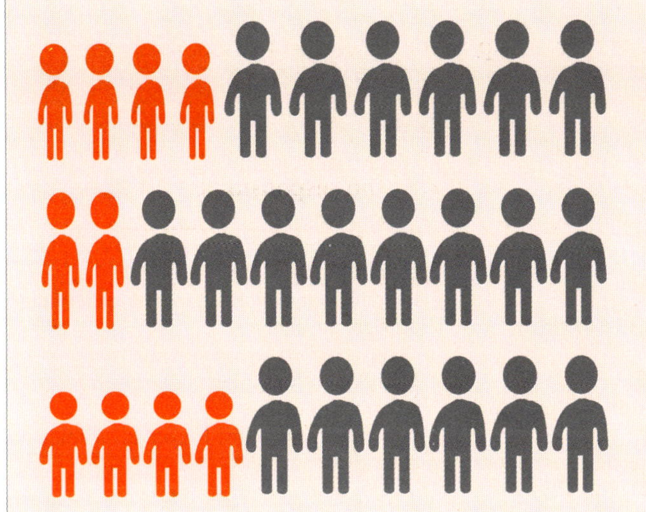

Fig 11: Burden of Malnutrition in India as per NFHS-4 data.
Source: National Family Health Survey (NFHS-4).

- More than half the children between 6 months and 59 months of age are anemic (hemoglobin level less than 11.0 g/dL).

Domain-specific Actions under Home-based Care for Young Child

Holistically considering the various paramount issues dominating health, nutrition, and development of children under 3 years of life, the HBYC programs lay down four domains **(Table 2)** which can promote hygiene, growth, and development and prevent childhood illnesses such as diarrhea and pneumonia.

The objectives of HBYC are to:
- Reduce child deaths and illnesses
- Improve nutritional status of young children
- Ensure proper growth and early childhood development of young children.
  Roles of ASHA and AWW in HBYC during different home visits are given in **Table 3**.[8]

Additional Incentives of Home-based Care for Young Child

Amount:
- Extra ₹ 50 per visit (incentive of INR ₹ 250/- for five additional home visits for each young child)
- In case of more than one child such as twins/triplets, the amount of incentive will be provided per child.

The process and outcome indicators: out of ASHA's home visit:
- Number of home visits conducted
- HBYC card filled
- Age-appropriate activities recorded in the MCP card.

■ CONCLUSION

HBNC and HBYC thus provide the newborn, postpartum mothers, family, and community in totality a complete window of care where a friendly neighborhood ASHA is the contact point to health-seeking behavior changes,

Table 2: Four domains of HBYC programs.

Key domains	Specific actions
Nutrition	Exclusive breastfeeding for 6 months Adequate complementary feeding from 6 months and continued breastfeeding up to 2 years of age Iron and folic acid (IFA) supplementation Promote use of fortified food
Health	Full immunization for children Regular growth monitoring Appropriate use of oral rehydration solution (ORS) during diarrhea episodes Early care seeking during sickness
Child development	Age-appropriate play and communication for children
Wash	Appropriate hand washing practices

(HBYC: Home-based care for young child)

Table 3: Roles of ASHA and AWW in HBYC during different home visits.

Home visits	ASHA	AWW

At 3 months	• Support exclusive breastfeeding
	• Ensure recording/plotting of growth chart for weight-for-age and weight-for-length/height by AWW; identify growth faltering
	• Check immunization status
	• Counsel for the following:
	  – Exclusive breastfeeding (birth to 6 months)
	  – Hand washing practices
	  – Family planning
	  – Parenting ensuring appropriate play and communication
	If the child is sick, has developmental delay or danger signs, provide counseling, first contact care, and refer if required
		• Weigh infants monthly
		• Record weight of the child and plotting on growth chart (weight-for-age)
		• Record length/height of the child and plotting on growth chart (weight-for-length/height)
		• Identify underweight and wasting in children and take appropriate action
		• Counsel regarding growth monitoring
		• Counsel mothers for exclusive breastfeeding from birth to 6 months of age
		• Distribute "Take Home Ration" to lactating mothers and counsel for nutrition
		Check for developmental delay

At 6th, 9th, 12th, and 15th months	All above activities *Plus:* • Ensure that age-appropriate complementary food is given on completion of 6 months • Ensure measles vaccine and vitamin A dose is given as per schedule • Counsel for age-appropriate complementary feeding on completion of 6 months • Provide oral rehydration salt (ORS) packet at home; demonstrate how to prepare ORS and give to the child when required • Provide IFA syrup at home • Teach mother/caregiver regarding IFA syrup administration; ensure that IFA syrup is given to the child by the mother/caregiver on a bi-weekly basis • Provide first contact care and referral for illness	All above activities *Plus:* • Distribute "Take Home Ration" and provide nutrition-specific counseling to mothers/caregivers for their children • Provide supplementary food from anganwadi center (AWC) • Counsel regarding age-appropriate complementary feeding on completion of 6 months of age • Counsel for deworming of children above 1 year of age

(ASHA: Accredited Social Health Activist; AWW: anganwadi worker; HBYC: Home-based care for young child; IFA: iron-folic acid)

prevention of illnesses, early diagnosis of serious illness, nutrition, and development.

■ REFERENCES

1. Ministry of Health and Family Welfare, Government of India. Home Based Newborn Care. Operational guidelines (Revised 2014). Available from: http://www.nihfw.org/pdf/NCHRC-Publications/Operational%20Guidelines%20on%20Home%20Based%20Newborn%20Care%20(HBNC).pdf. [Last accessed on December, 2019].

2. Neogi SB, Sharma J, Chauhan M, et al. Care of the newborn in community and at home. J Perinatol. 2016;36(Suppl 3);S13-7.

3. Bang AT, Bang RA. Background of the field trial of home-based neonatal care in Gadchiroli, India. J Perinatol. 2005;25 (Suppl 1):S3-10.

4. Bang AT, Bang RA, Reddy HM. Home-based neonatal care: summary and applications of the field trial in rural Gadchiroli, India (1993–2003). J Perinatol. 2005;25(Suppl 1):S108-22.
5. Mavalankar DV, Raman P. ANKUR Project: A Case Study of Replication of Home Based Newborn Care. [online] Available from: http://www.srujan.info/resource/50/hbnc—ankur.pdf. [Last accessed on December, 2019].
6. National Health Mission, Ministry of Health and Family Welfare, Government of India. ASHA Training Modules (1 to 7). [online] Available at https://nhm.gov.in/index1.php?lang=1&level=3&sublinkid=184&lid=257.
7. Home Based Care for Young Child (HBYC). Strengthening of Health and Nutrition through home visits. Operational Guidelines, April 2018. A joint initiative of Ministry of Health & Family Welfare and Ministry of Women and Child Development. [online] Available from: https//www.aspirationaldistricts.in/wp-content/uploads/2019/02/Home-Based-Care-for-Young-Child-Guidelines.pdf. [Last accessed on December, 2019].
8. Child Health Division, Ministry of Health and Family Welfare, Government of India. Handbook for ASHA on Home Based Care for Young Child, Additional home visits to address the young child. [online] Available from: http://nhsrcindia.org/sites/default/files/Handbook%20for%20ASHA%20on%20Home%20Based%20Care%20for%20Young%20Child-English.pdf. [Last accessed on December, 2019].

Neonatal Intensive Care Unit Graduate in the Tropics

Viraraghavan VR, Srinivas Murki

INTRODUCTION

Neonatal intensive care unit (NICU) graduates are a heterogenous group of high-risk infants discharged from an NICU who because of their biological, medical or social characteristics are at high risk of short-term and long-term health and developmental problems.[1] Though preterm infants form the predominant subgroup of these high-risk infants, some of the term infants with a variety of risk factors also come under this category.[2-4] There are mainly four categories of high-risk infants:

1. Infants with biological risk factors
2. Infants who required significant interventions during NICU stay
3. Infants who have special care needs or are dependent on technology at discharge
4. Infants with social and environmental risk factors.

Many of the tropical countries have made significant progress in neonatal care resulting in an improved survival rate of these high-risk infants and thus making their follow-up care more important than ever. However, follow-up care of high-risk infants requires a multidisciplinary team and extensive resources. In cost-constrained tropical countries, it is vital to identify infants who are at the highest risk for neurodevelopmental impairment and follow them in the high-risk clinic while the well-to-do infants are in follow-up with a general physician or a pediatrician. **Table 1** illustrates the types of high-risk infants discharged from an NICU.[4]

DISCHARGE PLANNING AND PREDISCHARGE CHECKLIST FOR HIGH-RISK INFANTS

The planning of discharge for a high-risk neonate should ideally start early in the course of NICU stay. Every NICU should have an individualized protocol for planning the discharge and should develop a predischarge checklist that could be easily administered by their doctors and nurses alike.

The most important components of discharge planning are given in the following text.[3]

Assessment of Infant Readiness for Discharge

Many units follow weight-based criteria for discharge of a very preterm or very low birth weight (VLBW) infant from the NICU, but multiple studies show that discharging preterm infants based on physiological criteria rather than on a weight-based criterion ensures an early discharge with no associated increase in adverse outcomes after discharge.[5-7] Physiological criteria are also useful for all at-risk infants. There are three main components in the physiological criteria:

1. The infant should be on oral feedings and should be gaining adequate weight, i.e. 15 g/kg/day for 3 consecutive days.
2. The infant who is adequately clothed should be able to maintain normal body temperature in an open cot at an environmental temperature of 25°C.
3. The infant should have a mature respiratory control and breathing room air.

Most infants qualify these criteria once they are 34–36 weeks postmenstrual age (PMA). However, a mature respiratory control may not be reached until 44 weeks PMA in extreme preterm infants born at less than 28 weeks and in infants with bronchopulmonary dysplasia (BPD). Many tertiary care centers in tropical countries such as India assess for discharge readiness at a PMA of 34 weeks when caffeine therapy is stopped. Although it is ideal to wait for more than a week after cessation of caffeine therapy and/or to assess for caffeine levels (level should be less than

Table 1: NICU graduates requiring follow-up in a high-risk clinic.

Infants with biological risk factors	Infants who required significant interventions during NICU stay	Infants with special care needs	Infants with social and economic risk factors
Prematurity (≤32 weeks) and/or VLBW (<1,500 g)	Mechanical ventilation for > 7 days	Home oxygen/home ventilation	Teen mother
Severe IUGR (<3rd centile)	High-frequency ventilation	Tracheostomy	Low socioeconomic status
Monochorionic twin with intrauterine death of the co-twin or twin-to-twin transfusion	Postnatal steroids within 14 days of life	Gastrostomy tube/gavage feeding	Substance abuse in the family
Chromosomal abnormalities	Surgical intervention for NEC, PDA, shunt		Low maternal education
Major malformations	Bronchopulmonary dysplasia		Infant born to retroviral-positive mother
Inborn errors of metabolism	Meningitis/culture proven sepsis		
TORCH infection	Neonatal hyperbilirubinemia >20 mg/dL or requiring exchange transfusion		
	Symptomatic hypoglycemia/hypocalcemic seizures		
	Symptomatic polycythemia		
	Neonatal seizures		
	Abnormal neurological examination at discharge		
	Hypoxic-ischemic encephalopathy state 2 and more		
	Shock requiring vasopressors		

(IUGR: intrauterine growth restriction; NEC: necrotizing enterocolitis; NICU: neonatal intensive care unit; PDA: patent ductus arteriosus; TORCH: Toxoplasmosis, Other, Rubella, Cytomegalovirus, and Herpes; VLBW: very low birth weight)

2 µg/mL) prior to discharge, in resource-limited settings most infants are discharged after an observation of 5–7 days for the recurrence of apnea.[8]

Parental Education

The parents should be involved in the care of their infants from hospital admission to discharge. They should be made to understand the nature of illness of their infant and that the care beyond the NICU stay at home plays a vital part in improving the outcomes of their baby. Mothers should learn to express breast milk for their sick infant. Mother/caregivers should manage day-to-day care of the neonate such as spoon-feeding, identifying the cues for feeding, diaper change, and hygiene precautions. Kangaroo mother care (KMC) is a cost-effective, high-impact intervention that has shown to improve the survival rates of low birth weight (LBW) infants, improve exclusive breastfeeding rates at discharge as well as 6 months postdischarge, and reduce the risk of infection and hypothermia.[9] The mother as well as other family members should be involved in KMC once the infant is stable and should be encouraged to continue it after discharge at home. The parents of those high-risk infants who need assistance even at discharge such as those on gavage feeding, those with a tracheostomy who require tracheostomy care, and those planned for home oxygen therapy should be well trained in taking care of their babies. It is important that the competency of these parents to take care of their high-risk infants at home be assessed prior to discharge. The caregivers should also be informed about the pending medical issues and the plan regarding the same. Finally, evaluation of the five important danger signs that might indicate a serious underlying condition—fever (temperature >37.5°C), hypothermia (axillary temperature <35.5°C), poor feeding, lethargy, and convulsions—should be taught to the parents.[10]

Completion of Other Elements of Care: Immunization and Routine Screenings

The infant should have been immunized for its chronological age prior to discharge. Other routine screening tests are as follows:

- Retinopathy of prematurity (ROP) screening
- Hearing screening
- Screening for congenital hypothyroidism

- Screening for metabolic disorders
- Pulse oximetry screening for critical congenital heart disease
- Screening for nutritional disorders such as anemia of prematurity and osteopenia of prematurity
- Screening for intraventricular hemorrhage and periventricular leukomalacia (PVL) should have been completed.

It is also vital to do a baseline neurological and a neurobehavioral assessment prior to discharge.

Plan for Unresolved Medical Issues

A clear plan for certain unresolved medical issues and other pending tests or reports should be clearly documented in the discharge proforma as well as conveyed to the caregivers.

Plan for Follow-up Care

The parents should be informed about the follow-up care of their neonates. For those residing at a far away distance from the tertiary care center, an appropriate primary care physician or a pediatrician should be identified to whom the family may consult in case of an emergency. The parents should also be aware of the high-risk clinic follow-up dates and timings. All efforts should be made to club the follow-up visits with the immunization schedule and/or with ROP and other screening schedules.

The discharge checklist should include the following:[3]

- On oral feeding with adequate weight gain of 15 g/kg/day or more for at least 3 consecutive days
- Maintain normal body temperature when fully clothed in an open cot at an ambient temperature of 25°C
- No episodes of apnea or bradycardia for at least 5 days after stopping caffeine therapy
- Immunized for the infant's chronological age
- Screened for congenital hypothyroidism and other metabolic disorders
- Screened for hearing either by otoacoustic emission (OAE) or brainstem evoked response audiometry (BERA) as appropriate or date assigned
- Screened for ROP screenings and follow-up visits and dates assigned
- Screened for anemia of prematurity and osteopenia of prematurity (OOP) and/or dates assigned
- Assessed for parental education and competency
- A complete discharge summary documenting the hospital course along with plans for unresolved medical issues and follow-up care handed over to the caregiver
- All assigned dates cross-checked and signed.

What is the Follow-up Schedule?

The follow-up schedule for a high-risk infant varies as per the risk profile of the infant. Preterm infants require more frequent follow-up (weekly) after hospital discharge till they attain a weight of 3 kg and subsequently their follow-up schedule becomes similar to their term counterparts. An appropriate follow-up schedule for high-risk infants is given in **Table 2**.

Follow-up of a Preterm Infant

The gestational age and birth weight threshold below which preterm infants are included in a high-risk follow-up clinic varies widely across tertiary care institutions based on their available resources. Usually, preterm infants less than or equal to 32 weeks and/or less than or equal to 1,500 g are enrolled in a high-risk follow-up clinic.[4] The corrected age (postnatal age minus the extent of prematurity) up to which these infants are followed also varies. But many high-risk clinics do longitudinal follow-up till these infants are 24 months of corrected age. Historically, it was believed that developmental assessment at 24 months corrected age was a good predictor of future outcomes. However, recent studies have pointed the opposite and thus many of the high-risk clinics are enrolling infants beyond this age.[11] Most comprehensive follow-up programs enroll infants until they are 8–10 years of age. The checklist for assessment of a high-risk preterm infant during follow-up is given in **Table 3**.

The following are monitored during the follow-up of a preterm infant.

Table 2: Follow-up schedule for high-risk infants.	
Type of high-risk infant	*Follow-up schedule*
Preterm infants ≤32 weeks and/or <1,500 g	*Initial visits*: 2 days after discharge and then every 2 weeks till 3 kg *Subsequent visits*: 3, 6, 9, 12, 15, 18, 24, 30, and 36 months corrected age and subsequent visits as per the local logistics
All other high-risk infants	*Initial visit*: 1 week after discharge *Subsequent visits*: 6 weeks, 10 weeks, 14 weeks, 6 months, 9 months, 12 months, 15 months, 18 months, 24 months, 30 months, 36 months

Table 3: Checklist for parameters to be assessed for a high-risk preterm infant during follow-up.

Parameter	When
Growth	Every visit
Nutrition	Every visit
Immunization	As per the existing immunization schedule
ROP	Refer to Table 5
Hearing evaluation	Infant should have crossed 34 weeks PMA, to be done prior to discharge. Rescreening every 6 months till 3 years
Neurological examination	3, 6, 9, 12, 15, 18, 24 months corrected age. Refer to Table 6
Developmental assessment	3, 6, 9, 12, 15, 18, 24 months corrected age. Refer to Table 6
Early stimulation	Every visit and continued at home
Any abnormal physical examination	*Every visit*: Look for anemia, hernia, rickets, hemangioma, deformation plagiocephaly
Pending tests/reports	• Congenital hypothyroidism and other metabolic diseases screening • Calcium, inorganic phosphorus and alkaline phosphatase for OOP • Complete blood count for anemia of prematurity • Echocardiogram for BPD with pulmonary hypertension • MRI brain/neurosonogram at 40 weeks PMA

(BPD: bronchopulmonary dysplasia; MRI: magnetic resonance imaging; OOP: osteopenia of prematurity; PMA: postmenstrual age; ROP: retinopathy of prematurity)

- *Growth:* Majority of the VLBW infants who are born AGA (appropriate for gestational age, weight for gestational age >10th centile) end up growth retarded and are classified as EUGR (extra uterine growth retardation, defined as weight for gestational age <10th centile at 36 weeks PMA).[12] Hence, it is vital that the growth of these vulnerable, already growth-restricted infants is monitored, and appropriate nutritional interventions are administered so that adequate catch-up growth occurs after discharge. Growth monitoring encompasses measurement of weight, length, mid-arm circumference, and head circumference. The weight should be measured after undressing the baby. These preterm infants grow at a rate of 15 g/kg/day till 40 weeks PMA beyond which they grow at a rate of 25–30 g/day.[13] These neonates are expected to catch up with their term counterparts by 24 months corrected age. Recumbent length should be measured using an infantometer till 24 months corrected age. The head circumference is measured as the maximal occipitofrontal diameter. The expected increment in head circumference is 0.9 cm/wk till 40 weeks PMA and 0.5 cm/wk since then.[13] Head "catchup" occurs early by around 8 months corrected age.[14] All these parameters should be plotted longitudinally on a growth chart. Different growth charts are available for monitoring the growth of a preterm infant and the recent addition to this is the INTERGROWTH-21 charts.[15] Fenton's growth chart is frequently used.[15] The anthropometric parameters of a preterm infant should be plotted till 50 weeks PMA in Fenton's chart beyond which WHO Multicenter Growth Reference Study (MGRS) charts have to be used. The growth should be plotted for the corrected age, i.e. after correcting for prematurity.

- *Nutrition:* The assessment of nutritional intake is a very critical aspect of follow-up of preterm infants. The feeding history should be elicited by documenting the type of feeds (exclusive breastfeeding, fortified total breast milk feeding, formula feed, animal milk along with dilution if used) and the mode of feeding (spoon, paladai, bottle). Animal milk should be discouraged till at least 1 year of chronological age. All efforts should be made to discharge the preterm infant on total breast milk feeding. This is more relevant in tropical countries where exclusive breastfeeding decreases the risk of morbidities such as diarrhea and pneumonia requiring hospitalization and eventually reduces the risk of mortality.[16] Fortification is an essential part of preterm infant nutrition and is advised till 40 weeks PMA or 2 kg, whichever is later.[17] Human milk fortifiers (HMFs) are available and usually 1 g (one sachet) is added to 25 mL of expressed breast milk. Most HMFs available in the market supply adequate amounts of calcium, phosphorus, iron, vitamin D, and other fat-soluble/water soluble vitamins needed for the preterm infant. The nutritional requirements for such preterm infants who are not on HMF or whose HMF has been stopped at 40 weeks PMA or 2 kg are summarized

Table 4: Nutritional requirements for a high-risk infant.

Birth weight	Nutritional intervention
<1,500 g	*HMF*: Started at 80–100 mL/kg enteral feeds and continued till 2 kg or 40 weeks PMA, whichever is later. 1 g sachet added to 25 mL mother's milk. Those infants on at least 10 HMF sachets per day do not require any addition of supplements. Target daily calories of 130–150 kcal/kg/day and protein of 3.5–4 g/kg/day *Calcium/phosphate:** Calcium supplemented at 150–220 mg/kg/day and phosphate at 75–140 mg/kg/day. Started at 100 mL/kg/day enteral feeds and stopped at 40 weeks PMA or 2 kg whichever is later *Multivitamins:** Standard formulation supplemented at 1 mL/day. Started at 100 mL/kg/day enteral feeds and stopped at 40 weeks PMA or 2 kg, whichever is later *Iron:** Supplemented at 2–3 mg/kg/day. Started at 2 weeks of age and stopped at 1 year *Vitamin D:** Supplemented at 400 IU/day. Started at 100 mL/kg/day enteral feeds and stopped at 1 year *Started only after HMF has been stopped/not used or if the neonate is on preterm formula fortified breast milk.
1,500–2,499 g	*Iron*: Supplemented at 2–3 mg/kg/day. Started at 4 weeks of age and stopped at 1 year *Vitamin D*: Supplemented at 400 IU/day. Started at 1 week and stopped at 1 year
≥2,500 g	*Iron*: Supplemented at 2–3 mg/kg/day. Started at 4 months of age if the infant is exclusively breastfed and stopped at 6 months of age once complimentary feeds rich in iron are introduced *Vitamin D*: Supplemented at 400 IU/day. Started at 1 week and stopped at 1 year

(HMF: human milk fortifiers; PMA: premenstrual age)

in **Table 4**. Introduction of complimentary feeds should be advised from 6 months chronological age in these preterm infants. Direct breastfeeding should be encouraged as early as 32 weeks PMA and once the infant is capable of complete breastfeeding, stop the fortification and continue breastfeeding for as long as 3 years if possible.[16]

- *Immunization:* Preterm infants should be immunized according to their chronological age like the term infants. Prematurity or LBW is not a contraindication for any of the vaccines. Apart from the routine vaccines, additional vaccination with pneumococcus vaccine should be offered to all VLBWs.[18] Respiratory syncytial virus (RSV) prophylaxis (Synagis) which is routinely given to certain high-risk preterm infants in developed nations is not feasible in tropical countries due to cost constraints and nonavailability.[19] Influenza vaccine should be offered to all these preterm infants and their contacts at 6 months of chronological age.[20] There is an emerging concept of cocoon vaccination of family members for influenza prior to hospital discharge of a VLBW infant.

- *Physical examination:*
  - *Vitals:* All preterm infants should have their vitals, i.e. temperature, heart rate, respiratory rate, pulse volume, and capillary refilling time monitored during each follow-up visit. Blood pressure monitoring is vital in preterm infants with a history of BPD, umbilical arterial lines, urinary tract infection, or acute kidney injury. Saturation (SpO$_2$) should also be checked as and when indicated, especially in preterm infants on home oxygen therapy or those who are on pulmonary vasodilator therapy for pulmonary hypertension.

  - *Inguinal hernia:* Inguinal hernias are common in preterm infants. The usual age of appearance is at 40 weeks PMA and is more common in males. The risk of incarceration is also high in preterm infants compared to term infants.[21] The timing of surgery is controversial with some pediatric surgeons opting for surgery immediately after diagnosis while others delaying it till a later date.[22]

  - *Anemia:* Anemia of prematurity is a common occurrence in these infants. Preterm infants can be discharged at a hemoglobin level of 8 g/dL and reticulocyte count of >3%.[20] All preterm infants with a hemoglobin of <9.5 g/dL at discharge should have a complete blood count done at 2 weeks post-discharge and again at 1–2 months later.[20] A hemoglobin level of less than 7 g/dL is an indication for transfusion in an otherwise asymptomatic infant.[23]

  - Capillary hemangiomas are common in these infants and the parents should be counseled about their benign course.[24] Teeth eruptions at appropriate corrected age should be looked for. Deformation plagiocephaly is very common and it corrects on its own by 3–4 years of age. Tiny hard whitish lesions which are calcium deposits seen in preterm infants who had multiple heel pricks or IV cannula for a long time are benign and can last for years.[24]

- *Retinopathy of prematurity/eye evaluation:* The incidence of ROP in tropical countries such as India is quite different from that in developed nations where even bigger infants are affected by this ophthalmological complication in tropics.[25] Hence, Indian guidelines advise screening for all preterm infants less than or equal to 34 weeks and/or less than or equal to 2,000 g.[26] Those infants who were born at 34–36 weeks and who had other significant risk factors during the NICU stay such as requirement of mechanical ventilation, prolonged oxygen use, neonatal sepsis, poor postnatal weight gain, and blood transfusion also need to be screened for ROP. ROP screening and further follow-up visits are summarized in **Table 5**.[27,28] Preterm infants are also prone to a variety of other ophthalmological complications such as myopia, amblyopia, and strabismus. Hence, a repeat ophthalmological evaluation should be done after 12 months corrected age. The decision for glasses, patching, or corrective surgery will be taken by the ophthalmologist depending upon the ophthalmological issue that the infant has.[20]

- *Hearing evaluation:* Hearing evaluation is indicated in all newborns irrespective of their medical condition.[29] Universal hearing screening has become a part of many of the health programs in tropical countries such as India [Rashtriya Bal Swasthya Karyakram (RBSK)]. Preterm infants who are NICU graduates have a higher risk of hearing loss due to a myriad of reasons such as aminoglycoside/diuretics use, meningitis, noise pollution, and mechanical ventilation.[20] An automated brainstem evoked response test is used to screen for hearing. The 1-3-6 rule advocated by Joint Committee on Infant Hearing (JCIH) is usually followed.[29] All infants are to be screened for hearing loss by at least 1 month of chronological age (preterm infants should have crossed 34 weeks PMA), referred to a specialist for confirmation by at least 3 months of age, and interventions such as cochlear implants be done by at least 6 months of age. Earlier identification and intervention are shown to improve hearing outcomes. Those with normal hearing screen should be screened periodically at 6 monthly intervals till 3 years.

- *Osteopenia of prematurity:* The incidence of osteopenia of prematurity has come down significantly in the recent decades. However, its incidence in extreme premature infants and in infants with certain risk factors such as BPD, prolonged parenteral nutrition use, and those who had received diuretics is still high. All VLBW infants should be screened at 4 weeks of chronological age for OOP.[30] A blood sample for ionic calcium, inorganic phosphorus (iP), and alkaline phosphatase (ALP) should be sent for the same. An iP value of <4.0 mg/dL and ALP >800 IU/L is highly suggestive of OOP.[30] In such cases, further evaluation with urine calcium and phosphorus and wrist radiograph is indicated. In preterm infants with normal values, repeat screening is advised every 2 weekly till ALP values stabilize below 800 IU/L.

- *Gastroesophageal reflux disease (GERD):* GERD is very common in preterm infants. GERD should be

Table 5: ROP screening and follow-up for high-risk neonates.

Who requires screening?	• Infants <34 weeks and/or <2,000 g • Infants 34–36[6/7] weeks with risk factors such as requirement of mechanical ventilation/oxygen therapy/blood transfusion/culture proven sepsis
When to screen?	• <28 weeks—3 weeks postnatal age • 28–32 weeks—4 weeks postnatal age • ≥33 weeks—2 weeks postnatal age
When to treat?	• Zone I: Any stage ROP with plus disease • Zone I: Stage 3 ROP without plus disease • Zone II: Stage 2 or 3 with plus disease
When can anti-VEGF be used?	Zone I: Stage 3 ROP with plus disease
How to follow-up?	• *1 week or less follow-up*: Zone I immature vascularization, Zone I—stage 1 or 2, Zone II— Stage 3, any zone—suspected aggressive posterior ROP • *1–2 weekly follow-up*: Zone I—unequivocally regressing ROP, Zone II—stage 2, Zone II—posterior zone immature vascularization • *2 weekly follow-up*: Zone I—stage 1, Zone II—immature vascularization, Zone II—unequivocally regressing ROP • *2–3 weekly follow-up*: Zone III—stage 1 or 2 or regressing ROP
When to stop screening?	• Zone III—Vascularization attained without any previous Zone I or Zone II top • 45 weeks PMA and no prethreshold disease (stage 3 ROP in Zone II, any ROP in Zone I) or any worse ROP • 65 weeks PMA if anti-VEGF was used (in such cases, maximum risk of reactivation is at 45–55 weeks PMA) • Equivocally regressing ROP

(PMA: postmenstrual age; ROP: retinopathy of prematurity; VEGF: vascular endothelial growth factor) differentiated from physiological reflux. It should be treated if there are respiratory complications such as aspiration pneumonia, inadequate weight gain or if symptoms of esophagitis are present. Esophagitis presents as irritability and arching of head and back during feeding and feed aversion, eventually resulting in poor weight gain.[21] Both pharmacological and nonpharmacological interventions may be tried. Prone positioning as a nonpharmacological measure should not be advised in such infants as it increases the risk of sudden infant death syndrome (SIDS).[21]

- *Infantile colic:* The incidence of colic is much higher in preterm infants than terms. It starts around 1 month of age and resolves by 3 months.[21] It is characterized by excessive crying and irritability usually lasting for more than 3 hours per day, 3 days a week, and for more than 3 weeks.[31] It is a benign condition and antispasmodic medications which can cause serious side effects should not be used. Techniques such as decreasing stimulation, swaddling, and placing warm water bottles might be helpful. In resistant cases, cow milk protein intolerance should be considered.

- *Neurodevelopmental evaluation and neuroimaging:* Neurodevelopmental evaluation of a high-risk preterm should start during the course of stay of the infant in the NICU. A basic neurological and neurobehavioral examination should be done at discharge. There are various tools to assess the neurological status (Amiel Tison Neurological Evaluation of Newborn, Prechtl's Examination) as well as neurobehavior [Neonatal Behavioral Assessment Scale (NBAS), assessment of preterm infants' behavior (APIB)] during the NICU stay.[32] Some of these tools require formal training.

- During follow-up, screening should be done to detect any developmental delay. Many screening tools are available for the same. Some of the commonly used screening tools are Trivandrum Development Screening Chart (TDSC), Denver Development Screening Test (DDST) II, and Bayley Infant Neurodevelopmental Screener (BINS). Out of these, TDSC is a cheap and user-friendly assessment tool that might be appropriate for resource-constrained tropical countries. BINS is a modified version of Bayley Scale of Infant Development (BSID) III and is costly and requires training. An exhaustive developmental assessment is usually performed if the developmental screening reveals any abnormality. It is also routinely done at certain time frames for most of these high-risk infants by trained professionals by using specific tools such as Gross Movement Assessment (GMA) at 3–4 months

corrected age and BSID III at 12 months and 18–24 months corrected age.[33,34] Similar to developmental assessment, a neurological assessment is also performed using tools such as Hammersmith Infant Neurological Examination (HINE) and Amiel Tison at 3, 6, 9, 12, 15, 18, and 24 months corrected age.[35] Many of these NICU graduates are also at a high risk of autism, attention deficit hyperactive disorder, anxiety, and depression which should be assessed at appropriate ages. It should be noted that like growth, development is also adjusted for the degree of prematurity and corrected age is used rather than chronological age. **Table 6** summarizes the appropriate assessments for corrected age along with appropriate tools.

- Neuroimaging with magnetic resonance imaging (MRI) with or without diffusion-weighted images is usually advised in these neonates at 40 weeks PMA.[36] This can put a lot of burden on the existing system as well as on the parents in a tropical country due to cost and other logistic issues. In such a scenario, at least a neurosonogram should be performed to identify PVL, ventriculomegaly, intraparenchymal hemorrhage/cysts which might be useful to predict long-term neurodevelopmental outcomes.[37,30] It should be noted that a neurosonogram is not a sensitive tool to diagnose certain pathologies such as white matter injury, basal ganglia lesions, and small cerebellar hemorrhages, all of which have shown to affect the neurodevelopment of a preterm infant in an adverse way.[39]

- *Early intervention:*

What is early intervention?
Early intervention is a program directed at a high-risk infant along with his/her parents with an aim of improving the neurodevelopmental outcome of the susceptible infant.[2] The involvement of the parents is vital for the success of an early intervention program. Also, these programs have been found to be beneficial in improving maternal anxiety, depression, and parent-infant relationship, eventually having a positive outcome on the infant itself. Early intervention includes teaching the parent about general cognitive stimulation of the infant by using age-appropriate activities along with the stimulation of visual, auditory, and tactile systems. It also encompasses occupational therapy, physical therapy, and speech therapy. These are started early during the NICU stay.

What is the evidence for early intervention?
The largest randomized controlled trial (RCT) Infant Health and Development program enrolled infants

Table 6: Neurodevelopmental assessment during follow-up.

Corrected age	Parameters to be assessed	Tools for assessment	Who will administer?
3, 6, 9, 12, 15, 24 months	Screening for developmental delay	• Trivandrum Developmental Screening Chart (TDSC) or • Bayley Infant Neurodevelopmental Screener (BINS) or • Denver Development Screening Test II (DDST II)	Primary physician/pediatrician/neonatologist
3, 6, 9, 12, 15, 24 months	Neurological examination	• Amiel tison • Hammersmith Infant Neurological examination	
>2 years	Functional classification of children diagnosed with cerebral palsy	• Gross Motor Function Classification system (GMFCS)	
12, 18–24 months	Complete assessment of all spheres of development (gross motor, fine motor, social, language milestones)	• Developmental assessment of Indian Infants (DASII) • Bayley Scales of Infant Development III (BSID III)	These tools require adequate training and are labor intensive. A certified physician/pediatrician/neonatologist/developmental pediatrician can administer
18, 24 months	Autism risk	Modified-Check list for Autism in Toddlers-Revised (M-CHAT-R)	Primary physician/pediatrician/neonatologist. This is a questionnaire that can be easily administered by a primary physician, pediatrician, or a neonatologist. Based on the score, the child is either re-screened at a later age or directly referred to a child psychologist for complete evaluation

less than 2,500 g born during 1985–1988 after NICU discharge till 36 months corrected age.[40] Though improvements in IQ and cognitive function were seen at 3 years corrected age in those infants who received early intervention compared to the control group, these were not seen in the subgroup of infants with a birth weight of less than 1,000 g who are at the highest risk for neurodevelopmental impairment. Also, though evaluation of these infants at 8 years of age showed some improvement in growth outcomes, the initial improvements in IQ and cognitive function that were seen at 3 years were not observed.[41] When outcomes were assessed at the adolescent stage, findings similar to those seen at 3 years of age were noted and likewise in mature preterm infants only.[42] The meta-analysis of RCTs on early intervention shows similar results with improvements in growth and cognitive outcomes at preschool age but not persisting at school age or adolescence.[43] Despite such mixed results from RCTs, early intervention is still widely practiced by leading tertiary care units and should be implemented as a part of high-risk follow-up clinic for NICU graduates as absence of evidence is not the same as no evidence of benefit.

Follow-up of Preterm Very Low Birth Weight Infants with Specific Issues

Preterm Infant with Bronchopulmonary Dysplasia

Preterm infants with BPD are more prone to growth failure, ROP, apnea prolonging beyond 34 weeks PMA, OOP, systemic hypertension, pulmonary hypertension, GERD, readmission for respiratory illnesses, and neurodevelopmental impairment. These have been discussed in the previous section. Some of the preterm infants with BPD might be discharged on home oxygen therapy or might even require tracheostomy with or without invasive ventilation. Though home oxygen therapy is increasingly used in tropical countries, home ventilation is a very rare phenomenon. A saturation target of 93–95% for infants with BPD with or without coexisting pulmonary hypertension is advised.[44] Follow-up of such infants require adequate knowledge on tapering oxygen therapy, diuretics, and pulmonary vasodilator therapy. These infants who are planned to be discharged on home oxygen therapy need to satisfy certain predetermined criteria for discharge in addition to those in the routine discharge checklist. The infant should be at a low-flow oxygen flow rate of 0.5 L/min, should maintain a saturation of at least

80% on room air for 30 minutes (safeguard for accidental dislodgement at home), and should not have had any cyanotic or apneic spells in the previous 2 weeks. During follow-up, diuretics are initially weaned off to once-daily dosing and then stopped. Then, home oxygen is weaned at the rate of 0.1 L/min per month.[13,21] These should be done under supervision of a physician in the follow-up clinic. A 20-minute period of SpO_2 monitoring postweaning is done and if the infant maintains more than 93% during this period, the infant is sent home at the weaned rate.[45] A trial for stopping home oxygen should be done at 0.1 L/min in a similar fashion. Weaning from pulmonary vasodilator therapy is done after discussing with the cardiologist. Apart from SpO_2, the other major parameters that have to be taken into consideration before weaning are optimal growth and normalization of pulmonary pressures.[45]

Preterm Infant with Persisting Apnea of Prematurity beyond 34–36 Weeks Post-menstrual Age

Apnea of prematurity usually resolves by 33–34 weeks PMA. However, in a subset of preterm infants who are extremely preterm (<28 weeks) with or without BPD, it might persist for a longer duration of time, i.e. till PMA 44 weeks. In such infants, caffeine therapy can be continued along with an apnea monitor at home. Caffeine can be stopped by 40 weeks PMA in such babies. Home monitoring with an apnea monitor should be continued for another 4 weeks and can be stopped if there are no apneas during this time period.[21] Implementing this strategy is very challenging in tropical countries as affording an apnea monitor is very difficult for the parents. Newer monitoring devices with pulse oximeters incorporated in the mobile phones are available and hence remote monitoring is a possibility for such infants. When home monitoring is not available and the infant is having significant apnea, caffeine can be continued till 44 weeks PMA beyond which the risk of apnea is almost nil.[46]

Preterm Infant with Severe Intraventricular Hemorrhage (Grade III/IV) and/or Cystic Periventricular Leukomalacia

The monitoring of such infants should include a neurosurgical team also. Head circumference and ventricular diameters along with resistive index of anterior cerebral artery should be monitored with frequent neurosonograms. Lack of head growth (<0.8 cm/wk) as well as rapid head growth (>1.25 cm/wk) are both worrisome. The parents should be educated on the signs and symptoms of raised intracranial tension for which emergency care is to be sought. Depending on the head growth and features of *intracranial pressure* (ICP), requirement for a ventriculosubgaleal (VSG) or a ventriculoperitoneal (VP) shunt should be assessed. VSG shunt insertion is relatively less invasive compared to VP shunt and might buy some time for VP shunt insertion. The parents of those infants with a VP shunt should be educated about its associated complications such as shunt infection and shunt blockage. Preterm infants with cystic PVL are at a very high risk of developing cerebral palsy and hence require close follow-up as well as early intervention.[47]

Follow-up of Other High-risk Neonates

The follow-up schedule for other categories of high-risk neonates is almost similar to that of a preterm infant except that the timing of the first visit after discharge from the NICU is at a later period and further initial visits are planned coinciding with the vaccination schedule. This is summarized in **Table 2**. All these infants should also be monitored for growth, nutrition, and neurodevelopmental delay. Also, hearing evaluation, ophthalmic evaluation, and early intervention as done for preterm infants are vital in these infants too.

Follow-up of Neonates with Hypoxic-Ischemic Encephalopathy

The use of clinical staging systems such as Sarnat and Sarnat to prognosticate infants with HIE is widely used in tropical countries. The other parameters used to predict neurodevelopmental impairment in such infants such as amplitude electroencephalography (EEG) patterns in the initial course of the illness and MRI with or without diffusion-weighted imaging and magnetic resonance spectroscopy are minimally utilized in many of the tropical countries due to cost constraints. While all of the surviving infants with a Sarnat and Sarnat HIE stage III will end up with severe neurodevelopmental impairment, most with HIE stage I would have a normal neurodevelopmental outcome.[48] Poor head growth, feeding difficulties, excessive crying spells, and altered sleep rhythms are predictive of abnormal long-term neurological deficits in these infants. As some of these infants are discharged on antiepileptic drug (AED) therapy, the follow-up of these infants requires the treating physician to be aware as to when and how these medications are to be tapered and stopped. A neurological examination should be done for those infants who are discharged on AED at 1 month of age and if it is normal, AED can be stopped without tapering. If the neurological examination at 1 month of age is abnormal, an EEG should be obtained. If the EEG is normal, then AED should be tapered over 2 weeks and stopped. In case the EEG is also abnormal, AED should be continued and a review at 3 months of age is done and the same sequence of steps should be followed.[49] These infants might have other issues related to feeding such as oral aversion, swallowing difficulties, and GERD eventually resulting in growth failure which would require oromotor stimulation assisted by a speech pathologist and dietary modification advised by a dietician. Many might end up requiring gastrostomy secondary to severe GERD. The follow-up care of these infants is given in the following section.

Follow-up of Infants with Bilirubin Values of more than 20 mg/dL or Those Who had Required Exchange Transfusion or Those with Kernicterus

Unlike the developed nations, severe hyperbilirubinemia and kernicterus are still a major public health problem in the tropics. Genetics, early discharge from the hospital after birth (<48 hours) coupled with inadequate risk assessment for neonatal hyperbilirubinemia at discharge, poor follow-up, poor quality of phototherapy, inadequate access to blood exchange, and inadequate prophylaxis of Rh-negative mothers with anti-D are the possible reasons for the high incidence of severe jaundice and kernicterus in the tropics. These infants are prone to developing hearing loss, and hence the importance of hearing screening before the age of 1 month in this subgroup cannot be overstated.[50] Also, MRI changes of basal ganglia are evident within a short duration after the insult and hence MRI should be obtained prior to hospital discharge if feasible.[51] Infants who do develop kernicterus will require early stimulation and development monitoring like the other high-risk infants. Hearing deficits need early correction with hearing aids or stimulation as appropriate. These infants who later on might develop severe dystonia will require the active involvement of a pediatric neurologist for instituting medications directed at reducing dystonia. Most of these infants have either a normal or only mildly impaired intellect.

Follow-up of Infants with Tracheostomy Tube

Some infants with BPD might require a tracheostomy in view of prolonged mechanical ventilation. The other common indications for tracheostomy in NICU are congenital upper airway malformation such as severe laryngotracheomalacia, congenital subglottic stenosis, and bilateral vocal cord palsy. The parents should be proficient in the various aspects of tracheostomy care such as identifying blockage, suctioning, and replacement of a dislodged tracheostomy tube.[20] They should have a spare tracheostomy tube of a smaller size, suction apparatus, suction catheters, and self-inflating bag at home and should also be well versed with their use prior to discharge. The parents should be advised to do tracheostomy care at least twice daily using a clean technique. Sterile technique is not known to decrease the risk of infections.[13]

Follow-up of Infants with a Gastrostomy Tube

Gastrostomy tube (GT) is inserted in certain infants in whom oral feeding could not be established at discharge such as infants with GERD, tracheoesophageal fistula with a long gap, and severe neurological insults such as HIE III. The parents of these infants should be trained for taking care of their babies during the hospital stay. The skin around the GT insertion site should be washed with soap and water once daily. Also, the skin should be inspected for leakage and signs of infection such as erythema. Local skin erythema might be because of irritation due to leakage or due to infection.[13] Local infection with fungus is common and can be treated with topical ointments. The presence of concomitant fever should alert the physician toward bloodstream infections. It is important to assess the competency for oral feeding in some categories of infants with GT at each follow-up visit. Some types of swallowing studies might aid in decision making toward oral feeding. Feeds are slowly introduced orally once it is felt that the infant is fit for accepting orally and then slowly advanced. Accidental dislodgement of GT is frequent and might require hospital visits for replacement of GT. The GT button should be replaced every 3 months.[13]

Follow-up Outcomes

Though most of the data on long-term neurodevelopmental outcomes of preterm infants have been published from developed nations (EPICURE I and EPICURE II studies, EPIPAGE study, EXPRESS study), some literature from tropical countries such as India are also available.[52-57] It is important for the physician in charge of a high-risk follow-up clinic to know the risk of neurodevelopmental delay in different categories of high-risk infants and especially in those who are preterm. It aids not only in explaining the prognosis to the parents, but also in intervening at the right time to improve their outcomes. The long-term outcomes of preterm infants from different countries are summarized in **Table 7**.

Table 7: Follow-up outcomes of high-risk preterm infants.

Study/country/year/sample size	Gestational age/assessment age	Outcomes
EPICure2/United Kingdom/2012/*n* = 584	<27 weeks/3 years	Moderate disability (including cerebral palsy)—12% Severe disability (including cerebral palsy)—13% Severe visual impairment—1% Severe hearing impairment—0.2%
EPIPAGE 2/France/2017/ *n* = 4199	22–34 weeks/2 years	*24–26 weeks:* • Cerebral palsy—6.9% • Moderate neuromotor disability—3.1% • Severe neuromotor disability—2.9% • Blindness—0.7% • Deafness—1.4% *27–31 weeks:* • Cerebral palsy—4.3% • Moderate neuromotor disability—1.7% • Severe neuromotor disability—1.6% • Blindness—0.3% • Deafness—0.6 %
EXPRESS/Sweden/2014/ *n* = 445	<27 weeks/6.5 years	• Cerebral palsy— 9.2% • Moderate neurodevelopmental disability—19% • Severe neurodevelopmental disability—11% • Blindness—0.7% • Deafness—2%
Mukhopadhyay K/India/ 2010/*n* = 101	≤ 34 weeks and ≤ 1,500 g/year	• Cerebral palsy—3% • Mild hypotonia—3% • Gross motor delay—11% • Language abnormality—8%
Lakshmi CVS/India/2012/ *n* = 220	VLBWs with absent/reversed end-diastolic umbilical artery Doppler flow (AREDF) *vs.* those with forward end-diastolic flow (FEDF)./12–18 months corrected age	• AREDF—Cerebral palsy—7% • FEDF—Cerebral palsy—1%
Oommen SP/India/2019/ *n* = 422	<1,500 g	• Cerebral palsy—1.7% • Poor neurodevelopmental outcome—10.3% • Visual impairment—0.3% • Hearing impairment—0.3%

(VLBW: very low birth weight)

▪ REFERENCES

1. Orton JL, Olsen JE, Ong K, et al. NICU graduates: The role of the allied health team in follow-up. Pediatr Ann. 2018;47(4): e165-71.
2. Allen MC. The high-risk infant. Pediatr Clin North Am. 1993; 40(3):479-90.
3. American Academy of Pediatrics Committee on Fetus and Newborn. Hospital discharge of the high-risk neonate. Pediatrics. 2008;122(5):1119-26.
4. Follow-up care of high-risk infants. Pediatrics. 2004;114 (Suppl 5):1377-97.
5. Davies DP, Haxby V, Herbert S, et al. When should pre-term babies be sent home from neonatal units? Lancet. 1979;1(8122): 914-5.
6. Brooten D, Kumar S, Brown LP, et al. A randomized clinical trial of early hospital discharge and home follow-up of very-low-birth-weight infants. N Engl J Med. 1986;315(15):934-9.
7. Casiro OG, McKenzie ME, McFadyen L, et al. Earlier discharge with community-based intervention for low birth weight infants: a randomized trial. Pediatrics. 1993;92(1):128-34.
8. Spitzer AR. Evidence-based methylxanthine use in the NICU. Clin Perinatol. 2012;39(1):137-48.
9. Conde-Agudelo A, Díaz-Rossello JL. Kangaroo mother care to reduce morbidity and mortality in low birthweight infants. Cochrane Database Syst Rev. 2016;(8):CD002771.
10. Young Infants Clinical Signs Study Group. Clinical signs that predict severe illness in children under age 2 months: a multicentre study. Lancet. 2008;371(9607):135-42.
11. Hintz SR, Newman JE, Vohr BR. Changing definitions of long-term follow-up: Should "long term" be even longer? Semin Perinatol. 2016;40(6):398-409.
12. Ruth VA. Extrauterine growth restriction: a review of the literature. Neonatal Netw. 2008;27(3):177-84.
13. Goldstein RF, Malcolm WF. Care of the Neonatal Intensive Care Unit Graduate after Discharge. Pediatr Clin North Am. 2019; 66(2):489-508.
14. Viswanathan S, Khasawneh W, McNelis K, et al. Metabolic bone disease: a continued challenge in extremely low birth weight infants. JPEN J Parenter Enteral Nutr. 2014;38(8):982-90.
15. Tuzun F, Yucesoy E, Baysal B, et al. Comparison of INTERGROWTH-21 and Fenton growth standards to assess

size at birth and extrauterine growth in very preterm infants. J Matern Fetal Neonatal Med. 2018;31(17):2252-7.

16. Victora CG, Bahl R, Barros AJ, et al., Lancet Breastfeeding Series Group. Breastfeeding in the 21st century: epidemiology, mechanisms, and lifelong effect. Lancet. 2016;387(10017): 475-90.

17. Gupta V, Rebekah G, Sudhakar Y, et al. A randomized controlled trial comparing the effect of fortification of human milk with an infant formula powder versus unfortified human milk on the growth of preterm very low birth weight infants. J Matern Fetal Neonatal Med. 2018;28:1-171.

18. Saari TN. American Academy of Pediatrics Committee on Infectious Diseases. Immunization of preterm and low birth weight infants. Pediatrics. 2003;112(Pt 1):193-8.

19. Committee on Infectious Diseases. From the American Academy of Pediatrics: Policy statements—modified recommendations for use of palivizumab for prevention of respiratory syncytial virus infections. Pediatrics. 2009;124(6):1694-1701.

20. Andrews B, Pellerite M, Myers P, et al. NICU follow-up: Medical and Developmental Management age 0 to 3 years. NeoReviews. 2014;15(4):e123-32.

21. Verma RP, Sridhar S, Spitzer AR. Continuing care of NICU graduates. Clin Pediatr (Phila). 2003;42(4):299-315.

22. Masoudian P, Sullivan KJ, Mohamed H, et al. Optimal timing for inguinal hernia repair in premature infants: a systematic review and meta-analysis. J Pediatr Surg. 2019;54(8):1539-45.

23. Whyte R, Jefferies AL. Canadian Paediatric Society, Fetus and Newborn Committee. Red blood cell transfusion in newborn infants. Paediatr Child Health. 2014;19(4):213-7.

24. Ritchie SK. Primary care of the premature infant discharged from the neonatal intensive care unit. MCN Am J Matern Child Nurs. 2002;27(2):76-85.

25. Vinekar A, Dogra MR, Sangtam T, et al. Retinopathy of prematurity in Asian Indian babies weighing greater than 1250 grams at birth: ten year data from a tertiary care center in a developing country. Indian J Ophthalmol. 2007;55(5): 331-6.

26. Ministry of Health and Family Welfare. Government of India. Guidelines for Universal Eye Screening in Newborns including Retinopathy of Prematurity. Rashtriya Bal Swasthya Karyakram. (2017). [online] Available from: https://www.nhm.gov.in/images/pdf/programmes/RBSK/Resource_Documents/Revised_ROP_Guidelines-Web_Optimized.pdf. [Last accessed on October, 2019].

27. Wilson CM, Ells AL, Fielder AR. The challenge of screening for retinopathy of prematurity. Clin Perinatol. 2013;40(2):241-59.

28. Fierson WM. American Academy of Pediatrics Section on Ophthalmology, American Academy of Ophthalmology, American Association for Pediatric Ophthalmology and Strabismus, American Association of Certified Orthoptists. Screening examination of premature infants for retinopathy of prematurity. Pediatrics. 2018;142(6):e20183061.

29. Joint Committee on Infant Hearing. Year 2007 Position Statement: Principles and Guidelines for Early Hearing Detection and Intervention Programs. Pediatrics. 2007;120(4): 898-921.

30. Abrams SA. Osteopenia of prematurity. In: Martin RJ, Fanaroff AA, Walsh MC (Eds). Fanaroff and Martin's Neonatal-Perinatal Medicine. 10th edition. St. Louis: Elsevier; 2015. pp. 1485-7.

31. Wessel MA, Cobb JC, Jackson EB, et al. Paroxysmal fussing in infancy, sometimes called colic. Pediatrics. 1954;14(5):421-35.

32. Lehtonen L. Assessment and optimization of neurobehavioral development in preterm infants. In: Martin RJ, Fanaroff AA, Walsh MC (Eds). Fanaroff and Martin's Neonatal-Perinatal Medicine. 10th edition. St. Louis: Elsevier ; 2015. pp. 1004-8.

33. Bayley N. Bayley Scales of Infant and Toddler Development. 3rd edition. San Antonio, TX: Harcourt Assessment; 2006.

34. Einspieler C, Prechtl HF, Bos AF, et al. Prechtl's Method on the Qualitative Assessment of General Movements in Preterm, Term and Young Infants. London, UK: Mac Keith Press; 2004.

35. Romeo DM, Ricci D, Brogna C, et al. Use of the Hammersmith Infant Neurological Examination in infants with cerebral palsy: a critical review of the literature. Dev Med Child Neurol. 2016;58(3):240-5.

36. Skiöld B, Eriksson C, Eliasson AC, et al. General movements and magnetic resonance imaging in the prediction of neuromotor outcome in children born extremely preterm. Early Hum Dev. 2013;89(7):467-72.

37. Wood NS, Costeloe K, Gibson AT, et al. EPICure Study Group. The EPICure study: associations and antecedents of neurological and developmental disability at 30 months of age following extremely preterm birth. Arch Dis Child Fetal Neonatal Ed. 2005;90(2):F134-40.

38. Ment LR, Bada HS, Barnes P, et al. Practice parameter: neuroimaging of the neonate: report of the Quality Standards Subcommittee of the American Academy of Neurology and the Practice Committee of the Child Neurology Society. Neurology. 2002;58(12):1726-38.

39. de Vries L, Eken P, Groenendaal F, et al. Correlation between the degree of periventricular leukomalacia diagnosed using cranial ultrasound and MRI later in infancy in children with cerebral palsy. Neuropediatrics. 1993;24(5):263-8.

40. Enhancing the outcomes of low-birth-weight premature infants. A multisite, randomized trial. The Infant Health and Development Program. JAMA. 1990;263(22):3035-42.

41. McCarton CM, Brooks-Gunn J, Wallace IF, et al. Results at age 8 years of early intervention for low-birth-weight premature infants. The Infant Health Development Program. JAMA. 1997;277(2):126-32.

42. McCormick MC, Brooks-Gunn J, Buka SL, et al. Early intervention in low birth weight premature infants: results at 18 years of age for the Infant Health and Development Program. Pediatrics. 2006;117(3):771-80.

43. Spittle A, Orton J, Anderson P, et al. Early developmental intervention programmes post-hospital discharge to prevent motor and cognitive impairments in preterm infants. Cochrane Database Syst Rev. 2012;12:CD005495.

44. Fitzgerald DA, Massie RJ, Nixon GM; Thoracic Society of Australia and New Zealand. Infants with chronic neonatal lung disease: recommendations for the use of home oxygen therapy. Med J Aust. 2008;189(10):578-82.

45. Rhein L. Discharge and transition to home care. In: Goldsmith JP, Karotkin EH, Kezler M, Suresh KG (Eds). Assisted Ventilation of the Neonate—An Evidence-Based Approach to Newborn Respiratory Care. 6th edition. St. Louis: Elsevier; 2017. p. 450.

46. Miller MJ, Martin RJ. Apnea of prematurity, apnea and SIDS. Clin Perinatol. 1992;19(4):789-808.

47. Ancel PY, Livinec F, Larroque B, et al. EPIPAGE Study Group. Cerebral palsy among very preterm children in relation to gestational age and neonatal ultrasound abnormalities: the EPIPAGE cohort study. Pediatrics. 2006;117(3):828-35.

48. Robertson C, Finer N. Term Infants with hypoxic ischemic encephalopathy: outcome at 3.5 years. Dev Med Child Neurol. 1985;27(4):473-84.

49. Murki S, Jain N, Venkataseshan S, et al. National Neonatology Foundation's evidence based clinical practice guidelines

2010. Management of Seizures in the Newborn (NNF India, Guidelines). Barwala (Haryana, India): Chandika Press Pvt Ltd; 2010. pp. 115-27.

50. Shapiro SM. Kernicterus. In: Stevenson DK, Maisels MJ, Watchko JF (Eds). Care of the jaundiced neonate. New York: McGraw Hill; 2012. pp. 229-42.

51. Govaert P, Lequin M, Swarte R, et al. Changes in globus pallidus with (pre)term kernicterus. Pediatrics. 2003;112 (6 Pt 1):1256-63.

52. Pierrat V, Marchand-Martin L, Arnaud C, et al. EPIPAGE-2 Writing Group. Neurodevelopmental outcome at 2 years for preterm children born at 22 to 34 weeks' gestation in France in 2011: EPIPAGE-2 cohort study. BMJ. 2017;358:j3448.

53. Serenius F, Ewald U, Fellman V, et al. Neurodevelopmental Outcome of Extremely Preterm Infants At 6.5 Years of Age; Extremely Preterm Infants Study in Sweden (express). Arch Dis Child. 2014;99(Suppl 2):A131.

54. Moore T, Hennessy EM, Myles J, et al. Neurological and developmental outcome in extremely preterm children born in England in 1995 and 2006: the EPICure studies. BMJ. 2012;345:e7961.

55. Mukhopadhyay K, Malhi P, Mahajan R, et al. Neurodevelopmental and behavioral outcome of very low birth weight babies at corrected age of 2 years. Indian J Pediatr. 2010;77(9):963-7.

56. Lakshmi CV, Pramod G, Geeta K, et al. Outcome of very low birth weight infants with abnormal antenatal Doppler flow patterns: a prospective cohort study. Indian Pediatr. 2013;50(9):847-52.

57. Oommen SP, Santhanam S, John H, et al. Neurodevelopmental outcomes of very low birth weight infants at 18-24 months, corrected gestational age in a tertiary health centre: a prospective Cohort Study. J Trop Pediatr. 2019;65(6):552-60.

4

Bacterial and Rickettsial Infections

Abhay K Shah

Typhoid and Nontyphoidal Salmonellosis

Jaydeep Choudhury

INTRODUCTION

Typhoid fever is an endemic disease in developing countries. Poor sanitation and impure water supply are the two most important factors for endemicity. The disease is caused due to infection by the genus *Salmonella* which comprises *Salmonella typhi*, *S. paratyphi A*, *S. paratyphi B*, and *S. paratyphi C*. Among these organisms, *S. typhi* causes typhoid fever while the rest causes paratyphoid fever. Human is the only reservoir of typhoid in the form of either cases or carriers. The bacteria are excreted by the infected patients for a long period. About 3–5% of the typhoid fever cases excrete *S. typhi* bacilli for more than 1 year after clinical or subclinical typhoid infection and they are classified as chronic carriers.

EPIDEMIOLOGY

The typhoid endemicity has been categorized as high (>100 cases/100,000/year), medium (10–100 cases/100,000/year), and low (<10 cases/100,000/year) incidence settings. India including South Central Asia has an incidence setting of roughly 622 cases/100,000/year, which suggests that it is in the high-incidence setting group.

Typhoid fever is relatively more prevalent in children and young adults. The peak incidence is in children aged 5–15 years. The incidence is less in older children and adults as the person becomes relatively immune due to the acquired immunity by repeated subclinical exposure to typhoid bacilli. Most of the cases occur in monsoon and perimonsoon seasons—July to September. But typhoid infection may occur at any time of the year in endemic countries.

CAUSATIVE ORGANISM

Salmonella is a gram-negative bacillus. The organism survives intracellularly. It grows rapidly on ordinary media under aerobic and anaerobic conditions. *S. typhi*, *S paratyphi A*, *S paratyphi B*, and *S paratyphi C* organisms have three main antigens O, H, and Vi. *S. typhi* has more than 80 phage types.

Salmonella may remain viable at ambient temperatures and also in various food items for many weeks. It may remain viable in foods, especially after cooking at low heat (<140°C) and cooked for less than 12 minutes. *Salmonella* may survive for a few hours in the hands of food handlers. It may also survive in refrigerated food.

INCUBATION PERIOD

The incubation period of *Salmonella* is 10–14 days with a range from 3 days to 3 weeks. The incubation period often depends on the load of the bacillus ingested. *S. typhi* divides rapidly in less than 30 minutes. After 1–2 weeks of incubation, the amount of bacilli that results from even a single bacillus are large. Normal intestinal flora is an important defense against invasion by *Salmonella* and not all persons who get infected would get the disease.

SOURCE OF INFECTION

The primary source of *Salmonella* infection is the feces and sometimes urine of cases and carriers. The secondary sources are contaminated water, unsafe food, and dissemination by hands and flies. *S. typhi* can survive for more than a month in refrigerated food, ice, and ice-creams. It can grow rapidly in milk without altering its taste or appearance. Vegetables can be a source of infection if taken raw without being washed properly and grown on sewage-irrigated land. Other food sources such as meat products (when not cooked well) and untreated shellfish can commonly lead to infection. *Salmonella* remains viable on the external surface of houseflies for as long as 20 days. The flies carry the bacillus from the feces to food.

Defecation and urination in open spaces, improper hand washing after toilets, poor standard of food and kitchen hygiene, washing infected material near kitchen, illiteracy, and lack of health education are the various personal and social factors or practices which are facilitators for the spread of infection. Patients with parasitic infestations such as roundworms or schistosomiasis are also easily infected with *S. typhi* as the organism gets adhered to the surface of the parasites.

PATHOGENESIS

Salmonella typhi has to survive the gastric acid barrier to reach the small intestine. Low gastric pH is an important defense mechanism. Increased susceptibility to *Salmonella* is seen in conditions that decrease stomach acidity and also conditions that decrease intestinal integrity (inflammatory bowel disease, gastrointestinal surgery, alteration of intestinal flora by antibiotic administration). The invasiveness of *Salmonella* depends on the growth state of the bacteria, high osmolarity, low oxygen tension, and pH.

The bacteria colonize in the small intestine. It adheres to the intestinal epithelia, mainly to Peyer's patches. The easy access of *Salmonella* through the bowel may be due to the bacteria's ability to invade the gut without stimulating an acute inflammatory response or recruitment of neutrophils.

After passing through the intestinal epithelial cells, *Salmonella* reaches the lamina propria where it is phagocytosed by macrophages. The bacteria are conveyed to the draining mesenteric lymph nodes and from there reach the bloodstream via the thoracic duct. This is the stage of transient primary bacteremia. It is followed by seeding of the reticuloendothelial cells of different organs such as liver, spleen, and bone marrow.

The onset of symptoms of typhoid correlates with the secondary persistent bacteremia into the blood of a large number of organisms from primarily infected sites. The gallbladder is particularly susceptible to being infected and constantly delivers more bacilli to the intestine via the bile.

ORGAN INVOLVEMENT

The organism is widely disseminated throughout the body in the bacteremic phase. The most common sites of secondary infection are liver, spleen, bone marrow, gallbladder and Peyer's patches of the terminal ileum. Gallbladder invasion occurs either directly from the blood or by retrograde spread from the bile. Organisms excreted in the bile either reinvade the intestinal wall or are excreted in the feces. Proliferation of bacilli, which is enhanced by bile, continues in the bile ducts and especially in the gallbladder, from where large numbers of bacteria pass into the gut and may be cultured from a duodenal aspirate.

The hepatosplenomegaly is due to recruitment of mononuclear cells and the development of a cell-mediated immune response to *S. typhi* colonization. The recruitment of additional mononuclear cells and lymphocytes to Peyer's patches afterward can result in marked enlargement of Peyer's patches, with right lower quadrant abdominal pain. Erosion of blood vessels may cause intestinal hemorrhage, and extension of necrosis through the bowel wall may result in perforation.

Many tissues of the body can be affected, including liver, spleen, kidney, heart, and lungs.

Typhoid nodules, which are foci of macrophages and lymphocytes, can be detected in a large number of internal organs.

CLINICAL FEATURES

The clinical features of typhoid vary with the age group, from patient to patient and in different geographical locations. The disease often does not have any definite distinguishing feature and the diagnosis is sometimes made by exclusion.

The clinical features usually manifest in children toward the end of the first week or second week after the infection. The typical clinical features are fever, chills, malaise, anorexia, nausea, poorly localized abdominal discomfort, myalgia, and dry cough. Physical signs develop later. Toxic features with coated tongue, tender abdomen, hepatomegaly, and splenomegaly are manifestations in the later phase of illness.

Fever

Fever is the most constant presentation of typhoid fever. The onset of fever is gradual. Though initially the fever is low grade, it rises progressively in a stepwise manner and by the second week it is often high and sustained at 39–40°C (102–104°F). In most cases, there is no definite pattern of fever. This typical pattern may not be found in some patients. One should consider enteric fever if there is fever without focus for more than 4 days. Older children may complain of body ache, headache, and anorexia.

Gastrointestinal Manifestations

The most common gastrointestinal manifestations are abdominal pain, splenohepatomegaly, anorexia, vomiting, and sometimes diarrhea. A soft spleen becomes palpable by the end of the first week. Hepatomegaly is more common in children below 2 years of age. Abdominal symptoms such as distension, tenderness, and cecal gurgling (typhlitis) are sometimes seen in children.

Though diarrhea is common in typhoid fever, it usually does not cause dehydration. It generally starts 3 days after the onset of fever and lasts for a few days. Constipation is more likely in older children and in later course of the disease.

Skin Manifestations

Rose spots, typically blanching erythematous maculopapular lesions approximately 2–4 mm in diameter on the abdomen and chest, are rare findings. They leave a slightly brownish discoloration of the skin on healing.

Other Manifestations

During the second week of illness, high fever is sustained and prostrations, fatigue, anorexia, cough, and abdominal symptoms increase in severity. Inflammation may be observed in the form of cholecystitis, localized abscesses, pneumonia, bronchitis, septic arthritis, osteomyelitis, pyelonephritis, glomerulonephritis, endophthalmitis, and meningitis. *S. typhi* osteomyelitis is commonly associated with sickle cell disease. Meningism may be seen in some children.

■ DIFFERENTIAL DIAGNOSIS

Malaria

Features such as high fever with chills and rigors, and splenohepatomegaly often mimic malaria. But fever is usually of abrupt onset in malaria and fever pattern is erratic.

In typhoid usually eosinopenia is seen whereas in malaria, being a parasitic infection, eosinophilia is common.

Viral Hepatitis

Reduced appetite, fever, and hepatomegaly may be the initial presentation of viral hepatitis. Jaundice is not common in typhoid fever and SGPT (serum glutamic pyruvic transaminase) levels are restricted to few hundreds only.

Pneumonia

The presentation of fever, cough, and chest findings may mimic pneumonia. Presence of associated abdominal findings indicates typhoid fever.

■ COMPLICATIONS

Typhoid fever is known for various complications, which occur mostly after the first week of illness. The main complications which endanger life are intestinal perforation and hemorrhage. Relapse occurs in 5–10% of patients, usually 2–3 weeks after the resolution of fever. Reinfection may also occur and can be distinguished from relapse by molecular typing.

Mortality is highest among children under 1 year of age. The most important contributor to a poor outcome is delay in starting effective antibiotic.

Severe Typhoid Fever

Patients with severe typhoid fever present with marked mental confusion, delirium, obtundation, stupor or coma, and shock.

Gastrointestinal Complication

Intestinal Hemorrhage

It is caused by erosion of a blood vessel by the ulcerating Peyer's patches. It is rare in children under 10 years of age. Bleeding may be frank or presence of altered blood in stool. It is a self-limiting process and does not need surgery.

Intestinal Perforation

It is the most dreaded complication of typhoid and the leading cause of mortality in children suffering from typhoid fever. It is not related to the severity of disease and is seen in the third week of illness. The presentation may be acute or subacute. Patients present with severe abdominal pain localized mainly in the right lower quadrant, vomiting, guarding, rebound tenderness, and rigidity. Occurrence of sudden onset pain along with rise in pulse rate and fall in blood pressure is the characteristic presentation. Free fluid in the abdomen and gas under the diaphragm establishes the diagnosis. Antibiotics form the mainstay of therapy along with conservative management. The usual site of perforation is terminal ilium.

Cardiovascular Complications

Nonspecific electrocardiogram changes are the most common cardiovascular complication. Myocarditis, arrhythmias, pericarditis, and venous thrombosis are other complications.

Pulmonary Complications

Bronchitis is quite common in children and manifests as dry cough. Lobar pneumonia may be seen in the second week of illness.

Neuropsychiatric Complications

About 50% of patients of typhoid fever are associated with a variety of neuropsychiatric complications. The most frequent complication is disturbance in the level of consciousness. It may range from disorientation, delirium, obtundation, stupor to coma. Of these, delirium is the earliest neurological symptom observed. Post typhoid, confusion may persist for weeks to months, but recovery is the rule.

The factors responsible for neurological manifestation of typhoid fever are hyperpyrexia, fluid and electrolyte disturbance, release of typhoid neurotoxin, vasculitis and autoimmune mechanism.

Typhoid state or typhoid encephalopathy may be found in the second week of illness. It is an acute confusional state characterized by disorientation, delirium, and restlessness. Delirium, stupor, and coma are associated with poor prognosis with a high case-fatality rate.

Other rare neurological complications are typhoid meningitis, seizures, cerebellar ataxia, brain abscess, depression, schizophrenic states with catatonic encephalomyelitis, transverse myelitis, peripheral neuropathy, cranial neuropathy, acute disseminated encephalomyelitis, and Guillain-Barré syndrome.

Genitourinary Complications

Asymptomatic excretion of *S. typhi* in urine is present in 25% cases in various stages of typhoid fever. There may be transient proteinuria, rarely immune-complex mediated glomerulonephritis presenting as renal failure or nephrotic syndrome, cystitis, and orchitis.

Hepatobiliary Complication

Jaundice and acute and chronic cholecystitis are various manifestations.

Hematological Complications

Anemia is almost universal in children suffering from typhoid fever, especially in children below 2 years of age. The various causes for anemia may be hemolysis, bone marrow suppression, intestinal hemorrhage, or disseminated intravascular coagulation (DIC). Hemolytic-uremic syndrome with a mild form of DIC has also been described.

Leukopenia with neutropenia, eosinopenia, and relative lymphocytosis is a common finding.

Musculoskeletal Complications

Periostitis involving tibia and ribs, arthritis, polymyositis, and Zenker's degeneration of muscles are various manifestations.

Others

Complications like parotitis and typhoid abscess are rare. Due to sustained bacteremia, focal infection can develop at any site. The common sites are bone, brain, liver, spleen, etc.

■ RELAPSE

Relapse with an intervening normal period described as short as 1 day to as long as 70 days has been reported. It manifests clinically by a recurrence of fever and other symptoms. Fever generally reappears about 2 weeks after the completion of antibiotic therapy, but it may also occur in the convalescent period during antibiotic therapy. Rarely a chronic relapsing form has been found lasting for many months, especially after treatment with insufficient doses of antibiotics. Relapses are usually milder but not always. Relapse typhoid fever is definitive when the clinical symptoms reappear along with culture positive infection with an antibiogram similar to the initial isolate within 8 weeks of completion of successful therapy of initial infection. Relapse typhoid fever should be treated with the same antibiotics with proper dose and duration. Relapse is more common in young children who are less than 2 years.

■ INVESTIGATIONS

Complete Blood Count

Complete blood count (CBC) in typhoid is nonspecific. The hemoglobin drops with advancing illness. Severe anemia if present should make one suspect intestinal hemorrhage. Leukopenia has been reported in some children. Eosinopenia, often absolute, may be present in some.

■ CULTURES

Blood Culture

Blood culture is the gold standard diagnostic for diagnosis of typhoid. The sensitivity of blood culture is highest in the first week of illness and decreases with advancing illness. The sensitivity drops considerably with prior antibiotic therapy. Failure to isolate the organism may be caused by inadequate laboratory media, less volume of blood taken for culture, presence of antibiotics, and time of blood collection. For blood culture, it is essential to inoculate media at the time of drawing blood.

Salmonella can be easily cultured in routine culture media such as Hartley's media, blood agar, and MacConkey agar. Automated blood culture systems such as BACTEC™

enhance the recovery rate. In children, at least 5 mL blood is to be collected for culture. A ratio of 1:5–1:10 of blood to broth is recommended.

There are considerable advantages of blood cultures in investigation as they also provide information on the antimicrobial sensitivity of the isolate.

Bone Marrow Cultures

Salmonella typhi/paratyphi is an intracellular pathogen in the reticuloendothelial cells of the body including the bone marrow. The overall sensitivity of bone marrow cultures is high and is good even in the late stage of disease and despite prior antibiotic therapy.

The invasive nature of bone marrow aspiration deters from its use as a first-line investigation for diagnosis of typhoid.

Antimicrobial Sensitivity Testing

Salmonella culture should always be complemented by sensitivity testing. The crucial issue here pertains to fluoroquinolone-susceptibility testing.

■ EPIDEMIOLOGY OF MULTIPLE DRUG RESISTANT TYPHOID FEVER

Multiple drug resistant *S. typhi* are those strains of *Salmonella* which have resistance to all the three first-line antibiotics (chloramphenicol, ampicillin, and trimethoprim-sulfamethoxazole). It not only has assumed a massive proportion in many developing countries but is also being increasingly seen in the developed countries.

Chloramphenicol was the treatment of choice for typhoid in the initial period after its discovery in 1947. Major resistance to it developed in 1972 and outbreaks occurred in many countries including India. Toward the end of 1990s, typhoid was resistant to all the first-line drugs. Infections with these drug-resistant strains were reported from India also.

Fluoroquinolones was the next drug to be introduced in the treatment of typhoid. But soon fluoroquinolone resistance was also reported. Resistance to fluoroquinolones may be total or partial. Though nalidixic acid is not used for the treatment of typhoid, nalidixic acid-resistant *S. typhi* (NARST) is a marker of reduced susceptibility to fluoroquinolones. NARST isolates are susceptible to fluoroquinolones in current disk sensitivity test. The clinical response to treatment with fluoroquinolones of NARST is inferior to the nalidixic acid-sensitive strains.

Third generation cephalosporins including oral cefixime and parenteral ceftriaxone are now effective in children for the treatment of typhoid. There are sporadic reports of high-level resistance to ceftriaxone, though very rare. Recently, azithromycin is also used for the treatment of uncomplicated typhoid fever.

■ SEROLOGIC TESTS

Widal Test

Widal test detects agglutinating antibodies against O and H antigens of *S. typhi* and H antigens of paratyphi A and B. The "O" antigen is the somatic antigen of *S. typhi* and is shared by *S. paratyphi* A, paratyphi B, other *Salmonella* species, and other members of the Enterobacteriaceae family. Antibodies against the O antigen are predominantly IgM. It rises early in the disease and disappears fast. The H antigens are flagellar antigens of *S. typhi*, paratyphi A, and paratyphi B. Antibodies to H antigens are both IgM and IgG; these antigens rise late in the illness and persist for a longer time. Usually, O antibodies appear on days 6–8 and H antibodies on days 10–12 after the onset of disease. Ideally, the test should be performed on both an acute serum (at first contact with the patient) and a convalescent serum so that paired titration can be performed.

Antibiotics may dampen the immune response and prevent a rise in titers even in truly infected individuals. The Widal test as a diagnostic modality has suboptimal sensitivity and specificity. Various studies show that it can be negative in many culture-proven cases of typhoid fever. Poor specificity is a consequence of the preexisting baseline antibodies in endemic areas, cross reactivity with other Gram-negative infections and nontyphoidal *Salmonella* (NTS), and anamnestic reactions in unrelated infections. For practical purpose, the Widal test should be done only after 5–7 days of fever by the tube method where levels of both O and H antibodies with 1 in 160 dilution (fourfold rise) or more should be taken as a cutoff value for diagnosis.

Other Serologic Tests

Enzyme Immunoassay Test or Typhidot® Test

Typhidot® is a dot enzyme immunoassay (EIA) that detects IgG and IgM antibodies against a 50 KD outer membrane protein distinct from the somatic (O), flagellar (H), or capsular (Vi) antigen of *S. typhi*. The dot EIA test offers early diagnosis and high negative and positive predictive values. Simple method and quick result are the characteristic features of this test. The detection of IgM reveals acute typhoid in the early phase of infection while the detection of both IgG and IgM suggests acute typhoid in the middle phase of infection. The original Typhidot® test was modified by inactivating the total IgG in the serum samples. The Typhidot M that detects only IgM antibodies of *S. typhi* has been reported to be more specific.

IDL Tubex® Test

Tubex® test is easy to perform. It is based on detecting antibodies to a single antigen in *S. typhi* only. The O9 antigen used in this test is very specific. A positive result always suggests a *Salmonella* infection. Infection by other serotypes such as *S. paratyphi* A gives negative result. This test detects IgM antibodies but not IgG which is further helpful in the diagnosis of current infections.

IgM Dipstick Test

The test is based on the binding of *S. typhi*-specific IgM antibodies to *S. typhi* lipopolysaccharide antigen and the staining of the bound antibodies by an antihuman IgM antibody conjugated to colloidal dye particles. This test will be useful in places where culture facilities are not available.

◼ MOLECULAR METHODS

Polymerase chain reaction (PCR) methods target the flagellin gene, somatic gene, Vi antigen gene, 5S-23S spacer region of the ribosomal RNA gene, invA gene, and hilA gene of *S. typhi* for diagnosis of typhoid fever. This method has good sensitivity and specificity when compared to positive blood culture. The turnaround time for diagnosis has been less than 24 hours. But there are various limitations of diagnosis by PCR.

Amongst all the available tests, blood culture is the gold standard and should be offered upfront, before starting antibiotic as soon as typhoid is suspected on clinical grounds. Due to poor specificity and issues of paired sera and rising titers, the Widal test is no more a preferred test. Typhidot also lacks specificity and in a country like ours, false positives are real issues and hence should not be practiced.

◼ TREATMENT

Supportive management such as use of antipyretics, adequate hydration, nutrition, and prompt recognition and treatment of complications is important for a favorable outcome of typhoid fever. A stable child should have normal diet.

Most of the patients can be effectively managed at home with proper oral antibiotics and nursing care. Patients with persistent vomiting, inability to take oral feed, severe diarrhea, dehydration, and abdominal distension usually require parenteral antibiotics and need hospital admission.

Antimicrobial Therapy

The drug of choice as empiric therapy in uncomplicated typhoid fever is oral third-generation cephalosporin, e.g. cefixime. Clinical improvement usually occurs by days 5–7 or at times longer. If a child is improving otherwise in terms of toxemia, oral intake, and decreasing trend of fever, there is no need to change the antibiotic. If there is no clinical improvement, the child remains unwell, and the culture report is inconclusive, then look for other complications and search for an alternative diagnosis. In some rare situations, a second-line drug such as azithromycin or any other drug effective against *S. typhi* depending upon the sensitivity pattern of the area may be substituted.

For complicated typhoid parenteral third-generation cephalosporin, ceftriaxone is the drug of choice. In severe life life-threatening infection fluoroquinolones may be used as the last resort. Aztreonam and imipenem may also be used in these situations.

Typhoid fever usually responds to monotherapy. Combination therapy though practiced in some places needs substantiation with adequate data from studies.

Treatment of Uncomplicated Typhoid

Oral: Fully sensitive
- Third-generation cephalosporins, cefixime—15–20 mg/kg/day for 14 days
- Chloramphenicol—50–75 mg/kg/day for 14–21 days
- Amoxicillin—100 mg/kg/day for 14 days
- Trimethoprim—8 mg/kg/day; Sulfamethoxazole—40 mg/kg/day for 14 days.

Oral: Multidrug resistant
- Third-generation cephalosporins, cefixime—15–20 mg/kg/day for 14 days
- Azithromycin—15–20 mg/kg/day for 7 days.

Treatment of Severe Typhoid

Injectable: Fully sensitive
- Ceftriaxone—60–80 mg/kg/day or cefotaxime—100–150 mg/kg/day for 14 days
- Chloramphenicol—100 mg/kg/day for 14–21 days
- Ampicillin—100 mg/kg/day for 14 days.

Injectable: Multidrug resistant
- Ceftriaxone—60–80 mg/kg/day or cefotaxime 100–150 mg/kg/day for 14 days
- Aztreonam—50–100 mg/kg/day for 7 days.

Imipenem and aztreonam are potential second-line drug and fluoroquinolones can be used in life-threatening infection resistant to other recommended antibiotics.

There are some reports of ceftriaxone-resistant typhoid fever from various parts of the world. But these were not a major problem as they neither caused any epidemic nor did they lead to widespread disease. Multiple drug-resistant *Salmonella* is resistant not only to first-line antibiotics such as chloramphenicol, ampicillin, and cotrimoxazole but also to newer drugs such as fluoroquinolones and third-generation cephalosporins like ceftriaxone. They carry both plasmid and chromosome-borne resistance genes to oral first-line antibiotics, fluoroquinolones, and injectable ceftriaxone. So the only reliable option left to treat uncomplicated typhoid fever is oral azithromycin and for complicated disease the injectable carbapenems. These resistant organisms are known as extensively drug-resistant typhoid.

Treatment of Severe Typhoid Fever

Management of hospitalized patients requires:

- Use of antibiotics in appropriate doses
- Nursing care
- Adequate nutrition
- Proper fluid and electrolyte balance
- Prompt diagnosis and management of complications such as intestinal perforation
- Use of corticosteroids in severely ill patients.

■ SUPPORTIVE MEASURES

Supportive measures are important in the management of severe typhoid fever, such as oral or intravenous hydration, nutrition, and use of appropriate antipyretics. Patients with persistent vomiting, severe diarrhea, and abdominal distension may require hospitalization and parenteral antibiotic therapy.

■ STEROIDS IN SEVERE TYPHOID FEVER

Typhoid fever patients with altered mental status should be evaluated for meningitis by cerebrospinal fluid examination. If the findings are normal and typhoid meningitis is suspected, children should be treated with high-dose intravenous dexamethasone in addition to antimicrobials. Dexamethasone is given in an initial dose of 3 mg/kg by slow IV infusion over 30 minutes followed by 1 mg/kg every 6 hourly for 48 hours.

■ MANAGEMENT OF INTESTINAL PERFORATION

Generalized peritonitis and large amount of pus are seen in patients with perforation of intestine. Proper antibiotics, nasogastric suction, resuscitation with IV fluids, blood transfusion if required, and oxygen should be administered. Corticosteroids should be given in severely toxic children. Antibiotic should cover Gram-negative rods and anaerobes of intestinal flora apart from *Salmonella*. If perforation is confirmed, surgical repair should not be delayed. Metronidazole and gentamicin or ceftriaxone should be administered before and after surgery if a fluoroquinolone is not being used to treat leakage of intestinal bacteria into the abdominal cavity.

■ MANAGEMENT OF INTESTINAL HEMORRHAGE

Most cases of intestinal hemorrhage are not severe and do not require blood transfusion. Surgical consultation should be sought if intestinal perforation is suspected.

■ MANAGEMENT OF RELAPSE

Blood cultures should be obtained and standard antibiotic treatment should be administered. They are sensitive to the same antibiotics which were given for the first episode and should be given for a period of 5–7 days.

■ NONTYPHOIDAL SALMONELLOSIS

Typhoid fever is caused by *S. typhi* and *S. paratyphi*. Other serotypes of *Salmonella* are collectively known as nontyphoidal salmonellae (NTSs). NTS characteristically induces an early inflammatory reaction in the intestinal mucosa. It leads to the infiltration of polymorphonuclear leukocytes into the intestinal lumen and cause diarrhea. NTS causes intestinal inflammation and does not reach the systemic circulation as it is prevented by the intestinal defense mechanism in an immunocompetent individual. NTS gastroenteritis is of rapid onset, brief duration, and self-limited. NTS is a major cause of bacteremia in HIV-positive children where it causes invasive disease.

Clinical Features

Gastroenteritis due to *Salmonella* infection typically occurs 8–72 hours following exposure. Ingestion of contaminated food or water is the main source of infection.

Diarrhea, nausea, vomiting, fever, and abdominal cramping are the usual presenting features. There are no clinical characteristics that distinguish *Salmonella* infection from other forms of gastroenteritis. Enteric infection with NTS may be clinically mild or even asymptomatic. The classical "pea soup" stool is rarely seen. Blood in stools is also rare. A larger amount of ingested bacteria correlates with the severity of diarrhea and duration of illness. NTS is usually self limited. Fever generally resolves within 48–72 hours and diarrhea within 4–10 days. Constitutional symptoms such as fatigue, malaise, chills, weight loss, and headaches are sometimes present.

Complications

Very few individuals with NTS gastroenteritis develop bacteremia. It can lead to some extraintestinal manifestations such as endocarditis, mycotic aneurysm, visceral abscesses, and osteomyelitis. *S. choleraesuis* and *S. heidelberg* are more invasive than others. Antibiotic-resistant strains of *S. typhimurium* are associated with an increased risk of bacteremia.

Investigation

Definitive diagnosis of NTS gastroenteritis requires stool cultures for isolation of the pathogen. Indications for stool cultures in a patient presenting with acute diarrhea include severe illness, immunocompromised conditions, and comorbidities.

Treatment

Fluid and electrolyte replacement is the main therapy. The illness is usually self-limited. Antimicrobial therapy may be warranted for those with severe disease or risk factors for invasive disease. Third-generation cephalosporins such as oral cefixime or parenteral cefotaxime may be used for 5–14 days depending on the severity.

Many patients with salmonellosis have occult blood in stool. The presence of bloody diarrhea does not necessarily indicate the need for antimicrobial treatment. Overtly bloody stools are likely to be due to *Shigella* or enterohemorrhagic *Escherichia coli*.

Preemptive therapy is indicated in patients at high risk for complications of NTS infection:

- Young infants < 12 months
- HIV-infected patients
- Other immunocompromised patients
- Other individuals with cardiac, valvular, endovascular abnormalities, or rheumatological conditions.

■ SUGGESTED READING

1. Bhutta ZA, Khan M, Soofi SB, et al. New advances in typhoid fever vaccination strategies. Adv Experimen Med Biol. 2011; 697:17-39.
2. Choudhury J, Kundu R. Enteric fever. In: Choudhury J, Kundu R (Eds). Pediatric Infectious Diseases, 1st edition. New Delhi: Jaypee Brothers Medical Publishers; 2012. pp. 308-20.
3. Kundu R, Ganguly N, Ghosh TK, et al. IAP Task Force Report: diagnosis of enteric fever in children. Indian Pediatr. 2006;43:875-83.
4. Kundu R, Ganguly N, Ghosh TK, et al. IAP Task Force Report: management of enteric fever in children. Indian Pediatr. 2006;43:884-7.
5. McKinney JS. Enteric fever (typhoid fever). In: Kliegman RM, Blum NJ, Shah SS, St Geme JW, Tasker RC, Walson KM (Eds). Nelson Textbook of Pediatrics, 21st edition. Philadelphia: Elsevier; 2020. pp. 1502-7.
6. Ochoa TJ, Santisteban Ponce J. Salmonella. In: Cherry JD, Steinbach WJ, Harrison GJ, Hotez PJ, Kaplan SL (Eds). Feigin and Cherry's Textbook of Pediatric Infectious Diseases, 8th edition. Philadelphia: Elsevier; 2019. pp. 1066-80.
7. Roy K, Kundu R. Typhoid fever. In: Parthasarathy A, Menon PSN, Nair MKC (Eds). IAP Textbook of Pediatrics, 7th edition. New Delhi: Jaypee Brothers Medical Publishers; 2019. pp. 407-11.
8. Shastri D, Singhal T. Antimicrobial therapy in enteric fever. In: Singhal T, Shah N, Prabhu S, Yewale V (Eds). Rational Antimicrobial Practice in Pediatrics (IAP Specialty Series), 3rd edition. New Delhi: Jaypee Brothers Medical Publishers; 2019. pp. 252-9.

Diarrheal Illness and Dysentery

Ketan H Shah

INTRODUCTION

Diarrhea is a common cause of death below 5 years of age. It is defined as any type of liquid stool which takes shape of container. The frequency of stool may be three or more than three per day. Recent change in color and consistency of stool is important. This terminology usually denotes infectious causes of diarrhea. However several noninfectious causes of gastrointestinal illnesses are well known. In newborn yellow color stool is normal. It may be many in numbers, with perianal rash and quantity may be small. If newborn child is not thriving well with diarrhea and other associated sign and symptom are present then diarrhea becomes important. Hygiene, correction of malnutrition, promotion of breastfeeding, and treatment with ORS and zinc has improved the outcome of the acute diarrheal diseases.

TERMINOLOGY

Acute diarrhea: Diarrhea lasting for less than 14 days. It is usually infective. It has self-limited course. Sometimes it becomes protracted.

Chronic diarrhea: It is defined as stool volume of more than 10 g/kg/day in toddler and infant and greater than 200 g/day in older children, that last for more than 14 days or more. It is usually noninfectious and associated with malabsorption. Awakening at night to pass stool is often a sign of organic cause of diarrhea.[1]

Persistent diarrhea: Diarrhea lasting for more than 14 days. It has probably infectious cause.

Protracted diarrhea: This terminology now a day is not used. However it is characterized by diarrhea lasting for more than 2 weeks, starting before 3 months of age with severe nutritional disturbances and negative stool culture for enteropathogens. This has likely to be one of the congenital causes of diarrhea.[2] However, it is often difficult to differentiate between chronic diarrhea and protracted diarrhea.

Traveler's diarrhea: During visit to another country person may experience diarrheal illness. It is due to higher prevalence of indigenous infectious causes.

Dysentery: This term is used to describe the syndrome of bloody diarrhea with fever, abdominal cramps, rectal pain, and mucoid stools. It is either bacillary dysentery caused by *Shigella* or amoebic caused by *Entamoeba histolytica*.

EPIDEMIOLOGY

Diarrheal disease is the second leading cause of death in children under 5 years. It is both preventable and treatable. Each year diarrhea kills around 525,000 children under 5 years. A significant proportion of diarrheal disease can be prevented through safe drinking water and adequate sanitation and hygiene. Globally, there are nearly 1.7 billion cases of childhood diarrheal disease every year. Diarrhea is a leading cause of malnutrition in children under 5 years.

Causes

Acute diarrhea: Infectious and noninfectious diseases can cause acute diarrhea. They are listed in **Table 1**.[3] Many infectious causes from food and water can cause diarrheal illness. Incubation period may be variable. Preformed toxins, or toxins produced after ingestion can cause disease. In developing countries rotavirus remains main cause of disease. Many noninfectious causes are related to heavy metal and toxins. Common eatable fish can also cause diarrheal disease. Certain pesticide ingestion, heavy metal from tin, container, and stored food can also cause diarrheal disease. Many times it is difficult to identify the causative agent. Treatment remains same in majority of the cases. Few patients need antibiotic (dysentery) or antitoxins (antibotulin toxin).

Dysentery: Bacillary dysentery is caused by four strain of Shigella: *S. dysenteriae, S. flexneri, S. boydii,* and *S. sonnei,* they can cause bacillary dysentery. Infection by *Campylobacter jejuni, Salmonella* spp., enteroinvasive *Escherichia coli,* Shiga toxin-producing *E. coli, Yersinia enterocolitica, Clostridium difficile,* and *E. histolytica* can also cause dysentery.

Other differential diagnosis of acute dysentery includes inflammatory enterocolitis and proctitis. In case of long duration, chronic inflammatory processes like intestinal tuberculosis, mycosis, parasitic enteritis inflammatory bowel disease (ulcerative colitis, Crohn's disease), and allergic enteritis are considered.

Chronic diarrhea: Etiology is variable according to the age. It is due to persistent disturbance in digestive process. It could be due to abnormal digestion, defective absorption, altered gut transit, various secretory tumors, metabolic diseases, drugs, and chemical.[2] Various causes are listed in **Tables 2 and 3**.[1]

Tropical sprue: This entity is not well defined. In south Indian population it is common. It follows acute outbreak of diarrheal disease. With possible suspicion of infectious agent antibiotic is given. Diarrhea improves but malabsorption continues. Clinical presentation is with low grade fever, malaise, anorexia, intermittent diarrhea, glossitis, cheilosis, night blindness, hyperpigmentation and edema. It reflects various nutrient deficiencies. Small bowel biopsy will show villous flattening, crypt hyperplasia, and chronic inflammation. Treatment requires nutritional supplementation. Six months of therapy with folic acid, tetracycline or sulfonamides is recommended.[4]

■ PATHOPHYSIOLOGY

Usual mode of transmission is fecal-oral route. In warm and tropical climate transmission of disease is very common. Incidence increases in rainy season. Poor handling of food, poor personal hygiene, and person to person transmission are responsible factors for many pathogens. In warm climate food contamination is responsible for disease. Rapid spread in family, institute is known. Some organism needs small inoculums size.

Primary mechanism is divided into secretory and osmotic diarrhea. However, often it is overlapping. It is described in **Table 4**.[5]

Table 1: Causes of acute diarrhea (gastroenteritis).[3]	
Infectious	*Noninfectious*
Foodborne bacterial illness:	*Heavy metal poisoning:*
• *Bacillus anthracis*	• Antimony
• *Bacillus cereus* (preformed enterotoxin, diarrheal toxins)	• Arsenic
• *Brucella (abortus, melitensis, suis)*	• Cadmium
• *Campylobacter jejuni*	• Copper
• *Clostridium botulinum*	
• *Clostridium perfringens*	*Other toxin:*
• EH *Escherichia coli* (enterohemorrhagic *E. coli*)	• Ciguatera fish poisoning
• Enterotoxigenic *E. coli*	• Mushroom toxins
• *Listeria monocytogenes*	• Organophosphate poisoning
• *Salmonella* spp.	• Puffer fish
• *Shigella* Spp.	• Shellfish toxins
• *Staphylococcus aureus*	• Sodium fluoride
• *Vibrio cholerae, V. parahaemolyticus, V. vulnificus*	• Thallium
• *Yersinia enterocolitica, Y. pseudotuberculosis*	• Tin
	• Zinc
Foodborne viral illness:	• Vomitoxin
• Hepatitis A	
• Caliciviruses	
• Rotavirus	
• Other viral agents (astrovirus, adenovirus, and parvovirus)	
Foodborne parasitic illnesses:	
• *Angiostrongylus cantonensis*	
• *Cryptosporidium*	
• *Cyclospora cayetanensis*	
• *Entamoeba histolytica*	
• *Giardia lamblia*	
• *Trichinella spiralis*	

Table 2: Causes of chronic diarrhea: Infectious.[1]	
Developed country	*Underdeveloped country*
• *Clostridioides difficile*	• *E. coli* (enteroaggregative)
• *Escherichia coli* (enteroaggregative)	• Atypical *E. coli*
• Astrovirus	• Shigella
• Norovirus	• *E. coli* (enterotoxin producing)
• Rotavirus	• Rotavirus
• Small intestinal bacterial overgrowth	• Cryptosporidium
• Postenteritis diarrhea syndrome	• *Giardia lamblia*
	• Tropical sprue

Table 3: Noninfectious causes of chronic diarrhea.[1]

Etiology	Less than 2 years	Older than 2 years
Abnormal digestive process	Related to pancreatic dysfunction and biliary dysfunction, e.g. Shwachman-Diamond syndrome	Cystic fibrosis, terminal ileum resection
Nutrient malabsorption	Congenital enzyme deficiency or malabsorption of molecule like glucose-galactose malabsorption, lactase deficiency	Hypolactasia; acquired short bowel
Immune/inflammatory	Immunodeficiency and food allergy related causes	Celiac disease, eosinophilic gastroenteritis, inflammatory bowel diseases
Structural defects	Microvillus inclusion disease, lymphangiectasis and related diseases	Rare
Defects of electrolytes and metabolite transport	Example, congenital chloride diarrhea, sodium diarrhea, acrodermatitis enteropathica, etc.	Late onset chloride diarrhea
Motility disorder	Hirschsprung's disease, chronic intestinal pseudo-obstruction	Thyrotoxicosis
Neoplastic diseases	APUDomas like VIPoma, etc.	Same
Diarrhea associated with exogenous substances	Excessive intake of carbonated fluid, foods or drink, containing sorbitol, etc.	Excessive intake of carbonated fluid, foods, drink; excessive intake of antacid or laxative, excess cola, coffee, tea intake
Chronic nonspecific diarrhea	Functional diarrhea	Irritable bowel syndrome

Table 4: Pathophysiology of diarrhea.

Type	Osmotic	Secretory
Stool volume	Moderate	Very large
Response to fasting	Diarrhea stops	Continues
Stool osmolality	Normal to increased	Normal
Ion gape	≥100 mOsm/kg	<100 mOsm/kg
Mechanism	Due to nonabsorbed nutrients in the intestinal lumen as a result of: • Reduced absorptive surface area (e.g. celiac disease) • Defective digestive enzyme (e.g. lactase deficiency) • Nutrient overload (e.g. sorbitol in fruit juices) • Intestinal damage (e.g. infection)	Electrolytes and water efflux from wall to lumen Toxins bind to cell wall or toxins are produced in intestine by the infecting organism

Pathogenesis depends on etiological agent also. In virus it may be enterocyte lysis, brush border damage leading to impaired electrolytes absorption, stimulation of various channels like cyclic adenosine monophosphate, and others. In bacterial disease either production of toxins by enterotoxigenic bacteria, or invasion and inflammation of mucosa by enteroinvasive bacteria. In parasites invasion of epithelia cells leads to villous atrophy and eventually malabsorption.

■ CLINICAL MANIFESTATION

Clinical presentation may be variable from acute life-threatening event to mild disease. Chronic diarrhea usually present with ongoing symptoms and associated other systemic features also. There is no clinical diagnostic feature of any pathogen.

History

Clinical history of type, duration, associated gastrointestinal tract symptoms, and other associated systemic symptoms like cough, cold, urinary problem will give clue for secondary causes. Stool type, presence of blood, tenesmus, and symptoms of dehydration will help in overall assessment of patient. Epidemiological history like recent history of travelling, food ingestion, and family clustering of cases will give clue to the possible etiological agent. Underlying medical conditions like human immunodeficiency virus and immunocompromised disease need special attention. History of taking excessive cold drink, tea coffee, and junk food may be responsible for chronic diarrhea. In some patient cow's milk protein allergy may be causing chronic diarrhea.

Clinical Findings

The degree of dehydration is rated on a scale of severe, some, and no dehydration.

- *Severe dehydration* (at least two of the following signs):
  - Lethargy or unconsciousness
  - Sunken eyes
  - Unable to drink or drink poorly
  - Skin pinch goes back very slowly (≥2 seconds)
  - Weight loss greater than 10% and fluid deficit greater than 100 mL/kg.
- *Some dehydration* (two or more of the following signs):
  - Restlessness, irritability
  - Sunken eyes
  - Drinks eagerly, thirsty
  - Weight loss (5–10%) and fluid deficit 50–100 mL/kg.
- *No dehydration* (not enough signs to classify as some or severe dehydration): Weight loss of less than 5% and fluid deficit less than 50 mL/kg.

As the level of dehydration increases, level of consciousness, urine output, pulse volume, capillary refill time decreases. Pulse becomes feeble, skin elasticity is decreasing, and blood pressure falls down rapidly.

Fever, pain in abdomen, borborygmi, and perianal rash, may occur. Stool may show blood and mucus. In chronic diarrhea other signs of malnutrition may be seen.

Red Flags[5]

Prematurity, infancy, malnutrition, chronic medical disease, and immunocompromised statuses are red flag signs in management of diarrheal disease. High fever, severe dehydration, bloody stool, high purge rate, persistent vomiting, severe dehydration, poor response to ORS, etc. are also important consideration in management.

■ DIAGNOSIS

In case of acute diarrhea microbiological diagnosis is not required. Persistent and chronic symptoms call for investigations. Stool routine examination and stool culture in selected cases is advised. For chronic diarrhea investigations are directed depending upon suspected etiology.

■ TREATMENT

Fluid Management

Child needs plenty of fluid. Recommended fluid is ORS (oral rehydration solution: WHO formulation). Homemade ORS is prepared with pinch of salt, one spoon of sugar, and glass of water. This can also be recommended. Canned juices, glucose-containing powder, energy drink, and soft drinks are not to be prescribed. They rather increase purge rate due to high osmolarity and presence of caffeine in it. WHO formulation includes: Sodium 75 mEq/L, potassium 20 mEq/L, chloride 64 mEq/L, glucose 75 mmol/L with osmolarity of 245 mOsm/L. Addition of amino acids, flavoring agents, etc. are not recommended. Various misleading formulations are available with name of ORS, they should be banned. After each loose stool under 2 years of age 50–100 mL and between 2–10 years 100–200 mL extra fluid is needed. For adult and older children as much fluid as they want can be given. Coffee, tea, and caffeine-containing beverages should be avoided.

If patient comes with no dehydration, information about the disease, extra liquid, nutrition, and ORS is advised. For some dehydration ORS is given under observation in OPD. Reassessment is done after sometime. If child vomits ORS, extra amount of ORS 120–240 mL is given. If he/she does not retain and clinical condition worsens then intravenous (IV) fluids management is planned. Preferred IV fluid is normal saline (NS) or Ringer's lactate (RL). 75 mL/kg over 4 hours and additional ORS with antiemetic drug is given. If after 4 hours clinical condition improves ORS and normal diet is advised. If stool output is more like in cholera and severe watery diarrhea, maintenance fluid with 5% glucose saline is given and additional NS/RL as per requirement is given. Sometime IV line is not accessible then with nasogastric tube ORS is given.

Diet

Breastfeeding is continued with other treatment. There is no contraindication of breastfeeding in diarrheal disease. Proper diet with some extra calorie is recommended. As mentioned sweetened, caffeinated beverages are not recommended. Energy intake is aimed at 100 kcal/kg/day and protein intake of 2–3 g/kg/day. Sometime addition of amylase from homemade germinated food will help. In spite of damage to brush border and loss of luminal enzymes, there is sufficient evidence that satisfactory food digestion takes place.

Acute lactose intolerance occurs in some group of diarrheal disease. Avoiding lactose-containing diet is not recommended. Milk-based diet like milk-cereal diet (usually rice based), comminuted chicken or elemental diet is recommended in persistent diarrhea. Addition of green banana or pectin to the diet has also been shown to be effective.

In malnourished child proper diet plan is very important. Education of mother and community health

Table 5: Use of antibiotics in diarrhea and dysentery-like illness.

Organism	Drug of choice
Shigella	Ciprofloxacin, ampicillin, ceftriaxone, azithromycin or TMP-SMX
EPEC, ETEC, EIEC	Ciprofloxacin, TMP-SMX
Nontyphoidal *Salmonella*	• In normal host not needed • In immunocompromised and in infants younger than 3 months treat like *Shigella* • Resistance to antibiotic is concern
Campylobacter jejuni	Erythromycin or azithromycin
Yersinia Spp.	For immune-compromised doxycycline, aminoglycoside, TMP-SMX, and fluoroquinolones
Clostridium difficile	Metronidazole, vancomycin (second line)
Entamoeba histolytica	Metronidazole followed by iodoquinol or paromomycin
Giardia lamblia	Furazolidone, metronidazole, or albendazole
Cryptosporidium spp.	In normal host not needed. In immunocompromised aggressive treatment
Vibrio cholerae	Single oral dose of doxycycline (2–4 mg/kg/day), azithromycin (20 mg/kg) or ciprofloxacin (20 mg/kg)

Doses:
- *Ceftriaxone*: 50–100 mg/kg/day qid/bid intravenous/intramuscular × 7 days
- *Ciprofloxacin*: 20–30 mg/kg/day PO bid × 7–10 days (drug authority has not approved in pediatric patients)
- *Azithromycin*: 5–10 mg/kg/day qid PO × 5 days
- *Erythromycin*: 50 mg/kg/day divided tid PO × 5 days
- *Trimethoprim/sulfamethoxazole (TMP-SMX)*: TMP 10 mg/kg/day and SMX 50 mg/kg/day bid PO × 5/7/10 days depending upon etiology
- *Metronidazole*: 30–40 mg/kg/day tid PO × 7–10 days
- *Iodoquinol*: 30–40 mg/kg/day tid PO × 20 days
- *Paromomycin*: 25–35 mg/kg/day tid PO × 7 days
- *Albendazole*: 200 mg bid PO × 10 days
- *Nitazoxanide*: Children 1–3 years 100 mg bid PO × 3 days, children 4–11 years: 200 mg bid PO

(EIEC: enteroinvasive *Escherichia coli;* EPEC: enteropathogenic *E. coli*; ETEC: enterotoxigenic *E. coli*)

worker is also very essential. Various commercial available formulas are not recommended.

Zinc and Vitamin A

This is standard recommended treatment for diarrhea. All varieties of diarrheas need zinc supplement for 14 days. It prevents recurrence, reduces mortality, and prevents hospitalization also. Dose will be 20 mg/day for above 6 months of age. It is given for 10–14 days. In developed country its exact role is less certain. Vitamin A supplementation does reduce morbidity. In malnourished and 6–59 months child it is needed.[6]

Antibiotics

In selected cases of diarrhea antibiotic is needed. **Table 5** gives information on uses of antibiotics in diarrhea and dysentery like illness. All severely malnourished children, immunocompromised host, persistent diarrhea with diagnosed infection outside gut (e.g. pneumonia, otorrhea, urinary tract infection—treat the cause), and child having systemic sepsis should receive antibiotics.

■ ROLE OF PROBIOTICS AND PREBIOTICS

Although the evidence is inconclusive, lactobacillus, *Saccharomyces boulardii*, and *Bifidobacterium* have good safety record. *S. boulardii* is effective in antibiotic-associated diarrhea. *Lactobacillus rhamnosus* GG is associated with reduced diarrheal duration and severity. However Indian trials are limited and no conclusive evidence is available.

Antimotility drugs in acute diarrheal diseases have no role. Racecadotril has limited experience and is not recommended. Antiemetic drugs like phenothiazine are contraindicated. Ondansetron-like drugs are more preferred as antiemetic drug.

■ PREVENTION

- Contact tracing and source identification
- Proper hand hygiene
- Proper food hygiene and improving water and sanitation facility
- Breastfeeding
- Avoiding use of contaminated food

224

- Improving complementary feeding practice
- Immunization (rotavirus vaccination, cholera vaccine, etc.)
- Proper case management.

CHRONIC DIARRHEA MANAGEMENT

Chronic diarrhea associated with malnutrition needs proper evaluation. Treatment includes general supportive measures, nutritional support, medications, and elimination diet when indicated. Sometimes parenteral nutrition is also required. Micronutrient and vitamin supplementation is required. Functional diarrhea can be reduced by reducing fructose, fluids, and increasing fat and fiber. Pharmacologic therapy depends on identified bacterial agent, antiparasite agent, probiotics, and human serum immunoglobulin 300 mg/kg single dose for severe persistent rotavirus diarrhea.[7] Specific etiology is addressed, like malabsorption due to pancreatic disease, absorption defect or due to neuroendocrine tumors.

REFERENCES

1. Guarino A, Branski D, Winter HS. Chronic diarrhea. In: Kliegman RM, Stanton B, St Geme J, Schor N (Eds). Nelson Textbook of Pediatrics, 1st South Asia edition. India: Elsevier; 2016. pp. 1875.
2. Paul S, Matthai J. Chronic and persistent diarrhea. In: Sibbal A, Gopalan S (Eds). Textbook of Pediatric Gastroenterology, Hepatology and Nutrition. New Delhi: Jaypee Brothers Medical Publishers (P) Ltd. 2015. pp. 119-23.
3. Bhutta ZA. Acute gastero-enteritis in children. In: Kliegman RM, Stanton B, St Geme J, Schor N (Eds). Nelson Textbook of Pediatrics. First South Asia edition. Elsevier; 2016. Table 340-1. Food born bacterial illness. pp. 1855-63. [From Centers for Disease Control and Prevention: Diagnosis and Management of Food Borne Illness. MMWR. 2004;53(RR-4):1-33.]
4. Shamir R, Branski D. Intestinal infections and infestations associated with malabsorption. Tropical sprue. In: Kliegman RM, Stanton B, St Geme J, Schor N(Eds). Nelson Textbook of Pediatrics, 1st South Asia edition. India: Elsevier; 2016. pp. 1841-2.
5. Bharadva K. Infective diarrhea. In: Kundu R, Yewale V (Eds). Textbook of Pediatric Infectious Diseases. Indian Academy of Pediatrics. Infectious Disease Chapter. 2nd edition. Jaypee Brothers Medical Publishers. 2019, Table 3.9-2: Primary mechanism responsible for acute diarrhea. pp. 205-13.
6. Lakshminarayanan S, Jayalakshmy R. Diarrheal diseases among children in India: Current scenario and future perspectives. J Nat Sci Biol Med. 2015;6(1);24-8.
7. Guarino A, Branski D, Winter HS. Chronic diarrhea. In: Kliegman RM, Stanton B, St Geme J, Schor N (Eds). Nelson Textbook of Pediatrics. First South Asia edition. Elsevier; 2016. Table: 341-7. Treatment of infectious persistent diarrhea. p. 1882.

Diphtheria

Ashok Rai

INTRODUCTION

Diphtheria is an acute infectious, communicable disease caused by *Corynebacterium diphtheriae*. This name was derived from Greek "diphthera," meaning leather hide, described by Hippocrates in the 5th century. It is known as "Ghatsarpa" in Ayurveda, which means a snake winding tightly around the neck of a pot. In the prevaccine era, this disease has killed thousands of children, but after the vaccination, the death rate has reduced significantly. Many developed countries have almost eradicated this disease due to effective vaccine program.

The incidence has significantly declined in developing countries but still accounts for major global burden (80–90%). In 2015, 52.21% (2,365 cases) of diphtheria were reported from India only as compared to 4,530 cases globally. Re-emergence of diphtheria with widespread mortality and morbidity was reported in both developed and developing countries. Outbreaks have been reported in Brazil, Haiti, India, Indonesia, Laos, Nepal, Pakistan, South Africa, Thailand, Venezuela, and Vietnam in the last 5 years.

Introduction of diphtheria antitoxin (DAT) for the treatment and development of effective vaccine had a significant impact on the incidence and mortality of this disease. Young children were protected due to effective National Immunization Program. But the age shift to adolescent and young adults has been reported due to waning immunity and inadequate coverage with booster vaccination.

A significant decline was reported for the most of the vaccine-preventable diseases, after introduction of Expanded Program on Immunization in 1978 and Universal Immunization Programme in 1985. Diphtheria is still endemic in India.

ETIOLOGY

Diphtheria is caused by *Corynebacterium*, an aerobic Gram-positive, nonsporulating, unencapsulated, nonmotile, pleomorphic bacillus. Four main biotypes of *C. diphtheriae* have been reported: gravis, intermedius, mitis and belfanti. Globally, the intermedius strain is most often linked with exotoxin production, though all strains produce exotoxins. Exotoxin produced by these bacteria is lethal to humans, causing death with a dose of 130 μg/kg/body weight.

Von Behring discovered diphtheria toxin in 1890. Diphtheria toxin is a single, polypeptide chain of 535 amino acids consisting of two subunits linked by disulfide bridges known as A and B toxins. Both subunits A and B are responsible for various local and systemic effects. Humans are the only known natural host for *C. diphtheriae*. It is usually transmitted by direct contact or by sneezing or coughing.

This disease usually affects children below 5 years of age. In population with high coverage of immunization, age shift was seen in this disease affecting unimmunized or poorly immunized adults.

PATHOGENESIS

Human are the natural host for *C. diphtheriae*. The organism colonizes in the nasopharynx of the host and produces a toxin which inhibits cellular protein synthesis. This toxin causes the local tissue necrosis and edema of the affected tissue and forms a pseudomembrane. This toxin is also absorbed in the bloodstream and causes major complications such as myocarditis and peripheral neuritis. Rarely, it is responsible for distant systemic infections such as bacteremia, endocarditis, and septic arthritis.

Nontoxin-producing strain does not form a pseudomembrane but is responsible for mild-to-moderate pharyngitis, chronic skin ulcerations, and rarely invasive diseases such as endocarditis and osteomyelitis.

CLINICAL FEATURES

The incubation period of diphtheria is usually 2–5 days (range 1–10 days). Any mucous membrane can be affected due to diphtheria but usually nasal, pharyngeal, and laryngeal mucous membranes and skin are involved.

Nasal Diphtheria

This disease usually presents with mucopurulent nasal discharge, sometimes blood tinged also. A white membrane is usually seen on the nasal septum. Characteristically, there is history of unilateral nasal discharge from the affected side.

Pharyngeal and Tonsillar Diphtheria (Fig. 1)

This is the most common site of diphtheria lesion. Malaise, sore throat, anorexia, and low-grade fever usually occur in the initial 2–3 days, followed by pseudomembrane formation, usually on the tonsils and cover most of the soft palate. This membrane is usually white and glossy but turns into dirty grey-white. Necrotic green or black patches may be seen on the membrane. The membrane is firmly adherent to mucosa and may bleed on attempt to scrap or dislodge.

Patients with severe disease develop severe edema of the submandibular region, and anterior neck with cervical lymphadenopathy, giving a characteristic bull neck appearance.

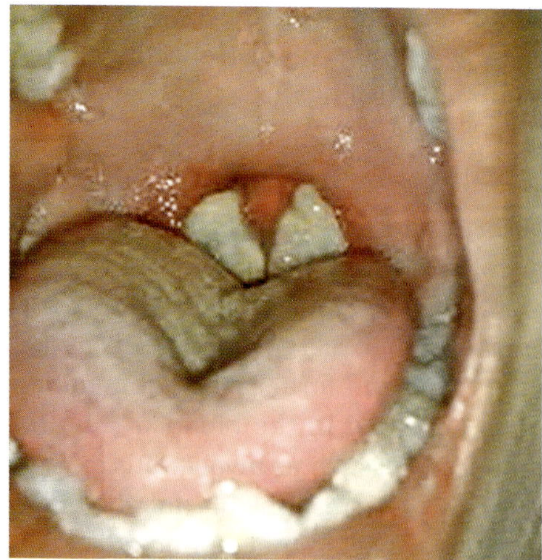

Fig. 1: Tonsillar diphtheria.
(*Source*: Centers for Disease Control and Prevention)

Laryngeal Diphtheria

Fever, hoarseness, and barking cough are the usual features of laryngeal involvement. Either this can be extension of the pharyngeal form or only larynx is involved. Stridor, airway obstruction, and dyspnea can occur with involvement of larynx.

Cutaneous Diphtheria

It is not uncommon in the tropics and manifests as scaling rash or by ulcers with a clearly demarcated edge termed "Ecthyma diphtheriticum." It usually presents as a vesicle or pustule field with straw-colored fluid which breaks down easily. Cutaneous lesions are usually caused by nontoxigenic strains. Lower legs, feet, and hands are the common sites for diphtheric lesions. The lesions are usually painful and may be covered with an adhering eschar. Conjunctiva, vulvovaginal area, and external auditory canal are rarely involved in diphtheria.

COMPLICATIONS

Most complications occur due to toxin, which affects organs and tissues distant from the site of involvement. Common complications of diphtheria are myocarditis and peripheral neuritis.

Myocarditis is the most known complication of diphtheria. It usually occurs after 7–14 days of the onset of illness. It may present as abnormal cardiac rhythms. Electrocardiogram (ECG) changes such as ST-T wave changes, QTc prolongation, and first-degree heart block were reported in as many as two-third of patients. It is very important to monitor ECG changes in patients of diphtheria. Usually, 10–25% develop clinical cardiac dysfunctions though subtle evidence of myocarditis can be detected in two-third of patients. It may also present as acute congestive failure and circulatory collapse or progressive dyspnea, weakness, diminished heart sounds, cardiac dilatation, and gallop rhythm. Patients with bundle branch blocks and complex dissociation carry a poor prognosis and survivors may develop a permanent conduction defect.

Neurological complications are reported in 5% cases, but up to 75% of patients with severe diphtheria develop some manifestations of neurological involvement. Paralysis of soft palate and posterior pharynx are the most common notable complications, which manifest as regurgitation of swallowed fluids through nose and change in voice. Palatal palsy usually occurs in the second and third weeks of illness and it is the earliest neurological complication. Cranial nerve palsies such as those involving oculomotor, facial, or laryngeal nerve may occur later in the course of the disease. Demyelinating peripheral neuritis is a delayed complication, which usually occurs weeks to months after the illness. It may present as mild weakness with diminished reflexes to total paralysis. Neurological complications usually resolve completely but may be slow with prolonged convalescence. Renal failure may occur due to direct effect of toxin on the kidney.

LABORATORY DIAGNOSIS

It is usually diagnosed clinically along with throat swab culture for the organism. Swab should be taken from the pharyngeal area, especially any discolored area, ulcerations, or pseudomembrane.

Tellurite culture medium is the preferred one as it provides a selective advantage for the growth of this organism.

Gram stain and Kenyon stain of the materials are also helpful to confirm the clinical diagnosis. The Gram stain shows multiple, club-shaped forms **(Fig. 2)** which look like Chinese characters, but they are not sufficiently sensitive nor specific in the diagnosis of diphtheria.

Diagnosis is done mainly by detection of *C. diphtheriae* through culture or by polymerase chain reaction (PCR) detection of the TOX gene. The presence of the TOX gene does not necessarily indicate that the toxin is being produced and PCR does not distinguish between *C. diphtheriae* and *C. ulcerans*. Elek's test should be done to confirm the toxin production of the *Corynebacterium* species.

DIFFERENTIAL DIAGNOSIS AND PROGNOSIS

Diphtheria should be detected and treated early, otherwise it can cause significant mortality and morbidity. A high index of suspicion is must for early detection. Exclude the other causes of pharyngo-tonsillar disease such as streptococcal pharyngitis, infectious mononucleosis, Vincent's angina, and candida, which may form pseudomembrane in throat. Streptococcal pharyngitis usually manifests as high-grade fever, tonsillar exudates, and tender and enlarged anterior cervical nodes and is diagnosed by throat swab culture. Infectious mononucleosis presents as fever, sore throat, rashes, tonsillopharyngitis, hepatosplenomegaly, and lymphadenopathy. Vincent's angina is characterized by gingival pain, foul breath, and pseudomembrane formation.

Delayed diagnosis and initiation of treatment, laryngeal infection, airway compromise, cardiac involvement, and neurological involvement (phrenic nerve involvement or vasomotor center involvement) carry poor prognosis. Overall, the case-fatality rate of diphtheria is 5–10%.

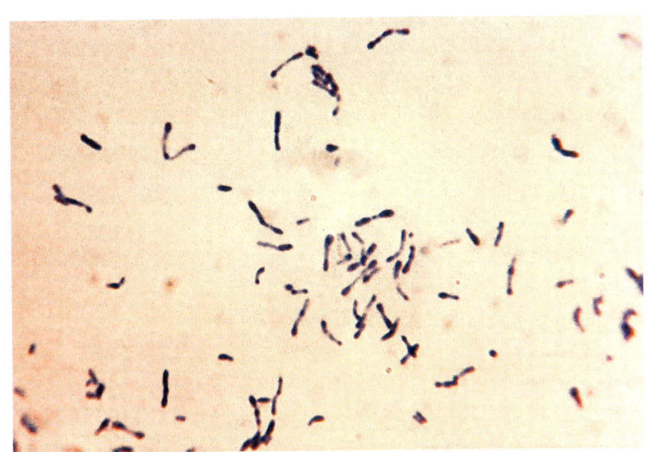

Fig. 2: *Corynebacterium* diphtheria.
(*Source*: Centers for Disease Control and Prevention)

MEDICAL MANAGEMENT

The patient should be kept in an isolated ward as the disease spreads through air and personal contacts. DAT is the mainstay of therapy in suspected diphtheria patients. This should be administered on a strong suspicion of case as DAT neutralizes the toxins before its entry into cells. Appropriate antibiotics to eradicate carriage of the organisms and supportive care should also be given.

Diphtheria Antitoxin

Diphtheria antitoxin neutralizes the unbound toxin and prevents the progression of the disease. It does not neutralize the toxin that is already bound to tissues. It should be administered to all strongly suspected cases in a hospital setting. However, it is not indicated in cutaneous diphtheria without systemic manifestation.

Sensitivity test should be done before administration of antitoxins. It is done by 1:1,000 dilution of antitoxin on the ventral aspect of the forearm. The antitoxin doses are empirical and vary from 20,000 units to 120,000 units depending on the duration and severity of the disease. DAT should be administered by the intravenous route in severe cases. The antitoxin dose should be mixed in 250–500 mL normal saline and administered slowly over 2–4 hours, with a close monitoring for anaphylaxis. Antitoxin may be given intramuscularly (IM) in mild or moderate cases.

Antibiotics

Antibiotics are given to eradicate the organism from nasopharynx and limit the transmission of organism. Recommended antibiotics are macrolides (erythromycin, azithromycin, or clarithromycin) or benzyl penicillin. Erythromycin [40–50 mg/kg/day divided every 6 hours

Table 1: Doses of diptheria antitoxin in various types of diptheria

Diphtheria clinical presentation	DAT dose (units)
Pharyngeal or laryngeal of 2 days' duration	20,000–40,000
Nasopharyngeal disease	40,000–60,000
Extensive disease of 3 or more days' duration or patient with diffuse swelling of neck	80,000–100,000
Skin lesions only rare case where treatment is indicated)	20,000–40,000

(DAT: diphtheria antitoxin)

by mouth or intravenously (IV); maximum 2 g/day], aqueous crystalline penicillin G (100,000–150,000 U/kg/day divided every 6 hours IV or IM), or procaine penicillin (25,000–50,000 U/kg/day divided every 12 hours IM) for 14 days are also recommended.

SUPPORTIVE TREATMENT

Hydration and nutrition of the patients should be maintained. Airway should be managed properly. Tracheostomy and mechanical ventilation may be required, if there is airway obstruction by diphtheritic membrane. Myocarditis and neurological complications usually need critical care support. Bed rest is advised during the acute phase usually for 2 weeks, until the risk of symptomatic cardiac damage diminishes.

CONTROL AND PREVENTION OF DIPHTHERIA

The diphtheria vaccine was developed in 1920 and WHO recommended its use since 1974. The recommended schedule for the primary series is 6, 10, and 14 weeks of age followed by two boosters at 18 months and 5 years. The schedule for catch-up vaccinations is 0, 1, and 6 months. Tdap (tetanus–diphtheria–acellular pertussis) vaccine should be used for children above 7 years for catch-up vaccination. This contains 2 Lf (Limits of Flocculation) of diphtheria toxoid. The Indian Academy of Pediatrics recommends Tdap at 10–12 years of age for children who have received the full course of diphtheria–pertussis–tetanus (DPT) vaccination. All diagnosed diphtheria causes should receive a booster dose of diphtheria-containing vaccine once they are clinically stable, as infection does not reliably induce protective antibody levels.

Chemoprophylaxis for Contacts

All the contacts should be screened for diphtheria by nasal swab or throat swab culture. Chemoprophylaxis should be started in all close contacts of index case with appropriate antimicrobials irrespective of their immunization status. A single dose of benzathine penicillin (600,000 U children <30 kg) and 1.2 million units for >30 kg or erythromycin (40 mg/kg/day) should be given for 7 days as chemoprophylaxis.

The asymptomatic individuals, where organisms are detected in throat swab, must be treated like index case with isolation, antibiotics, and supportive care.

Both contacts and index case should be given a booster dose of diphtheria-containing vaccine if they have received DPT 5 years ago.

Follow-up

Repeat culture should be performed after 2 weeks of completion of therapy to patients and carriers. If the organism is detected in swab, then an additional course of oral erythromycin should be given for 10 days and follow-up culture should be done.

SUGGESTED READING

1. Balasubramanian S, Shah A, Pemde HK, et al. Indian Academy of Pediatrics (IAP) Advisory Committee on Vaccines and Immunization Practices (ACVIP) Recommended Immunization Schedule (2018-19) and Update on Immunization for Children Aged 0 Through 18 Years. Indian Pediatr. 2018;55(12):1066-74.
2. Besa NC, Coldiron ME, Bakri A, et al. Diphtheria outbreak with high mortality in northeastern Nigeria. Epidemiol Infect. 2014;142(4):797-802.
3. du Plessis M, Wolter N, Allam M, et al. Molecular characterization of Corynebacterium diphtheriae outbreak isolates, South Africa, March-June 2015. Emerg Infect Dis 2017; 23(8):1308-15.
4. Efstratiou A, Engler KH, Mazurova IK, et al. Current approaches to the laboratory diagnosis of diphtheria. J Infect Dis. 2000;181(Suppl 1):S138-45.
5. Garib Z, Danovaro-Holliday MC, Tavarez Y, et al. Diphtheria in the Dominican Republic: reduction of cases following a large outbreak. Rev Panam Salud Publica. 2015;38(4):292-9.
6. Ledbetter MK, Cannon AB, Costa AF. The electrocardiogram in diphtheritic myocarditis. Am Heart J. 1964;68:599-611.
7. MacGregor RR. Corynebacterium diphtheriae. In: Mandell GL, Bennett JE, Dolin R. (Eds). Principles and Practice of Infectious Diseases, 7th edition. Philadelphia, PA: Churchill Livingstone; 2010. pp. 2687-94.
8. Reynolds GE, Saunders H, Matson A, et al. Public health action following an outbreak of toxigenic cutaneous diphtheria in an Auckland refugee resettlement centre. Commun Dis Intell Q Rep. 2016;40(4):E475-81.
9. Santos LS, Sant'anna LO, Ramos JN, et al. Diphtheria outbreak in Maranhão, Brazil: microbiological, clinical and epidemiological aspects. Epidemiol Infect. 2015;143(4):791-8.
10. Sein C, Tiwari T, Macneil A, et al. Diphtheria outbreak in Lao People's Democratic Republic, 2012-2013. Vaccine. 2016;34(36):4321-6.
11. Wagner KS, White JM, Lucenko I, et al. Diphtheria in the postepidemic period, Europe, 2000-2009. Emerg Infect Dis. 2012;18(2):217-25.

Pertussis

Meenakshi Sesama, Piyush Gupta

INTRODUCTION

Pertussis, also known as whooping cough, is caused by bacterium *Bordetella pertussis*. It is an acute, highly infectious respiratory disease. The illness affects all ages, but the clinical spectrum and duration and severity of illness are more serious in young infants. The disease is characterized by inexorable bouts of cough which often make it hard to breathe. Following the introduction of pertussis vaccine, there was worldwide decline in the number of cases of pertussis but in the recent era, the disease has re-emerged, cause being largely enigmatic.

ETIOLOGY

Bordetella pertussis, a Gram-negative coccobacillus, is the most common cause of pertussis. *B. parapertussis and B. bronchiseptica* are other species implicated as the causative pathogens. *B. holmesii* is also reported to cause pertussis-like cough.

Prolonged episodes of paroxysmal spasmodic cough can be due to many other causes. Protracted paroxysmal coughing may be caused by *Mycoplasma*, parainfluenza viruses, influenza viruses, enteroviruses, respiratory syncytial viruses, or adenoviruses. Endobronchial tuberculosis, inhaled foreign body, and reactive airway disease are other conditions presenting with prolonged episodes of spasmodic cough.

EPIDEMIOLOGY

Pertussis is endemic worldwide. With the development and subsequent introduction of whole-cell pertussis vaccine (wPV) in late 1940s in national immunization programs, there was marked decline in the incidence of the disease but still it remained a major public health challenge. However, due to the side effects reported after immunization with wPV, less reactogenic acellular pertussis vaccine (aPV) was developed from *B. pertussis* components that induced protective immune responses with less side effects. These aPVs contained pertussis antigens, such as pertussis toxin (PT), pertactin (PRN), fimbrial proteins 2 (FIM2) and 3 (FIM3), and filamentous hemagglutinin (FHA). But several trials on efficacy demonstrated that the aPVs were able to confer short-term protection compared to wPVs as well as no herd immunity.

Disease rates are highest among young children in developing countries and where vaccination coverage is low. According to the 2013 WHO estimates, pertussis caused around 63,000 deaths in under-five children worldwide.[1] The disease is reemerging universally,[2,3] but the cause remains unclear. Switching from wPVs to aPVs is the major reason behind resurgence of pertussis cases in developed nations, whereas low vaccination coverage, particularly not giving timely booster dose during adolescents, adults, and during pregnancy being among the few possible reasons for resurgence of the disease in developing countries. From India, in the year 2015, nearly 25,000 cases of pertussis were reported while nearly 37,000 cases were reported in 2016.

The disease spreads by aerosol droplets from an active case and the attack rate is almost 100% in susceptible individuals. Adolescents and adults who have not received a booster dose of vaccination can become infected or reinfected with pertussis as protection from infection or vaccine-derived immunity wanes over time. An endemic pool of adults is generated due to the waning of the immunity with time and they act as a reservoir of transmission to young children.[4-6] Therefore, emphasis must be on timely booster doses of vaccination.

Because of the complex immune response to the many virulence factors expressed by *B. pertussis*, no reliable serological marker of protection has been identified.[7] Malnourishment and overcrowding help in the spread of the disease. Pertussis exhibits no uniform pattern of seasonality.[8,9]

CLINICAL FEATURES

The incubation period of pertussis on an average is 3–14 days. Symptoms of pertussis in young infants extend from a mild illness, mimicking common cold, to severe illness resulting in hospitalization and even death. Classically, pertussis is a prolonged illness, divided into three stages:

1. Catarrhal
2. Paroxysmal
3. Convalescent.

In a typical case of pertussis, after 3–14 days of exposure to infectious source, mild upper respiratory tract symptoms such as low-grade fever or no fever, sneezing, lacrimation, and conjunctival suffusion begin similar to common cold and often parents do not seek medical intervention during this stage (*catarrhal* stage lasting for 1–2 weeks). The patient is highly contagious/infectious during this stage. Disease in young infants can be atypical, with a short catarrhal stage which might go unnoticed. This is followed by cough which starts as dry, hacking, and intermittent and evolves into episodic paroxysms ending with high-pitched inspiratory whoop (*paroxysmal* stage lasting for 2–6 weeks). The classical cough with whoop is most common in children but may not be present in young infants. In between the paroxysmal coughing episodes, the patient has generally no complains. Severe inexorable coughing can lead to post-tussive vomiting, bulging eyes, lacrimation, salivation, and engorged neck veins. In infants, this can lead to apnea, cyanosis, or poor feeding. The apneic episodes may result in seizures.

The paroxysmal coughing spells gradually resolve into milder and less frequent coughing and wane over many weeks (*convalescent* stage). If the patient develops another respiratory illness during this time, the symptoms of pertussis get exacerbated and duration of this stage might get prolonged. The clinical spectrum and the duration of illness are influenced by many factors such as age of patient, immunization status, prior history of pertussis, and maternal immunization status during pregnancy with Tdap (tetanus, diphtheria and acellular pertussis).

Physical examination of a patient of pertussis is generally uninformative in between the coughing spells.

COMPLICATIONS

Complications vary with the age of patient and the immunization status against pertussis or previous infection with the disease. Young infants have partial immunity against pertussis as the vaccine series is not yet complete. Hence, the complications are more severe in them, such as apnea, convulsions, pneumonia, respiratory failure, or even death. Infants with pneumonia can also develop pulmonary hypertension, which can rapidly progress and is life threatening if refractory to treatment.[10] Mortality and morbidity are high in infant.

In adults and adolescents, the chronic cough can cause sleep disturbances, subconjunctival bleeds, abdominal hernias or even intracranial bleeds, and vertebral artery dissection leading to stroke.[11] Due to inexorable coughing, conjunctival hemorrhages and petechiae on upper body are common.

Secondary infections such as otitis media and pneumonia, and neurological complications such as seizures and encephalopathy might occur. Weight loss, urinary incontinence, and syncopal attacks are other complications of inexorable prolonged coughing.

RECOMMENDED CASE DEFINITION[12]

Clinical Case Definition

A case diagnosed as pertussis by a physician or a person with a cough lasting for at least 2 weeks with at least one of the following symptoms:

- Paroxysms (i.e. fits) of coughing
- Inspiratory whooping
- Post-tussive vomiting (i.e. vomiting immediately after coughing) without other apparent cause.

Criteria for laboratory confirmation:

- Isolation of *B. pertussis*
- Detection of genomic sequences by means of the polymerase chain reaction (PCR)
- Positive paired serology.

Case Classification

Clinically confirmed: A case that meets the clinical case definition but is not laboratory-confirmed.

Laboratory confirmed: A case that meets the clinical case definition and is laboratory-confirmed.

DIAGNOSIS

Pertussis is a clinical diagnosis, suspected in any individual who has a chief complaint of cough (>2 weeks), especially if fever, malaise, and sore throat are absent. Lymphocytic leukocytosis is characteristic in catarrhal stage. In a clinical setting of pertussis, a high leukocyte count with lymphocytic predominance must be evaluated further for possibility of pertussis. Exception to this are young infants who might not have the elevated leukocyte findings due to transplacentally acquired antibodies to pertussis. Definitive confirmation of pertussis cases can be done by culture, PCR, or positive paired serology.

Culture of nasopharyngeal aspirate or nasopharyngeal swabbing with Dacron swabs on Bordet-Gengou culture medium is diagnostic. The sample should be stored and transported into specialized transport media in case of delayed inoculation. In general, PCR is more sensitive and rapid test compared to culture. It takes only 1–2 days in providing results compared to culture which might take more than a week. Moreover, prior antibiotic treatment does not affect PCR results.

Serological testing or direct fluorescent antibody test is not routinely recommended for diagnostic confirmation.[13]

■ TREATMENT

Antibiotics

Antibiotics reduce the transmission of disease to other persons by eradicating the bacteria from the nasopharynx and causing microbiological cure.[14-16] The CDC (Centers for Disease Control and Prevention) guidelines recommend a macrolide antibiotic (azithromycin, clarithromycin, or erythromycin) or trimethoprim-sulfamethoxazole, in case of macrolide intolerance, as an alternative for pertussis. Ideally, antibiotics should begin within 1–2 weeks of the onset of symptoms.[17] Azithromycin is typically administered in doses of 10 mg/kg/day orally for 5 days. Azithromycin is the preferred antibiotic for infants below 1 month due to the risk of infantile hypertrophic pyloric stenosis with oral erythromycin. Due to the shorter duration of antibiotic course and once-a-day administration, compliance is more likely with azithromycin compared with erythromycin. Corticosteroids, bronchodilators, antitussives, and antihistamines are not generally recommended for the symptoms of pertussis.[18]

Isolation

Suspected cases should be placed in isolation with droplet precautions to reduce contact with respiratory secretions. They should be isolated from general population until 5 days after initiation of macrolide therapy.

Care of Close Contacts

Postexposure prophylaxis is recommended within the first 21 days of illness for all household and other close contacts of cases irrespective of age, symptoms, and previous immunization history.[19] The recommended drugs and dosing regimens are the same for postexposure prophylaxis and for the treatment of pertussis.

■ PREVENTION

Neither natural disease nor immunization against pertussis provides lifelong immunity against the disease. Vaccine-induced immunity wanes after 4–12 years shifting the bulk of pertussis cases in adolescent and adults. Hence, apart from primary immunization schedule, timely booster doses of vaccination against pertussis are required.

Whole-cell pertussis vaccine was introduced in 1948; the incidence and outbreaks declined significantly after that, but the resurgence of pertussis cases in recent years in both developed and developing nations is a big concern and a major public health challenge. The temporal relation between the wPVs and neurological complications lead to the introduction of aPVs. Acellular vaccine is less reactogenic, hence lesser side effects, but the effectiveness and duration of protection is less compared to wPV. Therefore, the switch to aPV for primary immunization has been associated with resurgence of disease in developed nations.[20,21] Therefore, in primary series, wPV is recommended. Low vaccination coverage, particularly not giving timely booster dose during adolescents, adults, and pregnancy, is among the few possible reasons for resurgence of the disease in developing countries.

As per the IAP (Indian Academy of Pediatrics) guidelines (2018–19) on vaccines, all infants and children should receive pertussis vaccine in combination with vaccines against diphtheria, tetanus, hepatitis B, and *Haemophilus influenzae type b* at ages 6, 10, and 14 weeks in primary series and booster doses of DwPT/DaPT (Diphtheria, whole/acellular pertussis and tetanus vaccine) 15–18 months and 5 years.[22]

- Persons aged ≥7 years should receive only acellular vaccine (Tdap). The schedule for catch-up vaccination below 7 years is DTwP/DaPT at 0, 1, and 6 months while above 7 years is Tdap, Td (tetanus and diphtheria toxoids), Td at 0, 1, and 6 months.
- Persons aged >10 years should receive Tdap vaccine, if not received earlier followed by Td booster every 10 years.

The most cost-effective additional strategy for preventing disease in infants too young to be vaccinated is vaccination of pregnant women with Tdap during each pregnancy, irrespective of their history of receiving prior Td/Tdap (preferably in 27–36 weeks of gestation). This strategy appears to be more effective than cocooning.[1]

CONCLUSION

Pertussis is a highly contagious but vaccine-preventable respiratory illness. There is resurgence of the disease in recent era in both developed and developing countries. Hence, emphasis has to be on high vaccination coverage and timely booster doses administration, of not only infants and young children but of the adults, adolescents, and pregnant females to eliminate the pool of reservoirs.

REFERENCES

1. World Health Organization (WHO). Pertussis Vaccines: Who Position Paper, August 2015. Weekly Epidemiological Record. 2015;90:433-60.
2. Libster R, Edwards KM. Re-emergence of pertussis: what are the solutions? Expert Rev. Vaccines. 2012;11(11):1331-46.
3. Plotkin SA. The pertussis problem. Clin Infect Dis. 2014;58: 830-3.
4. Wendelboe AM, Van Rie A, Salmaso S, et al. Duration of immunity against pertussis after natural infection or vaccination. Pediatr Infect Dis J. 2005;24(Suppl 5):S58-61.
5. Cherry JD. Epidemiological, clinical, and laboratory aspects of pertussis in adults. Clin Infect Dis. 1999;28(Suppl 2):S112-7.
6. von König CH, Halperin S, Riffelmann M, et al. Pertussis of adults and infants. Lancet Infect Dis. 2002;2(12):744-50.
7. Higgs R, Higgins SC, Ross PJ, et al. Immunity to the respiratory pathogen Bordetella pertussis. Mucosal Immunol. 2012;5(5): 485-500.
8. Edwards KM, Decker MD. Pertussis vaccines. In: Plotkin SA, Orenstein WA, Offit PA (Eds). Vaccines, 6th edition. Philadelphia, PA: Elsevier, Saunders; 2013. pp. 447-92.
9. Cherry J, Heininger U. Pertussis and other Bordetella infections. In: Cherry J, Demmler-Harrison GJ, Kaplan S, Steinbach W, Hotez P (Eds). Feigin and Cherry's textbook of pediatric infectious diseases. Philadelphia, PA: Saunders/Elsevier; 2014. pp. 1616-39.
10. Namachivayam P, Shimizu K, Butt W. Pertussis: severe clinical presentation in pediatric intensive care and its relation to outcome. Pediatr Crit Care Med. 2007;8(3):207-11.
11. Singh M, Lingappan K. Whooping cough: the current scene. Chest. 2006;130(5):1547-53.
12. World Health Organization (WHO). Who-recommended surveillance standard of pertussis. [online] Available from: https://www.who.int/immunization/monitoring_surveillance/ burden/vpd/surveillance_type/passive/pertussis_standards/ en/[Last accessed on December, 2019].
13. Menzies SL, Kadwad V, Pawloski LC, et al. Development and analytical validation of an immunoassay for quantifying serum anti-pertussis toxin antibodies resulting from Bordetella pertussis infection. Clin Vaccine Immunol. 2009; 16(12):1781-8.
14. Altunaiji S, Kukuruzovic R, Curtis N, et al. Antibiotics for whooping cough (pertussis). Cochrane Database Syst Rev. 2007;(3):CD004404.
15. Langley JM, Halperin SA, Boucher FD, et al. Azithromycin is as effective as and better tolerated than erythromycin estolate for the treatment of pertussis. Pediatrics. 2004;114(1): e96-101.
16. Wood N, McIntyre P. Pertussis: review of epidemiology, diagnosis, management and prevention. Paediatr Respir Rev. 2008; 9(3):201-11.
17. Centers for Disease Control and Prevention. Pertussis (whooping cough): treatment. [online] Available from: https://www.cdc.gov/pertussis/index.html. [Last accessed on December, 2019].
18. Bettiol S, Wang K, Thompson MJ, et al. Symptomatic treatment of the cough in whooping cough. Cochrane Database Syst Rev. 2012;(5):CD003257.
19. Centers for Disease Control and Prevention. Guidelines for the control of pertussis outbreaks. 2000 (amendments made in 2005 and 2006). [online] Available from: http:// www.cdc. gov/pertussis/outbreaks/guide/index.html. [Last accessed on December, 2019].
20. Warfel JM, Zimmerman LI, Merkel TJ. Acellular pertussis vaccines protect against disease but fail to prevent infection and transmission in a nonhuman primate model. Proc Natl Acad Sci USA. 2014;111(2):787-92.
21. Smallridge WE, Rolin OY, Jacobs NT, et al. Different effects of whole-cell and acellular vaccines on Bordetella transmission. J Infect Dis. 2014;209:1981-8.
22. Balasubramanian S, Shah A, Pemde HK, et al. Indian Academy of Pediatrics (IAP) Advisory Committee on Vaccines and Immunization Practices (ACVIP) Recommended Immunization Schedule (2018-19) and Update on Immunization for Children Aged 0 Through 18 Years. Indian Pediatr. 2018;55(12):1066-74.

Pneumococcal Disease in Tropics

Shyam Kukreja, Tapisha Gupta

INTRODUCTION

Pneumococcus (*Streptococcus pneumoniae*) is an important cause of community-acquired pneumonia and meningitis as well as of invasive bacterial infections in children worldwide. Recently, drug resistance to penicillin has been an important development. Also, newer vaccines with wider serotype coverage are currently undergoing trials. These issues will be reviewed in the chapter.

HISTORY

Pasteur and Sternberg simultaneously in 1880 and 1881 discovered pneumococcus. In 1884, Friedlander first isolated pneumococci from blood. In 1919, Neufeld and Haendel classified the bacteria serotypes based on capsular swelling or Quellung reaction. This classification paved the way for further epidemiologic studies and vaccine development. Currently, 90 serotypes have been recognized. In 1930, Francis and Tillett found capsular polysaccharide to be immunogenic for humans and in 1945, for the first time, evidence of serotype-specific protection by vaccine was obtained in a trial by Macleod and associates on USA Army and Air Force recruits.[1]

MICROBIOLOGY

Ninety serotypes of pneumococcus consist of 25 individual serotypes and 65 serotypes grouped into 21 serogroups. Each has a specific polysaccharide capsule. The capsule is the major virulence factor, as it prevents phagocytosis. Capsular-specific antibodies are protective.[2] Many new virulence factors have been identified, e.g. Immunoglobulin A (IgA) protease, hyaluronidase, and surface-located choline-binding proteins. The pneumococcal histidine triad (Pht) proteins such as Pht A, Pht B, Pht D, and Pht E may be potential vaccine candidates.[3]

Streptococcus pneumoniae is a lancet-shaped, Gram-positive coccus, usually found in pairs and chains. Isolates are facultative anaerobes and grow in blood and chocolate agar media as well as liquid culture media. Using antibiotic-containing media (blood agar with gentamicin) improves isolation of pneumococcus.

The fact that bacteria can exchange DNA (deoxyribonucleic acid) was first discovered in pneumococcus. These bacteria are fascinating as they can sense pneumococcal density in the environment, communicate through small peptides, and signal for DNA transformation together. This process is called transformational recombination.[4]

HOST DEFENSE MECHANISMS

Anticapsular serum IgG antibody provides maximum protection against systemic infection and also prevents colonization to some extent. This phenomenon was first discovered in pneumococcus, hence paving the way for development of bacterial vaccines.

Respiratory viral infections, such as influenza, predispose to secondary bacterial pneumonia. The neuraminidase uncovers receptors for pneumococci on lung cells, thus increasing bacterial density.[5] Pneumococcal cell wall components induce cytokines such as interleukin-1 (IL-1) and tumor necrosis factor alpha (TNF-alpha) that mediate inflammatory response in bacterial meningitis and pneumonia.

Spleen is responsible for clearing pneumococci from bloodstream. Children who have undergone splenectomy or those with splenic dysfunction as in sickle cell anemia, thalassemia, chronic liver disease, HIV/AIDS (human immunodeficiency virus/acquired immunodeficiency syndrome), malignancies, etc. suffer from overwhelming pneumococcal infection. Deficiency of the second component of complement (C2) is also associated with recurrent pyogenic infections by encapsulated bacteria.

Interestingly, in a study in south India, neonatal vitamin A supplementation delayed the age at which nasopharyngeal colonization with *S. pneumoniae* occurred in infants. Vitamin A may play a role in host defense.[6] Also, basic fibroblast growth factor levels in cerebrospinal fluid (CSF) can be a good prognostic marker in the future, for pneumococcal meningitis. Poor outcomes such as sequelae or death occurred at higher CSF levels, while levels significantly fell after 24–48 hours of effective antibiotic therapy.[7]

PATHOGENESIS

Nasopharyngeal colonization is followed by the development of type-specific anticapsular antibody. The colonization usually does not progress to disease. Disease occurs when there is exposure to a serotype to which the host is nonimmune along with a condition, such as allergy and viral infection, that predisposes the host to infection by pneumococci.

A preceding viral infection causes cytokine activation of respiratory epithelium cells followed by upregulation of the PAF (platelet activating factor) receptor on their surface. This increases pneumococcal density and causes infection. Spread into bloodstream causes bacteremia and infection in distant sites such as meningitis and joint spaces. Pneumococci cause disease by replication in most tissue and activation of complement pathway pneumolysin, a potent cytotoxin, is associated with disease severity. It can form pores in cells and cause active killing. Pneumococci most commonly cause otitis media, pneumonia, meningitis, and bacteremia but have the capacity to produce disease in any organ of the body.

LABORATORY DIAGNOSIS

Direct Microscopy

Samples such as CSF, pus, or sputum show lancet-shaped, Gram-positive cocci in pairs, surrounded by a halo (due to capsule). CSF Gram stain positivity is especially useful while starting the treatment of meningitis. India ink staining of CSF can help as capsules are better seen.

Antigen Detection

Cerebrospinal fluid latex agglutination test to detect capsular antigen should be done, if the initial Gram stain is negative, especially if the patient has taken antibiotics prior to lumbar puncture.[8] Pneumococcal antigen detection in urine has also been developed though it is not yet available in India. As the test can come positive in healthy carriers, its use in diagnostics of disease is questionable.[9]

Antigen detection in pleural fluid by latex agglutination where available can confirm the diagnosis in children with parapneumonic effusion or empyema. It has high sensitivity and specificity.[10] Antigen testing of blood culture broth from cultures flagged positive by BACT/ALERT (but negative on growth) is currently undergoing trial. A positive result can help to detect bacteremia when Gram stain is positive, but culture is negative.[11] However, more studies are needed before antigen testing on blood culture samples can be used as a diagnostic test. Antibody detection to *S. pneumoniae* is not advisable as there are numerous infecting serotypes, and hence the specificity is poor.

Culture

Streptococcus pneumoniae growth on blood culture or on culture of body fluids such as CSF confirms the diagnosis. This organism is extremely rarely a skin contaminant and it grows only in enriched media in the presence of 5–10% CO_2. Isolation from respiratory secretions is better when blood agar containing gentamicin is used. It is an aerobe and a facultative anaerobe.

On blood agar, after an incubation of 18 hours, the colonies become small with alpha hemolysis around them and may resemble those of *S. viridans*. After further incubation, they are described to have a "carrom coin" appearance.

Another interesting feature of the organism is production of Lyt A, an autolytic intracellular enzyme. When grown in artificial media, unless picked up fast on the blood culture systems, the organism can autolyze rapidly.

Drug Susceptibility Testing

This may be performed by MIC (minimal inhibitory concentration) determination or by disk diffusion. For testing penicillin and beta lactams, disk diffusion with 1 µg oxacillin disk is used as a screening method, where a cutoff zone of 20 mm or more is taken as susceptible, whereas for strains with zones less than 20 mm, MIC needs to be determined.

Prior to 2007, CLSI (Clinical and Laboratory Standards Institute) breakpoints for MIC interpretation were based on antibiotic concentrations reached in CSF so that meningitis could be treated successfully. It was however found that nonmeningeal pneumococcal infections such as pneumonia could be treated successfully with penicillin even if the pre-2008 breakpoints suggest nonsusceptibility. Hence, in 2008, CLSI published new breakpoints.[12] These are as follows:

- For—non-CNS (central nervous system) isolates, the definition of sensitivity to penicillin (parenteral) is as follows:
    - Susceptible—MIC ≤ 2 µg/mL
    - Intermediate—MIC 4 µg/mL
    - Resistant—MIC ≥ 8 µg/mL
- For CNS isolates, these are as follows:
    - Susceptible—MIC ≤ 0.06 µg/mL
    - Resistant—MIC ≥ 0.12 µg/mL
- There is no intermediate category for meningeal isolates.

ANTIBIOTIC RESISTANCE IN PNEUMONOCOCCUS

Isolates resistant to beta lactams and several antibiotic classes were first reported in 1977 in South Africa. The foremost risk factor for acquiring antibiotic-resistant strain is recent antibiotic use. Other risk factors are age less than 5 years, recent respiratory infections, and day-care attendance. Introduction of pneumococcal conjugate vaccine (PCV) has significantly reduced antibiotic resistance in USA.[13] A higher incidence of penicillin resistance is noted in countries that do not have significant conjugate vaccine coverage.[14]

Penicillin-binding proteins (PBP) or enzymes are present on the pneumococcal cell surface. These enzymes synthesize peptidoglycan, the major cell wall constituent. Beta lactams bind irreversibly to it and inhibit bacterial growth. The resistance mechanism in pneumococcus is alteration of these PBP. The organism does not produce beta lactamase.

Antibiotic Resistance in the World

Multiresistant strains have now spread to many parts of the world and are also being reported from India. Currently in North America, as per the data of isolates collected in 2015–2016, penicillin susceptibility for non-CNS infections was seen in 96.7% (using parenteral nonmeningitis breakpoints). Using meningitis breakpoints, for ceftriaxone, the susceptibility was 43.3% in the same set of 6,135 isolates from North America.[15]

In the data collected from 60 hospitals in 11 Asian countries from 2008 to 2009 by the Asian Network for Surveillance of Resistant Pathogens (ANSORP), it was found that in nonmeningeal isolates penicillin nonsusceptible or intermediate pneumococci prevalence

(MIC ≥ 4 µg/mL) was 4.6% while penicillin resistance (MIC more than or equal to 8 µg/mL) was very rare, 0.7% only.[16]

Antibiotic Resistance in India

The Indian data available in 1993–1997 showed a penicillin intermediate resistance in 1.8% isolates. This figure was 3.8% in 1996–1997 and went up to 7.8% in 2000–2001.[17] Once the new CLSI 2008 breakpoints were applied to the nonmeningitis isolates, these percentages changed to less than 1%.[18]

In another study from South India published in 2015, penicillin nonsusceptibility was 5.2%, in 6 out of 114 isolates from blood, CSF, and pleural fluid.[19] A surveillance study by Alliance for Surveillance of Invasive Pneumococci (ASIP) network, India in 2017 showed that penicillin nonsusceptibility was seen in 8%, that is, in 29 out of 361 isolates.[20] In another study published in 2017, 830 invasive pneumococcal isolates were studied over a period of 8 years from January 2008 to August 2016; 167 out of 830 were meningeal isolates. The meningeal isolates showed 43.7% and 14.9% nonsusceptibility to penicillin and cefotaxime, respectively. Serotypes 14, 19F, 6B, 6A, 23F, 9V, and 5 were the most common serotypes causing meningitis. The first five serotypes were responsible for 75% of the resistant isolates. This indicates that guidelines for effective treatment of meningitis may have to evolve if similar data appears in the coming years from our country. However, in nonmeningeal isolates, the penicillin nonsusceptibility was less than 1% in an Indian setting.[21]

Implications of Antibiotic Resistance in India

It is important to understand that while treating nonmeningeal infections such as pneumonia, resistance to penicillin/cephalosporin is extremely rare in our country and if at all found in an isolate, it can be overcome by using higher concentrations of beta lactams, at maximum doses possible with appropriate pharmacokinetics like 8-hourly dosing. Oral drugs, where indicated such as amoxicillin in high doses at 90 mg/kg/day, or intravenous cephalosporins, such as cefotaxime, ceftriaxone, or cefuroxime, may be used.

In meningeal isolates, higher rates of antibiotic resistance have been reported; therefore, it is imperative that in suspected cases of pneumococcal bacterial meningitis, an effective antibiotic must be started. Ceftriaxone along with vancomycin may be started at the outset with judicious downgrade, if the isolate is found to be penicillin susceptible. Hence, an attempt must be made to isolate the organism by sending paired blood cultures in appropriate volume and by early lumbar puncture, preferably prior to antibiotics.

Cross-resistance to other antibiotic classes increases with increasing penicillin MICs. Also, whether resistance to these antibiotics can be overcome by increasing drug concentration is controversial. Strains with multiple antibiotic resistance have greater selective advantage. Researchers have postulated that rampant use of macrolides (azithromycin and clarithromycin) may promote beta-lactam resistance among pneumococcal strains.

Use of PCV reduces the carriage and disease incidence caused by the vaccine serotypes. However, replacement strains emerge, which are often antibiotic resistant. After PCV-7 use, serotype 19 A emerged which was then included in PCV-13. Now, serotypes 15 F, 23 A, 23 B, and 35B are being reported which are not present in either PCV or pneumococcal polysaccharide vaccine (PPSV) 23.

NASOPHARYNGEAL CARRIAGE

Pediatric serotypes that cause nasopharyngeal colonization of infants and young children in most parts of the world are serotypes 6A, 6B, 9V, 14, 18C, 19A, 19F, and 23F. Whether carriage leads to infection is unclear. Many prospective, longitudinal studies have shown that infections such as otitis media or pneumonia develop frequently following colonization with a new serotype. However, carriers develop circulating antibodies that protect them from invasive disease.

Viral infections, crowding, and day-care attendance increase carriage rates. In a study in India published in July 2019, 54.5% healthy children between 2 months and 59 months of age had nasopharyngeal colonization with pneumococcus.[22] The most common serotypes were 6A, 6B, 14, 19A, 19F, and 23F.

Another study in South India found the median age of acquisition of pneumococci to be 8 weeks, by which 53.9% of infants tested had nasopharyngeal colonization by pneumococci.[23] Colonization peaks in the second to third year of life and falls with increasing age. The role of innate immunity with increasing age is unclear. However, everyone carries pneumococci of different serotypes during their lifetime. Vaccination with PCV reduces the nasopharyngeal carriage of vaccine serotypes but it does not change the overall carrier rate.

CLINICAL SYNDROMES

Streptococcus pneumoniae causes two types of infections—invasive pneumococcal disease or mucosal infections. An invasive pneumococcal disease is defined as an infection in which the pneumococcus has been isolated from a normally sterile site, e.g. CSF, blood, pleural joint or peritoneal fluid, but not sputum. The high-risk conditions for an invasive pneumococcal disease are as follows:

- Age less than 2 years or male sex
- Recent viral respiratory infection
- Chronic liver disease
- Chronic renal disease such as nephrotic syndrome
- Chronic pulmonary disease such as asthma
- Chronic cardiovascular disease such as cardiomyopathy
- Diabetes mellitus
- Functional or anatomic asplenia (splenectomy)
- Inflammatory bowel disease
- CSF leaks or cochlear implants
- Immunosuppressive conditions (HIV/immuno-deficiency)
- Glucocorticoid use.

Bacteremia is a prerequisite for invasive pneumococcal disease to occur. In children less than 3 years of age, the most common clinical presentation of invasive pneumococcal disease is occult bacteremia. This is defined as a positive blood culture without a known focus of infection. Usually, bacteremia presents as fever without focus with temperature up to 40°C and a total leukocyte count of more than 15,000 cells/mm^3. About 75% of all cases with bacteremia are between 3 months and 24 months of age. About 6–10% of occult bacteremia may progress to complications such as sepsis meningitis, pneumonia, cellulitis, or osteomyelitis.

Meningitis

Streptococcus pneumoniae is the most common pathogen causing meningitis in infants and children above 1 month of age. The bacteria most commonly reach the meninges via bloodstream; however, at times meningitis may follow traumatic injury to the skull. Following introduction of PCV, the incidence of meningitis has decreased, though cases caused by nonvaccine serotypes are proportionately higher. Children usually present with the typical signs of meningitis, i.e. fever with irritability, confusion, headache, lethargy, photophobia, and vomiting. The average duration of meningitis like signs before admission is 28 hours, but it may range from 4 hours to 52 hours. About 20% of children may get a seizure. Infants may not show signs of meningismus. In a multicenter pneumococcal meningitis surveillance study, 11–16% children presented with shock or disseminated intravascular coagulation and 11% were comatose at the time of admission.[24] During therapy, children may develop raised intracranial pressure

(ICP), subdural effusion, and cerebral edema. Hearing loss is two to three times more common in pneumococcal meningitis.

Evaluation of CSF gives a clue to the etiology. CSF pleocytosis with neutrophilia, low CSF glucose with high CSF protein, and presence of Gram-positive diplococci on Gram stain of CSF suggest pneumococcus. Rapid diagnostic tests such as latex agglutination may be performed, if the initial Gram stain is negative. A positive blood culture in a patient with CSF pleocytosis can also clinch the diagnosis; hence, paired aerobic blood cultures of appropriate volume should be sent in all cases. Management involves supportive care, intravenous fluids, and prompt antibiotic therapy.

In view of rising antibiotic resistance noted in meningeal isolates, it may be prudent to treat suspected pneumococcal meningitis initially with both ceftriaxone and vancomycin, till the culture and sensitivity reports are available. Children who receive multiple antibiotic courses or those in child care facilities are often carriers of resistant strains.

Pneumonia

Streptococcus pneumoniae causes classic lobar consolidation; however, it may also cause bronchopneumonia. Children present with fever, cough, breathlessness, and lethargy. Around 40% may present with vomiting and up to 20% may present with abdominal pain and thus occasionally confound the clinician. On examination, crepts and bronchial breath sounds over the affected lobe may be heard. Almost half of the children may have hypoxemia at presentation. Complications may be seen in up to half of hospitalized patients. These are pleural effusion, empyema, collapse, necrotizing pneumonia, or lung abscess. Frequency of parapneumonic effusions/ empyema has decreased after the introduction of PCV vaccine. Strains that are penicillin intermediate or resistant more frequently cause parapneumonic effusion at a younger age and these are usually bacteremic, though the prognosis is good. Rarely, pneumatocele or pneumothorax may occur. Some children may also develop hemolytic uremic syndrome.

Diagnosis is usually made by history, physical examination, and on X-ray chest, as it is the most common cause of lobar pneumonia. The most important investigation for etiologic diagnosis is blood or pleural fluid culture, though the positivity rates may be less than 5%. In children who have received prior antibiotics, pneumococcal antigen detection in pleural fluid, where available, can be confirmatory. Pleural fluid polymerase chain reaction (PCR) may also help in diagnosis; however, it is not available widely. Sputum Gram stain showing predominant Gram-positive diplococci (>10 per oil immersion field) with less than 10 epithelial cells per low-power field is diagnostic; however, most children are not able to produce sputum.

Children who are stable, without oxygen requirement or hemodynamic instability, can be treated with oral antibiotics. Those who are toxic or of young age with poor oral intake must be admitted and provided prompt antibiotic therapy. Antibiotic sensitivity pattern guides therapy. For isolates with penicillin MIC ≤2 µg/mL, ampicillin or amoxycillin is the drug of choice. Alternative drugs are cefotaxime or ceftriaxone. Clindamycin may be used in those with penicillin hypersensitivity; if the isolate is resistant to clindamycin, vancomycin is the drug of choice. For isolates with MIC >2 µg/mL, ceftriaxone or cefotaxime is recommended. Clindamycin may be an alternative if there is drug hypersensitivity. Multidrug-resistant serotypes if isolated may be treated with vancomycin, linezolid, or levofloxacin. Treatment is continued for 7 days in uncomplicated pneumonia or up to 5 days after fever resolves in complicated cases. Children usually respond to therapy in 48 hours. Failure to improve should raise concern for resistant strains, development of complications, or alternative diagnosis.

Sinusitis

Acute bacterial rhinosinusitis mimics viral upper respiratory infection. Persistence and symptom severity distinguish the two. Nasal discharge which may be purulent, nocturnal cough, fever upto 102°F for at least 3 days later in the illness are pointers to the diagnosis. Headache and facial pain may or may not be present. Untreated bacterial sinusitis may progress to serious complications such as preseptal or orbital cellulitis or cavernous sinus thrombosis. *S. pneumoniae* is an important cause of acute bacterial rhinosinusitis. The risk factors for penicillin nonsusceptibility are age less than 2 years, day-care attendance, antibiotic therapy within 1 month, hospitalization in the last 5 days, and unimmunized with PCV vaccine. For children without risk factors, the drug of choice is amoxicillin clavulanate in standard dose (45 mg/kg/day in two divided doses) for 10 days. For children with any risk factor for antibiotic resistance, high-dose amoxicillin clavulanate (90 mg/kg/day of amoxycillin component) in two divided doses should be used. Broad-spectrum antibiotics which cover in addition *Haemophilus influenzae* and *Moraxella catarrhalis* must be used to treat sinusitis.

Otitis Media

Streptococcus pneumoniae is one of the three most common bacteria that cause acute otitis media (AOM). The other two are nontypeable *H. influenzae* and *M. catarrhalis*. Postlicensure surveillance of PCV13 has shown a fall in AOM episodes and prevalence of nasopharyngeal colonization due to PCV13 serotypes. Otitis media caused by *S. pneumoniae* tends to be more severe with high fever and severe otalgia and is associated with peripheral leukocytosis. Infants may lack specific symptoms and present with excessive irritability, fever, poor feeding, etc. Children more than 2 years of age may present with otalgia. Diagnosis of AOM is clinical and requires visualization of a fullness or a bulge in the tympanic membrane along with marked redness. Redness alone has a positive predictive value of 15% only for AOM. Otitis media with effusion (OME) must be distinguished from AOM; in the former, the tympanic membrane is usually retracted and antibiotics are not necessary. Treatment of AOM is analgesics such as acetaminophen or ibuprofen; at times, tympanocentesis may be necessary if the otalgia is severe. Topical anesthetics such as benzocaine or antihistamines and decongestants have no role in the management. Febrile children less than 6 months old diagnosed with AOM need to be evaluated to rule out other invasive bacterial infections and then need to be treated promptly with antibiotics. Children more than 6 months old with unilateral AOM and mild symptoms (ear pain >48 hours and temperature <102.2°F) may be observed initially, after shared decision-making with parents. Those with bilateral AOM, who look toxic and have severe symptoms (otalgia <48 hours and temperature <102.2°F), need to be treated with antibiotics. The initial therapy in children at low risk for amoxycillin resistance (no beta-lactam antibiotic in the last 30 days or history of recurrent AOM) is amoxycillin at a dose of 40 mg/kg/day for 10 days in children less than 2 years and a total of 7 days in those more than 2 years. Children who are at high risk of beta-lactam resistance may be treated with amoxicillin clavulanate at a dose of 90 mg/kg/day of amoxicillin in two divided doses for 10 days in children less than 2 years and 7 days in those more than 2 years.

Osteomyelitis and Septic Arthritis

Children older than 2 years with underlying medical conditions (chronic heart or lung disease, splenic dysfunction, sickle cell disease, diabetes mellitus, or immunodeficiency) and children less than 2 years who are unimmunized or partially immunized by PCV vaccine are susceptible to bone and joint infections by *S. pneumoniae*.

■ REFERENCES

1. Macleod CM, Hodges RG, Heidelberger M, et al. Prevention of pneumococcal pneumonia by immunization with specific capsular polysaccharides. J Exp Med. 1945;82(6):445-65.
2. Musher DM. Streptococcus pneumoniae. In: Mandell GL, Bennett JE , Dolin R (Eds). Principles and practice of infectious disease, 5th edition. Philadelphia: Churchill Livingstone; 2000. pp. 2128-46.
3. Adamou JE, Heinrichs JH, Edwin AL, et al. Identification and characterization of a novel family of pneumococcal proteins that are protective against sepsis. Infect Immun. 2001;69(2):949-58.
4. Mortier-Barriere I, Humbert O, Martin B, et al. Control of recombination rate during transformation of *Streptococcus pneumoniae*: an overview. Microb Drug Resist. 1997;3(3): 233-42.
5. LeVine AM, Koeningsknecht V, Stark JM. Decreased pulmonary clearance of S. pneumoniae following influenza A infection in mice. J Virol Methods. 2001;94(1-2):173-86.
6. Coles CL, Rahmathullah L, Kanungo R, et al. Vit A supplementation at birth delays pneumococcal colonization in young south Indian infants. Pediatr Infect Dis J. 2001;20:289-95.
7. Huang CC, Liu CC, Wang ST, et al. Basic fibroblast growth factor in experimental and clinical bacterial meningitis. Pediatr Res. 1999;45(1):120-7.
8. Tunkel AR, Hartman JB, Kaplan SL, et al. Practice guidelines for the management of bacterial meningitis. Clin Infect Dis. 2004;39(9):1267-84.
9. Dominguez J, Gali N, Blanco S, et al. Detection of Streptococcus pneumoniae antigen by a rapid immunochromatographic assay in urine samples. Chest. 2001;119(1):243-9.
10. Le Monnier A, Carbonnelle E, Zahar JR, et al. Microbiological diagnosis of empyema in children: comparative evaluations by culture, polymerase chain reaction, and pneumococcal antigen detection in pleural fluids. Clin Infect Dis. 2006;42(8):1135-40.
11. Baggett HC, Rhodes J, Dejsirilert S, et al. Pneumococcal antigen testing of blood culture broth to enhance the detection of Streptococcus pneumoniae bacteremia. Eur J Clin Microbiol Infect Dis. 2012;31(5):753-6.
12. Weinstein MP, Klugman KP, Jones RN, et al. Rationale for revised penicillin susceptibility breakpoints versus *Streptococcus pneumoniae*: coping with antimicrobial susceptibility in an era of resistance. Clin Infect Diseases. 2009;48(11):1596-600.
13. Centers for Disease Control and Prevention (CDC). (2019). Antibiotic resistance threats in the United States, 2019. [online] Available from: https://www.cdc.gov/drugresistance/pdf/threats-report/2019-ar-threats-report-508.pdf. [Last accessed on December, 2019].
14. Song JH, Lee NY, Ichiyama S, et al. Spread of drug-resistant *Streptococcus pneumoniae* in Asian Countries: Asian Network for Surveillance of Resistant Pathogens (ANSORP) Study. Clin Infect Dis. 1999;28(6):1206-11.
15. Sader HS, Mendes RE, Le J, et al. Antimicrobial Susceptibility of *Streptococcus pneumoniae* from North America, Europe, Latin America and the Asia-Pacific Region: Results From 20 years of the SENTRY Antimicrobial Surveillance Program (1997-2016). Open Forum Infect Dis. 2019;6(Suppl 1): S14-23.

16. Kim SH, Song JH, Chung DR, et al. Changing trends in antimicrobial resistance and serotypes of *Streptococcus pneumoniae* isolates in Asian countries: an Asian Network for Surveillance of Resistant Pathogens (ANSORP) study. Antimicrob Agents Chemother. 2012; 56(3):1418-26.

17. Song JH, Ko KS, Kim NY, et al. High prevalence of antimicrobial resistance among clinical Streptococcus pneumoniae isolates in Asia (an ANSORP study). Antimicrob Agents Chemother. 2004;48(6):2101-7.

18. Veeraraghavan B, Kurien T. Penicillin resistant Streptococcus pneumoniae in India: effects of new clinical laboratory standards institute breakpoint and implications. Indian J Med Microbiol. 2011;29(3):317-8.

19. Balaji V, Jayaraman R, Verghese VP, et al. Pneumococcal serotypes associated with invasive disease in under five children in India implications for vaccine policy. Indian J Med Res. 2015;142(3):286-92.

20. Manoharan A, Manchanda V, Balasubramanian S, et al. Invasive pneumococcal disease in children aged younger than 5 years in India: a surveillance study. Lancet Infect Dis. 2017; 17(3):305-12.

21. Varghese VP, Veeraraghavan B, Jayaraman R, et al. Increasing incidence of penicillin- and cefotaxime-resistant *Streptococcus pneumoniae* causing meningitis in India: Time for revision of treatment guidelines? Indian J Med Microbiol. 2017;35(2):228-36.

22. Sutcliffe CG, Shet A, Varghese R, et al. Nasopharyngeal carriage of *Streptococcus pneumoniae* serotypes among children in India prior to the introduction of pneumococcal conjugate vaccines: a cross-sectional study. BMC Infect Dis. 2019; 19(1):605.

23. Coles CL, Rahmathullah L, Kanungo R, et al. Nasopharyngeal carriage of resistant pneumococci in young South Indian infants. Epidemiol Infect. 2002;129(3):491-7.

24. Arditi M, Mason EO Jr, Bradley JS, et al. Three-year multicenter surveillance of pneumococcal meningitis in children: clinical characteristics, and outcome related to penicillin susceptibility and dexamethasone use. Pediatrics. 1998;102(5):1087-97.

Meningococcal Diseases

Jijo Joseph John, Piyush Gupta

INTRODUCTION

Gaspard Vieusseux from Geneva was the first to describe epidemic meningococcal meningitis in 1805. *Neisseria meningitidis* (*Meningococcus*) is a commensal of the human nasopharynx in 10% of the world population. Although a rare endemic disease in most parts of the world, hyperendemic and epidemic disease patterns are also seen.

BURDEN OF MENINGOCOCCEMIA

There are 13 known serotypes of meningococci, and six of these (A, B, C, Y, X, and W) have been associated with the majority of worldwide epidemics. Serogroup W-135 is now renamed as W.[1] The relative importance of various serogroups varies with age. Serogroup B causes more than 60% of cases in children <5 years of age, while C, Y, and W cause more than 75% cases among children older than 11 years.[2] The highest incidence of serogroup A disease is seen in the sub-Saharan meningitis belt with annual endemic rates of 10–25 per 100,000 population.[3] In recent times, a surge in serogroup W disease has been associated with Hajj pilgrimage.[4] According to the centers for disease control and prevention (CDC), the disease has a cyclical pattern with peaks in incidence every 7–10 years.[2]

Since the early 2000s, the incidence of invasive meningococcal disease (IMD) is declining steadily. In 2012–2015, the incidence was 0.1–0.2 cases per 100,000 population in USA with about 350–550 cases being reported annually. The decline in incidence of disease preceded the introduction of conjugate vaccines in the immunization schedule and may be postulated to be due to circulating antibodies to existing strains in the population and modification of behavioral risk factors such as smoking.

In Asia, six countries have had major meningococcal epidemics in the last 30 years, which were mostly due to serogroups A and C. However there is a lot of under-reporting in the area and most countries rely on passive reporting and anecdotal reports. Official figures from most south Asian countries is lacking.[5]

India has had serogroup A epidemics, most recently in 2005, in Delhi and surrounding regions. Between March and July 2005, 444 cases and 62 deaths with a case fatality rate of 16.9% were recorded. Between January and March 2006, another 177 cases were reported. During the epidemic, our peak attack rate was 13/100,000 population.[5] In 2008–2009, Northeast India had an isolated outbreak with about 2,000 cases and 250 deaths. But burden of disease in non-outbreak setting in India is low. In a 10-year retrospective analysis of acute bacterial meningitis cases from Bangalore, *N. meningitidis* accounted for only 1.4% of culture proven cases.[6] Invasive meningococcal disease is a notifiable disease in India and data from Ministry of Health and Family Welfare (MoHFW) show a declining trend in the total number of IMD cases. In 2016, there were 3,034 meningococcal cases reported, as against 5,609 cases in 2012.[7]

EPIDEMIOLOGY

Humans are the only natural reservoir of *Meningococcus* and asymptomatic nasopharyngeal carriage of disease is seen in 5–10% of population. Carriage is highest in adolescents and young adults. Only a small percentage of carriers develop disease, while the rest develop protective antibodies. By adulthood, almost 65–85% of population have protective antibodies against the disease.[2] Bimodal age peak for disease frequency is seen, with highest frequency during infancy and a second peak in adolescents and young adults.

Disease is transmitted from person to person by direct contact with droplets or respiratory secretions. Disease can be transmitted by both asymptomatic carriers and persons with invasive disease. The organism does not survive for long periods in the environment. *Meningococcus* has an incubation period of 1–10 days, usually less than 4 days.

Risk factors for the disease can be classified as factors related to the organism, host factors and environmental factors. Historically, blacks and people from lower socioeconomic status (SES) groups had highest prevalence of the disease, however, in recent times, this sociocultural gap seems to be decreasing. Other risk factors include anatomical/functional asplenia, persistent complement deficiencies (C3, C5-9, properdin deficiency), human immunodeficiency virus (HIV), and overcrowding. Active and passive smoking and recent upper respiratory tract seem to predispose to IMD. There has been an association between influenza season and IMD, with peak influenza season being seen about 2 weeks prior to surges in meningococcal disease.[8]

MICROBIOLOGY

Gonorrhea causing *Neisseria* was first described by Dr. Albert Neisser in 1879, and the genus was named after him. The important pathogens in this genus are *Neisseria gonorrhoeae* and *N. meningitidis*. *N. meningitidis* was first described by Weichselbaum in 1887, in the specimens of six patients who died of meningitis. He called the organism *diplococcus intracellularis meningitidis*.

Neisseria meningitidis is a Gram-negative diplococcus, usually less than 1 µm in size **(Fig. 1)**. The organisms are usually arranged as pairs, with adjacent sides flattened, similar to kidney beans. They can occasionally be seen as tetrads. They are aerobic (facultative anaerobic), non-motile, produce oxidase and catalase and may be encapsulated. *N. meningitidis* oxidizes glucose and maltose, while *N. gonorrhoeae* oxidizes only glucose. *Neisseria* grow best on chocolate or blood agar, and growth is enhanced when incubated in humidified 10% carbon dioxide. After 48–72 hours of incubation, bluish gray colonies, producing beta-hemolysis on blood agar can be seen.

Similar to other Gram-negative bacteria, *Neisseria* has outer and inner cell membranes composed of phospholipid bilayers, which sandwich a layer of peptidoglycan. Outer membrane has lipooligosaccharide (LOS) and outer membrane protein (OMP), which function as porins. A polysaccharide capsule external to the outer membrane protects the organism from phagocytosis. Meningococci have pili, which helps in adherence to host cells, colonization and invasion. The bacterium evades host defenses by altering the antigenic expression of pili. Also LOS and OMP display antigenic differences by phase variation.

Based on differences in capsular polysaccharides, OMP and LOS, meningococci are classified into serogroups, serotypes and subtypes. Presently, 13 serogroups are identified, viz. A, B, C, D, H, I, K, L, X, Y, Z, W, and 29E. Serogroups A, B, C, Y, and W are the most common causes of invasive disease worldwide.

PATHOPHYSIOLOGY

The human nasopharynx is the only natural reservoir for *N. meningitidis*. Bacteria adhere to the nonciliated columnar epithelial cells in the nasopharynx via pili, which interact with host CD46 molecule or an integrin. Internalization of meningococci by epithelial cell is followed by transcytosis to basolateral membrane and dissemination into the bloodstream. Immunoglobulin A1 (IgA1) protease secreted by the bacteria, breaks down the host surface IgA.[3] Following bacteremia, seeding of meninges with subsequent meningitis can occur.

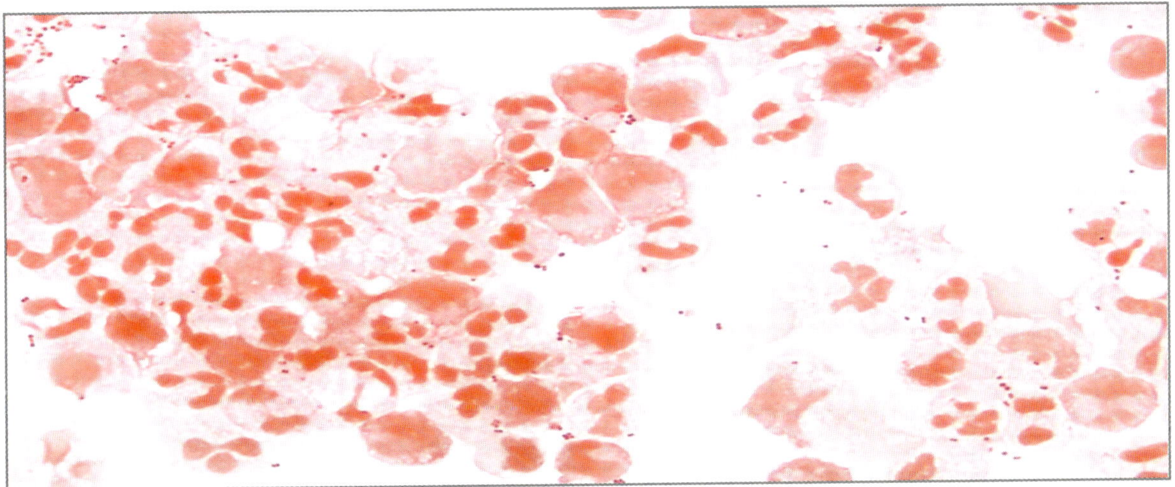

Fig. 1: Gram-negative diplococcus.

Meningococci release blebs from their surface containing OMP and LOSs. These LOS are potent endotoxins and they induce release of a host of proinflammatory cytokines in the body. TNF-α, IL-1, IL-6, IL-8, and IL-10 are released and their levels correlate with disease severity. These chemokines induce a procoagulant state in the body, and directly or indirectly lead to the formation of microthrombi, found in the skin, digits, and extremities.

Release of cytokines also causes activation of neutrophils, and upregulation of adhesion molecules, which lead to endothelial damage and capillary leakage. There is increased production of nitric oxide by the endothelial cells, leading to vasodilation and the initial presentation of warm shock. Subsequently, cytokine-mediated cardiac dysfunction, cardiac failure, hypotension, and irreversible shock ensues. Capillary leakage in the pulmonary bed can lead to acute respiratory distress syndrome (ARDS). Endotoxins also lead to activation of the coagulation system, causing consumptive coagulopathy and disseminated intravascular coagulopathy (DIC). Hypoxia, acidosis, hypokalemia, hypoglycemia, hypocalcemia, and hypophosphatemia are all common in severe sepsis and further depress cardiac function.

CLINICAL FEATURES

Meningococcus can cause a wide spectrum of disease, ranging from asymptomatic transient bacteremia, to fulminant sepsis, causing death in a few hours. Meningitis is the most common clinical manifestation, followed by bacteremia. More than half the children with IMD have skin rash in the form of petechiae, purpura or most characteristically, purpura fulminans.

Meningococcemia/Meningitis

Serious meningococcal disease usually occurs as either meningococcemia or meningitis. The initial clinical presentation is similar to common respiratory or viral infections of childhood, such as coryza, pharyngitis or tonsillitis. Progression of disease is rapid and death can occur within a few hours after disease onset.

Meningitis presents with headache associated with fever, lethargy and vomiting. They may have neck stiffness, photophobia and meningeal signs. Young infants can present with lethargy, irritability and/or bulging fontanels. The most common neurological complication of meningitis are hydrocephalus, cranial nerve palsies, subdural empyema, cortical venous thrombosis, cerebral edema or cerebral infarction. Neurological sequelae can be seen even without meningitis, in children with meningococcemia and shock.

Meningococcemia presents as fever with nonspecific signs such as upper respiratory tract infection, myalgia, muscle tenderness or skin rash. Even though purpura is the rash classically described with meningococcemia, maculopapular rash, petechial rash, pink macular salmon rash, or a varicella-like rash have all been described with IMD **(Figs. 2 and 3)**.[9] Finding of purpuric rash in a febrile child greatly increases the suspicion of meningococcemia, especially if the rash has an acral distribution. Rapid deterioration with circulatory collapse, shock, ARDS, DIC leading to multiple organ dysfunction syndrome (MODS) can happen.

In a retrospective case analysis of IMD from a tertiary care center in Northeast India, Hazarika et al. found that meningitis was seen in 61% of children, meningococcemia was in 20% and 18% had both. One-fourth of the patients had rash and blood culture was positive in 35%. Mortality was found to be 6.4%.[10] Prior to the era of antibiotics, case fatality rate (CFR) for *Meningococcus* was 70–85%. Now, with widespread use of antibiotics, CFR has been brought down to 10–15%.[2] Even with prompt initiation of therapy, CFR remains high.

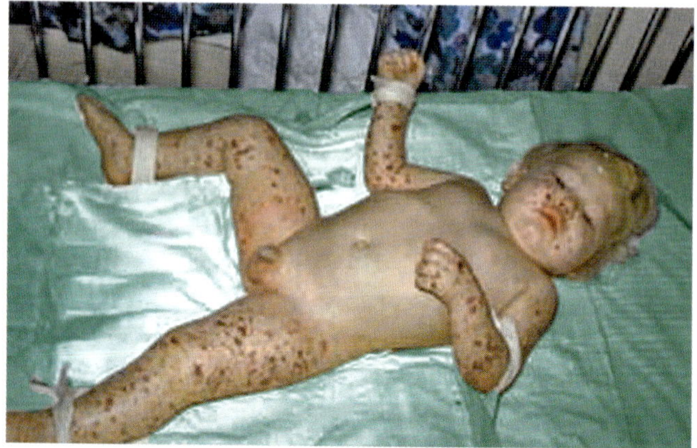

Fig. 2: Young boy with meningococcemia.

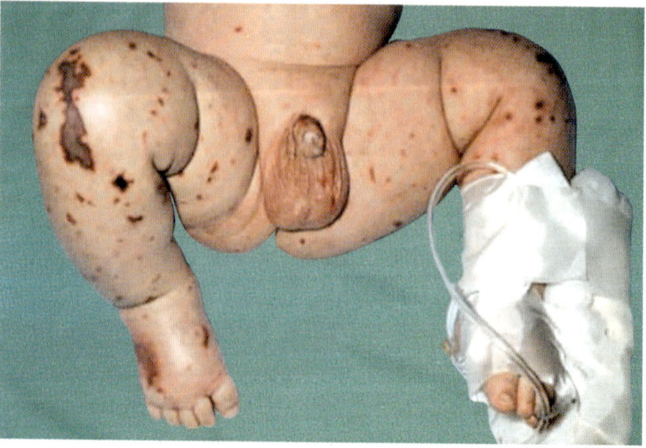

Fig. 3: Purpura fulminans.

Chronic Meningococcemia

It is defined as meningococcal sepsis without meningitis, in which fever has persisted for a week before antibiotics are initiated. Common symptoms are usually fever with chills, rash, arthralgia, headache, and splenomegaly. Symptoms are intermittent and may last up to 8 weeks before the diagnosis is made. Bacteremia is also intermittent in chronic meningococcemia and patients appear well in between fever spikes. In a study conducted by Benoit et al. an average of five blood cultures were taken before meningococci were isolated.[11] Localization of infection may occur later, leading to meningitis, carditis, nephritis, conjunctivitis, epididymitis, and retinitis.[9] Identification of the organism on blood culture is the gold standard for diagnosis. Effective treatment leads to prompt defervescence and dramatic recovery. The pathophysiology of chronic meningococcemia remains unclear, as the organisms are no less virulent. Defects in the host immunity have been suggested as cause. Hypersensitivity basis for this disease is being evaluated.

Meningococcal Pneumonia

Though meningococcal pneumonia is seen mostly in conjunction with meningococcemia or meningitis, primary meningococcal pneumonia can occur. Patients with preceding viral pneumonias are considered at greater risk. The diagnosis of meningococcal pneumonia is difficult as isolation of the organism from sputum does not establish *Meningococcus* as the cause for pneumonia. Blood cultures are positive in only 15% of cases. Most cases have a history of antecedent upper respiratory infection, with pharyngitis found in almost 80% of cases. Rales and fever is the most common presentation. X-ray chest shows involvement of predominantly lower lobes with patchy alveolar infiltrates. Pleural effusions can be seen in 25%.

Other Meningococcal Syndromes

Meningococcal infection can present with pharyngitis, conjunctivitis, and arthritis. Adrenal hemorrhage is a dreaded complication seen with meningococcal disease **(Fig. 4)**. Meningococcal arthritis is mostly seen in adults and is usually oligoarticular in nature. Pericarditis and myocarditis are reported in 3–5% as a complication of meningococcal infection. Pericardial effusions develop late in the disease and pericardial fluid is usually sterile. Hence, it is thought to be an immune complex-mediated process. Studies have reported the successful use of steroids in the treatment of meningococcal pericarditis. Rare complications such as peritonitis, mesenteric adenitis and genitourinary infections have been reported in literature.

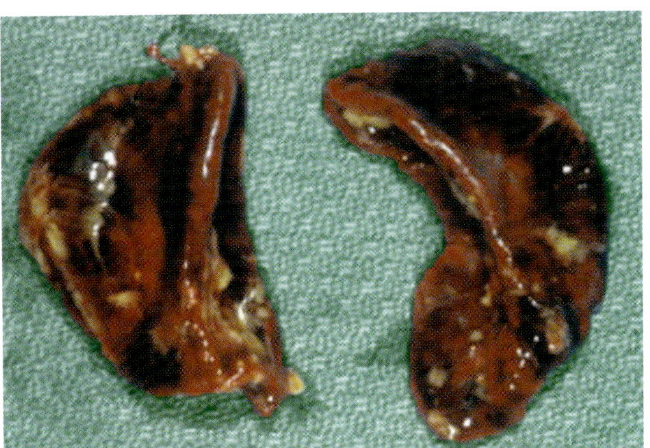

Fig. 4: Adrenal hemorrhage in a child with Gram-negative sepsis— a major complication of meningococcal disease.

■ DIFFERENTIAL DIAGNOSIS

Meningococcal disease can appear similar to sepsis or meningitis caused by various other Gram-negative bacteria, *Streptococcus pneumoniae*, *Staphylococcus aureus*, Rocky mountain spotted fever or epidemic typhus. Petechial rash can be seen in various viral infections such as enterovirus, measles, cytomegalovirus (CMV), parvovirus. Petechial rash can also be the presenting features in protein C or S deficiency, platelet disorders, Henoch-Schönlein purpura (HSP), connective tissue disorders.

■ DIAGNOSIS

Surveillance Case Definitions

- *Confirmed*: A clinically compatible case and isolation of *N. meningitidis* from a normally sterile site such as blood, cerebrospinal fluid (CSF), synovial fluid, pericardial fluid, pleural fluid or isolation from skin scraping of petechial or purpuric lesions.
- *Probable*: A clinically compatible case with either a positive result of antigen test or immunohistochemistry (IHC) of formalin fixed tissue or a positive polymerase chain reaction (PCR) of blood or CSF without a positive sterile site culture.
- *Suspect*: A clinically compatible case and Gram-negative diplococcic in any sterile fluid such as CSF, synovial fluid or scraping from a petechial or purpuric lesion.
- Clinical purpura fulminans without a positive blood culture.

Laboratory Diagnosis

Detection of organism in blood culture, CSF, or from petechiae remains the gold standard for diagnosis of

N. meningitidis. Gram stain of CSF can help in rapid diagnosis in children with meningitis. Other laboratory features include leukopenia, thrombocytopenia, hyponatremia (secondary to SIADH), deranged coagulation parameters, deranged liver or renal function tests, hypokalemia, hypocalcemia, and acidosis. In patients with skin lesions, a rapid presumptive diagnosis can be made by needle aspiration and Gram stain of a skin lesion. Needle aspiration yields Gram-negative diplococci in almost 50% of patients.

Counterimmunoelectrophoresis and latex agglutination are used to detect circulating antigens in blood and CSF. Latex agglutination tests in CSF can support the diagnosis of partially treated meningitis, where Gram stain and culture may be negative. However, in clinical practice, these tests have poor sensitivity and cross react with *Escherichia coli* K1 antigen.

Once antibiotics have been given, the yield of blood culture decreases to less than 50%. In such cases PCR tests have proven helpful in establishing the diagnosis. PCR using primers for meningococcal genes (e.g. *ctrA*) has a high sensitivity of 97%, and specificity of 99.6% in detecting *Meningococcus*, and results are rapidly available.[12]

MANAGEMENT

Prompt institution of therapy for children with suspected meningococcal disease may prove to be lifesaving. Broad spectrum antibiotics should be started early, after drawing blood for culture. A lumbar puncture may be performed in stable patients, but procedure should not delay the administration of antibiotics. The clinical features of meningococcal meningitis are like those caused by *S. pneumoniae* or *Haemophilus influenza*. Hence, empiric antibiotic therapy should cover the most likely pathogens till definitive culture report is available. In children older than 1 month, cefotaxime plus vancomycin is an appropriate empiric regimen. Similarly in neonates, ampicillin and cefotaxime is the empiric antibiotic cover of choice, with consideration for addition of vancomycin. For penicillin-sensitive meningococcemia or meningitis, IV penicillin G, 250,000–300,000 U/kg/day given in 4–6 divided doses for 7 days, is effective.

Administration of steroids in children with severe meningococcal disease is controversial and no clear guidelines exist. Steroids may decrease incidence of adrenal insufficiency and neurological sequelae, but they can also cause decreased penetration of antibiotics into CSF (decreased meningeal inflammation) and increased incidence of gastric ulceration. If steroids are being considered, they should be administered as close to the first dose of antibiotics as possible.[9]

There are various novel experimental therapeutics being investigated for the management of IMD. Few of these include antiendotoxin therapy, tissue plasminogen activator, antithrombin III infusion, topical nitroglycerin, plasmapheresis, and infusion of recombinant protein C. However, none of these have been found to be consistently beneficial in human trials so far and larger trials are required to establish benefit.

Additional supportive measures such as low-dose heparin infusion can be used, however, benefits of therapy have not been consistently proven.

PREVENTION

Chemoprophylaxis

Neisseria meningitidis is a highly virulent organism and secondary attack rates among household contacts have been found to be approximately 1,000 times the attack rate in the general population. Chemoprophylaxis is indicated for household contacts and for young daycare contacts. Prophylaxis is also indicated for healthcare professionals who had close contact with nasopharyngeal secretions (e.g. mouth-to-mouth resuscitation). Persons in contact with the patient for up to 7 days before onset of illness should be given prophylaxis. The various chemoprophylaxis drugs used are highlighted in **Table 1**. Rifampicin is not recommended for pregnant women. Ciprofloxacin is not recommended in children, pregnant, and lactating women. In pregnant women, single dose ceftriaxone is the prophylaxis of choice. Azithromycin is not currently recommended in CDC recommendation for prophylaxis.

Table 1: Chemoprophylaxis for eradication of *Neisseria meningitidis.*

Drug	Age	Dose/duration
Rifampicin	• Age < 1 month • Age ≥ 1 month • Adults	• 5 mg/kg/dose PO BID for 2 days (4 doses) • 10 mg/kg/dose PO BID for 2 days • 600 mg PO BID for 2 days
Ceftriaxone	• <15 years • ≥15 years	• 125 mg IM single dose • 250 mg IM single dose
Ciprofloxacin	• Children • Adults	• Not recommended • 500 mg single dose
Azithromycin	Adults	500 mg single dose (only studied in adults)

(PO: per orally; IM: intramuscular)

Table 2: American Academy of Pediatrics (AAP) recommendations for meningococcal vaccines.

General population		
<2 years	*2–10 years*	*11–21 years*
Not recommended	Not recommended	Single dose MenACWY at 11–12 years or 13–18 years. Single booster dose 5 years later.

Meningococcal Vaccines

Primary prevention of meningococcal disease is essential as the disease has a rapid and fulminant course. Antibiotic resistant strains of meningococci are now being recognized and chemoprophylaxis is cumbersome. Two vaccines—(1) meningococcal polysaccharide vaccine and (2) meningococcal conjugate vaccine (MCV) are currently licensed for prevention of meningococcal disease in the US. Both are quadrivalent and contain antigens from serotypes A, C, Y, and W-135.

Meningococcal polysaccharide vaccine has capsular polysaccharide antigens and is licensed for use in children older than 2 years who are at high risk of acquiring meningococcal disease. Though the vaccine is available and licensed for use, conjugate vaccine has greater immunogenicity, and lesser hyporesponsiveness and is preferred over the polysaccharide vaccine.

The first meningococcal conjugate vaccine was a serogroup C monovalent vaccine, which was licensed in 1999, in the UK. Quadrivalent ACWY vaccine has been widely available since 2005. Recommendations from the American Academy Pediatrics (AAP), for the use of meningococcal vaccine are given in **Table 2**.

In India two types of conjugate vaccines are licensed for use. Menactra™ (Sanofi-Pasteur) is licensed for use in India from 2012, for age groups 2–55 years. Menactra is a quadrivalent vaccine containing 4 µg of A, C, Y, and W polysaccharide each, conjugated to diphtheria toxoid. A single intramuscular dose of 0.5 mL is recommended. Within 3–4 years of vaccination, the effectiveness of the vaccine was found to be 80–85%. MenAfriVac™ (Serum Institute, India) is a monovalent serogroup A polysaccharide vaccine, conjugated to tetanus toxoid, which is licensed but not freely available in the market. According to Indian Academy of Pediatrics (IAP) position paper, meningococcal vaccine is recommended only for use in high-risk individuals, aged 2 years or more, and conjugate vaccine is preferred over polysaccharide vaccine due to better immunogenicity and provision of herd immunity. During disease outbreak polysaccharide vaccines can be used in countries with limited resources. In children with terminal complement deficiencies, functional/anatomical asplenia or hyposplenia and in people living with HIV and acquired immunodeficiency syndrome (AIDS), two doses of conjugate vaccine with 8 weeks interval is recommended. In laboratory personnel and healthcare workers routinely exposed to *N. meningitidis* in solutions, a single dose of MCV is recommended. In close contacts of cases with meningococcal disease, a single dose of MCV can be given as an adjunct to chemoprophylaxis.[13]

■ REFERENCES

1. Harrison OB, Claus H, Jiang Y, et al. Description and Nomenclature of Neisseria meningitidis Capsule Locus. Emerg Infect Dis. 2013;19(4):566-73.
2. CDC. VPD surveillance manual, MacNeil J, Patton M. Chapter 8: Meningococcal Disease. [online] Available from: https://www.cdc.gov/vaccines/pubs/surv-manual/chpt08-mening.pdf [Last accessed on November, 2019].
3. Kliegman RM, Stanton B, Schor N, et al. Nelson Textbook of Pediatrics, 20th edition. Philadelphia, Pennsylvania: Elsevier; 2016.
4. American Academy of Pediatrics. Meningococcal Infections. In: Pickering LK, Baker CJ, Kimberlin DW, Long SS (Eds). Red Book: 2012 Report of the Committee on Infectious Diseases. Elk Grove Village, IL: American Academy of Pediatrics; 2012. pp. 500-9.
5. Vyse A, Wolter JM, Chen J, et al. Meningococcal disease in Asia: an under-recognized public health burden. Epidemiol Infect. 2011;139(7):967-85.
6. Mani R, Pradhan S, Nagarathna S, et al. Bacteriological profile of community acquired acute bacterial meningitis: a ten-year retrospective study in a tertiary neurocare centre in South India. Indian J Med Microbiol. 2007;25(2):108-14.
7. Central Bureau of Health Intelligence. (2016). National Health Profile, India 2012-2016. [online] Available from: www.cbhidghs.nic.in [Last accessed on November, 2019].
8. Jacobs JH, Viboud C, Tchetgen ET, et al. The association of meningococcal disease with influenza in the United States, 1989-2009. PLoS One. 2014;9(9):e107486.
9. Anderson MS, Glodé MP, Smith AL. Meningococcal Infections. In: Feigin RD, Cherry JD, Kaplan SL, Demmler-Harrison GJ (Eds). Textbook of Pediatric Infectious diseases, 6th edition. Philadelphia: Saunders Elsevier, pp. 1350-62.
10. Dass Hazarika R, Deka NM, Khyriem AB, et al. Invasive meningococcal infection: analysis of 110 cases from a tertiary care centre in North East India. Indian J Pediatr. 2013;80(5):359-64.
11. Benoit FL. Chronic meningococcemia. Case report and review of the literature. Am J Med. 1963;35:103-12.
12. Richardson DC, Louie L, Louie M, et al. Evaluation of a rapid PCR assay for diagnosis of meningococcal meningitis. J Clin Microbiol. 2003;41(8):3851-3.
13. Indian Academy of Pediatrics, Advisory Committee on Vaccines and Immunization Practices (ACVIP), Vashishtha VM1, et al. Indian Academy of Pediatrics (IAP) recommended immunization schedule for children aged 0 through 18 years, India, 2013 and updates on immunization.

Sanjay Krishna Ghorpade

INTRODUCTION

Human brucellosis is one of the emerging infections. Most common source of infection in pediatrics is consumption of unpasteurized milk and milk products. The disease is having prolonged incubation period with disease course and sometimes may lead to fetal complications also. Other names for this disease are undulant fever, Malta fever or Mediterranean fever. This is one of the major bacterial zoonoses. Many times it transmits in the human being accidently. The disease is predominantly common in males and *Brucella melitensis* is common in pediatrics. Once it becomes chronic it leads to multisystemic involvement. It is difficult to diagnose due to nonspecific clinical presentation, prolonged incubation period which delays blood culture growth, difficult serological diagnosis, and its interpretation.

EPIDEMIOLOGY

The disease is prevalent in various parts of the globe which includes India, some of parts of Asia, Europe, and America. The disease is more common in rural population. The incidence of human brucellosis is ranging from <0.01 to >200 per 100,000 population. Due to missing diagnosis and underreporting real incidence may be 25 times high.

More than 80% of the population in India lives in villages. *B. melitensis* and *B. abortus* are two species common in India. As per review of literature the prevalence of human brucellosis varies from 3% to 34%.

Consumption of unpasteurized milk and milk products and travel to endemic regions are the factors responsible for the endemicity of the disease pertaining to the species *B. melitensis*. In developed countries the disease is less common due to regular animal vaccination and screening of domestic livestock.

ETIOLOGY

Agent: *Brucella* is gram-negative coccobacilli. This includes four species which are *B. melitensis, B. abortus, B. suis,* and *B. canis*. Most virulent and invasive species is *B. melitensis* **(Table 1)**.

Reservoir of infections: Cattle, goats, sheep, swine, buffaloes, horse, and dogs are main reservoirs of infection. The animals excrete organisms in the urine, milk, placenta, and uterine and vaginal discharges particularly during a birth or abortion. They may remain infected throughout life.

Mode of transmission: Infection transmits from animal to human. Human-to-human transmission is quite rare.

The following are routes of spread:
- *Foodborne infections*: Consumption of unpasteurized milk and milk products plays key role. Raw vegetables and contaminated water also become source of infection.

Table 1: Brucellosis: Brucella species and host affected.

Species	Natural host	Human pathogen
Brucella abortus	Cattle	Yes
B. melitensis	Goats, sheep	Yes
B. suis	Swine	Yes
	Hares	Yes
	Reindeer, caribou	Yes
	Rodents	Yes
B. canis	Dogs, other canids	Yes
B. ovis	Sheep	No
B. neotomae	Desert wood rat	No
B. maris (?)	Marine mammals	?

- *Contact infection*: It occurs by direct contact with infected tissues through abraded skin, mucosa, conjunctiva (mucocutaneous route), etc.
- *Airborne infections*: In slaughter houses and laboratories the infection mainly occurs by this route, i.e. inhalation of infected dust or aerosols.
- *Transplacental infections*: This includes congenital and neonatal infections.
- *Person-to-person infection*: It is extremely rare but basic precautions must be taken.

Incubation period: It ranges from 1 to 3 weeks but may go as long as 6 months or more. When the disease is suspected, the clinical laboratory should be informed so that cultures can be maintained for >21 days to ensure growth if the organism is present.

PATHOGENESIS

Brucella is an intracellular organism. Human being is end host. The transmission of organism occurs via ingestion or inhalation. Other routes are through conjunctiva, skin abrasions, contaminated meat or dairy products.

The nutrition and immune status of the host are important factors and the species of *Brucella*, *B. melitensis* and *B. suis,* are more virulent than *B. abortus* or *B. canis*. The cell wall of the organism is made up of lipopolysaccharide. Smooth lipopolysaccharide suggests more virulent and resistant strains. These organisms are facultative intracellular pathogens that can survive and replicate within the mononuclear phagocytic cells (monocytes, macrophages) of the reticuloendothelial system. The remaining organisms not phagocytosed by leukocytes are ingested by the macrophages which ultimately form granuloma in the organs such as liver, spleen, lymph nodes, and bone marrow (**Fig. 1**).

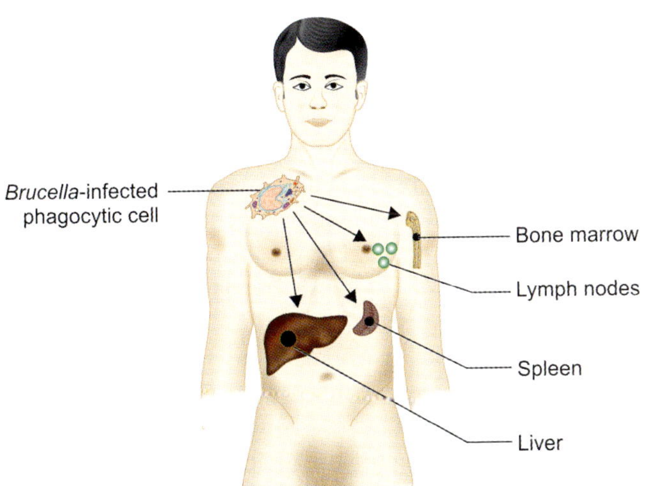

Fig. 1: Spread of *Brucella* in the body.

Antibodies produced against the lipopolysaccharide and other cell wall antigens are useful for long-term immunity as well as diagnosis of the disease.

The strains having smooth, nonendotoxic lipopolysaccharides block the development of innate and specific immunity during the early stage of infection, and protect the pathogen from the microbicidal activities of the immune system so they are more virulent. The strains having lipopolysaccharide lacking the O-side chain are less virulent because of their inability to overcome the host defense system.

CLINICAL MANIFESTATIONS

Brucellosis is many times missing diagnosis. History of animal and food exposure is very important. The disease can present with acute or subacute clinical manifestations including fever which may persist and progress to chronicity with complications. The disease course may prolong from weeks to months. The incubation period may range from 2 to 4 weeks. The classic triad of the disease is *fever, arthralgia/arthritis,* and *hepatosplenomegaly.* Fever of unknown origin is one more form of clinical presentation.

The disease if not treated in time may spread to various systems which include central and peripheral nervous system, gastrointestinal, hepatobiliary, genitourinary, musculoskeletal, cardiovascular, and integumentary systems. The major causative organisms in the human brucellosis are two species: *B. melitensis* and *B. abortus*. One-third of patients present with either hepatomegaly, splenomegaly or hepatosplenomegaly. About 10% patients present with lymphadenopathy.

Gastrointestinal and Hepatobiliary Manifestations

Liver is a most commonly involved organ. Abdominal pain, constipation, hepatomegaly, jaundice, and splenomegaly are also seen.

Osteoarticular Manifestations

About 50% focal clinical manifestations include sacroiliitis, spondylitis, peripheral arthritis, and osteomyelitis.

Cardiovascular Manifestations

The cardiac involvement includes mainly valvular. The aortic valve is most commonly affected valve. It is the most serious problem, accounting for 5% total mortality rate. Cardiac murmur is rare.

Genitourinary Manifestations

This is in terms of glomerulonephritis and orchie-pididymitis.

Neurological Manifestations

The clinical presentation includes meningoencephalitis, cranial nerve involvement, peripheral neuropathies, chorea, transient ischemic attacks, neuropsychiatric manifestations, etc.

Skin Manifestations

This includes erythematous papular lesions, purpura, dermal cysts, and Stevens–Johnson syndrome.

Pulmonary Manifestations

About 16% cases of brucellosis with complications present with pneumonias and pleural effusion.

Congenital and Neonatal Manifestations

Congenital and neonatal infections with these organisms have also been described but clinical features are nonspecific.

■ DIAGNOSIS

A history of consumption of unpasteurized milk and milk products is very important. For the definitive diagnosis culture of the organisms from blood, bone marrow aspiration or other tissues must be obtained. Regular blood examination may show thrombocytopenia, neutropenia, anemia, or pancytopenia. Leukocytosis is present in about 9% of patients. These patients less likely having possibility of focal disease. On the other hand leukopenia (11%) and thrombocytopenia (10%) are seen in some of the cases. Anemia is seen more common and affecting about 26% of patients **(Fig. 2)**.

Culture

Blood culture plays key role in the diagnosis. Now automated culture systems are available which give result very fast. Blood culture sensitivity depends upon stage of the disease as well as previous use of antibiotics. For acute case sensitivity ranges from 80% to 90% while for chronic cases it comes down to 30–70%. Due to prolonged incubation period we must advise microbiologist to keep sample of blood culture up to 4 weeks in the suspected case of *Brucella* infection.

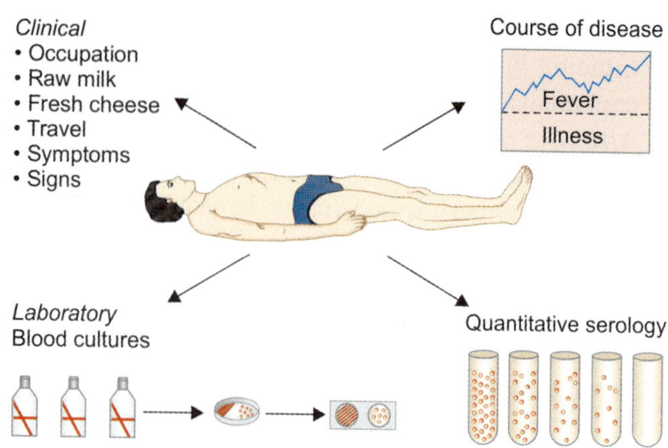

Fig. 2: History and physical examination.

Yield of organisms is more from bone marrow. It can also be cultured from pus, tissue samples, cerebrospinal, pleural, joint, or ascitic fluid.

Serodiagnosis

Agglutination Tests

This is one of the methods for the serodiagnosis of the disease which includes detection of antibodies against *B. melitensis*, *B. abortus*, and *B. suis*. This method does not detect antibodies against *B. canis* because this organism lacks the smooth lipopolysaccharide. This is another option where culture facilities are not available. Other agglutination tests are also available which include Rose Bengal test, the serum agglutination test, and the antiglobulin or Coombs test.

The Rose Bengal test is a screening test and positive results are confirmed by the serum agglutination test. These agglutination tests are based on the reactivity of antibodies against smooth lipopolysaccharide. In endemic areas, high background values could occur that may affect the diagnostic value of the test which is called as *prozone effect*. The prozone effect can give false negative result in the presence of high titers of antibodies and to avoid this serum that is being tested should be diluted to ≥1:320. The *Brucella* smooth lipopolysaccharide antigen tends to show cross reactivity with other gram-negative bacteria such as *Yersinia enterocolitica* O:9, *Vibrio cholerae*, *Escherichia coli* O:157, and *Francisella tularensis*, increasing the possibility of false positive results.

No single titer is ever diagnostic, but most patients with acute infections have titers of ≥1:160 is considered to be positive. Low titers may be found early in the course of the illness, requiring the use of acute and convalescent sera testing to confirm the diagnosis. Coombs test may be more suitable for confirmation of brucellosis in relapsing patients or patients with persisting disease.

Enzyme-linked Immunosorbent Assay

Now enzyme-linked immunosorbent assay (ELISA) becomes more useful test as compare to other tests. The sensitivity of ELISA is quite high as compare to other tests but its specificity is low. The result of ELISA depends upon detection of immunoglobulin M (IgM) and IgG antibodies against smooth polysaccharide and it must be interpreted carefully in the endemic area.

Rapid point-of-care assays: These tests include the fluorescent polarization immunoassay (FPA), immuno-chromatographic *Brucella* IgM/IgG lateral flow assay (LFA), and simplified version of ELISA. The sensitivity of these tests is 96% and the specificity is 98% for samples from healthy blood donors. These tests are useful tool for screening of brucellosis contacts.

Molecular Detection

As per various studies polymerase chain reaction (PCR) is found to be 100% sensitive and 98.3% specific to *Brucella* species, compared with 70% sensitivity for blood culture. PCR is found to be useful in patients with specific complications such as neurobrucellosis or other localized infections as serological testing often fails in such patients. PCR could be useful as a diagnostic test in relapsing brucellosis.

Other applications of PCR: PCR also appears to be useful in species differentiation and biotyping of isolates. PCR was recently used to assess treatment efficacy.

Sonography of Abdomen

Microabscesses in spleen may be found in *Brucella* infection.

■ DIFFERENTIAL DIAGNOSIS

Differential diagnosis in brucellosis includes tularemia, cat scratch disease, typhoid fever, and fungal infections due to histoplasmosis, blastomycosis or coccidioidomycosis. Infections caused by *Mycobacterium tuberculosis*, atypical mycobacteria, rickettsiae, and Yersinia can present in a similar fashion to brucellosis.

■ TREATMENT

The principles of treatment in human brucellosis include combination therapy (no monotherapy) and prolonged course. Relapses are mainly due to inadequate treatment in terms of number of drugs or duration of course. Prolonged antimicrobial therapy is imperative for achieving a cure. Doxycycline is one of the important drugs in the combination therapy **(Table 2)**.

The drugs that provide intracellular killing are required for eradication of this infection. Relapse is confirmed by isolation of *Brucella* within weeks to months after therapy has ended and is usually not associated with antimicrobial resistance.

Table 2: Recommended therapy for the treatment of brucellosis.

Age and condition	Antimicrobial agent	Dose	Route	Duration
≥8 years	Doxycycline	2–4mg/kg/day; maximum: 200 mg/day	PO	6 weeks
	+			
	Rifampin	15–20 mg/kg/day; maximum: 600–900 mg/day	PO	6 weeks
	Alternative:			
	Doxycycline	2–4 mg/kg/day; maximum: 200 mg/day	PO	6 weeks
	+			
	Streptomycin	15–30mg/kg/day; maximum: 1 g/day	IM	2 weeks
	or			
	Gentamicin	3–5 mg/kg/day	IM/IV	2 weeks
<8 years	Trimethoprim-sulfamethoxazole (TMP-SMZ)	TMP (10 mg/kg/day; maximum: 480 mg/day) and SMZ (50 mg/kg/day; maximum: 2.4 g/day)	PO	4–8 weeks
	+			
	Rifampin	15–20 mg/kg/day	PO	6 weeks
Meningitis, osteomyelitis, endocarditis	Doxycycline	2–4 mg/kg/day; maximum: 200 mg/day	PO	4–6 months
	+			
	Gentamicin	3–5 mg/kg/day	IV	2 weeks
	±			
	Rifampin	15–20 mg/kg/day; maximum: 600–900 mg/day	PO	4–6 months

(IM: intramuscular; IV: intravenous; PO: per oral)

Those patients having persistent symptoms and signs or recurrent disease, current recommendation is to give extended course of treatment. The surgical interventions may be required in abscesses and specific focalized forms of brucellosis which includes endocarditis, cerebral, epidural or splenic abscess as these forms are resistant to antibiotics.

COMPLICATIONS

If the disease is not diagnosed and treated in time with proper treatment these patients can land up with complications such as sacroiliitis, spondylitis, peripheral arthritis, osteomyelitis, and endocarditis—with the aortic valve being the most commonly affected structure.

Around 10% of patients present with complications such as orchiepididymitis, glomerulonephritis, and renal abscesses. Neurological complications include meningoencephalitis, cranial nerve involvement, peripheral neuropathies, chorea, transient ischemic attacks, neuropsychiatric manifestations, etc. Mucocutaneous complications are erythematous papular lesions, purpura, dermal cysts, and Stevens–Johnson syndrome.

Pulmonary complications such as pleural effusions and pneumonias are seen in 16% of complicated cases of brucellosis.

PROGNOSIS

The prognosis of human brucellosis after specific therapy is excellent. Early diagnosis, early treatment, prolonged therapy, and compliance of patient are important factors. If not treated properly in time the course of brucellosis often prolonged and may lead to death.

PREVENTION

Isolation of the Hospitalized Patient

This is restricted to patients with draining wounds.

Control Measures

- *In the humans*:
  - *Early diagnosis and treatment*: Combination and prolonged therapy are important factors.
  - *Pasteurization of milk*: Using pasteurized milk and milk products for consumption is important part for prevention of the disease.
  - *Protective measures*: This includes personal hygiene to prevent direct contact with infected animal and animal products.
  - *Vaccination*: No vaccine currently is available for use in children.
- *In the animals*: The most rational approach for preventing human brucellosis is the control and eradication of the infection from animal reservoirs which is based on the combination of the following measures:
  - *Test and slaughter*: This is one of the ways of control over infected animals.
  - *Vaccination*: Use of available animal vaccines must be promoted.
  - *Hygienic measures*: This includes mainly animal hygiene and veterinary care of the animals.

CONCLUSION

Human brucellosis is an emerging zoonosis. Because of nonspecific clinical features the diagnosis of disease becomes a challenge. Prolonged incubation period makes diagnosis difficult. High index of suspicion, proper history, and endemicity of the disease are helpful for the diagnosis. Early diagnosis and combination and prolonged drug therapy give excellent prognosis of the disease. The compliance of patient plays a key role in the treatment. Undiagnosed and neglected case of the disease may lead to complications making prognosis fetal.

SUGGESTED READING

1. Abdoel TH, Smits HL. Rapid latex agglutination test for the serodiagnosis of human brucellosis. Diagn Microbiol Infect Dis. 2007;57:123-8.
2. Agasthya AS, Isloor S, Prabhudas K. Brucellosis in high risk group individuals. Indian J Med Microbiol. 2007;25(1):28-31.
3. Almuneef M, Memish ZA. Persistence of Brucella antibodies after successful treatment of acute brucellosis in an area of endemicity. J Clin Microbiol. 2002;40:2313.
4. Almuneef MA, Memish ZA, Balkhy HH, et al. Importance of screening household members of acute brucellosis cases in endemic areas. Epidemiol Infect. 2004;132:533-40.
5. Araj GF. Enzyme-linked immunosorbent assay, not agglutination, is the test of choice for the diagnosis of neurobrucellosis. Clin Infect Dis. 1997;25:942.
6. Chahota R, Sharma M, Katoch RC, et al. Brucellosis outbreak in an organized dairy farm involving cows and in contact human beings, in Himachal Pradesh, India. Vet Arh. 2003;73:95-102.
7. Ewals JA, Brucellosis as an imported disease in a young man with arthritis. Ned Tijdschr Geneeskd. 2005;149(50):2810-4.
8. Giannacopoulos I, Eliopoulou MI, Ziambaras T, et al. Transplacentally transmitted congenital brucellosis due to Brucella abortus. J Infect. 2002;45:209-10.
9. Gogia A, Dugga L, Dutta S. An unusual etiology of PUO. J Assoc Physicians India. 2011;59:47-9.
10. Gokhale YA, Ambardekar AG, Bhasin A, et al. Brucella spondylitis and sacroiliitis in the general population in Mumbai. J Assoc Physicians India. 2003:659-66.

11. Gur A, Geyik MF, Dikici B, et al. Complications of brucellosis in different age groups: a study of 283 cases in southeastern Anatolia of Turkey. Yonsei Med J. 2003;44:33-44.

12. Kadri SM, Rukhsana A, Laharwal MA, et al. Seroprevalence of brucellosis in Kashmir (India) among patients with pyrexia of unknown origin. J Indian Med Assoc. 2000;98(4):170-1.

13. Kochar DK, Gupta BK, Gupta A, et al. Hospital-based case series of 175 cases of serologically confirmed brucellosis in Bikaner. J Assoc Phys India. 2007;55:271-5.

14. Kochar DK, Kumawat BL, Agarwal N, et al. Meningoencephalitis in brucellosis. Neurol India. 2000;48:170-3.

15. Kumar S, Tuteja U, Sarika K, et al. Rapid multiplex PCR assay for the simultaneous detection of the *Brucella Genus*, *B. abortus*, *B. melitensis*, and *B. suis*. J Microbiol Biotechnol. 2011;21(1):89-92.

16. Mangalgi S, Sajjan A, Mohite ST. Seroprevalence of brucellosis among Blood Donors of Satara District, Maharashtra (original article) Department of Microbiology, Krishna Institute of Medical Sciences University, Karad, (Maharashtra), India JKIMSU. 2012;1(1):55-60.

17. Mantur B, Parande A, Amarnath S, et al. ELISA versus conventional methods of diagnosing endemic brucellosis. Am J Trop Med Hyg. 2010;83(2):314-8.

18. Mantur BG, Amarnath SK, Parande AM, et al. Comparison of a novel immunocapture assay with standard serological methods in the diagnosis of brucellosis. Clin Lab. 2011;57(5-6):333-41.

19. Mantur BG, Mangalgi SS. Evaluation of conventional castaneda and lysis centrifugation blood culture techniques for diagnosis of human brucellosis. J Clin Microbiol. 2004;42(9):4327-8.

20. Mirnejad R, Doust RH, Kachuei R, et al. Simultaneous detection and differentiates of Brucella abortus and Brucella melitensis by combinatorial PCR. Asian Pac J Trop Med. 2012;5(1):24-8.

21. Palanduz A, Palanduz S, Guler K, et al. Brucellosis in a mother and her young infant: probable transmission by breast milk. Int J Infect Dis. 2000;4:55-6.

22. Purwar S, Metgud SC, Darshan A, et al. Infective endocarditis due to brucella. Indian J Med Microbiol. 2006;24(4):286-8.

23. Rahman AK, Dirk B, Fretin D, et al. Seroprevalence and risk factors for brucellosis in a high-risk group of individuals in Bangladesh. Foodborne Pathogens and Disease. 2012; 9(3):190-7.

24. Renukaradhya GJ, Isloor S, Rajasekhar M. Epidemiology, zoonotic aspects, vaccination and control/eradication of brucellosis in India. Vet Microbiol. 2002;90(1-4):183-95.

25. Roth F, Zinsstag J, Orkhon D, et al. Human health benefits from livestock vaccination for brucellosis: case study. Bull World Health Organ. 2003;81:867-76.

26. Ruiz-Mesa JD, Sanchez-Gonzalez J, Reguera JM, et al. Rose Bengal test: diagnostic yield and use for the rapid diagnosis of human brucellosis in emergency departments in endemic areas. Clin Microbiol Infect. 2005;11:221-5.

27. Sen MR, Shukla BN, Goyal RK. Seroprevalence of brucellosis in and around Varanasi. J Commun Dis. 2002;34:226-7.

28. Tikare NV, Mantur BG, Bidari LH. Brucellar meningitis in an infant—evidence for human breast milk transmission. J Trop Pediatr. 2008;54(4):272-4.

Tetanus

Abhay K Shah

INTRODUCTION

Tetanus is a noncommunicable disease contracted through exposure to toxigenic strains of spores of the bacterium, *Clostridium tetani*, that exists worldwide in soil and in animal intestinal tracts and as such can contaminate many surfaces and substances. Tetanus has been known since antiquity having been described by Hippocrates and Areatus. Tetanus has been described as "Dhanur" in most Indian languages meaning arching of the body due to stiffening of the body muscles. The disease remains an important public health problem in many parts of the world where immunization programs are suboptimal, particularly in the least developed districts of low-income countries. As a result of the ubiquity of the bacterium causing tetanus, the disease cannot be eradicated.

EPIDEMIOLOGY AND DISEASE BURDEN

Tetanus occurs worldwide and is more common in warmer climates and during warmer months, in part because of higher frequency of contaminated wounds associated with those locations and seasons. Tetanus is not transmitted from person to person. People of all ages can get tetanus, but the disease is particularly common and serious in newborn babies and their mothers when the mothers are unprotected from tetanus by the vaccine, tetanus toxoid (TT).

Tetanus occurring during pregnancy or within 6 weeks of the end of pregnancy is called "maternal tetanus," while tetanus occurring within the first 28 days of life is called "neonatal tetanus." Neonatal tetanus is common in many developing countries where pregnant women are not immunized appropriately against tetanus and nonsterile umbilical cord care practices are followed.

Non-neonatal cases of tetanus are associated with traumatic injuries, roadside injuries, and penetrating wounds following injury with dirty objects such as nail, splinter fragment of glass, or unsterile injections. Less commonly otorrhea, dental abscesses, chronic skin ulcerations, burns, compound fractures, gangrene, etc., are predisposing conditions for tetanus.

In many countries, tetanus disease surveillance is not well established and its incidence is not known accurately. Historically, surveillance systems have focused on detection of neonatal tetanus cases in health facilities. However, many cases occur outside the reach of the health system and are not reported. There are no global estimates of tetanus deaths beyond 5 years of age, including for maternal tetanus. In 2014, the total reported tetanus incidence in the European Union (EU) was 0.01 per 100,000 population, with 65% of cases aged ≥65 years. The average annual incidence in the United States of America (USA) from 2001 to 2008 was 0.01 per 100,000 population. During that period, 30%, 60%, and 10% of reported cases were in persons aged ≥65 years, 20–64 years, and <20 years, respectively. WHO estimates that in 2015, approximately 34,000 neonates died from neonatal tetanus. This represents a 96% reduction since 1988 and demonstrates significant progress toward the global maternal and neonatal tetanus elimination (MNTE) goal of <1 neonatal tetanus per 1,000 live births in every district of every country.

Worldwide, all countries are committed to "elimination" of MNT, i.e. a reduction of neonatal tetanus incidence to below one case per 1,000 live births per year in every district. While progress continues to be made, by July 2019, 12 countries have still not reached the MNTE status. Activities to achieve the goal are on-going in these countries, with many likely to achieve MNTE in the near future.

INDIAN SCENARIO

India has reduced neonatal tetanus mortality by 99.76% since the early 1980s, when tetanus claimed up to 204,380 babies within their first year of life. During 2000–2013, the global mortality rates for tetanus declined by more than 30% with an impressive annual rate reduction of 8.9% for neonatal tetanus. In 2013, the number of neonatal tetanus deaths across India fell to 415, and in 2014, the country recorded 492 such deaths. Three successive years of meeting the neonatal tetanus elimination threshold of less than one case in 1,000 live births in every district led the *WHO to declare India free of neonatal tetanus in May 2015.*

In May 2015, India achieved the landmark of elimination of neonatal and maternal tetanus, certification of which requires incidence of less than one case per 1,000 live births in all districts of the country for 2 consecutive years. This has been possible due to the sustained and diligent efforts in improving the vaccination coverage in pregnancy, rate of institutional deliveries, and promoting clean delivery and cord-care practices.

ETIOLOGICAL AGENT

Tetanus is caused by *C. tetani*, a gram-positive, noncapsulated, strictly anaerobic, spore-forming organism. They are motile and occur singly or occasionally in chains. Spores are prevalent in the environment, particularly in the soil of warm and moist areas, and may be carried in the intestinal tracts and feces of humans and animals. Manure-treated soil may also contain a large number of spores. The spores are wider than the bacillary body giving the bacillus a swollen spindle-like appearance, hence the name clostridium (Kloster = spindle).The bacilli are spherical, with terminal bulging giving the characteristic "drum stick" appearance.

Clostridium tetani produces three types of toxins:
1. *Tetanolysin or hemolysin*: It is heat labile and oxygen labile.
2. *Neurotoxin (tetanospasmin):* It is actually responsible for tetanus. The toxin is oxygen stable, relatively heat labile, being inactivated at 65°C in 5 minutes. It is antigenic and specifically neutralized by the antitoxin. It also gets toxoided spontaneously or with low concentration of formaldehyde. It is plasmid coded and is a simple protein composed of a single polypeptide chain.
3. *Nonspasmogenic toxins*: It is peripherally active neurotoxin and its role in tetanus is not known.

PATHOGENESIS

Clostridium tetani enters the human body through contaminated wounds or tissue injuries including those resulting from unclean deliveries, burns, surgery, and dental extractions. The site of entry is in some cases unknown or no longer visible at the onset of symptoms.

Under favorable anaerobic conditions, such as in devitalized or necrotic tissue, or dirty wounds, the dormant spores germinate, multiply, and convert to active toxin-producing tetanus bacilli. The most important toxin of *C. tetani* is the highly potent tetanospasmin. Tetanospasmin is one of the most potent known poisons on a weight basis (estimated minimum human lethal dose 2.5 ng/kg). This toxin blocks inhibitory neurotransmitters in the central nervous system and causes the muscular rigidity and spasms typical of generalized tetanus. Tetanus toxin binds to neuromuscular junctions and enters the motor nerves and exits in the spinal cord and adjacent spinal inhibitory interneurons, where it prevents release of gamma amino butyric acid (GABA). This results into normal inhibition of antagonistic muscles, resulting into sustained contractions of the affected muscle. The autonomic nervous system is also rendered unstable. The sensory nervous system is not affected in tetanus.

Disease

The incubation period of non-neonatal tetanus usually varies between 3 days and 21 days after infection. The median interval between entry of the organism and onset of symptoms is 7 days, but tetanus can develop up to 178 days after infection. In general, the further the injury site from the central nervous system, the longer the incubation period. Shorter incubation periods are associated with higher mortality rates. In neonatal tetanus, symptoms usually present 3–14 days, averaging 7 days, after birth in 90% of cases.

Painful body spasms lasting for several minutes, typically triggered by minor occurrences, such as a draft, loud noise, physical touch, or light, are highly diagnostic.

Three clinical presentations are characteristic of tetanus infection—localized, cephalic, and generalized tetanus.
1. *Localized tetanus* is uncommon; it is characterized by sustained contraction of the muscles in the same area as the injury site. Case-fatality rates for localized tetanus are <1%.
2. *Cephalic tetanus* is a rare form of the disease associated with ear infections (otitis media) or head lesions. It presents clinically as cranial nerve palsies. This form of tetanus has a short incubation period of only 1–2 days and a case-fatality rate of 15–30%. Cephalic tetanus can progress to generalized tetanus, in which case it has a similar poor prognosis.
3. *Generalized tetanus* occurs in >80% of cases, presenting as a generalized spastic disease. The overall severity of generalized tetanus disease and the case-fatality rate

are highly variable. Case-fatality rates vary from 10–% to 70% depending on treatment, age, and general health of the patient. Among patients are the youngest and oldest age groups. Without intensive care, case-fatality rates approach 100%. In settings where intensive care units (ICUs) are available, the case-fatality rate can be reduced to 10–20% in both neonatal and older patients.

Generalized Tetanus

The characteristic features of disease onset are early spasms of the muscles of the jaw, known as trismus or lockjaw (inability to open the mouth). Spasm of the facial muscles produces *risus sardonicus*, a distinctive facial expression that resembles a forced grin. Subsequently, sustained spasm of the muscles of the back leads to *opisthotonos*, the backward arching of the head, neck, and spine, and to sudden generalized seizure-like spasms, frequently in response to stimuli. Spasm of the glottis may cause sudden death. Tetanic seizures are the hallmark of the disease and are characterized by sudden, severe, tonic spasms of muscles, associated with clinching of face. They are provoked by smallest stimuli such as sound, light, touch or wind. Laryngeal and respiratory muscle involvement leads to airway obstruction and asphyxiation. Autonomic disturbances are seen in the form of tachycardia, hypertension, cutaneous vasoconstriction, urinary retention, etc.

Tetanus toxin does not affect sensory and cortical systems; hence, the patient remains conscious and in extreme pain and agony with a fearful anticipation of next tetanic seizures.

Neonatal Tetanus

Neonatal tetanus is a form of generalized tetanus that occurs in newborns. Infants who have not acquired passive immunity from the mother having been immunized are at risk. It usually occurs through infection of the unhealed umbilical stump, particularly when the stump is cut with a nonsterile instrument. In neonatal tetanus, generalized spasms are commonly preceded by the inability to suck or breastfeed and excessive crying. Typically, it appears between 3 days and 14 days of birth. Excessive crying and progressive increase in difficulty in feeding are the most common early features. An attempt to open the mouth or feed the child leads to reflex spasms of masseters leading to lock jaw. It is also associated with reflex spasm of pharyngeal muscles, dysphagia, and choking. Generalized muscle spasms are induced by sound, touch, or bright light. The spasms are more severe due to

the absence of inhibitory impulses from higher centers. Respiratory distress and accumulation of secretions in airways are due to involvement of tonic contractions of diaphragm, abdominal muscles, neck retraction, etc. Fever, tachycardia, and hyperpnea due to acidosis are due to increased sympathetic activity and profound muscle spasms. Cyanosis and apnea have also been reported. If fever is present, it is due to autonomic dysfunction, infection of the cord, or aspiration.

■ DIAGNOSIS

- Case definitions
  - The WHO definition of a confirmed neonatal tetanus case is an illness occurring in an infant who has the normal ability to suck and cry in the first 2 days of life, but who loses this ability between days 3 and 28 of life and becomes rigid or has spasms.
  - The WHO definition of adult tetanus requires at least one of the following signs: trismus or *risus sardonicus*; or painful muscular contractions. Although this definition requires a history of injury or wound, tetanus may also occur in patients who are unable to recall a specific wound or injury.
- Diagnosis is mainly clinical. Presence of four "S" in an unimmunized child, i.e. spasms, seizures, spasticity, and clear sensorium, with trismus are classical features for the diagnosis of tetanus.
- A clinical test, the "spatula test," may be performed, in which tetanus is diagnosed by reflex spasm of the jaw in response to touching the posterior wall of the pharynx with a soft instrument. This test has high specificity (100%) and sensitivity (94%).
- Blood counts, acute phase reactants, and cerebrospinal fluid (CSF) examination are usually noncontributory.
- *C. tetani* may be isolated from wound material by culture on blood agar but is positive only in one-third cases.
- Microscopic examination may reveal bacilli with a typical drumstick appearance but is not always diagnostic.

■ DIFFERENTIAL DIAGNOSIS

- Trismus may be seen with dental, retropharyngeal, and parapharyngeal abscesses.
- Rabies may present with trismus and seizures but hydrophobia is predominant and clonic seizures and dysphagia are very characteristic.
- Viral encephalitis may present with tonic seizures and facial spasms, but here the sensorium is altered, the

patient may be in coma, and CSF examination is often abnormal.

- Hypocalcemia may have tonic convulsions with laryngeal and carpopedal spasm, but here trismus is absent.
- Strychnine poisoning may produce tonic muscle spasm but here again trismus is absent.

COMPLICATIONS

Aspiration of secretions leading to aspiration pneumonia is the most common complication.

Severe seizures may cause tongue bite, body injuries, and intramuscular (IM) hematomas and even spinal fractures. Myoglobinuria following severe and long-standing muscle contractions may occur and is followed by renal failure. Venous thrombosis, pulmonary embolism, paralytic ileus, gastric ulcers, and urinary retention may be seen. Autonomic nervous system involvement leads to cardiac arrhythmias, unstable blood pressure, and unstable thermoregulation. Iatrogenic apnea may occur following use of excessive muscle relaxants. Endotracheal intubation and mechanical ventilation may have their own complications.

PROGNOSIS

- Localized tetanus with a long incubation period carries good prognosis.
- Generalized tetanus with a short incubation period of 3–7 days or less has poor prognosis.
- Tetanus in old age and neonatal age carries high mortality.
- Mortality is highest in the first week of illness.
- Neonatal tetanus carries mortality in the range of 10–75% and in general the mortality is 5–35%.

MANAGEMENT

It includes four principles:

1. *Wound management and eradication of C. tetani*:
   - Surgical wound excision and debridement is often needed to remove foreign body, dead, and devitalized tissue. It will not provide an anaerobic condition favorable for the growth of tetanus bacilli.
   - Surgery if needed should be promptly performed after the administration of antibiotics and tetanus immunoglobulins.
2. *Neutralization of tetanus toxin*:
   - Administration of human tetanus immune globulin (TIG) is recommended to prevent further

progression of the disease by removing unbound tetanus toxin but is unlikely to influence existing pathology. It should be instituted before tetanus toxin fixes to the spinal cord axons as TIG cannot neutralize the toxin, once it fixes to the axons.

- A single IM dose is recommended as soon as possible.
- Dose of TIG: 500 U IM. In severe cases, high doses of 3,000–6,000 U can be given.
- If human or equine TIG is not available, intravenous immune globulin may be used in a dose of 800–1,000 mg/kg.
- Intrathecal administration and local instillation of TIG in a wound are not effective.
- If TIG is not available or feasible, equine or bovine derived tetanus antitoxin (ATS) should be given in a dose of 50,000–100,000 U IM or IV after negative sensitivity test dose. Equine-derived ATS is associated with serious allergic reactions and should only be used in a single large dose after conducting hypersensitivity testing.

3. *Antibiotics*:
   - Metronidazole (30 mg/kg/day, given at 6-hour intervals; maximum 4 g/day) is effective in decreasing the number of vegetative forms of *C. tetani* and is the antimicrobial agent of choice.
   - Parenteral penicillin G (100,000 U/kg/day, given at 4– 6-hour intervals; maximum 12 million U/day) is an alternative treatment. Therapy for 7–10 days is recommended.
4. *Supportive care*:
   - Maintenance of airway, breathing, and circulation with cardiorespiratory monitoring are a must and topmost priorities.
   - Meticulous supportive and nursing care in a quiet, dark secluded environment with least disturbances, minimal handling, and maneuvering is most important. Triggers such as sound, light, and touch are strictly avoided as they will precipitate tetanus spasms. Benzodiazepines are the preferred treatment to control muscle spasms. The dose should be adjusted to achieve spasm control without excessive sedation and hypoventilation. The child may be sedated with diazepam with a dose of 0.1–0.2 mg/kg every 4–6 hourly and then as and when needed. This will provide efficient sedation, seizure control, and much needed muscle relaxation.
   - Drugs such as magnesium sulfate, midazolam, and chlorpromazine, can be used only in an ICU setup. Neuromuscular blocks such as pancuronium

are used to achieve flaccid paralysis and then managed by mechanical ventilation. Endotracheal intubation may be required to prevent aspiration of secretions and laryngospasm.

- Fluid, electrolytes, and calories management; care of skin, bowel, and bladder function including gentle suctioning; and intense nursing care should be an important integral part of the comprehensive management of tetanus.
- Tracheostomy may be required in an unintubated patient with severe laryngospasm.

TETANUS PREVENTION FOLLOWING EXPOSURE

The type of tetanus prophylaxis that is required following injury depends on the nature of the lesion and patient's immunization history. To prevent the development of tetanus after contaminated wounds or tissue injury, all wounds should be cleaned and debrided promptly and appropriately.

Passive immunization using TIG, preferably of human origin, is recommended for prophylaxis in the case of dirty wounds in incompletely vaccinated individuals and in those with uncertain vaccination history. Age-appropriate TT containing vaccine booster doses are recommended for those with incomplete vaccination. The full vaccination schedule should be completed as soon as possible for those who had not received all doses of the basic schedule,

in order to provide long-term protection against tetanus. In the unusual circumstance where an infant is born outside the hospital and the umbilical cord likely is contaminated (e.g. cut with nonsterile equipment), the maternal history of tetanus immunization should be confirmed. If the mother's tetanus immunization status is unknown and she is unlikely to have been immunized, TIG should be administered to the neonate unless tetanus serostatus can be confirmed quickly.

Infant diphtheria and TTs and acellular pertussis vaccine (DTaP)/diphtheria tetanus toxoids and whole cell vaccines (DTwP) should be given on a standard schedule.

The use of TT with or without TIG in management of wounds depends on the nature of the wound and the history of immunization with TT, as described in **Table 1**.

Passive Immunization

Human tetanus hyperimmunoglobulin is best for passive immunization. The dose is 250–500 IU. It gives longer protection of 30 days or more as compared to 7–10 days with ATS and has no risk of serum reaction.

- *Equine ATS*: If TIG is not available, equine ATS should be used in a dose of 1500 U subcutaneously after negative test dose.
- *The drawbacks with ATS are as follows*:
  - It causes sensitivity reaction and the incidence of serious reaction is 5–10%.
  - A person may tolerate it for the first time but with subsequent horse serum exposure may

Table 1: Tetanus prophylaxis in wound management.

History of adsorbed tetanus toxoid (doses)	Clean, minor wounds		All other wounds*	
	DPT/DTaP, Tdap or Td[†]	TIG[‡]	DPT/DTaP, Tdap, or Td[†]	TIG[‡]
Fewer than three or unknown	Yes	No	Yes	Yes

Three or more	• No
	  if <10 years since last tetanus-containing vaccine
	• Yes
	  if ≥10 years since the last tetanus-containing vaccine dose
		No
		
		No
			• No[§]
			  if <5 years since the last tetanus-containing vaccine dose
			• Yes
			  if ≥5 years since the last tetanus-containing vaccine dose
				No
				
				No

Notes:
- Tdap indicates booster tetanus toxoid, reduced diphtheria toxoid, and acellular pertussis vaccine
- DTaP, diphtheria, and tetanus toxoids and acellular pertussis vaccine
- Td, adult-type diphtheria, and tetanus toxoids vaccine
- TIG, Tetanus immune globulin (human).

*Such as, but not limited to, wounds contaminated with dirt, feces, soil, and saliva (e.g. following animal bites); puncture wounds; avulsions; and wounds resulting from missiles, crushing, burns, and frostbite.

†DTaP is used for children younger than 7 years. Tdap is preferred over Td for underimmunized children 7 years and older who have not received Tdap previously.

‡Immune globulin intravenous should be used when TIG is not available.

§More frequent boosters are not needed and can accentuate adverse effects.

Source: Adapted from Red Book: 2015 Report of committee on infectious diseases, Illinois: American Academy of Pediatrics; 2015.

cause serious systemic side effects including anaphylactic shock.

- Local sensitivity skin tests are quite unreliable to predict general sensitivity reactions.

Active Immunization

Fortunately, tetanus is completely vaccine-preventable disease. TT is available as a single-antigen vaccine and also as a combination vaccines to protect against other vaccine-preventable diseases including diphtheria, pertussis, poliomyelitis, hepatitis B, and illness caused by *Haemophilus influenzae* type b (Hib). The pentavalent vaccine, which provides protection against diphtheria, tetanus, pertussis, Hib, and hepatitis B (DTP-Hib-Hep B), is the most commonly used childhood vaccine worldwide, but other acellular pertussis containing pentavalent (DTaP-IPV/Hib) and hexavalent (DTaP-IPV/Hib-Hep B) combinations are also available.

All the children should be protected by active immunization with three primary doses of TT-containing vaccine (TTCV) with pentavalent or hexavalent vaccine at the age of 6–10–14 weeks as recommended by the Advisory Committee on Vaccines and Immunization Practices (ACVIP), Indian Academy of Pediatrics (IAP). These primary doses will be followed by booster doses at the age of 18 months and 5 years and at the age of 10 years.

All the pregnant women should be immunized with two doses of TTCV in the form of two doses of dT (diphtheria and tetanus) or Tdap (tetanus-diphtheria-acellular pertussis) (first dose) and dT (second dose) between 16 weeks and 36 weeks of gestation for the prevention of neonatal tetanus.

For primary immunization in adults, manufacturers recommend three doses and state that the first two doses should be administered 1–2 months apart and the third dose administered 6–8 months after the second dose, in series of Tdap, Td and Td.

For booster dosing, a tetanus–diphtheria combination with lower concentration of diphtheria antigen (d) is available as dT vaccine. Use of TTCV combinations with diphtheria toxoid is strongly encouraged and single-antigen vaccines should be discontinued whenever feasible to help maintain both high diphtheria and high tetanus immunity throughout the life course.

Tetanus-diphtheria-acellular pertussis formulations are licensed for use from 5 years of age. ACVIP recommends it after a minimum age of 7 years.

Duration of Protection and Booster Requirements in Children

Antibody concentration, avidity, and the duration of protection depend on a number of factors including the age of the vaccinees, the number of vaccine doses, and interval between them. Data from serological studies suggest that a primary series of three TTCV doses in infancy plus a booster during the second year of life will provide 3–5 years of protection. A further booster dose (e.g. in early childhood) will provide protection into adolescence, and another booster during adolescence will induce immunity that lasts through much of adulthood, thus protecting women through their childbearing years.

■ WORLD HEALTH ORGANIZATION POSITION PAPER

The aims of tetanus vaccination are: (1) to achieve global elimination of MNT and (2) to ensure lifelong protection against tetanus in all people by attaining and sustaining high coverage of six doses (three primary plus three booster doses) of TTCV through routine childhood immunization schedules. All children worldwide should be immunized against tetanus. Every country should seek to achieve early and timely infant vaccination initiated from 6 weeks of age and maintain high coverage of the complete three-dose primary series plus three-dose booster series prior to adolescence. In countries where MNTE has not yet been achieved, and in areas where MNT remains a public health concern, special attention is needed to ensure immunization of woman of reproducing age.

■ SUGGESTED READING

1. World Health Organization. (2018). Immunization, vaccines and biological and tetanus vaccines. [online] Available from: http://www.who.int/immunization/diseases/tetanus/en/ [Last accessed November, 2019].
2. Roper MH, Wassilak SGF, Tiwari TSP, et al. Tetanus toxoid. In: Plotkin S, Orenstein W, Offit P (Eds). Vaccines, 6th edition. Philadelphia: Saunders; 2013. pp. 447-92.
3. Liu L, Oza S, Hogan D, et al. Global, regional, and national causes of under-5 mortality in 2000–15: an updated systematic analysis with implications for the Sustainable Development Goals. Lancet. 2016;388(10063):3027-35.
4. Centers for Disease Control and Prevention (CDC). Tetanus surveillance—United States, 2001-2008. MMWR Morb Mortal Wkly Rep. 2011;60(12):365-9.
5. WHO. Global Vaccine Action Plan 2011–2020. Available at: http://www.who.int/immunization/global_vaccine_action_plan/GVAP_doc_2011_2020/en/ [Last accessed on November 2016].

6. IndiaSpend (2015). How India cut neonatal tetanus mortality by 99.76%. [online] Available from: https://archive.indiaspend.com/cover-story/how-india-cut-neonatal-tetanus-mortality-by-99-76-22329.

7. Liu L, Oza S, Hogan D, et al. Global, regional, and national causes of child mortality in 2000–13, with projections to inform post-2015 priorities: An updated systematic analysis. Lancet. 2015;385(9966):430-40.

8. Cousins S. India declared free of maternal and neonatal tetanus. BMJ. 2015;350:h2975.

9. Schiavo G, Matteoli M, Montecucco C. Neurotoxins affecting neuroexocytosis. Physiol Rev. 2000;80(2):717-66.

10. Roper MH, Vandelaer JH, Gasse FL. Maternal and neonatal tetanus. Lancet. 2007;370(9603):1947-59.

11. WHO-recommended standards for surveillance of selected vaccine-preventable diseases. World Health Organization, Geneva; 2003. Available at: http://apps.who.int/iris/bitstream/10665/68334/1/WHO_V-B_03.01_eng.pdf [Last accessed on November, 2016].

12. WHO. Current recommendations for treatment of tetanus during humanitarian emergencies. Technical Note 2010. Available at: http://www.who.int/diseasecontrol_emergencies/publications/who_hse_gar_dce_2010.2/en/; [Last accessed on October, 2016].

13. Indian Academy of Pediatrics. IAP Guidebook on immunization 2013-14.

14. Red Book 2015. Report of Committee on Infectious Diseases. Illinois: American Academy of Pediatrics.

15. WHO. Prequalified Vaccines. Available at: http://www.who.int/immunization_standards/vaccine_quality/PQ_vaccine_list_en/en/; [Last accessed on November, 2016].

16. World Health Organization. Tetanus. [online] Available from: https://www.who.int/immunization/policy/position_papers/pp_tetanus_2017_summary.pdf?ua=1.

Mycoplasma

Upendra Kinjawadekar, Shilpa Aroskar

INTRODUCTION

Mycoplasmas are small prokaryotic cells and absence of rigid cell wall makes them different from other bacteria. They are classified under mollicutes and belong to Mycoplasmataceae family. It was first isolated by Nocard and Roux in the year 1898, but was bovine pleuropneumonia. Dienes and Edsall did isolation of first human *Mycoplasma* in 1937 from a Bartholin's gland abscess. In 1944, Eaton et al. isolated another *Mycoplasma* from the sputum sample of a patient with primary atypical pneumonia and it was labeled as Eaton agent. Finally in 1962 Chanok et al. proposed taxonomic designation to Eaton agent as *Mycoplasma pneumoniae*.

EPIDEMIOLOGY

Mycoplasma bacteria are one of the common causes of community-acquired pneumonia (CAP) in children. Because of the paucity of clinical signs and variable or nonspecific radiological picture it is often described as "walking pneumonia" or "atypical pneumonia". Around 10–40% of CAP cases are caused by *M. pneumoniae*. The infection occurs all around the year. The mode of transmission is by infected respiratory droplets from an infected individual with an incubation period of about 2–3 weeks. It causes disease in all age groups, but a predilection for school going children above 5 years of age. Community outbreaks have been described in closed settings-colleges, schools, summer camps, and military base. High transmission rates have been documented within families with up to 40% of household contacts developing lower respiratory infections. The occurrence of *mycoplasma* infection is related to two factors—age and immunity.

PATHOGENESIS

Mycoplasma pneumoniae does not have a cell wall which makes it insensitive to beta-lactam antimicrobial agents. *M. pneumoniae* adheres to the ciliated cells of the epithelial lining of the respiratory tract with the help of an attachment organelle after inhalation. The absent cell wall also helps the organism to adhere to the membrane with the host cell easily. A toxin is produced by the bacteria community-acquired respiratory distress syndrome toxin (CARDS toxin) which causes ciliostasis resulting in airway inflammation and damage. Cilia and epithelium of the airways are also affected by hydrogen peroxide, which is produced locally and has a cytopathic effect. This typically causes persistent cough. Lack of protective immunity allows recurrent infections over time. Clinical manifestations are due to immunopathogenic and inflammatory effects by the host and not the organism itself. Autoimmunity has an important role to play in the extrapulmonary involvement.

CLINICAL FEATURES

Respiratory Tract Diseases

Upper as well as lower airways can be affected. Though initially the symptoms may manifest slowly and evolve over a period of few days, it has a tendency to persist for weeks or even months, if left untreated. Fever, sore throat, body ache, malaise, and persistent cough are the common clinical features of presentation in first week.

The clinical hallmark of *M. pneumoniae* infection is cough, usually worsens during the first week of illness and symptoms generally dissolve within 2 weeks. Cough can last up to 4 weeks. Children less than 5 years commonly present with coryza and wheezing and rarely develop pneumonia. On the contrary, bronchopneumonia or interstitial pneumonia more commonly in lower lobes is typically seen in age group 5–15 years. Chest auscultation shows scattered rales and expiratory wheeze.

Other respiratory illnesses caused by *M. pneumoniae* include pharyngitis (without cervical lymphadenopathy mostly), sinusitis and bronchitis, otitis media, and bullous myringitis.

Mycoplasma Infection and Asthma

Recently a link has been found between atypical pathogens like *M. pneumoniae* and asthma. *Mycoplasma* infection may precede the onset of a trigger an acute exacerbation in a child with asthma. Though many reasons have been postulated, it is mainly due to:

- *Mycoplasma* infection triggers airway inflammation via T-helper T2 pathway.
- Hypersensitivity due to immunoglobulin E (IgE).

In children with sickle cell disease, *Mycoplasma* infection may lead to acute chest syndrome.

Extrapulmonary Manifestations

Extrapulmonary involvement is seen in around 25% of children with *Mycoplasma* infections **(Table 1)**. Of this central nervous system (CNS) involvement is the most common of all. Sometimes the CNS involvement may outweigh the respiratory symptoms, making diagnosis a challenge.

The CNS symptoms occur after 3 days of onset of respiratory involvement and may persist for 2–3 weeks even after the resolution of the respiratory symptoms.

The common CNS presentations are encephalitis, meningoencephalitis, polyradiculitis, and aseptic meningitis. Complications may be either from direct invasion into the brain or by a neurotoxin produced by the organism or an immune mediated damage. CNS disease manifestations can occur 3–23 days (mean 10 days) after onset of respiratory symptoms. *Mycoplasma* encephalitis accounts for 5–15% of all childhood encephalitis.

Dermatological—Skin and Mucosa

While 10% patients may present with a maculopapular rash, 25% of patients are may have erythema multiforme, Stevens–Johnson syndrome (SJS), and toxic epidermal necrolysis.

Hematological

Autoimmune hemolytic anemia, thrombocytopenia, and disseminated intravascular coagulation (DIC) may be seen as complications of *M. pneumoniae* in few patients. This

Table 1: Extrapulmonary manifestations of *Mycoplasma*.

Neurological manifestations	• Aseptic meningitis • Meningoencephalitis • Cerebrovascular accidents • Hemiplegia • Transverse myelitis and ascending paralysis • Cerebral palsy and cerebellar ataxia • Optic neuritis and polyradiculopathy • Peripheral neuropathy • Guillain–Barré syndrome
Musculoskeletal	• Arthralgias and myalgias • Septic arthritis • Polyarthritis • Acute rhabdomyolysis
Hematological	• Hemolytic anemia • Thrombotic thrombocytopenia • Intravascular coagulation • Hemophagocytic syndrome
Cardiovascular	• Pericarditis and myocarditis • Endocarditis and CCF • Pericardial effusion • Raynaud's phenomenon
Dermatological	• Skin rashes • Stevens–Johnson syndrome • Erythema nodosum • Bullous erythema multiforme
Gastrointestinal	• Diarrhea and pancreatitis • Cholestatic hepatitis • Hypoechoic lesions in the spleen
Renal	• Acute glomerulonephritis and IgA nephropathy • Tubulointerstitial nephritis and renal failure

(CCF: congestive cardiac failure; IgA: immunoglobulin A)

occurs due to cross-reaction to cold agglutinins. Hemophagocytosis syndrome is not uncommon too.

Other extrapulmonary manifestations, though not so common, can be gastrointestinal tract (GIT) like hepatitis and pancreatitis, renal like glomerulonephritis, cardiac—pericarditis, myocarditis, rheumatic fever, and occasionally arthritis and arthralgia.

■ DIFFERENTIAL DIAGNOSIS

Mycoplasma pneumoniae and *Chlamydia pneumoniae* CAP closely resemble each other in their clinical manifestations, but have some important distinguishing features. *M. pneumoniae* is an acute infectious disease, while in contrast, *C. pneumoniae* may be acute but is typically a chronic disease. *M. pneumoniae*, like other atypical pneumonias, is characterized by its pattern of extrapulmonary organ involvement. *Mycoplasma* has a predilection for the upper, as well as the lower, respiratory tract, and thus patients with CAP who have upper respiratory tract involvement are most likely to have *M. pneumoniae*. Common upper respiratory tract manifestations of *M. pneumoniae* in a patient with CAP

Table 2: Differentiating features of pneumonia.		
Disease/ condition	*Differentiating signs/ symptoms*	*Differentiating tests*
Typical bacterial pneumonia	Acute onset with high fever with or without rigors. X-ray helpful in severe pneumonia	WBC count may be high. Blood culture positive in about 10% patients
Viral pneumonia	Coryza, GI symptoms, and radiologic findings could be nonspecific	Positive nasopharyngeal viral cultures; relative lymphocytosis in WBC
Tuberculosis	History of fever and/or unremitting cough for >2 weeks, history of TB contact, etc.	Sputum cultures and acid-fast bacillus stains positive; typical X-ray features

(GI: gastrointestinal; WBC: white blood cell; TB: tuberculosis)

include otitis, bullous myringitis, and mild nonexudative pharyngitis. These findings are less frequent with *C. pneumoniae* CAP. The most important clinical finding to differentiate *mycoplasma* from *C. pneumoniae* is the presence or absence of laryngitis.

Even very young children can become ill from *M. pneumoniae* even though it is less common. The differential diagnosis of respiratory viral infections and exacerbation of asthma-like symptoms must be considered.

The clinical presentation with a cough wheezing, gradual onset low-grade-fever, and rhonchi on auscultation in 33% of the youngest children can also be considered as a childhood asthma-like exacerbation, primarily due to viral infection in preschool children. Minor degree of mixed viral coinfections can also confound the clinical presentation. It can only be speculated in what pathogen was the primary cause of disease in these cases.

Viral infections like influenza, parainfluenza virus infection, respiratory syncytial virus (RSV), and rhinovirus infection can mimic *M. pneumoniae*. **Table 2** describes the differentiation between *Mycoplasma*, bacterial and tuberculous pneumonia.

LABORATORY STUDIES

Only when confronted with fulminant pulmonary disease or a severe extrapulmonary complication like SJS/CNS involvement/hemolytic anemia in a hospitalized child, a diagnostic laboratory test would be useful to diagnose *Mycoplasma* infection. Otherwise a gradual onset pneumonia presenting with cough as main feature in a child more than 5 years suggests *Mycoplasma* infection.

Various Laboratory Tests for *Mycoplasma*

A definite and specific diagnostic test is lacking forcing clinicians to use clinical judgment for the diagnosis. Currently serology based on acute and convalescent sera and combining it with polymerase chain reaction (PCR) from the respiratory secretions is the best tool available for the laboratory diagnosis.

Bacterial culture, which is a gold standard in the diagnosis of many infectious diseases, has become almost impractical in *Mycoplasma* diagnosis due to fastidious nature and slow growth (incubation of 2–4 weeks). Serologic diagnosis has been the mainstay of laboratory testing.

Cold agglutinating antibodies being positive in only 50% of individuals with *M. pneumoniae*, being observed in many other viral infections also being nonspecific are no longer tests of choice for the diagnosis.

Paired acute and convalescent sera are best for complement-fixation serology. IgM antibiotics rise only after the first week of illness and high false positivity as well as false negativity is associated with them. They may also persist for a long time even after the complete recovery. Therefore IgG antibiotics are more useful. A positive result requires a more than fourfold rise in IgG titer between acute and convalescent sera obtained 2–4 weeks apart.

Enzyme immunoassay (EIA) has largely replaced complement fixation test (CFT) and it can be performed on single serum specimen obtained on sixth or seventh day of acute infection.

Semi-nested PCR assay using 16S ribosomal deoxyribonucleic acid (rDNA) as a target and real-time PCR assays targeting the gene for P1 adhesion protein are available. Real-time PCR assays have the advantage of speed and the ability to analyze numerous samples with better sensitivity and specificity over serology.

They do not rely on an immunologic response; therefore, relatively early detection is possible. Although asymptomatic individuals may have positive PCR, positive nasopharyngeal PCR in a symptomatic child suggests causation.

RADIOGRAPHIC FEATURES: PLAIN RADIOGRAPH

No pattern is pathognomonic for *M. pneumoniae*. Even the most experienced clinician can sometimes find it difficult to differentiate between a viral or bacterial cause from *mycoplasma* as the features are mostly nonspecific and variable. The common patterns are peribronchial and perivascular interstitial infiltrates—reticular densities most common ~49%, consolidation ~38%, reticulonodular opacification ~8%, and nodular or mass-like opacification ~5%. Very rarely a necrotizing pneumonia (in sickle cell disease) or bronchiolitis obliterans (healthy child) could be observed. Pleural effusion (uncommon in ~25% of cases) and hilar lymphadenopathy ~30%. Computed tomography (CT), though not required for a routine case, certain radiologic features are commonly associated with *M. pneumoniae* areas of ground-glass attenuation and air-space consolidation are frequent on high-resolution computed tomography (HRCT) (~80% of cases).

Areas of consolidation may have a lobular distribution evident on CT in about 60% of cases.

■ TREATMENT OF *MYCOPLASMA PNEUMONIAE* RESPIRATORY INFECTIONS

Although bactericidal antibiotics like fluoroquinolones and bacteriostatic antibiotics like macrolides, ketolides, and tetracyclines have been used to treat *Mycoplasma* infection, actually the evidence to reach to some specific conclusion about its utility in clinical practice is lacking after Cochrane review was published on the similar lines. Absence of specific clinical features and full proof, easily available, and affordable diagnostic test further compounds the problem.

Due to good safety data, effectiveness against the organism, easy availability as well as low minimum inhibitory concentration (MIC), macrolide group of antibiotics have become the first choice of antibiotics. Amongst them azithromycin can be used for a duration of 5 days whereas clarithromycin is usually preferred for a course of 7–14 days while treating CAP. Although there are no head-to-head trials amongst various macrolides about therapeutic failure, adverse effects are definitely more with erythromycin. Absence of cell wall makes *mycoplasma* inherently resistant to beta-lactam antibiotics. There is some symptomatic relief despite persistent shedding of the organism (which is roughly 7 weeks after the disease onset) once put on treatment.

To what extent the immunomodulatory or anti-inflammatory actions of macrolides are beneficial is not yet proven. Apart from pneumonia, there is no benefit of treating with antibiotics in other respiratory tract infections, *mycoplasma* and to a lesser extent chlamydia may precipitate an attack of asthma or exacerbate existing asthma. Some patients who have recently had *M. pneumoniae* CAP develop post-CAP asthma which may be permanent. It would seem that *M. pneumoniae,* which resides on the surface of the respiratory epithelium, is in a perfect position to cause bronchial or hyperreactivities and/or bronchospasm. The treatment of *M. pneumoniae* and *C. pneumoniae* CAP is important, not because of the severity of the illness, but if for no other reason, to decrease communicability and to decrease post-CAP asthma.

Recommended regimens include:
- Azithromycin 10 mg/kg in one dose (maximum dose 500 mg) on the first day and 5 mg/kg in one dose (maximum dose 250 mg) for the next 4 days, or
- Clarithromycin 15 mg/kg per day in two divided doses (maximum daily dose 1 g) for 10 days.

It is important to remember that macrolide resistance is on the rise, especially mutations in 23S ribosomal ribonucleic acid (rRNA) strains. While on one side countries like Japan and China have reported it to the tune of 90%, Holland has reported no resistance at all. In India we do have some sporadic case reports related to it. As it is difficult to prove resistance in laboratory, in practice whenever on a strong clinical background patient fails to respond to macrolide in 48 hours it is prudent to switch to either doxycycline/levofloxacin suspecting resistance. The doses are:
- Doxycycline 2–4 mg/kg orally or intravenously per day in one or two divided doses (maximum daily dose 200 mg) for 10 days.
- Levofloxacin ≥6 months and <5 years—8–10 mg/kg per dose every 12 hours for 10 days (maximum daily dose 750 mg/day) for 10 days. ≥5 years—10 mg/kg per dose once per day (maximum daily dose 750 mg/day) for 10 days.

Adjunctive Therapy

Though conventionally never recommended, there is no way to disprove the direct involvement of the organism in the protean severe extrapulmonary manifestations of *mycoplasma* disease forcing us to rethink about using antibiotics in such cases. Corticosteroids and intravenous immunoglobulins along with antibiotics are most commonly used in treating mucositis/CNS involvement rash, etc.

■ SUGGESTED READING

1. Eaton MD, Meiklejohn G, van Herick W. Studies on the etiology of primary atypical pneumonia: a filterable agent transmissible to cotton rats, hamsters, and chick embryos. J Exp Med. 1944; 79:649-68.
2. Kashyap S, Sarkar M. Mycoplasma pneumoniae clinical features. Lung India. 2010;27:75-85.
3. Kliegman RM, Geme JS. Nelson Textbook of Pediatrics, 21st edition. Amsterdam, Netherlands: Elsevier; 2019.
4. Kumar S. Mycoplasma pneumonia: A significant but underrated pathogen in paediatric community-acquired lower respiratory tract infections. Indian J Med Res. 2018;147:23-31.
5. Lee KY. Pediatric respiratory infections by Mycoplasma pneumoniae. Expert Rev Anti Infect ther. 2008; 6:509-21.
6. Shah S. Mycoplasma Pneumoniae: Principles and Practice of Infectious Diseases, 3rd edition. London, United Kingdom: Churchill Livingstone; 2009. pp. 979-84.

Leptospirosis

Dhanya Dharmapalan

INTRODUCTION

Leptospirosis is an important zoonotic disease in the tropical and subtropical countries. The true incidence is not known as it is heavily underreported and a neglected public health problem in developing countries. The incidence is estimated at 10 or more per 100,000 population in tropical countries with rise to 100 or more per 100,000 population in an epidemic setting.[1]

It is caused by spirochetes which belong to the genus *Leptospira*. These are highly motile, thin, and helicoidal bacteria. The leptospires are visible on dark-field microscopy. They are obligate aerobes with an optimum growth temperature of 28–30°C. Leptospires are present in the blood and cerebrospinal fluid (CSF) during the first week of illness and later appear in the urine.

Serovar is the basic systematic unit in the classification of *Leptospira*. Currently there are over 250 serovars identified. The major antigen considered for serological classification is lipopolysaccharide (LPS). Pathogenic and nonpathogenic serovars have been identified as serovars of L. interrogans and L. biflexa respectively. The predominant serovars in India are L. andamana, L. pomona, L. grippotyphosa, L. hebdomadis, L. semaranga, L. javanica, L. autumnalis, L. canicola.[2]

TRANSMISSION

Humans are incidental hosts and do not transmit to other humans/animals. The mammalian reservoirs, most commonly rodents, cattle, horses, sheep, goat, pigs, and dogs carry the bacteria in the proximal tubules of their kidneys, which get excreted into urine. Rodents have the longest carrier state which spans throughout their life time. Serovars have been associated with reservoirs such as rats and serovar Icterohemorrhagiae, mice and serogroup Ballum, dogs and serovar Canicola, cattle with serovar Hardjo, or pigs with serogroup Australis.[3]

The spirochetes can survive for weeks to several months in the environment. Moisture helps in the environmental survival of these spirochetes. An accidental contact with *Leptospira* contaminated water or soil facilitates transmission to humans. Seasonal outbreaks occur following heavy rainfalls and flooding. Also there is increased occupational risk for agricultural workers, veterinarians, sewer workers, meat handlers, etc.

The common route of entry into human body is through cut and abrasions in the skin. The flagella help the motile *Leptospira* to invade the tissues. They can also penetrate through mucous membranes of nose, mouth and eyes. The incubation period is generally 7–10 days.

CLINICAL PRESENTATION

The clinical presentation can be divided into septicemic phase which is followed by the immune phase.

The anicteric leptospirosis presents as flu-like illness with sudden onset of high fever, headache, bodyache, nausea, abdominal pain. This lasts between 4 days and 7 days. In the immune phase the child can have headache, conjunctival effusion, hepatomegaly and features of aseptic meningitis. Initial CSF examination may initially show polymorphic or lymphocytic predominance but is lymphocytic in later stages. The proteins may be raised and glucose is usually normal.

Weil's syndrome presents with jaundice, renal failure, and hemorrhage. It can be progressive through the second week of illness and has mortality rate of 5%. Jaundice occurs due to hepatic dysfunction and affects the synthetic functions of the liver. Therefore, there is rise in liver enzymes with reduced serum albumin and vitamin K-dependent clotting factors. Renal impairment can be severe and occurs to tubular damage. In majority, the urine routine tests will be abnormal with proteinuria, hyaline or granular casts, hematuria, or pyuria. Oliguria, anuria and azotemia can occur and may need dialysis for management.

Weil's disease is a common presentation in children with lower fatality rates than adults. The nonicteric forms can be missed and therefore high index of suspicion is required.[4]

■ CLINICAL DIAGNOSIS

There is paucity of data regarding the application of modified Faine's criteria used in adults for clinical diagnosis of leptospirosis in children.

The following is the clinical case definition for leptospirosis as per National Centre for Disease Control (NCDC).[2]

Suspected Case

Acute febrile illness with headache, myalgia and prostration associated with a history of exposure to infected animals or an environment contaminated with animal urine with one or more of the following:

- Calf muscle tenderness
- Conjunctival suffusion
- Anuria or oliguria and/or proteinuria
- Jaundice
- Hemorrhagic manifestations (intestines, lung)
- Meningeal irritation
- Nausea, vomiting, abdominal pain, and diarrhea.

Probable: Suspected case with positive presumptive laboratory diagnosis.

Confirmed: Suspect/probable case with confirmatory laboratory test.

■ LABORATORY DIAGNOSIS

Complete blood count (CBC) may show normal to raised leukocyte counts. Leukocytopenia is not a feature of leptospirosis. There may be thrombocytopenia in the first week of illness. The lower values of hemoglobin and hematocrit between 3 days and 5 days can help differentiate from dengue.[5]

The various methods available to detect *Leptospira* are as follows:

Culture: Blood culture should be taken early in illness and if possible multiple cultures should be taken. CSF culture can also be used for isolation during the first week, while urine specimen can be cultured after 1 week of illness.

Cultures can confirm the diagnosis and also help identify the serovar. The most widely used culture medium is the oleic acid-albumin medium EMJH and contains Tween 80 and bovine serum albumin. However, the technique is complex and time consuming and also requires biosafety II facilities. The antibiotic susceptibility testing is also challenging due to several limitations which include long incubation period and inability to quality growth.[6]

Microscopic: Dark-field microscopy can identify leptospires during the septicemic phase. But it has low sensitivity and specificity. Sensitivity can be increased with use of special staining methods.

Immunologic: Leptospiral antigens can be detected by radioimmunoassay (RIA), enzyme-linked immunosorbent assay (ELISA), and chemiluminescent immunoassay (with greater specificity than dark-field microscopy).

Antibodies become detectable after 6 days of onset of illness and peaks by 3–4 weeks.

Microscopic agglutination test (MAT) is the reference method for serological diagnosis. A fourfold rise in titers on paired samples taken 2 weeks apart or seroconversion is confirmatory for the diagnosis. The disadvantage of MAT includes complexity of the technique and high risk of contamination. Therefore, the test is available only in few centers.

Immunoglobulin M (IgM) test by ELISA is widely available commercially. A systemic review with meta-analysis has reported sensitivity of IgM ELISA as 84% and specificity as 91%.[7] Other antibody detecting tests like slide agglutination, latex agglutination or immuno-chromatographic tests are also useful for serological screening.

Molecular: Molecular methods using polymerase chain reaction (PCR) is gaining popularity due to its scope for early detection (within 5 days of illness). Also the test has faster turnaround time, less contamination, and does not require a reference of hyperimmune antisera to determine the identity of the cultured organism. Studies have shown higher sensitivity of PCR compared to conventional serological tests.[4]

A limitation of PCR-based diagnosis of leptospirosis is the inability of most PCR assays to identify the infecting serovar,[8] this has relevance for epidemiological studies.

The following are the laboratory criteria for diagnosis:[2]

- *Presumptive diagnosis:*
  - A positive result in IgM-based immunoassays, slide agglutination test or latex agglutination test or immunochromatographic test.

- A MAT titer of 100/200/400 or above in single sample based on endemicity.
- Demonstration of leptospires directly or by staining methods.
- *Confirmatory diagnosis*:
  - Isolation of leptospires from clinical specimen.
  - Fourfold or greater rise in the MAT titer between acute and convalescent phase serum specimens run in parallel.
  - Positive by any two different types of rapid test.
  - Seroconversion.
  - PCR test.

The National referral laboratories in India for leptospirosis are listed below:

- Regional Medical Research Center (ICMR), Port Blair (A and N)
- National Centre for Disease Control, 22-Sham Nath Marg, Delhi
- National Institute of Epidemiology, Chennai
- Government Medical College, Surat
- BJ Medical College, Ahmedabad
- Madurai Medical College, Madurai
- National Institute of Veterinary Epidemiology and Disease Informatics (NIVEDI), Bengaluru, Karnataka
- Bacteriology and Mycology Division, IVRI, Izatnagar, UP - 243122
- DRDE, Gwalior (MP)
- Tamil Nadu Veterinary and Animal Sciences University, Chennai.

TREATMENT

Early antibiotic therapy is crucial to prevent complications. WHO recommends rapid presumptive antibiotic treatment so that antibiotic can be introduced before the fifth day of disease. Amoxicillin 30–50 mg/kg/day in three divided doses for 7 days is recommended for children less than 8 years. For older children, doxycycline 100 mg twice a day for 7 days is recommended.

For children requiring hospitalization, crystalline penicillin is the first-line agent for leptospirosis as dose of 2–4 lacs IU/kg/day for 7 days. Other effective antibiotics are third-generation cephalosporins (ceftriaxone/cefotaxime). Erythromycin (30–50 mg/kg/day) can be used in children with penicillin allergy.

Initiation of antibiotics can trigger a rare adverse event in the form of an acute febrile inflammatory reaction called Jarisch–Herxheimer reaction due to the cytokine release resulting from clearance of spirochetes from the circulation.

COMPLICATIONS

Septic shock is a frequent complication requiring the use of inotropes and intravenous therapy. Renal failure may need the use of hemodialysis. Peritoneal dialysis is also beneficial if hemofiltration is not available at the health center. In case of hemorrhage, blood transfusion with packed cells or platelets may be needed. Mechanical ventilation can be lifesaving in event of a pulmonary hemorrhage.

PREVENTION

Personal protection with rubber boots and gloves is needed among workers with high risk for occupational hazard. People should be warned against wading through flooded waters unprotected. Swimming pools must be chlorinated regularly.

In case of flooding, postexposure chemoprophylaxis with single dose doxycycline 4 mg/kg (max 200 mg) or alternatively azithromycin (10 mg/kg) has been found to be beneficial for preventing clinical disease. A large scale community chemoprophylaxis for high-risk individuals during Mumbai 2017 floods had shown favorable outcome or reduced incidence of disease and associated mortality and morbidity.[9]

REFERENCES

1. World Health Organization (2010). The Global Burden of Leptospirosis. [online] Available from: http://www.who.int/zoonoses/diseases/lerg/en/index2.html [Last accessed on November, 2019].
2. National Centre for Disease Control (2015). National Guidelines Diagnosis, Case Management Prevention and Control of Leptospirosis. [online] Available from: https://ncdc.gov.in/WriteReadData/l892s/File558.pdf [Last accessed on November, 2019].
3. Goarant C. Leptospirosis: risk factors and management challenges in developing countries. Res Rep Trop Med. 2016;7: 49-62.
4. Narayanan R, Sumathi G, Prabhakaran SG, et al. Paediatric leptospirosis: A population based case-control study from Chennai, India. Indian J Med Microbiol. 2016;34(2):228-32.
5. De Silva NL, Niloofa M, Fernando N, et al. Changes in full blood count parameters in leptospirosis: a prospective study. Int Arch Med. 2014;7:31.
6. Ahmad SN, Shah S, Ahmad FM. Laboratory diagnosis of leptospirosis. J Postgrad Med. 2005;51(3):195-200.
7. Rosa MI, Reis MFD, Simon C, et al. IgM ELISA for leptospirosis diagnosis: a systematic review and meta-analysis. Cien Saude Colet. 2017;22(12):4001-12.
8. Ahmed SA, Sandai DA, Musa S, et al. Rapid diagnosis of leptospirosis by multiplex PCR. Malays J Med Sci. 2012;19(3): 9-16.
9. Supe A, Khetarpal M, Naik S, et al. Leptospirosis following heavy rains in 2017 in Mumbai: Report of large-scale community chemoprophylaxis. Natl Med J India. 2018;31(1):19-21.

Rickettsial Infections

4.11 CHAPTER

Atul Kulkarni, Ashutosh V Yajurvedi

INTRODUCTION

Rickettsia is a group of infections caused by a family of organisms having common biology and interesting history. They are phylogenetically placed between bacteria and viruses and belong to genus *Rickettsia* within family Rickettsiaceae in order Rickettsiales. These are mainly arthropod-borne diseases, ticks being the most common vector but some are transmitted by lice, flea, or mites.

Though the disease has been known to clinicians for more than a century, it is one of the most common re-emerging infections of recent times. Even though amenable to cheap and easily available therapy in the early phase, rickettsial infections pose a diagnostic difficulty in this phase due to similarity with other acute febrile illnesses which makes identification and treatment challenging.

HISTORICAL ASPECTS

The earliest record of the disease dates back to 1873 when physicians used to call this life-threatening disease as "Spotted fever" or "Black measles" due to the presence of dark petechial rash. It was Howard T. Ricketts who in the early 20th century described the epidemiological characteristics of the Rocky Mountain spotted fever when he did extensive research in Bitterroot Valley in Montana (USA). It was he who demonstrated the transmission of the disease via ticks. While doing a study on typhus in Mexico, unfortunately, he contracted the same disease and died. Ricketts could not isolate or identify the organism causing spotted fever or typhus and ascribed the disease to be of viral origin. It was in 1916 when Simeon Burt Wohlbach identified the organism and named it after Ricketts.

The disease peaked during the times of wars. The winning streak of Napoleon was halted in Moscow when a large number of his troops got infected with typhus. During 1917–1925 around 25 million cases of epidemic typhus were documented, out of which 3 million deaths were reported. Hence, there goes the famous saying by Lenin that "Either socialism will defeat the louse or the louse will defeat the socialism."

During World War II, multitude of cases as well as deaths due to scrub typhus were seen in the Asia-Pacific region when the understanding of the disease increased enormously.

CLASSIFICATION

The Rickettsial infections were initially classified into "spotted fever" and "typhus" groups depending on the presence or absence of outer membrane protein A (*omp* A) gene. It is seen in the spotted fever group while it is absent in the typhus group. Further research led to the finding that there are several other species that have *omp* A gene but are genetically not the same as the spotted fever group. These species were later classified as the transitional group. Later it was found that scrub typhus, caused by *Orientia*, has many similarities but was antigenically different from the typhus group of rickettsia. Hence, it was considered a different group. The classification of the rickettsial diseases along with its vector, host, and reservoir is summarized in **Table 1**.

EPIDEMIOLOGY

Rickettsial infections are seen all over the world. Rickettsial infection was first documented in India from the Kumaon region in the foothills of Himalaya in 1930s. Since then, many reports of this disease from different parts of India followed. Even though initially it was thought to be the disease of rural population, a considerable number of

Table 1: Classification of rickettsial infections.

Disease	Rickettsial agent	Insect vector	Mammalian reservoir
• Typhus group			
– Epidemic typhus	*Rickettsia prowazekii*	Louse	Humans
– Murine typhus	*R. typhi*	Flea	Rodent
• Scrub typhus	*O. tsutsugamushi*	Mite	Rodent
• Spotted fever group*			
– Indian tick typhus	*R. conorii*	Tick	Dog/rodents
– Rocky mountain spotted fever	*R. rickettsii*	Tick	Dogs/rodents
• Others			
– Rickettsial pox	*R. akari*	Mite	Mice
– Q fever	*Coxiella burnetii*	Nil	Cattle sheep goat
– Trench fever	*Rochalimaea quintana*	Louse	Humans
– Ehrlichioses	*Ehrlichia*	Tick	Deer/dog
– Anaplasmosis	*Anaplasma phagocytophilum*	Tick	Deer/dog

*More than 19 types of spotted fever varieties are described depending upon the geographical area where these are prevalent.

cases are being detected in urban parts of India, possibly due to increasing ecotourism, trekking, and camping activities of the urban population. The type of infection prevalent in a particular region depends on the temporal distribution of the vectors which cause it.

India, being the part of the famous Tsutsugamushi triangle, is endemic to scrub typhus. It is the most common type of rickettsial infection found in India. Some regions report that up to 50% of all undifferentiated fevers constitute scrub typhus.

The next in the frequency of prevalence is Indian Tick Typhus (ITT). It is reported from many districts of Maharashtra, Karnataka, Tamil Nadu, Telangana, and Kerala. Murine typhus is also reported from Madhya Pradesh and Kashmir. Other rickettsial infections are rarely reported in India.

Rickettsial infections are seen throughout the year and do not have any specific seasonal variations although immediately after the rains due to increase in grass, there can be an increased number of cases. But it is said that the transmission of infection seizes when temperature falls below 25°C. It has been seen in all age groups with equal frequency of distribution and has been reported in neonates also.

■ THE ORGANISM

Rickettsia is a group of nonmotile, nonspore-forming, and highly pleomorphic organisms. They are an obligate intracellular organism as they need the cytoplasm of the cell they invade to survive and replicate. Rickettsia can be present as cocci (0.1 μ), rods (1–4 μ), or thread-like structures (10 μ). The cytoplasm of rickettsia is covered by the trilaminar membrane consisting of outer bilayer, peptidoglycan layer, and inner bilayer. The cytoplasm consists of ribosomes and a few strands of DNA. The genome of rickettsia is small and consists of 1–1.5 million bases. The organisms divide by binary fission. The major antigens of the rickettsia consist of lipopolysaccharides, lipoproteins, outer membrane proteins (omp A and omp B), and heat shock proteins. The cross reactivity of these antigens, especially with the antigens of the *Proteus mirabilis* and *Proteus vulgaris*, is the basis of the Weil-Felix test.

Etiopathogenesis

The target site of rickettsia is the vascular endothelial cell of medium- and small-sized blood vessels. There are three steps in the pathogenesis of the rickettsial infections: (1) adherence to the host cell, (2) invasion and multiplication, and (3) release from the host cell.

Adherence to the Host Cell

This is the first step in the pathogenesis of rickettsial infection. After the bite by vector or exposure to the feces of lice or fleas over denuded skin, rickettsia gets inoculated into the dermis of the host. Further, rickettsia travel through the bloodstream and reach the vascular endothelium.

Invasion of the Host Cell

Viability of rickettsia and effector function of the host cell cytoskeletal actin are essential conditions for the invasion of rickettsia into endothelial cells. The organism induces phagocytosis for its entry into the host cell. This is a unique finding as the phagocytosis is seen even in the cell that usually does not phagocytose the particles. Activation of phosphoinositide 3-kinase, Cdc42 (a small GTPase), src-family tyrosine kinases, and tyrosine phosphorylation of focal adhesion kinase (FAK) and cortactin are the signaling pathways that enable the rickettsial organism to enter the host vascular endothelium.

After the invasion of the host cell, the organism needs to be in the cytoplasm of the host cell as it will avoid formation of the phagolysosome which eventually leads to killing of the organism. This is carried out by the secretion of phospholipase D and hemolysin C, encoded by the rickettsial genes *pld* and *thyC* which have the ability to disintegrate the phagosomal membrane. Also, rickettsial organisms lack the intrinsic ability to metabolize carbohydrates and amino acids and hence are entirely dependent on the host cytoplasm containing nutrients, adenosine triphosphate, amino acids, and nucleotides required for their growth.

Release from the Host Cell

Rickettsia expresses a surface protein named Sca2. This protein causes mobilization of the Arp2/3 complex which results in host actin polymerization. The filaments of actin push rickettsia to the surface of the host cell, where lies the membrane. This membrane is bent outward invaginating into the adjacent cell. Destruction of the membrane between the two will lead to movement of rickettsia into the adjacent cell without exposing it to the extracellular environment.

The final mechanism through which the rickettsia cause host cell destruction and leave the cells differs between the typhus group, spotted fever group, and scrub typhus group. In the typhus group, there occurs cell lysis. After the infection with *Rickettsia prowazekii*, there occurs multiplication of the organism until the cell is packed with it and then bursts. In the spotted fever group, the organism does not accumulate in large numbers. The rickettsial organisms are propelled through cytoplasm into the tips of membrane extrusions. There is focal lysis of these extrusions and the organism leaves the cell. In scrub typhus, the organism leaves the host cell by budding.

It is obscure how rickettsia causes cellular damage and denudation of the endothelium of host endothelial cells. It is speculated that this cellular damage is caused by oxidative stress. This finding is supported by the evidence of accumulation of reactive oxygen species and altered levels of antioxidant enzymes, which are superoxide dismutase, glutathione peroxidase, glutathione reductase, glucose-6-phosphate dehydrogenase (G6PD), and catalase. Among other possible mechanisms, rickettsial phospholipase A2 activity leads to direct damage of host cells which is also important in the entry of organism into the host cell.

As the cells of vascular endothelium are the chief targets of the rickettsia, there is significant damage to the endothelial integrity leading to increased vascular permeability. This is an important pathophysiological effect leading to edema, loss of circulating fluid volume, hypoalbuminemia, reduced oncotic pressure, and hypotension. Aggregation of the platelets occurs due to injured endothelium leading to platelet consumption and thrombocytopenia. Proliferation of polymorphs and monocytes in vessel walls causes occlusive endarteritis which results in microinfarcts. These are named as "typhus nodules of Wohlbach." The endarteritis occurs in different organs such as brain, heart, kidney, liver, and lungs, which is the pathophysiological basis of different clinical manifestations of rickettsial fever.

The pathogenesis of rickettsial infections is summarized in **Flowchart 1**.

Mode of Transmission

The natural hosts of the rickettsial organism are ticks, mites, flea, and louse. They are also the reservoirs and vectors of the infection (except Q fever). These maintain infection naturally by transovarian transmission (passage of organism from infected ticks to their progeny) and trans-stadial passage. The organisms are found in the

Flowchart 1: Pathogenesis of rickettsial fever.

alimentary canal of these arthropods. Transfer of the organism to mammals such as rodents, dogs, and cats as well as humans occurs by bite of these insects following regurgitation of the saliva during their blood meal. Dogs and rodents serve as the reservoir of the host for these vectors.

Inoculation of the soil infected with the feces of lice or fleas on denuded skin is another mode of transmission of the organism.

Clinical Features

There is no specific clinical manifestation of rickettsial fever during the initial phase of illness. It resembles like any other acute febrile illness posing a diagnostic dilemma. The incubation period ranges from 2 days to 14 days with a median of 7 days. It can extend up to 28 days. A history of contact with the infested pet animal or tick may be given by parents on asking, but only half of the patients remember. This may be due to the ability of ticks to obtain a blood meal efficiently without significant pain as well as the attachment of the tick in the areas which are not easily seen. Thus, it is important for the physicians to not only depend on the history of tick bite but also enquire about the behavior that puts them at the risk of tick bite, like walking in woods or high grass or history of travel to the endemic area or the presence of domestic animals in the vicinity. At times, multiple family members may also be affected.

The clinical manifestations vary in severity from a mild, self-limiting illness to life-threatening catastrophe. Initially, patients present with headache, fever, anorexia, restlessness, and myalgia. Fever is abrupt and high grade at the onset and is associated with chills. The core body temperature sometimes exceeds 40°C. Headache is excruciating, unabating, and usually does not budge to common analgesics. Gastrointestinal symptoms are also found in the form of nausea, vomiting, and diarrhea. Abdominal pain is often complained in the initial phase of illness. Younger infants, who cannot verbalize about headache, have irritability as the manifestation of headache. Irritability can also be due to myalgia associated with the disease.

Usually, rickettsial fever is described as the triad of fever, headache, and rash which is seen only in 44% of the patients. Rash that is contemplated to be the characteristic finding in rickettsial infections can be absent at times. The skin rash is usually evident after the 2–4 days of onset of illness. Rash is discrete to start with. It is pale, rose red, blanching macular to start with, and becomes more petechial **(Fig. 1)** or hemorrhagic with progress

of the disease. During the initial phase, rash may not be evident in dark-skinned patients. Sometimes, there can be palpable purpura **(Fig. 2)**. The type of rash and its pattern of distribution vary from types of rickettsial fever. The rash is virtually present in all cases with ITT (up to 90%). The rash first develops on peripheries involving palm and sole **(Figs. 1 and 3)** and spreads rapidly toward the trunk (Centripetal). Around the sixth day, the rash becomes generalized petechial and the child becomes extremely sick. Recovery from this phase is usually gradual even after institution of correct treatment. Rash in rickettsial pox appears early and progresses rapidly. It starts on trunk and spreads all over the body, sparing palms and soles. Rash is seen in only 40–50% of the patients in scrub typhus. It starts from trunk, sparing the extremities. In epidemic typhus the rash appears late (5–8 days), seen first on the trunk and then spreads to peripheries. It typically spares face, palm,

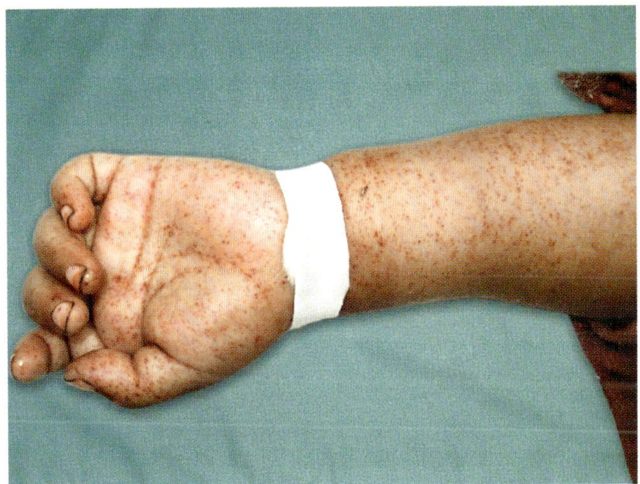

Fig. 1: Petechial rash.

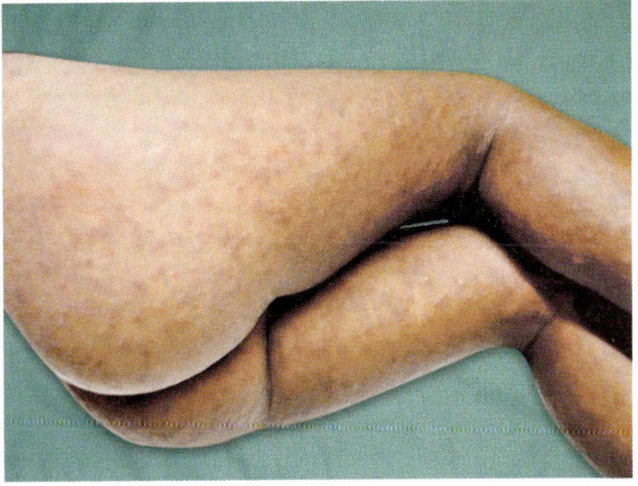

Fig. 2: Palpable purpura.

and sole. The rash is less frequent in murine typhus as it appears very late in the course of illness (10–12 days) and before the appearance of the rash, patients usually seek medical attention and are put on treatment.

Eschar is the initial site of the attachment of the chigger. Initially, it looks like a papule which later on becomes necrotic in the center, finally becoming a characteristic black crusted lesion **(Fig. 4)**. Eschar looks like a skin burn of cigarette butt. It is painless and rarely pruritic. The common sites are inguinal folds, buttocks, axillae, below the breast, and head and neck region. There is associated regional lymphadenopathy. If regional lymphadenopathy is found at examination, an eschar should be actively searched. Eschar is pathognomonic of scrub typhus but it can be missed if not actively looked for. Around 5–80% of the children with scrub typhus have eschar, while it is an uncommon feature of ITT (only 3–5%).

A severe vaso-occlusive disease following rickettsial infection due to vasculitis or thrombus formation is quite rare. But gangrene of the digits, toes, earlobes, skin, scrotum, or nose has been observed **(Figs. 5 to 8)**. Because of the autoamputation of the part of earlobe, sometimes this disease is referred to as Kan-Kapya disease (the disease that cuts one's ear in local spoken language).

Edema is seen over the dorsum of hands or feet, periorbital region, and sometimes it can be generalized. Leaky vessels following the inflammation inflicted by rickettsia and associated hypoproteinemia lead to edema. Organomegaly is one of the consistent features seen in many children.

There can be hepatosplenomegaly and conjunctival hyperemia.

The chief differentiating features of common rickettsial infections in India are summarized in **Table 2**.

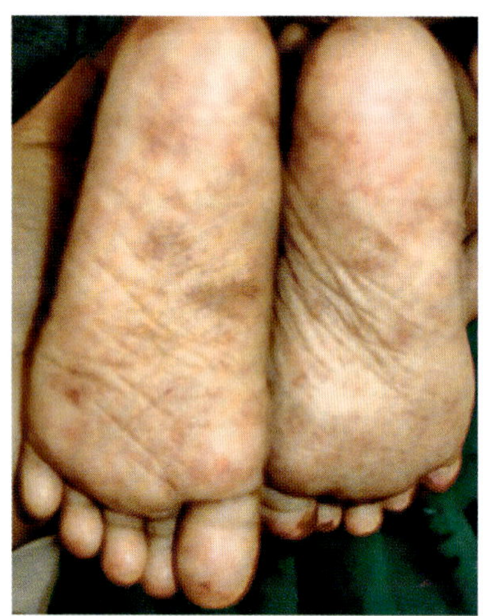

Fig. 3: Sole involvement.

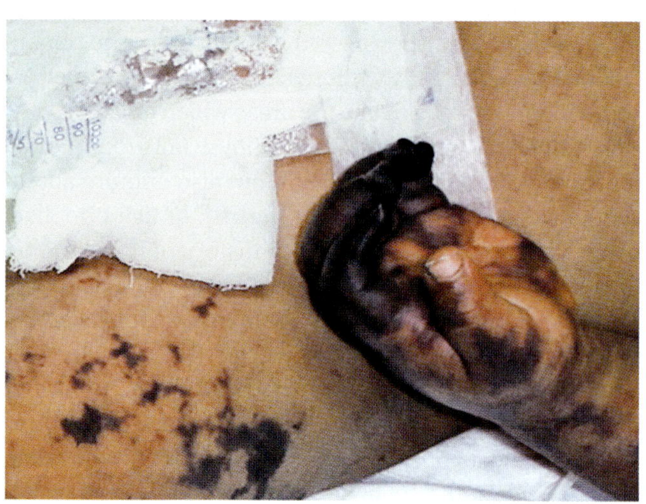

Fig. 5: Gangrene of digits.

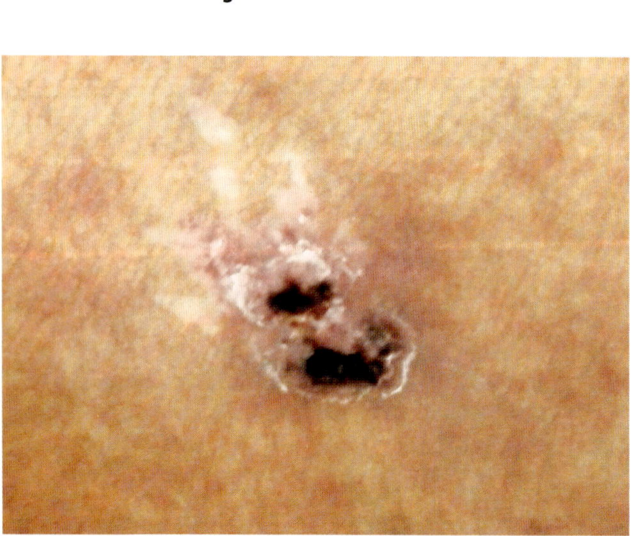

Fig. 4: Eschar.

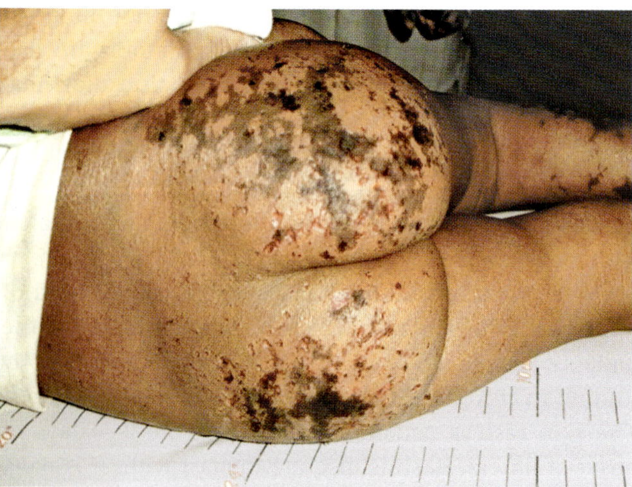

Fig. 6: Gangrenous rash over skin.

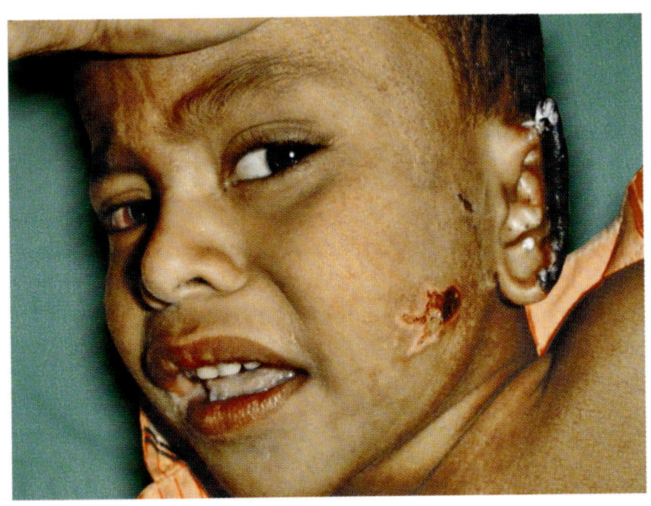

Fig. 7: Gangrene of earlobe (Kan-Kapya disease).

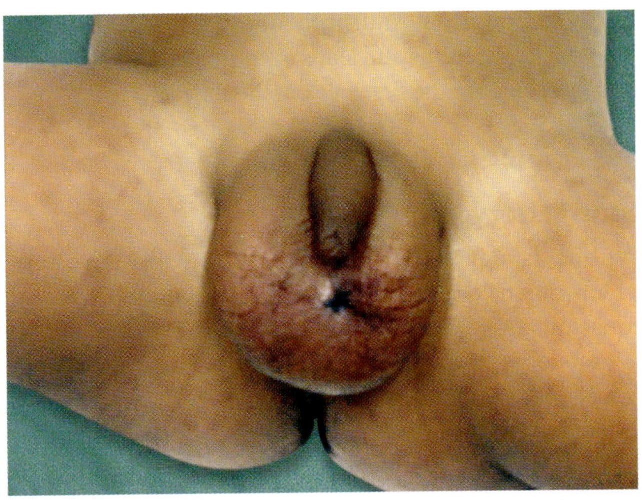

Fig. 8: Necrosis of scrotum.

Table 2: Differentiating features of common rickettsial infections in India.

Feature	Indian tick typhus	Scrub typhus	Murine typhus
Causative organism	*Rickettsia conorii*	*Orientia Tsutsugamushi*	*Rickettsia typhi*
Vector	Various tick genera (*Rhipicephalus, Ixodes, Boophilus*)	Trombiculid mite/chiggers	Flea (*Xenopsylla cheopis* in rats; *Ctenocephalides felis* in cats)
Mammalian host/reservoir	Dogs/rodents	Rodents	Rodents/cats
Epidemiological risk	Endemic in Maharashtra, Karnataka, Tamil Nadu, Telangana, and Kerala Woodlands Large domestic animals in vicinity	Endemic India (Tsutsugamushi triangle) Any terrain from sea levels to Himalayan foothills Woods and clearings	Rat infestations, especially near granaries and ports Cat as pet
Rash morphology	>90% have appearance on 2–4 days Begins as faint macule and becomes petechial later First appears on extremities and spreads centrally Involves palm and soles	40–50% appearance on day 5–8 Macular/maculopapular Rarely petechial Starts on trunk and spreads to peripheries Spares extremities	Rarely reported Present vary late in course of illness
Eschar	3–5% (uncommon)	5–80% (pathognomonic) Needs to be actively searched for	Not seen
Other significant findings	Gangrene of digits/earlobes leading to autoamputation Gastrointestinal symptoms (diarrhea/abdominal pain) Peripheral edema	Regional lymphadenopathy CNS involvement (*Typhos*: Clouding of sensorium) Sensorineural hearing loss	Self-limited with recovery within 1–2 weeks Very low rate of complications
Weil-Felix test	OX 2 Positive OX 19 Positive OX K Negative	OX 2 Negative OX 19 Negative OX K Positive	Not used OX 2 Positive OX 19 Negative OX K Negative
Treatment of choice	Doxycycline	Doxycycline	Doxycycline

Involvement of multiple organs occurs due to generalized vasculitis and leads to complications. They are usually seen after the first week of the illness.

COMPLICATIONS

Central Nervous System

Typhus is derived from the Greek word "typhos" which means smoky and refers to the altered state of consciousness seen in typhus and other life-threatening rickettsioses. Vasculitis of the central nervous system vessels leads to meningoencephalitis. It starts as confusion or lethargy and progresses to seizures, stupor, or delirium and coma. Involvement of the blood vessels contiguous to cerebrospinal fluid (CSF) leads to pleocytosis (10–100 cells/cu mm) with lymphocyte and macrophage predominance. Occasionally, polymorphonuclear pleocytosis with a cell count of more than 100 is seen. Seizures or coma usually denote a fatal outcome. Rickettsial meningoencephalitis should always be considered as the differential diagnosis of every patient with aseptic meningitis or meningoencephalitis or acute encephalitic syndrome with compatible epidemiological history. The Rickettsial encephalitis may have long-term neurological sequelae.

Sensorineural hearing loss has also been documented in scrub typhus which is reversible with treatment. It is seen in about one-third of the children and can be a diagnostic clue. Hearing loss due to nasal congestion must be differentiated from true hearing loss.

Cardiovascular

Pericarditis and myocarditis can sometimes complicate the disease. Pericardial effusion was seen in autopsy patients, but clinically significant pericardial effusion is a rare phenomenon. Relative bradycardia is a feature but other arrhythmias can be associated with cardiac involvement.

Pulmonary

Pneumonitis is a common complication and can be the presenting complaint of scrub typhus. Involvement of pulmonary microcirculation occurs in heavily infected, severely ill children. This leads to the development of noncardiogenic pulmonary edema, presenting as nonproductive cough and breathlessness. This pulmonary edema may sometimes end up into dreadful acute respiratory distress syndrome (ARDS).

Renal

Even though many of the children with rickettsial fever have normal renal function, nephritis and renal failure have been reported. Acute kidney injury (AKI) in rickettsial infection is thought to be the bad prognostic factor.

Others

Involvement of liver in the form of altered levels of transaminases is seen. The rickettsial fever may progress to disseminated intravascular coagulation and irreversible shock leading eventually to death. Other complications such as hemophagocytic lymphohistiocytosis, purpura fulminans, and gangrene of digits, earlobes, buttocks, and scrotum may also be seen. Gangrene of digits and earlobe may progress to autoamputation.

DIFFERENTIAL DIAGNOSIS

Rickettsial infection can be a differential diagnosis for any acute febrile illness or any exanthematous fever. The most important differential diagnoses include meningococcemia, measles, and enteroviral exanthemas. Other diseases included in the differential diagnosis are typhoid fever, secondary syphilis, leptospirosis, toxic shock syndrome, scarlet fever, rubella, Kawasaki disease, parvoviral infection, idiopathic thrombocytopenic purpura, thrombotic thrombocytopenic purpura, hemolytic uremic syndrome, Henoch-Schönlein purpura, acute abdomen, aseptic meningitis, hepatitis, dengue fever, infectious mononucleosis, drug reactions, malaria, tularemia, anthrax and other causes of pyrexia of unknown origin.

DIAGNOSIS

Lack of any specific clinical finding along with lack of a specific and sensitive test early in the course of the illness makes diagnosing rickettsial infection a challenging task. A high index of suspicion is the key to diagnosis of the rickettsial infection. It should be suspected when:

- Tick bite/ticks seen on clothes, in and around homes, or in areas where children play
- Visit to areas which are common habitats of vectors such as high uncut grass, weeds, bushes, rice fields, woodlands (where rodents share habitats with animals), grassy lawns, river banks, or poorly maintained kitchen gardens
- Animal sheds in the proximity of homes or contact with pet or stray dog infested with ticks
- Living in or travel to areas endemic for rickettsial diseases
- Occurrence of similar clinical cases simultaneously or sequentially in family members, co-workers, and neighborhood

- Undifferentiated fever of >5 days
- Dengue-like disease
- Aseptic meningitis/meningoencephalitis/acute encephalitic syndrome
- Sepsis of unclear etiology
- Fever with rash
- *Fever with*:
  - Edema
  - Headache and myalgia
  - Hepatosplenomegaly and/or lymphadenopathy
  - Cough and pulmonary infiltrates or community-acquired pneumonia
  - Acute kidney injury
  - Acute gastrointestinal or hepatic involvement.

Laboratory Diagnosis

The test to confirm the diagnosis of rickettsial infection early in the course of the illness is unavailable. There are few pointers in the investigations that increase the probability of rickettsial fever. The total white blood cell count is normal or low initially and later with progression of the disease there will be leukocytosis. Thrombocytopenia is because of consumption of the platelets due to vasculitis. Hypoproteinemia, hyponatremia, and elevated transaminases are some of the other features. Markers of acute inflammation such as erythrocyte sedimentation rate (ESR) and C-reactive protein (CRP) are often elevated. CSF findings are usually normal, but some may have pleocytosis (10–300 cells/µL) and about 20% may have elevated CSF proteins (200 mg/dL).

Multiple serological tests are available and all of them have one or other constraints. Physicians must be aware of these constraints before asking and interpreting the results.

Weil-Felix Test

It is a heterophile agglutination test. Antigenic cross reactivity between the species of rickettsia with certain serotypes of nonmotile Proteus species is the principle of this test. It was invented by Edmund Weil and Arthur Felix in 1916. OX 2 and 19 antigen of *Proteus vulgaris* and OX K of *P. mirabilis* are used. A type of specific rickettsial disease is suspected depending on agglutination with these antigens of *Proteus* species which is summarized in **Table 3**. A titer of more than 1:80 is considered significant but local titers must be defined. This is a cheap, easily available, and rapid diagnostic test, but lacks sensitivity and specificity. Rising titers have a better predictive value than a single value; hence diagnosis is retrospective, which

Table 3: Differentiating rickettsial infections by Weil-Felix test.

Disease	Weil-Felix		
	OX 19	OX 2	OX K
Epidemic typhus	++	+/–	–
Endemic typhus	++	–	–
Scrub typhus	–	–	++
Rocky Mountain spotted fever	+	+	–
Rickettsial pox	–	–	–
Q Fever	–	–	–

is another disadvantage. In spite of these disadvantages, it is still the most widely relied test where other tests are not available. The reports of this test must be interpreted with utmost caution taking history and clinical examination into consideration.

ELISA

Strain-specific immunoglobulin M (IgM) ELISA (enzyme-linked immunofluorescent assay) testing has high sensitivity and specificity; hence, it can be of choice test. Detection of IgM antibodies confirms about the recent rickettsial infection. The cutoff value taken is an optical density of 0.5. Baseline titers for a particular geographical region need to be defined.

Immunofluorescence Assay

Immunofluorescence assay (IFA) is considered as a gold standard test. The titer starts rising on 5–10 days of illness and peaks around 2–3 weeks. This test has several disadvantages. The exorbitant cost, sparse availability, and need of expertise make it less useful in clinical practice.

Indirect Immunoperoxidase Assay

Indirect immunoperoxidase assay (IPA) is similar to IFA in all respects such as sensitivity, specificity, and disadvantages.

Polymerase Chain Reaction

Polymerase chain reaction (PCR) based tests detect the rickettsial DNA in a given sample. These tests are useful diagnostic tests during the first week of the illness before there is seroconversion as well as even after the antibiotic usage. They have good specificity as well as sensitivity. Apart from blood, they can be done on CSF and eschar. Other advantages are rapidity, reproducibility, quantitative capability, and low risk of contamination. But the major disadvantage is availability at only a handful research labs.

CASE DEFINITIONS

A *suspected case* is the one which has a compatible case scenario with the patient coming from the endemic region in the absence of definitive alternate diagnosis.

If there is rapid (<48 hours) defervescence of illness with antirickettsial therapy or eschar, suggestive laboratory evidence, positive Weil-Felix test, or positive rickettsia IgM in a suspected case, it is termed as *probable case.*

A *suspected case* is said to be a confirmed case, when it shows a four-fold rise on acute and convalescent sera detected by IFA or immunoperoxidase assay (IPA) or detection of the rickettsial DNA in whole blood or tissue samples.

TREATMENT

Antibiotics are the mainstay of the treatment. Institution of treatment should never be withheld while awaiting results of investigations. A delay in starting treatment is associated with a significant increase in complications and mortality.

Doxycycline is the drug of the choice for all types of rickettsial infections. It is given in the dose of 2.2 mg/kg twice daily (max 200 mg) IV or orally. The IV route is preferred in comatose patients or patients with altered gastrointestinal (GI) aspirates or vomiting. The duration is usually 5–7 days or minimum 3 days after the subsidence of the fever. Response to treatment is dramatic and fever abates in less than 48 hours. This is another retrospective evidence of the correct diagnosis. A delayed response is usually seen in children in whom treatment is started late or there are associated complications. Persistence of fever even after 48 hours of starting therapy should prompt the physician to revise his/her provisional diagnosis of rickettsial fever. Rarely, there can be doxycycline resistance where alternate drugs can be used. The use of doxycycline in younger children is safe and is proven in recent studies.

Chloramphenicol is the alternate drug most commonly used when the child is allergic to doxycycline. On rare occasions, there can be bone marrow depression. Other alternatives are azithromycin and clarithromycin. Fluoroquinolones are not used in the pediatric population.

Antirickettsial antibiotics are summarized in **Table 4.**

Treatment of the Complications

Meningoencephalitis needs treatment with antiepileptics, anticerebral edema measures, and maintenance of airway. ARDS needs mechanical ventilation with smaller tidal volumes, judicial use of positive end-expiratory pressure (PEEP), and tight fluid balance. Bleeding manifestations may be because of thrombocytopenia or coagulopathy. Appropriate blood component replacement should be done. Packed red blood cell transfusion should be done to maintain Hb above 10 g/dL. AKI should be treated with fluid restriction or resuscitation depending on the type of AKI. The child may need hemodialysis or peritoneal dialysis. There is no specific treatment for myocarditis and should be treated with inotropes and other symptomatic measures.

Table 4: Summary of antirickettsial drugs.

Name of drug	Dose, route, and duration	Comments
Doxycycline	2.2 mg/kg/dose BD per oral or IV (max 200 mg) 5–7 days or for at least 3 days until the patient is afebrile	• Drug of choice • Rapidly defervesce within 48 hours • IV formulation for sick patients
Tetracycline	25–50 mg/kg/dose every 6 hourly per oral (max 2 g/day) 5–7 days or for at least 3 days until the patient is afebrile	• Rapidly defervesce within 48 hours • IV formulation for sick patients
Chloramphenicol	50–100 mg/kg/day every 6 hourly (max 3 g/day) 5–7 days or for at least 3 days until the patient is afebrile	• Most common alternative for tetracycline • Most common adverse effect is agranulocytosis
Azithromycin	10 mg/kg/day once daily (max 500 mg) 5–7 days or for at least 3 days until the patient is afebrile	• Preferred drug in pregnancy • Recommended when doxycycline resistance is present
Clarithromycin	15 mg/kg /day BD 5–7 days or for at least 3 days until the patient is afebrile	
Rifampicin	10 mg/kg Maximum is 300 mg 5–7 days or for at least 3 days until the patient is afebrile	• Doxycycline resistance cases • Shorter duration of fever with rifampicin in northern Thailand when compared with doxycycline
Fluoroquinolones	Not recommended in the pediatric age group	

PROGNOSIS

The earlier the diagnosis and institution of the treatment, the better he prognosis. A delay in diagnosis or treatment invariably means a complication, death, or long-term sequelae. The markers of poor prognosis are as follows:

- Age of the patient (younger age)
- Male gender
- Shorter incubation period
- Absence of rash
- *Comorbidities such as*:
  - Diabetes
  - Cardiovascular disease
  - G6PD deficiency
- Treatment with sulfonamides.

Oxidative stress is one of the mechanisms of cellular damage in rickettsial infection. Poor prognosis is seen with the drugs that cause increase in oxidative stress like sulfonamides. G6PD is a component of protective mechanism that handles antioxidant stress and its deficiency leads to fulminant disease.

PREVENTION

Availability of effective chemotherapy made scientist lose interest in the development of vaccine and hence no effective vaccine is available. There is no role of postexposure prophylaxis. The mainstay of the prevention is control of the vectors, prevention of bites, and prompt removal of the vector. The vectors can be controlled by controlling the rodents, chopping or burning the vegetations, and spraying of insecticides. Vector bite can be prevented by avoiding the visit to the endemic area. Other measures can be using long sleeves and light-colored clothes, spraying clothes with insecticides, and regularly inspecting for attachment of vectors. Tucking pants inside the shoes is not a fashion statement but a preventive measure from tick bites. Hot water bath removes ticks. Ticks require minimum 4–6 hours of attachment before they can transmit infection; hence, removing the tick immediately after its attachment is important. A tweezer should always be used for removal and should be done by holding the head of the tick as close to skin as possible. Washing the area with soap and water is recommended as the residual part or saliva of tick can be infective and can transmit the infection.

SUGGESTED READING

1. Biggs HM, Behravesh CB, Bradley KK, et al. Diagnosis and management of tickborne rickettsial diseases, CDC. MMWR Recomm Rep. 2016;65(2):1-44.
2. Dasari V, Kaur P, Murhekar MV. Rickettsial disease outbreaks in India: a review. Ann Trop Med Public Health. 2014;7(6): 249-54.
3. Kulkarni A, Vaidya S, Kulkarni P, et al. Rickettsial disease: an experience. Pediatr Infect Dis. 2009;1:118-24.
4. Kulkarni A. Childhood rickettsiosis. Indian J Pediatr. 2011; 78(1):81-7.
5. Kulkarni A. Rickettsial infections. IAP Textbook of Infectious Diseases, 1st edition. New Delhi: Jaypee Brothers Medical Publishers; 2013. pp. 376-85.
6. Mahajan SK. Rickettsial diseases. J Assoc Physicians India. 2012;60:37-43.
7. Martinez JJ, Cossart P. Early signaling events involved in the entry of Rickettsia conorii into mammalian cells. J Cell Sci. 2004;117(Pt 21):5097-106.
8. Paul ML, Ross MJ. Rickettsial and ehrlichia diseases. In: Cherry J, Demmler-Harrison GJ, Kaplan SL, Steinbach W, Hotez P (Eds). Feigin and Cherry's Textbook of Pediatric Infectious Diseases, 7th edition. New York: Saunders Elsevier; 2013. pp. 2647-66.
9. Prakash JA, Sohan Lal T, Rosemol V, et al. Molecular detection and analysis of spotted fever group Rickettsia in patients with fever and rash at a tertiary care centre in Tamil Nadu, India. Pathog Glob Health. 2012;106(1):40-5.
10. Rahi M, Gupte MD, Bhargava A, et al. DHR-ICMR guidelines for diagnosis and management of rickettsial diseases in India. Indian J Med Res. 2015;141(4):417-22.
11. Rathi N, Kulkarni A, Yewale V. IAP guidelines on rickettsial diseases in children. Indian Pediatr. 2017;54(3):223-9.
12. Rathi N, Maheshwari M, Khandelwal R. Neurological manifestations of rickettsial infections in children. Pediatr Infect Dis. 2016;7:64-6.
13. Rathi N, Rathi A. Rickettsial infections: Indian perspective. Indian Pediatr. 2010;47(2):157-64.
14. Todd SR, Dahlgren FS, Traeger MS, et al. No visible dental staining in children treated with doxycycline for suspected Rocky Mountain spotted fever. J Pediatr. 2015;166(5):1246-51.

5

Mycobacterial Infections

Abhay K Shah

Tuberculosis in Children

Varinder Singh, Vijay Yewale

INTRODUCTION

Tuberculosis (TB) is one of the top 10 causes of death worldwide. Nearly one fourth of the world's population is infected with *Mycobacterium tuberculosis* (*MTB*) and at risk of developing disease. The target 3.3 of the Sustained Development Goals (SDGs) is to end TB endemic by 2030 by reducing TB deaths by 90% and TB incidence rate by 80%. India has set an ambitious agenda of TB elimination by 2025.[1]

BURDEN OF DISEASE

It is estimated that world had 10 million TB cases in year 2018, of which 11% were among children and 8.6% among people living with HIV. About 2.2 lakh new cases are estimated to be occurring in children as per the Global TB report 2018 with a slightly higher burden among males. India contributes 27% of the global TB burden, while 10% of cases reported to the RNTCP (Revised National Tuberculosis Control Program) occur in children below 14 years. The exact burden of TB among children is not known. Direct measurements of TB incidence at national levels are challenging and cost intensive requiring enrolment and follow-up of hundreds of thousands of people. Notified cases can be taken as a proxy indicator of TB incidence, provided the surveillance system is of high performing standards. About 55% of estimated TB in children is not reported to the national TB programs and thus the estimates are likely to be underestimates. However, there has been an increase in reporting of cases to the RNTCP in the recent years. Though pulmonary TB is the most common form in children, extrapulmonary TB (EPTB) forms a larger proportion of cases than in adults.[2]

THE *BACILLUS*

Tubercle bacilli belong to the order Actinomycetales and family Mycobacteriaceae. There are five bacilli closely related to mycobacteria—*MTB, M. bovis, M. africanum, M. microti, and M. canetti. MTB* is the most common cause of human disease, and *M. bovis* and *M. africanum* are other rare causes. The aerobic, nonspore forming, nonmotile, acid-fast, slow-growing bacillus of *MTB* has a generation time of 12–24 hours. It can survive under adverse environmental conditions.

NATURAL HISTORY OF DISEASE

Tuberculosis is an airborne disease which is transmitted by inhalation of airborne mucus droplet nuclei of 1–5 µm size usually containing 1–10 bacilli. The number and virulence of bacilli of the source case determines the spread of disease. About 5–200 inhaled bacilli are usually needed for transmission of infection. Cavitary lesions have highest bacillary load while it varies with the type of lesion in the source case. Thus, the risk of infection is higher in persons in contact with a sputum smear-positive case as compared to a sputum smear-negative case. Poor air circulation and overcrowded environment facilitate transmission. Young children with primary form of TB may have very few bacilli in the respiratory secretions. Similarly, antitubercular treatment reduces the bacillary load thereby reducing the risk of transmission of infection to the contacts. *M. bovis* infection can occur following the consumption of large bacillary load in unpasteurized milk through oropharyngeal lymphoid tissue or gastrointestinal mucosa.[3]

There are three stages of TB, namely exposure, infection, and disease. In children, the infection to disease may be a continuum and clinical manifestation can vary. The outcome of tubercular infection is largely determined by the interplay between the mycobacterial virulence and the host immunity. The cell-mediated immunity (CMI) enhances intracellular killing and hypersensitivity promotes extracellular killing. The disease process varies as low bacillary load (antigen load) with high CMI leads to granuloma formation, high degree of tissue sensitivity in presence of high antigen load promotes caseation, and low tissue hypersensitivity in infants and immunocompromised children leads to failure of containment of the disease. The complex interaction between the bacillus and the host immunity determines the transition from a latent infection to a primary complex to a progressive disease and/or reactivation of the latent infection to disease as the child grows.

The risk of progression of the TB infection to disease decreases with age. There is a life-time risk of 5–10% with the highest risk of >50% in infants and 25% in 1–5 years. The least risk of breakdown is during the school age and it again increases during adolescence. Apart from the age, malnutrition, HIV–TB coinfection, post-measles state, and diabetes result in an increased risk of progression. Lack of treatment of latent infection and absence of BCG vaccination also increase the risk of disease in an individual.[3]

Inhaled bacilli multiply in the alveoli; most of them get killed but a few survive in the macrophages. Macrophages are activated by CD4 helper T and bacilli are killed with epithelioid granuloma formation. Caseation occurs when CD8 suppressor T cells lyse the macrophages infected with the mycobacteria. Bacilli are carried to the regional lymph nodes and tissue hypersensitivity sets in 2–12 weeks. Healing in the regional lymph nodes is less complete as compared to the parenchymal lesion. The affected lymph nodes can enlarge and compress the bronchus leading to hyperinflation or atelectasis or it may erode into the bronchus and cause endobronchial spread of disease leading to bronchopneumonia, consolidation, and/or collapse. Subpleural focus rupturing into the pleural space may lead to pleural effusion or empyema. Lymphohematogenous dissemination of the mycobacteria leads to involvement of other lymph nodes, the kidney, epiphyses of long bones, vertebral bodies, and juxta-ependymal meninges adjacent to the subarachnoid space and, occasionally, to the apical posterior areas of the lungs. Disseminated TB disease manifests when the bacillary load is very high and the host immune response is inadequate. Mycobacteria is a very recalcitrant agent and may remain dormant in these foci for years and can cause reactivation disease later in life.

In endemic regions, recurrent infection is probably more common than reactivation of old primary disease.

◼ DIAGNOSIS OF TUBERCULOSIS

Like for any other infectious disease, the early and accurate diagnosis followed by prompt appropriate treatment is crucial to control and end TB. Demonstration of acid-fast bacilli (AFB) under the microscope by Ziehl-Neelsen (ZN) staining of smear of an appropriate sample such as sputum or GA or isolation of the *MTB* on culture has been the conventional gold standard tools for TB diagnosis. Low sensitivity of these tests, difficulty in obtaining appropriate specimen, and lack of adequate laboratory facilities made these tools less useful in diagnosis of Pediatric TB. This has more recently changed with the availability of faster turnaround liquid cultures such as *Mycobacterium* Growth Indicator Tube™ (MGIT™) and development of newer generation rapid molecular tests such as cartridge-base Xpert Rif™ (Cepheid Inc USA) and chip-based nucleic acid amplification test TrueNAT™ (Molbio, India). The molecular tests also make it possible to identify the presence of rifampicin resistant when *MTB* is detected in a specimen, thus guiding the choice of therapy. The tests for resistance to other drugs remains technically more challenging.

When Do We Suspect TB Disease?

Pediatric TB can have symptoms overlapping with other common illnesses. Proper symptom characterization is the important initial step in the diagnosis of TB.

Presumptive pulmonary TB refers to children with persistent documented fever and/or unremitting cough for more than 2 weeks, loss of weight/no weight gain (5% or more as compared to the highest weight recorded in past 3 months) and/or history of contact with infectious TB cases. In a symptomatic child, contact with a person with any form of active TB within last 2 years may be a significant clue.

Presumptive EPTB refers to the presence of organ-specific symptoms and signs such as swelling of lymph nodes, pain and swelling in joints, neck stiffness, and disorientation and/or constitutional symptoms such as significant weight loss, persistent fever for >2 weeks, and night sweats.

Presumptive drug-resistant (DR) TB refers to those TB patients who have failed treatment with first-line drugs, pediatric TB nonresponders, previously treated cases, or cases who are exposed to a source with known DR TB (or rifampicin resistance) or likely DR TB (death of the source case due to TB).

In children with presumptive pediatric TB, every attempt must be made to microbiologically prove diagnosis through examination of appropriate respiratory/nonrespiratory specimens with quality-assured diagnostic tests. RNTCP-approved rapid tests such as cartridge- or chip-based nucleic acid amplification test (NAAT) is preferred over the conventional ZN staining due to its almost three times higher sensitivity. In addition, as the country is moving toward elimination of TB, optimized therapy based on drug sensitivity to key drug such as rifampicin is the current standard of care (called strategy of universal drug sensitivity testing or U-DST).

Xpert Rif[TM] is a nested NAAT which provides information about both the presence of the bacilli and the resistance to rifampicin. With a turnaround time of less than 2 hours, and higher sensitivity than ZN smear (100 bacilli per mL vs 1,000 bacilli per mL), it has added an important tool for the definitive diagnosis. It can be used on respiratory as well as nonrespiratory specimens [gastric aspirate (GA), bronchoalveolar lavage (BAL), induced sputum (IS), pleural fluid, cerebrospinal fluid (CSF), lymph node aspirate, etc.]. The sensitivity and specificity of cartridge based nucleic acid amplification test (CBNAAT) in sputum samples is around 98% and 99%, respectively, for smear-positive patients and 72% for smear-negative culture positive patients. The sensitivity and specificity on GA have been 68% and 99%, respectively. Xpert Ultra[TM] has sensitivity higher than the Xpert Rif[TM] equaling the yield of TB culture. However, this still falls short for the expectations of a clinician as TB culture has a sensitivity of 40–50% and sensitivity of CBNAAT is close to culture, and hence a negative test does not rule out TB. Further, CBNAAT performs equally well with CSF and lymph node aspirates but its yield is very poor with pleural or ascitic fluid.[4]

Liquid cultures by MGIT[TM] have reduced the time to grow TB bacilli (10–15 days to grow and 10–14 days for drug sensitivity) and have replaced the traditional solid culture on LJ (Löwenstein–Jensen) media. They are done for all presumptive DR TB cases at present and where resources permit, may be done on all CBNAAT-negative clinically diagnosed TB cases too. Line probe assays (LPAs) for first-line as well as second-line drugs can be used for drug sensitivity once the organism is isolated for rapid turnaround. Phenotypic drug sensitivity testing can also be carried out on the bacilli grown on liquid cultures. LPA approved by the WHO (World Health Organization) and used under RNTCP is GenoType MTBDR plus[TM] (Hain Lifescience, Germany). It can simultaneously detect presence of *MTB* and mutations associated with resistance to rifampicin and isoniazid (INH) (*katG* as well as *inhA*). It offers a rapid turnaround time of about 2 days on smear-positive samples or on culture isolates from any sample. The WHO-approved LPA testing for second-line drugs (GenoType MTBDRsl[TM], Hain Lifescience, Germany) primarily tests for class resistance to fluoroquinolones and second-line injectable drugs. It is recommended for all specimens showing rifampicin resistance.[5]

Unfortunately, despite the gains in sensitivity with newer tests, it can still miss a little over 50% of cases.

Conventional chest imaging is an important tool in TB diagnosis, especially when there is no microbiological confirmation of the disease. A good quality well-centralized inspiratory film with proper exposure without motion artefact can be a good aid in the diagnosis of TB. Miliary pattern, hilar and/or paratracheal lymphadenopathy, and fibrocavitary lesions are highly suggestive of TB in a presumptive TB setting. All presumptive TB cases with these X-ray features are probable TB cases and must be subjected to microbiological testing. The yield to effort improves considerably if the microbiological testing of respiratory specimens is directed by the presence of lesion on chest skiagram. Consolidations, nonhomogeneous opacity/infiltrates, thin-walled cavities, etc. are considered nonspecific shadows and are subjected to a trial of appropriate antibiotic. Nonresolving lesions despite appropriate antibiotic treatment in a child with TB suggestive symptomatology should further be subjected to molecular or bacteriological testing on another appropriate sample such as (induced or self-expectorated) sputum or GA.[6]

Other imaging techniques such as ultrasonography (USG) of chest have a place in diagnosing the presence and localization of pleural fluid. This tool can also be used for guided aspiration of a peripheral or deep-seated lymph node. It is a useful tool to differentiate thymic shadow from a mediastinal lymph node.

Computed tomography (CT) scan is requisitioned when evaluating a persistent pneumonia and yields information such as necrotic mediastinal lymph node, cavity with surrounding consolidation, or centrilobular nodules with a tree-in-bud pattern suggesting bronchiectasis highly indicative of TB. Mediastinal lymph node biopsy can be done under CT guidance. This tool should be used judiciously when conventional modalities with much less radiation fail to help. Neuroimaging with CECT (contrast-enhanced CT) and/or MRI (magnetic resonance imaging) play a more critical role for intracranial TB and is recommended.

Revised national tuberculosis control program–Indian academy of pediatrics algorithm[6] for diagnosis of intrathoracic TB among children is given in **Flowchart 1**. Important companion notes to the RNTCP–IAP diagnostic algorithm are listed in **Box 1**.

Diagnosis of Extrapulmonary Tuberculosis

Extrapulmonary TB is more common in children and develops in 25–30% of children with TB. Appropriate specimens from the sites of involvement must be obtained from all the presumptive EPTB patients for CBNAAT/smear microscopy/culture and drug-susceptibility testing (DST) for *MTB* and/or histopathological examination (HPE), etc. based on type of specimen and availability of facilities.

Sensitivity of CBNAAT is lower in pericardial, ascitic, and synovial fluid samples and more lower in pleural fluid. Examination of the body fluids such as pleural, or pericardial, or CSF fluid is important to make diagnosis of the TB in the involved organ system. Aspirated fluid should be examined for biochemical, cytological, and AFB smear by ZN stain to confirm the diagnosis. Typically, a tubercular effusion fluid is straw colored and has large numbers of cells (in hundreds; predominantly mononuclear) with high proteins (>3 g/dL) that are responsible for cobweb formation on standing.

Adenosine deaminase activity (ADA) has limited utility in the diagnosis of any effusion in children as data on comparison of ADA between tubercular and other bacterial effusion indicate a significant overlap in ADA values.

Culture yield of pleural fluid is very low, 5%, but about 28% of pleural effusion patients grow TB bacilli on culture of GA or IS. CBNAAT on pleural fluid has low sensitivity. Pleural biopsy with Cope's needle or Abraham's biopsy needle may be done and the tissue is examined for histopathology, AFB staining, and MGIT culture. It has a high sensitivity of 80%. The findings of granulomas with caseous necrotic tissue in the pleural biopsy make the diagnosis of TB highly probable.

Flowchart 1: RNTCP–IAP algorithm for diagnosis of intrathoracic TB among children.[6]

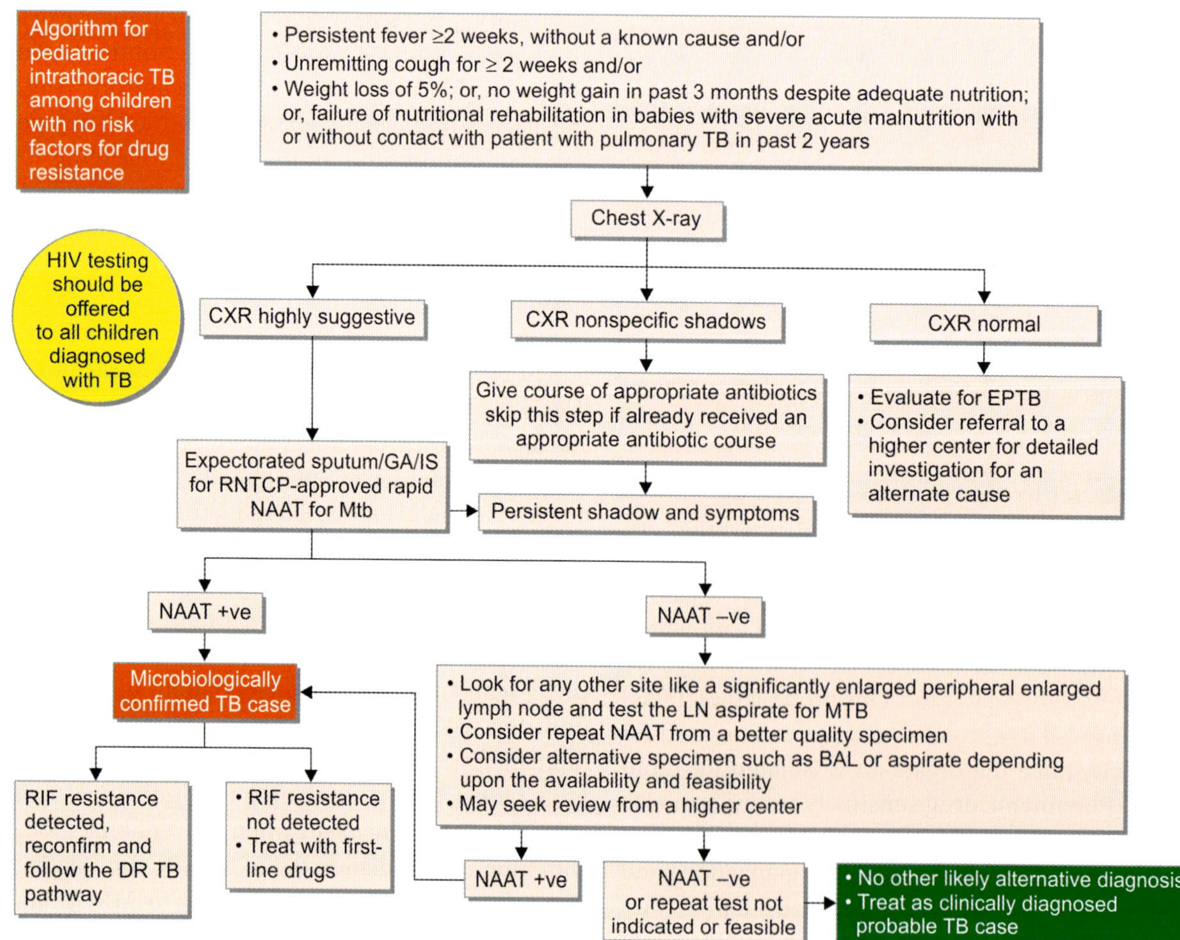

(CXR: chest X-ray; DR TB: drug-resistant TB; EPTB: extrapulmonary TB; GA: gastric aspirate; IS: induced sputum; LN: lymph node; NAAT: nucleic acid amplification test; *MTB: Mycobacterium tuberculosis*; RNTCP-IAP: Revised National Tuberculosis Control Program-Indian Academy of Pediatrics; TB: tuberculosis; BAL: bronchoalveolar lavage; RIF: rifampicin)

> **Box 1:** Important companion notes to the RNTCP-IAP diagnostic algorithm.
>
> - Chest X-ray shall be done upfront in cases who are suspected to have TB:
>   - If a recent good quality chest X-ray is available, it need not be repeated
> - Highly suggestive chest X-ray refers to miliary shadows, or lymphadenopathy (hilar or mediastinal), or chronic fibrocavitary shadows
> - Nonspecific chest X-ray: Refer to patterns other than highly suggestive like consolidations, in-homogenous shadows or bronchopneumonia, etc.
> - Molecular methods such as RNTCP-approved NAAT shall be preferred over smear examination in all childhood specimens:
>   - Available RNTCP-approved NAAT includes cartridge or chip-based rapid tests [Xpert Rif™ and TrueNAT™] and line probe assays [GenoType MTBDRplus™]
>   - If a specimen is positive by any of these methods, the case is labeled as microbiologically confirmed TB
>   - At the initial step, If self-expectorated sputum is available and imaging/RNTCP-approved NAAT test is not available or delayed, smear may be done (for ease of availability and low cost). However, these patients still need further testing for drug sensitivity
>   - Whenever smear is used for diagnosis at least two samples should be tested while a single sample is sufficient for more sensitive NAAT
>   - If a specimen is negative by RNTCP-approved NAAT (or smear), the second aliquot or a fresh good quality specimen should be submitted for a repeat NAAT and liquid culture
>   - In case of rifampicin resistance is detected on NAAT, in a new case without any risk factors, reconfirmation by same or different method is desirable
> - Antibiotics of choice include amoxicillin or co-amoxiclav:
>   - Antibiotics like linezolid or any quinolone should not be used as they have anti-TB action
>   - In case antibiotic trial has already been done in adequate dose and duration, it may not be repeated
> - *Clinically diagnosed probable TB case*: Is a patient with a high clinical suspicion for TB disease based on suggestive symptoms, radiology, and often supportive circumstances (history of exposure to a TB case) or evidence of infection (positive skin test for TB or positive IGRA) *but* the rapid microbiological tests are negative. Such a case may be treated as clinically diagnosed patient provided common alternative diagnoses have been ruled out:
>   - Where facilities exist, send one aliquot of the specimen for liquid culture, if the CBNAAT is negative for *MTB*.

(CBNAAT: cartridge-based nucleic acid amplification test; TB: tuberculosis; *MTB: Mycobacterium tuberculosis;* RNTCP: Revised National Tuberculosis Control Program; NAAT: nucleic acid amplification test; IAP: Indian Academy of Pediatrics; IGRA: interferon gamma release assays)

Tubercular Meningitis

Diagnosis of tubercular meningitis (TBM) can be challenging and requires a high index of suspicion. CSF picture may resemble that of aseptic meningitis in stage 1. Later, the CSF shows a cell count of 10–500 cells/mm^3. Polymorphonuclear (PMN) cells may be seen early in the illness but it is mainly lymphocytic. CSF glucose usually remains below 40 mg/dL (CSF glucose/blood glucose below 0.5, protein is elevated (more than 100 mg/dL). Tuberculin skin test (TST) may be nonreactive in half of the cases and about 20–50% cases have a normal X-ray chest. MRI is the preferred neuroimaging modality, but when not available, CECT head may be done. The neuroimaging may be normal in initial stages but as the disease progresses, basilar enhancement, communication hydrocephalus, cerebral edema, and focal ischemia may be seen. *Cryptococcal meningitis, cytomegalovirus (CMV) encephalitis, toxoplasmosis, sarcoidosis, meningeal metastases, and lymphoma* can have similar radiological findings.

Abdominal Tuberculosis

Abdominal TB is caused by hematogenous dissemination or swallowing of TB bacilli from the active lung lesion, by ingestion of contaminated milk, or from contiguous spreads from adjacent organs. Lymphadenopathy, peritoneal thickening, omental thickening and bowel wall thickening,

and ascites may be seen on USG abdomen. A reactive TST and mesenteric lymphadenopathy in a child with recurrent abdominal pain are not to be taken as confirmatory diagnosis of abdominal TB as they usually do not cause isolated recurrent or chronic abdominal pain without any other clinical feature. CECT and CT enterography give useful information on the different organ involvement. However, tissue diagnosis is the gold standard and can be achieved by various endoscopic procedures.

Others

In Pott's spine, plain X-ray of the spine may be abnormal only when 30–50% of bone loss has occurred. It shows endplate erosion, decreased height of vertebra, and collapse and narrowing of discal space and paravertebral soft tissue shadow. MRI is most sensitive (nearly 100%). The features in MRI are marrow edema, destruction of adjacent vertebral bodies, and opposing endplates, destruction of intervening disk, occurrence of prevertebral, paravertebral, and epidural abscesses. Microbiology should always be attempted for definitive diagnosis and to pick up multidrug-resistant (MDR)-TB.

In all cases of EPTB, one should look for coexistence of pulmonary TB. If surgery is not planned, then CT-guided biopsy of the paravertebral soft tissue/vertebral body

Table 1: Recommended drug regimens for managing childhood tuberculosis (TB).

Type of patient*	Regimen
New microbiologically confirmed pulmonary TB New clinically diagnosed pulmonary TB New microbiologically confirmed extrapulmonary TB New clinically diagnosed extrapulmonary TB Drug-sensitive previously treated TB[‡] (recurrence, treatment after loss to follow-up, and treatment after failure)	2HRZE+4HRE[†]

*Molecular testing shall be done in all new cases in children with suspected TB at diagnosis
[†]In case of neuro and spinal TB the continuation phase is extended to 10 months
[‡]All these category of children shall be evaluated as DR TB suspects and evaluated as per DR TB algorithm. DST based treatment shall be followed. In case they are found to be drug sensitive they shall be started on the above regimen as for a new case. This group was earlier treated with CAT II regimen which is now withdrawn

Table 2: Antituberculosis drug dosages for children.

		Range (mg/kg/d)	Average (mg/kg/d)	Maximum dose (mg)
Rifampicin	R	10–20	15	600
Isoniazid	H	7–15	10	300
Pyrazinamide	Z	30–40	35	2,000
Ethambutol	E	15–25	20	1,500
Streptomycin	S	15–20	20	1,000

Table 3: Regimens for drug-resistant tuberculosis (TB) case (0–18 years).

Type of TB case	Treatment regimen	Special considerations
RR/MDR-TB without additional drug-resistance to FQ and/or SLI (conventional short regimen—initial regime for pulmonary and isolated PE or LN TB)	*Intensive phase:* (4–6) Mfx[h] Km Eto Cfz Z H[h] E *Continuation phase:* (5) Mfx[h] Cfz Z E	• For pulmonary cases or isolated lymph node disease or pleural effusion • Nonexposure to reserve drugs
MDR TB/MDR TB + FQ resistance/XDR-TB (all oral regime for children above 6 years)	*Intensive phase:* 6–8 Dlm (Bdq) (6) Lf (Mfx[h]) Lzd Cfz Cs *Continuation phase:* 12 Lf (Mfx[h]) Lzd (l) Cfz Cs	• Not for EPTB other than isolated lymph node disease or pleural effusion • Not for children under 6 years • Bdq to be replaced by Dlm between 6 years and 17 years age • Lf to be replaced by Mfxh if FQ class resistance
MDR TB(EP)/MDR TB + FQ resistance/XDR-TB and Not eligible for all oral regime above	*Intensive phase:* (6–9) Amika, Mfx[h] Lzd Cfz Eto Cs *Continuation phase:* (18) Mfx[h] Lzd (l) Cfz Cs	Disseminated or severe extrapulmonary disease
Resistance to INH with or without any nonrifampicin first-line drug-resistance	(6) Lfx R E Z Uniphasic regime	• Can be extended to 9–12 months in • Extensive pulmonary disease • Extensive pulmonary • Extrapulmonary disease such as bone or intracranial

Note: Levofloxacin (Lf) 15–20 mg/kg/d; Moxifloxacin (Mfx) 10 mg/kg/d and high dose (Mfx[h]) 15 mg/kg/d; Linezolid (LZ) <6 years age: 10–12 mg/kg/d; >6 years age: 15 mg/kg/d; Clofazimine (Cfz) 2–5 mg/kg/d; Ethionamide (Eto) 15–20 mg/kg/d; Cycloserine (Cs) 15–20 mg/kg/d; High dose INH (H[h]) 15–20 mg/kg/d; Delamanid (Dlm) 6–11 years: 50 mg BD, 12–17 years: 100 mg BD; Ethambutol (E) 15–25 mg/kg/d; Pyrazinamide (Z) 30–40 mg/kg/d
(FQ: fluoroquinolones; MDR: multidrug-resistant; RR: rifampicin resistant; SLI: second-line injectable drugs; XDR: extensively drug-resistant; LN: lymph node; EPTB: extrapulmonary tuberculosis)

should be carried out and should be subjected to HPE, or culture, or CBNAAT. Diagnostic yield will vary in various methods from 50% to 70%.

■ TREATMENT OF TUBERCULOSIS

Conventionally, the treatment of TB is done with standardized regimes for new and retreatment cases. But currently as every case of childhood TB now gets upfront testing for rifampin resistance under the U-DST and all retreatment cases get tested for at least INH resistance in addition, the standardized regimes have now undergone a change. The currently recommended treatment[5,6] regimens for drug-sensitive disease (rifampicin and/or INH) or a new case with low probability of drug-resistant TB are as given in **Table 1**. Drug dosages for the first-line drugs for treating children with TB are given in **Table 2**.

A note should be made that now fixed-drug combinations (FDCs) with revised proportions are recommended and many of the existing FDC products may not provide the right rational dose.

Further, the experts recommend pyridoxine supplementation (10 mg/d) to all those receiving INH therapy. Low cost, safety, and lack of any interference with INH action in the small prophylactic dose used favor its use for its potential benefit for covering the risk of babies getting peripheral neuropathy with INH with a coexisting malnutrition. Otherwise, no supplemental treatment in form of multivitamin or multimineral is advised as there is no evidence of any of these improving the outcome among these patients. The recommended regimens for drug-resistant TB among children are detailed in **Table 3**.

■ REFERENCES

1. World Health Organization. (2019). Global Tuberculosis Report 2019. [online] Available from: https://www.who.int/tb/global-report-2019. [Last accessed on December, 2019].
2. World Health Organization. New roadmap towards ending TB in children and adolescents; 2018. [online] Available from: https://www.who.int/tb/features_archive/new-roadmap-to-end-child-adolescent-TB-deaths/en/. [Last accessed on December, 2019].
3. Marais BJ, Schaaf HS. Tuberculosis in children. Cold Spring Harb Perspect Med. 2014;4(9):a017855.
4. World Health Organization. Automated real-time nucleic acid amplification technology for rapid and simultaneous detection of tuberculosis and rifampicin resistance: Xpert MTB/RIF assay for the diagnosis of pulmonary and extrapulmonary TB in adults and children. Policy update; 2013. [online]. Available from: https://apps.who.int/iris/handle/10665/112472. [Last accessed on December, 2019].
5. Central Tuberculosis Division, Ministry of Health & Family Welfare. Government of India. Technical and Operational Guidelines for TB Control in India 2016. [online] Available from: https://tbcindia.gov.in/index1.php?sublinkid=4573&level=2&lid=3177&lang=1. [Last accessed on December, 2019].
6. Indian Academy of Pediatrics. (2019). RNTCP-IAP Updated Pediatric Tuberculosis Guideline 2019. [online] Available from: https://indianpediatrics.net/aug2019/692-693.pdf. [Last accessed on December, 2019].

Nontuberculous Mycobacterial Infection in Children

Tanu Singhal

CASE VIGNETTE

A 10-year-old previously healthy girl presents with a rapidly enlarging right submandibular swelling for the past 1 month. The family of Indian origin has recently relocated from the US about 6 months ago. She does not have any systemic complaints. The fine-needle aspiration cytology (FNAC) shows some ill-defined granulomas. She undergoes excision biopsy of one node which shows necrotizing granulomas that are smear positive for acid-fast bacilli (AFB). The Xpert Mycobacterium tuberculosis/rifampicin (MTB/RIF) is negative. The chest X-ray (CXR) is normal and Mantoux is positive with 12-mm induration. Eight days later, the MGIT (mycobacterial growth indicator tube) culture grows AFB that are MPT64 negative. The Hain line probe assay identified the mycobacteria as *M. abscessus*. It was sent for susceptibility testing and the patient was started on treatment with clarithromycin and linezolid. Susceptibility testing showed that the isolate was sensitive to only clarithromycin, amikacin and linezolid and resistant to other drugs including imipenem, quinolones and tetracyclines. There was complete resolution of the adenitis over 1 month of therapy and treatment was stopped at 3 months.

This case describes a child with nontuberculous mycobacterial (NTM) lymphadenitis, an infrequently reported cause of cervical adenitis in India. The species of NTM implicated is also an unusual cause of NTM adenitis. This case sets the scene for discussing NTM infections in children.

INTRODUCTION

The mycobacterial genus is divided into three main categories: *M. tuberculosis* complex (MTB complex) (comprised mainly of *M. tuberculosis* and *M. bovis*), *M. leprae* and the nontuberculous mycobacteria. NTM previously termed as atypical mycobacteria/environmental mycobacteria are acid-fast bacilli commonly found in the environment and infrequently cause human disease. There is limited knowledge and awareness about their role as human pathogens as a result of which they are often confused with *M. tuberculosis* and treated as such. Paradoxically, there is also a risk of overdiagnosis since they may contaminate clinical samples. This chapter gives a bird's eye view of their clinical importance in children.

ETIOLOGY

There are more than 180 species of NTM discovered till date and new ones are constantly being identified. There is geographical variation in the distribution of NTM with different species predominating in different countries, *M. kansasii*, *M. scrofulaceum*, *M. fortuitum*, *M. abscessus* among many others. These organisms are found in the environment, most commonly water and soil, and also infect birds, reptiles, and fish. They are sturdy and resistant to common disinfectants including chlorination. They are transmitted to humans by inhalation, ingestion, injection, or inoculation and cause disease only in a fraction of the infected hosts. Person-to-person transmission is very rare and thus they are not usually an infection control issue unlike *M. tuberculosis*.

CLINICAL FEATURES, EPIDEMIOLOGY, AND PATHOGENESIS

Nontuberculous mycobacteria cause specific clinical syndromes in children, namely lymphadenitis, skin and soft-tissue infections, pulmonary disease, and disseminated disease. Lymphadenitis is the most common clinical presentation in children and usually affects immunocompetent children. Skin and soft-tissue infections can occur due to natural infection as in the case of *M. ulcerans* and *M. marinum* or more commonly as surgical site infections/procedure-related infections due to use of inadequately sterilized instruments, needles, and laparoscopes. Pulmonary disease usually affects children with underlying lung disease including bronchiectasis and cystic fibrosis and is relatively less common as compared to their adult counterparts. Disseminated disease is seen in children with advanced HIV infection, cancer, immunocompromised children and those with Mendelian susceptibility to mycobacterial disease (MSMD). Besides this, pseudo-outbreaks due to contamination of bronchoscopes and endoscopes with tap water are not uncommon.

Data about the prevalence and incidence of NTM infection is grossly lacking. This is often because it is not a reportable disease. Most data pertains to adults and not children. Data from highly tuberculosis (TB) endemic and low-resource settings is scarcer. Developed countries including Australia, Sweden, Canada, Netherlands, and Finland have reported an incidence of NTM lymphadenitis as 0.8–1 case/100,000 children. Data from low-resource countries comprises mainly of NTM isolation in respiratory samples tested for TB and here studies indicate that 10–15% of isolates obtained from sputum, gastric lavage of children with suspected TB are NTM. The usual species causing disease in children from developed countries include *M. avium intracellulare complex*, *M. malmoense*, *M. haemophilum*, and *M. lentiflavum* while common species reported from low-resource countries include *M. fortuitum*, *M. szulgai*, and *M. gordonae*.

Transmission to humans is most commonly through inhalation of aerosols contaminated; NTM are frequently isolated from public, hospital and home water systems and shower biofilms. Exposure also occurs through soil and animals. Innate cell-mediated immunity plays an important role in protection against NTM as it is true for TB.

DIAGNOSIS

The diagnosis of NTM is complicated. A single isolation from a sterile site such as blood, body fluid, tissue, lymph node, and surgical specimen should be considered pathogenic. However, if the sample is a nonsterile site such as sputum and bronchoalveolar lavage, only repeated isolation is considered significant. The specimen should be subjected to microscopy, culture, and molecular methods. If the organism burden exceeds 10,000 bacteria per mL, microscopy can show acid-fast bacilli. Though

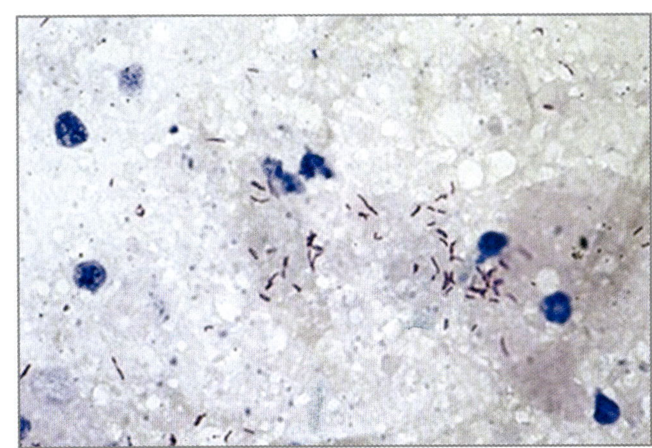

Fig. 1A: Zn stain appearance of NTM. (NTM: nontuberculous mycobacteria)

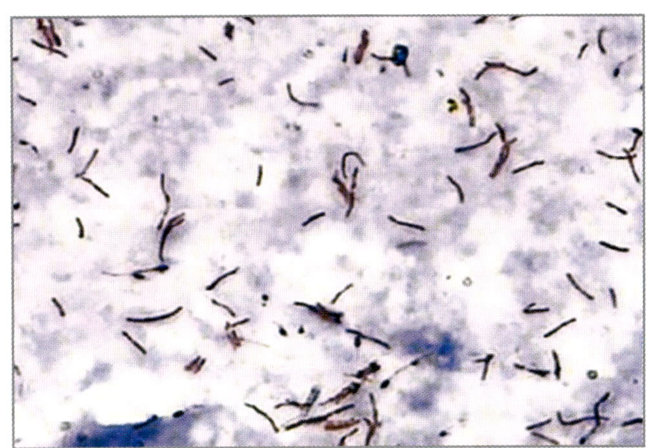

Fig. 1B: Zn stain appearance of MTB. (MTB: *Mycobacterium tuberculosis*)

they are short, thick, and nonbeaded **(Fig. 1A)** unlike MTB which is long and beaded **(Fig. 1B)**, accurate distinction is generally not possible. The sample should be inoculated into both liquid and solid media. The NTM can be separated on the basis of their growth characteristics into rapid grower mycobacteria (RGM, grow within 7 days) or slow growers (those that take more than 7 days). The NTM have exacting growth requirements and some like *M. haemophilum* may need incubation at low temperature of 30°C for isolation. The laboratory must be alerted if NTM are suspected. Once the bacteria grow, the MPT64 can be used as a test to differentiate between MTB complex and NTM (positive in former). The species identification of NTM is challenging. Earlier this was on the basis of colony morphology, pigment, and biochemical characteristics and then by high-performance liquid chromatography (HPLC). Now, species identification is mostly based on molecular methods including use of probes, PCR amplification-restriction analysis, and DNA sequencing. Commercial systems such as Hain's have probe-based assays for identification of the common NTM species and are commonly used in India. Identification of rare species needs DNA sequencing. Another emerging method for NTM identification is MALDI-TOF (Matrix-assisted laser desorption ionization-time of flight analysis). Identification of NTM directly from clinical specimens by molecular methods is also possible and is more sensitive than culture.

Drug susceptibility testing for NTM is still in infancy. It is only validated for certain species and for certain drugs. It is important to test *M. avium* complex (MAC) for macrolide susceptibility and *M. kansasii* for rifampicin susceptibility. Antibiotic susceptibility testing for rapidly growing mycobacteria is also recommended especially to clarithromycin, amikacin, imipenem, doxycycline, quinolones, linezolid, clofazimine, etc.

Tuberculin skin test (TST) may be positive in patients with NTM infection since there is antigenic cross-reactivity between NTM and MTB. However, the interferon gamma release assays (Elispot assay/Quantiferon Gold test) are usually negative in patients with NTM infections. However, *M. kansasii, M. szulgai, M. marinum,* and *M. riyadhense* also express ESAT-6 and CFP-10 antigens and may cause false-positive interferon gamma-release assays. None of these tests (TST/gamma interferon assays) should, however, be used to confirm or refute the diagnosis of NTM infection.

■ TREATMENT

Treatment of NTM infections is multimodality and includes watchful waiting, surgical excision, and medical management. Medical therapy depends on the site of disease and the species. Macrolides, particularly clarithromycin, are the most important component of therapy. Other drugs with efficacy include isoniazid, rifamycins (rifampicin/rifabutin), ethambutol, amino-glycosides, quinolones, linezolid, clofazimine, etc.

■ SYNDROME COMPLEXES

Lymphadenitis

As mentioned earlier, lymphadenitis is the most common manifestation in children. In countries with low TB endemicity, it causes up to 90% of all mycobacterial adenitis; while in highly TB endemic areas such as India, studies show that NTM cause only 10% of all mycobacterial cervical adenitis. The most common causes of NTM lymphadenitis in the developed world are MAC complex,

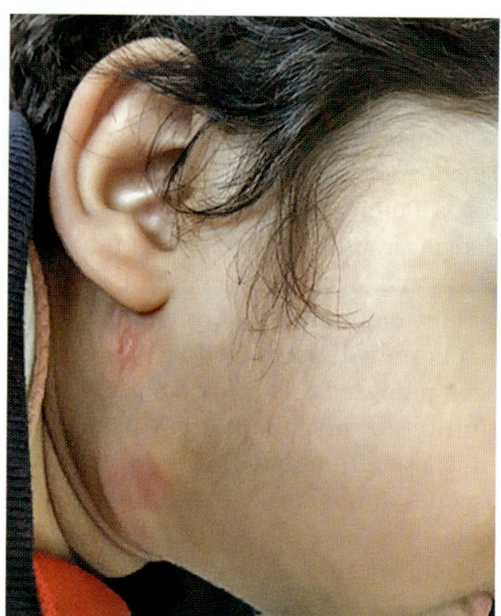

Fig. 2: NTM lymphadenitis.
(NTM: nontuberculous mycobacteria)

M. kansasii, M. scrofulaceum, M. haemophilum, and others. Children infected with *M. haemophilum* tend to be older than those with the MAC. However, in a study from Taiwan, the most common isolates from NTM adenitis were RGM. The index case discussed in the beginning of this chapter also had an RGM, *M. fortuitum* isolated from the lymph node.

The peak age of affection is between the ages of 2 years and 5 years with 50% of children being below 3 years and 80% below 5 years. This is often due to the habit of young children putting objects contaminated with NTM into their mouth. There is usually unilateral involvement of the jugulodigastric **(Fig. 2)**, parotid, preauricular, submandibular, and posterior triangle nodes. There are no systemic symptoms. In contrast, tubercular lymphadenitis usually presents in older children, can be bilateral and may be associated with systemic symptoms. The adenitis may persist for a long time and then regress or may go through the changes seen with tubercular lymphadenitis, namely stage 1 (firm node with increased vascularity), stage 2 (liquefaction), stage 3 (violaceous discoloration over the skin with thinning), and finally stage 4 (fistulization).

Differential diagnosis includes MTB lymphadenitis, nonspecific reactive lymphadenitis, bacterial lympha-denitis, toxoplasma lymphadenitis, lymphoma, and Kikuchi disease.

The diagnosis is established by FNAC or biopsy of the involved nodes. The histopathology shows caseating granulomatous inflammation. The smear may be positive for AFB. The Xpert MTB/RIF is negative. A positive MTB smear with a negative Xpert should make one suspect NTM since the sensitivity of Xpert for MTB in smear-positive samples is more than 99%. Definitive diagnosis is by culture. However, some of the NTM have exacting nutritional requirements and often need to be incubated at low temperatures (30°C), especially for *M. haemophilum*. The sensitivity of cultures is only 50–60%. Molecular diagnosis on the tissue has higher sensitivity but is currently not available in India.

Treatment of choice of NTM adenitis is surgical excision of the nodes. In a randomized controlled trial conducted on 100 children with proven NTM lymphadenitis, surgical excision resulted in cure in 96% of the patients as against 66% who were treated with a medical regime of clarithromycin, rifampicin, and ethambutol. However, surgical excision was associated with certain complications including facial palsy, scar, and disease recurrence. In another large series of NTM lymphadenitis in 107 children from Australia, where 104 children underwent complete excision of the nodes, the incidence of facial palsy was 7.5%. Recurrence rate in the series was almost 20% (2–4 recurrences). The authors demonstrated zero rates of recurrence when children were treated with clarithromycin and rifampicin combination after surgical excision as compared to children who were not given medical therapy or those treated with clarithromycin alone following surgery. The authors postulated that the role of conservative medical treatment as an alternative to surgical excision or as an adjuvant to complete/partial excision should be evaluated further.

The author has experience in treating five children with clinical picture resembling NTM lymphadenitis with histopathology showing caseating granulomas and negative Xpert and culture. These children were treated with a combination of isoniazid, rifampicin, ethambutol, and clarithromycin. This regime was chosen since it would be effective against both MTB and NTM. All children responded with no drug-induced adverse effects and treatment was stopped at 6 months. Three of five children needed a repeat needle aspiration of the node.

Disseminated Disease

Disseminated disease is usually seen in the immuno-compromised including advanced HIV and MSMD. Most MSMD disorders are associated with mutations in IL-12 and gamma interferon pathway. Many of these children die in infancy.

Disseminated NTM infection in HIV-infected children has reduced over time due to advances in antiretroviral therapy (ART) unlike in the pre-ART era where it was only second to *P. jiroveci* as an opportunistic infection in HIV-infected children. The infection usually occurs in older children with severe immunocompromise. It can sometimes affect young children with high CD4 counts. The most common NTM here is MAC complex but can also include *M. simiae* and other NTM. The patients present with a chronic illness including fever, weight loss, night sweats, recurrent or persistent diarrhea, abdominal pain (mimicking appendicitis due to mesenteric lymphadenitis), anemia, hepatosplenomegaly, and generalized lymphadenopathy. The lung is usually spared and respiratory manifestations are infrequent. Investigations reveal pancytopenia, hepatitis [with marked elevation of alkaline phosphatase (SAP) and gamma-glutamyltransferase (GGT) and lesser elevation of aspartate transaminase (AST) and alanine transaminase (ALT)]. Diagnosis can be established by blood/bone marrow cultures or cultures from lymph node/liver/colon biopsies. Blood cultures are positive in >90% of patients with disseminated disease and recovery enhanced by repeated testing, using special Myco/F lytic media and techniques such as lysis centrifugation. Identification can be done by HPLC or molecular probes. Susceptibility testing of MAC to clarithromycin should be done if available. Treatment with combination therapy of macrolide (clarithromycin 7.5–15 mg/kg twice daily, maximum 500 mg twice daily/azithromycin 5 mg/kg once daily, maximum 250 mg) and ethambutol (15–25 mg/kg once daily, maximum 2.5 g) is usually recommended. Studies show that clarithromycin is more efficacious than azithromycin in clearing bacteremia. Azithromycin should only be substituted for clarithromycin if drug interactions or intolerance is a problem. Clarithromycin interacts with many ART regimens. Rifabutin (5 mg/kg once daily with food, maximum 300 mg) is also weakly effective against MAC but is not usually recommended upfront due to its toxicity and interaction with ART. It may be considered in very sick patients with continued immunosuppression and high mycobacterial load. Other drugs that are effective and can be used include quinolones and aminoglycosides in sick/intolerant patients or those with clinical failure/resistance to the first-line drugs. Immune reconstitution syndrome can occur after initiating treatment particularly when ART is started. For this reason, ART should be withheld for at least 2 weeks after initiating anti-NTM therapy. Treatment duration is usually for at least 12 months. For patients with persistent immunosuppression, therapy with the same combination should be continued as secondary prophylaxis. Secondary prophylaxis can be discontinued if all the following criteria are met:

- Aged ≥2 years and have completed ≥12 months of treatment for MAC
- Remain asymptomatic for MAC
- Receiving stable ART (i.e. ART not requiring change for virologic or immunologic failure)
- Have sustained (≥6 months) CD4 count recovery well above the age-specific target for initiation of primary prophylaxis (>100 cells/mm^3 for children aged ≥6 years and >200 cells/mm^3 for children aged 2–6 years).

Primary prophylaxis is indicated for children with low CD4 counts. This cutoff for initiating prophylaxis is 50 in children more than 6 years, 75 in children between 2 years and 6 years, 500 in children aged from 1 to <2 years and 750 in infants below 1 year. Options include weekly azithromycin (20 mg/kg, maximum 1,200 mg) or daily azithromycin (5 mg/kg, maximum 250 mg) or daily clarithromycin (7.5–15 mg/kg twice daily, maximum 500 mg twice daily). Primary prophylaxis can be discontinued in children with HIV infection aged ≥2 years receiving stable ART for ≥6 months and experiencing sustained (>3 months) CD4 count recovery well above the age-specific target for initiation of prophylaxis >100 cells/mm^3 for children aged ≥6 years, and >200 cells/mm^3 for children aged 2–6 years).

Disseminated disease can also be seen in children with cancer/organ transplant with indwelling central venous catheters. Here infection occurs due to contamination of the central catheter and the usual agents are RGM. These children present with fever and sometimes multiple skin nodules. Treatment involves removal of the catheter and combination antimicrobial therapy depending on the susceptibility of the bacteria.

Pulmonary Disease

Pulmonary NTM disease is common in adults where it generally affects patients with previously diseased lungs such as TB and bronchiectasis. The usual offenders are MAC, *M. kansasii,* and *M. abscessus* and the clinical presentation is indistinguishable from TB. Many adults with pulmonary NTM infection are treated as tuberculosis/ multidrug-resistant tuberculosis before the diagnosis is made, if ever.

In children pulmonary disease due to NTM is mainly found in children with cystic fibrosis (CF). Studies reveal a prevalence ranging from 3% to 13% in children with CF. The usual NTM are MAC complex and *M. abscessus.* Furthermore, the prevalence has increased over the years. This may be due to increased longevity of patients with

CF, more awareness, and better methods for culture and identification. The main problem here is differentiating colonization from infection. A single isolation of NTM from the sputum of children with CF may just indicate colonization. However, if NTM are repeatedly isolated (2 or more times) with clinical symptoms, radiologic findings, and rapid decline in lung function, treatment should be considered.

The clinical presentation of NTM in children with CF usually is cough with sputum production, hemoptysis, chest pain, dyspnea, fatigue, weight loss, and fever. These manifestations are indistinguishable from other infections in CF. The CXR is not specific; high-resolution computed tomography (HRCT) of chest may show tree in bud nodules, parenchymal opacities, consolidation, and cavitation. These too are not specific for NTM. The usual decline in lung function in children with CF is 1–3% of forced expiratory volume in 1 second (FEV1) per year. NTM infection particularly due to *M. abscessus* is associated with a more rapid decline in lung function and is associated with a poor prognosis.

Children with suspected NTM infection should undergo solid and liquid mycobacterial cultures of sputum/bronchoalveolar lavage samples. The isolates should be identified to the species level since treatment and prognosis depends on the species isolated. The isolates should be tested for macrolide susceptibility whenever possible (excess use of macrolides in patients with CF has also been associated with increased resistance which in turn is associated with poor prognosis).

If decision is taken to initiate therapy, then combination therapy based on the species isolated is used. Treatment comprises an initial intensive phase of 3–4 months with 4–5 drugs and then a maintenance phase for around 12 months. MAC complex is treated with combination of rifampicin, clarithromycin, and ethambutol and in severe disease amikacin in the initial phase (nebulized/ systemic). In *M. abscessus*, treatment depends on susceptibility and includes clarithromycin/azithromycin, amikacin (nebulized/systemic), clofazimine, imipenem, tigecycline among other drugs. Treatment is associated with resolution of symptoms and improvement of lung function. Duration of therapy is usually 18 months and at least 12 months after culture conversion. Treatment has often to be interrupted due to drug adverse effects. The outcome of treatment in patients with NTM infection in CF is worse as compared to NTM infection in non-CF patients with only 50%, especially those with *M. abscessus* infection achieving culture clearance. Adjuvant surgery can be considered for localized disease. Nutritional support is crucial. Care should be taken to prevent transmission of NTM infection among hospitalized cystic fibrosis patients by using appropriate infection control measures. Previous NTM infection is not a contraindication for lung transplantation with some centers taking patients who have become smear negative whereas others who only take patients once they have become culture negative.

In India, CF is uncommon. Pulmonary NTM infection is more commonly found in children with lungs diseased from other causes such as bronchiectasis and tuberculosis. We describe here a 16-year-old girl who was a known case of tricuspid atresia and underwent a palliative Fontan surgery in early childhood. She continued to be hypoxic and polycythemic and presented with weight loss of 5–6 kg over past 5 months and high-grade fever and cough for 5 days. A chest X-ray (CXR) showed a large cavitary consolidation **(Fig. 3A)** and CT confirmed the findings **(Figs. 3B and C)**. The sputum was 3+ smear positive for AFB and Xpert MTB/RIF was negative. The MGIT (Mycobacteria Growth Indicator Tube) cultures grew on day 8 AFB which was identified by line probe assay as MAC. Treatment was initiated with rifampicin, ethambutol, and clarithromycin with which there was gradual improvement. Treatment is planned for 18 months.

Skin and Soft-tissue Infections

These have become increasingly common in current-day practice. These may be community acquired such as those due to *M. marinum* and *M. ulcerans* or nosocomially acquired. *M. marinum* causes fish tank granuloma and *M. ulcerans* causes Buruli ulcer, both of which are not commonly reported from India.

More common in the Indian setting are nosocomial skin and soft-tissue infections are seen after surgical procedures where asepsis is not maintained and instruments are not adequately sterilized. These infections are particularly common after laparoscopic surgeries since laparoscopes may not have been completely dismantled for cleaning and disinfection. If the time between two cases is short, contact time with the disinfectant (Cidex) is less and thus failures happen. These infections have also been seen following use of unsterile needles for vaccination/injections. Stent-related endocarditis is a unique problem seen in India due to reuse of balloons with incomplete sterilization. The usual culprits are the RGM including *M. chelonae*, *M. fortuitum* group, and *M. abscessus*. Of these, *M. abscessus* is the most drug resistant. The illness usually presents with local site redness, induration, discharge, and sinus

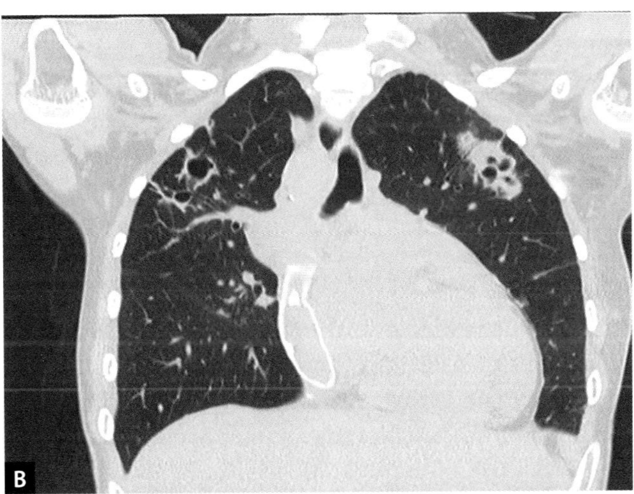

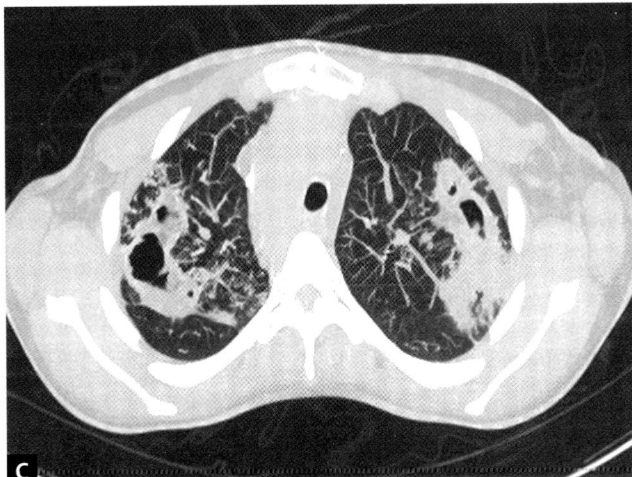

Figs. 3B and C: CECT of a patient with pulmonary NTM.
(CECT: contrast-enhanced computed tomography; NTM: nontuberculous mycobacteria)

Fig. 3A: CXR of a patient with pulmonary NTM.
(CXR: chest X-ray; NTM: nontuberculous mycobacteria)

formation. There are no systemic symptoms. The infection is usually indolent and presents late that differentiates it from the usual bacterial pathogens. Surgical debridement helps both in treatment and diagnosis. The tissue shows granulomatous inflammation and can sometimes be smear positive for AFB. Cultures in both solid and liquid media are recommended. Cultures in aerobic media can also grow RGM, if the plates are not discarded on day 5. Identification of NTM species is important and so is susceptibility testing. The most effective drugs are clarithromycin, linezolid, amikacin, and imipenem. There is rising resistance to quinolones and doxycycline/ minocycline. Drugs such as tigecycline and clofazimine also have good activity against RGM. Combination therapy can be started empirically but should be later modified depending on susceptibility results. If cultures are negative or if susceptibility testing is not possible, a combination of clarithromycin with clofazimine and linezolid can be initiated. The dose of linezolid is 10 mg/kg per day and the patient should be monitored for adverse effects. Amikacin may also need to be administered in the initial treatment regime. The duration of therapy varies from 6 weeks to even 12 months depending on the extent of disease, adequacy of surgical debridement, and response to therapy. Repeated surgical debridement may be sometimes needed.

A problem unique to children is injection site abscesses due to NTM. These babies present with thigh swelling after diphtheria tetanus and pertussis vaccine (DTP) injections that are usually indolent. They are drained and if smear is positive for AFB they are mistaken for tuberculous pyomyositis and treated as such. Abscesses following accidental intramuscular injection of Bacillus Calmette-Guérin (BCG) in the thigh due to mixing up of syringes are also not uncommon. These children also present with abscesses and are smear positive for AFB and show granulomatous inflammation. However, the Xpert MTB/RIF is positive in children with BCG-related abscesses but negative in those due to NTM. Clinicians should be aware of these two entities to diagnose and treat them appropriately. For both NTM- and BCG-related abscesses, surgical excision is usually curative and antimycobacterial treatment is rarely needed.

Prevention of RGM entails proper infection control techniques including use of properly sterilized instruments, disposable needles, appropriate skin cleaning prior to injections, proper dismantling and disinfection of laparoscopes, and avoiding reuse of single-use devices.

The author has seen dozens of nosocomial RGM infections following liposuction and cosmetic surgery, arthroscopic knee surgery, laparoscopic appendicectomy, dental extraction, MMR and DTP injection, placement of intravascular stent, chemotherapy ports, and cesarean section. The most commonly isolated species was *M. abscessus* which showed susceptibility to only linezolid, clarithromycin and amikacin. The patients needed surgical debridement with prolonged medical therapy and significant morbidity. The patient with intravascular stent-related infection died.

Pseudo-nontuberculous Mycobacterial Infections

Since NTM are common inhabitants of the environment including water, contamination of medical equipment and samples can occur. Most common are contamination of bronchoscopes and endoscopes with NTM during the terminal tap water rinse. Since cultures for TB are usually sent when these procedures are performed, positive results are obtained. These AFB should be differentiated from MTB on the basis of the morphology, negative Xpert, and negative MPT64 and not treated. The disinfection procedure for the scopes should be reviewed and corrected and the terminal rinse should be with sterile water or alcohol instead of tap water.

CONCLUSION

Nontuberculous mycobacteria are relatively uncommon but an important cause of infections in children and are often missed or misdiagnosed as TB. They should be suspected in children presenting with cervical adenopathy, as cause of respiratory infections in children with underlying lung disease or those with cystic fibrosis, disseminated disease in immunocompromised children and infections following surgery/injections. Clues to diagnosis include indolent nature, granulomatous inflammation on histopathology, presence of AFB on smear with a negative Xpert MTB/RIF, and positive mycobacterial cultures with negative MPT64. Care should be taken to exclude colonization and contamination. If the isolate is considered significant, it should be sent to a reference laboratory for species identification and susceptibility testing. Treatment depends on site, species, and severity and includes combination of medical and surgical methods and sometimes just watchful waiting. Patients with severe disseminated disease should be investigated for an underlying immunodeficiency. Prevention entails good infection control practices, thorough disinfection and sterilization, avoiding reuse of single-use devices, and chemoprophylaxis when indicated.

SUGGESTED READING

1. Devi DR, Indumathi VA, Indira S, et al. Injection site abscess due to Mycobacterium fortuitum: a case report. Indian J Med Microbiol. 2003;21(2):133-4.

2. Diagnosis and treatment of disease caused by nontuberculous mycobacteria. This official statement of the American Thoracic Society was approved by the Board of Directors, March 1997. Medical Section of the American Lung Association. Am J Respir Crit Care Med. 1997;156(2 Pt 2):S1-25.

3. Ding LW, Lai CC, Lee LN, et al. Lymphadenitis caused by non-tuberculous mycobacteria in a university hospital in Taiwan: predominance of rapidly growing mycobacteria and high recurrence rate. J Formos Med Assoc. 2005;104(12):897-904.

4. Kannaiyan K, Ragunathan L, Sakthivel S, et al. Surgical site infections due to rapidly growing mycobacteria in Puducherry, India. J Clin Diagn Res. 2015;9(3):DC05-8.

5. Lindeboom JA, Kuijper EJ, Bruijnesteijn van Coppenraet ES, et al. Surgical excision versus antibiotic treatment for nontuberculous mycobacterial cervicofacial lymphadenitis in children: a multicenter, randomized, controlled trial. Clin Infect Dis. 2007;44:1057-64.

6. López-Varela E, García-Basteiro AL, Santiago B, et al. Non-tuberculous mycobacteria in children: muddying the waters of tuberculosis diagnosis. Lancet Respir Med. 2015;3(3):244-56.

7. Lu M, Saddi V, Britton PN, et al. Disease caused by non-tuberculous mycobacteria in children with cystic fibrosis. Paediatr Respir Rev. 2019;29:42-52.

8. Saeed DK, Shakoor S, Irfan S, et al. Mycobacterial contamination of bronchoscopes: Challenges and possible solutions in low resource settings. Int J Mycobacteriol. 2016;5(4):408-11.

9. Siberry GK, Abzug MJ, Nachman S, et al; Guidelines for the prevention and treatment of opportunistic infections in HIV-exposed and HIV-infected children: recommendations from the National Institutes of Health, Centers for Disease Control and Prevention, the HIV Medicine Association of the Infectious Diseases Society of America, the Pediatric Infectious Diseases Society, and the American Academy of Pediatrics. Pediatr Infect Dis J. 2013;32(Suppl 2):i-KK4.

10. Soman R, Gupta N, Suthar M, et al. Intravascular Stent-related Endocarditis due to Rapidly Growing Mycobacteria: A New Problem in the Developing World. J Assoc Physicians India. 2015;63(1):18-21.

11. Tebruegge M, Pantazidou A, MacGregor D, et al. Non-tuberculous Mycobacterial Disease in Children - Epidemiology, Diagnosis and Management at a Tertiary Center. PLoS One. 2016; 11(1):e0147513.

Leprosy in Children

Rajeshwar Dayal, Madhu Singh

INTRODUCTION

Leprosy has tormented humanity throughout history, leaving a long-lasting impact on religion, literature, and art. The first description of leprosy dates back to the 6th century BC from India and China. The spread of disease from India to Europe took place around the 4th century BC. In "*Sushruta Samhita*", which dates back to 600 BC, it was described as "Kushtha Roga". The word "kushtha" in Sanskrit means eating away. In ancient times, it was popularly believed that the disease was a wrath of God on those who had done some evil deeds (Paap) in their present and past life; as a result, the poor survivors were abandoned by the family and society.

In 1873, a Norwegian physician, Dr. Gerhard Henrik Armauer Hansen discovered *Mycobacterium leprae* as a causative agent of leprosy; therefore, leprosy was known as Hansen's disease in ancient times. Among all the illnesses that still scourge humanity, leprosy has the worst reputation as a cause of the deformity and disability. Until the recent past, leprosy was considered both highly infectious and incurable.

EPIDEMIOLOGY

The annual figures on leprosy [derived from 150 countries in the six WHO (World Health Organization) regions], revealed the registered global prevalence of 192,713 cases (0.25/10,000 population) at the end of 2017. During the same year, 210,671 new cases of leprosy were reported accounting for the new case detection rate of 2.77 per 100,000 population **(Fig. 1)**.

Southeast Asian regions accounted for nearly 73% of the total leprosy burden. The countries with the highest burdens in descending order were India, Brazil, and Indonesia (80.2% of the total new cases). In 2017, the total number of new cases with grade-2 disabilities were 12,189, which depicted a decrease of about 14% in the last 10 years.

Around, 126,164 new cases of leprosy (60% of the global burden) were residing in India in the year 2017.

Childhood leprosy accounts for 8% of the total disease burden. Of the total 16,979 new pediatric cases detected in 2017, 39% and 61% were of multibacillary (MB) and paucibacillary (PB) variety, respectively.

In the pediatric leprosy population, children between 5 years and 14 years are most commonly affected, though, in very high endemic countries, the prevalence in children between 0 year and 4 years is also significant. Leprosy affects males more than females. Since the disease is nonhereditary, infants born to leprous parents can be protected from the exposure and subsequent disease development if they are separated soon after birth. Concomitant human immunodeficiency virus (HIV) infection does not alter the risk of leprosy.

ETIOLOGY

Leprosy is a mycobacterial disease caused by *M. leprae*, which is an acid-fast and nonsporing bacillus, found both intracellularly as well as extracellularly. In a stained smear, it lies singly, as rods or in clumps called globi. *M. leprae* has an affinity for Schwann cells and cells of the reticuloendothelial system. It cannot be grown in any artificial media.

SOURCE OF INFECTION AND MODE OF TRANSMISSION

The infected human being is the only source of leprosy infection. MB leprosy patients have 4–11 times higher infective potential as compared to patients with PB leprosy.

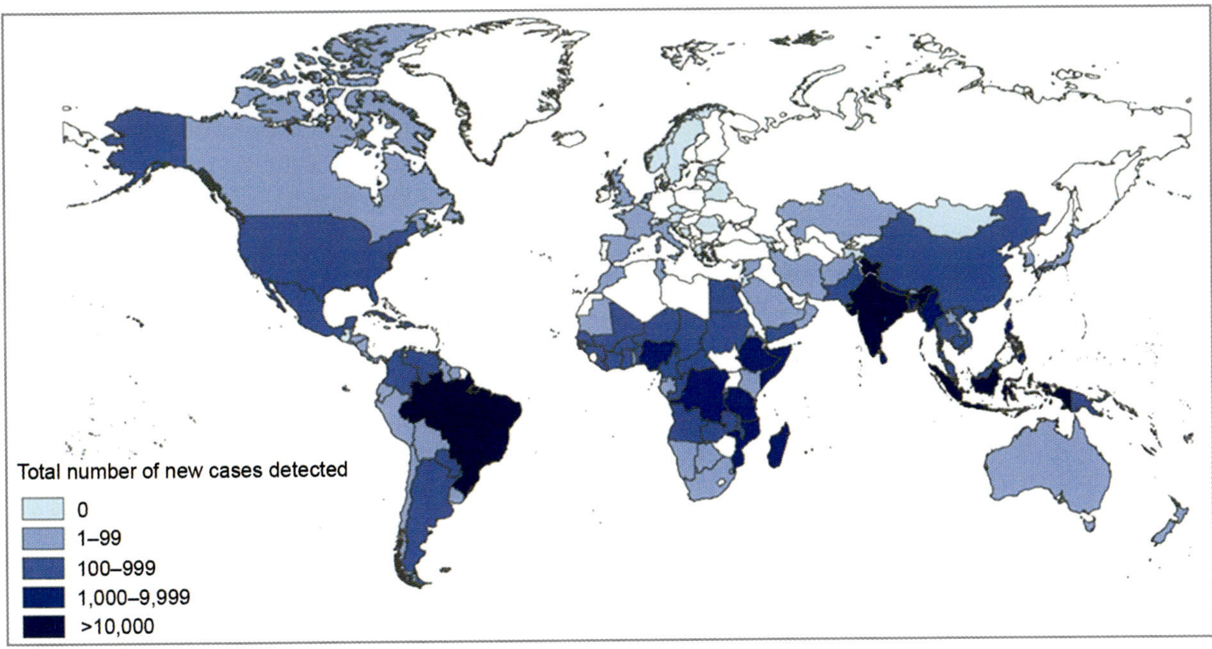

Fig. 1: Global geographical distribution of new leprosy cases, 2017.
Source: World Health Organization: Weekly Epidemiological Record, 2018.

Direct Transmission

For direct transmission, prolonged and close contact is required. An "intrafamilial" contact carries a greater risk of infection than an "extrafamilial" one.

Untreated lepromatous patients can discharge as many as 100 million bacilli per day from their nasal secretions. The inhalation of these bacilli, via droplets, is the most common mode of entry of leprosy bacilli into the contact person. After inhalation, the bacilli enter the respiratory system and transverse via blood to skin and peripheral nerves where depending on the host immune response, the disease may manifest either as tuberculoid leprosy (where there is good cell-mediated immune response to *M. leprae*) or may manifest at lepromatous leprosy (LL) (where there is anergy to *M. leprae*).

Other portals of entry include scratched, abraded, or insect bitten skin (which facilitates passage of organism via the droplets laden with leprosy bacilli through the epidermis into the dermis), and ingestion of infected breast milk.

Indirect Transmission

Mycobacterium leprae can easily remain viable for several days even outside the human body. Occasionally, leprosy may spread by fomites used by the patient suffering from MB leprosy. Localized infections via infected syringes and tattooing needles can also occur.

CLINICAL MANIFESTATIONS

Incubation Period

The incubation period for leprosy varies from a few months to as long as 20 years (average between 2 years and 5 years). The onset is usually gradual but may be sudden in highly susceptible people.

Early Signs of Childhood Leprosy

- A hypopigmented nonirritating patch in the skin, present for a long duration, with loss of sensation to touch, pain, and temperature.
- Thickening of the skin, which also becomes more red and shiny as compared to the surrounding areas, prominently on the face and hands.
- Loss of sensation, numbness, feeling of "pins and needles" or "crawling of ants", tingling sensation in the affected areas, especially in hands and feet. There may be paresis in hands or feet. Fine movements of fingers are also affected.
- Spontaneous blisters and ulcers may occur, especially in the fingers.

CLASSIFICATION

According to the Indian Association of Leprologists classification, leprosy is subdivided into five major groups: (1) indeterminate, (2) borderline, (3) tuberculoid,

(4) lepromatous, and (5) polyneuritic. The borderline group is further classified into borderline lepromatous (BL), borderline (BB), and borderline tuberculoid (BT) types.

Indeterminate Leprosy

It is the earliest detectable form of leprosy which is seen in only 10–20% of infected individuals and it is characterized by the presence of a single hypopigmented macule with ill-defined border, measuring around 2–4 cm in diameter. Erythema or induration is characteristically absent. Anesthesia may be minimal or even absent. The biopsy can show a granuloma but bacilli are very rarely seen. In 50–75% of patients, the lesion heals spontaneously; however, in the remaining cases, it gradually progresses to other classic forms.

Tuberculoid Leprosy

In this subtype, single or few asymmetrical, well-defined, hypopigmented, erythematous or copper-colored patches with sensory loss are characteristically present. The patch or only its margins are raised above the level of the surrounding skin.

Initially, a single nerve trunk in close relation to the lesion is affected. The nerve trunk becomes enlarged, hard, and tender and sometimes transforms into a nerve abscess. Lepromin test is positive. Skin smear shows no bacilli. Biopsy shows foci of lymphocytes, epithelioid cells, and Langhans giant cells. It is the most common subtype of leprosy, especially in children. The course of the disease is relatively benign and stable and carries a good prognosis.

Borderline Leprosy

Borderline leprosy is further divided into three subtypes based on clinical and histological criteria. These subtypes are as follows:

1. *Borderline tuberculoid leprosy*: In this subtype, the lesions are greater in number but smaller in size as compared to tuberculoid leprosy. The margins of the BT lesions are less distinct and the center is less atrophic and anesthetic. There may be small satellite lesions around older lesions. Thickening of two or more superficial nerves is frequently seen.
2. *Mid borderline leprosy*: In this subtype, the lesions are more numerous and heterogeneous. The lesions may become confluent. Plaques may be present. The borders are poorly defined and the erythematous rim fades into the surrounding skin. Hyperesthesia is a common finding than anesthesia.
3. *Borderline LL*: In borderline LL, there are a large number of heterogeneous asymmetrically distributed lesions. Macules, papules, plaques, and nodules may all coexist. Usually, the individual lesions are small unless confluent. Anesthesia is mild and superficial nerve trunks are spared.

Lepromatous Leprosy

Almost all cases of LL begin as borderline leprosy forms, i.e. BB or BL. LL form of leprosy is seldom seen in childhood. Classical skin lesions are usually preceded by the nasal symptoms (stuffiness, crust formation, and blood-stained discharge) and bilateral edema of legs and ankles (prominent in the late evening and disappears after overnight rest). The latter should be looked for to diagnose leprosy infection at the earliest.

Numerous symmetrically distributed erythematous or coppery, shiny, macules with ill-defined margins are usually the first skin lesions to appear. Other skin lesions are also seen namely macules, papules, nodules or a combination of them. Patients may have a leonine facies characterized by absent eyebrows and eyelashes. There is no sensory impairment in these lesions in early disease. Disease progression may show the symmetrical involvement of many peripheral nerves. The affected nerves are initially softer and larger than normal and are painful to touch. As the illness advances, fibrosis develops and a result of which the nerves become thin and hard resulting in extreme anesthesia. The skin smear is almost always positive but the lepromin test is negative. It is the most infectious form and frequently associated with lepra reactions if left untreated. The prognosis is quite poor.

The characteristic features of these varieties of leprosy are summarized in **Table 1**.

Neuritic Leprosy

These cases show only nerve involvement without any skin lesions. Neuritic leprosy may be of primary or secondary variety. In the primary subtype, the nerves are directly involved without any skin lesion while in the secondary neuritic variety, the infection spreads into the nerves from leprous skin lesions. The affected nerves become thickened and tender, producing sensorimotor and trophic changes in their respective areas of distribution. Nerve involvement may lead to deformities, neuropathic ulcers, and lagophthalmos leading to serious eye complications. Ulnar, median, lateral popliteal, tibial, great auricular, and rarely radial nerves are involved. V and VII cranial nerves may also be affected.

Table 1: Clinical aspects of tuberculoid, borderline and lepromatous leprosy.

Features	Types of leprosy				
	TT	BT	BB	BL	LL
Number of lesions	Single usually	Single or few	Several	Many	Very many
Size of lesions	Variable	Variable	Variable	Variable	Small
Surface of lesions	Very dry, sometimes scaly	Dry	Slightly shiny	Shiny	Shiny
Sensation in lesions	Absent	Markedly diminished	Moderately diminished	Slightly diminished	Not affected
Hair growth	Absent	Markedly diminished	Moderately diminished	Slightly diminished	Not affected
AFB in lesions	Nil	Nil or scanty	Moderate numbers	Many	Very many (plus globi)
AFB in nasal scrapings/in nose blows	Nil	Nil	Nil	Usually nil	Very many (plus globi)
Lepromin test	Strongly positive (+++)	Weakly positive (+ or ++)	Negative	Negative	Negative

(AFB: acid–fast bacilli; TT: tuberculoid; BT: borderline tuberculoid; BB: borderline; BL: borderline lepromatous; LL: lepromatous leprosy)

■ REACTIONS

Reactions are acute exacerbations due to changes in the host-parasite immune relationship. These are common during the initial years of multidrug therapy. Two types of reactions are seen which are as follows:

- *Type 1 reversal reaction*: These reactions are seen in borderline cases. There is acute tenderness and swelling at the site of the lesion. This reaction requires urgent intervention to avoid irreversible nerve injury.
- *Type 2 erythema nodosum leprosum (ENL) reactions*: Type 2 reactions are seen in lepromatous and BL cases as a systemic inflammatory response. The patient presents with high-grade fever, lymphadenitis, migrating polyarthralgia, orchitis, and iridocyclitis. Tender red papules or nodules resembling erythema nodosum are pathognomonic of type 2 reactions.

■ DIAGNOSIS

Childhood leprosy can be diagnosed if any one of the following cardinal signs is present:

- A definite loss of sensation in a pale (hypopigmented) or reddish skin patch
- Thickened or enlarged peripheral nerve, with loss of sensation and/or weakness of the muscles supplied by that nerve
- Presence of acid-fast bacilli in a slit-skin smear.

Smear Examination

Sample for bacteriological examination is usually taken from the most affected parts of the lesion. The smear should be taken from ear lobules and buttocks if there are no definite patches. Smears are prepared using the "slit and scrape" method and stained by Ziehl–Neelsen staining. Smears are positive for *M. leprae* in LL, BL, and some BB and BT cases. It is of limited utility in tuberculoid and indeterminate lesions and patients with early atypical clinical presentation.

Histopathology

Histopathology is used to diagnose and classify indeterminate lesions.

Bacillary Index

Bacillary index (BI) is a semi-quantitative estimation of bacillus density in skin smears and biopsies. It is measured on two scales, namely (1) Dharmendra scale and (2) Ridley scale. It determines a total load of acid-fast bacilli in the microscopic field, including both live and dead bacilli.

Patients are labeled as PB leprosy when there are less than or equal to five skin lesions and no bacilli on skin smears. They are labeled as MB leprosy when there are more than or equal to six skin lesions and bacilli are present on skin smears. The bacterial index ranges 0, i.e. no bacilli present in 100 oil immersion fields to 6, where >1,000 bacilli are seen per oil immersion field.

Footpad Culture

The inoculation of material into the mouse footpad is the only certain way to demonstrate the multiplication of bacilli. This method is 10 times more sensitive at detecting *M. leprae* than slit skin smear examination.

Immunological Methods

Test for Cell-mediated Immunity

Lepromin test: In this test, 0.1 mL of lepromin (Dharmendra or Mitsuda antigen) is injected intradermally into the inner aspect of the forearm. The reaction is read at 48 hours (Fernandez reaction) and 21 days (Mitsuda reaction) to stage leprosy. This test is based on the cell-mediated immunity of an individual. Lepromin test is not a diagnostic test, but it is essential for disease classification. The test is positive in cases of tuberculoid and BT leprosy, negative in LL, BL leprosy, and weakly positive/variable in BB leprosy. The lepromin negative contacts have a higher risk of developing the disease when compared with lepromin positive contacts. Two kinds of lepromin antigen are commonly used in the test:

1. The crude antigen of Mitsuda
2. The refined antigen of Dharmendra.

The test is outdated and currently, not recommended for the diagnosis of leprosy.

Serological Assays

Serological tests can be used for detecting subclinical infection. The major serological assays include the following:

- *Fluorescent leprosy antibody absorption (FLA-ABS) test*: This highly sensitive test based on immunofluorescence technique detects the antibodies against *M. leprae*. It can be used to identify healthy contacts of leprosy patients who are at risk of developing the disease.
- *Radioimmunoassay*: It detects antibodies against the cell wall antigen of *M. leprae* bacillus.
- *Enzyme-linked immunosorbent assay (ELISA)*: Phenolic glycolipid-enzyme-linked immunosorbent assay (PGL-ELISA) is an ELISA-based technique that shows positivity in MB cases. However, it lacks positivity in PB and subclinical leprosy cases.

Most serological tests are not useful for diagnosing childhood leprosy as they miss most PB leprosy cases and continue remaining positive even after the completion of treatment in MB cases.

Molecular Biological Approaches

Recombinant deoxyribonucleic acid (DNA) technology is a rapid modality to identify the organisms. It uses probes based on specific gene sequences of *M. leprae*. Recently, several gene amplification techniques [polymerase chain reaction (PCR)] for amplifying *M. leprae* specific sequences from a variety of specimens have been developed. The diagnostic advantage of these PCR techniques lies in their high sensitivity and specificity.

In Situ Polymerase Chain Reaction

In situ PCR, or slide PCR, is a method in which PCR is run directly on small tissue samples, tissue microarrays, or other small cell samples rather than extracting DNA or RNA (ribonucleic acid) first, and then performing PCR, real-time PCR, or quantitative PCR from the extracted material. A positivity of 57.1% in the early or localized form of leprosy, i.e. indeterminate/BT and 61.5% in BB or BL group is shown in our series. We have also found that as a diagnostic modality, it is superior to histopathological examination (significant enhancement of 15% as compared to histopathological examination). It improves diagnostic yield in early doubtful cases of childhood leprosy and in cases where histopathology is nonspecific.

In Situ Hybridization

In contrast to *in situ* PCR, *in situ* hybridization technique uses a labeled complementary DNA/RNA strand to localize specific DNA/RNA in a portion or section of tissue. *In situ* hybridization significantly enhances early diagnosis of leprosy. In our series, it has shown a positivity of 42.8% in early leprosy (I/BT) and 46.7% in the BB/BL group, thus enhancing the diagnosis of leprosy by 18.1%.

In Situ PCR on Slit-skin Smears

Another molecular biological approach is *in situ* PCR on the slit-skin smears with an added advantage of being minimally invasive and less cumbersome. It can be performed at those sites where skin biopsy is difficult to perform. *In situ* PCR on slit-skin smears is better than that on skin biopsies (average positivity of 72% vs. 60%).

M. Leprae-specific Repetitive Element PCR

The *M. leprae*-specific repetitive element *(RLEP)* amplicon of *M. leprae* is very specific for the organism and thus RLEP PCR is a better diagnostic tool than conventional PCR. Our studies based on *RLEP PCR* techniques showed that it was significantly better than the Ziehl-Neelsen staining.

◼ MANAGEMENT

Childhood leprosy should be treated with the utmost patience and perseverance. Along with antibacterial therapy, the patients and their guardians require moral support and reassurance. Parents should be informed about the importance of hygiene, nutritious diet, and regular treatment.

Multidrug Therapy

The simultaneous administration of different antibacterial agents prevents the emergence of drug-resistance. This forms the basis of multidrug therapy in leprosy cure. The standard treatment regimen for children (10–14 years) is as follows:

- Multibacillary leprosy (Duration: 12 months)
  - *Rifampicin*: 450 mg once a month
  - *Clofazimine*: 150 mg once a month, and 50 mg every other day
  - *Dapsone*: 50 mg daily.
- Paucibacillary leprosy (Duration: 6 months)
  - *Rifampicin*: 450 mg once a month
  - *Clofazimine*: 150 mg once a month, and 50 mg every other day
  - *Dapsone*: 50 mg daily.

The WHO treatment regimen for children below 10 years of age is listed in **Table 2**.

Rifampicin-resistant Leprosy

Rifampicin-resistant leprosy can be effectively treated using at least two second-line drugs (clarithromycin, minocycline, or a quinolone) plus clofazimine daily for 6 months, followed by clofazimine plus one of these drugs for an additional 18 months. The total duration of therapy is 2 years (24 months).

When ofloxacin resistance is also present, a fluoroquinolone should not be used as part of second-line treatment. The regimen in such cases consists of 6 months of clarithromycin, minocycline, and clofazimine followed by clarithromycin/minocycline plus clofazimine for an additional 18 months.

Chemoprophylaxis

For adults and children (aged 2 years of age and above), single-dose rifampicin (SDR) is used in contacts of leprosy patients, after excluding leprosy and tuberculosis and in the absence of other contraindications **(Table 3)**. A prospective seroepidemiological study on contact transmission and chemoprophylaxis in leprosy found that SDR is highly cost-effective, and is associated with a 57% reduction in the risk of leprosy after 2 years and 30% after 5–6 years.

Treatment of Reactions

Drugs that are frequently used to treat leprosy reactions are oral antimalarials like chloroquine, antimonials [intravenous (IV) potassium antimony tartrate and intramuscular (IM) fantosin], clofazimine, corticosteroids, and thalidomide. Iritis and neuritis should be promptly treated to avoid deformities and neuropathic ulcers.

◼ PROPHYLAXIS

Leprosy Vaccine

National Leprosy Eradication Program (NLEP) has introduced the *Mycobacterium indicus pranii* (MIP) vaccine in a project mode in India from the year 2016. Hospital and population-based trials conducted in MB leprosy patients and their contacts showed that the vaccine has both immunotherapeutic and immunoprophylactic effects. Postvaccination it has shown a reduction of the bacillary load and histopathological upgradation of the lesions, facilitating the complete clearance of granuloma, and reduction in reactions, neuritis, and the total duration of multidrug therapy.

Under the new field project, operated in certain regions of India by Indian Council of Medical Research and NLEP, all index leprosy cases will be receiving the MIP vaccine. Family members and contacts of these index cases would be immunized with MIP twice (at an interval of 6 months). In an index case, it facilitates the rapid clearance of bacteria and clinical lesions whereas, in contacts, MIP vaccination

Table 3: Rifampicin dose for single-dose rifampicin.

Age/weight	Rifampicin single dose
15 years and above	600 mg
10–14 years	450 mg
Children 6–9 years (weight ≥20 kg)	300 mg
Children <20 kg (≥2 years)	10–15 mg/kg

Table 2: WHO multidrug therapy regimens.

Age group	Drug	Dosage and frequency	Duration	
			Paucibacillary	Multibacillary
Children <10 years old or <40 kg	Rifampicin	10 mg/kg once a month	6 months	12 months
	Clofazimine	100 mg once a month, 50 mg twice weekly		
	Dapsone	2 mg/kg daily		

(WHO: World Health Organization)

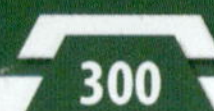

enhances immunity, thereby resisting the development of clinical disease on exposure to cases suffering from leprosy.

Bacille Calmette Guerin Vaccine

Bacille Calmette Guerin Vaccine (BCG) booster vaccination, which comprises a two-dose BCG regimen given at 0 and 3 months of age provides 50–75% protection against leprosy infection.

■ CONCLUSION

Globally, maximum number of patients of leprosy reside in India. For early diagnosis, a high index of suspicion is required when confronted with a child presenting with hypopigmented skin lesions. Histopathology and molecular techniques confirm the diagnosis. Multidrug therapy and chemoprophylaxis are very effective.

■ SUGGESTED READING

1. Dayal R, Agarwal M, Natrajan M, et al. PCR and in-situ hybridization for diagnosis of leprosy. Indian J Pediatr. 2007; 74:645-8.
2. Dayal R, Singh SP, Mathur PP, et al. Diagnostic value of in situ polymerase chain reaction in leprosy. Indian J Pediatr. 2005; 72:1043-6.
3. Gupta P. Textbook of Preventive and Social Medicine, 4th edition. New Delhi: CBS; 2013.
4. Kamal R, Dayal R, Gaidhankar K, et al. RLEP PCR as a definitive diagnostic test for Leprosy from skin smear samples in childhood and adolescent leprosy. Indian J Lepr. 2016;88:193-7.
5. Kamal R, Pathak V, Kumari A, et al. Addition of Mycobacterium indicus pranii (MIP) vaccine as an immunotherapeutic with standard chemotherapy in borderline leprosy: A double-blind study to assess clinical improvement (A preliminary report). Br J Dermatol. 2016;176(5):1388-9.
6. Leprosy. In: Park K (Ed). Textbook of Preventive and Social Medicine, 23rd edition. India: Bhanot Publishers; 2015. pp. 314-30.
7. Powell DA. Hansen disease (Mycobacterium leprae). In: Kliegman R, Behrman R, Jenson H, Stanton B, (Eds). Nelson Textbook of Pediatrics, 18th edition. Philadelphia, Elsevier Saunders; 2008. pp. 1255-8.
8. World Health Organization: Weekly Epidemiological Record. 2018;35:445-56.
9. Yan W, Xing Y, Yuan LC, et al. Application of RLEP real-time PCR for detection of M. leprae DNA in paraffin-embedded skin biopsy specimens for diagnosis of paucibacillary leprosy. Am J Trop Med Hyg. 2014;90(3):524-9.

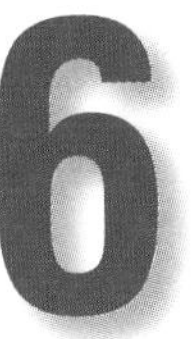

SECTION 6

Viral Infections

S Balasubramanian

Epidemiology of Viral Infections in Tropics

Preeti Malhotra, Piyush Gupta

INTRODUCTION

Epidemiology is the study of the determinants, dynamics, and distribution of diseases in the population. Medical science branch which deals with the control and transmission of infections in human beings is known as epidemiology. The same holds true for the viral diseases. In times of disease outbreak of viral diseases, epidemiology can help us disrupt this cycle of infection in the community.

Tropical diseases are infectious diseases which thrive in hot, humid conditions. Flies and mosquitoes are the most common insects acting as carriers for the spread of diseases in the subtropical and tropical regions. Majority of the disease burden is seen during the rainy season and the subsequent season. But certain viral infections remain prevalent throughout the year. The geographical condition of India is such that it is one of the world's largest tropical countries having the prevalence of viral diseases.

The reason for the viral diseases being more prevalent is due to their inherent property of mutation as compared to other organisms such as bacteria. Viruses can infect both human beings and livestock with equal virulence. Another unique property of viruses is the biodiversity and crossing-over of the species barrier leading to the amalgamation of the signs and symptoms. It is of paramount importance to study the viral epidemiology as the load of viral infections and the resulting morbidity and mortality from them are very high. Clinicians need to have a high index of suspicion for the diagnosis of viral infections as the symptomatology may be misleading or overlapping with other diseases, and their empirical therapy may not be effective in alleviating of the symptoms.

Children living in the tropics and subtropics continue to be at risk for endemic diseases. Compared to industrialized countries, the under-five and infant mortality rates in developing countries remain high. Infections are still high on card as the cause of mortality. Due to changes in food chain and increase in travel and transport internationally, there is increased biologic interaction. Due to ecological changes and man-made transformations, the organisms have undergone changes including genomic mutations. As a result of these complex interactions, the epidemiology and geographical distribution of infectious diseases have changed, e.g. the shift of measles from children to unvaccinated young adults following childhood immunization and changes in the geographic distribution of disease vectors (spread of *Aedes* spp., vector of dengue). An example associated with successful control program is the disappearance or sharp decline of poliomyelitis. There is change in the epidemiology of diseases with the reemergence of diseases in epidemics such as dengue and Ebola.

The three major determinants of the change in the epidemiology of infectious diseases are (1) changes in the susceptibility to infectious diseases, (2) increased opportunities for infection, and (3) the rapid adaptation of the microbial world. These factors have increased the threat globally for infectious diseases.[1,2]

CHARACTERISTIC FEATURES OF VIRUSES

Viruses are smallest, obligate infective agents containing only one type of nucleic acid (DNA or RNA). They have no metabolic activity outside the living cells. They do not possess a cellular organization and lack the enzymes necessary for protein and nucleic acid synthesis. Progeny of virus for its production requires macromolecules specific for the virus, which are synthesized by host metabolism once it is diverted by the virus genome. Viruses multiply by complex process. They do not grow in inanimate media. They are resistant to antibiotics. Viruses may have icosahedral symmetry, helical symmetry, or complex symmetry. They multiply only in living cells. Three methods are employed for cultivation of viruses, namely animal inoculation, embryonated egg inoculation, and tissue culture. Virus-host interaction may cause different effects, ranging from no apparent cellular damage to rapid cell destruction. Some viruses (e.g. polioviruses) cause cell death (cytocidal infection); others may cause cellular proliferation or malignant transformation (oncogenic viruses). In some cases, viruses remain as latent infection (herpes simplex virus), whereas other produce some morphological changes in cells to form inclusion bodies (rabies virus). Viruses may enter the body through respiratory tract, alimentary tract, skin, genital tract, conjunctiva or congenitally. As viruses are strict intracellular parasites, they absolutely depend on the biosynthesis mechanisms of the host cell for their replication. Antiviral agents block the replication of viruses by various mechanisms.[3,4]

CHARACTERISTICS OF RESPIRATORY VIRUSES

Etiology of Common Respiratory Illnesses

The most common etiology for the respiratory infections are the viruses. These viruses infect and reinfect without any change in antigenicity and do not result in long-lasting immunity being surface infections, the exceptions being parainfluenza and respiratory syncytial virus (RSV) in young children as they can cause severe infection which on initial presentation may appear like common cold or mild infection. Older brothers or sisters in the family might get a mild infection which can get transmitted to a younger sibling in the form of pneumonia or bronchiolitis. Children born to mothers having high titers of maternal antibody are at the lowest risk to develop severe disease. Influenza belonging to orthomyxoviruses is another exception causing severe infection in older children and adults.

The most common cause of laryngotracheobronchitis (croup) is parainfluenza virus types 1 and 2 in the older age group. In comparison to RSV and parainfluenza virus, coronaviruses and rhinoviruses (picornaviruses) are responsible for symptoms resembling cold in both children and adults. The most common cause for the common cold is rhinoviruses, which can affect individuals many times throughout their life span. Respiratory viral infections differ in their seasonality, but their frequency increases during the winter seasons in most of the places in the world. Different regions in the world can have different time periods for the spread of these virus illnesses

throughout the year. For example, parainfluenza infection occurs more during the spring and late autumn while RSV affects the individuals more during the winter season.

Influenza or flu is an acute, contagious, viral respiratory illness and is mostly ignored. But in certain cases, this can lead to serious infections ultimately leading to the demise of the patient. It is estimated that all over the world, 3–5 million suffer from seasonal influenza and 300,000–500,000 die every year. Children and elderly suffer more. Different areas in the world can have the disease at different seasons like in equatorial regions the disease is prevalent throughout the year, but in the northern and southern hemispheres the disease occurs during the winter months. People with flu can spread the infection while talking, coughing, and sneezing in the form of droplets. Seasonal human influenza outbreaks or epidemics are due to circulating influenza type A or B viruses undergoing drift in the virus. The seriousness of the disease and outbreak depends on the amount of the drift. A minor drift in the surface antigen of influenza virus [hemagglutinin (H) and neuraminidase (N)] is the reason for yearly outbreak of the disease. Whenever there is a shift in the surface antigenicity, pandemic results. The Indian scenario is very precarious. The disease load **(Fig. 1)** is showing an increasing trend which can be seen from the fact that till the beginning of April 2019, the cases were more than the total number of cases seen in the year 2018. Rajasthan topped the list of

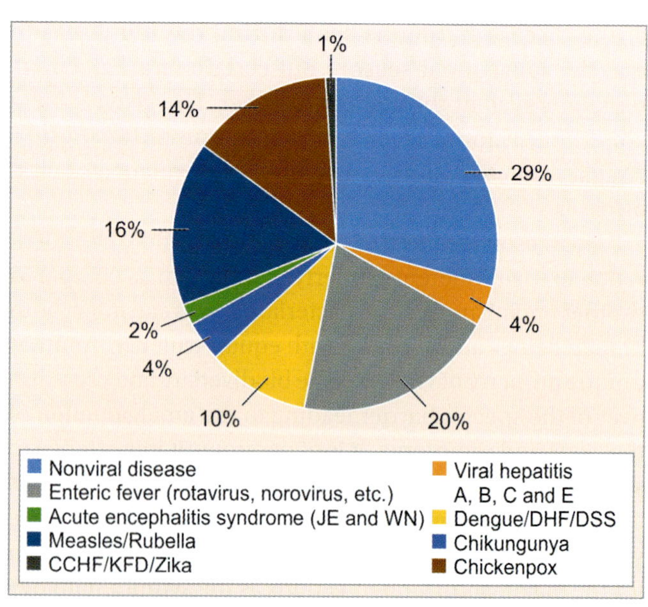

Fig. 1: Disease-wise outbreaks in India.
(CCHF: Crimean-Congo hemorrhagic fever; DHF: dengue hemorrhagic fever; DSS: Dengue Shock syndrome; JE: Japanese encephalitis; KFD: Kyasanur forest disease; WN: West Nile)
Source: Mourya DT, Yadav PD, Ullas PT, et al. Emerging/re-emerging viral diseases and new viruses on the Indian horizon. Indian J Med Res. 2019;149(4):447-67.

the states affected by the disease having the mortality of 192 patients and almost double the number of patients till April 2019 in comparison to 2018. The crucial virological and epidemiological data is being generated by the Indian Council of Medical Research through its sentinel surveillance at 12 surveillance sites pan India.[5-7]

■ VIRUSES INFECTING THE GASTROINTESTINAL TRACT

- Agents of diarrheal disease
- Poliovirus
- Enteric hepatitis virus.

Etiology of Diarrheal Disease

Industrialized countries have a different etiology for the diarrheal diseases. During the outbreaks of diarrheal diseases, etiological agents may be bacterial or parasites rather than virus in comparison to the respiratory illnesses. During the winter season, most of the diarrheal diseases are of viral origin and can have a greater preponderance for spread in the family. Worldwide rotavirus is the most common organism for diarrheal disease leading on to dehydration. The rotavirus resembles the respiratory virus in its pattern of infection as being the surface infection, the reoccurrences are common. Initial infection may be severe in infants, but reinfections are usually of milder nature and may even be asymptomatic in their presentation. The route of transmission of rotavirus is feco-oral. Stool of the infected patient carries a large amount of viral load. Rotavirus vaccines prepared from live-attenuated strains are used in infants for vaccination. The reason for vaccination is that it appears as reinfection, thus reducing the severity of disease. The rotavirus strains show a lot of diversity and thus higher incidence of mixed infections. G6, G8, G10, and G9P strains have been responsible for human infection while Kolkata and Pune have reported group B rotavirus. Other viruses such as *Norvovirus*, Norwalk, and adenovirus are difficult to grow in cell culture. Norvovirus causes water-related outbreaks, especially while swimming in the contaminated water or by drinking the contaminated water, consumption of virus infested sea food has also been implicated.[2,5,6]

Poliovirus

Polio or enteroviruses are responsible for causing a serious and crippling disease. Poliovirus has three serotypes, namely P1, P2, and P3, but immunity to one serotype does not protect against infection with other serotypes. Live-attenuated vaccine was used universally and repeatedly in young children to globally eliminate the polio. The method

is based on the known transmission pattern of the vaccine virus, which resembles that of the wild virus in being shed in large quantities and for long periods in the stool of inoculated children. The shed virus can be transmitted to contacts, especially other children and to adults in the family. Therefore, when the Pulse Polio Programme is being conducted as part of immunization to cover large masses, it indirectly protects the unimmunized children from the virus in the environment. This approach is called herd immunity. It increases the level of antibodies in the population so that susceptible people are less in number and transmission is interrupted. Usually, poliovirus spreads from person to person via the fecal-oral route but droplet spread may also occur. Seasonal variation is not seen in tropics, but incidence increases in the summer months in temperate zones.[2,7]

Hepatitis A

Hepatitis A is also grouped under *Enterovirus* sharing similar epidemiology to other enteroviruses, but it has unusually longer incubation period. In developing countries, spread can be from contaminated water or food with fecal contaminants. Infection in a developing country like India is often asymptomatic and presents at a younger age, whereas in the developed countries infection is rare and presentation can be delayed; about two decades ago, it was not uncommon to identify children with natural protection against HAV following exposure to this virus. Improvement in socioeconomic status has resulted in a shift of epidemiology of HAV with children not acquiring protective antibodies in childhood and therefore being more susceptible to the infection later in life. The recent introduction of vaccines has also changed the etiological profile of viral hepatitis. The relative incidence of HAV is probably less than before, although it may be still high in some parts of the country.[2,3,6]

Hepatitis E

Epidemiology-wise, hepatitis E resembles hepatitis A. It is more common in North India, especially in regions situated around the river Ganges.

■ VIRAL INFECTIONS WITH BLOOD-BORNE TRANSMISSION

Hepatitis B

Hepatitis B virus is the most common viral infection transmitted through blood and blood products. It was discovered much earlier than the HIV (human immunodeficiency virus) infection. The incubation period is variable from 1 month to 6 months. It can cause acute and chronic hepatitis. Blood-borne transmission is less likely when viremia is for few hours only but the rate of transmission increases when viremia persists for longer periods as in the case with someone infected with hepatitis B for years. Thus, perinatal infection results in chronic viremia. Hepatitis B virus is transmitted through blood and blood products, sexual contact, and other body fluids such as semen. A small amount of blood from minor abrasion may be responsible for transmission. Professional blood donors and certain professionals such as dentists and surgeons are major risk groups for hepatitis B. The average estimated carrier rate of hepatitis B in India is 4%, with a total pool of approximately 36 million carriers.[2,3,6]

Hepatitis C

Hepatitis C usually does not cause acute hepatitis in children but can be seen in children receiving multiple blood transfusion. Disease course is benign and mild; its progression to acute liver failure is less than 1%. Incidence of chronicity is more than that of hepatitis B virus infection.[2,7]

Human Immunodeficiency Virus

The epidemiology of HIV is like that of hepatitis B. In cases of hepatitis B, there is high load of viremia which leads to transmission of virus for a long period of time, whereas in cases of HIV the transmission of viruses takes place either in the early part of disease or later (development of AIDS) when viremia is high. The early part of the disease is probably more important for transmission as the individuals may not know that they are infected, and they remain sexually active. India is having epidemic of HIV with 2.40 million people suffering from HIV. About 0.31% are adults, 3.5% are children (<15 years), and 39% are women. The epidemic is concentrated among vulnerable populations at high risk for HIV. Unprotected sex and drug addiction play a major role in the spread of disease. The 2019 statistics states that Mizoram had the highest adult prevalence followed by Manipur and Nagaland. Earlier data reveals that southern states had higher incidence of HIV.[2,6,8]

■ ZOONOSES AND VECTOR-BORNE INFECTION

Viral infections transmitted to humans by animals (wild and domestic), birds, and reptiles where they act as the main reservoir of viral agents are known as zoonotic infections. Humans are infected accidentally but the infective cycle is maintained by these reservoirs. Zoonoses

are classified according to their reservoir hosts whether they are men or lower vertebrate animals. They can also be categorized based on the type of life cycle of the infecting organism as direct zoonoses (rabies), cyclozoonoses, metazoonoses (arbovirus), and saprozoonoses. The zoonotic diseases have reached to a point of concern in India as majority of its population (80%) live in close proximity with domestic animals and the wild animals are also not very far off from the human habitat. Some of the important zoonotic viral diseases are Dengue fever, Chikungunya fever, rabies, Japanese encephalitis and sand fly fever, etc. Dengue, chikungunya fever, yellow fever, rabies, Japanese encephalitis (JE), Chandipura, West Nile fever, sandfly fever, etc. are the few important examples of zoonotic viral infections.

Rabies

Rabies affects the central nervous system and the causative organism is *Lyssavirus* type 1. The disease is highly fatal and is acute in nature. Only warm-blooded animals, especially carnivorous, are affected by this disease. Dogs, cats, wolves, and jackals are to name the few. In humans, it is transmitted by either the bite or the licks of rabid animals where the saliva comes in direct contact with the raw skin wounds or the mucosal membrane of the humans. The incubation period is not consistent; rather variability is the norm. Humans act as the dead end for this infection.

Yellow Fever

Yellow fever is a zoonotic disease caused by *Flavivirus fibricus*, formerly classified as group B arbovirus. It affects principally monkeys and other vertebrates in tropics. It is transmitted to man by certain culicine mosquitoes. It presents as viral hemorrhagic fever. It is a fatal disease and is characterized by severe hepatic and renal involvement. Certain environmental factors such as humidity, temperature of 24°C or more, urbanization, industrialization, and increasing travel have led to spread of disease from infected people to nonimmune community in large number and also the *Aedes* mosquitoes. Person-to-person infection is then transmitted by these infected mosquitoes.

Japanese Encephalitis

Culicine mosquitoes are responsible for the transmission of this type of encephalitis and the virus causing belongs to group B arbovirus (*Flavivirus*). Since the transmission is from mosquitos to humans, it is classified as zoonotic disease. Different geographical regions have different major genotypes of this virus but have the same serotype and their preference for the host and virulence is same. Once bitten by an infected mosquito, the virus initially replicates in local and regional lymph nodes. The virus spreads to the central nervous system through blood. In Asia, JE is the leading cause of encephalitis. The annual incidence ranges between less than 10 and more than 100 per 100,000 population in different geographical locations both within the country and outside the country. The disease peaks during the rainy season as the mosquitoes have a plenty of breeding ground and conducive weather during this time. The irrigation programs associated with agricultural development are also linked with the spread of JE in new areas.

Kyasanur Forest Disease

Kyasanur forest disease is caused by arbovirus (*Flavivirus*) and is transmitted to man by the bite of ticks. The presentation is with fever and hemorrhage. The Shimoga district of the Karnataka state was the first to detect this disease. Locally, it was known as the monkey disease as people living there associated it with the death of monkeys.

Measles (Rubeola)

Measles is caused by the specific virus of the group myxovirus (paramyxovirus). It is highly infectious disease of childhood. The virus can be grown in cell culture and it has one serotype. It occurs only in humans. There is no animal source of infection. The only source of infection in a case of measles is the secretions from the respiratory tract and throat and nasal secretions from the person suffering from measles during the prodromal phase and the stage of rash.

Rubella (German Measles)

The RNA virus belonging to the Toga family is the causative organism for rubella. There is only one antigenic type of the virus of the Togavirus family. Nasopharynx, throat, blood, cerebrospinal fluid (CSF), and urine harbor the virus. It can be propagated in cell culture. Postnatally acquired rubella does not show any carrier state. Infants having congenital rubella may keep on shedding the virus for many months. As compared to measles, rubella is less communicable since the symptoms of cough are not present. The infection occurs mainly when the rashes are erupting. The vaccine virus is not communicable.

Varicella (Chickenpox)

Varicella is a highly infectious disease caused by varicella zoster (VZ) virus. VZ virus, also known as "Human virus 3," is the causative agent for chickenpox. In temperate climates and tropical settings, there is a seasonal trend. In tropics, it is during coolest and driest months, while in temperate climates peak incidence is during winter and spring. Transmission is by droplet infection and by droplet nuclei from person to person. Congenital varicella is caused when the virus crosses the placental barrier infecting the fetus.

Roseola Infantum (Exanthem Subitum)

Roseola infantum is caused by human herpes virus (HHV-6), and less commonly by HHV-7 and echovirus 16, and is also called sixth disease. HHV-6 and HHV-7 are DNA viruses that target the CD4 T cells, and like herpes viruses, can remain latent in the body for several year after acute infection.

Erythema Infectiosum (Fifth Disease)

Erythema infectiosum is a common exanthematous illness, caused by a small DNA virus, parvoviruses B19. This virus has tropism for cells of the erythroid lineage at the pronormoblast stage. Transmission of infection is by the respiratory route. The characteristic rash first appears as erythematous flushing on the face in a "slapped-cheek" appearance.

Hand-Foot-Mouth Disease

Hand-foot-mouth disease is caused by viruses of the genus *Enterovirus* belonging to family Picornaviridae. The most common causes of this disease are *Coxsackievirus* A16 and *Enterovirus* 71. The disease usually presents as outbreak, often in preschool children, and transmission is by direct contact with an affected patient or infected fomites.[3,7]

Zika Virus

Zika virus has recently been recognized as a global serious disease and is transmitted by *Aedes* mosquito. It belongs to Flaviviridae group. It was first isolated from rhesus monkey in the Zika forest in Uganda. Humid areas of tropical Africa and southeast Asia have more disease prevalence. The main symptoms are fever, rash, arthralgia, headache, and myalgia resembling dengue.[7]

■ EMERGING AND REEMERGING VIRAL DISEASES

Any infectious disease which has appeared and affected the community for the first time or previously present but has started increasing rapidly or has spread to new geographical areas is known as emerging or reemerging disease. Recently, many of the viral zoonotic diseases are having huge outbreaks in India and the factors responsible for this emergence are increased trade and travel activities. Internationally, war causing mass migration of people, natural calamities, advances in medical care, rural urbanization, human encroachment on wildlife habitats, wildlife trade, ecotourism, etc. lead to viral zoonotic diseases. Some of the several viral infections reported are *Nipah virus*—a zoonotic paramyxovirus; *Hantavirus*—enveloped, ssRNA family Bunyaviridae; *Chikungunya*—enveloped ssRNA, Togaviridae; *Human enterovirus 71*—nonenveloped ssRNA, Picornaviridae; *Chandipura*—enveloped ssRNA, Rhabdoviridae; *Pandemic influenza 2009 H1N1*—enveloped ssRNA Orthomyxoviridae; *Avian influenza H5N1*—enveloped ssRNA Orthomyxoviridae; *Crimean Congo virus*—enveloped ssRNA, Bunyaviridae; *SARS*—enveloped ssRNA Coronaviridae; and *Buffalopox*—enveloped dsDNA Poxviridae.[9,10]

VIRAL SEPSIS (A NEW ENTITY VIRAL SEPTICEMIA)

Sepsis is a life-threatening condition in which there is organ dysfunction caused by unregulated host response to infection. Majority of sepsis is caused by bacteria but other pathogens such as viruses and fungi can also cause sepsis. Up to 42% of sepsis are culture-negative, suggesting a nonbacterial cause. But still diagnosis of viral sepsis remains obscured. Any virus can cause sepsis-like illness in vulnerable patients such as neonates, infants, and immunosuppressed groups. Actual incidence and prevalence of viral sepsis is not known. The initial standard of care for all septic cases is the immediate usage of broad-spectrum antibiotics, irrespective of their culture result.

Since there are no definitive criteria to diagnose viral sepsis or means to exclude bacterial sepsis, under such circumstances in tropical areas viral sepsis may be underdiagnosed. This leads to unnecessary use of antimicrobial agents, eventually leading to antimicrobial resistance and increasing healthcare cost.[11,12]

CONCLUSION

Children living in tropical and subtropical areas are at risk of infectious diseases. Clinicians need to have high index of suspicion for the diagnosis of viral infections as the symptomatology may be misleading or overlapping with other infections. The effective management of the disease may not be possible without the prior knowledge of epidemiology of viruses and this knowledge will help them in diagnosing and managing these cases.

REFERENCES

1. Rodier GR, Ryan MG, Heymann DL. Global epidemiology of infectious diseases. In: Strickland GT (Ed). Strickland Hunters Tropical Medicine and Emerging infectious Diseases, 8th edition. Philadelphia: WB Saunders Company; 2000. pp. 1071-104.
2. Monto SA. The epidemiology of viral infections, In: Brain WJ, Meulen VT (Eds). Topley and Wilson's Microbiology and Microbial infections, Virology (1), 10th edition. USA: Wiley; 2007. pp. 353-74.
3. Baveja CP. Virology. In: Baveja CP (Ed). Textbook of Microbiology, 6th edition. Delhi: Arya Publications; 2018. pp. 423-44.
4. Harvey AR, Cornelissen CN, Fisher BD. Introduction to the viruses. In: Harvey AR (Ed). Microbiology Lippincott's illustrated Reviews. 3rd South Asian edition. New Delhi: Wolters Kluwer Lippincott Williams & Wilkins; 2017. pp. 233-43.
5. American Society of Tropical Medicine and Hygiene, Advancing Global Health Science. Tropical Diseases. [online] Available from: www.astmh.org. [Last accessed on December, 2019].
6. Brachman PS. Epidemiology. In: Baron S (Ed). Baron S, Medical Microbiology, 4th edition. Galveston: University of Texas Medical Branch at Galveston; 1996. p. 9.
7. Shastri D. Common viral infections. In: Parthasarathy A (Ed). Textbook of Paediatric Infectious Diseases IAP, 2nd edition. New Delhi: Jaypee Brothers; 2019. pp. 287-379.
8. Park K. Zoonoses: Epidemiology of communicable diseases. In: Park K (Ed). Park's Textbook of preventive and social medicine, 23rd edition. Jabalpur: Bhanot; 2015. pp. 276-89.
9. Sejvar J, Tselis AC, Boos J. Handbook of Clinical Neurology, 1st edition. China: Elsevier; 2014. pp. 67-87.
10. Mani RS, Ravi V, Desai A, et al. Emerging Viral Infections in India. Proceedings of the National Academy of Sciences, India Section B: Biological Sciences. 2012;82(1):5-21.
11. Patel S. Integration of HIV and other health programmes: Implications and challenges. Int J Med Sci Public Health. 2014;3(6):643-8.
12. Lin G, McGinley JP, Drysdale SB, et al. Epidemiology and Immune Pathogenesis of Viral Sepsis. Font Immunol. 2018; 9:2147.

Human Immunodeficiency Virus and Acquired Immunodeficiency Syndrome

Amarnath Saran, Prachi Jain, Piyush Gupta

INTRODUCTION

HIV-1 and HIV-2 viruses were identified as cause of human immunodeficiency virus (HIV) infection and acquired immunodeficiency syndrome (AIDS) more than three decades ago. Advancements in diagnosis and early initiation of treatment have improved the survival in this disease; however, it continues to be one of the most dreaded infections faced by mankind. Higher viral burden and faster depletion of infected CD4 lymphocytes in infants and children lead to faster progression of the infection with nearly 50% of the untreated children dying within the first 2 years of life.[1] HIV infection also has a large social, psychological and economic impact on the affected individuals and their families, especially children who end up missing out on proper schooling, living in poverty, and suffering from depression, apart from also being at a higher risk of exposure to HIV.

MAGNITUDE OF THE PROBLEM

According to the UNAIDS (United Nations Program of HIV/AIDS) 2019 fact sheet, 37.9 million people were living with HIV in 2018, of which 1.7 million were children <15 years of age.[2] Improved healthcare system has resulted in significant reduction in new infections as well as mortality associated with HIV/AIDS, changing its perception to a chronic manageable disease now. In 2018, 62% of all people living with HIV and 54% of all children with HIV had access to treatment. About 82% of pregnant women with HIV could get treated for the prevention of mother to child transmission. Since 2010 there has been 16% reduction in new infections, from 2.1 million to 1.7 million in 2018. HIV/AIDS-related deaths have seen a bigger decline, by 33% since 2010 (from 1.2 million to 770,000 in 2018). Similar trend is seen in pediatric age group where the new infections have declined by 41% (from 280,000 to 160,000 in 2018). AIDS-related mortality in children also reduced from 210,000 in 2010 to 120,000 in 2018.[2]

India has the third highest burden of HIV in the world. In 2017, there were 2.14 million people living with HIV, of which 61,000 were children <15 years of age.[3] Since the identification of first few cases of HIV in the country, India has been contributing majorly in bringing down the burden of HIV/AIDS globally. India's antiretroviral treatment (ART) program is the second largest in the world with an estimated coverage of 56% of all cases of HIV.[4] About 60% of all pregnant women living with HIV in India received antiretroviral treatment (2017). Early infant diagnosis has improved from 6% in 2010 to 23% in 2017.[3]

The number of new infections in children <15 years of age has reduced from 13,000 in 2005 to 3,700 in 2017. Similar trend can be seen in AIDS-related mortality in children <15 years of age, which has come down from 11,000 in 2005 to 2,600 in 2007.[4] AIDS-related deaths have decreased in major part of India, except states of Assam, Bihar, Jharkhand, Haryana, Delhi, and Uttarakhand.[5]

EPIDEMIOLOGY

Agent Factors

Human immunodeficiency virus is a nontransforming, spherical virus that belongs to *Lentivirus* genus of *Retroviridae* family and contains a cone-shaped core surrounded by a lipid envelope that is derived from the host cell membrane.

The core contains:

- The major capsid protein p24
- Nucleocapsid protein p7/p9
- Two copies of viral genomic RNA

- The three main viral enzymes (reverse transcriptase, protease, and integrase)

P24 is the viral antigen that is detected by ELISA (enzyme-linked immunosorbent assay) based tests used routinely for diagnosis of HIV.

The viral core is surrounded by a matrix protein called p17, followed by an envelope that is studded with two important glycoproteins, gp120 and gp41. Inside the envelope lies the RNA genome. Three important regions of the genome are the gag, pol, and env genes. Gag encodes for the viral core proteins (like p24), Pol is for production of viral enzymes (reverse transcriptase, integrase, and protease) and Env region encodes the envelope proteins (e.g. gp41, gp120). A unique enzyme called reverse transcriptase is used to produce DNA from the RNA genome which is then translated into viral proteins, hence the name retrovirus.

There are two types of HIV identified—HIV-1 and HIV-2. HIV-1 is the most common serotype worldwide. There are three major groups of HIV-1, designated as M (major), O (outlier) and N (non-M/non-O). Group M includes nine subtypes, or "clades", A to K, which have spread with specific geographic distribution in the worldwide pandemic. HIV-1 subtype C is the most widespread in India with almost 6 million persons infected. HIV-2 is endemic in West Africa, but has spread to Europe and India.

Modes of Transmission

Transmission of HIV can occur through sexual contact, parenteral exposure to infected blood (needle sharing by drug abusers, multiple blood/blood product transfusions) or vertical transmission from mother to child. The primary mode in pediatric population (<15 years) is vertical transmission, which can occur before delivery (intrauterine), during delivery (intrapartum) or after delivery (postpartum). Presence of laboratory evidence of infection [polymerase chain reaction (PCR) or positive viral culture] in the first week of life suggests that 20–30% of infected neonates are infected in utero.[1] Majority of in utero infection occurs in late pregnancy when integrity of placental vasculature weakens allowing microtransfusions between fetal and maternal circulations. Intrapartum infection is more common and occurs because of mucosal exposure to infected blood, vaginal secretions or increased microtransfusions due to uterine contractions during labor. The overall risk of vertical transmission before or during delivery is 15–25%. The risk of mother to child infection through breastfeeding is 9–16%, however if breastfeeding is continued till 18–24 months, the risk increases to 30–45%. The risk is highest in breastfeeding mothers who acquire HIV postnatally (29–53%). Maternal viral load, preterm delivery and maternal antenatal CD4 count affect vertical transmission.

PATHOGENESIS

The HIV replication cycle is composed of the following main steps: (1) entry into host cell, (2) uncoating, (3) integration with host DNA and dormant phase, and (4) virus particle formation and release of new virus particle by budding.[6]

Entry into the host cell: The viral envelope has a trimeric complex, composed of transmembrane protein gp41, and gp120 on the surface of the cell. This complex is essential for recognition of the host cell by the virus and its entry into target cells. HIV targets the CD4 positive cells in our body. Gp 120 selectively binds to CD4 protein, which is expressed on the surface of T-lymphocytes, T-cell precursors within the bone marrow and thymus, on monocytes/macrophages, eosinophils, dendritic cells, and microglial cells of the central nervous system (CNS). This binding allows the gp41-gp120 envelope complex to undergo a structural change, exposing a specific domain in the gp120 that binds to specific chemokine coreceptors, the most common being CXCR4 and CCR5. CXCR4 is found on T-lymphocytes, while CCR5 is present on monocytes/macrophages, dendritic cells, and activated T-lymphocytes. The presence of these coreceptors is essential for binding of HIV and plays an important role in affinity of different strains of HIV-1 toward specific cells. Practically, the chemokines RANTES, MIP-1-α and MIP-1-β, ligands for the CCR5 receptor and α-chemokine SDF-1, and a ligand for CXCR4 have been used to suppress HIV-1 infection in vitro, because they inhibit the binding of HIV to CCR5 by competitive inhibition. A stable bond thus formed between gp120, CD4, and CCR5/CXCR4 receptor allows the HIV particle to penetrate and enter through the cell membrane.

Uncoating and integration: Then the virus core uncoats inside the cytoplasm of the host cell freeing the viral RNA. Viral RNA is converted into DNA with the help of enzyme *reverse transcriptase* which gets incorporated into host cell DNA with the help of *integrase* resulting in formation of *provirus DNA*. Monocytes/macrophages, microglial cells, and other quiescent CD4+ T-cells thus contain integrated provirus and become long-living reservoirs of HIV, that upon activation transcribe and produce virus particles in large numbers.

Upon activation of host cell, precursor molecules are synthesized by various genes and are cleaved by HIV *protease* enzyme, resulting in formation of HIV particles.

In infected individuals, approximately 100 billion new viral particles are produced and 1–2 billion CD4+ T cells die each day.

B-cell dysfunction: Although β-cells are not directly infected by HIV, they show profound abnormalities. There is acquired inability to mount specific antibody responses to newly encountered antigens, while at the same time paradoxically increased B-cell production and hypergammaglobulinemia.

HIV variability: Variability of HIV is a major tool that allows it to evade the host immunity and the effects of drugs and vaccines. This variability is achieved with the help of three peculiar features: (1) the "error-prone" nature of the enzyme reverse transcriptase, that leaves, on average, one substitution mutation per genome per replication cycle (2) the rate of viral replication being exceptionally high generating a large number of virions per day, and (3) the occurrence of recombination processes between two or more different HIV strains within the same individual.

NATURAL COURSE OF HIV INFECTION

Like other members of *Lentivirus* family, HIV has a chronic natural history of illness, a long clinical latent period characterized by persistent viral replication, followed by overt clinical disease and also direct involvement of CNS. The pathogenesis of HIV infection is based on the direct effects of the virus along with the host immune response.

After transmission of HIV through infected body fluid into dendritic cells and CD4+ lymphocytes through receptor-dependent mechanisms, the virus spreads to regional lymph nodes. There is extensive viral replication in the lymphatic tissue of infected mucosae and regional lymph nodes in the early stages of the infection. The infected cells either undergo lysis or become a center of latent infection. The presence of latent HIV infection in lymphatic tissues is the barrier that prevents complete eradication of the infection despite receiving adequate ART.

Viremia is detectable in the plasma 10–12 days after the primary infection. This high level of viremia is however short-lived, since the host generates humoral and cellular immune responses that partially curbs viral replication. Over the next few weeks, viremia steadily declines and reaches a low or undetectable steady state. Virus specific CD8+ T-cell cytotoxic activity seem to play the central role in this initial control of virus replication, and is followed by the appearance of anti-HIV antibodies. Seroconversion usually occurs between 3 weeks and 5 weeks, but may take up to 3 months. The time period during which the individual is infected but antibodies are not yet detectable in the serum is called the "window period".

The initial clinical manifestations are usually that of a flu-like illness in the form of fever, pharyngitis, lymphadenopathy, arthralgia, malaise, maculopapular rash, and oral ulcers. These symptoms are heterogeneous in severity and duration between different patients, usually lasting 7–10 days. This acute illness coincides with the phase of viremia and dramatic fall in CD4+ T-cell count. With the onset of host immune response HIV viremia declines and CD4+ T cells rise again, although the preinfection levels are not reached. At this time, serology also becomes positive.

Latent phase: After this acute phase has subsided, the infected individuals enter an asymptomatic period wherein there is ongoing continuous viral replication in the lymphatic tissues of the body, but without overt clinical features. In many individuals, HIV viremia is not detectable for many years. There is a slow but progressive ongoing loss of CD4+ lymphocytes and functional impairment of the persisting cells.

Low CD4 counts imply poor host immunity and become the harbinger of opportunistic infections (OIs) by bacteria, viruses, fungi and parasites, and tumors, which are the presenting symptoms in most patients when HIV is diagnosed. Depending on the rate of progression of disease from the time of infection, patients are classified into "elite controllers", who can adequately control HIV infection, "progressors", "rapid progressors", "nonprogressors", and "long-term nonprogressors".

CLINICAL MANIFESTATIONS

Clinical manifestations of HIV are mostly linked to the OIs and neoplasms associated with the impaired immune status. Overt clinical manifestations in the form of generalized lymphadenopathy, unexplained fever and significant weight loss, persistent diarrhea and respiratory symptoms appear initially.

The most common OIs are caused by pneumocystis carinii pneumonia (PCP), oral and esophageal candidiasis, *Cytomegalovirus* (CMV) and hematopoietic stem cell (HSC) infection, chronic diarrhea caused by *Cryptosporidium*, *Giardia*, and *Isospora* and pulmonary and extrapulmonary tuberculosis (TB). Opportunistic infections are responsible for the majority of deaths in untreated patients with HIV. Many of these infections represent reactivation of latent infections, which are normally kept in check by our robust immune system.

A progressive encephalopathy induced by HIV itself or other OIs may also be the presenting manifestation. Neoplastic diseases such as Kaposi's sarcoma and lymphomas are rare manifestations as far as children are concerned.

Lymphocytic interstitial pneumonia (LIP) is a special entity described in stage 3 HIV disease. It is a lymphoproliferative, noninfectious pulmonary disorder characterized by diffuse infiltration of CD4 lymphocytes, plasma cells, and histiocytes in the alveolar septa and along the lymphatics. It is most common in children infected with HIV, especially those aged >2–3 years. It has an insidious onset of mild but persistent cough, with or without exertional dyspnea, and breathing difficulty. It should be suspected in patients who have associated clubbing with respiratory illness and the child does not respond clinically or radiologically despite appropriate antibacterial and antituberculosis treatment (ATT). Treatment of LIP includes bronchodilators and corticosteroids. The World Health Organization (WHO) clinical staging is described in **Box 1**.[7]

DIAGNOSIS OF HIV IN CHILDREN

The National AIDS Control Program (NACP) offers services of integrated counseling and testing centers (ICTC) for early diagnosis of HIV and effective streamlining of patients to the treatment centers. Rapid diagnostic tests (RDTs) are used for diagnosis of HIV in all individuals who are more than 18 months of age.[8] These RDTs detect antibodies to HIV and are based on the principle of enzyme immunoassay, immunoconcentration, and particle agglutination. They have a sensitivity of >99.5% and a specificity of >98%.

Two situations in which serological tests for antibodies prove ineffective in diagnosis are patients less than 18 months of age, because maternal antibodies will be found both in the presence and absence of active HIV infection, and in the 6–12 weeks "window period" of patients who have recently acquired HIV infection but have not yet developed antibodies against the same. These situations warrant the use of PCR analysis for direct detection of viral replication or waiting until the appropriate time for serological tests to become positive.

All testing should follow five C's of counseling: Consent, confidentiality, counseling, correct test results and immediate connection to services for HIV prevention, treatment, and care.

Box 1: Clinical staging of human immunodeficiency virus (HIV) infection in children.

Stage 1:
- Asymptomatic
- Persistent generalized lymphadenopathy

Stage 2:
- Unexplained persistent hepatosplenomegaly
- Recurrent or chronic upper respiratory tract infections (otitis media, otorrhea, sinusitis, tonsillitis)
- Herpes zoster
- Lineal gingival erythema
- Recurrent oral ulceration
- Papular pruritic eruption
- Fungal nail infections
- Extensive wart virus infection
- Extensive molluscum contagiosum
- Unexplained persistent parotid enlargement

Stage 3:
- Unexplained moderate malnutrition not adequately responding to standard therapy
- Unexplained persistent diarrhea (14 days or more)
- Unexplained persistent fever (above 37.5°C, intermittent or constant, for longer than one 1 month)
- Persistent oral candidiasis (after the first 6 weeks of life)
- Oral hairy leukoplakia (OHL)
- Lymph node tuberculosis
- Pulmonary tuberculosis
- Severe recurrent bacterial pneumonia
- Acute necrotizing ulcerative gingivitis or periodontitis
- Unexplained anemia (<8 g/dL), neutropenia (<0.5 × 10^9/L) or chronic thrombocytopenia (<50 × 10^9/L)
- Symptomatic lymphoid interstitial pneumonitis
- Chronic HIV-associated lung disease, including bronchiectasis

Stage 4:
- Unexplained severe wasting, stunting or severe malnutrition not responding to standard therapy
- Pneumocystis (jiroveci) pneumonia
- Recurrent severe bacterial infections (such as empyema, pyomyositis, bone or joint infection, meningitis, but excluding pneumonia)
- Chronic herpes simplex infection (orolabial or cutaneous of more than 1-month duration or visceral at any site)
- Esophageal candidiasis (or candidiasis of trachea, bronchi or lungs)
- Extrapulmonary tuberculosis
- Kaposi's sarcoma
- *Cytomegalovirus* infection (retinitis or infection of other organs with onset at age more than 1 month)
- Central nervous system toxoplasmosis (after the neonatal period)
- HIV encephalopathy
- Extrapulmonary cryptococcosis, including meningitis
- Disseminated mycobacterial (NTM) infection
- Progressive multifocal leukoencephalopathy (PML)
- Chronic cryptosporidiosis (with diarrhea)
- Chronic isosporiasis
- Disseminated endemic mycosis (extrapulmonary histoplasmosis, coccidioidomycosis, penicilliosis)
- Cerebral or B-cell non-Hodgkin lymphoma
- HIV-associated nephropathy or cardiomyopathy

Diagnosis of HIV Infection in Infants and Children Aged More Than 18 Months of Age

Symptomatic patients: A patient whose clinical profile warrants evaluation of HIV is referred to the ICTC for testing. The patient is declared HIV-negative if the first test is nonreactive. No second test is applied. However, in case one sample yields a positive result, a second test with a different antigen or principle is applied to confirm the diagnosis. Two tests must show reactive results to declare a patient HIV-positive. A third test is needed when the first test is positive but the second one is negative. If the third test is negative the patient is reported as negative, but if it is reactive, the result is reported as indeterminate and the individual is retested after 14–28 days.

Asymptomatic patients: For clinically asymptomatic patients including blood donations and pregnant females, three separate tests must be found positive to declare a person HIV positive. In case of any disparity, indeterminate status is declared and patient retested after few weeks.

Diagnosis of HIV Infection in Infants and Children Aged Less Than 18 Months of Age

Infants and children less than 18 months of age who have had perinatal exposure to HIV are expected to have maternally acquired antibodies and hence positive serology even in the absence of active HIV infection. Hence, they need another mode of testing that directly detects virus replication. DNA-PCR on dried blood spot (DBS) sample is recommended for infants born to HIV positive mothers, at 6 weeks or the earliest opportunity after that.

After 6 months of age: Screening with antibody tests, if positive, should be followed by a DNA-PCR.

Breastfeeding: Since breastfed babies are exposed to infection till a later stage, they are to be retested with DNA-PCR 6 weeks after cessation of breastfeeding, even if a prior test was nonreactive. The diagnostic algorithm for HIV infection is shown in **Flowcharts 1 and 2**.

HIV-2 Infection

HIV-1 is the most common serotype in India. But few cases of HIV-2 have been reported. HIV-2 infection is inherently resistant to nonnucleoside reverse transcriptase inhibitors (NNRTIs). Thus, there are both epidemiological and treatment implications of presence of HIV-2 infection. The RDTs being used by ICTCs do differentiate the presence of HIV-1 and 2 infection, but diagnosis of HIV-2 cannot be definitively based on these.

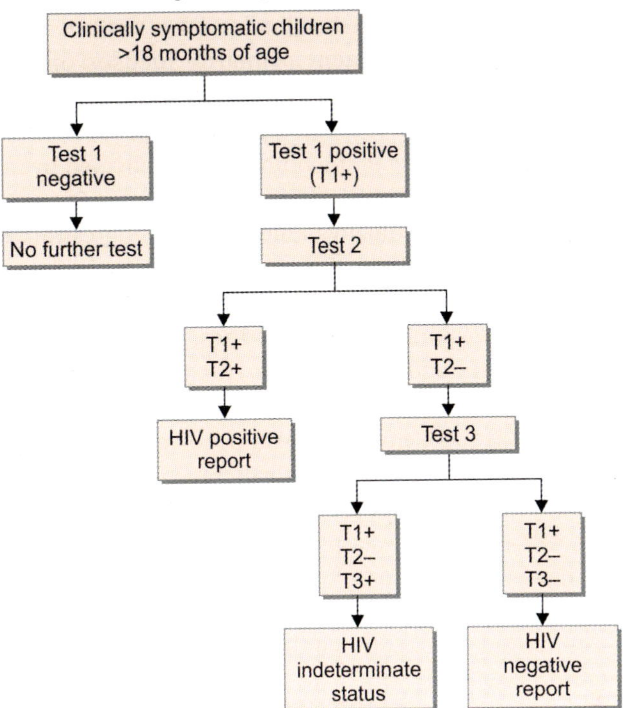

Flowchart 1: Diagnostic algorithm for children >18 months age.

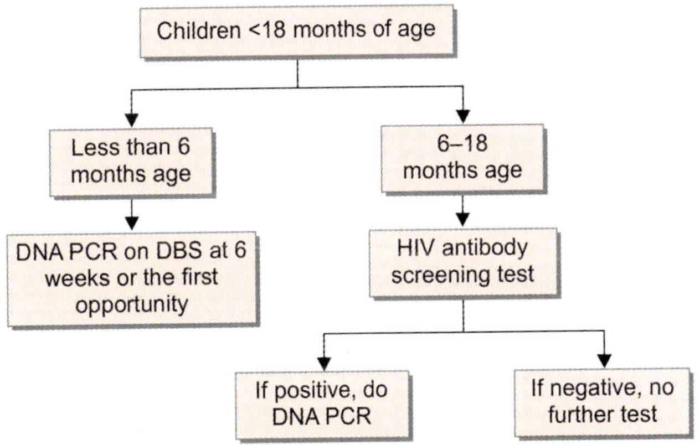

Flowchart 2: Diagnostic algorithm of human immunodeficiency virus (HIV) for children <18 months age.

(DBS: dried blood spot; PCR: polymerase chain reaction; DNA: deoxyribonucleic acid)

Patients with a HIV-2 reactive report need to be referred to the nearest State Reference Laboratories (SRLs) and National Reference Laboratories (NRLs) that are responsible for confirmation of HIV-2 infection.

■ TREATMENT

General Principles of Treatment

Currently available antiretroviral (ARV) drugs cannot eradicate the virus from the human body. This is because a reservoir of latently infected CD4 cells gets established during the earliest stages of HIV infection. This pool persists within lymphoid tissue, liver and brain despite suppression of viremia in the blood.

Antiretroviral treatment primarily focuses on the maximal and sustained reduction of number of viral copies and replication in the blood and restoration of immunological status of the body. This is reflected by an increase in the CD4 count, reduced frequency of OIs, and improvement in the quality of life. Disease progression to AIDS is prevented despite the presence of HIV infection.

Treatment is started after a parent's/guardian's informed decision and preparedness to initiate ART with an understanding of the benefits of the treatment, lifelong medication, and issues related to adherence. Need for adequate nutritional support, vaccination and social wellbeing play a major role in the overall treatment success and must be reinforced to caregivers on regular visits. ART is not to be started in the presence of an active OI. In general, OIs should be treated or stabilized before commencing ART. Baseline investigations to be done before starting ART is given in **Box 2**.

Antiretroviral treatment uses a combination of at least three ARV drugs with different mechanisms of action to achieve this purpose.[8]

The various points in the replication cycle of HIV at which ARV drugs are designed to act are:

- *Fusion inhibitors and CCR5 coreceptor blockers*: Block binding of HIV to the host cell.
- *Reverse transcriptase inhibitors*: Block the conversion of viral RNA into DNA [non-nucleoside reverse transcriptase inhibitors (NNRTIs)]

- *Integrase inhibitors*: Block the enzyme integrase, which helps in incorporation of the proviral DNA into the host cell chromosome.
- *Protease inhibitors (PIs)*: Block enzyme protease. Classification of ARV drugs is summarized in **Table 1**.

First-line ART Regimen in Children

NRTI: Zidovudine (AZT) or abacavir (ABC) are the first choice NRTIs in the absence and presence of anemia (Hb < 9 g/dL) respectively.

For children above 10 years and 30 kg body weight, tenofovir (TDF) is the preferred drug. Stavudine (d4T) is phased out from pediatric first-line regimen; however, its use may be considered in case of dual toxicity for both AZT and ABC.

Lamivudine is the second drug that is a part of all first-line regimens.

NNRTI: Efavirenz (EFV) is the preferred drug in >3 years and 10 kg weight.

Integrase inhibitor: Lopinavir/ritonavir (LPV/r) is the third drug recommended in all children less than 3 years of age. For children older than 3 years, EFV is used.

Basic principles of first-line ART regimen is summarized in **Table 2**.

Adverse Effects of ART

Patients should be monitored clinically and biochemically for adverse effects of the various ARV drugs being taken. In case of side effects significantly affecting quality of life or organ functions, change in drugs should be considered. Adverse effects of different ARV drugs are summarized in **Table 3**.

When to Change ART?

Substitutions versus switch: When an adverse reaction or toxicity to a certain drug is identified, it is *substituted* for another drug. But if clinical features or laboratory evidence are suggestive of treatment failure, it warrants change or *switch* of the entire treatment regimen.

Treatment failure: The prerequisites for considering treatment failure on any ART regimen in any patient include:

- Child should have received the regimen for at least 6 months.
- Adherence to therapy should be assessed and should be optimal.
- Any acute or OIs should be treated and resolved before interpreting CD4 counts.

Box 2: Baseline workup to be done prior to starting antiretroviral treatment (ART).

- *Blood investigations*:
  - CBC
  - LFT
  - KFT
  - Lipid profile
  - Fasting blood sugar
  - HBsAg, anti-HCV
  - VDRL
  - CD4 count and CD4%
  - rK39 strip test to rule out leishmaniasis (especially in patients with HIV infection who live in Bihar, Eastern UP, Jharkhand, and West Bengal)
- Urine routine microscopic examination
- *Radiological examination*:
  - Chest X-ray P/A view
  - USG abdomen

(CBC: complete blood count; HBsAg: hepatitis B surface antigen; HCV: hepatitis C virus; HIV: human immunodeficiency virus; KFT: kidney function test; LFT: liver function test; VDRL: venereal disease research laboratory test; USG: ultrasonography)

Table 1: Classification of antiretroviral (ARV) drugs.

Nucleoside reverse transcriptase inhibitors (NRTIs)	Nonnucleoside reverse transcriptase inhibitors (NNRTIs)	Protease inhibitors (PI)	Integrase inhibitors	Nucleotide reverse transcriptase inhibitor (NtRTI)	Fusion inhibitor (FI)	CCR5 entry inhibitor
Zidovudine (AZT)	Nevirapine (NVP)	Saquinavir (SQV)	Raltegravir (RGV)	Tenofovir (TDF)	Enfuvirtide (T-20)	Maraviroc
Stavudine (d4T)	Efavirenz (EFV)	Ritonavir (RTV)	Elvitegravir (EVG)			
Lamivudine (3TC)	Delavirdine (DLV)	Nelfinavir (NFV)	Dolutegravir (DTG)			
Abacavir (ABC)	Rilpivirine (RPV)	Amprenavir (APV)				
Didanosine (ddI)	Etravirine (ETV)	Indinavir (INV)				
Zalcitabine (ddC)		Lopinavir (LPV)				
Emtricitabine (FTC)		Fosamprenavir (FPV)				
		Atazanavir (ATV)				
		Tipranavir (TPV)				
		Darunavir (DRV)				

Table 2: Basic principles of first-line antiretroviral treatment (ART) regimens in children.

Drug 1 (NRTI)	Hb >9 g%	AZT
	Hb < 9 g%	ABC
Drug 2 (NRTI)	3TC	
Drug 3 (NNRTI)	Age > 3 years	EFV
	Age < 3 years	L/R

(ABC: abacavir; EFV: efavirenz; AZT: zidovudine)

- Immune reconstitution inflammatory syndrome (IRIS) and malnutrition must be excluded.
- Possibility of adverse effects of the drugs manifesting like clinical treatment failure should be ruled out.

Virological failure: It is defined as presence of 1,000 copies/mL of virus present in the blood after at least 6 months of ART. It is the most sensitive indicator of treatment failure.

Immunological failure: It almost always precedes clinical failure. In the situation of any new clinical event occurring after 6 months of appropriate ART, immunological criteria help to differentiate between treatment failure and other overlapping conditions like IRIS, OIs and drug toxicities.

Clinical failure: The development of new or recurrent clinical event belonging to WHO clinical stage 3 and 4 disease (with the exception of TB) after 6 months of effective treatment is considered evidence of the progression of HIV disease. TB can occur at any CD4 level and does not necessarily indicate ART failure.

Table 3: Important side effects of major antiretroviral (ARV) drugs.

Drug	Adverse effect
Zidovudine (AZT)	• Severe anemia • Neutropenia • Lactic acidosis • Hepatotoxicity • Lipoatrophy • Lipodystrophy • Myopathy
Abacavir (ABC)	• Hypersensitivity reactions
Nevirapine (NVP)	• Hepatotoxicity • Severe skin rash and hypersensitivity reaction, including Stevens-Johnson syndrome • Chronic kidney disease • Acute kidney injury and Fanconi syndrome
Efavirenz (EFV)	• Neuropsychiatric symptoms such as dizziness, insomnia, abnormal dreams or anxiety, depression, mental confusion • Seizures • Hepatotoxicity • Skin and hypersensitivity reactions • Gynecomastia • ECG abnormalities (PR and QRS interval prolongation, torsades de pointes)
Lopinavir/ ritonavir (L/R)	• Hepatotoxicity • Pancreatitis • Dyslipidemia • Diarrhea

(ECG: electrocardiogram)

All children with suspected treatment failure should be referred to State AIDS Clinical Expert Panel (SACEP), Pediatric Centers of Excellence (pCoE) or ART plus center

Table 4: Criteria for treatment failure on a particular antiretroviral treatment (ART) regimen.	
Virological failure	*Plasma viral load above 1,000 copies/mL after 6 months of ART*
Immunological failure	*Between 1–3 years:* • CD% falls below 15% • Persistent CD4 level below 200 cells/mm^3 *Between 3–5 years:* • CD% falls below 10% • Persistent CD4 levels below 200 cells/mm^3 *5 years and above:* • Fall of CD4 count to pretherapy baseline • 50% fall from peak "on treatment" level • Persistent CD4 levels below 100 cells
Clinical failure	New or recurrent clinical event belonging to WHO clinical stage 4 after 6 months of ART

for targeted viral load assessment. Criteria of treatment failure are summarized in **Table 4**.

Malnutrition and HIV Treatment

Human immunodeficiency virus and associated infections increase the need for energy, proteins and micronutrients like iron, zinc, and vitamin C. Failure to meet these increased needs in the form of malnutrition leads to further weakening of the immune system. This makes the child more vulnerable to OIs like TB, pneumonia, diarrhea. A vicious cycle is formed between HIV infection and malnutrition when accelerated disease progression further increases the nutritional demands of the body. The growth of these children is monitored regularly and classified based on standard WHO recommended anthropometric criteria. They are examined for visible signs of malnutrition like loss of subcutaneous fat and muscles and bipedal edema. Children without visible signs of malnutrition should be given nutritional support at home, with early follow-up (5–7 days).

Practically, asymptomatic children with adequate growth require 10% additional energy. Those with poor weight gain require 20–30% additional energy and severely malnourished children have 50–100% additional energy requirements per day.[8]

Micronutrient intake at the recommended dietary allowance (RDA) should be ensured through a balanced diet. If the child's diet does not contain a variety of fruits, vegetables, and food from animal sources give a daily supplement that provides RDA of vitamins and other micronutrients. Investigate for the presence of anemia and give iron supplements if needed. Vitamin A, zinc supplementation and routine deworming strategies should be followed similar to the general population.

PREVENTION AND CONTROL OF HIV/AIDS

HIV and Pregnancy

All pregnant women enrolled into antenatal care (ANC) should be offered HIV counseling and testing. HIV positive women presenting in labor or breastfeeding should be immediately started on ART. Promoting institutional deliveries, additional screening for associated conditions (TB, sexually transmitted infections and other OIs), psychological support, nutritional, and breastfeeding counseling should be done for all HIV-infected pregnant women. In India, vaginal delivery is recommended unless there is an obstetric indication for cesarean section. Wiping the nose and mouth of the baby as soon as the head is delivered and early cord clamping should be practiced.

HIV and Breastfeeding

Three drug ART significantly reduces the risk of vertical transmission through breastfeeding (from 30–45% to 2%). Infected pregnant women should be counseled regarding breastfeeding during the ANC visits, so that they can take informed decision regarding the feeding options. According to WHO, in developing countries where other diseases like diarrhea, pneumonia and malnutrition contribute majorly to infant mortality, the benefit of breastfeeding is many times higher than the risk of HIV transmission. HIV-infected mothers should exclusively breastfeed their infants for first 6 months and continue breastfeeding for at least 1 year. Similar to general population, breastfeeding can be continued for 24 months and beyond, ensuring ART adherence of the mother.[9] Breastfeeding should be stopped only when safe and nutritionally adequate alternative can be provided.

Infant Prophylaxis

All infants born to HIV-infected mothers should receive prophylaxis. The drug and duration of prophylaxis depends on the type of HIV infection in mother, duration of ART received by the mother during antenatal period and breastfeeding status.[8]

For HIV-1 infection which constitute majority of cases in India, infants should be started on daily nevirapine (NVP) prophylaxis at their first encounter with the health services. NVP can be started even after more than 72 hours since birth and should be continued. Summary of NVP prophylaxis is given in **Table 5**.

For mothers with HIV-2 infection, which is very less and seen primarily in western India, daily AZT prophylaxis is given to the infant for 6 weeks. Infants born to mothers

Table 5: Duration of infant prophylaxis.

Mother's ART status	Breastfeeding	Duration of NVP prophylaxis
Received for at least 24 weeks	+ / –	6 weeks
Not received/received for <24 weeks	+	12 weeks
Not received/received for <24 weeks	–	6 weeks

(ART: antiretroviral treatment; NVP: nevirapine)

Table 6: Dosage of drugs for infant prophylaxis.

Birth weight	Drug	Dosage
<2 kg	NVP	2 mg/kg OD
	AZT	10 mg BD
2–2.5 kg	NVP	10 mg OD
	AZT	10 mg BD
>2.5 kg	NVP	15 mg OD
	AZT	15 mg BD

(AZT: zidovudine; NVP: nevirapine)

with combined HIV-1 and HIV-2 infection should receive the recommended AZT prophylaxis till minimum 6 weeks of age.[7] Dosage of ARV drugs for prophylaxis is summarized in **Table 6**.

Postexposure Prophylaxis

Postexposure prophylaxis (PEP) is instituted to minimize the risk of infection following exposure to blood borne pathogens (including sexual assault). It includes providing first aid, risk assessment, investigations after informed consent of the source and exposed person, and providing short-term ARV drugs with proper follow-up.

Postexposure prophylaxis is most beneficial when started within 2 hours of exposure and has less benefit when started >72 hours postexposure but can still be started. PEP is given for 4 weeks.[8]

Drugs used for PEP in pediatric age group include:

- Zidovudine—preferred choice (abacavir if AZT is contraindicated)
- Lamivudine
- Lopinavir/ritonavir (Efavirenz in children >3 years and >10 kg).

■ OPPORTUNISTIC INFECTIONS (OIs)

Human immunodeficiency viruses infection being an immunodeficiency disorder is marked by OIs which can be bacterial, viral, fungal or protozoal. OIs contribute heavily to the mortality and morbidity in HIV-infected patients. In developing countries like India, where diagnostic tests may not be available or affordable for the patients, clinical diagnosis based on high index of suspicion should be kept for identifying them at the earliest.[10]

Pneumocystis carinii (jiroveci) Pneumonia (PCP)

In infants, PCP is the most common OI with a peak incidence at 3–6 months of age. Tetrad of fever, tachypnea, dyspnea, and cough is seen in HIV-infected children. Reticulonodular/ground-glass pattern on chest X-ray, hypoxia, and high lactate dehydrogenase form the basis of presumptive diagnosis. Definitive diagnosis is based on demonstration of P. carinii in sputum sample (Sn-50%, Sp-90%) or bronchoalveolar lavage (BAL) (Sn-90%, Sp-99%, even 72 hours postinitiation of treatment). Treatment of PCP is IV trimethoprim-sulfamethoxazole (TMP-SMX) (15–20 mg/kg/day in four divided doses), severe cases may also require steroid administration.

Cotrimoxazole (TMP-SMX) preventive therapy (CPT) reduces the incidence of PCP, also protects from other bacterial infections and toxoplasmosis. Dapsone (2 mg/kg OD, max 100 mg/day) is the alternative drug for children with severe adverse reaction to TMP-SMX or other sulfa drugs and G6PD deficiency. CPT is summarized in **Table 7**.

Mycobacterium Avium Complex

These nontubercular mycobacteria are commonly associated OIs in children with low CD4 counts (<50 cells/mm^3), high plasma RNA levels (>100,000 copies/mL), previous OIs, and previous colonization in respiratory or GI tract. *M. avium* is associated predominantly with a disseminated disease and *Mycobacterium intracellulare* mainly causes respiratory manifestations. They can present with isolated lymphadenitis, recurrent fever, failure to thrive, night sweats, fatigue, chronic diarrhea, and recurrent abdominal pain. Presence of organism in stool or respiratory samples indicate colonization and does not mark active infection. Isolation or culture of organism in blood or biopsy specimen form the basis of diagnosis. Treatment recommendation includes two or more drugs for at least 18 months. Clarithromycin (7.5–10 mg/kg/day PO BD) or azithromycin (10–12 mg/kg/day PO OD) with ethambutol (15–20 mg/kg/day PO OD) is commonly used combination. Disseminated disease requires 3 or 4 drug combination with addition of rifabutin to the above combination. Alternatively, levofloxacin, ciprofloxacin and/or amikacin, and streptomycin can be used if rifabutin is not available.

Table 7: Indications of cotrimoxazole preventive therapy (CPT).

Patient profile	When to start?	When to stop?
All HIV-exposed infants/children	Start at 6 weeks or first encounter with health services	Stop when HIV infection is ruled out (negative antibody test at 18 months), regardless of ARV initiation
All HIV-exposed infants/children up to 5 years of age	Start irrespective of CD4 count/ WHO staging/CD4%	Can be stopped in a child >5 years of age with WHO clinical stage 1 or 2 and with CD4 count >350 cells/mm^3 on two occasions minimum 6 months apart
All HIV-exposed infants/children >5 years of age	WHO stage 3 or 4 Or CD4 < 350 cells/mm^3 irrespective of WHO staging	Can be stopped when child >5 years of age is clinically stable with WHO clinical stage 1 or 2 and with CD4 count > 350 cells/mm^3 on two occasions minimum 6 months apart
As secondary prophylaxis	After completion of PCP treatment	• Not to be stopped in children < 5 years of age • Can be stopped in children > 5 years of age with WHO clinical stage 1 or 2 and with CD4 count > 350 cells/mm^3 on two occasions minimum 6 months apart

(ARV: antiretroviral; HIV: human immunodeficiency virus; PCP: pneumocystis carinii pneumonia)

Candidiasis

Candidiasis is the most common fungal infection in children with HIV. In infants with HIV, >8 weeks of age, oral thrush is the most common and recurrent presentation. Treatment includes topical clotrimazole (4–6 hourly for 1–2 weeks) or oral nystatin suspension. Oral antifungal drugs (fluconazole, ketoconazole, and itraconazole) may be used if topical treatment is ineffective. Patients with low CD4 count (<100 cells/mm^3), high viral load, neutropenia and coexisting oropharyngeal candidiasis may end up into esophageal candidiasis. The treatment includes IV fluconazole (3–6 mg/kg/day for 21 days), made oral once child is able to swallow. Alternatively, IV amphotericin blue can also be used. The systemic manifestations of candidiasis can lead to endophthalmitis, sepsis or shock. Management includes IV amphotericin B (0.5–1.5 mg/kg/day over 1–2 hours) or IV fluconazole (10–12 mg/kg/day IV or oral BD) for 14–21 days. Flucytosine is added in severe disease. Children with recurrent mucocutaneous candidiasis or esophageal candidiasis should be started on prophylaxis with fluconazole (3–6 mg/kg/day OD) or itraconazole (5 mg/kg/day OD) and can be stopped once CD4 count is ≥15% on more than two occasions.

HIV and Tuberculosis

Tuberculosis is the leading cause of death in people living with HIV, accounting for nearly one-third of AIDS related deaths. According to UNAIDS, 10 million people were diagnosed TB in 2017, of which 9% were HIV infected.[3] The disease manifests more severely in HIV cases, with extrapulmonary manifestations, drug resistance and association with atypical mycobacteria encountered

Table 8: ATT regimen for HIV and TB coinfection.

Case type	Treatment regimen
New case (never taken ATT or taken for <1 month)	2 HRZE + 4 HRE
Previously treated (received ATT for 1 month or more)	2 HRZES + 1 HRZE + 5 HRE

(ATT: antituberculosis treatment; HIV: human immunodeficiency virus; TB: tuberculosis)

frequently. Children infected with HIV should be screened for TB during every visit to ART centers using the four symptoms complex which includes current cough, fever, poor weight gain, and history of contact with TB. Presence of any of the four symptoms (4S+) warrants investigation for TB.[8]

As per revised National TB Control (RNTCP) guidelines, cartridge-based nucleic acid amplification test (CBNAAT) (Sn-84%) is the investigation of choice for diagnosis of TB in HIV-infected individuals compared to smear microscopy (Sn-52.8%). Sputum microscopy has poor sensitivity in HIV cases as there are fewer organisms in sputum. CBNAAT detects bacterial DNA and has added advantage of faster result and detection of rifampicin resistance. All HIV cases diagnosed with TB should be started on daily ATT at the ART center. Recommended treatment schedule is summarized in **Tables 8** and **9**.

Rifampicin being an enzyme inducer, alters the hepatic clearance of NNRTIs and PIs and therefore dose of EFV and NVP require adjustment when used concomitantly with rifampicin. In children <3 years age and weighing <10 kg where EFV (preferred NNRTI) cannot be used, either rifampicin is substituted with *rifamycin* or *rifabutin* or *ritonavir super boosting* is used. Ritonavir super

Table 9: Timing of starting ART in relation to initiation of ATT.

HIV-TB coinfection	Start ATT first followed by ART (irrespective of CD4 count) as soon as ATT is tolerated (between 2 weeks and 2 months)
HIV-TB coinfection with CD4 count < 50 cells/mm³	Start ATT first then ART within 2 weeks

(ART: antiretroviral treatment; ATT: antituberculosis treatment; HIV: human immunodeficiency virus; TB: tuberculosis)

boosting implies the use of L:R ratio of 1:1 instead of the conventional ration of 4:1. For patients who are already on ART at the time of diagnosis of TB, modification of ART is needed to maintain efficacy of both treatment regimens.

All children >12 months age living with HIV who are unlikely to have active disease on screening or contact with TB should be started on isoniazid preventive therapy (IPT) for 6 months. Below 12 months of age IPT should be started only in those cases who came in contact with TB case but do not have active disease. Besides, secondary IPT for 6-month duration is indicated for all children of HIV and TB who have completed course of ATT. Pyridoxine (vitamin B6) should be given in case of appearance of any symptoms of peripheral neuropathy.

■ REFERENCES

1. Yogev R, Chadwick EG. Acquired Immunodeficiency Syndrome (Human Immunodeficiency Virus). In: Kliegman RM, Stanton BF, St Geme III JW, Schor NF, Behrman RE (Eds). Nelson Textbook of Pediatrics, 20th edition (Vol. 2). Philadelphia: Elsevier; 2016. pp. 1645-66.
2. United Nations Programme on HIV and AIDS. Global HIV and AIDS statistics 2019 fact sheet; 2019. [online] Available from: https://www.unaids.org/en/resources/fact-sheet [Last accessed on December, 2019].
3. United Nations Programme on HIV and AIDS. Data 2018. [online] Available from: https://www.unaids.org/sites/default/files/media_asset/unaids-data-2018_en.pdf [Last accessed on December, 2019].
4. National AIDS Control Organisation. Annual report 16-17: Department of AIDS control (Ministry of Health and Family Welfare); 2017. [online] Available from: http://naco.gov.in/documents/annual-reports [Last accessed on December, 2019].
5. National AIDS Control Organisation. National strategic plan, 2017-24: Department of AIDS control (Ministry of Health and Family Welfare); 2017. [online] Available from: http://naco.gov.in/national-strategic-plan-hivaids-and-sti-2017-24 [Last accessed on December, 2019].
6. Naif HM. Pathogenesis of HIV infection. Infectious disease reports. Infect Dis Rep. 2013;5(Suppl 1):e6.
7. World Health Organization. WHO case definitions of HIV for surveillance and revised clinical staging and immunological classification of HIV-related disease in adults and children; 2007. [online] Available from: https://www.who.int/hiv/pub/guidelines/HIVstaging150307.pdf [Last accessed on December, 2019].
8. National AIDS Control Organisation. National Technical Guidelines on Anti-retro viral treatment NACO Care Support and Treatment Services; 2018. [online] Available from: http://naco.gov.in/sites/default/files/NACO%20-%20National%20Technical%20Guidelines%20on%20ART_October%202018%20%281%29.pdf. [Last accessed on December, 2019].
9. World Health Organization and United Nations Children's Fund (UNICEF). Guideline: updates on HIV and infant feeding: The duration of breastfeeding and support from health services to improve feeding practices among mothers living with HIV; 2016. [online] Available from: https://apps.who.int/iris/bitstream/handle/10665/246260/9789241549707-eng.pdf;jsessionid=65E0316D918D4FFA83EBE4C81EB682B1?sequence=1 [Last accessed on December, 2019].
10. AIDSinfo. Panel on opportunistic infections in HIV-exposed and HIV-infected children. Department of Health and Human services; 2019. [online] Available from: https://aidsinfo.nih.gov/contentfiles/lvguidelines/oi_guidelines_pediatrics.pdf [Last accessed on December, 2019].

Subramanya NK, Sarika Gupta

6.3 CHAPTER

Viral Respiratory Infections

INTRODUCTION

Respiratory tract infections (RTIs) contribute as a leading cause of childhood morbidity and mortality. Worldwide, RTI accounts for 2 million expiries in children less than 5 years of age. However, the National Family Health Survey (NFHS) reports show that prevalence of acute respiratory tract infections has reduced from the level of 5.6% in NFHS-3 to 2.7% in NFHS-4. Though the statistics are rapturous, we must strive to maintain it and abate it further to contain the risk associated with multidrug-resistant bacteria and unique respiratory viruses with pandemic prospective. Such viruses are the severe acute respiratory syndrome corona- virus (SARS-CoV), swine-origin influenza A (H1N1), Middle East respiratory syndrome coronavirus (MERS-CoV), and resistant *Cytomegalovirus* (CMV) strains in immunocompromised. Other threatening viruses include avian influenza A H7N9, influenza A swine H3N2 and H1N1, human adenovirus 14p1, and rhinovirus (RV) group C.

The nonspecific clinical picture of RTI creates questions in the accurate diagnosis of causative bacteria/virus. Timely and pristine etiological diagnosis in respiratory infections is crucial to decide about correct antiviral or antibacterial therapy, start infection control measures, public health surveillance, and lessen the hospital stay duration.

DIAGNOSTIC TESTS FOR VIRAL INFECTIONS

Potential specimens for detection of respiratory viruses, include bronchoalveolar lavage (BAL), throat swab, nasopharyngeal (NP) swab/washes/aspirates, and lung aspirates.

Available older generation tests for detection of viral infection include complement fixation tests demonstrating antibody rise, immunofluorescence, or colorimetric tests to detect viral antigen, and cell culture to isolate virus, followed by immunofluorescence or hemadsorption on the same sample. Limitation of these test includes time constraint to result.

Rapid immunoassays (RIAs) have the potential to find the place in clinical decision-making algorithm as it can provide result in less than 30 minutes. The lateral flow immunoassay (LFIA) is the widely held immunochromatographic method.

Direct fluorescent antibody (DFA) testing of NP wash specimens is a rapid and reliable method for detecting respiratory viral infections. It has high sensitivity and specificity in the range of 90–100%, for common respiratory viruses including human metapneumovirus (hMPV), adenovirus, respiratory syncytial virus (RSV), and parainfluenza viruses. The high specificity of DFA indicates that the test can be used in the initial days of the illness as a reliable detection method. The newer advanced tests include multiplex polymerase chain reaction (PCR) tests that use several primer sets running within a single PCR mixture, with short throughput time compared with multiple single-target PCRs. They provide rapid detection of respiratory viruses in clinical specimens and are used for identifying the epidemiology of new emerging viruses. Multiplex PCR has the advantage of identifying several different viruses in a single test.

The newer advanced colorimetric tests for direct antigen detection offer amplification of up to 20 viral pathogens from a clinical sample in a shorter turnaround time.

Clinical Potential

Despite the advantage, the difficulty lies with interpreting the findings in relation to a patient's clinical status. Detection of a weak signal of one virus may represent a commensal or the tail end of a previous infection, although it may also show that the infection is recent and evolving. Another possibility is that the weaker signal is a pronounced viral infection in the lower respiratory tract, but the virus is not yet well represented in the upper respiratory tract, where there is a different viral infection present. The issue of which clinical sample will generate the highest diagnostic yield is also dependent on the pathogenesis of the virus.

Challenges

A major challenge of implementation of molecular testing technology will be the ability of the test to distinguish between microbial colonization, infection, and disease causation. Respiratory tract specimens often contaminated with colonizing organisms from the nasopharynx give false-positive detection of these colonizers because of increased sensitivity of molecular techniques. Multiple pathogenic species can be present in one specimen. Whether they represent coinfections or a mixture of infection and colonization needs to be determined. Inability to distinguish between infection and colonization creates a dilemma as to whether such results should be used to guide treatment. This problem can be rectified by the use of quantitative PCR.

Viral respiratory tract infections are typically divided into two subgroups:

1. *Upper respiratory tract infections*: Symptoms occur mainly in the nose and throat. Viral upper respiratory tract infections may occur at any age and include the common cold and influenza.
2. *Lower respiratory tract infections*: Symptoms occur in the airways and lungs. Viral lower respiratory tract infections include croup, bronchiolitis, and pneumonia.

The common respiratory viral pathogens include RVs, influenza viruses, parainfluenza viruses, RSV, enteroviruses, coronaviruses, and certain strains of adenovirus. RV is the most commonly identified virus in upper RTI. RSV, hMPV, influenza, and adenovirus are the commonly identified viruses in cases of community-acquired pneumonia.

Most often, viral RTIs spread when children's hands come into contact with nasal secretions from an infected person. When the children touch their nose or eyes, the viruses gain entry and produce a new infection. Less often, infections spread when children breathe air-containing droplets that were coughed or sneezed out by an infected person.

Nasal or respiratory secretions from children with viral respiratory tract infections contain more viruses than those from infected adults. This increased output of viruses, along with typically lesser attention to hygiene, makes children more likely to spread their infection to others. The possibility of transmission is further enhanced when many children are gathered together, such as in child care centers and schools.

■ PATHOPHYSIOLOGY OF CLINICAL FEATURE OF VIRAL RESPIRATORY TRACT INFECTION

The pathophysiology of clinical feature of viral RTI is given in **Flowchart 1**.

■ COMMON COLD

The common cold is an acute, self-limiting viral infection of the upper respiratory tract. Incidence of common cold in young children is 6–8 colds per year, which decreases with age, with 2–3 illnesses per year by adulthood. RVs (>100

Flowchart 1: Pathophysiology of clinical feature of viral respiratory tract infection.

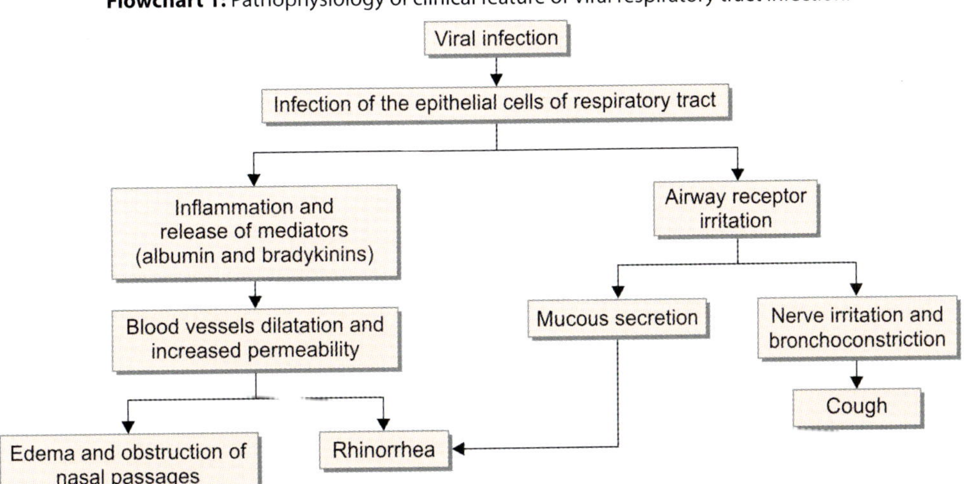

serotypes), accounts for up to 50% of colds in children. Other causative viruses include human coronaviruses, RSV, hMPV, parainfluenza viruses, and adenoviruses, influenza viruses, non-polio enteroviruses, and human coronaviruses.

The common cold may occur at any time of year, but there is typically a high prevalence during the fall and winter months. However, enteroviruses mostly cause cold in the summer with low rate throughout the year.

The clinical manifestations include nasal obstruction and rhinorrhea, sore throat, cough, headache, hoarseness, irritability, difficulty sleeping, or decreased appetite. Influenza viruses, RSVs, hMPV, and adenoviruses are more likely than RVs or coronaviruses to be associated with fever and other constitutional symptoms.

The most important task of the physician caring for a patient with a cold is to exclude other conditions that are potentially more serious or treatable which include allergic rhinitis, rhinitis medicamentosa, foreign body, vasomotor rhinitis, and sinusitis.

Treatment is symptomatic relief. Maintain adequate oral hydration. For the relief of congestion, topical or oral adrenergic agents (not recommended for use in children younger than 6 year) can be used. Saline nose drops is another alternative. For rhinorrhea, first-generation antihistamines are used and to relive cough, first-generation antihistamines/bronchodilators are used. Antipyretics are used to control the fever.

■ INFLUENZA

Every year, influenza infection causes a substantial encumbrance of disease in the pediatric population worldwide. Both healthy and chronically ill children may suffer complications either due to the virus itself or due to secondary bacterial infection.

Influenza infection is caused by influenza virus types A and B. Although the prevalence of influenza C usually is lower, it may cause infection, in young children. Influenza type C usually causes sporadic mild upper respiratory symptoms. There are two influenza A subtypes circulating in humans—A/H1N1 and A/H3N2—and two influenza B subtypes—the Yamagata and Victoria lineages.

Since the viral shedding persist for about 10 days, patients can be contagious before the onset of symptoms and for several days after. For the same reason, children with mild symptoms remain an important reservoir of disease.

Influenza outbreaks of varying extension and intensity occur every year. This epidemiologic pattern of influenza reflects multiple factors such as the changing nature of the antigenic properties of the virus, transmissibility power of the virus, and the susceptibility of the population.

Influenza classically begins with the abrupt onset of high-grade fever, myalgia, headache, and malaise, accompanied by symptoms of nonproductive cough, sore throat, and nasal discharge. Myalgia is most prominent in the calf muscle, paravertebral and back muscles, and the extraocular muscle, which causes painful eye movement.

Influenza also has the potential to affect other organs such as the lungs, brain, and heart more than it can affect the respiratory tract and cause hospitalization. Young children (6 months to 5 years) and those with underlying medical conditions are at increased risk for hospitalization or severe or complicated influenza infection though this phenomenon may also occur in healthy children. Groups at risk of influenza complication include children with asthma, neurodevelopmental delay, congenital heart disease, sickle cell disease or other hemoglobinopathies, chronic kidney disease, and children with cancer. Apart from younger age and underlying medical condition, factors associated with increased mortality include bacterial coinfection with *Staphylococcus aureus* or *Streptococcus pneumoniae* and increased circulation of influenza A H3N2 strains.

Patients with uncomplicated influenza usually improve over approximately 1 week; however, convalescent period may last for some weeks, during which dry cough and malaise persist.

Complication includes pneumonia which may be either a continuum of the acute influenza syndrome or secondary bacterial pneumonia. Other respiratory complications include exacerbation of asthma, respiratory failure, and croup. Nonrespiratory complications include myocarditis, pericarditis, myositis, Guillain-Barré syndrome, encephalitis, acute liver failure, and the Reye syndrome.

During the influenza season, majority of influenza cases are diagnosed by their clinical manifestations and there is no need for laboratory tests. It should also be considered at other time of year in children with febrile respiratory illness who are epidemiologically linked to an outbreak of influenza. Laboratory confirmation of influenza is not necessary for initiation of antiviral therapy and it should not delay initiation of antiviral therapy in children for whom it is indicated.

During the influenza season, indications for laboratory testing in children include suspected influenza in patients with high risk of complications or underlying medical conditions and age < 2 years, hospitalization and acute febrile respiratory illness or severe respiratory illness, neurologic complications of influenza, or acute worsening of chronic cardiopulmonary disease.

Laboratory confirmation of influenza virus infection requires detection of viral proteins or viral RNA by nucleic acid tests, or rapid diagnosis kits or rarely virus isolation by culture methods. Rapid influenza diagnostic tests [reverse transcriptase (RT)-PCR] is preferred to detect influenza viral antigens and screen patients with suspected influenza in a timely manner. Rapid tests provide results within 30 minutes. Antigen detection tests (direct and indirect immunofluorescence assays) and traditional rapid influenza diagnostic tests can be used if molecular assays are not available.

Currently, three classes of antiviral drugs are available for the prevention and treatment of influenza in children: Neuraminidase inhibitors (oseltamivir, zanamivir, peramivir, and laninamivir), selective inhibitors of influenza cap-dependent endonuclease (baloxavir), and adamantanes (M2 inhibitors, amantadine, and rimantadine). Since the majority of influenza strains are susceptible to neuraminidase inhibitors, it is recommended for treatment. The greatest effect is classically seen when therapy is started in the first 24 hours.

Treatment Indications

- Any child hospitalized with presumed influenza
- Children with confirmed or suspected influenza who have severe, complicated, or progressive illness
- Influenza infection of any severity in children of high-risk group
- Any otherwise healthy child with influenza infection for whom a decrease in duration of clinical symptoms is felt to be warranted by his or her provider (particularly if treatment can be initiated within 48 hours of illness onset).

Vaccination

The most important strategy for the prevention of influenza and its severe outcomes is annual vaccination against seasonal influenza.

The recommended vaccine structure for 2019–2020 influenza season in Northern hemisphere for children <18 years of age is quadrivalent vaccine including A/Brisbane/02/2018 (H1N1), A/Kansas/14/2017 (H3N2), B/Colorado/06/2017, and B/Phuket/3073/2013.

For the 2019 southern hemisphere influenza season (April to September), World Health Organization (WHO) recommends the following strains—A/Michigan/45/2015 (H1N1), A/Switzerland/8060/2017 (H3N2), B/Colorado/ 06/2017), and B/Phuket/3073/2013.

■ CROUP

Croup is also named as laryngotracheobronchitis. Croup is an upper respiratory illness characterized by inspiratory stridor, barking cough, and hoarseness due to inflammation in the larynx and subglottic airway.

Viral croup is an early childhood viral syndrome, occurring in the age group of 3 months to 5 years. It is more common in boys. Most cases of croup occur in winter season.

The parainfluenza viruses (type 1, 2, and 3) account for 75% of cases of croup. Other viruses implicated are influenza A, B, adenovirus, measles, RSV, RV, coronavirus, and hMPV. Croup also may be caused by bacteria. *Mycoplasma pneumoniae* has been associated with mild cases of croup.

The hallmark of croup is narrowing of the subglottic airway. In addition to fixed obstruction of cricoid cartilage, dynamic obstruction of the extrathoracic trachea below the cartilaginous ring may occur when the child is agitated. Host factors predisposing to clinically significant narrowing of the upper airway include congenital subglottic stenosis, hyperactive airways, and acquired airway narrowing from a postintubation subglottic stenosis.

The clinical course starts with rhinorrhea, pharyngitis, mild cough, and low-grade fever for 1–3 days followed by characteristic barking cough, hoarseness, and inspiratory stridor. Symptoms are more during the early hours of morning. Examination findings include inflamed pharynx, increased respiratory rate, nasal flaring, stridor, and suprasternal, infrasternal, and intercostal retractions.

The diagnosis of croup is clinical. The severity of croup is assessed by "Westley croup score."

- *Mild croup (Westley score of ≤2)*: No stridor at rest (stridor present when upset or crying), a barking cough, hoarse cry, and negligible chest wall/subcostal retractions.
- *Moderate croup (Westley score of 3–7)*: Stridor at rest, mild retractions, with other symptoms or signs of respiratory distress, but little or no agitation.
- *Severe croup (Westley score of ≥8)*: Significant stridor at rest, (intensity of stridor decreases with worsening upper airway obstruction and decreased air entry). Severe retractions along with sternal indrawing and the child may appear anxious, agitated, or pale and fatigued.
- *Impending respiratory failure (Westley croup score of ≥12)*: Signs of impending respiratory failure, including fatigue, striking retractions, decreased or absent breath sounds, depressed level of consciousness, tachycardia out of proportion to fever, and cyanosis.

Treatment

Management of children with croup begins with an assessment of severity at first. Children with mild croup are managed at home. It consists of supportive care (reduction of agitation and discomfort) and single dose of dexamethasone orally. All other categories are treated in hospital setting with supportive care (relieving the agitation, humidified oxygen, antipyretics and hydration), single dose of dexamethasone intravenous (IV), nebulized epinephrine, and airway management with increasing severity. Antibiotics, antitussives, and decongestants are of unproven benefit in croup.

Most of the children with croup recover uneventfully.

PNEUMONIA

Most of the children younger than 5 years of age who are admitted to the hospital with pneumonia have viral pneumonia. Viral etiology is implicated in about 14–50% of pneumonia. The most common virus isolated in children younger than 5 years is RSV. Other viral pathogens include influenza A and B viruses, hMPV, parainfluenza virus, coronaviruses, adenovirus, enterovirus D68, RV, human bocavirus, and human parechovirus types 1, 2, and 3.

The two major patterns of viral pneumonia include interstitial pneumonitis and parenchymal infection with viral inclusions. Presence of lobar pneumonia and pleural effusion denotes absence of viral pneumonia though similar presentation may be there in viral pneumonia with superimposed bacterial pneumonia. Viral pneumonia does not require antibiotic therapy unless a mixed infection or secondary bacterial infection is suspected.

There are no specific and effective antivirals available for most of the viral pneumonias. However, there are some exclusions which include specific therapy for influenza, herpes simplex virus (HSV), or varicella zoster virus (VZV).

Viral causes of pneumonia may be life-threatening in the immunocompromised host. Immunocompromised children require attention to antiviral therapy. It includes ribavirin for RSV or parainfluenza and cidofovir for adenovirus. Simultaneous administration of immunoglobulin therapy is an additional consideration including palivizumab for RSV, CMV immunoglobulin for CMV, and IV immunoglobulin for the other viral etiologies.

BRONCHIOLITIS

Bronchiolitis is virus-induced inflammation of small bronchioles and their surrounding tissue. Bronchiolitis typically occurs in children less than 2 years of age.

Clinically, bronchiolitis is characterized by expiratory breathing difficulty in infants. Other symptoms include cough, tachypnea, hyperinflation, chest retraction, widespread crackles, and wheezing. Bronchiolitis is diagnosed clinically. Chest radiographs and laboratory tests are needed to evaluate complications, comorbid infections, or differential diagnosis.

It is characterized by viral infection of terminal bronchiolar epithelial cells, causing direct damage and inflammation in the small bronchi and bronchioles. Edema, excessive mucus, and sloughed epithelial cells lead to obstruction of small airways and atelectasis.

Respiratory syncytial virus is the most common cause of bronchiolitis followed by RV. Other viruses include human bocavirus, hMPV, parainfluenza virus, adenovirus, coronavirus, and influenza virus.

Main risk factors for bronchiolitis include prematurity, chronic lung disease (low lung function), congenital heart disease, and other underlying medical conditions, anatomic defects of the airways, immunodeficiency, neurologic disease, and young age (1–6 months of age).

Environmental factors, including passive smoking, crowded household, daycare attendance, being born around the period of epidemic, concurrent birth siblings, older siblings, and high altitude, are other factors contributing to more severe disease.

Infants and children with moderate-to-severe respiratory distress (nasal flaring, retractions, grunting, respiratory rate > 70 breaths per minute, dyspnea, cyanosis, toxic appearance, poor feeding, lethargy, apnea, and/or hypoxemia) require hospitalization for supportive care and monitoring.

Supportive care (maintenance of adequate hydration, provision of oxygen and respiratory support as necessary, and monitoring disease progression) and anticipatory guidance are the mainstays of management of severe bronchiolitis. One-time trial of inhaled bronchodilators may be done for infants and children with bronchiolitis and severe disease. Systemic glucocorticoids, nebulized hypertonic saline or heliox are not recommended for the treatment of bronchiolitis.

SUGGESTED READING

1. Barr R, Green CA, Sande CJ, et al. Respiratory syncytial virus: diagnosis, prevention and management. Ther Adv Infect Dis. 2019;6:2049936119865798.
2. Everard ML. Paediatric respiratory infections. Eur Respir Rev. 2016;25(139):36-40.
3. Jartti T, Smits HH, Bønnelykke K, et al. Bronchiolitis needs a revisit: Distinguishing between virus entities and their treatments. Allergy. 2019;74(1):40-52.
4. le Roux DM, Zar HJ. Community-acquired pneumonia in children—a changing spectrum of disease. Pediatr Radiol. 2017;47(11):1392-8.
5. Moghadami M. A Narrative Review of Influenza: A Seasonal and Pandemic Disease. Iran J Med Sci. 2017;42(1):2-13.

Acute Encephalitis Syndrome

Puneet Kumar, Vipin M Vashishtha

INTRODUCTION

Acute encephalitis is an important cause of morbidity and mortality in children in tropical countries. The etiological agents are varied and often clinically indistinguishable. The lack of availability and high cost of diagnostic testing for specific agents in resource-limited countries add further to the limitations faced by the treating physicians. While some of the cases such as herpes simplex encephalitis (HSE) occur sporadically, others such as Japanese encephalitis (JE) often occur in epidemics. JE has been a major public health problem in many parts of Asia, claiming thousands of lives every year and leaving many others with permanent sequelae. The term Acute Encephalitis Syndrome (AES) was coined by the World Health Organization (WHO) in context of surveillance for JE for syndromic case-finding. It is defined as the acute onset of fever and a change in mental status (including signs and symptoms such as confusion, disorientation, delirium, or coma) and/or new onset of seizures (excluding simple febrile seizures) in a person of any age at any time of the year.[1] However, this broad definition of AES includes acute encephalitis cases due to other viruses; other central nervous system (CNS) infections such as bacterial meningitis, tubercular meningitis, and cerebral malaria; other systemic infections with complications involving CNS such as dengue, scrub typhus, and influenza; and even other etiologies such as acute disseminated encephalomyelitis (ADEM) and heat stroke. One needs to be acutely aware of such heterogeneous entities grouped under one umbrella whenever one is involved in studying/researching/managing/classifying cases of AES. The use of other terms such as "acute febrile encephalopathy" and even using terms such as "brain fever", "infectious encephalitis", or "viral encephalitis" loosely in the literature and relative lack of consensus in definition of "acute" add

further to the cauldron. This chapter would provide a brief overview of this syndrome.

ETIOLOGY

Neurotropic viruses are the most common etiological agents for AES. **Table 1** lists the viruses that cause AES in epidemic and sporadic forms. The incidence of AES ranges from 10.5 to 13.8 per 100,000 children as concluded from various prospective studies from the Western world.[2] JE is the single most important cause of outbreaks of AES worldwide, especially Eastern and Southeastern Asia, accounting for 30,000–50,000 cases with 10,000–15,000 deaths globally every year.[3] Till the turn of this century, most epidemics of AES in JE-endemic regions were presumed to be JE outbreaks, even before investigations were initiated.[4] In India, the largest epidemic outbreak in the last three decades occurred in Gorakhpur (Uttar Pradesh), through November 2005 killing 1,344 people.[2] However, many epidemics of AES in the last two decades have been attributed to other viruses such as Chandipura virus (rhabdovirus)[5,6] and enteroviruses (especially EV71).[7] Chikungunya virus, dengue virus, and Nipah virus have also caused some outbreaks. In fact, some of these outbreaks have been recorded even in JE-endemic regions and in the same season. There has been significant fall in percentage of AES cases that are caused by JE virus in the last two decades. This decrease has been attributed to JE-control strategies [vaccination, control of vector (mosquito), and amplifier host (pig) population] and periodic fluctuation of the virus circulation and/or vector leading to true epidemiological shift. In addition, advances in molecular diagnostics, viral culture and isolation, as well as use of an extended panel of tests for potential etiological agents has also "unmasked" other agents causing AES outbreaks.[4] The viruses that cause AES outbreaks are also responsible

Table 1: Viruses causing AES.

AES outbreaks	Sporadic cases of AES
JE virus*	All viruses causing outbreaks
Enteroviruses* (especially Enteroviruses 71, 89, 76)	Enteroviruses (Coxsackie A and B viruses, Echovirus 7, etc.)
Chandipura virus*	*Herpes simplex* virus*
Chikungunya virus*	Varicella Zoster virus*
Nipah virus*	Mumps virus*
Dengue virus*	Rubella virus
Measles virus*	Human herpes virus (HHV) 6 and 7*
West Nile virus*	Human Parvovirus 4
	Epstein-Barr virus (EBV)*
	Bagaza virus
	Influenza viruses
	Human immunodeficiency virus (HIV)
	Kyasanur Forest disease virus*
	Rabies virus*
	Adenovirus (for example, serotypes 1, 6, 7, 12, 32)
	Human metapneumovirus
	Respiratory syncytial virus
	Rotavirus
	Cytomegalovirus (CMV)
	Human parechovirus
	Lymphocytic choriomeningitis virus
	La Crosse strain of California virus
	St Louis virus
	Powassan encephalitis virus
	Venezuelan, Eastern, and Western equine encephalitis viruses
	Louping ill virus
	Rift valley fever virus
	Colorado tick fever virus
	Crimean–Congo hemorrhagic virus
	Murray Valley encephalitis virus*
	Yellow fever virus

Note: The viruses marked with asterisk (*) are common in Asia.
(AES: acute encephalitis syndrome; JE: Japanese encephalitis)

for some of the sporadic cases of AES. Among other viruses that cause AES sporadically **(Table 1)**, herpes simplex virus (HSV) is significant for several reasons. First, it is the most important cause of sporadic fatal AES worldwide with an incidence of 1–3/million in western countries (such data from India is lacking). Second, it carries very high mortality (~70%) in untreated cases. Third, unlike most other viral AES cases, specific antiviral treatment is available and appropriate treatment brings down mortality from ~70% to ~30%.[8]

In exceptionally rare situations, live virus vaccines against polio, measles, mumps, or rubella can also cause encephalitis.[9]

Rickettsiae, especially those of the typhus fever group (*Rickettsia prowazekii* and *R. typhi*) and scrub typhus (*Orientia tsutsugamushi*), are known to cause AES[10] as one of the severe manifestations. In fact, many JE-endemic areas are actually reporting more cases of scrub typhus encephalitis than JE. For example, a study of 2015 outbreak of AES in Gorakhpur (Uttar Pradesh), revealed that 65% cases were positive for scrub typhus while only 10% were positive for JE.[11]

Streptococcus pneumoniae, Neisseria meningitidis, and *Haemophilus influenzae are the most common causes of bacterial meningitis globally[12,13] that also presents as AES.* *Staphylococcus epidermidis* and other coagulase-negative staphylococci cause meningitis and cerebrospinal fluid (CSF) shunt infection in patients with hydrocephalus or in those who have undergone neurosurgical procedures. Immunocompromised children can develop meningitis caused by *Pseudomonas, Serratia, Proteus,* and diphtheroids. A comprehensive list of bacteria causing meningitis is published elsewhere in the textbook. *Mycobacterium tuberculosis* causes tubercular meningitis. Parameningeal bacterial infections such as brain abscess, subdural, or epidural empyema may also sometimes present as AES.

Plasmodium falciparum causes cerebral malaria that also presents as AES. Rarely, even P. vivax can cause cerebral malaria.[14] The endemic regions and seasonality for malaria often overlap with those of JE, making it very significant epidemiologically. *Trypanosoma brucei, Toxoplasma gondii, Naegleria fowleri, Echinococcus granulosus,* and *Schistosomia* are rare parasitic causes of AES.[15]

Fungi (such as *Cryptococcus neoformans* and *Coccidioides immitis) and prions* (Creutzfeldt-Jakob prion disease) are rare possible causes of AES.[16]

Acute encephalitis syndrome can also occur without direct brain infection, for example in acute disseminated encephalomyelitis (ADEM), its more severe form, and acute hemorrhagic leukoencephalitis (AHLE), anti-N-Methyl-D-Aspartate (NMDA) receptor encephalitis. Other noninfective causes of AES include plant toxins (such as *Cassia occidentalis*), heat stroke, nutritional encephalopathies, rheumatological conditions such as systemic lupus erythematosus (SLE) and Sjögren syndrome, Hashimoto encephalopathy, Reye and MELAS (Mitochondrial myopathy, Encephalopathy, Lactic acidosis, and Stroke) syndromes, inborn error of metabolism, nonconvulsive status epilepticus, intracranial hemorrhage, and CNS neoplasms.[15,17-22] "Outbreaks" of some of these noninfective AES have also been recorded.

EVALUATION AND MANAGEMENT

Acute encephalitis syndrome is a medical and neurological emergency, requiring immediate efforts to stabilize, evaluate (clinically and diagnostic), and start empirical treatment proceed almost simultaneously. A stepwise approach, as recommended by the Indian Academy of Pediatrics (IAP),[8] is described in the following text.

Step 1: Raid Assessment and Stabilization

As in any emergency, initial steps are directed toward ensuring adequacy of airway, breathing, and circulatory functions. Airway management is of paramount importance in children with altered sensorium, as their protective reflexes are obtunded and they are more prone to aspiration. The standard recommendation is to intubate children with Glasgow Coma Score (GCS) less than 8; mechanical ventilation is to be provided in case the breathing efforts are not adequate. Appropriate oxygenation is ensured. The next important step is establishment of vascular access. If there is evidence of circulatory failure, fluid bolus (20 mL/kg-normal saline) is administered and repeated if necessary. Samples are drawn for various investigations. If hypoglycemia is present, intravenous dextrose is administered. If the child is having seizures, or there is history of a seizure preceding the encephalopathy, anticonvulsant (intravenous midazolam/diazepam followed by loading dose of phenytoin (20 mg/kg)

is administered. In case there are features of raised intracranial pressure (asymmetric pupils, tonic posturing, papilledema, evidence of herniation), measures to decrease intracranial pressure are immediately instituted (head elevation, minimal disturbance, normothermia, hyperventilation, pharmacotherapy, etc.). Acid–base and electrolyte abnormalities are corrected. Normothermia is maintained.

Step 2: Detailed History and Examination

A careful history should be taken with special emphasis on onset and duration, and other features such as fever, headache, vomiting, irritability, seizures, and rash. There may be a prodrome of upper respiratory illness, flu-like illness or diarrhea. Detailed history (including history of past illness, family and contact history, and travel history) and thorough examination throw up several pointers that can help suspecting specific etiological diagnosis **(Table 2)**. Differentiation between inflammatory AES (encephalitis) and noninflammatory AES (encephalopathy) is also possible to some extent. Most encephalopathies do not come under ambit of AES, since fever is absent in most of them. However, fever can be precipitated in some encephalopathies by systemic infection/sepsis even

Table 2: Pointers in history and physical examination toward etiological diagnosis of AES.

Pointer	Possible etiology
History of contact with an infectious cause of AES (e.g. JE, chickenpox, and mumps)	Respective infectious agent
History of travel to an endemic region (e.g. JE-endemic region)	Respective infectious agent
Associated gastrointestinal symptoms	Enteroviruses, rotavirus, Human parechovirus, *Shigella* (encephalopathy), encephalopathy due to dyselectrolytemia
Associated respiratory illness	Influenza and parainfluenza viruses, *mycoplasma* and other respiratory pathogens
History of drug/toxin exposure	Respective drug/toxin
History of head trauma	Traumatic brain injury
Past history of similar illness	Inborn error of metabolism (urea cycle defects, organic acidemias and fatty acid oxidation defects), but may also be present in migraine, epilepsy, substance abuse, and Munchausen syndrome by proxy
History of animal bite	Rabies virus
Risk factors for immunodeficiency [Human immunodeficiency virus (HIV) risk factors, cancer treatment, steroid/immunosuppressant treatment]	Atypical pathogens known to infect immunocompromised hosts
Family history of infant/child deaths	Inborn errors of metabolism
Pallor	*Plasmodium falciparum*, intracranial bleed
Icterus	*Plasmodium falciparum*, *Leptospira*, *Coxiella burnetii*, hepatic encephalopathy
Skin rashes	*Neisseria meningitides*, *Varicella zoster* virus (VZV), measles virus, rubella virus, dengue virus, rickettsia, arboviruses, enteroviruses, HHV-6

Contd...

Contd...

Pointer	Possible etiology
Enanthems	Enteroviruses, VZV, measles virus, rubella virus, and WNV
Lymphadenopathy	HIV, Epstein-Barr Virus (EBV), measles virus, rubella virus, West Nile virus
Hemorrhagic conjunctivitis	Enterovirus, dengue and other hemorrhagic fever viruses
Parotid swelling and/or orchitis	Mumps virus
Labial herpes	Herpes simplex encephalitis
Herpangina	Enteroviruses
Mutism	JE virus
Progressive symmetrical external ophthalmoplegia (especially if associated with ataxia)	*Mycoplasma pneumoniae* (Bickerstaff brainstem encephalitis)
Personality changes, confusion and disorientation (frontotemporal lobe dysfunction)	Herpes simplex encephalitis
Features of brainstem dysfunction	Enterovirus 71, mumps virus, rabies virus
Associated acute flaccid paralysis	Enteroviruses (anterior horn cell involvement), poliomyelitis (anterior horn cell involvement), acute disseminated encephalomyelitis (due to myelitis) and rarely JE virus/West Nile virus/tick borne encephalitis virus
Myoclonic jerks	Enterovirus
Dystonia or extrapyramidal movements (choreoathetosis/ballism)	JE virus, West Nile virus, and Nipah virus
Associated neuritis or myeloneuritis or sensory/autonomic neuropathy	EBV
Subacute onset with movement disorder, orofacial dyskinesia and refractory seizures	Autoimmune encephalitis
Cerebellar ataxia	Varicella zoster virus
Dementia	HIV, measles virus
Retinal hemorrhages	Plasmodium falciparum
Retinitis	Cytomegalovirus (CMV), West Nile virus
Meningeal signs (neck rigidity, Kernig's sign, and Brudziński's sign)	*Streptococcus pneumoniae, Neisseria meningitides, Haemophilus influenza, and other bacteria causing bacterial meningitis*
Signs of myocarditis	*Enterovirus 71*
Signs of pulmonary edema/pleurodynias	*Enterovirus 71*

(AES: Acute encephalitis syndrome; JE: Japanese encephalitis)

without cerebral inflammation per se. Focal seizures and focal neurological signs are pointers toward true encephalitis although hypoglycemic encephalopathy is an important exception. A steady deterioration of mental status is a clue to suggest encephalopathy.[15]

The neurological examination is targeted to document the degree and localization of brain dysfunction. Level of consciousness is usually recorded in form of Glasgow Coma Scale or modified GCS score in infants and young children. However, a more detailed description of the child's clinical findings is often more useful for relaying detailed information and detecting changes over time. Pupillary size, shape, symmetry, and response to light provide valuable clues to brainstem and third nerve dysfunction and unilateral pupillary dilatation in the comatose patient should be considered as evidence of oculomotor nerve compression from ipsilateral uncal herniation, unless proved otherwise. The presence of oculocephalic (doll's eye), oculovestibular, corneal, cough and gag reflexes are checked for brainstem function. Brainstem herniation syndrome requires prompt treatment to prevent permanent damage. The trunk, limb position, spontaneous movements, response to stimulation and involvement of bladder and bowel control are observed to look for any focal deficits, and posturing (decerebrate or decorticate). The focal neurological signs may even be fluctuating or migratory. The cranial nerve examination along with tone, power of the limbs, and deep tendon reflexes help further in localization of lesion.

Step 3: Investigations

Basic investigations: Complete blood count, blood glucose, serum electrolytes, liver and kidney function tests, blood culture, arterial blood gas, and lactate (if available) are done in all cases of AES. A peripheral smear for malarial parasite, rapid diagnostic test for malaria and a chest X-ray are also done.

Lumbar puncture: If the patient is hemodynamically stable, and there are no features of raised intracranial pressure, a lumbar puncture is performed straight away. If lumbar puncture is contraindicated, a neuroimaging study should be obtained prior to the lumbar puncture. Empirical treatment (Step 4) should be started pending the results of lumbar puncture and/or neuroimaging studies. CSF is examined for cytology, biochemistry, Gram stain, Ziehl-Neelsen stain for acid-fast bacilli (AFB), bacterial culture, latex agglutination, polymerase chain reaction (PCR) for HSV 1 and 2, enterovirus and parechovirus,[22] and IgM antibodies for JE and for dengue virus (if suspected). Concurrent blood sugar is also measured to look for the CSF to blood sugar ratio. 1–2 mL CSF is stored for other virological studies, if needed. The storage is to be at 4°C if testing is likely to be within 24 hours or frozen at -80°C for longer term storage. Usual CSF findings in viral encephalitis include lymphocytic pleocytosis (>5 lymphocytes/mm^3), mild to moderately elevated protein, and normal CSF sugar. Similar findings may occur in tubercular meningitis and partially treated pyogenic meningitis; however, the CSF sugar is likely to be low in these situations. In cases with extensive brain destruction as in HSV encephalitis, the protein concentration may be very high. With certain viruses such as mumps virus, the CSF glucose might be significantly low. With parechovirus and Chandipura virus (and sometimes measles virus), CSF glucose, protein, and cell counts all might be normal. This happens possibly due to fulminant course of illness so that child presents with AES before development of CSF abnormalities.

Neuroimaging: Except in cases such as cerebral malaria where the diagnosis is clear by other investigations, neuroimaging is required in almost all cases of AES. Although the modality of choice is magnetic resonance imaging (MRI), but often the patients of AES are too unstable and restless for it and a computerized tomography (CT) scan is done initially. Even a CT scan may give valuable information such as presence of bleed, cerebral edema, temporal lobe hypodensities in herpes simplex encephalitis, thalamic abnormalities in JE, and basal exudates and hydrocephalus in tubercular meningitis. It may also show brain herniation, effacement of cisterns, and infective collections such as brain abscesses and subdural empyema. MRI scan [including diffusion-weighted imaging (DWI) and contrast-enhanced images] is done as soon as the patient is stable enough for it, as it gives very valuable information regarding the etiology and neuropathology of the case. Nonspecific features of viral encephalitis (such as cortical hyperintensities and cerebral edema) help in differentiating these cases from other forms of AES such as encephalopathies and ADEM. Some specific findings in MRI can help further in suspecting the specific etiology of viral encephalitis **(Table 3)**. MRI spectroscopy, positron emission tomography (PET), and single photon emission computed tomography (SPECT) are not indicated in suspected viral encephalitis,[22] but newer modalities such as gradient echo imaging can detect small areas of hemorrhage. DWI can distinguish old from new insults.[23]

Microbiological investigations: These are required when the etiology is not clear. These may not be required in all the cases in epidemic situations, once the etiology has been determined in first few cases. These samples include urine, throat swab, nasopharyngeal aspirate, serum (acute and convalescent after 2 weeks), and swab from vesicles or rash, if present. Antigen detection from throat samples can also be attempted using immunofluorescence and ELISA (enzyme-linked immunosorbent assay) to detect HSV, varicella zoster virus (VZV), influenza A and B, and parainfluenza viruses. Virus type can also be identified from cell cultures by electron microscopy. The tests for specific etiologies are described in **Table 4**. Availability of tests is a challenge in resource-limited tropical countries such as India. Tests for JE, HSV 1 and 2, dengue, poliovirus, measles, mumps and rubella are available in selected government and private laboratories. Tests for Nipah virus, VZV, Epstein-Barr virus (EBV), adenovirus, and enterovirus are not easily available. There are commercially available tests, which test for a panel of viruses [HSV1, 2, VZV, Human herpes virus (HHV)-6, Measles, Mumps, Rubella, Chandipura, Chikungunya, Nipah, Rabies, Enteroviruses, Japanese B, Dengue, West Nile virus] and bacteria with 1–2 mL CSF sample, using DNA hybridization technique and very short turnaround time. The limitation of these are exorbitant cost and lack of published literature on their sensitivity and specificity. For viruses for which CSF PCR is available but was not done or negative, CSF can be tested for specific IgM antibodies 2 weeks after onset of illness. Serum is also tested for IgM antibodies (for HSV1 and 2, CMV, VZV, HHV-6, enterovirus, parvovirus, adenovirus, and influenza A and B viruses) in two samples 2–3 weeks apart.[22] Despite extensive testing, no pathogen is identified in up to 63% cases of encephalitis even in the developed

Table 3: MRI findings in various cases of AES.[8,15,22]

Etiology	Finding
Herpes simplex encephalitis	Abnormal signal intensity (significant edema and hemorrhage) in medial temporal lobe, cingulate gyrus, and orbital surface of frontal lobes. Meningeal and gyral enhancement after Gd-DTPA administration
Japanese B encephalitis	Abnormal signal intensity in thalami (87–94%), substantia nigra, and basal ganglia
EV 71	Abnormal signal intensity in the dorsal pons, medulla, midbrain, and dentate nuclei of the cerebellum; high-signal lesions can also be found in the anterior horn cells of spinal cord in patients with acute flaccid paralysis
Chandipura virus	Normal
Nipah virus and parechovirus	Focal subcortical and deep white matter and gray matter lesions; small hyperintense lesions in the white matter, cortex, pons, and cerebral peduncles have also been seen.
Varicella	Multifocal abnormalities in cortex, associated cerebellitis, vasculitis, and vasculopathy.
ADEM	Multifocal abnormalities in subcortical white matter; involvement of thalami, basal ganglia, and brainstem also seen
West Nile virus	Abnormalities in deep gray matter and brainstem (50%); white matter lesions mimicking demyelination may also be seen; meningeal involvement on contrast-enhanced images.
Rabies virus	Symmetrical thalamic and basal ganglia changes
Eastern equine encephalitis	Disseminated lesions in the brainstem and basal ganglia
H1N1 virus	Abnormalities in corpus callosum
Limbic encephalitis due to voltage-gated potassium channels (VGKC) antibodies	Abnormalities in hippocampal region

(AES: acute encephalitis syndrome; ADEM: acute disseminated encephalomyelitis; EV 71: enterovirus 71; Gd-DPTA: gadolinium-diethylenetriamine pentaacetic acid)

world,[9] the percentage is somewhat higher in developing world.

In patients having unexplained encephalopathy with fever and rash, testing for rickettsial infections (Weil-Felix test and rickettsial serology) must be performed. In cases of AES with atypical pneumonia, *Mycoplasma* and *Chlamydia* serology and cold agglutinins in serum should be sought. In cases of suspected AIDS, virus encephalitis, or in cases with unexplained encephalitis, HIV antibody testing is done. Additional tests required in immunocompromised patients are CSF AFB staining and culture for *Mycobacterium tuberculosis,* CSF culture for *Listeria monocytogenes*, Indian Ink staining and cryptococcal antigen testing in CSF, antibody testing and if positive then CSF PCR for *Toxoplasma gondii*, serum antibody testing and if positive then CSF for syphilis.[8,22]

Electroencephalography (EEG): It is another valuable test in AES. It is diagnostic for nonconvulsive status and helps to differentiate focal encephalitis from generalized encephalopathies. Some EEG changes might be relatively specific. For example, the presence of 2–3 Hz periodic lateralized epileptiform discharges (PLEDs) originating from temporal lobe may indicate underlying herpes simplex encephalitis, but their absence does not rule out the diagnosis, since these are limited to about half the cases in the later stages. Typical triphasic slow waves diffusedly are seen in cases of hepatic encephalopathy. EEG may also be helpful in patients with subtle and doubtful seizures to guide antiepileptic drug management, pick up a metabolic encephalopathy misdiagnosed as viral encephalitis and to exclude psychiatric causes of altered sensorium.[8,22]

Other tests: If the diagnosis is not clear with the above tests, then alternative etiologies must be explored. In young children with unexplained altered sensorium, especially with premorbid developmental delay, investigations for inborn errors of metabolism (plasma ammonia, blood tandem mass spectroscopy, urine gas chromatography-mass spectroscopy) must be carried out. In older children, especially in presence of psychiatric symptoms, intractable seizures or new-onset movement disorder with coma, the possibility of autoimmune disorders such as SLE (antinuclear antibodies, anti-dsDNA antibodies), Hashimoto encephalopathy [anti-TPO (Anti-thyroid peroxidase) antibodies], and anti-NMDA (N-methyl-d-aspartate) receptor and anti-VKGC (voltage-gated potassium channel-complex) antibody-mediated

Table 4: Microbiological tests in AES.[8,22]

Test	Comments
JE Virus Virus-specific IgM antibody in a single sample of CSF or serum, as detected by an IgM-capture ELISA specifically for JE virus	Since JE virus shares some antigens with other flaviviruses such as West Nile virus (WNV) and dengue virus, further confirmatory tests should be carried out: (1) When there is an ongoing dengue or other flavivirus outbreak; (2) when JE vaccination coverage is very high; or (3) in cases in areas where there are no epidemiological and entomological data supportive of JE transmission Large majority of JE infections are asymptomatic. Therefore, in areas that are highly endemic for JE, it is possible to have AES due to a cause other than JE virus and have JE virus-specific IgM antibody present in serum
Enterovirus encephalitis Detection of EV genome by reverse transcriptase polymerase chain reaction (RT-PCR) or an equally sensitive and specific nucleic acid amplification test (real time) in CSF	Highly specific for EV encephalitis. However, CSF positivity is very low, since the duration of time the virus remains in the CSF is brief Isolation of virus from serum/stool/throat swab establishes carriage or systemic infection, but not necessarily the cause of the CNS disease; hence suggestive overall clinical picture and neuroimaging are important in establishing etiology
Dengue viral encephalitis Dengue virus-specific IgM antibody in a single sample of CSF, as detected by an IgM-capture ELISA	CSF positivity establishes the diagnosis of dengue encephalitis. Serum positivity only confirms dengue infection
Herpes simplex virus (HSV) encephalitis Detection of HSV DNA in CSF by PCR HSV-specific antibody titers in serum and CSF	Most sensitive method for early diagnosis of HSE: Sensitivity>95%, specificity~100% IgG preferable to IgM, useful in cases where illness duration >10–12 days, initial PCR not done or negative
Mumps virus encephalitis Detection of mumps virus RNA in CSF by PCR	Sensitivity > 95% in patients with a clinical diagnosis of viral CNS disease
Varicella zoster virus (VZV) encephalitis Detection of VZV DNA by PCR in CSF	
Nipah virus Detection of Nipah virus-specific IgM antibodies in serum and CSF by IgM-capture ELISA PCR from CSF	*Sensitivity*: Serum, 70%; CSF, < one-third of cases –
Measles virus Appearance of measles virus specific IgM antibody in the CSF	Specificity of kit used should be checked; false positivity is a known issue
Chandipura virus Detection of specific IgM antibodies in CSF by ELISA PCR from CSF	– –
Human herpes virus 6 (HHV6) PCR in CSF	If positive, then serum PCR is done to exclude chromosomal integration
Rabies virus Corneal imprint smear Nuchal biopsy PCR in CSF	–
Mycoplasma pneumoniae Serology and PCR in CSF or respiratory tract	–

(AES: acute encephalitis syndrome; CNS: central nervous system; CSF: cerebrospinal fluid; ELISA: enzyme-linked immunosorbent assay; HSE: herpes simplex encephalitis; JE: Japanese encephalitis; PCR: polymerase chain reaction) encephalitis may be considered. A urine toxicology screen should be performed. Finally, stereotactic brain biopsy from nondominant frontal lobe may be needed to look for primary CNS vasculitis or neoplastic processes. Nuchal pad biopsy is a standard procedure in suspected rabies.[8,22]

Step 4: Empirical Treatment

Considering the fact that any delay in starting the treatment can have significant bearing on the outcome, empirical treatment is started in all the cases, while waiting reports of lab investigations. Broad-spectrum antibiotic such as ceftriaxone (100 mg/kg/day) and acyclovir (20 mg/kg 8 hourly in newborns and infants < 3 months of age, 500 mg/m^2 8 hourly in case of 3 months to 12 years, and 10 mg/kg 8 hourly in a child > 12 years with normal renal function) is started. The dose of acyclovir is to be adjusted in cases with deranged renal function. The antibiotic is discontinued if there is no evidence of pyogenic meningitis and acyclovir is stopped if an alternative diagnosis is confirmed, or if HSV PCR in the CSF is negative on two occasions (24–48 hours apart) and MRI imaging does not suggest HSE. Empirical antimalarial (artemisinin-based combination therapy) must be started if there is a suspicion of cerebral malaria. This should be stopped if the peripheral smear and rapid diagnostic tests are negative. Intravenous azithromycin is recommended in areas that are endemic for scrub typhus or when mycoplasma or ehrlichial infections are suspected.[8,22]

Step 5: Definitive Treatment

Definitive treatment is as per the confirmed etiology. The treatment for pyogenic meningitis, cerebral malaria, and other infections is described in detail elsewhere in the book. Antiviral therapy is indicated in some forms of viral encephalitis. This is listed in **Table 5**. Antiviral therapy is not needed in most of the other viral encephalitis cases, including VZV cerebellitis. Corticosteroids are indicated in ADEM, Hashimoto encephalopathy, and autoimmune encephalitis.[8,22] There is a role of intravenous immunoglobulin and plasmapheresis also in autoimmune and postinfectious encephalitis.[9]

Step 6: Supportive Care

Prompt institution of good supportive treatment (along with empirical treatment) is most crucial for optimum outcome in most case of viral encephalitis, the most common cause of AES. Many cases of AES (with GCS < 8, features of raised intracranial pressure, or status epilepticus) need intensive care, at least initially. Cases of rabies encephalitis and those with severe immunosuppression, exanthematous encephalitis or a potentially contagious viral hemorrhagic fever need to be under isolation. The following are the components of supportive care:

- *Maintenance intravenous fluids:* Fluid therapy should be targeted to maintain euvolemia, normoglycemia, and electrolyte balance. Normal daily maintenance requirement of fluids as per the weight of child is infused

Table 5: Antiviral drugs used in various forms of viral encephalitis.	
Virus	*Antiviral therapy*
Herpes simplex virus encephalitis	Intravenous acyclovir for 14–21 days. In young kids between 3 months of age and 12 months of age, the minimum duration is 21 days. After this, CSF PCR can be repeated weekly and acyclovir is continued till CSF PCR becomes negative. High incidence of recurrence (within weeks to three months) of HSE has been reported, if acyclovir is used for a shorter duration.[14] Some experts recommend oral acyclovir in dose of 300 mg/m^2 per dose 8 hourly for 6 months after 21-day course of intravenous acyclovir
Varicella zoster virus encephalitis	Acyclovir 10–15 mg/kg thrice daily for 3 weeks intravenously with or without a short course of steroids
Influenza virus encephalitis	Oseltamivir
Acute measles virus encephalitis	Ribavirin
Human herpes virus 6 encephalitis	Ganciclovir or foscarnet is indicated in immunocompromised; can be considered in immunocompetent cases also
Cytomegalovirus encephalitis	Combination therapy with ganciclovir (5 mg/kg intravenously twice daily) with or without foscarnet (60 mg/kg every 8 hours or 90 mg/kg every 12 hours) initially followed by ganciclovir (5 mg/kg/day) and foscarnet (60–120 mg/kg/day) for 3 weeks (6 weeks in immunocompromised). However, the response is not very dramatic
JE encephalitis	Minocycline has shown some experimental evidence of benefit

(CSF: cerebrospinal fluid; HSE: herpes simplex encephalitis; JE: Japanese encephalitis; PCR: polymerase chain reaction)
Source: Iype M. Viral Encephalitis. In: Gupta P, Menon PSN, Ramji S, Lodha R (Eds). PG Textbook of Pediatrics, 2nd edition. New Delhi: Jaypee Brothers Medical Publishers (P) Ltd.; 2018. pp. 2482-7.[22]

in form of isotonic fluid (hypotonic fluids are avoided). Serum sodium is monitored, and abnormalities of serum sodium are corrected slowly. If there are features of syndrome of inappropriate secretion of antidiuretic hormone, only then fluids should be restricted to two-thirds of the daily maintenance.

- *Management of raised intracranial pressure (ICP):* It is crucial to recognize and promptly manage signs of raised ICP, as it is a common cause of death in children with viral encephalitis. The patient should have adequate sedation and analgesia. Noxious stimuli should be avoided; nebulized lignocaine should be administered prior to endotracheal tube suctioning in intubated patients. The patient is intubated if the GCS is less than 8, or if there is evidence of herniation, or if the patient has irregular respirations and inability to maintain airway. In case of signs of impending herniation, hyperventilation to a target $PaCO_2$ of 30–35 mm Hg is done. Mannitol (0.25 g/kg bolus followed by 0.25 g/kg 6 hourly as per requirement, up to 48 hours) is given. Hypertonic (3%) saline infusion 0.1–1 mL/kg/hr) is preferable to mannitol in the presence of hypotension, hypovolemia, and renal failure. The serum sodium should be targeted to a level of 145–155 mEq/L.

- *Maintain euglycemia:* Identifying and treating hypoglycemia with intravenous dextrose (2 mL/kg 10% dextrose, then glucose infusion rate of 6–8 mg/kg/min) is another important step. Blood glucose is monitored to avoid and both hypo- and hyperglycemia.

- *Treatment and prevention of seizures:* If the child is having seizures, or has history of seizures, anti-convulsant should be administered. Midazolam (0.1 mg/kg) (diazepam 0.3 g/kg and lorazepam 0.1 mg/kg are other alternatives) is given followed by phenytoin loading dose (20 mg/kg). Even if there is no history or clinical evidence of seizures, empirical anticonvulsant therapy may be considered in children with GCS < 8, and features of raised intracranial pressure. This is because seizures may further raise the intracranial pressure and thus worsen the outcome.

- *Corticosteroids:* The role of large doses of corticosteroids (dexamethasone or methylprednisolone) in the setting of acute infective encephalitis is debatable and theoretically can increase viral replication. While some small studies such as that of Kamei et al.[24] showed that lack of administration of corticosteroids was a significant independent predictor of a poor outcome in cases of HSE, the evidence is not robust.

Recently, a multicentric randomized controlled trial was attempted in adults, but had to be terminated midway, as adequate number of patients could not be recruited.[25] However, steroids might be specifically indicated in certain other situations such as tuberculous meningoencephalitis or granulomatous angiitis after varicella zoster infection.[15] They are also indicated in ADEM, Hashimoto encephalopathy, and autoimmune encephalitis.

- *Monitoring/prevention/treatment of associated issues:* Careful monitoring is required to detect acid-base and electrolyte imbalance, neutropenia (due to acyclovir), associated bacterial infections (such as pneumonia), and organ dysfunction (myocarditis, pulmonary edema, acute kidney injury, etc.). Prompt and appropriate management of these is essential for optimal outcome. Careful monitoring is also required for changing level of consciousness, fever, seizures, autonomic nervous system dysfunction, increased intracranial pressure, and speech and motor disturbances. Regular change of body posture, good nursing care, and use of water/air bed (if available) is of paramount importance to prevent bedsores. Involvement of physiotherapist and dietitian early in the course of illness helps improve the outcomes significantly.

Step 7: Rehabilitation and Follow-up

Many cases of AES, especially encephalitis and meningitis, have many residual sequelae in a significant proportion of survivors, depending on age of child, causative agent, severity, course and promptness and appropriateness of treatment received. As in any critical illness, nutritional status is also affected. Motor incoordination, tremors seizures, total or partial deafness, visual disturbances (chorioretinopathy and perpetual amblyopia), intellectual and psychologic deficits/personality changes can occur. Recurrence (especially in suboptimally treated cases) and postinfective encephalitis are also known sequelae of infective encephalitis and meningitis. Some of the sequelae, on the other hand, may be very subtle, thus making neurologic, psychiatric, developmental, and audiological follow-up very important. A multidisciplinary team led by a pediatrician with involvement of dietitian, physiotherapist, occupational therapist, and speech therapist is ideal, wherever feasible.

■ REFERENCES

1. Solomon T, Thao TT, Lewthwaite P, et al. A cohort study to assess the new WHO Japanese encephalitis surveillance standards. Bull World Health Organ. 2008;86(3):178-86.

2. Roy A, Mandal K, Sen S, et al. Study of acute viral meningoencephalitis in children in sub-Himalayan Tarai region: Clinico-epidemiological, etiological, and imaging profile. Indian J Child Health. 2015;2(4):177-81.

3. Misra UK, Kalita J. Overview: Japanese encephalitis. Prog Neurobiol. 2010;91(2):108-20.

4. Joshi R, Kalantri SP, Reingold A, et al. Changing landscape of acute encephalitis syndrome in India: a systematic review. Nat Med J India. 2012;25(4):212-20.

5. Rao BL, Basu A, Wairagkar NS, et al. A large outbreak of acute encephalitis with high fatality rate in children in Andhra Pradesh, India, in 2003, associated with Chandipura virus. Lancet. 2004;364(9437):869-74.

6. Chadha MS, Arankalle VA, Jadi RS, et al. An outbreak of Chandipura virus encephalitis in the eastern districts of Gujarat state, India. Am J Trop Med Hyg. 2005;73(3):566-70.

7. Sapkal GN, Bondre VP, Fulmali PV, et al. Enteroviruses in patients with acute encephalitis, Uttar Pradesh, India. Emerg Infect Dis. 2009;15(2):295-8.

8. Sharma S, Mishra D, Aneja S, et al. Expert Group on Encephalitis, Indian Academy of Pediatrics. Consensus guidelines on evaluation and management of suspected acute viral encephalitis in children in India. Indian Pediatr. 2012;49(11):897-910.

9. Janowski AB, Hunstad DA. Viral meningoencephalitis. In: Kliegman RM, Geme III JW, Blum NJ, Shah SS, et al. Nelson Textbook of Pediatrics, 21st edition. Philadelphia: Elsevier; 2019. pp. 3232-4.

10. Rathi N, Rathi A. Rickettsial Infections: Indian Perspective. Indian Pediatr. 2010; 47(2):157-64.

11. Mittal M, Bondre V, Murhekar M, et al. Acute Encephalitis Syndrome in Gorakhpur (Uttar Pradesh), 2016: Clinical and Laboratory Findings. Pediatr Infect Dis J. 2018;37(11):1101-6.

12. Jayaraman Y, Veeraraghavan B, Chethrapilly Purushothaman GK, et al. Burden of bacterial meningitis in India: Preliminary data from a hospital based sentinel surveillance network. PLoS One. 2018;13(5):e0197198.

13. Oordt-Speets AM, Bolijn R, van Hoorn RC, et al. Global etiology of bacterial meningitis: A systematic review and meta-analysis. PLoS One. 2018;13(6):e0198772.

14. Thapa R, Patra V, Kundu R. Plasmodium vivax cerebral malaria. Indian Pediatr. 2007;44(6):433-4.

15. Chaudhuri A, Kennedy PGE. Diagnosis and treatment of viral encephalitis. Postgraduate Medical Journal. 2002;78: 575-83.

16. Glaser CA, Honarmand S, Anderson LJ, et al. Beyond Viruses: Clinical Profiles and Etiologies Associated with Encephalitis. Clin Infect Dis. 2006;43(12):1565-77.

17. Vashishtha VM, Kumar A, John TJ, et al. Cassia occidentalis poisoning causes fatal coma in children in western Uttar Pradesh. Indian Pediatr. 2007;44(7):522-5.

18. Sriramachari S. Heat hyperpyrexia: time to act. Indian J Med Res. 2004;119(6): vii-x.

19. Ghosh D, Dhadwal D, Aggarwal A, et al. Investigation of an epidemic of Reye's syndrome in northern region of India. Indian Pediatr.1999;36(11):1097-106.

20. John TJ, Date A, Patoria NK. Acute encephalopathy in children in Nagpur: similarity to Reye's syndrome. Indian J Pediatr. 1983;50(403):129-32.

21. John TJ. Outbreak of killer brain disease in children: mystery or missed diagnosis? Indian Pediatr. 2003; 40(9):863-9.

22. Iype M. Viral Encephalitis. In: Gupta P, Menon PSN, Ramji S, Lodha R (Eds). PG textbook of Pediatrics, 2nd edition. New Delhi: Jaypee Brothers Medical Publishers (P) Ltd.; 2018. pp. 2482-7.

23. Steiner I, Budka H, Chaudhuri A, et al. Viral meningo-encephalitis: a review of diagnostic methods and guidelines for management. Eur J Neurol. 2010;17(18):999-e57.

24. Kamei S, Sekizawa T, Shiota H, et al. Evaluation of combination therapy using aciclovir and corticosteroid in adult patients with herpes simplex virus encephalitis. J Neurol Neurosurg Psychiatry. 2005;76(11):1544-9.

25. Meyding-Lamadé U, Jacobi C, Martinez-Torres F, et al. The German trial on Aciclovir and Corticosteroids in Herpes-simplex-virus-Encephalitis (GACHE): a multicenter, randomized, double-blind, placebo-controlled trial. Neurol Res Pract. 2019.

■ INTRODUCTION

Hepatitis is characterized by inflammation of the liver and presence of inflammatory cells in the liver tissue. Hepatitis is acute when it lasts less than 6 months and chronic when it persists longer. Hepatic parenchymal fibrosis develops secondary to long-term wound healing process. Cirrhosis results from chronic insult to liver. The complications of cirrhosis are secondary to loss of hepatic function and portal hypertension.[1] Before liver failure is manifested clinically, liver parenchyma of approximately 80–90% must be lost. Further discussion in this chapter would be on hepatitis B and C.

■ HEPATITIS B

Epidemiology

Hepatitis B is one of the most common infectious diseases in the world. 30–40% of world's population of almost 350 million people are said to have had contact with hepatitis B or are carriers of hepatitis B virus (HBV). In sub-Saharan Africa and East Asia, there is highest prevalence of hepatitis B. The endemic rates of hepatitis are divided into high (>8%), intermediate (2–7%), and low (<2%), based on positive seroprevalence of HBsAg (hepatitis B surface antigen) in the population.[2] 2–5% of population of the Middle East and the Indian subcontinent are chronically infected, while chronically infected population in Western Europe and North America is less than 1%. This diversity in risk of chronicity is related to the age and the mode of acquisition of infection which also determines the HBV endemicity rate. Chronic HBV infection occurs in nearly 90% of infection acquired parentally but is as low as 5% when diagnosed in an adult.[3] Acute infection would more likely progress to chronic infection in immunosuppressed patients. 60% of the world's population lives in areas where HBV infection is highly endemic, such as China, Indonesia, Nigeria, and rest of Asia and Africa. Either due to acute or due to chronic hepatitis B, almost 300,000 people die annually. Hepatitis B definitely is a major global health problem, despite the availability of an effective vaccine, which is worse in developing countries.

Molecular Biology

Hepatitis B virus belongs to the Hepadnaviridae family and is a DNA virus. HBV is a small virus of 3.2 kilobase (kb) and contains a partially double stranded DNA genome with four open reading frames (ORFs). There are four viral genes, namely *surface*, *core*, *polymerase*, and *X* genes. The core gene encodes the core nucleocapsid protein and is responsible for production of HBeAg (hepatitis B envelope antigen). The surface gene encodes the pre-S1, pre-S2, and S proteins. X protein may be a major factor in hepatic carcinogenesis. The polymerase gene encodes a large protein which is involved in critical functions of DNA replication and packaging. The virion attaches to host cell membranes in HBV infection, and nucleocapsid is released into the cytoplasm. We poorly understand the mechanisms of intracellular transport of viral genome into the nucleus; however, conversion of the circular form of HBV DNA into a double-stranded, covalently closed circular form (cccDNA) appears to be the first step in genomic replication. The cccDNA serves as the template for viral transcription.

Hepatitis B Virus Genotypes

There are eight genotypes of hepatitis B virus—A to H. There is intergroup divergence of approximately 8% in the nucleotide sequence and genotypes. In northern Europe and the United States, genotype A is predominant;

while in eastern Asia and the Far East, genotypes B and C are common.[4] In the Mediterranean area, Middle East, and south Asia, genotype D is prevalent while in western sub-Saharan areas, genotypes E and G are indigenous and in central America, genotype F prevails. Mexico has prevalence of genotype H. HBeAg seroconversion is earlier in genotype B patients than in genotype C patients. Response to therapy with PEG (pegylated) interferon,[5] frequency of mutation, and probable risk of hepatocellular carcinoma (HCC) are different in various genotypes of hepatitis B.

Mutations of the Hepatitis B Virus Genome

Point mutations of 10^{10} to 10^{11} per day may occur in the HBV genome and binding of neutralizing antibodies may be prevented due to such point changes such as substitution of arginine by glycine at amino acid position 145.[6] As many as 50% patients of postliver transplant have escape mutations despite HBIG (hepatitis B immune globulin) which may result in recurrent HBV infection. Production of HBeAg may be influenced by mutation. Mutations in the basal core promoter and precore regions of the HBV genome have been seen in severe or fulminant hepatitis cases and are linked to increased risk of HCC. Recognition of HBV by cytotoxic T lymphocytes (CTLs) may be blocked by core gene mutation, thus interfering with response of interferon.

Mutations in the sequence of HBV polymerase can lead to drug resistance to nucleoside analogs used in treatment of HBV. For example, YMDD mutants in C domain (Y = tyrosine, M = methionine, D = aspartate) result in resistance to lamivudine; in almost 70% of the cases, resistance to lamivudine may be seen by 5 year of its usage. Similarly, nucleotide substitutions have been described that lead to resistance with other drugs such as entecavir, telbivudine, and rarely with tenofovir. Adefovir resistance is seen in up to 29% of the cases after 5 years. Entecavir and tenofovir have the least resistance.

Transmission and Pathogenesis

Hepatitis B virus is transmitted by perinatal, sexual exposure, percutaneous route, and by close contact of person to person. Survival of hepatitis B virus outside the body could be for a prolonged period.[7] The intensity of the host immunologic response to the virus, both the innate and the adaptive immune responses, determines the HBV-associated liver disease.

During acute HBV infection, both innate immune system (cytokine) and cell-mediated immune responses (Th1 cell) are vigorous, resulting in clearance of the

HBV DNA molecules from the liver.[8] Weak HBV-specific T-cell responses are seen in persons with chronic HBV infection. Apoptosis of infected hepatocytes is secondary to CTLs. Antiviral cytokines produced by CD4 cells help in neutralizing antibody production.

Perinatal Transmission

Perinatal transmission of HBV results in chronic infection. Infants born to HBeAg-positive women have a 90% incidence of developing chronic HBV infection. In about 80–95% infants, neonatal vaccination prevents newborn infection. Prompt immunization may not prevent transplacental transmission which makes a minority of infection. Maternal HBeAg positivity, HBsAg titer, and HBV DNA level are risk factors of HBV infection through the transplacental route.[2,9] Cesarean section as compared to normal vaginal delivery is assumed to have a less transmission rate. However, at this point, most obstetrical algorithms, regardless of the HBeAg status or level of viremia, do not include change in the planned mode of delivery for HBsAg-positive women.

Diagnosis (Fig. 1 and Table 1)

HBsAg: 2–10 weeks after exposure to the virus, HBsAg appears and it usually becomes undetectable after 4–6 months in those who recover. Persistence of HBsAg for more than 6 months implies progression to chronic HBV infection. Appearance of anti-HBs (antibody to hepatitis B surface antigen) confers long-term immunity, which is associated with disappearance of HBsAg. Anti-HBc

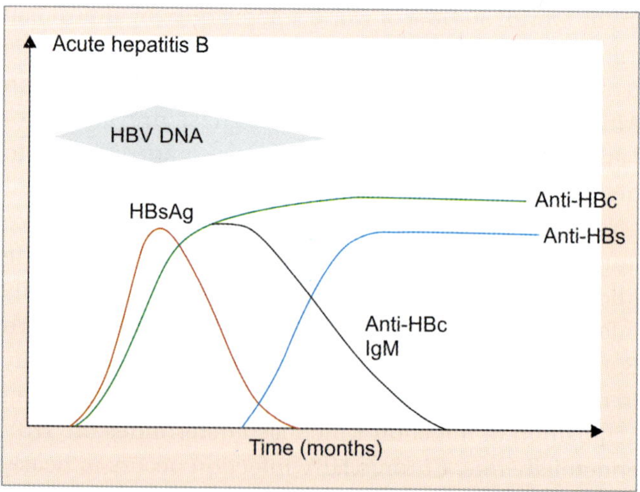

Fig. 1: Serologic markers during chronic hepatitis B virus infection. (Anti-HBc: antibody to hepatitis B core antigen; Anti-HBs: antibody to hepatitis B surface antigen; Anti-HBc IgM: IgM antibody to hepatitis B core antigen; DNA: deoxyribonucleic acid; HBsAg: hepatitis B surface antigen; HBV: hepatitis B virus)

Table 1: Diagnosis of hepatitis B virus infection.

	HBsAg	HBeAg	IgM anti-HBc	IgG anti-HBc	Anti-HBs	Anti-HBe	HBV DNA	Interpretation
Acute HCV infection	+	+	+		-		+	Early phase
Chronic HBV infection	+	+	-	+	-	-	+	Replicative phase (HBeAg-positive chronic hepatitis)
	+	-	-	+	-	+	-	Nonreplicative phase (HBeAb-positive chronic hepatitis B

HBV DNA detected by unamplified assay.
(Ab: antibody; DNA: deoxyribonucleic acid; HBV: hepatitis B virus; HCV: hepatitis C virus; HBc: hepatitis B core IgM immunoglobulin; HBeAg: hepatitis B envelope antigen; HBsAg: hepatitis B surface antigen)

(antibody to hepatitis B core antigen) is detectable in both acute and chronic HBV infections. Anti-HBc IgM (IgM antibody to hepatitis B core antigen) is predominant in acute infection while anti-HBc IgG (IgG antibody to hepatitis B core antigen) persists in those who recover from acute hepatitis B.[10]

HBeAg: It is found in serum early during acute infection. HBeAg, a soluble viral protein, positivity at 3 months and beyond after the onset of illness indicates a high likelihood of transition to chronic infection. HBeAg positivity is also to be considered as an indication of viral replication and infectivity. Seroconversion from HBeAg to anti-HBe (antibody to hepatitis B envelope antigen) is associated with disappearance of HBV DNA in serum and disease remission.

HBV DNA: HBV DNA estimation is required to assess the need of therapy and response to antiviral therapy, identify drug resistance, and diagnose occult/cryptic hepatitis B infection, when HBsAg is negative. HBV DNA is also used to diagnose hepatitis B infection in an anti-HBc-positive donor and in patients with fulminant hepatitis B who have cleared HBsAg.

The diagnosis of acute hepatitis B is based on the detection of HBsAg and anti-HBc IgM. Positive anti-HBs and anti-HBc IgG are suggestive of past HBV infection. However, immunity secondary to HBV vaccination is indicated by the presence of anti-HBs only with absence of anti-HBc IgG. The diagnosis of chronic HBV infection is based on HBsAg detection which could be low replicative when HBeAg/HBV DNA are negative or in replicative phase when the above two markers are positive. The severity of liver disease can be assessed by liver function tests, prothrombin time, alpha-fetoprotein, and baseline ultrasound. Besides assessment of viral replication, concomitant diseases such as hepatitis C and HIV should be ruled out. If anti-HAV antibody is negative, vaccinate for hepatitis A. In addition, one should vaccinate all family members with hepatitis B vaccine following their screening.

Management

The main aim of the treatment of chronic hepatitis B is to suppress HBV replication and prevent irreversible liver damage. The ultimate goals are to eliminate HBV, prevent progression to cirrhosis and HCC, and improve survival. Response is usually defined as sustained clearance of HBeAg with or without detectable anti-HBe, failure to detect HBV DNA in serum (with unamplified assays), and regression of liver disease [normalization of ALT (alanine aminotransferase) levels and decrease in necrotic inflammation on liver biopsy] **(Table 2)**.

Antiviral therapies are as follows:
- *Interferon α*:
  - Antiviral agents (nucleoside and nucleotide analogs): Lamivudine, adefovir, entecavir, tenofovir, tenofovir disoproxil, emtricitabine, clevudine, and β -l-thymidine (L-dT).
- *Immunomodulatory therapy*:
  - Interleukin 12
  - Thymosin.
- HBV-specific:
  - DNA vaccination.
- Combination treatment:
  - Interferon + Lamivudine
  - Lamivudine + adefovir dipivoxil.
- New immunomodulatory therapy.

Aims and Treatment

The primary treatment goal for children with hepatitis B is to strengthen the immune system so that it can effectively

Table 2: Definition of response to antiviral therapy of chronic hepatitis B.

Category of response	
Biochemical response (BR)	Decrease in serum level to within the normal range
Virological response (VR)	Decrease in serum HBV DNA to undetectable levels in unamplified assays ($<10^5$ copies/mL) and loss of HBeAg in patients who were initially HBeAg positive.
Histologic response (HR)	Decrease in histology activity index by at least 2 points in comparison with value on pretreatment liver biopsy
Complete response (CR)	Fulfillment of criteria of biochemical and virological response and loss of HBsAg
Time to assessment	
End of treatment	*At the end of a defined course of treatment*
Sustained response (SR-6)	6 months after discontinuation of therapy
Sustained response (SR-12)	12 months after discontinuation of therapy

(DNA: deoxyribonucleic acid; HBV: hepatitis B virus; HBeAg: hepatitis B envelope antigen; HBsAg: hepatitis B surface antigen)

prevent the virus from replicating, and hence achieve an undetectable HBV viral load, thus halting any liver damage. Unfortunately, treatment available for hepatitis B infection in children so far have had limited success. The only new drugs approved by the US Food and Drug Administration (FDA) to treat hepatitis B in children are standard interferon, lamivudine (>2 years), adefovir (> 12 years), entecavir (>2 years), telbivudine (> 16 years) and PEG interferon and tonoferon (>12 years). Majority of infected children are in the immune-tolerant phase, in which the presently available drug therapy is ineffective. Further research is needed to study the appropriate immunomodulatory therapy in the immune-tolerant phase.

Antiviral Therapy

Interferon has direct immunomodulatory properties. Because of its side effect, interferon acceptance is poor. The major disadvantage of interferon relates to its poorer acceptance because of side effects such as flu-like illnesses, bone marrow suppression, anorexia, nausea, depression, and fatigue. In decompensated liver disease, cytopenia, autoimmune disease, and severe renal or cardiac disease, interferon is contraindication. Its recommended dose is 0.1 MU/kg or 3–6 MU/m^2 three times a week for 4–6 months. The duration of treatment can be extended up to 12 months. Results of interferon varied from 20 to 60% in various studies. In a recent study of PEG interferon conducted in children from 3 years to <18 years with chronic hepatitis B, alfa 2a treatment for 48 weeks in the immune-active phase of children with chronic hepatitis B suggested that it was well tolerated and efficacious and was associated with higher incidence of HBsAg clearance than adults. Hence, FDA approval of PEG interferon alpha 2a for the treatment of chronic hepatitis B came in 2019.[11]

Nucleoside and Nucleotide Analogs

Nucleoside and nucleotide analogs act as a competitive inhibitor of the viral reverse transcriptase and DNA polymerase by replacing natural nucleosides during the synthesis of the HBV DNA.

These drugs have proved to be particularly useful in the management of patients with decompensated cirrhosis.

The major disadvantage of using nucleos(t)ide analogs is that due to its mechanism of action of partially suppressing viral replication, the treatment duration becomes prolonged and carries risk of development of drug resistance. With these agents, HBsAg clearance rarely occurs after 1 year of treatment. Serum ALT flares have been seen after discontinuation of nucleoside analog therapy in nearly 25% of cases.

Lamivudine: This drug is a potent inhibitor of viral replication. It is convenient to administer and free of severe adverse effects; it is recommended at the age of 2 years and above and in a dose of 3 mg/kg/day as a single dose (maximum dose 100 mg/kg). Its drawback is its need of prolonged duration of therapy and high incidence of viral resistance like YMDD mutations, virtually in three fourths of the patients by 5 years of therapy. *Adefovir dipivoxil* is recommended for use in more than 12 years of age in a daily dose of 10 mg/kg. Patients with lamivudine-resistant HBV may benefit from the use of adefovir. Potential nephrotoxicity is the major disadvantage with adefovir; therefore, it is no longer used in the present era due to the availability of newer oral antiviral therapy.

Entecavir, a guanosine nucleoside analog, is approved in children of 2 years and above with chronic hepatitis B. *Tenofovir disoproxil fumarate* is an acyclic nucleotide inhibitor of HBV polymerase and is approved by the FDA in 2017 for use in children of 12 years and above. It has least incidence of developing resistance.

There are few other drugs that are being used in adults, e.g. telbivudine, emtricitabine, and clevudine. These drugs are currently not recommended for use in children.

Combination Therapies

Comparisons between interferon and lamivudine plus interferon have been conducted in children but there have been no significant differences in the outcome measured. Further larger studies are required to test the various combination therapies for treatment of chronic hepatitis B infection in children. Research is needed to further study the immunological abnormalities in the immune-tolerant phase of hepatitis B and developing appropriate immunomodulatory therapies.

Prevention

Passive immunization: Immune globulin is an important tool for the prevention of HBV infection. When an individual is exposed to a person with acute hepatitis, immune globulin treatment should be given as soon as feasible; it should be given within 2 weeks of exposure. It should not be given if the delay is greater than 14 days. Postexposure prophylaxis with HBIG has been recommended for administration of the following: Perinatal exposure of an infant born to an HBsAg-positive woman (discussed later), percutaneous or mucosal exposure to HBsAg-positive products, sexual exposure to HBsAg-positive person, or household contact.[12]

Active immunization: In highly endemic areas, a very effective measure to prevent hepatitis B transmission is use of hepatitis B vaccination. The most recommended regimen for vaccination in newborn is the 0-, 1-, and 6-month schedule and this regimen appears to have a higher efficacy of more than 95%. For preterms < 2 kg birth weight, one extra dose is given. In high-risk population and immunocompromised individuals, postvaccination testing is recommended to check for a protective concentration of anti-HBs. The dose of vaccine is 10 µg for children < 18 years of age and 20 µg for adults. The recombinant and plasma vaccines are well-tolerated. In children, the middle third of anterolateral thigh is preferred. The vaccine in adults should be given in deltoid and not in the gluteal region for better immunogenicity. Transient pain and low-grade fever are only common side effects. Fatigue, headache, nausea, and skin rash can occur very rarely.

Hepatitis B vaccination is a good modality of preventing hepatitis B infection and thus eventually cirrhosis and HCC in adults. The major objective of hepatitis B vaccination is prevention of chronic infection, which leads to cirrhosis and HCC. One of the good modalities of preventing vertical transmission is to screen child-bearing women for hepatitis B and C. In addition, screening high-risk groups like immune-deficient patients such as malnourished and those receiving chemotherapy or on steroids or immunosuppression. It is crucial to increase the public awareness for hepatitis B and C and educate the masses through different modalities.

■ HEPATITIS C

Hepatitis C is the result of infection with hepatitis C virus (HCV). It is relatively less common infection in children than adults. It is estimated to affect 170–200 million people worldwide and is based on studies in blood donors who are approximately 1% of the population. There is no sufficient data on HCV in children. The published data suggest that most population in America, western Europe, and southeast Asia have a prevalence rate of antibody to HCV (anti-HCV) of <2.5%. In the Middle East and central Asia, anti-HCV prevalence varies from 1% to >12%. Eastern Europe has an average prevalence of 1.5–5%, while western Pacific region has 2.5–4.9%.

Genomic Organization and Viral Proteins

Hepatitis C virus consists of a 9.6-kb, positive (sense)-, single-stranded RNA genome that comprises a highly conserved 341-base 5′ noncoding region, a single long open reading frame (ORF) , and a 3′ noncoding region **(Fig. 2)**.[12]

Genotype 3 is common in the Indian subcontinent and Southeast Asia and six genotypes have been described

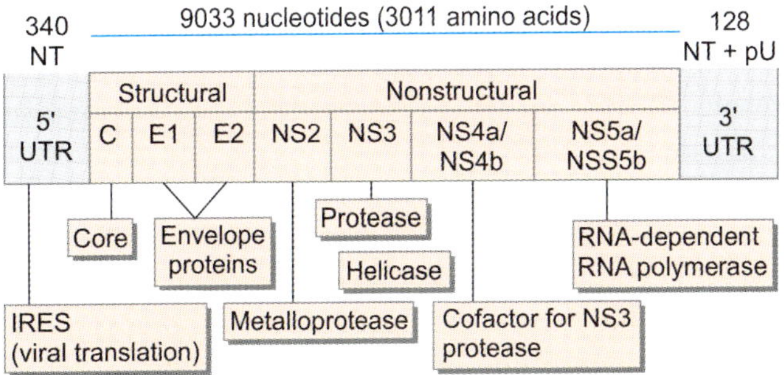

Fig. 2: Hepatitis C virus genome showing encoding region and functions.
(IRES: internal ribosome entry site; NT: nucleotide; UTR: untranslated region)

Box 1: The modes of transmission of hepatitis C.
- Blood transfusion
- Administration of blood products (antihemophilic factor, factor IX, intravenous immunoglobulin)
- Injection drug use
- Cocaine snorting
- Accidental occupational exposure (i.e. needlestick)
- Exposure to contaminated medical equipment (reusable syringes, inadequately sterilized medical instruments, contamination of intravenous fluids or injectable medications)
- Tattooing or body piercing
- Sexual spread
- Maternal-infant spread.

worldwide. Genotypes 1 and 2 are common in USA. The clinical relevance of genotypes is related to the response to antiviral therapy. Genotypes 1 and 4 have poor response to interferon-based therapy than patients with genotype 2 or 3.

Box 1 depicts the mode of transmission of hepatitis C.

Vertical transmission from an HCV-positive mother to a newborn is uncommon. In large prospective studies, 5–10% of infants born to anti-HCV-positive mothers acquire hepatitis C during the first 1–2 years of life. Passive transfer of anti-HCV may persist in a newborn for a year or longer, so testing for anti-HCV as source of infection is not reliable. Nearly 50% of infected newborns clear HCV RNA spontaneously. It is only when HCV RNA is positive as in 2–5% of children that maternal-infant transmission is considered and not on anti-HCV presence.

Clinical Course of Hepatitis C

The incubation period of acute hepatitis C is on average 50 days (range 15–75 days). The diagnosis of acute hepatitis C is suggested by positive HCV RNA in serum with biochemical evidence of acute hepatitis **(Fig. 3)**.

ELISA (enzyme-linked immunosorbent assay) immune assays are most widely used for anti-HCV testing. Immunoblot assays for anti-HCV are available for confirmation of EIA (enzyme immunoassay) test results. Testing for HCV RNA by the PCR (polymerase chain reaction) method is the most direct method of demonstrating active HCV infection. Genotype assay is done following a positive PCR test. HCV RNA is detectable by PCR within 2 weeks of exposure. ALT levels rise thereafter and symptoms appear 6–8 weeks after viremia. The chronic infection is shown by persistence of HCV RNA positivity with or without ALT elevations.

Liver Biopsy

Liver biopsy is useful to give information about the staging of fibrosis and the degree of hepatic inflammation. It also

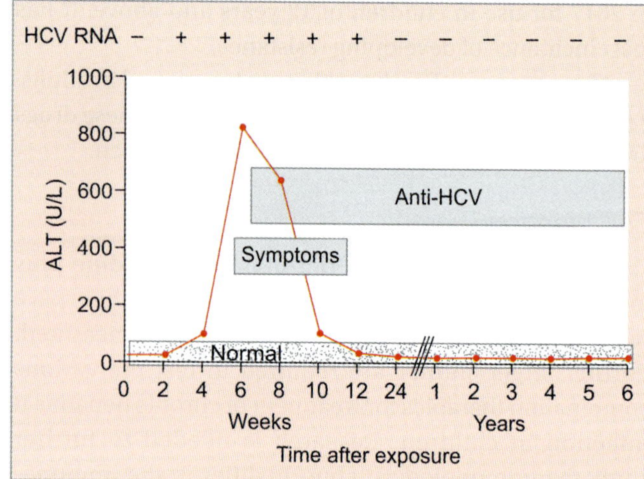

Fig. 3: HCV RNA is detectable by PCR within 2 weeks of exposure. ALT levels rise thereafter, and symptoms appear 6–8 weeks after viremia. Anti-HCV generally arises late, after onset of ALT elevations and symptoms. In self-limited disease, HCV RNA is cleared and ALT returns to normal levels with resolution of the clinical disease.
(ALT: serum alanine aminotransferase; HCV: hepatitis C virus; RNA: ribonucleic acid)

provides information on prognosis. However, liver biopsy is not mandatory in order to initiate therapy and with the availability of noninvasive elastography methods such as fibroscan, liver biopsy is rarely done.

Treatment

Eradication of infection is the goal of treatment which would prevent complications of HCV infection. Sustained virologic response (SVR) is defined as the absence of HCV RNA in serum by a sensitive test at the end of treatment and 6 months later. Nonresponders are those in whom HCV RNA levels remain stable on treatment and partial responders are those whose HCV RNA levels decline (e.g. by >2 logs), but never become undetectable.

The present treatment of hepatitis C infection consists of 6–12 months of combination of PEG interferon and ribavirin. Viral eradication can be achieved in >90% of patients with HCV genotype 2 or 3 and in only half of all of the patients with HCV genotype 1. Common side effects include pancytopenia, flu-like symptoms, or depression which could lead to early discontinuation of drugs and treatment failure.[13] Recent discovery of numerous potential targets for antiviral therapy, direct acting agent (DAA), such as inhibitors of the HCV NS3/4A protease and nucleotide inhibitors of the HCV NS5B polymerase, has shown variable antiviral activity against different HCV genotypes, but polymerase inhibitors show a higher genetic barrier to resistance than protease inhibitors.

Due to slow progression of fibrosis, rarely would children develop advanced disease or cirrhosis. However, a high-risk factor for early progression of disease includes children with comorbid diseases, such as obesity with nonalcoholic fatty liver disease, congenital heart disease with elevated right heart pressure, and those on hepatotoxic drug. As per AASLD (American Association for the Study of Liver Diseases) 2019, treatment with the newer approved DAAs for adolescents > 12 years—ledipasvir (90 mg)/sofosbuvir (400 mg); for patients with genotypes 1, 4, 5, and 6 with or when compensated cirrhosis for 12 weeks or glecaprevir 300 mg/pibrentasvir (120 mg) for patients with any genotype, who are treatment naive with/without cirrhosis for 8 weeks and 12 weeks for treatment experienced. Presently, oral antiviral therapy is not approved in children less than 12 years. In the near future, it is anticipated that additional DAA regimens will be available for children aged 3–11 years.

■ REFERENCES

1. Friedman S, Schiano T. Cirrhosis and its sequelae. In: Goldman L, Ausiello D (Eds). Cecil Textbook of Medicine, 22nd edition. Philadelphia, Pa: Saunders; 2004. pp. 936-44.
2. World Health Organization. (2000). Hepatitis B: World Health Organization Fact Sheet 204. [online] Available from: https://www.who.int/en/news-room/fact-sheets/detail/hepatitis-b. [Last accessed on December, 2019].:.
3. Tassopoulos NC, Papaevangelou GJ, Sjogren MH, et al Natural history of acute hepatitis B surface antigen positive hepatitis in Greek adults. Gastroenterology. 1987;92(6):1844-50.
4. Okamoto H, Tsuda F, Sakugawa H, et al. Typing hepatitis B virus by homology in nucleotide sequence: comparison of surface antigen subtypes. J Gen Virol. 1988;69 (Pt 10):2575-83
5. Janssen HL, van Zonneveld M, Senturk H, et al. Pegylated interferon alpha-2b alone or in combination with lamivudine for HbeAg-positive chronic hepatitis B: a randomised trial. Lancet. 2005;365(9454):123-9.
6. Hsu HY, Chang MH, Liaw SH, et al. Changes of hepatitis B surface antigen variants in carrier children before and after universal vaccination in Taiwan. Hepatology. 1999;30(5):1312-7.
7. Terrault NA, Lok ASF, McMahon BJ, et al. Update on prevention, diagnosis, and treatment of chronic hepatitis B: AASLD 2018 hepatitis b guidance. Hepatology. 2018;67(4):1560-99.
8. Ganem D, Prince AM. Mechanism of disease: hepatitis B virus infection-natural history and clinical consequences. N Engl J Med. 2004;350(11):1118-29.
9. McMahon BJ, Alward WL, Hall DB, et al. Acute hepatitis B virus infection: relation of age to the clinical expression of disease and subsequent development of the carrier state. J Infect Dis. 1985;151(4):599-603.
10. Hoofnagle JH, Di Bisceglie AM. Serologic diagnosis of acute and chronic viral hepatitis. Semin Liver Dis. 1991;11(2):73-83.
11. Efficacy and safety of peginterferon Alfa 2a (40KD in children with chronic hepatitis B: The PEG-B-ACTIVE study. Hepatology. 2018;68(5):1681-94.
12. Hochman JA, Balistreri F. Acute and chronic viral hepatitis. In: Suchy FJ, Sokol RJ, Balistreri FW (Eds). Liver diseases in children, 3rd edition. New York: Cambridge University Press; 2007. pp. 382-424.
13. Sroczynski G, Esteban E, Conrads-Frank A, et al. Long-term effectiveness and cost-effectiveness of antiviral treatment in hepatitis C. J Viral Hepat. 2010;17(1):34-50.

Dengue and Chikungunya

Kriti Mohan, Piyush Gupta

DENGUE FEVER

■ INTRODUCTION

Dengue fever (DF), a viral illness, was reported as one of the neglected tropical diseases among 17 diseases by World Health Organization (WHO) in its first report on neglected tropical diseases.[1] But now dengue is on the high priority in healthcare system as over the five decades it has become hyperendemic in many regions of the world as well as the virus gained its virulence tremendously with many reported severe cases from all over the world.

■ DISEASE BURDEN

Exact burden of the disease is unpredictable because cases reported are just a tip of the iceberg, and increasing number of cases with severity is a major concern for healthcare system. Annually, 50 million cases are estimated by WHO all over the world; out of them 500,000 need hospitalization due to severity while 20,000 lead to death.[2] Number of cases reduced in 2017–18, but there is resurgence of cases in 2019 again.[3] Dengue is being reported from 100 countries all over the world and Africa, the Americas, the Eastern Mediterranean, South-East Asia, and Western Pacific. South-East Asia and the Western Pacific carry nearly 75% of disease burden.[4] In India, dengue is endemic in all the states and union territories except West Bengal and Lakshadweep now. Many states such as Andhra Pradesh, Assam, Delhi, Goa, Haryana, Gujarat, Karnataka, Kerala, Maharashtra, Odisha, Puducherry, Punjab, Rajasthan, Tamil Nadu, Telangana, Uttar Pradesh, and West Bengal had recurrent outbreaks in last five decades.[5] In India, first epidemic of dengue-like illness was reported from Chennai in the year 1780 but virologically proven first epidemic was reported from Calcutta and Eastern coast of India in 1963–1964.[6] Largest outbreak of dengue from India was reported in 1996 from Delhi which was caused by serotype 2 of the virus.[7] All serotypes are reported from India. According to the National Vector Borne Disease Control Program (NVBDCP), India has reported more than 67,000 cases and 48 deaths of DF as of October in 2019 with Karnataka being the leading state in morbidity and mortality due to dengue with 12,756 reported cases. Apart from this, Karnataka, Maharashtra, Uttarakhand, Gujarat, Kerala, Bihar, and Delhi reported 7,863, 7,513, 5,819, 3,075, 1,588, and 1,431 cases, respectively, in 2019 **(Table 1; Figs. 1 and 2)**.[8]

■ EPIDEMIOLOGY

Dengue is now endemic in almost all countries and this is prevalent in urban as well as rural areas due to lifestyle changes of human beings such as urbanization, increasing constructions, stagnation of water after raining due to improper drainage, improper water supply, and water storage providing adequate breeding site for the vector.[9] Endemicity of dengue depends on complex relationship between host (man and mosquito), agent (virus), and environment (abiotic and biotic factors). For high vector density temperatures in the range of 25°C ± 5°C, relative humidity around 80% and many water collection sites are required. Monsoon and postmonsoon seasons provide suitable environment for the vector to survive well.[9] Dengue transmission is low with extreme temperatures and low relative humidity.[10]

Dengue Virus

The agent for dengue disease is dengue virus that belongs to genus *Flaviviridae*. They are small viruses (50 nm), having single-stranded RNA. They have antigenically similar four serotypes— DENV-1, DENV-2, DENV-3, and DENV-4—but

Table 1: Dengue serotypes in India.

Year	State	Serotype
1964	Tamil Nadu	2
1968	Tamil Nadu	1, 2, 3, and 4
1970	Uttar Pradesh	1, 2, 3, and 4
1996	Uttar Pradesh	2
1996	Delhi	2
1996	Haryana	3
1997	Delhi	1
2001	Madhya Pradesh	2
2003–2005	Delhi	1, 2, 3, and 4
2007–2009	Delhi	1, 2, 3, and 4
2009–2010	Maharashtra	4
2010–2011	Delhi	1
2009–2012	Uttar Pradesh	1, 2, and3
2011–2013	Telangana	1, 2, 3, and 4
2011–2012	Karnataka	1, 2, 3, and 4
2013	Manipur	1, 2, 3, and 4
2013	Madhya Pradesh	2
2013–2015	Kerala	1, 2, and 3
2003–2014	Uttar Pradesh	1, 2, 3, and 4
2014	Delhi	1, 2, and 3
2014	Andaman and Nicobar	3
2015	Delhi	1, 2, 3, and 4

Source: Ganeshkumar P, Murhekar MV, Poornima V, et al. Dengue infection in India: a systematic review and meta-analysis. PLoS Negl Trop Dis. 2018;12(7):e0006618.

they are different in providing cross protection to each other to the host after infection and this is also the reason that single or multiple serotype can be in circulation in any particular area at the same time.[10]

Molecular Epidemiology

The four serotypes (DENV 1–4) of dengue virus form a phylogenetic group, but their nucleotide sequencing is different. They are closely related to one another and form an antigenic complex of their own. Based on

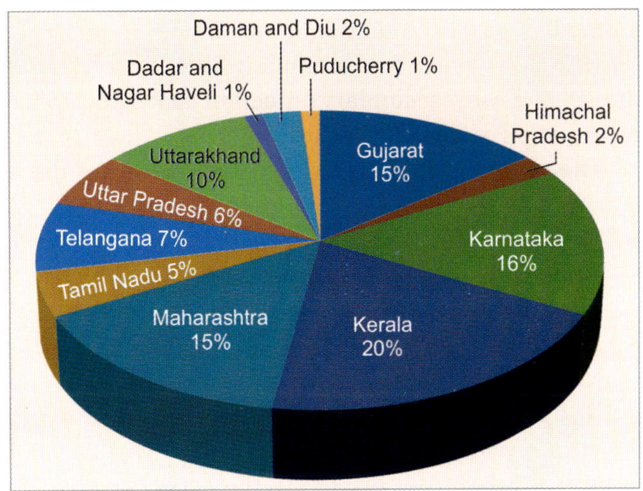

Fig. 2: Deaths due to dengue in India in 2019 in all age groups.
Source: Dengue/DHF situation in India. (NVBDCP) Available from: https://https://www.nvbdcp.gov.in/index4.php?lang=1&level=0&linkid=431&lid=3715. [Last accessed on November, 2019].

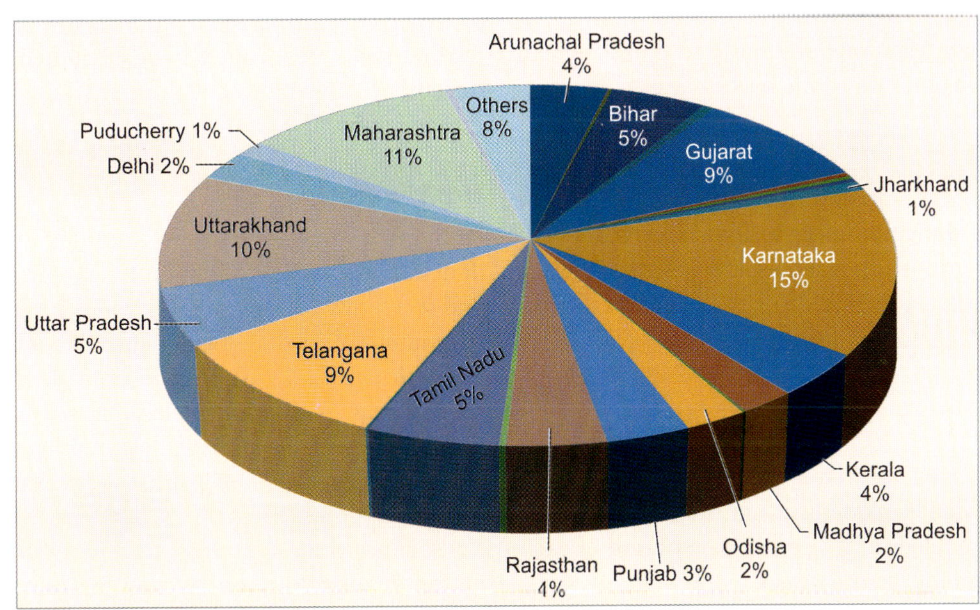

Fig. 1: Dengue cases in different states in India in 2019 in all age group.
Source: National Vector Borne Disease Control Programme. Dengue/DHF situation in India. [online]
Available from: https://www.nvbdcp.gov.in/index4.php?lang=1&level=0&linkid=431&lid=3715. [Last accessed on November, 2019].

their phylogenetic analysis of the genomic region in the envelope gene, each serotype has following subtypes or genotypes:

- DENV-1: Three
- DENV-2: Two (one nonhuman primate)
- DENV-3: Four
- DENV-4: Four (one nonhuman primate).[11,12]

Antibody response to the virus differs individual to individual. On the basis of antibody response, primary infection can be differentiated from secondary infection. Characteristic unique feature in dengue virus infection is that all serotypes have ability to utilized pre-existing antibodies produced during infection with heterotypic *Flavivirus* in past, for enhancing infection. This is the reason why secondary infection leads to severe presentation of illness in the host.

The genome of dengue virus is composed of three structural protein genes encoding for:

- The nucleocapsid of core protein (C)
- A membrane-associated protein (M)
- An envelope protein (E)
- Seven nonstructural (NS) proteins—NS1, NS2A, NS2B, NS3, NS4A, NS4B, and NS5.

NS1 is responsible for interacting with host immune system, especially T cell response, and its level in the blood is one of the diagnostic markers during acute infection.

Most of the infected patients with dengue are asymptomatic and some have severe life-threatening infection.[13] But cause for this various severity in different infected individuals is not clearly understood. Some studies suggest correlation of severity with particular serotype as hemorrhagic manifestations are found to be associated with serotype 4 in one study done by Kumaria.[14-16]

Vector

Female *Aedes* (*Ae.*) mosquitoes are responsible for transmission of dengue infection from infected person to others. The following species are responsible for transmission of dengue:

- *Ae. aegypti*
- *Ae. albopictus*
- *Ae. polynesiensis*
- *Ae. niveus.*

Aedes aegypti is considered as primary vector of dengue in urban areas, breeds in domestic man-made containers, and is a day-time feeder with peak biting period of early morning and evening, before sunset.[17]

Aedes albopictus is considered secondary vector of dengue and is prevalent in Asia and had largely spread to USA and many European countries, reason being

the international trade in used tires, the most common breeding habitat of this vector and having highly adaptive nature of eggs and adult of vector in terms of tolerance to cold.[18,19] In India though *Ae. aegypti* is primary vector and responsible for dengue in urban regions, *Ae. albopictus* is also responsible for transmitting the disease in many states.

The female *Aedes* lays eggs on the damp surface just above waterline. Adults come out of shell in favorable condition in 7 days, while in low temperature they may take several weeks. Eggs can survive for more than a year in dry conditions and adults can emerge within 24 hours whenever come in contact with water. This adaptation is a great hurdle for prevention and control of the disease.

Transmission of disease heavily depends on life cycle, breeding, and longevity of vectors, which further depends on climatic conditions. Life span of *Ae. aegypti* and *Ae. albopictus* are 30 days and 8 weeks, respectively and they can fly only 400 meters. So till the effectivity of the available vaccine is proven and specific treatment for dengue is found, vector control is a major target for preventing the disease.

Ae. polynesiensis and *Ae. niveus* are responsible for causing dengue in few countries.

Environmental Factors

Rainfall and water storage are important favorable factors for the growth of *Ae. aegypti*. Longevity of vector heavily depends on temperature and rainfall. Survival is best at temperature between 16°C and 30°C and a relative humidity of 60–80%. It can survive at altitude between sea level and 1,000 feet above sea level. *Ae. aegypti* is primarily an urban vector but recent reports show that it has spread to rural areas also. This may be attributed to lifestyle and developmental changes with improved transportation to these regions.[15,20]

Host Factors

Humans and several lower primates are the host for dengue virus. Pediatric age group is at high risk of mortality and morbidity in dengue infection, but recently there is a paradigm shift of high incidence of dengue infection from pediatric age group to adolescent and adult. Some studies suggest male predominance and most affected age group of 16–30 years for acquiring dengue infection which may be due to high exposure to the external environment and mosquito vector (**Fig. 3**).

Secondary dengue infection is the most important factor for development of dengue hemorrhagic fever (DHF). An infant can develop DHF commonly even with primary infection due to transplacental transmission of antibodies from mother. In nonendemic regions, traveling

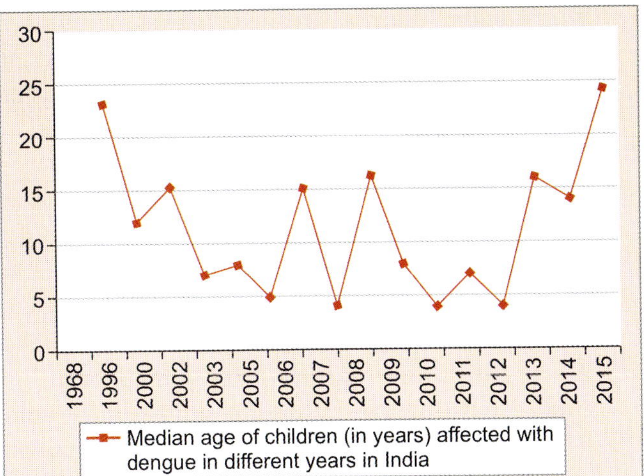

Fig. 3: Median age of the children affected due to dengue year-wise in India.

Source: Ganeshkumar P, Murhekar MV, Poornima V, et al. Dengue infection in India: a systematic review and meta-analysis. PLoS Negl Trop Dis. 2018;12(7):e0006618.

to endemic region is the single most factor for acquiring dengue infection. But in a person from nonendemic region who develops fever after 2 weeks of travel to endemic region, DF is least likely the possibility. Traveling is the most important responsible factor for geographical spread of the infection.

Transmission Cycle

The female *Aedes* mosquito becomes infected with dengue virus while taking the blood of the person in viremia phase of dengue illness. After an extrinsic incubation period of 8–10 days, the mosquito becomes infected and is now able to transmit infection. Now when the mosquito sucks the blood from human, it injects viruses with saliva into the bite wound. After the intrinsic incubation period of 3–14 days, symptoms of dengue start appearing. There is also evidence that the infected female mosquito can transmit viruses vertically to its offspring.

Though primary mode of transmission of dengue is through vector, other modes of transmission reported are through blood transfusion, organ transplantation, and pregnant mother to fetus (late in pregnancy).[21] Recent reports suggest transmission of dengue virus sexually.[22]

Vertical Transmission and Neonatal Dengue Infection

Incidence of transmission of dengue infection from pregnant women to their fetus is 1.6–64%.[23] Fetus and neonates are at great risk of bleeding and capillary leakage. Vertically infected neonates may have mild (fever with petechial rash, thrombocytopenia, and hepatomegaly) to severe illness, i.e. pleural effusion, gastric bleeding, circulatory failure, and massive intracerebral hemorrhage. Severity of illness in neonate does not depend on maternal disease severity, dengue immune status, or mode of delivery. Though the timing of getting the infection by the mother is important, if mother is infected during peripartum period, newborn poses a risk of developing severe manifestations and transfer of antibodies against dengue virus crossing the placenta is supposed to be responsible for this. Dengue illness in newborn may be confused with neonatal sepsis and other neonatal diseases.[23]

■ IMMUNOPATHOGENESIS

The exact mechanism for various manifestations is not clearly understood till now, but these manifestations are because of complex immune response of the host such as T cell-mediated antibodies, cross-reactivity with vascular endothelium, enhancing antibodies, complement and its products, and various soluble mediators including cytokines and chemokines. Unique feature of pathogenesis in dengue is "Cytokine Tsunami" due to enhancing antibodies and memory T-cells by virus strains in secondary infection. Target for these mechanisms is vascular endothelium, platelets and multiple organs that eventually lead to vasculopathy, coagulopathy, and multisystem organ dysfunction.[10]

Capillary Leakage and Shock

Fall in blood pressure occurs due to plasma leakage. Anti-NS1 antibody acts as autoantibodies that cross-reacts with platelets and endothelium and leads to capillary permeability. As a result development of hemo-concentration, and third space losses, i.e. pleural effusion or ascites occurs.

Coagulopathy in Dengue

Mechanism of coagulopathy in dengue is also not understood well but increase in activated partial thromboplastin time (aPTT) and reduction in fibrinogen concentrations are found consistently in dengue. In the pathogenesis of dengue heparin sulfate or chondroitin sulfate, similar molecules to heparin in structure, is released from the glycocalyx and mimics the function as an anticoagulant that contributes to coagulopathy.

Causes of bleeding in DF/DHF:
These are listed below.
- Abnormal coagulogram
- Thrombocytopenia and platelet dysfunction
- Prothrombin complex deficiency secondary to liver involvement

- Endothelial injury
- Disseminated intravascular coagulation (DIC) and prolonged aPTT
- Decreased fibrinogen level
- Increased level of fibrinogen degradation product (FDP)
- Increased level of D-dimer
- Consumptive coagulopathy (activation of mononuclear phagocytes)
- Sequestration of platelets.

Causes of thrombocytopenia:
- Destruction of platelet (antiplatelet antibodies)
- Disseminated intravascular coagulation
- Bone marrow suppression in early stage
- Peripheral sequestration of platelets.

■ CLINICAL MANIFESTATIONS

A dengue-affected person may be asymptomatic or may have symptoms ranging from undifferentiated fever to hemorrhage and shock.[24-26] These differences in various manifestations depend on the following factors:
- Age
- Immune status of the host
- The virus strain
- Primary or secondary infection.

Undifferentiated Dengue Fever

It is more common in infants and young children. Patient presents with mild-to-moderate grade fever with or without maculopapular rashes like any other viral illness. Bleeding manifestations and features of capillary leakage are absent.

Classic Dengue Fever

- *Febrile phase*: It is more common in older children, adolescents, and adults. It has three phases. It starts with sudden onset of high-grade fever and lasts for 2–7 days. This is characterized by flushing and erythema of skin, severe body ache and myalgia, arthralgia, headache, anorexia, nausea, and vomiting. Sometimes, sore throat and congestion in conjunctiva may be associated. Few patients may present with minor bleeding manifestations like petechial rashes, mucosal bleed, i.e. nasal and gum bleed and positive tourniquet test. Tender hepatomegaly may present indicating the risk of severe manifestations. White cell and platelet count are usually low. Dehydration due to high-grade fever, febrile convulsions, and rarely severe bleeding may be the complications in this phase.

- *Critical phase*: This most dreaded phase starts after 3–7 days of onset of fever when fever starts coming down. It lasts for 24–48 hours. Bleeding and shock are the major risks in this phase. Thrombocytopenia and increase in packed cell volume (PCV) due to plasma leakage are important features in this phase. Organ dysfunction such as severe hepatitis, encephalitis or myocarditis, severe bleeding, and shock are major complications in this phase.

- *Recovery phase*: This phase starts 24–48 hours after the onset of critical phase and lasts for 48–72 hours. In this phase, extravasated extravascular compartment fluid starts getting reabsorbed in the vascular compartment. Patient's symptoms improve, i.e. general condition and appetite of the patient improve, patient becomes hemodynamically stable and diuresis starts. Platelet count and white blood counts become normal and PCV becomes normal or low due to hemodilution. Main complication of this phase may be due to fluid overload, e.g. congestive cardiac failure and pulmonary edema.

Few children, especially immunocompromised children, may have extended course of illness like thrombocytopenia or multiple organ dysfunction may last for longer.

Dengue in Infants

Like the older children and adults, infants can have undifferentiated fever to severe dengue manifestations and infants of 4–9 months of age carry the major burden of dengue. There are few salient features which are found more commonly in dengue-infected infants. With high-grade fever, upper respiratory symptoms (cough, cold, nasal congestion, and dyspnea), gastrointestinal symptoms (vomiting and diarrhea), and febrile convulsions are more common in infants as compared to older children. Common childhood illnesses such as pneumonia, meningoencephalitis, measles, and rotavirus infections may often be confused with dengue infection in febrile phase in infancy. With the hepatomegaly, splenomegaly is found in 10% of infected infants. Shock occurs when significant amount of plasma is leaked out of capillary and temperature may be subnormal this time. Possibility of bacterial sepsis should always be kept in mind when fever is present at the onset of shock in infant. In infant, rise of hematocrit from baseline suggests severe plasma leakage as normal hematocrit in infant is relatively low and it may be lower further due to associated iron deficiency anemia, which is very common in infancy. Liver involvement is more common in infant as compared to older children and adults.

DIFFERENTIAL DIAGNOSIS

Dengue fever is often confused with following infections causing acute fever with or without bleeding manifestations:

- Chikungunya
- Influenza
- Malaria
- Enteric fever
- Leptospirosis
- Meningococcemia
- Rickettsiosis
- Zika infection.

DIAGNOSIS

ELISA-based NS1 Antigen Tests

Dengue NS1 antigen, a glycoprotein, is found in the serum of patients during the initial stages of dengue infection. Its presence in serum indicates acute infection. This test is highly specific and sensitive. Since due to detection of NS1, cases can be identified early in the viremic stage, this test has epidemiological significance.

MAC-ELISA

The anti-dengue immunoglobulin M (IgM) antibody is detectable by day 5 of the illness and persists up to 60–90 days usually in primary infection. MAC ELISA (IgM antibody capture enzyme-linked immunosorbent assay), a simple test, requiring very less sophisticated instruments, is very useful tool for surveillance of DF/DHF, especially for hospitalized patients in which fairly detectable IgM antibodies are present in serum.

Isolation of Dengue Virus

Dengue virus can be detected if the samples, i.e. acute phase serum, plasma or washed buffy coat from the patient, autopsy tissues from fatal cases, especially liver, spleen, lymph nodes, and thymus and mosquitoes collected in nature are collected within 5 days of illness and processed without any delay. Isolation of virus requires 7–10 days so it is not a very good tool for diagnosing DF/DHF in view point of management.

Polymerase Chain Reaction

This test has replaced the virus isolation methods due to fast results for genome detection of virus.

IgG-ELISA

In primary infection of dengue, IgG level rises slowly but in low titers and can be detected by days 9–10. These low IgG levels persist for many years and indicate a past dengue infection.[2,27-31] While in secondary infection, there is a rapid and higher increase of anti-dengue-specific IgG antibodies and slower and lower levels rise of IgM are found. These IgG levels remain high for 30–40 days. So this test can differentiate between primary and secondary infection but cannot be considered as diagnostic test as it does not rule out possibility of past infection.

Rapid Diagnostic Tests

There are many test kits available in market to detect IgM, IgG, and NS1 antigen that give results in 15–20 minutes. Accuracy is the problem with these kits as they are not validated properly. False positive results are very high with these kits and sensitivity and specificity vary from batch to batch. So WHO does not recommend these kits in clinical settings to decide management of suspected dengue patient.

National Vector Borne Disease Control Program and Government of India (GoI) recommended use of ELISA-based antigen detection test (NS1) for diagnosing the cases from the first day onward and antibody detection test MAC-ELISA for diagnosing the cases after the fifth day of onset of disease.

Nonspecific tests: Children with severe dengue infection show rising hematocrit and thrombocytopenia and low leukocyte counts with lymphocyte predominance. Liver enzymes are raised with more increase in serum glutamic oxaloacetic transaminase (SGOT) than serum glutamic-pyruvic transaminase (SGPT) that is suggestive of dengue infection.

MANAGEMENT

For the management of patients with dengue illness can be classified as:

- Undifferentiated fever
- Dengue without warning signs
- Dengue with warning signs
- Severe dengue infection.

Undifferentiated Fever

Antipyretic and monitoring for development of complication is the management in this phase.

Dengue Infection without Warning Signs

Patients in this phase are treated symptomatically. Paracetamol, monitoring for the warning signs by the healthcare worker, and serial hematocrit and platelet counts monitoring are main treatment.

Dengue with Warning Signs

Warning signs in dengue are:

- Abdominal pain or tenderness
- Persistent vomiting
- Clinical fluid accumulation
- Mucosal bleed
- Lethargy or restlessness
- Liver enlargement >2 cm
- Palpitation and breathlessness
- Decrease urine output
- Cold clammy extremities
- Narrow pulse pressure
- Rapid pulse
- Hypotension
- Laboratory features like increase in PCV (hematocrit) concurrent with rapid decrease in platelet count.

Pediatric age group itself is high risk for morbidity and mortality in dengue infection, but following are the risk factors in children for developing severe manifestations of dengue:

- Infancy
- Obesity
- G6PD deficiency
- Thalassemia
- *Chronic diseases*: Diabetes, bronchial asthma, and hypertension
- Patients on steroid or anticoagulant drugs
- HIV infection
- Immunocompromised children.

Any child who presents with suspected dengue and having any of the above warning sign, needs in patient care. Intravenous fluids are the mainstay of treatment in this phase. Ringer's lactate or normal saline infusion at a rate of 7 mL/kg over 1 hour should be started in all hospitalized children irrespective of hypotension. After 1 hour hematocrit and vital parameters are monitored, if hematocrit is decreasing and vitals are improving, fluid infusion rate tapered to 5 mL/kg over next hour and then to 3 mL/kg/hr for next 24–48 hours. Frequent hematocrit and vital parameter monitoring is must during this period. If child is stable in terms of good oral intake and urine output with normal blood pressure, he/she can be discharged.

In case after 1 hour, the hematocrit is rising and vital parameters are not improving, this is the time when fluid infusion rate should be increased to 10 mL/kg over next hour. If no further improvement, fluid infusion rate is further increased to 15 mL/kg over next hour (third hour). Colloids or plasma infusion is started in doses of 10 mL/kg

if at the end of third hour, there is no rise in hematocrit and improvement in vital. After stabilization of vital parameters and with rising hematocrit, fluid infusion rate is decreased slowly over 24–48 hours and discontinued.

Severe Dengue

Children having any of the following features are classified under severe DF:

- Severe plasma leakage leading to:
  - Shock
  - Fluid accumulation with respiratory distress
- Severe bleeding as evaluated by clinician
- Severe organ involvement:
  - *Liver*: Aspartate transaminase (AST) or alanine aminotransferase (ALT) ≥1,000 IU/L
  - *CNS*: Impaired consciousness
  - Heart and other organs.

Children should be hospitalized immediately, preferably in intensive care unit, and normal saline or Ringer's lactate solution should be started immediately at the rate of 10–20 mL/kg over 1 hour or given as a bolus if blood pressure is unrecordable. If there is no improvement in vital parameters and the hematocrit is rising; colloid 10 mL/kg is infused rapidly. Hematocrit and vitals should be monitored intensively; if hematocrit is falling with no improvement in vital parameters, blood transfusion should be started, keeping in mind the possibility of occult blood loss. If hematocrit starts falling with improvement in vitals, fluid infusion rate is gradually reduced.

Management of Severe Bleeding

If patient has minor bleeding, i.e. mild mucosal bleed or petechial spots, and hemodynamically stable, supportive care, e.g. bed rest, plenty of fluid ingestion, vital monitoring, and avoidance of any intramuscular injection or any procedure, is the treatment.

But if patient has severe bleeding, i.e. excessive mucosal bleed, internal gastrointestinal or intracranial bleed and hemodynamic instability, fresh blood/packed red blood cells transfusion should be started immediately with vital monitoring. When bleeding is not managed with this, fresh-frozen plasma and platelet-rich plasma may be considered keeping the possibility of DIC in mind.

■ PROGNOSIS

There is no doubt that dengue is one of the biggest health hazards as in severe dengue mortality is 20–30%. Though for dengue, case fatality rate (CFR) of the South-East Asian Region (SEAR) countries in 2006 was less than 1%, but India, Indonesia, Bhutan, and Nepal still have CFRs above

1%.[32] According to NVBDCP data in 2018, over 1 lakh people were diagnosed as having dengue and an estimated 172 died from it. The condition was worse in 2017 as 1.88 lakh people diagnosed with dengue and 325 died of it. Early diagnosis and management are the important steps to reduce the dengue CFR to <1%.

■ PREVENTION[33]

To achieve the target, reduction of dengue mortality and morbidity by 50% and 25% respectively by 2020, WHO is focusing on mosquito vectors management through the following:

- *Prevention of mosquito breeding*:
  - Reducing egg-laying habitats by environmental management and modification
  - Disposing of solid waste properly and removing artificial man-made habitats
  - Covering, emptying, and cleaning of domestic water storage containers weekly
  - Applying appropriate insecticides to water storage outdoor containers.
- *Personal protection from mosquito bites*:
  - Using of personal household protection measures such as window screens, repellents, insecticide-treated materials, coils and vaporizers, and wearing clothing that minimize skin exposure to mosquitoes are advised. These measures should be used both inside and outside home and at day time also.
- *Community management*:
  - Educating the community on the risks of mosquito-borne diseases
  - Engaging with the community to improve participation and mobilization for sustained vector control.
- *Reactive vector control*: Emergency vector control measures such as applying insecticides as space spraying during outbreaks may be used by health authorities.
- *Active mosquito and virus surveillance*:
  - Active monitoring and surveillance of vector abundance and species composition should be carried out to determine effectiveness of control interventions
  - Prospectively monitor prevalence of virus in the mosquito population, with active screening of sentinel mosquito collections.

■ WHO POSITION ON THE CYD-TDV VACCINE

In September, 2018, the-live attenuated dengue vaccine CYD-TDV was in clinical trials and found to be efficacious and safe in persons who have had a previous dengue virus infection (seropositive individuals), but it carries an increased risk of severe dengue in seronegative (at the time of vaccination) persons who will get natural primary infection after vaccination. WHO recommends prevaccination screening for countries considering vaccination as part of their dengue control program. With this strategy, only persons with evidence of a past dengue infection would be vaccinated (based on an antibody test or on a documented laboratory-confirmed dengue infection in the past). Vaccination should be considered as a part of an integrated dengue prevention and control strategy. But vaccination does not rule out the need of prompt medical care by the individual having DF/DHF, irrespective of vaccination status.

In India, in five centers (Delhi, Ludhiana, Pune, Bangalore, and Kolkata), an observer-blind, randomized, placebo-controlled, phase II safety and immunogenicity trial of dengue vaccine (CYD 47) was conducted in subjects of 18–45 years of age in 2016. Results showed that the dengue vaccine was well tolerated and produced antibodies against all four dengue serotypes in both dengue seropositive and seronegative Indian adults after three doses of 0.5 mL each administered subcutaneously at 0, 6, and 12 months. No single case of severe dengue reported, death or related serious adverse events reported during the trial. This phase 2 clinical trial results are consistent with the results of the global dengue vaccine clinical trials.[34]

■ REFERENCES

1. World Health Organization. First report on neglected tropical diseases: working to overcome the global impact of neglected tropical diseases. Geneva: World Health Organization; 2010.
2. Dengue Guidelines for Diagnosis, Treatment, Prevention and Control. Joint publication of the World Health Organization (WHO) and the Special Program for Research and Training in Tropical Diseases; 2009.
3. World Health Organization. (2019). Dengue and severe dengue. [online] Available from: https://www.who.int/news-room/fact-sheets/detail/dengue-and-severe-dengue. [Last accessed on November, 2019].
4. World Health Organization. Comprehensive Guidelines for Prevention and Control of Dengue and Dengue Hemorrhagic Fever. New Delhi: WHO, SEARO; 2011.
5. Disease Control Programme (NHM). (2017-18). [online] Available from: https://mohfw.gov.in/sites/default/files/05Chapter.pdf. [Last accessed on November, 2019].
6. Gunasekaran P, Kaveri K, Mohana S, et al. Dengue disease status in Chennai (2006-2008): A retrospective analysis. Indian J Med Res. 2011;133:322-5.
7. Gupta E, Dar L, Kapoor G, et al. The changing epidemiology of dengue in Delhi, India. Virol J. 2006;3:92.
8. National Vector Borne Disease Control Programme. Dengue/DHF situation in India. [online] Available from: https://www.nvbdcp.

gov.in/index4.php?lang=1 &level=0&linkid=431&lid=3715. [Last accessed on November, 2019].

9. Ganeshkumar P, Murhekar MV, Poornima V, et al. Dengue infection in India: A systematic review and meta-analysis. PLoS Negl Trop Dis. 2018;12(7):e0006618.

10. National Vector Borne Disease Control Programme. (2015). National Guidelines for Clinical Management of Dengue Fever. [online] Available from: http://pbhealth.gov.in/Dengue-National-Guidelines-2014%20Compressed.pdf. [Last accessed on November, 2019].

11. Dutta AK, Biswas A, Baruah K, et al. National guidelines for diagnosis and management of dengue fever/dengue hemorrhagic fever and dengue shock syndrome. J Ind Med Assn. 2011;109(1):30-5.

12. Dash AP, Bhatia R, Kalra NL. Dengue in South-East Asia: An appraisal of case management and vector control. Dengue Bulletin. 2012;36:1-12.

13. Simmons CP, Farrar JJ, Nguyen vV, et al. Dengue. N Engl J Med. 2012;366(15):1423-32.

14. Mehta TK, Shah PD. Identification of prevalent dengue serotypes by reverse transcriptase polymerase chain reaction and correlationwith severity of dengue as per the recent World Health Organization classification. Indian J Med Microbiol. 2018;36:273-8.

15. Kumaria R. Correlation of disease spectrum among four dengue serotypes: A five years hospital based study from India. Braz J Infect Dis. 2010;14:141-6.

16. Rocha BM, Guilarde AO, Argolo ALT, et al. Dengue-specific serotype related to clinical severity during the 2012/2013 epidemic in centre of Brazil. Infect Dis Poverty. 2017;6:116.

17. Trpis M, McClelland GA, Gillett JD, et al. Diel periodicity in landing of Aedes aegypti on man. Bull World Health Organ. 1973;48(5):623-9.

18. Medlock JM, Avenell D, Barrass I, et al. Analysis of the potential for survival and seasonal activity of Aedes albopictus (Diptera: Culicidae) in the United Kingdom. J Vector Ecol. 2006;31(2):292-304.

19. Romi R, Severini F, Toma L. Cold acclimation and overwintering of female Aedes albopictus in Roma. J Am Mosq Control Assoc. 2006;22(1):149-51.

20. Patankar M, Patel B, Gandhi V, et al. Seroprevalence of dengue in Gujarat, Western India: A study at Tertiary care hospital. Int J Med Sci Public Health. 2014;3:16-8.

21. Chen LH, Wilson ME. Non-vector transmission of dengue and other mosquito-borne flaviviruses. Dengue Bull. 2005;29:18-30.

22. Lee C, Lee H. Probable female to male sexual transmission of dengue virus infection. Infect Dis (Lond). 2019;51(2):150-2.

23. World Health Organization and Tropical Diseases Research. Handbook for Clinical Management of Dengue. Geneva: World Health Organization; 2012.

24. Kalayanarooj S. Clinical manifestations and management of dengue/DHF/DSS. Trop Med Health. 2011;39(Suppl 4):83-9.

25. Guzman MG, Halstead SB, Artsob H, et al. Dengue: a continuing global threat. Nat Rev Microbiol. 2010;8(Suppl 12):7-16.

26. Sharma S, Sharma SK, Mohan A, et al. Clinical profile of dengue hemorrhagic fever in adults during 1996 outbreak in Delhi, India. Dengue Bulletin. 1998;22:20-30.

27. Guzmán MG, Rosario D, Kouri G. Diagnosis of dengue virus infection. In: Kalitzky M, Borowski P (Eds). Molecular Biology of the Flaviviruses. United Kingdom: Bioscience Horizons; 2009.

28. Buchy P, Yoksan S, Peeling RW, et al. Laboratory Tests for the Diagnosis of Dengue Virus Infection. Geneva: TDR/Scientific Working Group; 2006.

29. Guzmán MG, Kourí G. Dengue diagnosis, advances and challenges. Int J Infect Dis. 2004;8:69-80.

30. Dengue and dengue hemorrhagic fever in the Americas: Guidelines for prevention and control. Washington DC: Pan American Health Organization; 1994. p. 548.

31. Vázquez S, Cabezas S, Pérez AB, et al. Kinetics of antibodies in sera, saliva, and urine samples from adult patients with primary or secondary dengue 3 virus infections. Int J Infect Dis. 2007;11:256-62.

32. Seneviratne SL, Malavige GN, de Silva HJ. Pathogenesis of liver involvement during dengue viral infections. Trans R Soc Trop Med Hyg. 2006;100(7):608-14.

33. World Health Organization. (2012). Global Strategy for dengue prevention and control, 2012-2020. [online] Available from: http://www.who.int/dengue control/9789241504034/en/. [Last accessed on November, 2017].

34. Dubey AP, Agarkhedkar S, Chhatwal J, et al. Immunogenicity and safety of a tetravalent dengue vaccine in healthy adults in India: A randomized, observer-blind, placebo-controlled phase II trial. Hum Vaccin Immunother. 2016;12:512-8.

CHIKUNGUNYA

■ INTRODUCTION

Chikungunya is a vector-borne acute viral disease characterized by fever usually >102°F, polyarthralgia, and skin rashes. Outbreaks of chikungunya fever have occurred in Caribbean islands, Central Africa, Europe, and Indian subcontinent. Chikungunya was first recognized in Tanzania in the early 1952 and has caused periodic outbreaks in Asia and Africa since 1960s. It has been reported in all age groups of population including neonates.[1]

■ ETIOPATHOGENESIS

Chikungunya virus is an alpha virus with single-stranded RNA as genetic material and belongs to the *Togaviridae* family, it carries approximately 11.8 kb genome with a capsid and a phospholipid envelope of 60–70 nm. Phylogenetic analysis has proposed three diverse groups based on partial sequences of *NS4* and *E1* genes: (1) West African, (2) East-Central-South African (ESCA), and (3) Asian or South-East Asia.[2,3] Chikungunya virus is transmitted to humans through day-biting mosquitoes which belong to the *Aedes* genus; *Aedes albopictus* and *Aedes aegypti* as the virus is arbovirus, the virus is sustained in the environment between humans or other animals and mosquitoes. Humans are major reservoirs during epidemics. The precise mechanism of its transmission into mammalian cells is still not clear.[4,5] Bernard et al. proposed that chikungunya virus enters mammalian epithelial cells via a clathrin-independent, esp-15-dependent, dynamin 2-dependent route which needs an endocytic pathway in combination with other unknown pathways.[6]

Some cases of blood-borne transmission have also been reported in laboratory personnel handling infected blood, and fetomaternal transmission has been documented during pregnancy mainly in perinatal period.[7]

EPIDEMIOLOGY

This mosquito-borne arboviral disease was discovered in 1952 in Tanzania and named after the classical symptom of joint pain which lead to stooped appearance due to severe arthralgia.[1] The disease is mainly localized to Africa, South-East Asia, and India, and as other arboviral diseases, it is also known for its reemergence. Second emergence occurred in 2005–2006 where outbreaks started in the Indian subcontinent with around 1.9 million reported cases.[1] Now the disease has spread to American subcontinent with frequent outbreaks in Brazil, Bolivia, and Columbia.[8]

After its discovery in 1952–1953, India has faced five major epidemics till 1973[9] after which the disease became sporadic with frequent outbreaks in Maharashtra till 2000. In last 5 years, around 2.6 lakh suspected cases and around 59,000 confirmed cases were reported by the National Vector Borne Disease Control Program, around 20% of the reported cases were reported in this period from Karnataka.[10]

CLINICAL FEATURES

About 3–28% population infected with chikungunya remain asymptomatic and symptomatic individuals present[11] with sudden onset of fever with polyarthralgia more often bilateral symmetric pattern, myalgia, headache, fatigue, and skin rashes, its incubation period ranges from 2 days to 12 days and peak viremia phase in humans occur in the first 2–6 days.[10]

Fever may rise up to 104°F and may be associated with rigors. Fever lasts up to 7 days. Joint pain is symmetric and small joints of hand and feet are more commonly involved and rashes usually appear over trunk and extremities after onset of fever.[1]

Atypical and Severe Manifestations[12]

Chikungunya fever also has some atypical and severe manifestations which occur due to viral genome or immune response of host or may be related to drug toxicity and unrelated causes to chikungunya fever. Neonates exposed during intrapartum and adults more than 65 years and individuals with comorbid medical conditions are prone for following atypical and severe manifestations:

- Vesiculobullous lesions, febrile seizures, and meningoencephalitis in infants and young children
- Optic neuritis and uveitis
- Guillain-Barré syndrome, seizures, encephalopathy, and cerebellar syndrome
- Pericarditis, myocarditis, and arrhythmias
- Photosensitive hyperpigmentation
- Acute renal failure
- Bleeding dyscrasias, respiratory failure, syndrome of inappropriate secretion of antidiuretic hormone, and hypoadrenalism.

DIAGNOSIS

Definitive diagnosis of chikungunya fever is based on clinical features, geographical area, and exposure with lab diagnosis that is done by testing the blood for the virus RNA through real-time polymerase chain reaction (PCR) or by sequencing or antibodies to the virus. Virus-specific IgM are initially not traceable, but in convalescence phase they become positive, so to rule out the diagnosis, blood sample should be tested in this phase of disease.[13,14]

Depending on clinical sign and symptoms, following differential diagnoses should be considered:

- Dengue
- Zika
- Malaria
- Leptospirosis
- Parvovirus and enterovirus
- Group A *Streptococcus*
- Measles, mumps, and rubella (MMR)
- Septic arthritis
- Rheumatological conditions.

TREATMENT

Antiviral treatment for chikungunya is not available yet. In view of no specific antiviral therapy, mainstay of treatment is symptomatic management:

- Assess hydration and hemodynamic status and provide supportive care as needed.

- Patients should be evaluated for other serious conditions (e.g. malaria, dengue, and bacterial infections) and treated or managed accordingly.
- Paracetamol should be used for initial fever and pain control.
- Dengue is a close differential diagnosis; aspirin or other nonsteroidal anti-inflammatory drug (NSAIDs) (e.g. ibuprofen and naproxen) should not be used until the patients have been afebrile ≥48 hours and have no warning signs for severe dengue.
- In case of persistent joint pain, use of NSAIDs, corticosteroids, or physiotherapy is considered.

■ PREVENTION[15,16]

Chikungunya virus was found for the first time in the Americas on islands in the Caribbean. There is a risk that the virus will be imported to new areas by infected travelers and there is no vaccine to prevent or medicine to treat chikungunya virus infection. Travelers can protect themselves by preventing mosquito bites when traveling to countries with chikungunya virus. Mosquito vector management is the key for prevention and vector management in chikungunya is identical to that in dengue mentioned earlier.

■ PROGNOSIS

As there is no reported mortality due to chikungunya disease, more research is needed to assess the burden as disability adjusted life years (DALYs) due to subacute and chronic complications of the disease in children. One study was done in India in 2009 in adults that assessed burden of disease during 2006 epidemic. It estimated 25,588 DALYs lost during 2006 epidemic, with an overall burden of 45.26 DALYs per million. Karnataka was the topmost bearer of this burden contributing 55% of national burden, persistent arthralgia imposed heavy burden accounting for 68%.[17]

■ REFERENCES

1. World Health Organization. (2017). Fact Sheet, Chikungunya. [online] Available from: www.who.int/news-room/fact-sheets/detail/chikungunya. [Last accessed on November, 2019].
2. Mohan A, Kiran DH, Manohar IC, et al. Epidemiology, clinical manifestations, and diagnosis of Chikungunya fever: lessons learned from the re-emerging epidemic. Indian J Dermatol. 2010;55(1):54-63.
3. Chhabra M, Mittal V, Bhattacharya D, et al. Chikungunya fever: a re-emerging viral infection. Indian J Med Microbiol. 2008;26(1):5-12.
4. Teo TH, Lum FM, Claser C, et al. A pathogenic role for CD4+ T cells during Chikungunya virus infection in mice. J Immunol. 2013;190(1):259-69.
5. Teo TH, Lum FM, Lee WW, et al. Mouse models for Chikungunya virus: deciphering immune mechanisms responsible for disease and pathology. Immunol Res. 2012;53(1-3):136-47.
6. Bernard E, Solignat M, Gay B, et al. Endocytosis of chikungunya virus into mammalian cells: role of clathrin and early endosomal compartments. PLoS One. 2010;5(7):e11479.
7. Erin Staples J, Hills SL, Powers AM, et al. Chikungunya: Traveler's health. CDC Yellow Book; 2020.
8. Centers for Disease Control and Prevention. Chikungunya Virus. [online] Available from: www.cdc.gov/chikungunya/geo/index.html [Last accessed on November, 2019].
9. National Vector Borne Disease Control Programme. Chikungunya, Facts. [online] Available from: https://nvbdcp.gov.in/index4.php?lang=1&level=0&linkid=488&lid=3764 [Last accessed on November, 2019].
10. National Vector Borne Disease Control Programme. Chikungunya Situation in India. [online] Available from: https://nvbdcp.gov.in/index4.php?lang=1&level=0&linkid=488&lid=3765. [Last accessed on November, 2019].
11. Centers for Disease Control and Prevention. Chikungunya fact sheet – General information. [online] Available from: https://www.cdc.gov/chikungunya/hc/resources.html. [Last accessed on November, 2019].
12. Centers for Disease Control and Prevention. Chikungunya fact sheet – Atypical and severe manifestations. [online] Available from: https://www.cdc.gov/chikungunya/hc/resources.html. [Last accessed November, 2019].
13. World Health Organization. Dengue Control. [online] Available from: https://www.who.int/denguecontrol/arbo-viral/other_arboviral_chikungunya/en/.[Last accessed on November, 2019].
14. Johnson BW, Russell BJ, Goodman CH. Laboratory diagnosis of chikungunya virus infections and commercial sources for diagnostic assays. J Infect Dis. 2016;214(Suppl 5):S471-4.
15. Centers for Disease Control and Prevention. Chikungunya virus. [online] Available from: https://www.cdc.gov/chikungunya/hc/index.html. [Last accessed on November, 2019].
16. World Health Organization. (2012). Global Strategy for dengue prevention and control, 2012-2020: WHO report. [online] Available from: https://www.who.int/denguecontrol/9789241504034/en/. [Last accessed on November, 2019].
17. Krishnamoorthy K, Harichandrakumar KT, Krishna Kumari A, et al. Burden of chikungunya in India: estimate of disability adjusted life years (DALY) lost in 2006 epidemic. J Vector Borne Dis. 2009;46(1):26-35.

Emerging and Re-emerging Viral infections

Ashwani K Sood, Sandesh Guleria

INTRODUCTION

Emerging viral infections affecting human beings have caused major epidemics in recent past and are major threats against humanity. The new appearance of a pathogen into a population is known as emergence, while the rapid increase in the incidence of endemic pathogen is called re-emergence.[1] Zoonotic viruses such as Arboviruses, Nipah virus, Zika virus, Ebola virus, and Hendra virus are the major emerging and re-emerging viral pathogens in humans. The emergence may be due to migration of insect vectors into other new regions, the affection of new vectors, and the presence of wild reservoirs.[2] The emerging viral infections, described in this chapter, can be a cause of major health concern in near future.

SWINE INFLUENZA VIRUS

Influenza virus is a common pathogen causing respiratory illnesses in humans and has the potential to cause pandemics. Swine influenza virus (H1N1) causes infection in pigs. It has recently been found a cause of epidemics world over in humans.[3,4]

Epidemiology

Epidemics of H1N1 virus infection are a cause of concern world over due to morbidities and mortality associated with it. H1N1 influenza affected cases were for the first time reported in March 2009 from Mexico and in next 6 months it spread to almost all countries including India with more than 18,000 deaths, two-thirds of that in the USA alone.[3] According to the Union Ministry of Health, Government of India data, in the year 2018, the total number of H1NI virus infected cases was 14,992 and out of these 1,103 died.[5]

Virus Genotype

H1N1 is a ribonucleic acid (RNA) virus, which belongs to the *Orthomyxoviridae* family of viruses.[6]

Transmission

H1N1 virus mainly transmits through contact with respiratory droplets by sneezing and coughing. Other body fluids and fomites also play a role in transmission. Viral shedding begins the day prior to symptom onset and often to persist for 5–7 days or even longer in children and in immunocompromised individuals.[4,7]

Clinical Features

The average incubation period is 1–3 days. Fever, cough, and coryza are most common clinical features, seen in >95% children. Other common clinical manifestations are myalgia, sore throat, headache, vomiting, and diarrhea.[4] The common life-threatening complications are progressive pneumonia, acute respiratory distress syndrome (ARDS), myocarditis, encephalitis, acute kidney injury, and rhabdomyolysis.[5,8] The risk factors for influenza complications are seen in children less than 5 years of age, elderly, obese individuals, pregnant ladies, and persons with asthma or chronic obstructive pulmonary disease (COPD) and other chronic illnesses.[8]

Diagnosis

Laboratory investigations may show leukopenia, thrombocytopenia, anemia, transaminitis, elevated serum bilirubin, and increased muscle enzymes. X-ray chest may reveal features of ARDS. Real time-polymerase chain reaction (RT-PCR) has high sensitivity and specificity and can confirm the diagnosis. Nasopharyngeal, throat swab, or tracheal aspirate samples can be used. Although viral culture has moderate sensitivity and high specificity but due to long turnaround time, it is not recommended in clinical settings. Similarly, rapid antigen tests have low sensitivity.[5,7]

Treatment

Severe or complicated disease, younger age, high-risk medical conditions, and obesity are the indications for treatment in children. Oseltamivir is the recommended drug for both prophylaxis and treatment. Dosages for children are according to weight band and duration of treatment is 5 days (weight: <15 kg—30 mg BD; 15–23 kg—45 mg BD; 24–40 kg—60 mg BD; >40 kg—75 mg BD). Oseltamivir is well tolerated; nausea and vomiting are common side effects. Bronchitis, insomnia, and vertigo are rarely reported.[9]

Prevention

The available vaccines for its prevention are inactivated influenza vaccine (most commonly used), recombinant influenza vaccine, and live attenuated influenza vaccine. The selection of vaccine subunits is based on the strain prevalence during the previous year influenza activity.[10]

■ NIPAH VIRUS

Nipah virus (NiV) has recently emerged as a new pathogen infecting humans. Initially, the manifestations of NiV infection were ascribed to Japanese B encephalitis (JE), but manifestations were found to be atypical of JE and later this virus was isolated.[11]

Epidemiology

First case of NiV infection was reported from Malaysia in 1998, since than there have been major outbreaks worldwide.[12] In 2001, an outbreak of NiV infection occurred in Bangladesh and later cases were reported from Siliguri in India which is in close proximity to Bangladesh.[13] There was an outbreak of NiV infection in Kerala, India, in 2018. In 2 months (June-July, 2018), 19 NiV cases, including 17 deaths, were reported.[14]

Virus Genotype

Nipah virus is a member of genus *Henipavirus* and family *Paramyxoviridae*.[11]

Transmission

Fruit bats are the main reservoir of NiV which can transmit disease to humans and animals. Human-to-human transmission has also been documented.[11]

Clinical Features

The incubation period is 4 days to 2 months and almost all present within 2 weeks of exposure.[15] The clinical manifestations may vary from asymptomatic infection to severe encephalitis. Fever, headache, dizziness, and vomiting are common symptoms. Many patients develop aseptic meningitis, encephalitis with altered sensorium, and prominent signs of brainstem dysfunction, cerebellitis, vasomotor changes, and seizures. These patients can develop relapse and late-onset encephalitis, which are unique features associated with this virus.[11,15,16]

Diagnosis

Virus isolation, serology, and PCR can be used for laboratory diagnosis of this virus. Serological tests are less sensitive. Serum immunoglobulin M (IgM) peaks at 9 days of illness and can persist for 3 months and IgM enzyme-linked immunosorbent assay (ELISA) can be used for NiV infection diagnosis. RT-PCR is a highly sensitive test for the diagnosis and specimen from nasal aspirate, cerebrospinal fluid, urine, and blood can be used.[11,17]

Treatment

Treatment of NiV infection is supportive with measures to control seizures, raised intracranial pressure, treatment of secondary infection, and ventilator support. Few studies have shown ribavirin to be effective due to its broad-spectrum activity and ability to cross the blood-brain barrier.[11,18] NiV infection is fatal most of the time with mortality rate ranging from 40% to 70%.[16]

Prevention

Prevention includes vector control and measures to prevent animals from acquiring NiV and avoid rapid spread of disease among animals. In preclinical studies on animals, a few vaccines have been found to be effective against NiV.[19]

■ HANTAVIRUS

Hantaviruses (HeV) infection is an emerging zoonotic disease that has increased the number of affected humans over the last few years and is involving new geographical regions. The viruses are endemic in many regions worldwide and has high mortality rates (12–60%).[20,21]

Epidemiology

The first outbreak of HeV occurred in Korea between 1950 and 1953, referred to as hemorrhagic fever with renal syndrome (HFRS), followed by another outbreak in the

United States in 1993, in which more than 2,000 cases were reported to be affected with different strains of HeV.[21] In India, cases of possible HeV infections were reported from Vellore, Tamil Nadu, in 2008. In this multi-institutional study, 28 seropositive cases were found among patients with chronic renal disease, warehouse workers, and tribal members by using combination of ELISA, indirect immunofluorescence (IIF), and Western blot.[22]

Virus Genotype

Hantavirus is a RNA virus of genus *Hantavirus* in the family *Bunyaviridae.*[20,23]

Transmission

Inhalation of aerosolized excreta among rodents and from rodents to humans is the main mode of transmission.[24]

Clinical Features

Hantavirus infections mainly involve respiratory and renal systems. Manifestations vary from asymptomatic infection to fatal outcome. In humans, however, hantaviruses primarily cause two diseases: HFRS and hantavirus (cardio) pulmonary syndrome.[20,23]

Diagnosis

Serological tests are commonly used diagnostic tests which detect IgM and IgG antibodies by IIF assays, strip immunoblot, or ELISA. Reverse transcription PCR, detecting viral genomes in blood, is a specific and sensitive test which can also differentiate between different species.[20,25]

Treatment

Treatment of HeV infection is only supportive therapy, as no effective antiviral therapy is available. Ribavirin has been shown to reduce mortality in patients with HFRS, but the usefulness in other patients is still controversial.[20,21,23]

Prevention

Four inactivated HeV vaccines are in use and have been shown to be safe and efficacious.

■ ZIKA VIRUS

Zika virus (ZIKV) is an arthropod-transmitted *Flavivirus.* It was first time isolated in monkeys in the year 1947 in Uganda and later found in humans in 1952 in Uganda and Tanzania. *Aedes* mosquitoes are the vector for transmission of ZIKV.[26,27]

Epidemiology

Outbreaks of ZIKV infection have been reported from Africa, the Americas, and Asia between 1960s and 1980s. In the year 2015, Brazil reported an association of ZIKV disease with microcephaly. Till now, a total of 86 countries have reported ZIKV infection.[26] In the year 2018, an outbreak occurred in Rajasthan, India. Prior to this outbreak, India reported four confirmed cases of ZIKV infection in 2017, three cases in Ahmadabad, Gujarat, and one case in Krishnagiri District of Tamil Nadu.[26,28]

Virus Genotype

Zika virus belongs to the family *Flaviviridae* and the genus *Flavivirus.*[26]

Transmission

The primary vector for ZIKV transmission is infected mosquito of genus *Aedes*, mainly *Aedes aegypti*. Other modes are vertical transmission (mother to fetus), sexual contact, and through blood and blood products.[26,29]

Clinical Features

The incubation period of ZIKV infection is 3–14 days. Common symptoms are fever, rash, conjunctivitis, myalgia, arthralgia, and headache. These manifestations usually subside in next 2–7 days. In most of the patients, ZIKV infections are subclinical. One of the dreaded complications of ZIKV infection is Zika syndrome which leads to microcephaly and other congenital malformations in infants after infection in pregnant women. Other complications of pregnancy after ZIKV infections are prematurity and abortion.[26,29]

Diagnosis

There is no gold standard diagnostic tool for ZIKV diagnosis. The laboratory diagnosis is based on detection of viral RNA by RT-PCR, but sensitivity of RT-PCR is only 40%.[27,29] In first 5 days of illness blood samples and after 5 days urine samples should be used. Serology-based test are used for the diagnosis, but are not specific due to cross reaction with other species.[29]

Treatment

There are no specific antiviral drugs effective against ZIKV. Treatment which is mainly supportive consists of analgesic, antipyretics, and antihistaminics.

Prevention

Vector control and prevention of mosquito bites are key measures to prevent ZIKV infection with special attention to pregnant women and children. No effective vaccine against ZIKV is yet available.[27,29]

DENGUE VIRUS

Dengue fever is a mosquito-borne tropical illness and a major arthropod-transmitted disease in the world. The manifestations may vary from subclinical infection to dengue hemorrhagic fever (DHF) and dengue shock syndrome (DSS) with fatal outcome.[30,31]

Epidemiology

Every year, more than 100 million cases of dengue fever and half a million cases of DHF occur worldwide and is endemic in more than 100 countries. About 90% of DHF patients are children <15 years of age.[30,32] In India, most of the states report dengue virus (DENV) infections, especially during rainy season. In 2010, 12,484 DENV infections were estimated in India which is 34% of global estimates.[33]

Virus Genotype

The DENV is a RNA virus belonging to the *Flaviviridae* family and has four serotypes—DENV-1 to DENV-4.[32,33]

Transmission

Mosquitoes belonging to the genus *Aedes* transmit DENV. *Aedes aegypti* is the most common vector in tropical and subtropical regions and is a day biting mosquito which breeds on small collection of water. Other species of *Aedes* may act as vector depending upon the geographic location.[34]

Clinical Features

The illness starts with high-grade fever, body aches, headache, arthralgia, abdominal pain, and maculopapular rash. The fever may last for 2–7 days. Flushing is a characteristic feature and is commonly seen on the face and neck.[35] DHF and DSS are two life-threatening manifestations of DENV infection associated with high mortality. Other complications are encephalitis, hepatitis, myocarditis, and disseminated intravascular coagulation (DIC).[30,31,35]

Diagnosis

Laboratory investigations show leukopenia, thrombocytopenia, hemoconcentration, and transaminitis. Leukopenia is usually seen in the first week of illness.

Dengue-specific IgM ELISA is the most common serological investigation used for the diagnosis which is quick and has good sensitivity, but in most patients IgM antibodies appear by fifth day of illness. Nonstructural protein 1 (NS1 antigen) through ELISA allows rapid detection of DENV in the first few days of illness. RT-PCR is a useful and sensitive test for the detection of dengue infection early in the disease.[30,36]

Treatment

There is no specific antiviral therapy effective against DENV. Treatment of DENV infection is only symptomatic with maintenance of fluid balance, early identification of shock, and prompt resuscitation. Outcome is better in patients who are admitted early to hospital before they develop shock.[30,31,37]

Prevention

Dengvaxia (CYD-TDV) was the first vaccine developed and used in 2015 in Mexico. CYD-TDV is a live recombinant dengue vaccine, used as a three-dose regimen in Phase III clinical studies and registered for use in individuals 9–45 years of age living in endemic areas.[38]

CHIKUNGUNYA

Chikungunya virus (CHIKV) is another mosquito-borne disease prevalent in tropical and subtropical regions. It is emerging as a major epidemic threat over the past 15 years. Debilitating chronic joint pain is unique manifestation of CHIKV infection.[39,40]

Epidemiology

Chikungunya virus infection has been reported from over 40 countries mainly from Africa and South East Asia. Periodic outbreaks have been reported from countries in this region since 1952.[39] In India, outbreaks of chikungunya occurred first time in 1960s and in the year 2006, an outbreak affected 1.4 million people in 13 states.[41]

Virus Genotype

Chikungunya virus is a single-stranded RNA virus of the genus *Alphavirus* and the family *Togaviridae*. CHIKV has three genotypes, named after their geographical distributions.[39,41,42]

Transmission

Chikungunya virus is transmitted to human by infected female *Aedes* mosquito. The two most common species transmitting CHIKV are *A. aegypti* and *A. albopictus*.[39,41]

Clinical Features

The incubation period is 4–7 days. The disease course is divided into an acute and chronic stage. Acute stage lasts for a week and has fever and arthralgia. Arthralgia is typically polyarthralgia seen in 30–90% of cases and is often bilateral and symmetric. Ophthalmic, neurological, and cardiac symptoms may occur.[41,43] The most prominent symptoms in chronic phase, which can last for months to years, are arthritis, fatigue, chronic pain, and neuritis.[40,44]

Diagnosis

Detection of CHIKV-specific IgM antibody by ELISA or IIF test is sensitive if samples are collected >5 days of illness. Detection of viral RNA by RT-PCR in the first week of illness is useful.[45]

Treatment

There are no specific antiviral drugs effective against CHIKV, so treatment is mainly supportive.

Prevention

No vaccine against CHIKV is available. Prevention and control of chikungunya relies on vector control measures.[46]

◼ CHANDIPURA VIRUS

Chandipura virus (CHPV) is a recently described neuro-tropic virus which leads to rapid clinical deterioration and high mortality, especially in children. CHPV outbreaks have been reported from Indian states of Andhra Pradesh and Gujarat with typical encephalitic manifestations.[47]

Epidemiology

Chandipura virus was first time isolated in 1965, during an febrile outbreak in Nagpur, Maharashtra.[48] Cases of CHPV are also being reported from other countries in Indian subcontinent and Africa.[49,50] During an outbreak of CHPV infection in 2003-2004 in central India, 322 child deaths with case fatality rate of 56–75% were reported.[51]

Virus Genotype

Chandipura virus is an arbovirus belonging to genus *Vesiculovirus* in the family *Rhabdoviridae*.[50,52]

Transmission

Chandipura virus is believed to be transmitted through mosquitoes, ticks, and sand flies. The important transmitters include two genera of sandflies: *Phlebotomus* and *Sergentomyia*. Laboratory studies have also documented vertical and venereal transmission of CHPV in *A. aegypti*.[50,53]

Clinical Features

The disease manifests with high-grade fever followed by seizures, altered sensorium, vomiting, and loose stools. There is rapid deterioration and death in majority of the patients.[50-52] The cause of death in most children is acute encephalitis.[52,54]

Diagnosis

Chandipura virus-specific IgM antibodies in the patient's serum and cerebrospinal fluid (CSF) can be used for the diagnosis but due to rapid deterioration and fatal course, serological tests are not useful. CHPV RNA RT-PCR assay has high specificity for the diagnosis of CHPV infection.[50,52]

Treatment

There is no specific treatment available for CHPV infection and symptomatic treatment includes measures to reduce raised intracranial pressure due to neurological involvement.[47,52]

Prevention

Containment of disease-transmitting vectors will help in controlling this highly fatal disease. Vero cell-based inactivated vaccine has shown promising results on mice and can be a future modality for prevention of CHPV infection.[55]

◼ JAPANESE ENCEPHALITIS VIRUS

Japanese encephalitis virus (JEV) is a flavivirus with distribution in many countries of Asia, Africa, Europe, and Australia. It is one of the most common cause of viral encephalitis world over and has a high mortality rate of up to one-third among those with clinical illness.[56]

Epidemiology

More than 20 countries from South-East Asia and Western Pacific regions are endemic for this disease and around 3 billion people are at risks of infection.[57] In India, periodic outbreaks of JE have been reported during monsoon and post-monsoon periods. The most affected states in India are Andhra Pradesh, Assam, Bihar, Karnataka, Kerala, Orissa, Uttar Pradesh, and West Bengal.[58]

Transmission

Various species of mosquito *Culex* are vector for JEV transmission. Pigs, birds, and bats are natural reservoirs, while human is a dead-end host. The most important vector is *Culex tritaeniorhynchus* which thrives in irrigated crop fields.[56,57]

Virus Genotype

Japanese encephalitis virus is single-stranded RNA virus, belongs to family *Flaviviridae*, and has five genotypes—G-I to G-V.[59,60]

Clinical Features

Japanese encephalitis virus has incubation period of 6–16 days. JEV infection is most often subclinical. In symptomatic children, it usually starts with abrupt onset of fever, chills, myalgias, and headaches accompanied by vomiting. Nausea, vomiting, and abdominal pains can be initial manifestations in children. Later, they develop seizures, altered sensorium confusion, abnormal posturing, and coma. Case fatality rate of 20–30% has been reported, especially in children with acute cerebral edema or ARDS. Those who recover from illness usually have serious behavioral and neurological sequelae.[57,58,61]

Diagnosis

The JEV-specific IgM ELISA is recommended investigation for detection of acute infections. Plaque reduction neutralization test is another option which can differentiate JEV from other flaviviruses. A fourfold increase in IgG titer in acute and convalescent sera can confirm the diagnosis. The RT-PCR also has high specificity and sensitivity and can detect low viral copies in early phase of illness.[57,62,63]

Treatment

There is no specific antiviral therapy against JEV and treatment is mainly supportive. Many antiviral drugs have been tried, but none of these have shown to be effective.

Prevention

Considering the burden of disease, Government of India has formulated a multipronged strategy which includes JE vaccination in affected districts, surveillance programs, vector control measures, and proper case management. The live-attenuated JE vaccine has been introduced into the national immunization programs recently in selected states.[56,61,64]

■ AVIAN INFLUENZA VIRUS

Avian influenza virus (H5N1), a highly pathogenic viral in poultry, has recently posed a major challenge to human and is potentially a serious pandemic threat.[65]

Epidemiology

H5N1 virus was first time found in diseased geese in Guangdong, China. It was first detected in humans in Hong Kong in 1997 in 18 patients. Since then outbreaks of H5N1 infection have been reported from Japan, South Korea, and China and in many South-East Asian countries including India. Fifty four countries reported this infection by 2006.[65-67]

Virus Genotype

H5N1 is an influenza A virus which is an enveloped RNA virus and belongs to *Orthomyxoviridae* family of viruses.[65]

Transmission

Transmission of H5N1virus occurs from infected birds to humans. Although it replicates in diseased humans but efficient person-to-person transmission is less often found.[68,69]

Clinical Features

H5N1 virus has incubation period of 2–4 days. The most common presenting symptoms are fever, cough, and shortness of breath. Chest X-ray often shows pneumonia or ARDS-like picture. Loose stools, vomiting, and abdominal pain are other frequently occurring manifestations. Abdominal symptoms may be presenting features in some patients. Few patients can develop acute encephalitis but neurological manifestations are not commonly reported.[70,71]

Diagnosis

Laboratory investigations usually show lymphopenia and mild-to-moderate thrombocytopenia. Virus isolation, detection of viral nucleic acids by RT-PCR, and serological test are used for the diagnosis of H5N1 viral infection. Virus culture on inoculation of embryonated eggs or Madin-Darby canine kidney is the gold standard for diagnosis and further viral genetic and antigenic characterization. But due to long turnover time for viral culture, RT-PCR and ELISA for detection of viral antigen are the first tests used for the diagnosis of H5N1 infection.[66,70,71]

Treatment

Amantadine, rimantadine, oseltamivir, and zanamivir are the drugs that are active against influenza viruses. Early use of these drugs may provide clinical benefit. Corticosteroids and interferon-α has been tried in these patients with some success but appropriately controlled trials are needed to document their beneficial role.[66,70]

Prevention

Seasonal influenza vaccine does not protect from avian influenza but can help reducing the complications associated with H5N1 infection. An inactivated influenza virus vaccine against H5N1 has been in use since 2007, first time approved and used in USA. This vaccine is currently only recommended for use by those at higher risk of exposure to H5N1 virus.[72]

■ SEVERE ACUTE RESPIRATORY SYNDROME–CORONAVIRUS

Severe acute respiratory syndrome–coronavirus (SARS-CoV) was isolated in 2003. SARS-CoV is thought to be zoonotic with bat as reservoir but there is still uncertainty over the animal reservoir of this virus.

Epidemiology

The first human infection of SARS-CoV was documented in Guangdong, China, in 2002 and later it spread rapidly to 30 countries across Asia, the Americas, and Europe, with more than 8,000 cases and more than 800 deaths in less than a year. Few probable and suspected cases have also been reported from India at that time.[73]

Virus Genotype

Severe acute respiratory syndrome coronavirus is a single-stranded RNA virus, which belongs to *Coronaviridae* family and *Nidovirales* order.[74]

Transmission

Transmission of SARS-CoV is primarily person to person, which occurs mainly in the healthcare setting, due to inadequate infection control measures.[73,75]

Clinical Features

The incubation period of SARS-CoV is 2–14 days. The typical illness begins with fever, rigors, myalgias, and cough and later evolves into pneumonia with rapid respiratory deterioration. Coryza and pharyngitis are less frequently reported clinical features. Fever is sometimes absent. Some patients deteriorate rapidly with progression to ARDS and requiring mechanical ventilation.[75,76]

Diagnosis

Virus culture and serological test with fourfold rise in the antibody titer are definitive evidence of infection. RT-PCR and antigen detection by ELISA are the alternative. RT-PCR on nasal swab is the most sensitive and rapid method of diagnosis.[74,76]

Treatment

There are no effective antiviral drugs for treatment of SARS-CoV infection so management is largely supportive with prompt diagnosis and respiratory support.

Prevention

A retrospective analysis have shown some benefit with passive immunization using convalescent plasma with neutralizing antibodies in SARS-CoV infected patients who continued to deteriorate.[77]

■ EBOLA VIRUS

Ebola virus (EBOV) infection is a zoonotic disease, with occasional infection of humans and other animals. It can spread from person to person with fatal outcome. World Health Organization has declared it as a public health emergency.[78,79]

Epidemiology

Ebola virus was discovered as hemorrhagic fever with fatal outcome in Zaire in 1976. Since then periodic small outbreaks have been reported from Africa. The largest outbreak occurred in West Africa in 2014–2016 with over 5,000 reported deaths.[80,81] Sporadic EBOV infection cases have also been reported from India.[80]

Viral Genotype

Ebola virus is a member of genus *Ebolavirus* and family *Filoviridae*.[79]

Transmission

Ebola virus is transmitted by direct contact with infected animals and also human-to-human transmission can occur after contact with infected person.[79,81]

Clinical Features

The incubation period of EBOV is 2–21 days. Fever is the most common symptom. Other clinical features are myalgias, headache, sore throat, vomiting, rash, and loose stools. Hemorrhagic manifestations are seen in 30–50% of patients. Later, as the disease progresses, multiorgan failure and hypovolemic shock may develop. The common neurologic manifestations are meningitis, encephalitis, neuropsychiatric manifestations, seizures, and cerebellitis. EBOV infection has high fatality rate with up to 90% reported mortality in epidemics.[78,79,81,82]

Diagnosis

Viral RNA detection in blood by RT-PCR helps in diagnosis in acute phase of illness. It is a sensitive test with high specificity. EBOV antigens or specific IgM or IgG antibody detection helps in the diagnosis.[79,83]

Treatment

No antiviral drugs are effective in treatment and decreasing mortality in EBOV infection and management of EBOV disease is mainly supportive.

Prevention

To control Ebola disease outbreaks, early case identification, rapid isolation, and clinical management of patients, health promotion and community engagement are essential.[83,84]

■ REFERENCES

1. Forum on Microbial Threats, Board on Global Health, Institute of Medicine. Emerging Viral Diseases: The One Health Connection: Workshop Summary. Washington (DC): National Academies Press (US); 2015.
2. Taylor LH, Latham SM, Woolhouse ME. Risk factors for human disease emergence. Philos Trans R Soc Lond B Biol Sci. 2001;356(1411):983-9.
3. ScienceDaily (2016). 2009 swine flu pandemic originated in Mexico, researchers discover. [online] Available from: https://www.sciencedaily.com/releases/2016/06/160627160935.htm.
4. Sriram P, Kumar M, Renitha R, et al. Clinical Profile of Swine Flu in Children at Puducherry. Indian J Pediatr. 2010;77(10):1093-5.
5. NewsClick (2019). Swine Flu Hits 'Epidemic' Proportions in India. [online] Available from: https://www.newsclick.in/swine-flu-hits-epidemic-proportions-india.
6. Bouvier NM, Palese P. The biology of influenza viruses. Vaccine. 2008;26(Suppl 4):D49-53.
7. Hackett S, Hill L, Patel J, et al. Swine flu in children: clinical presentations, treatment and outcome in Birmingham, UK. Arch Dis Child. 2010;95(Suppl 1):A23.
8. Centers for Disease Control and Prevention (2009). H1N1 Flu. People at High Risk of Developing Flu-Related Complications. [online] Available from: https://www.cdc.gov/h1n1flu/highrisk.htm. [Last accessed on November, 2019].
9. (2019). Clinical guidelines.pdf [online]. Available from: http://www.nrhmhp.gov.in/sites/default/files/files/Clinical%20guidelines.pdf. [Last accessed November, 2019].
10. Everyday Health (2019). Influenza virus vaccine, H1N1, live-Side Effects, Dosage, Interactions. [online]. Available from: https://www.everydayhealth.com/drugs/influenza-virus-vaccine-h1n1-live. [Last accessed on November, 2019].
11. Ang BSP, Lim TCC, Wang L. Nipah Virus Infection. J Clin Microbiol. 2018;56(6):e01875-17.
12. Semantic Scholar (2003). Epidemiological aspects of Nipah virus infection. [online] Available from: https://www.semanticscholar.org/paper/Epidemiological-aspects-of-Nipah-virus-infection-Tan-Tan/3735f4fd0619e58b422b7621299437bcc421f62d. [Last accessed on November, 2019].
13. Chadha MS, Comer JA, Lowe L, et al. Nipah virus-associated encephalitis outbreak, Siliguri, India. Emerg Infect Dis. 2006;12(2):235-40.
14. World Health Organization (2018). Nipah virus—India. [online]. Available from: https://www.who.int/csr/don/07-august-2018-nipah-virus-india/en/. [Last accessed on November, 2019].
15. Goh KJ, Tan CT, Chew NK, et al. Clinical features of Nipah virus encephalitis among pig farmers in Malaysia. N Engl J Med. 2000;342(17):1229-35.
16. World Health Organization (2019). Nipah virus outbreaks in the WHO South-East Asia Region [online]. Available from: http://www.searo.who.int/entity/emerging_diseases/links/nipah_virus_outbreaks_sear/en/. [Last accessed on November, 2019].
17. Mazzola LT, Kelly-Cirino C. Diagnostics for Nipah virus: a zoonotic pathogen endemic to Southeast Asia. BMJ Glob Health. 2019;4(Suppl 2):e001118.
18. Chong HT, Kamarulzaman A, Tan CT, et al. Treatment of acute Nipah encephalitis with ribavirin. Ann Neurol. 2001;49(6):810-3.
19. Satterfield BA, Dawes BE, Milligan GN. Status of vaccine research and development of vaccines for Nipah virus. Vaccine. 2016;34(26):2971-5.
20. Schmaljohn C, Hjelle B. Hantaviruses: a global disease problem. Emerg Infect Dis. 1997;3(2):95-104.
21. Jonsson CB, Figueiredo LTM, Vapalahti O. A Global Perspective on Hantavirus Ecology, Epidemiology, and Disease. Clin Microbiol Rev. 2010;23(2):412-41.
22. Chandy S, Yoshimatsu K, Ulrich RG, et al. Seroepidemiological study on hantavirus infections in India. Trans R Soc Trop Med Hyg. 2008;102(1):70-4.
23. Zhang Y-Z, Zou Y, Fu ZF, et al. Hantavirus Infections in Humans and Animals, China. Emerg Infect Dis. 2010;16(8):1195-203.
24. Plyusnin A, Morzunov SP. Virus Evolution and Genetic Diversity of Hantaviruses and Their Rodent Hosts. In: Schmaljohn CS, Nichol ST (Eds). Hantaviruses. Current Topics in Microbiology and Immunology, Volume 256. Berlin Heidelberg; Springer; 2001.
25. Evander M, Eriksson I, Pettersson L, et al. Puumala hantavirus viremia diagnosed by real-time reverse transcriptase PCR using samples from patients with hemorrhagic fever and renal syndrome. J Clin Microbiol. 2007;45(8):2491-7.
26. World Health Organization (2018). Zika virus. [online] Available from: https://www.who.int/news-room/fact-sheets/detail/zika-virus. [Last accessed on November, 2019].
27. Bordi L, Avsic-Zupanc T, Lalle E, et al. Emerging Zika Virus Infection: A Rapidly Evolving Situation. Adv Exp Med Biol. 2017;972:61-86.
28. World Health Organization (2017). Zika virus infection—India. [online] Available from: http://www.who.int/csr/don/26-may-2017-zika-ind/en/. [Last accessed November, 2019].
29. Falcao MB, Cimerman S, Luz KG, et al. Management of infection by the Zika virus. Ann Clin Microbiol Antimicrob. 2016;15:57.
30. Gurugama P, Garg P, Perera J, et al. Dengue viral infections. Indian J Dermatol. 2010;55(1):68-78.
31. Kalayanarooj S, Rothman AL, Srikiatkhachorn A. Case Management of Dengue: Lessons Learned. J Infect Dis. 2017;215(Suppl 2):S79-88.
32. Malavige GN, Fernando S, Fernando DJ, et al. Dengue viral infections. Postgrad Med J. 2004;80(948):588-601.

33. Bhatt S, Gething PW, Brady OJ, et al. The global distribution and burden of dengue. Nature. 2013;496(7446):504-7.

34. World Health Organization. Prevention and Control of Dengue and Dengue Haemorrhagic Fever. South-East Asia; WHO Regional Office; 1999.

35. Narayanan M, Aravind MA, Thilothammal N, et al. Dengue fever epidemic in Chennai--a study of clinical profile and outcome. Indian Pediatr. 2002;39(11):1027-33.

36. Guzmán MG, Kourí G. Advances in dengue diagnosis. Clin Diagn Lab Immunol. 1996;3(6):621-7.

37. Nguyen TH, Nguyen TL, Lei HY, et al. Volume replacement in infants with dengue hemorrhagic fever/dengue shock syndrome. Am J Trop Med Hyg. 2006;74(4):684-91.

38. World Health Organization (2017). Dengue vaccine research. [online] Available from: http://www.who.int/immunization/research/development/dengue_vaccines/en/. [Last accessed on November, 2019].

39. World Health Organization (2019). Chikungunya. [online] Available from: http://www.who.int/denguecontrol/arboviral/other_arboviral_chikungunya/en/. [Last accessed on November, 2019].

40. Brighton SW, Prozesky OW, de la Harpe AL. Chikungunya virus infection. A retrospective study of 107 cases. South Afr Med J Suid-Afr Tydskr Vir Geneeskd. 1983;63(9):313-5.

41. World Health Organization. chikungunya_factsheet.pdf [online]. Available from: http://www.searo.who.int/india/topics/chikungunya/chikungunya_factsheet.pdf.

42. Harapan H, Michie A, Mudatsir M, et al. Chikungunya virus infection in Indonesia: a systematic review and evolutionary analysis. BMC Infect Dis. 2019;19(1):243.

43. Bonifay T, Prince C, Neyra C, et al. Atypical and severe manifestations of chikungunya virus infection in French Guiana: A hospital-based study. PLoS One. 2018;13(12):e0207406.

44. Silva JVJ Jr, Ludwig-Begall LF, Oliveira-Filho EF, et al. A scoping review of Chikungunya virus infection: epidemiology, clinical characteristics, viral co-circulation complications, and control. Acta Trop. 2018;188:213-24.

45. Johnson BW, Russell BJ, Goodman CH. Laboratory Diagnosis of Chikungunya Virus Infections and Commercial Sources for Diagnostic Assays. J Infect Dis. 2016;214(Suppl 5):S471-4.

46. da Cunha RV, Trinta KS. Chikungunya virus: clinical aspects and treatment—a review. Mem Inst Oswaldo Cruz. 2017;112(8):523-31.

47. Sudeep AB, Gurav YK, Bondre VP. Changing clinical scenario in Chandipura virus infection. Indian J Med Res. 2016;143(6):712-21.

48. Bhatt PN, Rodrigues FM. Chandipura: a new arbovirus isolated in India from patients with febrile illness. Indian J Med Res. 1967;55(12):1295-305.

49. Kemp GE. Viruses other than arenaviruses from West African wild mammals. Factors affecting transmission to man and domestic animals. Bull World Health Organ. 1975;52(4-6):615-20.

50. Menghani S, Chikhale R, Raval A, et al. Chandipura virus: an emerging tropical pathogen. Acta Trop. 2012;124(1):1-14.

51. Rao BL, Basu A, Wairagkar NS, et al. A large outbreak of acute encephalitis with high fatality rate in children in Andhra Pradesh, India, in 2003, associated with Chandipura virus. Lancet. 2004;364(9437):869-74.

52. Sapkal GN, Sawant PM, Mourya DT. Chandipura Viral Encephalitis: A Brief Review. Open Virol J. 2018;12:44-51.

53. Mavale MS, Geevarghese G, Ghodke YS, et al. Vertical and venereal transmission of Chandipura virus (Rhabdoviridae) by Aedes aegypti (Diptera: Culicidae). J Med Entomol. 2005;42(5):909-11.

54. Tandale BV, Tikute SS, Arankalle VA, et al. Chandipura virus: A major cause of acute encephalitis in children in North Telangana, Andhra Pradesh, India. J Med Virol. 2008;80(1):118-24.

55. Jadi RS, Sudeep AB, Barde PV, et al. Development of an inactivated candidate vaccine against chandipura virus (Rhabdoviridae: Vesiculovirus). Vaccine. 2011;29(28):4613-7.

56. Kulkarni R, Sapkal GN, Kaushal H, et al. Japanese encephalitis: a brief review on Indian perspectives. Open Virol J. 2018;12:121-30.

57. Solomon T, Dung NM, Kneen R, et al. Japanese encephalitis. J Neurol Neurosurg Psychiatry. 2000;68(4):405-15.

58. Kabilan L, Rajendran R, Arunachalam N, et al. Japanese encephalitis in India: an overview. Indian J Pediatr. 2004;71(7):609-15.

59. Solomon T, Ni H, Beasley DWC, et al. Origin and evolution of Japanese encephalitis virus in Southeast Asia. J Virol. 2003;77(5):3091-8.

60. Li M-H, Fu S-H, Chen W-X, et al. Genotype V Japanese encephalitis virus is emerging. PLoS Negl Trop Dis. 2011;5(7):e1231.

61. Medhi M, Saikia L, Patgiri SJ, et al. Incidence of Japanese Encephalitis amongst acute encephalitis syndrome cases in upper Assam districts from 2012 to 2014: A report from a tertiary care hospital. Indian J Med Res. 2017;146(2):267-71.

62. Solomon T, Thao LTT, Dung NM, et al. Rapid Diagnosis of Japanese Encephalitis by Using an Immunoglobulin M Dot Enzyme Immunoassay. J Clin Microbiol. 1998;36(7):2030-4.

63. Centers for Disease Control and Prevention. (2019). Diagnostic Testing. Japanese Encephalitis. [online]. Available from: https://www.cdc.gov/japaneseencephalitis/healthcareproviders/healthcareproviders-diagnostic.html. [Last accessed on November, 2019].

64. Rustagi R, Basu S, Garg S. Japanese encephalitis: Strategies for prevention and control in India. Indian J Med Spec. 2019;10(1):12.

65. Peiris JSM, Jong MD de, Guan Y. Avian Influenza Virus (H5N1): a Threat to Human Health. Clin Microbiol Rev. 2007;20(2):243-67.

66. Malik Peiris JS, de Jong MD, Guan Y. Avian Influenza Virus (H5N1): a Threat to Human Health. Clin Microbiol Rev. 2007;20(2):243-67.

67. World Health Organization (2018). Influenza (Avian and other zoonotic) [online]. Available from: https://www.who.int/news-room/fact-sheets/detail/influenza-(avian-and-other-zoonotic). [Last accessed on November, 2019].

68. Centers for Disease Control and Prevention (2015). Transmission of Avian Influenza A Viruses Between Animals and People. Avian Influenza (Flu). [online]. Available from: https://www.cdc.gov/flu/avianflu/virus-transmission.htm. [Last accessed on November, 2019].

69. Hayden F, Croisier A. Transmission of Avian influenza viruses to and between Humans. J Infect Dis. 2005;192(8):1311-4.

70. The Writing Committee of the World Health Organization (WHO) Consultation on Human Influenza A/H5. Avian Influenza A (H5N1) Infection in Humans. N Engl J Med. 2005;353(13):1374-85.

71. Chotpitayasunondh T, Ungchusak K, Hanshaoworakul W, et al. Human disease from influenza A (H5N1), Thailand, 2004. Emerg Infect Dis. 2005;11(2):201-9.

72. US Food and Drug Administration (2018). H5N1 Influenza Virus Vaccine, manufactured by Sanofi Pasteur, Inc. Questions and Answers. [online] Available from: http://www.fda.gov/vaccines-blood-biologics/vaccines/h5n1-influenza-virus-vaccine-manufactured-sanofi-pasteur-inc-questions-and-answers. [Last accessed on November, 2019].

73. World Health Organization (2019). SARS (Severe Acute Respiratory Syndrome). [online]. Available from: https://www.who.int/ith/diseases/sars/en/. [Last accessed on November, 2019].

74. Satija N, Lal SK. The molecular biology of SARS coronavirus. Ann N Y Acad Sci. 2007;1102:26-38.

75. Cheng VCC, Lau SKP, Woo PCY, et al. Severe acute respiratory syndrome Coronavirus as an agent of emerging and reemerging infection. Clin Microbiol Rev. 2007;20(4):660-94.

76. Mehta S, Sashindran V, Kumar K, et al. Severe acute respiratory syndrome: an update. Med J Armed Forces India. 2007;63(1):52-5.

77. Cheng Y, Wong R, Soo YO, et al. Use of convalescent plasma therapy in SARS patients in Hong Kong. Eur J Clin Microbiol Infect Dis. 2005;24(1):44-6.

78. SEARO. World Health Organization (2019). India update on Ebola Virus Disease. [online] Available from: http://www.searo.who.int/india/areas/communicable_diseases/india_ebola/en/

79. Malvy D, McElroy AK, Clerck H de, et al. Ebola virus disease. Lancet. 2019;393(10174):936-48.

80. My India. (2014). Ebola Virus Outbreak—Is India Prepared? [online] Available from: https://www.mapsofindia.com/my-india/society/ebola-virus-outbreak-is-india-prepared. [Last accessed on November, 2019].

81. Centers for Disease Control and Prevention (Division of High-Consequence Pathogens and Pathology; Viral Special Pathogens Branch), National Center for Emerging and Zoonotic Infectious Diseases (2016). Outbreaks Chronology: Ebola Virus Disease. [online] Available from: https://www.cdc.gov/vhf/ebola/resources/outbreak-table.html. [Last accessed on November, 2019].

82. Outbreak of Ebola haemorrhagic fever in Yambio, south Sudan, April–June 2004. Wkly Epidemiol Rec. 2005;80(43):370-5.

83. Beeching NJ, Fenech M, Houlihan CF. Ebola virus disease. BMJ. 2014;349:g7348.

84. World Health Organization (2018). Ebola virus disease. [online] Available from: http://www.who.int/en/news-room/fact-sheets/detail/ebola-virus-disease. [Last accessed on November, 2019].

Antiviral Drugs in Office Practice

Jeeson C Unni

INTRODUCTION

Antiviral drugs used in commonly used in children include:

- Anti-herpes virus agents
- Antivirals for respiratory viral infections
- Antivirals for hepatic viral infections
- Antiretroviral (ARV) agents.

The drugs used and their antiviral spectrums are as follows:

- *Acyclovir*: Herpes simplex virus (HSV)-1, HSV-2, varicella zoster virus (VZV)—chickenpox, and herpes zoster
- *Ganciclovir/cidofovir*: *Cytomegalovirus* (CMV)
- *Famciclovir*: Herpes genitalis and herpes zoster—famciclovir is a prodrug of penciclovir—has greatest bioavailability (OD/BD dose)
- *Foscarnet*: HSV, VZV, CMV, and human immuno-deficiency virus (HIV)
- *Penciclovir*: Herpes labialis, CMV—poor bioavailability—only for topical use
- *Trifluridine*: Herpetic keratoconjunctivitis.

ACYCLOVIR

Uses

- *Herpes simplex*:
  - Eye
  - Skin (genital, labial)
  - Neonatal
  - Encephalitis
  - In the immunocompromised (prophylaxis)
  - Suppression of HSV infection in special situations.
- *Chickenpox and herpes zoster.*
- *Herpes labialis with gingivostomatitis:*
  Oral acyclovir: Gingivostomatitis—1 month to 2 years 100 mg; 2–18 years 200 mg 5 times daily for 7 days within 4 days of onset.

Oral antiviral, e.g. acyclovir, may reduce duration of pain and time to healing for a first attack of herpes labialis compared with placebo; however, evidence is limited. There are no randomized controlled trials (RCTs) comparing topical antiviral versus placebo and no treatment. Research in this area is difficult because people may not consult clinicians until they have experienced several attacks of herpes labialis.

Prophylactic oral antivirals may reduce the frequency and severity of attacks compared with placebo, but there are no recommendations regarding the best timing and duration of treatment. Acyclovir, famciclovir, and valacyclovir may reduce the duration of symptoms and the time to heal in recurrent attacks of herpes labialis. Limited evidence shows that topical antiviral agents may reduce pain and healing time in recurrent attacks which are inconsistent and of marginal clinical importance. Ultraviolet sunscreen may reduce recurrent attacks; however, evidence is limited. Topical anesthetic agents or zinc oxide are not useful. Zinc oxide cream may, in fact, increase skin irritation.

Drug treatment of recurrences:

Adolescents: To shorten duration of episode—

- Valacyclovir (2,000 mg bid PO for 1 day)
- Acyclovir (200–400 mg 5 times daily PO for 5 days)
- Famciclovir (1,500 mg once daily PO for 1 day).

Long-term prophylaxis for frequent or severe recurrences:

- Acyclovir (400 mg bid PO) or
- Valacyclovir (500 mg once daily PO).

- *Herpetic keratoconjunctivitis*: Application of 1 cm of acyclovir ointment 5 times daily (continue for at least 3 days after complete healing) is the treatment of choice. Topical trifluorothymidine, vidarabine, idoxuridine, or ganciclovir is also useful. Interferon (IFN) monotherapy has a slight beneficial effect on dendritic epithelial keratitis, but not better than other antiviral agents. There are studies that suggest that a combined IFN–nucleoside therapy improves healing. Children with HSV keratitis are at risk for recurrent keratitis and amblyopia. Prolonged systemic antiviral prophylaxis may help to prevent such consequences (1 year acyclovir/valacyclovir). Immune regulatory drugs, e.g. cyclosporine, present attractive alternative to managing HSV stromal keratitis, given the immune-mediated pathogenesis of stromal disease.

- *Herpes encephalitis*: There are limited studies in neonates/children. Poor prognosis and relapses despite treatment [antibodies against N-methyl-d-aspartate receptors (NMDARs)] are not uncommon.
  Intravenous acyclovir infusion: Neonate—3 months 20 mg/kg 8 hourly for 21 days; 3 months to 12 years 250 mg/m^2 8 hourly for 21 days. Confirm whether cerebrospinal fluid (CSF) is –ve for HSV before stopping. Doubling the dose is recommended in immunocompromised neonates and children.

- *Genital herpes*: It is a recurrent, incurable viral disease. Treatment of the initial infection reduces the severity and duration of subsequent recurrent infections but has no effect on the frequency of subsequent recurrent infections. Adolescent: Acyclovir at 400 mg tid; child: 10–20 mg/kg/dose qid × 7–10 days. Extend the treatment if the healing incomplete. Topical acyclovir has negligible or no clinical benefit.
  For episodic therapy for recurrent genital herpes: Adolescent—800 mg tid × 2 days (start within 1st day of onset or in prodrome). In HIV patients, imiquimod may be tried in episodic treatment of lesions thought to be acyclovir resistant or nonresponsive. Valacyclovir and famciclovir are also effective but clinical experience is lacking.

- *Herpes simplex prophylaxis in the immunocompromised*: *Oral acyclovir*: Child 1 month to 2 years: 100–200 mg 4 times daily and for children (2–18 years): 200–400 mg 4 times daily.

- *Herpes simplex suppression*: Suppressive therapy reduces frequency of recurrences by 70–80%.
  Oral acyclovir: Child 12–18 years 400 mg twice daily *or* 200 mg 4 times daily. The dose may be increased to 400 mg thrice daily if recurrences occur on standard suppressive therapy or for suppression of genital herpes during late pregnancy (from 36 weeks gestation). Therapy is interrupted every 6–12 months to reassess recurrence frequency; consider restarting after two or more recurrences.

- *Acyclovir in chickenpox*: Antiviral therapy modifies course in both varicella and herpes zoster.
  Neonates: Regardless of immune status and use of any immunoglobulins, acyclovir must be administered due to high risk of severe disease. Oral acyclovir is not recommended as absorption is variable. A healthy child from 1 month to 12 years need not be treated. Adolescent—treat within 24 hours.
  Immunocompromised children and those at special risk (severe CVS/respiratory disease/chronic skin disorder): 10 days of acyclovir with at least 7 days of parenteral treatment. It is preferable to start therapy for chickenpox within 1st 24 hours of onset of illness.
  Acyclovir in herpes zoster: Systemic antiviral treatment can reduce the severity and duration of pain, reduce complications, and reduce viral shedding. Treatment with the antiviral should be started within 72 hours of the onset of rash and is usually continued for 7–10 days. Immunocompromised patients at high risk of disseminated or severe infection should be treated with a parenteral antiviral drug.
  Dose of acyclovir in chickenpox and herpes zoster infection:
  Oral: 1 month to 2 years—200 mg; 2–6 years 400 mg; 6–12 years 800 mg 4 times daily for 5 days; 12–18 years 800 mg 5 times daily for 7 days (herpes zoster in the immunocompromised continue for 2 days after crusting of lesions).
  Intravenous (IV) infusion: Neonate-3 months 10–20 mg/kg 8 hourly for at least 7 days; 3 months to 12 years 250 mg/m^2; 12–18 years 5 mg/kg 8 hourly for 5 days. At all ages, double the dose in encephalitis or immunocompromised (given for 10–14 days in encephalitis, possibly longer if also immunocompromised). To avoid excessive dose in obese, IV dose is calculated on the basis of ideal weight for height.
  Prophylaxis of chickenpox after delivery—Intravenous infusion: Neonate 10 mg/kg 8 hourly; continued until serological tests confirm the absence of virus (VZ IgM).
  Attenuation of chickenpox if VZ immunoglobulin is not indicated or not available: *Oral*: 1 month to 18 years 10 mg/kg 4 times daily for 7 days starting 1 week after exposure *IV infusion*, reconstitute to 25 mg/mL with water for injection or normal saline then dilute to concentration of 5 mg/mL with normal saline *or* glucose saline and give over 1 hour; OR use infusion pump and central line to administer the 25 mg/mL solution over 1 hour.
  Resistance to acyclovir: It does occur in immuno-compromised. If HSV lesions are unresponsive,

worsening or there is frequent recurrence, the chances of acyclovir resistance is high. In such conditions, an attempt is to be made to isolate the virus for sensitivity testing. Foscarnet or cidofovir have been used in such situations with success.

VALACYCLOVIR

- *Herpes zoster in immunocompromised: Oral*: 12–18 years 1 g tid for 7 days (continue for 2 days after crusting of lesions)
- *Treatment of herpes simplex: Oral*: 12–18 years 1st episode, 500 mg BD for 5 days; recurrent infection, 500 mg BD for 3–5 days (double dose for 5–10 days in immunocompromised or HIV +ve)
- *Treatment of herpes labialis: Oral*: 12–18 years initially 2 g, then 2 g 12 hours after initial dose
- *Suppression of herpes simplex: Oral*: 12–18 years 500 mg OD in 1–2 divided doses (immunocompromised or HIV +ve 500 mg BD; interrupt every 6–12 months to reassess; consider restarting after 2 or more recurrences
- *Prevention of CMV following solid organ transplantation (within 72 hours): Oral*: 12–18 years 2 g 4 times daily usually for 90 days.

FOSCARNET

- *Cytomegalovirus* disease
- *Retinitis* (ganciclovir resistant/immunocompromised patient)
  IV infusion: 1 month to18 years induction 60 mg/kg q8h for 2–3 weeks, then maintenance dose of 60 mg/kg daily, increased to 90–120 mg/kg if tolerated; if disease progresses on maintenance dose, repeat induction regimen.
- *Mucocutaneous herpes simplex infection* (acyclovir resistant/immunocompromised patient):
  IV infusion: 1 month to 18 years—40 mg/kg q8h for 2–3 weeks or until lesions heal; give *IV infusion* as undiluted solution via a central venous catheter; alternatively dilute to a concentration of 12 mg/mL with 5% glucose or normal saline via a peripheral vein; give over at least 1 hour (give doses greater than 60 mg/kg over 2 hours).

GANCICLOVIR

It is a drug of choice for life- or sight-threatening CMV infection in immunocompromised.

Prevention of CMV during immunosuppressive therapy following organ transplantation:

- *IV infusion*: 1 month to18 years initially (induction) 5 mg/kg q12h for 14–21 days for treatment or for 7–14 days for prevention; maintenance (for patients at risk

of relapse of retinitis), 6 mg/kg daily on 5 days/week *or* 5 mg/kg daily until adequate recovery of immunity; if retinitis progresses, repeat initial induction treatment. CMV infection of the CNS.

- *IV infusion*: Neonate—6 mg/kg every 12 hours for 6 weeks.
  Close monitoring of full blood count (severe deterioration may require correction and possibly treatment interruption).

Other Rare Indications for Antivirals in Children

Orofacial HSV is reactivated after cosmetic facial lacer resurfacing—day before procedure, start oral valacyclovir/famciclovir.

HSV infection in burns patients: Severe/life-threatening—IV acyclovir.

HSV-associated erythema multiforma: Antivirals not effective—long-term herpes labialis prophylaxis prevents recurrences of erythema multiforme (EM).

CMV Retinitis and Acyclovir-resistant HSV 1 and 2 in Immunocompromised Patients

Foscarnet is not to be used for anything except CMV retinitis and/or acyclovir-resistant HSV in immunocompromised child.

Ganciclovir: Reserve for life- or sight-threatening CMV infection in immunocompromised; prevention of CMV during immunosuppressive therapy following organ transplantation and CMV infection of the CNS.

ANTIVIRALS FOR RESPIRATORY VIRAL INFECTIONS

Influenza

- Amantadine/rimantadine (No longer recommended).
- *Oseltamivir/zanamivir*: These *neuraminidase inhibitors* prevent the release of new virions and their spread from cell to cell. They are effective against both influenza A and B. They are used for both prophylaxis and treatment. For treatment and postexposure prophylaxis: Oseltamivir should be started within 48 hours and zanamivir within 36 hours of symptoms/exposure. In healthy individuals, it reduces illness duration by about 1–1.5 days. However, for severe influenza or in the immunocompromised children, these drugs may be effective even after the ideal time for initiating therapy, if viral shedding continues (unlicensed use).

Oseltamivir and zanamivir are also licensed for use in exceptional circumstances (e.g. when vaccination does not cover the infecting strain) to prevent influenza in an epidemic.

Evidence suggests that some strains of influenza A have reduced susceptibility to oseltamivir, but retain susceptibility to zanamivir. Resistance to oseltamivir may be greater in severely immunocompromised children. Zanamivir should therefore be reserved for patients who are severely immunocompromised, or when oseltamivir cannot be used, or when resistance to oseltamivir is suspected.

For those unable to use the dry powder for inhalation, zanamivir is available as a solution that can be administered by nebulizer or intravenously (unlicensed).

- *Oseltamivir*:
  Prevention of influenza: Oral 13–18 years —75 mg once daily for at least 7 days after exposure or for up to 6 weeks during an epidemic.
  Treatment of influenza: Oral—for children above 1 year age up to 16 kg: 30 mg, 16–23 kg: 45 mg, 23–40 kg: 60 mg, and >40 kg: 75 mg—every 12 hours for 5 days.
- *Zanamivir*: By inhalation of powder.
  Postexposure prophylaxis of influenza: 5–18 years 10 mg once daily for 10 days.
  Prevention of influenza during an epidemic: 5–18 years 10 mg once daily for up to 28 days.
  Treatment of influenza: 5–18 years 10 mg BD for 5 days (10 days if resistance to oseltamivir suspected).
  There is a risk of bronchospasm with use of zanamavir.

Respiratory Syncytial Virus Bronchiolitis

Ribavirin is a guanosine analog.

It inhibits a wide range of DNA and RNA viruses. Inhalation treatment of severe respiratory syncytial virus (RSV) bronchiolitis in infants, especially with other serious diseases. There is no evidence of clinically relevant benefit.

Ribavirin may also be used orally with peginterferon alfa/IFN alfa for the treatment of chronic hepatitis C infection, Lassa fever, and intravenously for the treatment of life-threatening RSV, parainfluenza virus, and adenovirus infections in immunocompromised (unlicensed indications).

Anemia and jaundice are adverse effects to be watched out for when ribavirin is administered.

■ HEPATIC VIRAL INFECTIONS

The drugs used are:
- Interferons

- *Lamivudine (3TC)*: Cytosine analog—hepatitis B virus (HBV)
- *Entecavir*: Guanosine analog—HBV lamivudine-resistant strains
- *Ribavirin*: Hepatitis C (with IFNs).

Chronic Hepatitis B

Recommendations are still in evolution; no one drug currently achieves reliably complete eradication of the virus. Treatment is individualized and done under the care of a pediatric gastroenterologist. Therapy may be indicated only in the immune active form of disease, with evidence of ongoing inflammation or fibrosis as in these children, there exists a higher risk for cirrhosis during childhood.

Treatment Strategies

- *Interferon-α-2b (IFN-α2b)* has immunomodulatory and antiviral effects, but its use is limited by cost; need for subcutaneous administration; prolonged therapy of 24 weeks therapy; and side effects such as marrow suppression, depression, retinal changes, and autoimmune disorders. *Interferon-α-2b* is contraindicated in decompensated cirrhosis.
- *Lamivudine* given to children more than 2 years for 52 weeks, resulted in HBeAg clearance in 34% of patients with an alanine transaminase (ALT) more than 2 times normal; 88% remained in remission at 1 year. Good safety profile was reported in this age group. The therapy was continued for 6 months or more after viral clearance. Emergence of a mutant viral strain (YMDD) poses a barrier to its long-term use. Combination therapy in children using IFN and lamivudine did not seem to improve the rates of response in most series.
- *Adefovir:* Adefovir dipivoxil is a prodrug that is rapidly converted to adefovir after oral administration. Adefovir, an analog of adenomonophosphate and an inhibitor of viral DNA polymerase, was approved by the Food and Drug Association (FDA) for treatment of chronic HBV infection in 2002 for adults and in 2008 for children aged 12–17 years.

Chronic Hepatitis C

In children with moderate or severe liver disease, the regimen is chosen according to the genotype of the infecting virus and the viral load. A combination of ribavirin with either IFN alfa or peginterferon alfa-2b is licensed for use in children over 3 years. A combination of peginterferon alfa and ribavirin is preferred.

Interferon alfa—dosage

Chronic Active Hepatitis B

Subcutaneous injection: Child 2–18 years: 5–10 million units/m^2 3 times weekly.

Chronic Active Hepatitis C (in Combination with Oral Ribavirin)

Subcutaneous injection: Child 3–18 years: 3 million units/m^2 3 times weekly.

In practice in India....IFN—very expensive (10-kg child for 6/12 – ₹1.5 lakh). Further, IFN is very toxic. Most of the chronic hepatitis B cases is due to transplacental infection and in these cases treatment with IFN is not very effective; most studies demonstrate an effectiveness of 10–15%.

Hepatitis C is not seen or recognized in children as it is asymptomatic and usually detected when screened for blood donation.

■ ANTIRETROVIRAL DRUGS

Antiretroviral medicines:
- NRTI (Nucleoside reverse transcriptase inhibitors)
- NtRTI (Nucleotide reverse transcriptase inhibitors)
- NNRTI (Non-nucleoside reverse transcriptase inhibitors)
- Protease inhibitors (PI)
- Entry inhibitors
- Integrase inhibitors.

Uses of ART (Antiretroviral therapy):
- PMTCT (Prevention of mother-to-child transmission)
- PEP (Post-exposure prophylaxis)
- PrEP (Pre-exposure prophylaxis)
- Treatment of established case of HIV/AIDS.

Antiretroviral Therapy

The currently available therapy does not eradicate virus or cure patient; it only suppresses virus for extended periods and changes course of disease to a chronic process. Decisions about ART for pediatric HIV are based on viral load/replication, CD4 count or percentage, and clinical condition.

Antiretroviral therapy: Reason for combining at least three ARVs from at least two different classes is for its synergistic effect and to prevent the development of resistance, possible when used in monotherapy.

It is important to note that combination therapy increases the rate of toxicity. Complex drug-drug interactions exist among many of the ARV drugs. Many protease inhibitor drugs are inducers or inhibitors of the cytochrome P450 system and are therefore likely to have serious interactions with multiple drug classes. Inhibitory effect of ritonavir (a protease inhibitor) on the cytochrome P450 system has been exploited, and small doses of the drug are added to several other protease inhibitors (lopinavir, tipranavir, and atazanavir).

The preferred ART combination is 2 NRTI (to suppress replication in both active and resting cells) and 1 NNRTI or 1 protease inhibitor (to produce prolonged viral suppression).

Additional alternate regimens:
- Triple NRTIs (i.e. abacavir, zidovudine, and lamivudine)
- *Boosted PI*: Lopinavir/ritonavir in combination with 2 NRTIs
- One NRTI and one NNRTI.

Prevention of mother-to-child transmission: Zidovudine (ZDV).

Zidovudine is given to the pregnant woman (100 mg 5 times/24 hour PO). A combination antiretroviral therapy (cART) containing ZDV should be preferred. Therapy should be started as early as 14 weeks gestation and continued during delivery or till the baby is exclusive breastfed or for the first 6 weeks of life (2 mg/kg q6h PO). In the developed world, this decreases perinatal HIV transmission rate to <1%.

A short-term regimen (300 mg BD from 36 weeks gestation and 300 mg every 3 hours during delivery) resulted in almost 50% reduction in transmission. Even if a mother receives no ART during gestation or delivery, a 6-week ZDV prophylaxis for the newborn as soon as possible after delivery and preferably within 6 hours of birth results in a meaningful reduction of transmission rate.

Full-term infants: ZDV—2 mg/kg q6h for 6 weeks.

Preterm infants: 1.5 mg/kg orally or IV q12h for the first 2 weeks (if available) and then increased to 2 mg/kg q8h.

Prevention of mother-to-child transmission: Nevirapine (NVP).

Oral nevirapine: One dose to women in labor and once to infant in the first 48–72 hours of life reduces perinatal transmission by 50%; effective because of prolonged half-life of nevirapine. This is a simple and highly cost-effective regimen for developing countries. But if ART is required for children more than 6 months age, a NVP-based regimen was found to have a high failure rate.

Indications of Antiretroviral Therapy

- Start before the immune system is irreversibly damaged
- All infants, regardless of clinical or immunological must receive ART

Table 1: Formulations of FDCs available for pediatric HIV use in India.

Formulation	Stavudine (d4T)	Lamivudine (3TC)	Nevirapine (NVP)
FDC 6 (baby tab)	6 mg	30 mg	50 mg
FDC 10 (tab)	10 mg	40 mg	70 mg
FDC 12 (junior tab)	12 mg	60 mg	100 mg
FDC 30 d4T (adult tab)	30 mg	150 mg	200 mg
FDC 30 AZT (adult tab)	300 mg	150 mg	200 mg

(FDC: fixed-dosed combinations; HIV: human immunodeficiency virus; AZT: zidovudine)

- *Child 36–59 months*: If CD4 < 350 cells/mm^3 (15%)
- *Child more than 5 years old*: Follow adult guidelines
- *Adult and adolescents*:
  - WHO clinical stage 1 or 2 and a CD4 count ≤350 cells/mm^3: Initiate ART before CD4 drops below 200 cells/mm^3
  - WHO clinical stage 3 or 4 regardless of CD4 count
  - HIV and TB coinfection regardless of the CD4 count
  - HIV/HBV coinfection with evidence of active liver disease.

What to Start (National AIDS Control Organization)?

Pediatric formulations will be provided at all ART centers. The drugs supplied are fixed-dosed combinations (FDC) available in India which are stavudine-based regimens. It has been recommended that in order to scale up the treatment of children, this will be used as long as zidovudine (AZT)-based regimens are available and recommended globally, as the preferred choice for children **(Table 1)**.

Choice of ART Drug

- <2-year-old exposed to NVP in mother or in infancy: Start boosted PI-based regimen (lopinavir/ritonavir, LPV/r)—because of concerns about persistence of resistant mutants to NVP
- >3 years: HIV+TB – 2NRTI+ Efavirenz (EFV) (avoid nevirapine /rifampicin interaction); If EFZ not possible: Triple NRTI regimen

- >12 years: HIV + hepatitis B: Tenofovir (TDF) + emtricitabine (FTC)/lamivudine (3TC) + NVP/EFV (benefit of providing two potent drugs against hepatitis B infection).

Efavirenz is not considered in <3-year-old because of inadequate information on dosage and in adolescent girls due to its teratogenic potential in the first trimester of pregnancy.

Toxicity of ARV Drugs

Hematological: With AZT (anemia, neutropenia, and thrombocytopenia).

Mitochondrial dysfunction: With other NRTI drugs—include lactic acidosis, hepatic toxicity, pancreatitis, and peripheral neuropathy.

Lipodystrophy and other metabolic abnormalities: More common with stavudine (d4T) and protease inhibitors, and to a lesser degree with other NRTI drugs. Abnormalities include fat maldistribution and body habitus changes, hyperlipidemia, hyperglycemia, insulin resistance, diabetes mellitus, osteopenia, osteoporosis, and osteonecrosis.

Allergic reactions: Include skin rashes and hypersensitivity reactions. These are more common with the NNRTI drugs, but also seen with certain NRTI drugs, such as abacavir (ABC).

Hepatic dysfunction: In children with hepatic dysfunction of any etiology, NVP requires careful consideration because of its potential life-threatening hepatotoxicity.

■ POINTS TO REMEMBER

- Anti-herpes virus agents—Know all about the prototype/first-line drug—ACYCLOVIR other anti-HSV drugs are rarely required.
- Antivirals for respiratory viral infection: Oseltamivir
- Antivirals for hepatic viral infections—used sparingly
- Antiretroviral therapy: Those dealing with HIV/AIDS need to know all the issues involved—drug resistance, issues with compliance/monitoring, dosages, etc.

Prevention of Viral Infections in the Tropics

Sachidananda Kamath, Anitha P Moorkoth, Geeta M Govindaraj

INTRODUCTION

Viral infections account for an increasingly high burden of disease, disability, and death in the tropics. Preventive measures for the individual as well as the community at large need to be prioritized and practiced on a war footing. The success stories of prevention of poliomyelitis and HIV (human immunodeficiency virus) infection need to be built upon and expanded to other viral infections, which take a heavy toll of lives and livelihoods in the tropics. The mode of transmission of the various viral infections determines the strategies most appropriate for their prevention. The preventive measures are hence discussed with reference to the modes of transmission.

MAJOR ROUTES OF TRANSMISSION

The major routes of transmission of viral infections include person-to-person transmission, which is the most worrisome in overcrowded settings; vector-borne transmission, which is increasing rapidly; and transmission due to contaminated food or water. Vector-borne diseases have increased due to several reasons including rapid urbanization and climate change.

Person to Person

Quarantine

The word "quarantine" has its origin in the Italian "quaranta giorni" which is based on the practice of having ships rest at anchor for 6 weeks in the Middle Ages after they had been thought to have arrived from infected ports. In the modern age of global travel, quarantine is now mainly used in the prevention of hemorrhagic fevers such as Ebola, Crimean Congo fever and acute respiratory syndromes, and quarantine stations exist mainly at airports and border crossings. It involves isolation and restriction of movement of humans and animals deemed to have come in contact with a communicable disease, but who do not have signs of infection.

Isolation

Isolation of patients suffering from infectious disease has stood the test of time and is still practiced. Isolation of patients suffering from measles, mumps, and varicella and those with respiratory viral syndrome is routine. Isolation may be contact isolation, droplet isolation, or airborne isolation depending on the disease involved and the mode of transmission. Contact isolation is required when transmission occurs from contact either with the patient or with immediate surroundings. Droplet isolation prevents deposition of large particles over mucosae from a relatively short distance of less than 3 feet. Airborne transmission occurs due to dissemination of evaporated droplet nuclei or dust particles of size 5 µm or less and often involves the use of negative pressure systems, special high-density masks or self-contained breathing systems.

Pre- and Postexposure Prophylaxis

Pre-exposure prophylaxis is mainly used for the prevention of HIV infection amongst the uninfected population indulging in unsafe practice including risky sexual behavior and drug abuse. Postexposure prophylaxis is effective by active immunization with hepatitis A vaccine and varicella vaccine within 10 days and 72 hours of exposure, respectively.

Vector Borne

Integrated Vector Management

The cornerstones of integrated vector management include:

- Advocacy, social mobilization, legislative measures
- Collaboration in the health sector and intersectoral

- Integrated approach
- Evidence-based decisions
- Capacity-building at all levels.

Outbreak Preparedness

There should be judicious use of insecticides along with other control measures.

Community action has a vital role to play in dengue and chikungunya prevention, by reducing mosquito-breeding sites at homes and institutions and preventing human contact with the vectors.

Source reduction in peridomestic areas by removal of stagnant water in all manner of receptacles, frequent changes of water in trays around potted plants and flower pots, and use of larvivorous fish such as gambusia and guppy in ornamental tanks is of prime importance. Prevention of contact with vectors is affected by use of mosquito nets, window mesh, mosquito repellents, and pyrethroid sprays.

Food Contamination

Good food hygiene practices are of utmost importance in preventing transmission of food borne viral illness especially viral Hepatitis A and Enteroviral infections.

■ INFECTION CONTROL PRECAUTIONS

It is important to follow standard precautions in all cases regardless of the infectious status of patients and additional transmission-based precautions. Contact/droplet/airborne precautions need to be followed depending on the modes of transmission of the infectious diseases.

Standard Precautions

These were previously referred to as "Universal precautions" and recognize the fact that healthcare personnel are at risk of being infected by pathogens from infected patients, who may not have manifested symptoms as yet. They should be in place in all healthcare facilities.

Standard precautions include:
- Hand hygiene
- Use of personal protective equipment (PPE)
- Prevention of needle sticks/sharp injuries
- Cleaning and disinfection of the environment and equipment
- Waste management
- Respiratory hygiene
- Safe injection practices

- Use of mask, e.g. when performing spinal or epidural procedures.

Hand Hygiene

It would be better if this information on Hand hygiene is given below Standard precautions prior to Transmission based precautions

Hands are an important mode of transmission of infection, and hence appropriate hand hygiene (HH) is of paramount importance and is the most essential standard precaution measure to prevent transmission of infections.

Hand hygiene includes hand wash with soap and water and use of alcohol hand rub.

Transient microbial flora contaminating the superficial layers of skin (Norovirus and other multidrug-resistant organisms) are more important in transmission of infections than the normal resident flora [coagulase-negative staphylococci (CoNS)/diphtheroids] of skin. The transient flora can be easily removed by effective HH.

For effective HH, it is necessary to use an effective compound in sufficient amount using the right technique and at the right indicated situations.

Alcohol-based hand rubs (ABHR) with 60%–80% ethanol and emollient are recommended by the World Health Organization (WHO). It is important to use adequate volume (3–5 mL) for 20–30 seconds and follow the steps of HH effectively. As per the WHO guidelines, the key indications for HH are given as "My 5 moments of Hand hygiene":

1. Before touching a patient
2. Before any clean/aseptic procedure
3. After a procedure or body fluid exposure
4. After touching a patient
5. After touching patient surroundings.

Both ABHR and hand wash with soap (plain neutral pH soap without added antimicrobials) and water are acceptable. ABHR are an effective and convenient alternative to hand wash; however, hand wash with soap and water is essential in certain situations such as before eating, after use of restroom, when hands are visibly soiled with dirt/blood/body fluids, when handling diarrheic patients, and when there is potential exposure to spore-forming organisms.

Transmission-based Precautions

They are used empirically, according to the clinical syndrome and the likely etiological agent **(Table 1)**:
- Contact
- Droplet
- Airborne.

Table 1: Precautions to be adopted for prevention of transmission of viral infection.

Activity	Standard	Contact	Droplet	Airborne
	For all patients irrespective of infectious status	Diarrheal pathogens	RSV Para influenza Influenza	VZV Measles SARS
Hand hygiene	Yes	Yes	Yes	Yes
Isolation room	Not required	Single room with toilet facility	Single room	Single room with negative pressure ventilation
Use of gloves	When likely to touch blood/body fluids	To wear gloves on entering room	When likely to touch blood/body fluids	When likely to touch blood/body fluids
Gown/Apron	Only if soiling is likely to occur	Wear on entering the room	Only if soiling is likely to occur	Only if soiling is likely to occur
Face mask	• Assess risk • Surgical mask used when aerosol-generating procedures are done	• Assess risk • Surgical mask used when aerosol-generating procedures are done	Wear surgical mask	Use N95 or FFP2 (high-efficiency filtration mask) on room entry
Eye protection	Use if splashes or aerosols are likely	Use if splashes or aerosols are likely	Use if splashes or aerosols are likely	Use if splashes or aerosols are likely
Additional remarks	If PPE used, it is to be removed after procedure followed by hand hygiene	Remove gloves and gown, hand hygiene before leaving room	Cough etiquette to be followed by patient. If cohorting is used provide separation of >3 feet between patients	Cough etiquette to be followed by patient

(PPE: personal protective equipment; RSV: respiratory syncytial virus; SARS: severe acute respiratory syndrome; VZV: varicella zoster virus)

Appropriate sterilization/decontamination of equipment and environmental cleaning and disinfection are applicable to all situations.

Respiratory Viral Infections

It is advisable to follow standard precautions with contact and droplet precautions initially.

Influenza

In addition to standard precautions such as HH, use of gloves and gown for patient care activity, adherence to droplet precautions too is necessary. All aerosol-generating procedures performed on patients such as endotracheal intubation, cardiopulmonary resuscitation (CPR), bronchoscopy, chest physiotherapy, and suctioning necessitate adoption of airborne precautions (use of appropriate PPE and N95 mask) in a negative pressure airborne infection isolation room. Patients should wear face mask and follow respiratory hygiene, cough etiquette, and HH. As per Centers for Disease Control and Prevention (CDC) recommendation, airborne precautions also need to be followed, when there is an ongoing pandemic influenza due to a novel strain. Precautions for other respiratory viral pathogens are given in **Table 2**.

Viral Diarrhea/Gastroenteritis

While dealing with patients with probable viral diarrhea (Rotavirus/Norovirus), it is preferred to wash hands with soap and water rather than use alcohol hand rub. In general, for viral gastroenteritis cases, standard with contact precautions are to be followed. Isolation of patients until 48–72 hours after symptoms have subsided is advisable **(Table 3)**.

Blood-borne Viral Infections

HIV, Hepatitis B, and Hepatitis C: Strict adherence to standard precautions including HH; use of PPE such as gloves, mask, and gown depending on the risk of exposure; safe use and disposal of sharps in puncture-proof containers; and prompt clearing of blood and body fluid spillage is mandatory to avoid transmission **(Table 4)**. Vaccination with Hepatitis B and ensuring adequate protective immunity are crucial. Prompt appropriate postexposure prophylaxis in indicated cases reduces the risk of transmission following exposure in HIV and Hepatitis B.

HIV Prevention from Mother to Child

Prevention of mother to child transmission of HIV infection by administering ART to the child for 6–12 weeks

Table 2: Precautions for respiratory viral pathogens.

Agents	Precautions	Remarks
Rhinovirus (common cold)	Standard + Droplet	Contact precautions to be added in young infants and when copious secretions are present
Influenza	Standard + Droplet + Contact	As per CDC recommendation, additional airborne precautions to be used when aerosol-generating procedures are performed or when there is an ongoing pandemic influenza due to a novel strain
Respiratory syncytial virus, para influenza virus, and *human metapneumovirus*	Standard + Contact	To be followed for the duration of illness
Severe acute respiratory syndrome (SARS)	Standard + Contact + Airborne	To be followed for 10 days after resolution of fever with improvement in respiratory symptoms
Adenovirus pneumonia	Standard + Droplet + Contact	

(CDC: centers for disease control and prevention)

Table 3: Precautions for viral diarrheal pathogens.

Aetiological agents	Precautions	Remarks
Rotavirus	Standard + Contact	Contact precautions are essential (virus is shed for up to a week after symptom onset)
Norovirus	Standard + Contact	• Contact precautions to be followed for a period of 48 hours after resolution of symptoms as virus shedding may continue • To wear mask while dealing with feces/vomitus as aerosolization is likely • Hypochlorite solution is essential for environmental cleaning
Adenovirus and other agents	Standard precautions	Contact precautions also in diapered and incontinent for the duration of illness
Enterovirus	Standard + Contact	

Table 4: Precautions for blood-borne viral infections.

Agent	Precautions	Remarks
HIV	Standard	No additional precautions are necessary
Hepatitis B virus	Standard	No additional precautions are necessary
Hepatitis C virus	Standard	No additional precautions are necessary

(HIV: human immunodeficiency virus)

and lifelong to the mother has been one of the biggest success stories of the last decade. Oral nevirapine is the drug of choice for the baby and is given for 12 weeks if the mother has not received at least 6 months of ART and has chosen to breastfeed the baby. Exclusive breastfeeding is the method of choice and prevention of mixed feeding is of paramount importance. Cesarian sections are performed only in case of obstetric indications. The other prongs of HIV prevention include prevention of unwanted pregnancies and screening of all pregnant mothers.

Prevention of Perinatal Transmission of Hepatitis B Infection

The birth dose of hepatitis B vaccine is administered within 24 hours of delivery to all newborn babies. This helps in prevention of infection from infected mothers, and is especially important since the risk of chronic infection and its consequences approaches 90% with perinatal transmission. In case of HBsAg positive mothers, the baby is given 0.5 mL of hepatitis B immunoglobulin along with the vaccine at a different site. This is ineffective if delayed beyond 7 days. The preferred schedule for vaccinating a baby born to a hepatitis B positive mother is 0, 1 and 6 months. If HBIG is unavailable, the vaccine may be given at 0, 1, 2 and 9 to 12 months.

Postexposure prophylaxis for Hepatitis B virus:
- For individuals who are vaccinated: Three doses
- Previously vaccinated and known responder with hepatitis B surface antibody (anti-HBs) levels ≥10 mIU/mL: No treatment

For individuals who are vaccinated but antibody response unknown:

Look for anti-HBs titer. If ≥10 mIU/mL: No action needed

If it is <10 mIU/L
- Administer both hepatitis B immunoglobulin (HBIg) (0.06 mL/kg) and vaccine, preferably within 12 hours
- The vaccine dose given at the same time but at a different site and complete the vaccine schedule.

If still undergoing vaccination/incomplete vaccination
- HBIg ×1 dose and complete series
- (HBIg dose 0.06 mL/kg intramuscularly)

Table 5: Precautions for common viral infections.

Viral infection	Precautions followed	Comments
Hepatitis A and E	Standard precautions	Additional contact precautions if diapered/incontinent
Dengue and other arthropod-borne viruses	Standard precautions	
Varicella zoster	Standard + Airborne + Contact	To be followed until lesions are dry and crusted. Airborne precautions are mandatory if its an immunocompromised host or disseminated disease in any patient
Measles	Standard + Airborne	
Polio	Standard + Contact	Precautions to be followed throughout the duration of illness
Rabies	Standard + Contact	
CMV and Epstein-Barr virus	Standard	
Congenital rubella	Standard + Contact	
Acute viral ocular infection (acute hemorrhagic)	Standard + Contact	To be followed for the duration of illness
Viral hemorrhagic fevers/Nipah virus Infection	Standard + Contact + Droplet	HCW to use complete PPE

(CMV: *Cytomegalovirus*; HCW: healthcare worker; PPE: personal protective equipment)

Table 6: Precautions to be followed for deceased bodies based on category of the infectious disease.

Categories	Infections	Body bag	Embalming	Autopsy	Final treatment
1	Rest of the viral infections	No	Allowed	Allowed	Any method
2	HAV/HEV	No	Allowed	Avoid	Cremation advisable
	HIV/HBV/HCV	Yes—one	Not allowed	Avoid	Cremation advisable
3	Nipah/Ebola/Rabies/Viral hemorrhagic fevers	Yes—two	Not allowed	Avoid	Cremation must

(HAV: hepatitis A virus; HBV: hepatitis B virus; HCV: hepatitis C virus; HEV: hepatitis E virus; HIV: human immunodeficiency virus)

Unvaccinated/nonimmune
- HBIg ×1; initiate HBV vaccine series

If previously vaccinated and is a known nonresponder (i.e. after six doses, the anti-HBs < 10 mIU/L)
- Two doses of HBIg 1 month apart.

Viral Hepatitis A and E

Standard with contact precautions if diapered/incontinent **(Table 5)**.

Varicella Zoster Virus Infection

All cases of chickenpox are to be kept in isolation rooms. Airborne precautions and contact precautions must be followed until lesions are dry and crusted.

Measles

Airborne precautions with isolation in negative pressure rooms must ideally be followed for all cases of measles. Also, PPE such as N95 mask need to be used when dealing with measles cases.

Arboviral Hemorrhagic Fever

Dengue fever and other arthropod-borne viral diseases require adherence to standard precautions.

Nipah Virus Infection

As most of the transmission from Nipah-infected patients occur within the healthcare facility, it is important to adhere to strict infection control measures that include standard, contact, and droplet precautions. All cases are to be treated in an isolation facility.

With regard to HH, being biosafety level 4 pathogen use of 70% alcohol with 2% chlorhexidine combination is advisable in high risk areas. A complete set of PPE is to be worn, including N95 mask, shoe cover, and goggles. Donning and Doffing is to be done with utmost care in the sequence recommended by CDC.

Standard infection control precautions need to be followed for all deceased bodies too. Precautions to be followed are based on the category of the infectious disease **(Table 6)**.

■ SUGGESTED READING

1. Bennett JE, Dolin R, Blaser MJ (Eds). Mandell, Douglas and Bennett's Principles and Practices of Infectious Disease, 8th edition. Philadelphia, PA: Elsevier; 2015.
2. Damani N. Manual of Infection Prevention and Control, 4th edition. Oxford: Oxford University Press; 2019.
3. Sastry AS, Deepashree R. Essentials of Hospital Infection Control. Delhi: Jaypee Brothers; 2019.

7

Parasitic and Protozoal Infections/Infestations

Jaydeep Choudhury

ECTOPARASITES

- **Scabies**
  Vijay Kulkarni, Maheshwari

- **Pediculosis, Myiasis, and Leeches**
  Subhasish Bhattacharyya, Mamta Kumari

PROTOZOAN INFECTIONS

- **Malaria**
  Ritabrata Kundu

- **Leishmaniasis (Kala-azar)**
  Nigam Prakash Narain, Rajesh Kumar

- **Ameba, Giardia, and Cryptosporidium**
  Kiranpreet Kaur, Piyush Gupta

- **Naegleria, Acanthamoeba**
  K Dhanalakshmi, Lakshan Raj

HELMINTHIC INFECTIONS

- **Schistosomiasis, Flukes, and Filariasis**
  Rajesh Kumar Meena, Piyush Gupta

- **Soil-transmitted Helminths**
  Shalu Jain, Dheeraj Shah

- **Echinococcosis (Hydatid Disease)**
  Baldev S Prajapati, Rajal B Prajapati

- **Tapeworms and Cysticercosis**
  Narayanappa D, Rujuni HS

7.1 CHAPTER

Scabies

Vijay Kulkarni, Maheshwari

INTRODUCTION

Scabies, a parasitosis, is a contagious skin disease caused by the infestation of mite sarcoptes scabiei var hominis that causes a pruritic skin eruption. It is an obligate human parasite measuring about 300–400 μm. Overcrowding is an important factor in the transmission of scabies and is most common in tropical, humid regions. In developing countries, scabies is commonly seen in the preschool children and adolescents and it decreases in mid-adulthood and increases in the elderly. The hallmark symptom of scabies infestation is pruritus, which can be debilitating. Disruption of the skin's protective barrier function promotes secondary bacterial infections, which can lead to additional, potentially life-threatening, complications.

DISEASE BURDEN

Scabies affects people from every country, accounting for a substantial proportion of skin disease in developing countries. Globally, it is estimated to affect more than 200 million people at any time, although further efforts are needed to assess this burden. Prevalence estimates in the recent scabies-related literature range from 0.2% to 71%. In 2015, it was estimated that the direct effects of scabies infestation on the skin alone led 0.21% of disability-adjusted life-years (DALYs) from all conditions globally.[1] Sambo et al. who mainly studied the prevalence of scabies in school-going children, reported that 55.8% patients were in the age 5–8 years, whereas 44.2% patients were in the age range from 9 years to 12 years. Recognition of scabies on the global health agenda would increase awareness, education, and research into diagnosis, treatment, and prevention. In recognition, WHO recently formally designated scabies as a neglected tropical disease.[2]

SCABIES MITE AND ITS LIFE CYCLE

The scabies mite is an obligate parasite that burrows in the epidermis of human skin, on average, within 30 minutes after the first contact.[3] The adult mite burrows at 0.5–5.0 mm/day into the stratum corneum and deposits feces in its path; female mites also lay eggs.[4] Eggs hatch into larvae within 2–3 days, which then leave the burrow to mature on the skin surface. In 10–11 days, females mature into egg-laying adults.[5] During maturation on the skin surface, larval mite forms are capable of burrowing into the patient's epidermis or moving to a different host. Mites can crawl as fast as 2.5 cm/min on warm skin.[6] The total life span of the adult female is approximately 5 weeks. Adult mites have eight legs, making them easily distinguishable from less mature larval forms, which have six legs.[6] Transmission is by direct skin-to-skin contact. Human scabies mites are capable of surviving in the environment, outside of the human body, for 24–36 hours in normal room conditions (21C and 40–80% relative humidity) and up to 19 days in a cool, humid environment; during this time, they remain capable of infestation.[3] Indirect transmission (via clothing, bedding, and other fomites) has been proposed; however, this has been difficult to prove experimentally.[7] Adult mites use odor and thermotaxis to identify a new host.[8]

CLINICAL PRESENTATION

Scabies can present as three basic presentations: classic, crusted, and nodular.

Classic Scabies

Classic scabies is the most common form, with the most common symptom being severe pruritis. In infants or small children, pruritus is particularly intense during the night and at naptime. Pruritus may be so severe that the child is persistently irritable and even refuses to eat. The nocturnal pruritus is usually intense and characteristic.[9] The reason for the nocturnal pruritus is not known, although increased mite activity with warmer skin temperatures may be an explanation.[10] Other symptoms include fatigue, irritability, and, in some children, fever from secondary impetigo or cellulitis. The mite density in classic scabies is usually low, with an average of 10–12 mites during the first 3 months of infestation.[11,12] The classic sign of scabies is the burrow, a serpiginous gray line in the skin formed by the digestive properties of secretions from the advancing mite.[13] Classical scabies affects the anterior axillary folds, nipple area, periumbilical skin, elbows, volar surface of the wrists, interdigital web spaces, thighs, buttocks, penis, scrotum, and ankles. This is referred to as the circle of Hebra.[14] In infants and young children, the palms, soles, and head (face, neck, and scalp) are more commonly involved.[15] Burrows may not be present in tropical climates and are not a requisite in children as burrows often are obliterated by bathing, scratching, crust formation, or superinfection.[4] Hypersensitivity of both immediate and delayed types has been implicated in the development of lesions other than burrows.[16]

Crusted Scabies

Crusted scabies occurs more commonly in immuno-compromised patients, such as those on long-term immunosuppressive therapy (i.e. organ transplant recipients) or those with human immunodeficiency virus (HIV) or human T-lymphotropic virus type 1 infection. Other susceptible groups are intellectually or physically handicapped patients, such as those who have paralyzed limbs, sensory neuropathy, or leprosy, because they may be unable to feel the itch or to scratch.[17] An older and now disfavored term for crusted scabies is "Norwegian scabies," a reference to affected Norwegian patients with leprosy. Crusted scabies can present in a generalized or focal manner, with manifestations limited to the scalp, face, nails, or soles. But about 50% of patients who develop crusted scabies report only mild pruritus or none at all.[18] Progression from classic scabies is uncommon. Clinically, crusted scabies presents as a hyperkeratotic dermatosis, typically involving the palms and soles, often with deep skin fissures. Generalized lymphadenopathy, peripheral blood eosinophilia,[19] and raised serum immunoglobulin E (IgE) levels[20] are frequently observed, and secondary bacterial infection is common and associated with a significant mortality.

The parasite burden in crusted scabies is much greater and can range from thousands to millions per patient.

Hence, it is more infectious since eradicating the mite and egg burden from heavily crusted areas of the skin is difficult. One study found that up to 4,700 mites per gram of skin were counted in skin shed from hyperkeratotic patients, suggesting that crusted scabies predisposes contacts of the patient to infection through infested fomites in addition to direct contact.[21]

Nodular Scabies

Nodular scabies is an uncommon form and is characterized by extremely pruritic reddish-brown nodules up to 2 cm in size that are typically found on the genitalia, buttocks, groin, and axillae. Nodules are considered to be the result of hypersensitivity reactions to mite products because mites almost never are identified in these lesions. Nodular scabies can create a treatment dilemma because nodules can persist for weeks after treatment and may require corticosteroid injections.[18] Often, patients will demand repeat therapy with scabicides, and overly aggressive repeat therapy must be tempered with reassurance that the nodules eventually will resolve with appropriate anti-inflammatory therapy.

◼ MODE OF TRANSMISSION

The incubation period before symptoms occur is 3–6 weeks in cases of primary infestation, but as little as 1–2 days in cases of reinfestation.[12] This clinically latent period is responsible for undetected transmission and is thought to be due to delayed type IV hypersensitivity reaction against mites and mite products.[18] The histologic examination of scabies lesions shows inflammatory cell infiltrates composed of eosinophils, lymphocytes, and histiocytes confirming the cell-mediated response.[22] Scabies theoretically can be contracted by the transfer of eggs, larvae, or mature mites to the skin of the new host; however, mature mites are the most likely culprits. Early studies by Mellanby[11] demonstrated that direct body contact was the predominant route for scabies transmission, and the number of scabies mites is directly proportional to risk of transmission. Transmission among family members is most common, supported by evidence from molecular studies that show that the genotype of mites from household members is more homogeneous than the genotypes of mites from separate households within a community.[21]

◼ COMPLICATIONS

The morbidity associated with scabies is frequently underestimated when considering the impact of the disease. The intense pruritis which causes discomfort and loss of sleep can become secondarily infected due to bacterial entry into excoriated skin. Sometimes, the mites itself can transmit bacteria like *Staphylococcus aureus* and nephritogenic strains of group A *Streptococcus*. These bacteria have been isolated from mites and fecal pellets.[23] This can lead to furuncle, impetigo, or cellulitis which can progress to acute poststreptococcal glomerulonephritis and rheumatic heart disease. Such conditions will require treatment with topical or systemic antibacterial agents.

Postscabies pruritis due to the hypersensitivity to mites and mite products can last for days to weeks after the primary infestation. This should not be confused with treatment failure leading to overprescribing scabicidal medication. Oral antihistamines or corticosteroids, and a trial of phototherapy may be warranted in resistant cases of postscabies pruritis.[24]

Serious psychological and emotional distress in some patients, including feelings of shame, guilt, and persistent delusions of parasitosis, are also seen in some.[24] Educating the patients and the family about the disease can help alleviate the fear and improve the compliance with treatment.

DIFFERENTIAL DIAGNOSIS

Almost all pruritic dermatoses must be considered in the differential diagnosis. Various infections, arthropod assault, bullous dermatoses, and cutaneous lymphoproliferative disorders can all mimic scabies. Of note, scabies can present like bullous pemphigoid, having bullae associated with eosinophils and a positive direct immunofluorescence.[25]

Scabies in children is often missed until close contacts present with similar symptoms. Typical and atypical scabies skin lesions are found more often in areas of the body that are historically spared in adults, including the scalp, face, palms, soles, and intertriginous areas.[8,11] In such cases, scabies can be easily confused with atopic dermatitis or infantile acropustulosis. Several case reports document misdiagnosis of scabies as Langerhans cell histiocytosis.

The potential for misdiagnosis in pediatric patients can lead to inappropriate long-term application of potent topical corticosteroids, which predisposes these already vulnerable populations to more severe forms of the disease, including crusted scabies. Long-term corticosteroid use can also affect the presentation of routine scabies, with vesicles, pustules, and nodules predominating over classic skin lesions.

DIAGNOSIS

Scabies is one of the easiest and yet most difficult diagnoses in dermatology. Epidemiological history, occurrence of itching, distribution of the lesions, and pruritus form the basis of the diagnosis. Scabies can be diagnosed by a variety of methods: potassium hydroxide (KOH) scraping of a burrow, dermoscopy, magnification of digital photography, and skin biopsy. The gold standard involves direct visualization of the mite or its eggs. Direct visualization can be achieved by KOH preparation of a skin scraping taken from a burrow or biopsy of a burrow demonstrating a mite. After scraping the skin, the sample is suspended in mineral oil or saline. The presence of the mite or egg casings under microscopy is considered to be the diagnostic criteria. KOH testing provides excellent specificity (few false-positives) but low sensitivity (many false-negatives) because of the small number of parasites found in a typical host who has classic scabies.[22] As the specimen debris can look like the scybala, it alone is not considered diagnostic. Biopsy showing only perivascular inflammatory cell infiltrates with numerous eosinophils, edema, and epidermal spongiosis is merely suggestive and not definitive.[26]

Dermoscopy was initially used for the diagnosis of skin tumors. Nowadays, it has gained popularity in the use of infectious and inflammatory skin disorders. It is less time-consuming and is more acceptable to patients than skin scrapings. It can be used to replace skin scrapings as it allows a quick screening of a large number of sites. Apart from that, it can also be used in therapeutic trials to select the site in patients where skin scrapings can be done. Dermoscopy has been found to be useful for the diagnosis of scabies incognito.[27] Closer examination with a handheld dermatoscope allows better visualization of the curvilinear scaly burrow, and the mite itself may be seen at the end of the burrow as a dark triangular structure, corresponding to the pigmented head and anterior legs of the scabies mite. This picture is often referred to as a "jet with contrail." Dermoscopy and magnification of high-resolution digital photography are good diagnostic methods, albeit less definitive than visualizing a mite on KOH preparation or biopsy. Also, the high cost of the dermatoscope is a disadvantage.

Alternative methods of diagnosis include the burrow ink test (BIT), in which suspicious papules are marked with ink and then wiped off with an alcohol pad to remove the surface ink from the lesion. A positive BIT result occurs when the ink tracks down the mite burrow, forming a characteristic dark, zig-zag gedline that is readily apparent to the naked eye. This test is useful if one does not have a digital camera, microscope, dermatoscope, or skin biopsy capabilities. Epiluminescence microscopy ("jet-with-contrail" pattern) and high-resolution video dermatoscopy are newer, noninvasive techniques that allow inspection of the skin *in vivo* from the surface to the superficial papillary dermis.[22] More advanced tests, such as polymerase chain reaction antigen detection, intradermal skin test, and enzyme linked immunosorbent assay antibody detection, are in progress.[22]

PRINCIPLES OF TREATMENT

The treatment of scabies is as important as making a correct diagnosis. The mainstay of treatment is topical scabicidal agents. Certain principles have to be followed to treat patients successfully. The choice of scabies treatment is based on effectiveness, potential toxicity, type of disease, and patient's age. An ideal scabicide should be effective against adult and egg, easily applicable, nonsensitizing, nonirritating, nontoxic, and economical; it should also be applicable in all ages.

General principles for treatment of scabies:

- Establish your diagnosis.
- Choose an appropriate medication.
- Treat the whole body from neck to toes in adults and head and face in babies.
- Treat all the contacts.
- Give a detailed verbal and written prescription.
- Fingernails should be cut and subungual debris should be cleaned.
- Treat secondary infection if present.
- Avoid over-treatment.
- Have a follow-up at 1 and 4 weeks after treatment.
- Launder clothing and bedding after completing treatment.

Patients should be properly instructed about the method of using the scabicide **(Box 1)**.

It is important to remember that pruritus can persist for up to 4 weeks after successful treatment as a result of hypersensitivity reactions and can be treated with antihistamines and anti-inflammatory agents, such as medium-potency topical corticosteroids. In the case of crusted scabies, crusts can harbor thousands of mites. Keratolytics should be added to the treatment regimen until the hyperkeratosis has resolved. Typically, cases of crusted scabies require more cycles of retreatment than classic scabies. When treating fomites and the home environment, all clothing, bedding, and towels can be decontaminated by drying them at 60°C for 10 minutes;

washing is not necessary.[6] Vacuuming the floors of the bedroom and bathroom, as well as heavily used couches and chairs, is prudent in all cases and integral in cases of crusted scabies.

PHARMACOTHERAPY IN SCABIES

Scabicidal drugs can be broadly divided into topical agents and oral agents **(Box 2)**.

Permethrin

Permethrin is a synthetic pyrethroid and potent insecticide. Permethrin is absorbed cutaneously only in small amounts, rapidly metabolized by skin esterases, and excreted in urine. Permethrin 5% cream is accepted as the current gold standard for scabies treatment because of an efficacy of 90% in most studies from the past two decades[23,28] and an excellent safety profile. Permethrin is labeled for application to the entire body for 8–12 hours, usually right before bedtime. In addition to its superior efficacy, permethrin also has an excellent safety profile. Permethrin is indicated and is safe for use in newborns, young children, and pregnant (category B)

Box 1: Instructions for the treatment of scabies.

Scabies is caused by itch mite and it can be easily cured if the following instructions are followed carefully:

- Start with a warm bath and dry thoroughly afterward.
- The medication provided should be rubbed into the skin. All parts of the body from chin downwards, whether involved or uninvolved, should be treated.
- Treatment is best done at night before going to bed.
- Avoid touching your mouth or eyes with your hands.
- If hands are washed before the typically recommended 8-hour application time, the topical agent should be reapplied to the hands.
- Change your underclothing and sheets the next day and launder them.
- You may itch for few days but do not repeat the treatment.
- Everyone in the house should be treated at the same time.
- Report to your doctor after 1 week.
- Modified from Alexander's Arthropods and Skin2

Box 2: Antiscabietic drugs.

Topical agents
- Permethrin 5% cream
- Lindane (gamma benzene hexachloride) 1% lotion or cream
- Benzyl benzoate 10% and 25% lotion or emulsion
- Malathion 0.5% lotion
- Monosulfiram 25% lotion
- Crotamiton 10% cream
- Precipitated sulfur 2–10% ointment
- Esdepallethrine 0.63% aerosol
- Ivermectin 0.8% lotion

Oral drug: Ivermectin

and lactating women.[24] The limiting factor in the use of permethrin is its cost as it is the most expensive of all the topical scabicides.

Malathion

In the United Kingdom, malathion is approved for scabies and is available over the counter. Malathion requires two applications 7 days apart.[29] Because malathion is available as a runny lotion, it may be more appropriate than scabicidal cream for treatment of hairy areas of the body, such as the scalp. Adverse effects of malathion include occasional skin irritation and conjunctivitis with eye contact.

Crotamiton

Crotamiton (crotonyl-N-ethyl-o-toluidine) is used as 10% cream or lotion. The best results have been obtained when applied twice daily for 5 consecutive days after bathing and changing clothes.[30] Safety for the use of crotamiton in newborns and infants has not been well established. Potential adverse effects from crotamiton cream include erythema and conjunctivitis. In addition, high-resistance rates have been reported after a single application of 8–12 hours.

Lindane

Lindane acts on the central nervous system of insects and leads to increased excitability, convulsions, and death. It is absorbed through all portals of entry including the lung mucosa, intestinal mucosa, and other mucous membranes and it is distributed to all body compartments with the highest concentration in lipid-rich tissue and the skin. It is metabolized and excreted in urine and feces. Lindane 1% cream or lotion has been found to be very effective in the treatment. Its use is greatly limited by safety concerns regarding its potential neurotoxicity. The spectrum of serious neurologic adverse effects includes irritability, vertigo, seizures, vomiting, diarrhea, and syncope.[18]

Benzyl Benzoate

Benzyl benzoate is a scabicide used alone or in combination with topical sulfiram. It is labeled for use in adults and in a diluted form for children, infants, and breastfeeding mothers.[18] Benzyl benzoate should be washed off within 24 hours after application because it is a known irritant that can cause contact dermatitis.[16] In developing countries where the resources are limited, it is used in the management of scabies as a cheaper alternative.

Ivermectin

Ivermectin acts via the suppression of conduction of nerve impulses in the nerve–muscle synapses of insects by stimulation of glutamate gamma-aminobutyric acid (GABA) from presynaptic nerve endings and enhancement of binding to postsynaptic receptors. One or two doses of ivermectin (200 mg/kg, 3–9 days apart) produced cure rates equivalent to treatment with conventional topical medications (benzyl benzoate, lindane, and permethrin) for classic scabies.[18] A single dose of ivermectin yielded a 70% cure rate, which increased to 95% with a second dose at 2 weeks.[31] The temporal and additive nature of this clinical response suggests that ivermectin may lack ovicidal properties and thus may not be effective during all stages of the mite lifecycle. Based on its route of administration, ivermectin holds the greatest potential for treating scabies in the context of epidemic or endemic outbreaks. Therapy with a tablet is relatively quick and efficient and virtually guarantees whole-body exposure. Hence, ivermectin has also been efficacious for the treatment of severe crusted scabies in older children, usually when given in multiple doses and in combination with topical permethrin.[18] Adverse effects of ivermectin include hepatotoxicity, tachycardia, and hypotension. It is also not indicated during pregnancy, lactation, and in children less than 5 years of age.

■ CLINICAL CONTEXTS

For a case of classic scabies in the outpatient setting, treatment is targeted toward the source patient and any close contacts, whether or not contacts exhibit symptoms (in light of the clinically latent period that can last up to 6 weeks). Because the commonly used topical scabicides are essentially innocuous, it is not necessary to examine close contacts before prescribing topical therapy.

Crusted scabies needs prolonged and persistent treatment. Oral ivermectin is effective but multiple doses plus topical agents may be required. The hyperkeratosis is treated with a keratolytic agent (5–10% salicylic acid in petrolatum). Nails are cut short and brushed with a scabicidal agent. A cure is obtained after a mean treatment of 3 weeks. Nodular scabies is treated with antiscabitics followed by intralesional steroids. A patient with classic scabies from an institutional setting must be put on contact isolation and all close contacts must be informed, educated about the delayed onset of symptoms, and offered treatment. Close contacts may be defined as those who have extended, nongloved physical contact, including visitors, doctors, phlebotomy, and radiology technicians, nurses, and other patients residing in the same room.

Causes of Treatment Failure

The treatment of scabies can fail because of various reasons:

- *Improper application*: The drug should be applied from the neck downward all over the body. The most common mistake is that the drug is applied only to the affected areas, which leads to a relapse of the disease.
- *Inadequate application*: The drug dispensed should be used and it should not be diluted. When drugs such as lindane are diluted, their efficacy is reduced.
- *Reinfestation*: Reinfestation is a common problem and it occurs because of failure to treat contacts. It can be avoided if the instructions are clearly followed.
- *Resistance*: Resistance has been reported with drugs such as lindane, permethrin, and crotamiton. Resistance to permethrin is very rare and only isolated reports exist. In such areas, the combination of lindane and benzyl benzoate or permethrin can be used. Resistance should be considered only if all the other causes for treatment failure are ruled out.

■ REFERENCES

1. Karimkhani C, Colombara DV, Drucker AM, et al. The global burden of scabies: a cross-sectional analysis from the Global Burden of Disease Study 2015. Lancet Infect Dis. 2017;17(12): 1247-54.
2. Engelman D, Fuller LC, Solomon AW, et al. Opportunities for integrated Control of Neglected Tropical Diseases that affect the Skin. Trends Parasitol. 2016;32(11):843-54.
3. Walton SF, Holt DC, Currie BJ, et al. Scabies: new future for a neglected disease. Adv Parasitol. 2004;57:309-76.
4. Heukelbach J, Feldmeier H. Scabies. Lancet. 2006;367(9524): 1767-74.
5. Arlian LG, Vyszenski-Moher DL. Life cycle of Sarcoptes scabiei var. canis. J Parasitol. 1988;74(3):427–30.
6. Arlian LG. Biology, host relations, and epidemiology of Sarcoptes scabiei. Annu Rev Entomol. 1989;34:139-61.
7. Mellanby K. Transmission of Scabies. Br Med J. 1941; 2(4211): 405-6.
8. Meinking T. Infestations. Curr Probl Dermatol. 1999;11(3): 73-120.
9. Shacter B. Treatment of scabies and pediculosis with lindane preparations: an evaluation. J Am Acad Dermatol. 1981;5(5): 517-27.
10. Pramanik AK, Hansen RC. Transcutaneous gamma benzene hexachloride absorption and toxicity in infants and children. Arch Dermatol. 1979;115(10):1224-5.
11. Mellanby K. Biology of the parasite. In: Orkin M, Maibach HI (Eds). Cutaneous Infestations and Insect Bites. New York: Marcel Dekker; 1985. pp. 9-18.
12. McCarthy JS, Kemp DJ, Walton SF, et al. Scabies: more than just an irritation. Postgrad Med J. 2004;80(945):382-7.
13. Burgess IF. Human lice and their management. Adv Parasitol. 1995;36:271-342.
14. Hicks MI, Elston DM. Scabies. Dermatol Ther. 2009;22(4): 279-92.
15. Heukelbach J, Wilcke T, Winter B, et al. Epidemiology and morbidity of scabies and pediculosis capitis in resource-poor communities in Brazil. Br J Dermatol. 2005;153(1):150-6.
16. Chosidow O. Scabies and pediculosis. Lancet. 2000;355(9206): 818-26.
17. Cargill CF, Pointon AM, Davies PR, et al. Using slaughter inspections to evaluate sarcoptic mange infestation of finishing swine. Vet Parasitol. 1997;70(1-3):191-200.
18. Hengge UR, Currie BJ, Jäger G, et al. Scabies: a ubiquitous neglected skin disease. Lancet Infect Dis. 2006;6(12):769-79.
19. Sluzevich JC, Sheth AP, Lucky AW. Persistent eosinophilia as a presenting sign of scabies in patients with disorders of keratinization. Arch Dermatol. 2007;143(5):670-3.
20. Arlian LG, Morgan MS, Estes SA, et al. Circulating IgE in patients with ordinary and crusted scabies. J Med Entomol. 2004;41(1):74-7.
21. Walton SF, McBroom J, Mathews JD, et al. Crusted scabies: A molecular analysis of Sarcoptes scabiei variety hominis populations from patients with repeated infestations. Clin Infect Dis. 1999;29(5):1226-30.
22. Walton SF, Currie BJ. Problems in diagnosing scabies, a global disease in human and animal populations. Clin Microbiol Rev. 2007;20(2):268-79.
23. Burgess I. Sarcoptes scabiei and scabies. Adv Parasitol. 1994;33:235-92.
24. Chouela E, Abeldaño A, Pellerano G, et al. Diagnosis and treatment of scabies: a practical guide. Am J Clin Dermatol. 2002;3(1):9-18.
25. Balighi K, Robati RM, Hejazi N. A dilemma: bullous-pemphigoid-like eruption in scabies or scabies-induced bullous pemphigoid. Dermatol Online J. 2006;12(4):13.
26. Falk ES, Bolle R. IgE antibodies to house dust mite in patients with scabies. Br J Dermatol. 1980;103(3):283-8.
27. Park JH, Kim CW, Kim SS. The diagnostic accuracy of dermoscopy for scabies. Ann Dermatol. 2012;24(2):194-9.
28. Zargari O, Golchai J, Sobhani A, et al. Comparison of the efficacy of topical 1% lindane vs 5% permethrin in scabies: a randomized, double-blind study. Indian J Dermatol Venereol Leprol. 2006;72(1):33-6.
29. Derbac M. Liquid [package insert]. Manchester, United Kingdom: SSL International; 2008.
30. Konstantinov D, Stanoeva L, Yawalkar SJ. Crotamiton cream and lotion in the treatment of infants with scabies. J Int Med Res. 1979;7(5):443-8.
31. Usha V, Gopalakrishnan Nair TV. A comparative study of oral ivermectin and topical permethrin cream in the treatment of scabies. J Am Acad Dermatol. 2000;42(2 Pt 1):236-40.

7.2 CHAPTER — Pediculosis, Myiasis, and Leeches

Subhasish Bhattacharyya, Mamta Kumari

PEDICULOSIS

Introduction

Lice are ectoparasites and belong to the arthropods of order Anoplura (sucking lice). Three species of louse are parasite to human—*Pediculus capitis* (head louse), *Pediculus humanus* (body louse), and *Pthirus pubis* (crab or pubic louse) **(Figs. 1A to C)**. Lice cannot fly; transmission is by human-to-human close contact. Lice spread readily and host response offers no protection against reinfestation. The lice saliva causes an intensely irritating maculopapular or urticarial rash. Although most infestations are merely bothersome, lice can act as a vector for disease such as epidemic typhus, trench fever, and louse-borne relapsing fever. Secondary infections with *Staphylococcus* or *Streptococcus* can enter through skin sores that result from scratching. Treatment can be pharmacological (topical or oral) or nonpharmacological. Resistance to chemical pediculicides is widespread, like knockdown resistance to permethrin and pyrethroid which is related to a double gene mutation and glutathione-S-transferase-based resistance respectively.

Life Cycle of Louse

Three species have a similar life cycle comprising eggs, nymphs, and adults. Female head pubic lice cement their eggs on hair and body lice on clothing. A fertilized female louse lays eggs which hatch in 7–9 days. The hatchling molts their exoskeleton three times in a 7–10-day period to develop into a mature adult which survives approximately 10 days. Each female may lay 50–300 eggs. The empty egg, also known as nit, may remain attached for months. Head lice can survive for about 24 hours outside the scalp.

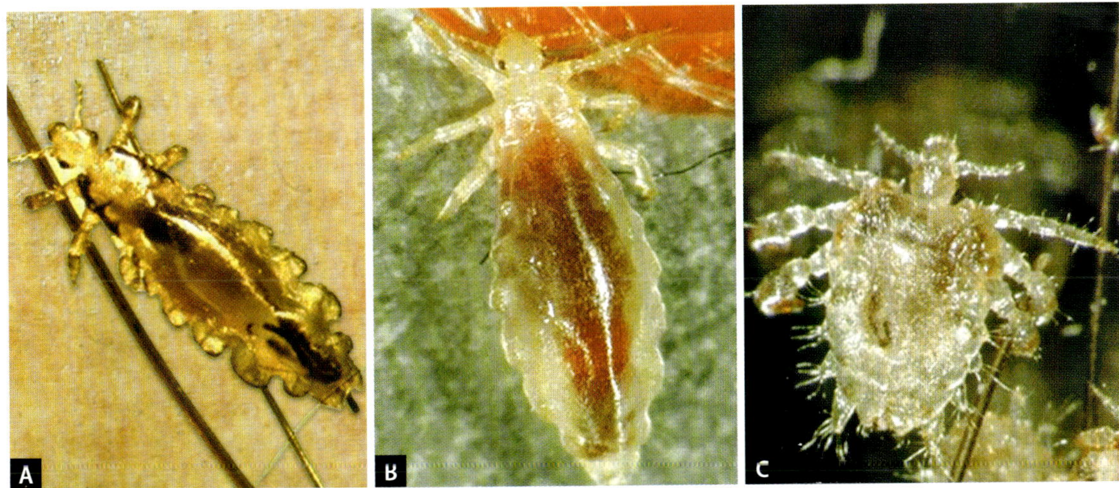

Figs. 1A to C: All types of lice. (A) Head lice, (B) body lice, and (C) pubic lice.
Source: Infectious Agent Surveillance Report. Lice infesting humans and louse-borne diseases. 2010;31:348-9.

Transmission

For all three types, transmission is through close contact with an infected person. Head lice are spread by fomites and head-to-head contact. Body lice are transmitted by direct contact and by sharing of bed and clothing. Pubic lice are usually transmitted during sexual contact but nonsexual transmission can occur and there is some evidence that fomites play a role.

Diagnosis

It is dependent on visual identification of at least one adult louse with detection of viable eggs on the hair shafts. Empty egg cases attached to hair shaft are not diagnostic of an active infection and it is important not to confuse live lice or nits with dandruff (seborrheic dermatitis), piedra, psoriasis, hair cast, or other debris **(Table 1)**.

Pediculosis Humanus var Capitis (Head Louse)

Head lice are dirty white to greyish-black in color. It is the most common form of lice to affect children. Translucent 0.5 mm eggs are laid near the proximal portion of hair shaft and become adherent to one side of the shaft. They can survive for 6–24 hours away from the human host, dying of dehydration at a rate dependent on the relative ambient humidity.

Epidemiology

Head lice infestation occurs throughout the world and affects population in every stratum of society. Children aged 3–11 years are most frequently affected with girls twice as likely to be infested probably as a result of social behavior (e.g. closer physical contact, sharing of hair accessories). Sociodemographic status and seasonality do not appear to affect prevalence. Head lice rarely infest Africans and Americans, and this is possibly related to the diameter, shape, or twisted nature of their hair shaft (which makes grasping of the shaft more difficult for the louse). Head lice are not a sign of poor hygiene; all socioeconomic groups are affected. Head lice are not a health hazard because they are not responsible for the spread of any disease.

Clinical Features

Pruritus is the most common symptom of infestation but many children are asymptomatic. Adult lice or eggs (nits) are found in the hair, usually near the nape of the neck and behind the ears. Lice deposit eggs on a hair shaft 3–4 mm from scalp skin. The duration of infestation can be estimated by the distance of nit from scalp as the rate of hair growth is approximately 1 cm per month. After a louse pierces the skin, a toxic salivary secretion is exuded resulting in pruritic dermatitis. Secondary pyoderma after trauma from scratching may result in matting together of the hair and posterior cervical and occipital lymphadenopathy. Rarely glomerulonephritis may occur as a consequence of Group A *Streptococcus* superinfection of the skin. Persistent infestation can lead to poor performance, secondary to sleep disturbance, and difficulty in concentration.

Pediculus Humanis (Body Louse)

The adult is greyish-white, reddish, or cream in color with thinner antennae, better developed abdominal muscle than the head louse. Females lay their nits in the seams or hems of clothes (especially underwear) that are adjacent to the surface of the skin. They feed only when the host is resting or sleeping. Unfed body lice rarely survive longer than 10 days, while those who have fed may survive in most clothing for 30–40 days away from the host.

Epidemiology

Body lice infestation is found worldwide, but generally limited to a person who lives in a crowded condition, owns just one set of clothes, and does not have access to hot water for regular bathing and laundering of clothes (refugees, victims of war or natural disasters, homeless people). Under these conditions, body lice can spread rapidly through direct contact or contact with contaminated clothing or bedding.

Table 1: Differential diagnosis of nits.	
Differential diagnosis	*Points in favors*
Nits	Firmly adhere to hair shaft and not easily removed with fingers
Seborrheic dermatitis	Diffuse scalp scaling with erythema. Scales occasionally adhere to hair but easy to remove from hair shaft
Hair cast	It is keratin protein that encircles hair shaft which can be easily removed
Piedra	It is fungal infection of the hair. Firm nodules attached to hair shaft which may be white or black in color
Psoriasis	Thick silvery scales, overlying red plaques on the scalp are often present

Clinical Features

The primary lesion is a small, intensely pruritic, red macular or papule with a central hemorrhagic punctum located on shoulder, trunks, or buttocks. Additional lesion includes excoriation, wheal, and eczematous, secondarily infected plaques. Massive infestation may be associated with constitutional symptoms of fever, malaise, and headache. Chronic infestation may lead to postinflammatory hyperpigmentation and thickening of the skin known as "vagabond's disease" and parasitic melanoderma which manifest as lichenified, scaling hyperpigmented plaques, most commonly on trunks.

Body lice are known vectors of epidemic or louse-borne typhus (*Rickettsia prowazekii*), trench fever (*Bartonella quintana*), and louse-borne relapsing fever (*Borrelia recurrentis*). Since 1995, louse-borne disease has had emergence and trench fever has been diagnosed in many developed and developing countries. The body louse has demonstrated the true vector of trench fever by using polymerase chain reaction to detect within them the *B. quintana* DNA (deoxyribonucleic acid) from the infected patient. Detection of rickettsial DNA in the body lice has confirmed the presence of typhus.

Phthirus Pubis (Crab or Pubic Lice)

Pubic lice are grey in color and their nits are oval, opalescent 0.5–0.8 mm in size and glued firmly to hair. Pubic lice most commonly infest pubic and perianal hair, but can be found in the hair of beard, moustache, eyelashes, armpits, chest, and abdomen. Maculae cerulea, similar to those seen in body louse infestation, can be found. Pubic lice are associated with but do not cause other sexually transmitted infections (STIs).

Epidemiology

Pubic louse infestation is common in adolescents and young adults. Infestation rates of around 2% are usually cited. Infestation in children can be indicative of sexual abuse. Infestation is uncommon in older age. Pubic louse can also be transferred by contaminated towels and shared cloths. Adolescents with pubic lice are twice as likely to have chlamydial or gonococcal infection as uninfested adolescents. An infested adolescent should be screened for STIs including chlamydia, gonorrhea, HIV (human immunodeficiency virus), hepatitis B, and syphilis.

Clinical Features

Puncture sites are red with swelling in the immediate area. Intense itching is common but is delayed until approximately 4 weeks after the initial infestation. A characteristic macule of 3 mm diameter with grey-blue pigmentation (maculae cerulae) appears at the site of bite, mainly over abdomen and thigh. This is thought to result from altered human blood pigments or a reaction to substance excreted in louse saliva. Underwear commonly is stained with bloody louse excrement. Pubic lice do not transmit disease, but excoriation and secondary infection can occur in those with symptoms. Many hairy areas of the body can be infested, i.e. eyebrows, beard, axilla, eyelashes, and perianal area. Blepharoconjunctivitis may be the presenting sign of the involvement of eyelashes.

Treatment of All Types of Lice

Head Lice

Shaving of head and pubic parasitized hair will eradicate head and pubic lice but it is not cosmetically acceptable. Mechanical removal by wet combing is labor intensive.

A systemic review (1995) concluded that sufficient evidence existed only for the use of pyrethroid insecticide (louse neurotoxin) as a 1% permethrin cream rinse. It acts on voltage-gated sodium channel resulting in paralysis (knockdown) and death. Knockdown resistance is widespread and identified by lack of initial immobilization which may cross over to other pyrethroids. This is biodegradable and generally a very safe product and remains the recommended first-line therapy. It should be applied to wet hair and left in the place for about 10 minutes before rinsing. Because of the variable reports of head lice resistance to 1% permethrin, the current recommendation is two treatment application 7–14 days apart or even three treatment 0, 7, 15 days based on the life cycle of head lice. Some success has been reported with the use of 5% permethrin preparation and wearing a shower cap overnight. To remove the firmly adherent nits, a fine-toothed stainless-steel comb (LiceMeister) has been recommended.

Malathion lotion 0.5%, a weak organophosphate (louse neurotoxin), has been an excellent alternative for those older than 6 years in the area where permethrin resistance has occurred. Recent studies showed no toxicity from 2 years onward, when applied to the hair and left in place for 8–12 hours to provide residual protection. Malathion is both pediculicidal and ovicidal and resistance is quite rare. Those treated should not use open flame or electric heat source, including hair dryer and electric curler as it is flammable.

Ivermectin has been used when other medications have failed. For those at least 6 months of age, ivermectin lotion 0.5% was approved by Food and Drug Administration (FDA) for the treatment of head lice; ivermectin in a single, oral dose of 200 µg/kg has been effective. If needed, a second dose of 400 µg/kg 9–10 days later can be given. The drug should be used cautiously in a patient weighing less than 15 kg or in those who are pregnant or breastfeeding. Ivermectin was reported to have superior efficacy than malathion.

Two other topical pediculicides that have received FDA approval as non-neurotoxic treatment for pediatric use are benzyl alcohol and spinosad. Benzyl alcohol (5% lotion) can be applied for 10 minutes in children more than 6 months and spinosad can be applied in the same way as benzyl alcohol in children 4 years of age or older. Benzyl alcohol occludes the respiratory spiracles of the louse. Due to this, a sufficient quantity must be applied to saturate the hair completely. This treatment achieved 100% efficacy in a phase-three trial. Retreatment after 9 days is recommended to kill newly hatched lice. Benzyl alcohol can induce histamine release and produce scalp itching and has been associated with neonatal gasping syndrome, and hence its use should be avoided in children below 6 months of age **(Table 2)**.

Dimeticones kill head lice by physical means and it is a new promising agent as an alternative to neurotoxic pediculicides. Crotamiton, an antiscabetic agent, has activity against louse. Lindane [gamma-BHC (benzene hexachloride)] is organochloride, a neurotoxin, that is used as single application but should be avoided in a child with a history of seizure disorder. Lindane should be avoided as long as it is effective and safer alternatives are available. Many botanical products and oils available through Internet may be effective, but most of them are common contact allergen.

The use of a high-volume, hot air blow dryer alone has been reported to have killed 94–98% of the live eggs and 76–80% of hatched lice. Virtually all of the patients were completely cured after 1 week. Although this approach is promising, it necessitates further testing. If proved efficacious, this modality can eliminate use of chemicals to which some lice are becoming resistance day by day.

Reports suggest a possible association between pyrethroids, other pesticides, and childhood leukemia. Congenital leukemia has been reported in a child whose mother had heavily abused permethrin during pregnancy. It may induce mixed-lineage leukemia (MLL) gene cleavage in cells. Some children are more susceptible to toxic effects of pesticides due to variations in cytochrome P450 monooxygenases, esterases, alcohol, and aldehyde dehydrogenases activity in the cells.

Body Lice

The general recommendation has been thorough washing of the body with soap water followed by application of pyrethrin or pyrethroid or malathion for 8–24 hours (should be used cautiously in a child). Decontamination of clothing and bed linens should be done either by washing them in heat soapy water at a temp of 54°C for 30 minutes or by placing them in a hot cloth dryer for 20 minutes.

Table 2: Treatment for *Pediculosis capitis*.

Name	Instruction for use	Points to note
Permethrin 1% cream rinse	Apply to damp hair after shampooing, leave on for 10 minutes, and then rinse	Pediculicidal and Ovicidal; repeat treatment in 7–10 days
Benzyl alcohol 5% lotion	Apply to dry hair; leave on for 10 minutes; rinse	Approved for children 6 months and older; pediculicidal only; repeat treatment in 7 days. Should not be used below 6 months because of gasping syndrome
Malathion 0.5% lotion	Apply to dry hair; rinse after 8–12 hours	Approved for children 6 years and older; ovicidal and pediculicidal; not first-line treatment; repeat therapy in 7–10 days if needed. It is a flammable liquid
Spinosad 0.9% suspension	Apply to dry hair; rinse after 10 minutes	Approved for children 4 years and older; ovicidal and pediculicidal; repeat therapy in 7 days if needed
Ivermectin 0.5% lotion	Apply to dry hair; rinse after 10 minutes	Approved for children 6 months and older. It is only pediculicidal
Ivermectin (3 mg/ 6 mg) oral tablets	200 µg/kg single dose; repeat in 1–2 weeks	Occasionally used for resistant cases. Side effects include nausea, vomiting, headache, dizziness. Not recommended in children weighing less than 15 kg
Manual nit removal	Comb with fine-toothed nit removal comb or fine-toothed stainless-steel comb (LiceMeister) should be used	Recommended by some in conjunction with pediculicides. Wet combing on damp hair, slow down live lice and facilitate removal. Vinegar loosens the nit

Pubic Lice

Treatment should be similar to that used for managing head lice. Cloths and bed linen should be decontaminated. In case of children, parents should also be treated and in the case of an adolescent, the sexual partner requires treatment. Pediculicides should not be used for infestation of eyelashes by pubic lice. Lice over eyelashes can be treated by applying petroleum jelly (Vaseline) applied two to four times daily for 8–10 days or oral cotrimoxazole for 10 days has been reported to be effective.

Control and Prevention

Regular surveillance, early detection, and treatment may reduce the burden of lice infestation. Washing of clothes, bed linen, and towels used by an infested individual using a hot water laundry cycle and a high heat drying cycle is recommended for body and pubic lice infestation but not for head lice infestation. Shaving pubic hair can be helpful and all the sexual contacts should be examined and treated empirically. Household contact should be treated only if infested.

In many cases, there is treatment failure due to misunderstanding of instruction, noncompliance, inappropriate preparation, resistance, reinfestation, and misdiagnosis.

■ MYIASIS

Introduction

Myiasis is the infestation of body tissues of animals by the larvae (maggots) of nonbiting flies from order Diptera. Animals are most commonly infested, but humans are sometimes infested depending on their behavior, environment, or clinical status. Myiasis is the fourth most common travel-associated skin disease and cutaneous myiasis is the most frequently encountered clinical form. In countries where myiasis is not endemic, it can present as the most common travel-associated skin disease. Parasitologically, flies may be classified into two main myiasis-producing groups: obligatory and facultative or accidental. Obligatory myiasis-producers always pass their larval stage parasitically in the body of an animal. Larvae of facultative myiasis-producers usually develop on decaying flesh or vegetable matter but may infest wound. In accidental myiasis, eggs or larvae reach the body opportunely, via natural orifices, traumatic wounds, or in the digestive tract based on the location of the affected area such as cutaneous, nasopharyngeal, ocular, intestinal, or urogenital.

Biology and Epidemiology

Myiasis is mostly found in humid and warm climates of tropical and subtropical regions. Female flies usually lay their eggs or larvae on the skin, inside wounds, or in the opening of body cavities. The hatching larvae undergo two molts and develop to second- and third-stage larvae. The latter penetrate the host in order to pupate in a dry environment and develop into adult fly.

Several species (nearly 50 species) are important in human disease. These include *Wohlfahrtia magnifica* (the spotted flesh fly), *Chrysomya bezziana* (the old world screwworm fly), *Cordylobia anthropophaga* (tumbu fly), and *Dermatobia hominis* (botfly). The latter two are the most common cause of human disease.

Marginal housing, poor disposal of refuse, and undernutrition are important factors of myiasis.

Pathogenesis and Clinical Presentation

Myiasis is classified based on Bishop's, James, and Zumpt's classification into sanguivorous or blood sucking, cutaneous myiasis, furuncular myiasis, migratory myiasis, wound myiasis, and cavitary myiasis and is also based on the organ involvement such as cerebral myiasis, aural myiasis, nasal myiasis, and ophthalmomyiasis.

The habits of the flies and their larvae determine the variations in the clinical manifestations for which they are responsible.

Cutaneous Myiasis

Traumatic or wound myiasis has been a serious complication of war wounds in tropical areas and is sometimes seen in neglected ulcers or wounds in most parts of the world. *Cochliomyia hominivorax, C. bezziana,* and *W. magnifica* are the most common flies, worldwide, that cause obligatory human wound myiasis. Wound myiasis is most often initiated when flies oviposit in necrotic, hemorrhaging, or pus-filled lesions. In the presence of an open wound, the most important predisposing factors for wound myiasis are a lack of hygiene and poor socioeconomic status. Obligatory cutaneous myiasis occurs in two main clinical forms (furuncular and migratory myiasis); in both there may be mild constitutional symptoms and eosinophilia. Both occur mainly on exposed skin, often on the face, scalp, arms, or legs. In the furuncular form, boil-like lesions develop gradually over a few days **(Fig. 2)**. Each lesion has a central punctum (central breathing pore) that emits bubbles when submerged in water which also discharges serosanguinous fluid **(Fig. 3)**. The posterior end of the larva, equipped with

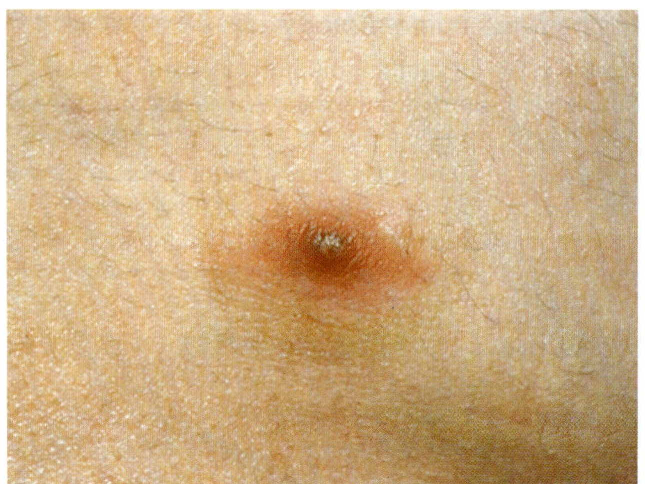

Fig. 2: *Furuncular myiasis* showing an initial lesion on the face.
Source: Francesconi F, Lupi O. Myiasis. Clin Microbiol
Rev. 2012;25(1):79-105.

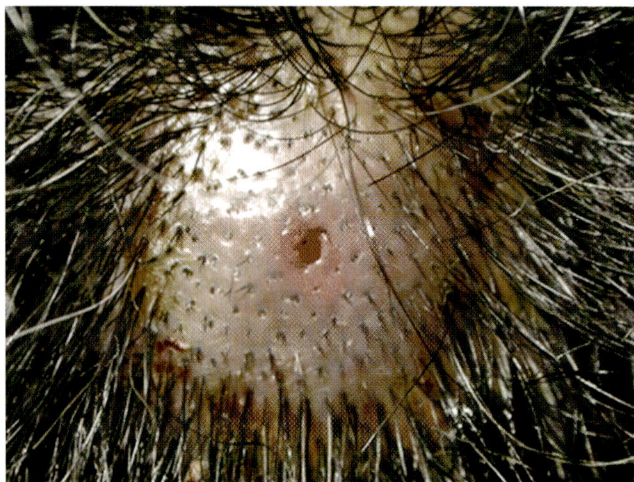

Fig. 3: *Furuncular myiasis* on the scalp due to *Dermatobia hominis*.
Note the bald area on the scalp with ulcer and punctum.
Source: Francesconi F, Lupi O. Myiasis. Clin Microbiol
Rev. 2012;25(1):79-105.

a group of spiracles, is usually visible in the punctum, and its movements may be noticed by the patient and may lead to severe emotional distress. The lesions are often extremely painful but sometimes not. The inflammatory reaction around the lesions may be accompanied by lymphangitis and regional lymphadenopathy and/or systemic symptoms. Secondary bacterial infection due to *Staphylococcus aureus*, Group A *Streptococcus*, and Gram-negative organism is a possible complication. Once the larva has emerged, or has been removed, the lesions rapidly resolve. The flies causing furuncular myiasis in humans are *D. hominis, Cuterebra, C. anthropophaga, Cordylobia (Stasisia) rodhaini, Wohlfahrtia* species, and *Hypoderma* species.

The second principal clinical form (migratory myiasis) is a creeping eruption, resembling cutaneous larva migrans, in which a tortuous thread-like red line with a terminal vesicle marks the passage of the larva through the skin. The larva lies ahead of the vesicle in apparently normal skin. The larva may live for months in human skin and may migrate 1–30 cm/day. Infestation may present with pustules, nodules, or recurrent swelling. This form of myiasis is produced by *Gasterophilus* larvae. The inflammatory nodular lesions produced by the *Hypoderma* species are migratory.

Body Cavity Myiasis

The infestation of natural body cavities is called cavitary myiasis. Cavitary myiasis receives specific names, depending on the anatomic region affected. Internal organs may also be affected. *Eristalis tenax*, a fly called "drone fly," can cause intestinal, gastric, or urinary myiasis. It is an accidental myiasis related to ingestion of contaminated uncooked food or water containing fly larvae. Abdominal pain, diarrhea, and anal bleeding are the symptoms of intestinal myiasis which may last for 2–6 weeks.

Oral Myiasis

Oral myiasis includes orofacial, oromaxillofacial, and orotracheal myiasis. It is rare and is often associated with poor oral hygiene (e.g. advanced periodontitis) or mental disability. It is most common in rural areas in the tropical and subtropical zones of Africa and America.

Ocular Myiasis

Ocular myiasis includes ophthalmomyiasis, orbital, and palpebral myiasis. It is characterized by catarrhal conjunctivitis with irritation and redness. There is infestation of the eye or periorbital tissue by larvae and represent less than 5% of human myiasis. When larvae remain outside the eye, it is called ophthalmomyiasis externa whereas penetration of the eye is called ophthal-momyiasis interna, a severe condition that can lead to retinal detachment, blindness, and destruction of globe. *D. hominis* very occasionally causes ophthalmomyiasis externa with eyelid and conjunctival involvement. The conjunctivitis may vary from mild to severe orbital cellulitis.

Nasal Myiasis

Nasal myiasis includes nasopharyngeal myiasis. Larvae of *Oestrus ovis* are deposited into the mouth and nostrils of human, where they usually survive only a few days without further development. Nasal symptoms such as sneezing, nasal discharge, and epistaxis may occur. Larva may invade meninges.

Aural Myiasis

Aural myiasis includes otomyiasis, myiasis of external and middle ear. It has been described in a child without underlying disease. It is relatively common in warm and humid climates. In such cases, larvae feed on necrotic and living tissue until metamorphosis.

Urogenital Myiasis

Urogenital myiasis includes vaginal myiasis, genital myiasis, myiasis of uterine cavity, pelvic organ myiasis, vulvovaginal, and vulvar myiasis. It has been observed due to infestation of *Piophila casei*, *Musca domestica*, and *Fannia canicularis*.

Gastrointestinal Myiasis

It is an accidental phenomenon, which occurs due to ingestion of food contaminated with eggs. Usually the patient is asymptomatic and sometimes may be associated with abdominal pain, diarrhea, nausea and vomiting and at times bleeding.

Diagnosis

Generally, diagnosis of myiasis depends upon the type of myiasis and is based on clinical features, visual inspection, and dermatoscopy. In some cases ultrasonography (USG) is required and when USG fails to detect larvae, color Doppler sonography is used to visualize the movement of internal fluid of the larvae. Whenever the patient presents with unusual pruritus or unresolving skin lesion, myiasis should be considered. Larvae can be demonstrated in the wound.

Prevention and Treatment

Cutaneous myiasis is usually a self-limiting clinical condition, as the third-stage larvae have to leave the skin and pupate outside the host. Spontaneous expulsion of the larvae may be precipitated by the use of an asphyxiating agent, which brings larvae deposited in deeper tissue layers to the surface, thereby facilitating their surgical removal. A cotton pellet soaked with an agent such as petroleum jelly, turpentine, liquid paraffin, or mineral oil should be applied in the opening and the larvae can be removed using forceps.

The larva of *Cordylobia* can often be expressed by firm pressure around the edges of the lesion, but sometimes the punctum may require enlargement surgically. The larva of *D. hominis* has a bulbous anterior end equipped with rows of spines that help to anchor it in the skin and make its removal by manual pressure difficult. Traditional methods of treatment include occluding the punctum with pork fat, blocking the spiracles of the larva, and stimulating premature extrusion. In some cases punctum can be enlarged by cruciate incisions, and this enables removal of an intact larva. However, in most cases, a surgical excision is necessary. Oral ivermectin or albendazole may be helpful, if extraction is not possible because the larva is too deep into the tissue.

Wound myiasis requires debridement and irrigation to remove larvae, and treatment of secondary infection by local and systemic antibiotic.

Ivermectin has been used both topically and orally in the management of myiasis. Different therapeutic schemes have been adopted for ivermectin use in the treatment of myiasis. Ivermectin is not recommended for furuncular myiasis, because it may kill the larva inside the lesion, with a consequent inflammatory reaction.

The prevention of human myiasis requires good wound care, adequate personal hygiene, screening to protect against flies, and prevention of myiasis in domestic animals. Flypapers, baited traps, and electrocutions to control fly population and keeping the area free of decaying organic matter and excreta decrease fly population. Insect repellents such as N,N-diethyl-meta-toluamide (DEET) and ethyl benzamide and avoiding exposures are good preventive measures.

◼ LEECH INFESTATIONS

Introduction

Out of 650 leech species, few are predator and mostly hematophagous. They are living in fresh water near forest and vegetation. Species such as *Haemadipsa zelanica*, *H. picta* and *H. sylvestris* attack human and feed on human blood. Some of the leeches are used for treatment of various conditions such as venous congestion in surgical flaps. This practice has been complicated by wound infections and myonecrosis caused by *Aeromonas hydrophila* (up to 20% secondary infection), a gut commensal of leech. Medicinal leeches are *Hirudo medicinalis*, *H. orientalis*, *Placobdella ornate*, etc.

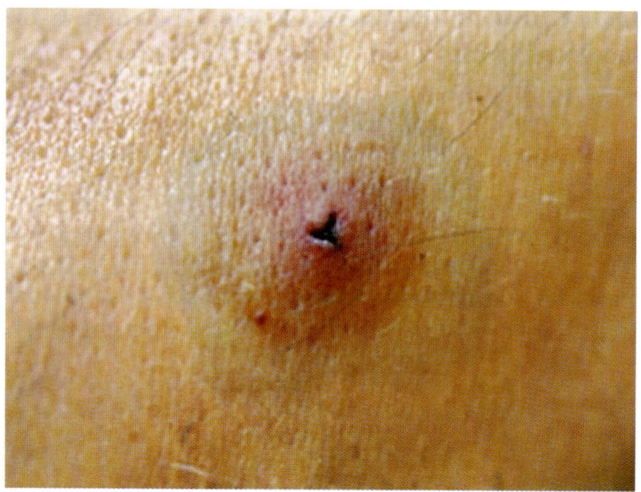

Fig. 4: Leech bites showing ecchymosis with "Y"-shaped mark. *Source*: Mumcuoglu KY. Recommendations for the use of leeches in reconstructive plastic surgery. Evid Based Complement Alternat Med. 2014;2014:205929.

They have an elongated, soft-segmented, flattened body with anterior and posterior suckers. Anterior suckers composed of three jaws, pointing in three different directions that make a bite mark, leave an inverted Y inside a circle and posterior suckers are used for attachment with skin **(Fig. 4)**. Leech saliva contains a number of compounds such as an anesthetic agent which limits the sensation felt by the host (that reduces the chance of the host trying to detach it); histamine like vasodilators and hyaluronidase cause the local blood vessel to become dilated to supply the leech with up to 150 mL of blood for up to 48 hours. Saliva also contains hirudin, which is a highly effective anticoagulant, and calin (a platelet aggregation inhibitor), which may remain active for more than 20 minutes and bleeding continues. Leech bites commonly occur while drinking, bathing, and swimming in contaminated water.

Clinical Features

Local pain at the bite site is short-lasting because analgesics are injected into the skin with saliva. Hirudin, a powerful anticoagulant secreted by leech, causes continued bleeding even after leech detachment. Wound healing is slow with greater chances of bacterial infections. Small ecchymosis, itching, and erythema may develop at the bite site. A small scar, if left undistributed, disappears by 3 weeks' time. Sometimes, there may be local allergic reaction, severe itching, and redness.

Rarely leech may lead to irritant dermatitis, follicular pseudolymphoma, and anaphylaxis particularly during repeated exposure, i.e. medicinal purpose. Sometimes, bleeding at the bite site can last for a longer period during

anticoagulant therapy and with bleeding disorders. Infestation may occur by drinking infested water and bathing in the pools, springs, and stagnant water by which leech enters through eyes, urethra, vagina, rectum, and nose and may lead to mucosal, orifical, and vesicle hirudiniasis. This kind of internal hirudiniasis may lead to epistaxis, otorrhagia, hemoptysis, coughing, dyspnea, hematuria, hematemesis, vaginal bleeding, and rectal bleeding. Leeches do not carry diseases, but they can cause death in some extreme situation. They enter the body by bathing or by drinking of infested water. When ingested, they attach themselves to the lining of the nose or throat. Leech endoparasitism may cause inspiratory stridor, acute laryngotracheal obstruction, lethal dyspnea, hemoptysis, and hematemesis. Diagnosis can be made by indirect or fiberoptic laryngoscopic examination under general anesthesia and surgical removal can be undertaken as an emergency procedure. Sometimes, X-ray, ultrasound, and computed tomography (CT) scan may be required to rule out leech infestation in nasal cavity, paranasal sinus, pharynx, and larynx.

Treatment and Prevention

Externally attached leeches drop off when they are engorged after blood meal. Extra caution should be exercised when removing the leech as not to have reflux of contents back into the wound for risk of infection as well as increased bleeding. One should not pull off leaches by force during blood feeding, as their jaws can remain on the skin which can cause secondary infections. Application of salt, alcohol, vinegar, lidocaine, and burning cigarette on the apical part of leeches can be used for the removal of the leeches. Washing the area with soap, water, and povidone iodine, if available, is required. Bleeding can be controlled by applying pressure over the area or applying tranexamic acid and silver nitrate. There are some case reports where even blood products' transfusion was required. Antibiotics are indicated if there is development of an ulcer or wound. There is a possibility of a serious allergic reaction and life-threatening anaphylaxis in some cases and which may be delayed even up to 2 hours of bite. Oral, rectal, and nasopharyngeal leech removal can be done by saline wash and saline gurgle. The application of traditional medicines may lead to dislodging of ingested leech deeper and results in suffocation and death. So the possibility of leech endoparasitism should be considered in endemic areas as a cause of unexplained bleeding from nose and throat, particularly with history of recent contact with streams and springs water. It is advisable to avoid application of traditional medication which may dislodge the leech and lead to obstruction of major airways that may result in death. Cystoscopic removal can be done for leech, into the urinary bladder. The management of leech bites is done by a multidisciplinary team which includes an emergency physician, nurse, surgeon, and infectious disease consultant.

Leech bite can be prevented by wearing clothing that covers lower extremity, avoiding fresh streams or springs water for drinking and bathing, and using insect repellants such as DEET or N,N-diethyl benzamide (Odomos) over skin.

Complications

Leeches are a carrier of bacteria and viruses. HIV and hepatitis C were isolated from live leech in Africa. The virus may remain in leech as long as 5 months. Studies have also shown possibility of malaria transmission from leech-ingested blood. *Aeromonas hydrophila* secondary infection is common which can be treated by fluoroquinolones.

■ SUGGESTED READING

1. Baker CJ. Red Book Atlas of Pediatric Infectious Disease, 2nd edition. Illinois: American Academy of Pediatrics; 2013.
2. Conley K, Juergens AL. (2019). Leech bite. [online] Available from: https://www.ncbi.nlm.nih.gov/pubmed/30085513. [Last accessed on November, 2019].
3. Currie MJ, Bowden FJ, McCarthy JS. Louse infestation. Manson's Tropical Diseases, 23rd edition. New York: Elsevier; 2014. pp. 839-42.
4. Drutz JE. Arthropods. Feigin and Cherry's Textbook of Pediatric Infectious Diseases, 8th edition. Philadelphia: Elsevier; 2019. pp. 2270-6.
5. Elston DM. Ectoparasites (lice and scabies). In: Long S, Pickering L, Prober C (Eds). Principles and Practice of Pediatric Infectious Diseases, 4th edition. New York: Elsevier; 2012. pp. 1257-60.
6. Francesconi F, Lupi O. Myiasis. Clin Microbiol Rev. 2012;25(1): 79-105.
7. Mekonnen D. Leech infestation: the unusual cause of upper airway obstruction. Ethiop J Health Sci. 2013;23(1):65-8.
8. Monsel G, Delaunay P, Chosidow O. Arthropods. In: Griffiths C, Barker J, Bleiker T, Chalmers R, Creamer D (Eds). Rook's Textbook of Dermatology, 9th edition. UK: John Wiley & Sons; 2016.
9. Mumcuoglu KY. Other ectoparasites: leeches, myiasis and sand fleas. Manson's Tropical Diseases, 23rd edition; New York: Elsevier; 2014. pp. 843-7.
10. Nadipuram S, Cherry JD. Aeromonas. Feigin and Cherry's Textbook of Pediatric Infectious Disease, 8th edition. Philadelphia: Elsevier; 2019. pp. 1101-5.
11. Paller AS, Mancini AJ. Infestation, bites and stings. Hurwitz Clinical Pediatric Dermatology, 5th edition. New York: Elsevier; 2016. pp. 428-47.
12. Pollack RJ, Norton SA. Ectoparasite infestations and arthropod injuries. In: Kasper DL, Hauser SL, Jameson JL, Fauci AS, Longo DL, Loscalzo J (Eds). Harrison's Principles of Internal Medicine, 19th edition. New York: McGraw Hill; 2015. pp. 2744-51.

7.3
CHAPTER

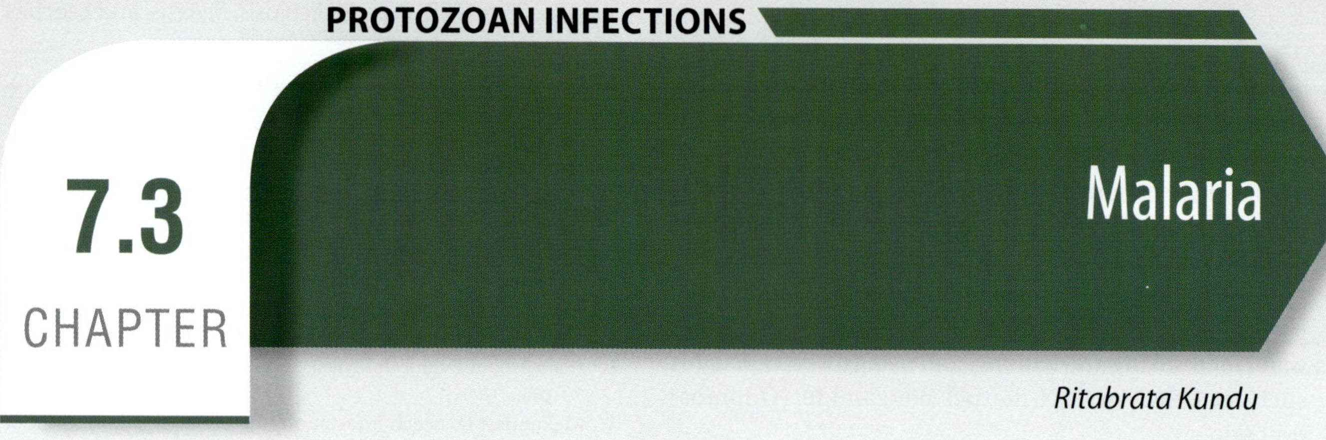

Malaria

Ritabrata Kundu

INTRODUCTION

Malaria is a major public health problem of developing countries like India which contributes to under five-mortality in children. These days, the number of *Plasmodium falciparum* cases is in rise. The problem of resistance is further enhanced by development of resistance to first-line antimalarial drugs like chloroquine (CQ). The cause of resistance is high drug pressure and haphazard use of antimalarials without a proper parasitological diagnosis. Considerable decrease in antimalarial drug use could be achieved through improving the diagnosis of malaria and hence rationalizing treatment.

Malaria thought to be restricted to low income rural areas of Eastern and North-Eastern states of India, does not hold true. It has been found in both central as well as more arid Western parts of the country. Urban malaria initially starting in large towns has spread to small cities and towns. The increasing problem of urban malaria is due to population migration from village to earn livelihood and better facility in the city. Unplanned urban growth has resulted in "urban slum" with poor housing and sewerage condition that facilitated mosquito breeding. Unplanned expansion has led to unplanned water storing practices favoring mosquito breeding.

Unstable transmission characteristic of malaria is seen in India. Most of the areas have low transmission with increased incidence during or following monsoon rains. This unstable transmission dynamics has resulted in little or no immunity against malaria in our country. Entire population including infants and children are at risk of developing serious malaria. Intense malaria transmission is seen in North-Eastern states, large areas of Odisha, Jharkhand, Chhattisgarh, Madhya Pradesh and Rajasthan. There rivulets, hilly tracts and forests provide proper support for malaria transmission throughout the year. In these regions, young children who have not yet developed immunity of their own and have lost the immunity transmitted from their mothers are subject to develop severe malaria. Also the nonimmune visitors, particularly army personnel and migratory labor in these areas are prone to severe malaria.

Anopheles culicifacies is the main vector in rural and periurban areas which breeds in natural and man-made breeding sites. It is highly zoophilic hence high cattle density may give some protection to man. *Anopheles stephensi* breeding in stagnant water bodies is responsible for malaria in urban and industrial areas. Vector in hilly areas, forests and forest fringe areas of Eastern parts of India is *Anopheles fluviatilis*. Vectors, transmitting malaria bites from dusk and continues till dawn. Resistance to dichlorodiphenyltrichloroethane (DDT) and malathion, the common insecticides are seen in both the important species.

The two most important species of malaria parasite in India are *P. falciparum* and *Plasmodium vivax*. *P. falciparum i*s more prevalent in some Northern states of India, Odisha, Jharkhand and Andhra Pradesh, where mortality from malaria is highest. So, malaria is dual species infection in India with different treatment regimen for each species. Hence, correct diagnosis of the species is extremely important to cure the patient and halt the spread of drug resistance.

Malaria is endemic in whole of India except at elevations above 1,800 m and in some coastal areas. It is heartening to note that from 2 million cases per year in the nineties has started to decline since the year 2002. According to Directorate of National Vector Borne Disease Control Programme (NVBDCP) year 2016 has reputed number of malaria cases just above million which declined to less than a million in the next year. Falciparum malaria which contributed to less than 50% of cases in nineties started showing increased incidence since the year 2000. In last few years, falciparum malaria contributed to more than 60% cases of malaria. It is of concern that falciparum has become the predominant species of malaria these days.

Resistance of *P. falciparum* to CQ is now common in practically all malaria endemic countries. Resistance to sulfadoxine-pyrimethamine (SP) is widespread in South-East Asia and South America. Mefloquine (MQ) resistance is now common in the border areas of Thailand with Cambodia and Myanmar. Resistance of *P. vivax* to CQ has now been reported from Indonesia, Myanmar, Papua New Guinea and Vanuatu. Fortunately vivax malaria is still sensitive to CQ in India.

■ CLINICAL DISEASE

Malaria in India is seasonal thereby the population lacks lasting immunity against it. All age groups suffer from acute malaria with chances of progression to severe malaria particularly in cases of *P. falciparum* infection.

It is crucial to distinguish uncomplicated from complicated or severe malaria as the later needs highest level of patient care for favorable outcome. Ineffective or delay treatment in early stages of uncomplicated falciparum malaria will result in resistance of the parasite mass to produce organ dysfunction resulting in severe malaria.

Symptoms of malaria are nonspecific and often resembling viral fevers like influenza. It may present with muscle ache, headache, lethargy and vague abdominal pain. The classical fever paroxysm described in the earlier textbooks are hardly seen these days. Fever with chills and rigors are more common with vivax malaria whereas falciparum may present with any type of fever. Both abdominal and respiratory symptoms like anorexia, nausea, vomiting or cough may be present. With passage of time, liver and spleen enlarge with gradual increasing pallor. Diagnosis of malaria on basis of signs and symptoms will invariably lead to over diagnosis.

Symptomatic malaria with signs of severity or evidence of vital organ dysfunction is known as complicated or severe malaria.

Plasmodium vivax occasionally produces severe malaria; common manifestations include severe anemia, splenic rupture, metabolic acidosis and shock with coma. Most of the complicated malaria is due to *P. falciparum* infection. Common manifestations of severe malaria in children include cerebral malaria, severe anemia, hypoglycemia and metabolic acidosis. Early detection and prompt treatment are extremely in the child. Following clinical or laboratory features are suggestive of complicated or severe malaria.

Cerebral Malaria

Three most common presentations are decreasing consciousness to unarousable coma, prostration and seizures. Unarousable coma is not attributable to any other cause in a patient with *P. falciparum* malaria is most common. Unlike febrile seizures, coma in cerebral malaria persists for 30 minutes to 1 hour following seizure. Convulsion generalized or focal may be often subtle to start with, like twitching in the corner of the mouth or intermittent nystagmus. Neurological features include symmetrical encephalopathy with no focal signs. Extreme agitation, decorticate and decerebrate rigidity and unarousable coma suggest poor prognosis.

Severe Anemia

Anemia is a common finding in severe malaria, particularly in children. Hemoglobin is often below 5 g/dL and hematocrit below 15%. Anemia is often microcytic hypochromic due to concurrent iron deficiency. Patients with severe anemia may have absent or low parasitemia where useful indicator of malaria is the presence of malaria pigments in neutrophilic leukocytes.

Children with severe anemia present with tachycardia and dyspnea. Restlessness and confusion are cerebral signs due to severe anemia along with gallop rhythm, heart failure, hepatomegaly and pulmonary edema.

Hypoglycemia

Whole blood glucose concentration less than 40 mg/dL (2.2 mmol/L) denotes hypoglycemia. It is particularly seen in young children, in patients with hyperparasitemia, convulsions or profound coma and those treated with quinine may also develop hypoglycemia due to quinine-induced hyperinsulinemia. Classic symptoms are anxiety, sweating and fainting but at times presents with altered consciousness and convulsion. Features are often confused with cerebral malaria.

Respiratory Distress (Acidosis)

Acidosis is defined as plasma bicarbonate concentration below 15 mmol/L or arterial or capillary pH below 7.35. Labored hyperventilation with retraction of the chest wall but without any localizing chest signs is usual presentation due to accumulation of lactic acid particularly in children with cerebral malaria or severe anemia who are also dehydrated and hypovolemic. Persistent respiratory distress has poor prognosis.

Circulatory Collapse or Shock (Algid Malaria)

It is defined as systolic blood pressure less than 50 mm Hg in children (1–5 years) or less than 80 mm Hg in adults. Listlessness accompanied by cold, clammy skin and feeble pulse is usual presentation. Recurrent vomiting with diarrhea along with dehydration and hypovolemia, gastrointestinal bleeding or ruptured spleen may pass into shock stage. Shock is often associated with gram-negative septicemia; the source of infection (meningitis, urinary tract infection, indwelling catheters) must be sought and treated.

Pulmonary Edema

Pulmonary edema is common in adults but less common in children. It may develop several days after initiation of treatment even when the parasite level is diminishing. Increased pulmonary capillary permeability and at times fluid overload usually causes it. Radiological sign of "bat wing edema" develops. Initially presenting with increase respiratory rate to be followed by distress. At times it may develop several days after the disease when the parasite count is coming down.

Abnormal Bleeding and Disseminated Intravascular Coagulation

Bleeding usually results from thrombocytopenia or disseminated intravascular coagulation (DIC). Thrombocytopenia is seen in patients treated with quinine and may also occur in those with cerebral malaria. Common findings are petechiae and subconjunctival hemorrhage. It is self-limiting and usually improves with successful treatment of malaria.

It is common in patients with cerebral malaria, secondary infection and malaria in pregnancy. DIC may produce bleeding from gums, epistaxis or severe gastrointestinal bleeding.

Renal Failure

It is defined as serum creatinine more than 3.0 mg/dL or urine volume less than 0.5 mL/kg/h in children despite normal hydration. Fortunately this complication is rare in children.

Acute tubular necrosis is the cause, presenting with acute metabolic acidosis, jaundice and pulmonary edema. Subacute presentation with gradually rising serum creatinine, oliguria and never anuric has better prognosis. Presentation may be late when the parasite mass has diminished. Renal failure is also seen in patients with massive hemolysis with hemoglobinuria.

Hemoglobinuria

Acute intravascular hemolysis is often accompanied by hemoglobinuria. It is usually seen in nonimmune people visiting malaria endemic regions and patients treated with quinine. It is also known as blackwater fever often associated with renal failure and hepatic dysfunction. Hemoglobinuria is also seen in Glucose-6-phosphate dehydrogenase (G6PD)-deficient patients treated with antioxidant drug like primaquine.

Jaundice

Jaundice in malaria is defined as serum bilirubin more than 3 mg/dL or presence of clinical icterus. If present with other signs of severe malaria then it is of greater significance.

Hyperparasitemia

In our setup, proportion of parasitized red cells is 5% or more is considered hyperparasitemia.

Hyperparasitemic patients may lead to severe malaria quickly and the chances of treatment failure are high. In low transmission areas of Thailand that mortality rate in uncomplicated malaria is only 0.1% but increases to 3% when parasite density is above 4%. Some patients can tolerate high parasite load without any complication.

◼ DIAGNOSIS OF MALARIA

All cases of malaria should have a parasitological diagnosis. Clinical diagnosis is nonspecific and will definitely lead to over treatment.

Microscopic Diagnosis

Thick and thin film microscopy still remains the "gold standard" for malaria diagnosis. Thick films are more sensitive for diagnosis of malaria as larger amount of blood are there in a given area. However, identification of species is better with thin films as shape of the parasite and red blood cells (RBCs) are well preserved.

Blood should be tested as soon as malaria is suspected irrespective of degree of fever. Definitely it should be done before administration of antimalarials.

Smear should be examined with 100× oil immersion objective and minimum 100 fields examined before discarding the slide.

Trained microscopist in proper condition is able to diagnose even if parasites are as low as 5–10 parasites/µL of blood.

As identification of species along with stage of parasite can be detected, it helps in adequate treatment and prognostication.

It can also determine the parasite density which helps to ascertain the severity of malaria along with prognosis and assessing the response to treatment.

Microscopy is time consuming and in certain places the slides have to be sent to distant central laboratory thereby delaying treatment.

At the periphery often skilled technicians, good microscope, proper reagents with proper infrastructure are unavailable.

Microscopy cannot detect parasite sequestered deep in the vascular compartment for which repeated blood smear examination is needed.

Rapid Diagnostic Tests

Unlike microscopy rapid diagnostic tests (RDTs) are immunochromatographic tests to detect malaria antigens which are cheap and rapid. These tests have poor sensitivity with low parasite density often unable, to distinguish between species accurately and not accurate in hot and humid tropical countries. Their main advantage is simple to perform, quick and does not require sophisticated devices.

Targeted antigens in currently available RDTs:
- *Histidine-rich protein II (HRPII)* is actively secreted by asexual stages and young gametocytes of *P. falciparum* but not by mature gametocytes.
- *Parasite lactate dehydrogenase (pLDH)* is produced by all four viable species of plasmodia, both asexual and sexual (gametocytes) stages.
- New antigens like *Plasmodium* aldolase an enzyme of the glycolytic pathway produced by all four species have been recently developed.

Plasmodium falciparum and *P. vivax* malaria are present in our country; typically producing a single species infection hence a RDT which can detect both *P. falciparum* and *P. vivax* malaria and distinguish between them is needed. As treatment of *P. falciparum* and *P. vivax* malaria is different in our country. So both species should be identified separately.

The World Health Organization (WHO) has recommended a minimum standard of 95% sensitivity for *P. falciparum* densities of 100 parasite/µL of blood and a specificity of 95%.

Rapid diagnostic tests using HRPII are generally more sensitive than RDTs detecting *P. falciparum*-specific pLDH. Independent peer reviewed evaluation for most commercially available RDTs are not available. With high parasite density, these tests are fairly sensitive but with low parasite load sensitivity decreases. False-positive result may also develop when gametocytes are present but asexual stage parasites are eradicated by therapy.

Histidine-rich protein II antigen persists at detectable levels for more than 28 days even after successful therapy.

Aldolase and pLDH rapidly fall to undetectable levels after initiation of effective therapy but these antigens are present in gametocytes which may appear after clinical infection is cleared. So none of the RDTs are useful for monitoring the response to treatment for which microcopy is the investigation of choice.

In areas with poor health infrastructure microscopic diagnosis is not available, the RDTs are helpful.

If both RDT and microscopy are available they can complement each other. RDTs used as screening test in suspected cases whereas microscopy reserved for confirmation of doubtful cases or confirmation of negative result in RDTs with high clinical suspicion of malaria.

National Drug Policy for Malaria (2013) has advocated that all fever cases clinically suspected of malaria should be investigated for confirmation of malaria by microscopy or RDT.

Rapid diagnostic tests that target HRPII of *P. falciparum* shows antigen to persist for a long time even after cure. So this test is unsuitable for assessment of treatment failure and monitoring of drug resistance.

Rapid diagnostic tests cannot distinguish new infection from a recent and effectively treated infection.

They are unable to quantify the parasite load so they have no prognostic value nor they can detect therapeutic efficacy of antimalarial drugs.

Detection thresholds of RDTs are 40–60 parasites/µL of blood, which are much higher than microscopy.

Gametocytes of *P. falciparum* can persist even after successful chemotherapy if gametocidal drugs are not given but they are nonpathogenic. RDTs will give false-positive result in such situation with chances of unnecessary treatment.

Rapid diagnostic test kits have to be stored at under 30°C but in places without electricity the temperature can soar to 40°C or more.

So in conclusion, RDTs permit on the spot confirmation of malaria even at the peripheral healthcare system, by unskilled health worker with minimal training. This will reduce unnecessary treatment based on symptomatic diagnosis hence in turn decrease drug pressure.

Molecular Methods of Diagnosis

- *Molecular probes*: DNA and RNA probes are used for diagnosis of malaria. Its use in field conditions is impractical.
- *Polymerase chain reaction*: This test can also be used for diagnosis of malaria particularly in cases of low parasitemia and mixed infection. This technique is expensive, needs expertise and time consuming. It is better suited for epidemiological monitoring.

Serology

Antibody detection by this method cannot differentiate between present and past infection and has no utility in routine practice.

Microscopy and RDTs are the mainstay for diagnosis of malaria. The other tests are not suitable for routine disease management and their use is currently for only research and epidemiological purpose.

■ TREATMENT OF UNCOMPLICATED MALARIA

Random *de novo* genetic mutations of malaria parasite result in development resistance to antimalarial drugs. Patients of our country are infected with large number of parasites as there mostly nonimmune hence the chances of development of resistance. Here lies the necessity of early effective treatment which will prevent development of resistance.

Few years back monotherapy in falciparum malaria resulted in failure with development of drug resistance. First falciparum was resistance to CQ following which SP was introduced but that fell rapidly to resistance in early 1980. Then soon after introduction of MQ monotherapy, it took 4–5 years to loose efficacy.

To stop this spread of resistance to falciparum due to monotherapies, WHO recommends combinations therapy for treatment of the same.

Drug Resistance in India

First reports of resistance of *P. falciparum* to CQ came from Diphu of Karbi Anglong district in Assam state. Thereafter, it spread rapidly throughout the country. Reports of resistance to SP are widely prevalent all along the North-Eastern part of our country.

Fortunately, in spite of few reports of emergence of CQ-resistant *P. vivax* still this drug has retained its efficacy against vivax malaria in our country.

Antimalarial Combination Therapy

To insure better treatment outcome and stop the spread of resistance, WHO suggests combination therapy for the treatment of all falciparum malaria. Combination therapy is use of two or more blood schizontocidal antimalarial drugs with independent mode of action and different biochemical target in the parasite.

Two drugs with different mode of action and different resistance mechanism, if used in combination then the probability of developing simultaneous resistance to both drugs is the product of their individual per parasite probabilities. The mutant parasite developing *de novo* resistance in the course of treatment to one drug it will be killed by the other drug. Drugs used in combination therapy should be individually effective. This mutual protection will prevent emergence of resistance or at least delay emergence of resistance. Increased risk of adverse effect and cost of therapy are the drawback.

One of the partners in combination therapy should be artemisinin or its derivatives hence known as artemisinin-based combination therapy (ACT). There are several reasons for choosing artemisinin, firstly its rapid clearance of parasitemia and resolution of symptoms. The second important reason is its rapid elimination of the drug so that the residual concentration of the drug does not provide a selective filter for the parasites to develop resistance. Thirdly, its lack of serious toxic effects and due to its gametocytocidal action.

Artemisinin if combined with slowly eliminated antimalarials like SP, MQ or lumefantrine shorter courses of treatment (3 days) will be effective which will ensure adherence.

In 3-day ACT regimen, artemisinin is present in the body during the two asexual parasite life cycles each lasting for 2 days thereby bringing down the parasite to very low level. The complete clearance of the remaining parasites will depend on the efficacy of partner medicine and its persistence at parasiticidal concentration until all the infecting parasites have been killed. Thus, the partner compound is to be relatively slowly eliminated.

As a result of combination therapy, the artemisinin is protected from resistance by the partner medicine and partner medicine is in turn protected by the artemisinin derivative. The following ACTs are currently available in our country.

- Artesunate (AS) + SP
- Artesunate + MQ
- Artemether-lumefantrine

Of these, artemether-lumefantrine is available as coformulated tablets and liquid preparation and lumefantrine

Box 1: Recommended treatment of uncomplicated *P. vivax* malaria.

Recommended treatment

Chloroquine 10 mg base/kg stat orally followed by 5 mg/kg at 6, 24 and 48 hours (total dose 25 mg/kg)

Or

Chloroquine 10 mg base/kg stat orally followed by 10 mg/kg at 24 hours and 5 mg/kg at 48 hours (total dose 25 mg base/kg)

Primaquine should be given in a dose of 0.25 mg/kg once daily for 14 days to prevent relapse

- Chloroquine should not be given in empty stomach and in high fever. Temperature should be brought down first. If vomiting occurs within 45 minutes of a dose of CQ that particular dose is to be repeated after taking care of vomiting by using antiemetic (domperidone/ondansetron).
- As primaquine can cause hemolytic anemia in children with G-6-PD deficiency, they should be preferably screened for the same prior to starting treatment. As infants are relatively G-6-PD deficient it is not recommended in this age group and children with 14 days regimen should be under close supervision to detect any complication. In cases of borderline G-6-PD deficiency once weekly dose of primaquine 0.6–0.8 mg/kg is given for 6 weeks.

is not available as monotherapy. Other combinations are available separately.

Treatment Regimen of Uncomplicated Malaria

Malaria needs early and effective treatment. It should not progress to severe disease and morbidity of treatment failure should be avoided.

Parasitological diagnosis is needed otherwise clinical diagnosis alone will increase the drug pressure and favor resistance.

Treatment regimens are designed according to the resistance pattern of the region from where the patient hails. It has been now decided that all falciparum cases should be treated with ACT both in public or private health care system. All cases of mixed infection, i.e. *P. vivax* and *P. falciparum* are to be treated as falciparum malaria along with primaquine for 14 days.

Treatment regimens are to be tailored specifically according to the resistance pattern of the region from where the patient hails **(Boxes 1 to 3)**.

Treatment of P. vivax malaria: In spite of some stray reports of CQ-resistant *P. vivax* infection but CQ is still the drug of choice for *P. vivax* malaria in our country. According to the NVBDCP and the National Institute of Malaria Research, CQ should be used in full therapeutic dose of 25 mg/kg divided over 3 days.

Box 2: Recommended treatment of uncomplicated *P. falciparum* malaria in all states other than North-Eastern states of India.

Recommended treatment

Artesunate 4 mg/kg of body weight orally once daily for 3 days and a single administration of SP as 25 mg/kg of sulfadoxine and 1.25 mg/kg of pyrimethamine on day 1

Or

Artesunate as above and mefloquine 25 mg/kg of body weight in two divided doses (15 mg/kg and 10 mg/kg) on day 2 and day 3

Or

Coformulated tablets containing 20 mg of artemether and 120 mg of lumefantrine can be used as a six-dose regimen orally twice a day for 3 days. For 5–14 kg body weight 1 tablet at diagnosis, again after 8–12 hours and then twice daily on day 2 and day 3. For 15–24 kg body weight same schedule with 2 tablets. For 25–35 kg body weight and above same schedule with 3 and 4 tablets, respectively

A single dose of primaquine (0.75 mg/kg) is given for gametocytocidal action.

- Currently there are insufficient safety and tolerability data on MQ at its recommended dosage of 25 mg/kg body weight in children. MQ shares cross resistance with quinine which is still a effective drug in our country. Health planners of our country do not advocate use of MQ.
- Advantage of artemether-lumefantrine combination is that lumefantrine is not available as monotherapy and has never been used alone for the treatment of malaria. Lumefantrine absorption is enhanced by coadministration with fatty food like milk.
- Artemether-lumefantrine is not recommended in children weighing less than 5 kg.

Box 3: Recommended treatment of uncomplicated *P. falciparum* malaria in North-Eastern states of India.

Recommended treatment

Coformulated tablets containing 20 mg of artemether and 120 mg of lumefantrine can be used as a six-dose regimen orally twice a day for 3 days. For 5–14 kg body weight 1 tablet at diagnosis, again after 8–12 hours and then twice daily on day 2 and day 3. For 15–24 kg body weight same schedule with 2 tablets. For 25–35 kg body weight and above same schedule with 3 and 4 tablets, respectively

Or

Artesunate 4 mg/kg of body weight orally once daily for 3 days and mefloquine 25 mg/kg of body weight in two divided doses (15 mg/kg and 10 mg/kg) on day 2 and day 3

A single dose of primaquine (0.75 mg/kg) is given for gametocytocidal action

- Currently there are insufficient safety and tolerability data on MQ at its recommended dosage of 25 mg/kg body weight in children. MQ shares cross resistance with quinine which is still a effective drug in our country. Health planners of our country do not advocate use of MQ.
- Advantage of artemether-lumefantrine combination is that lumefantrine is not available as monotherapy and has never been used alone for the treatment of malaria. Lumefantrine absorption is enhanced by coadministration with fatty food like milk.
- Artemether-lumefantrine is not recommended in children weighing less than 5 kg.

TREATMENT OF UNCOMPLICATED *P. FALCIPARUM* MALARIA

Problem started in the successful treatment of malaria with development of resistance of *P. falciparum* to the first-line drug CQ. The first resistance to the cheapest and the most used drug was reported from Diphu of Karbi Anglong district of Assam in the year 1973. Thereafter, it has spread throughout the country.

Plasmodium falciparum has developed resistance to almost all antimalarials currently used (CQ, SP, MQ, quinine and amodiaquine) except artemisinin and its derivatives. WHO has suggested combination of different antimalarials with different mode of action to ensure high cure rates through full adherence to correct dose regimens.

Therapeutic response is adequate if the patient shows clinical improvement without parasitemia from day 3 onward. If patient does not respond with parasite positive in peripheral blood after 3 days in spite of full therapeutic dose without vomiting or diarrhea suspect of resistance. Patient should be given alternative therapy as guided later.

If follow-up smear is not possible, on clinical follow-up if by day 5 after the initial treatment there is not clinical improvement a blood smear is to be repeated. In case it is positive then start alternative therapy.

Management of Treatment Failure

Reappearance of *P. falciparum* malaria is due to either a recrudescence or a reinfection that is treatment failure which may not be possible to distinguished in a individual patient. Failure of fever or parasitemia to resolve or recur within 2 weeks of treatment is considered as treatment failure.

Treatment failure must be confirmed by microscopic examination of blood. RDTs must not be done as antigenemia may remain positive for weeks after the initial infection.

Failure within 14 Days

Treatment failure within 14 days of ACT therapy is unusual. It should be treated with a second-line antimalarial drug.

Second-line antimalarial treatment: The choice of second-line drugs depends on the initial therapy.
- Artesunate was given initially—quinine plus tetracycline or doxycycline or clindamycin (given for total 7 days)
- Quinine was given initially—artesunate plus tetracycline or doxycycline or clindamycin (given for total 7 days)
- An alternate ACT known to be effective in the region may be given.

Failure after 14 Days

All treatment failures after 14 days of initial treatment should be considered as new infection, and should be treated with first-line ACT. MQ within 60 days of first treatment may be associated with an increased risk of neuropsychiatric problems hence avoided.

TREATMENT OF SEVERE AND COMPLICATED MALARIA

All cases of malaria presenting with severe manifestations are to be treated as complicated malaria with injectable antimalarials irrespective of the species. Mostly severe life-threatening malaria are due to *P. falciparum*.

Delay in starting treatment may be fatal and be treated at highest level of medical facility available, preferably in a intensive care setting. Do not withhold treatment if confirmation of diagnosis needs more than 1 hour. In cases of high index of suspicion, prompt antimalarial therapy should be started even if parasites are not found in the initial blood examination.

Any children with severe malaria need antimalarial chemotherapy, supportive management and management of complications. All these three interventions are equally important and to be taken care of simultaneously.

Antimalarial Chemotherapy of Severe and Complicated Malaria (Table 1)

Antimalarial drug should be given by intravenous (IV) infusion, at least to start with then be replaced by oral administration as soon as condition permits.

According to the National Anti-Malaria Programme (NAMP), in all cases of severe malaria require parenteral artemisinin derivatives or IV quinine irrespective of CQ resistance status.

Choice of Therapy

Artemisinin is the most rapidly acting antimalarial drug with highest killing rate thereby producing maximum reduction of parasites per asexual cycle. They have antimalarial effects in the tiny ring forms to early schizonts. Thereby parasite maturation from the less pathogenic early circulating ring stages to the more pathogenic cytoadherent stages are stopped.

It is extremely safe and treatment cost as compared to quinine is almost similar. There are few reports of resistance to artemisinin at present but declining sensitivity to quinine has been reported from some South-East Asian countries like Thailand.

Table 1: Recommended treatment of complicated and severe malaria.

Drug	Dosage
Quinine salt	• 20 mg salt/kg (loading dose) diluted in 10 mL of isotonic fluid/kg by infusion over 4 hours • Then give a maintenance dose of 10 mg salt/kg every 8 hours, calculated from beginning of previous infusion, until the patient can swallow, then quinine tablets, 10 mg salt/kg 8 hourly to complete a 7-day course of treatment (including both parenteral and oral). Tetracycline or doxycycline or clindamycin is added to quinine as soon as the patient is able to swallow and should be continued for 7 days • Tetracycline (above 8 years) or doxycycline (above 8 years) to be given for 7 days 4 mg/kg/dose four times daily or 3.5 mg/kg once a day respectively. Clindamycin to be given 20 mg/kg/day in two divided doses for 7 days • If controlled intravenous (IV) infusion cannot be administered, then quinine salt can be given in the same dosages by intramuscular (IM) injection in the anterior thigh (not in buttock) • The dose of quinine should be divided between two sites, half the dose in each anterior thigh. If possible IM quinine should be diluted in normal saline to a concentration of 60–100 mg salt/mL. (Quinine is usually available as 300 mg salt/mL). Tetracycline or doxycycline or clindamycin should be added as above Or
Artesunate	2.4 mg/kg IV stat then at 12 hours and 24 hours, then once a day. Once the patient is able to swallow oral medication, complete the treatment by giving a course of: • Artemether plus lumefantrine in North-Eastern states as shown in **Box 3** • Artesunate plus sulfadoxine-pyrimethamine in all states other than North-Eastern states of India as shown in **Box 2** Or
Artemether	3.2 mg/kg (loading dose) IM, followed by 1.6 mg/kg daily. Once the patient is able to swallow oral medication, complete the treatment by giving a course of: • Artemether plus lumefantrine in North-Eastern states as shown in **Box 3**. • Artesunate plus sulfadoxine-pyrimethamine in all States other than North-Eastern states of India as shown in **Box 2**. • Parenteral treatment in severe malaria should be continued at least for 24 hours irrespective of patient's ability to tolerate oral medication earlier than 24 hours. • Loading dose of quinine should not be used if the patient has received quinine, quinidine or MQ within the preceding 12 hours. Alternatively loading dose can be administered as 7 mg salt/kg by IV infusion pump over 30 minutes, followed immediately by 10 mg salt/kg diluted in 10 mL isotonic fluid/kg by IV infusion over 4 hours. • Quinine should not be given by bolus or push injection. Infusion rate should not exceed 5 mg salt/kg/hour. • If there is no clinical improvement after 48 hours of parenteral therapy, the maintenance dose of quinine should be reduced by one-third to one-half, i.e. 5–7 mg salt/kg. • Quinine should not be given subcutaneously as this may cause skin necrosis. • Artesunate, 60 mg per ampoule, is dissolved in 0.6 mL of 5% sodium bicarbonate diluted to 3–5 mL with 5% dextrose and given immediately by IV bolus (push injection). • Artemether is dispensed in 1 mL ampoule containing 80 mg of artemether in peanut oil. • Mefloquine should be avoided in cerebral malaria due to neuropsychiatric complications associated with it.

Randomized trials comparing artesunate and quinine from South-East Asia show clear benefit with artesunate.

Simultaneous use of quinine and artemisinin is not indicated as it may be harmful and there is no added advantage. In limited studies, available artesunate has been found to be better than artemether.

Supportive Management

All patients need rapid assessment with respect to level of consciousness, blood pressure, respiratory rate and depth, anemia, hydration and temperature.

Initial investigation should include blood film both thick and thin, hematocrit, blood glucose and lumbar puncture (LP) especially in cerebral malaria. Proper antibiotic cover for meningitis must be given if LP is delayed. Secondary infection is common in severe malaria and may be treated with antibiotics. IV antimalarials should be started after getting the blood samples. Proper fluid balance to be ensured, under- or overhydration should be avoided.

Good nursing care with positioning, attention to airways, eyes, mucosa and skin should be done.

Nasogastric tube is needed in unconscious to reduce the risk of aspiration.

Appropriate anticonvulsants to be given to control seizure.

High fever is treated with tepid sponging, fanning and paracetamol.

Blood smear examination every 6–12 hours for parasitemia for first 48 hours is needed.

With quinine therapy, parasite count may remain unchanged or even rise in first 18–24 hours which should not be taken as an indicator of quinine resistance. However, parasite count should fall after 24 hours of quinine therapy and should disappear within 5 days.

With artemisinin derivatives, usually the parasite count comes down within 5–6 hours of starting therapy. Asexual parasitemia generally disappears after 72 hours of therapy.

Management of Complicated and Severe Malaria

Following are the important complications of *P. falciparum* malaria in children.

- Cerebral malaria
- Severe anemia
- Respiratory distress (acidosis)
- Hypoglycemia
- Hyperparasitemia
- Circulatory collapse (algid malaria)
- Spontaneous bleeding and coagulopathy (DIC).

Cerebral Malaria

Mostly present with extreme prostration unable to eat or drink. The progression to coma or convulsion may be rapid within 1 or 2 days. Convulsions are of various types. Irrespective of height or duration of fever and age of the child is also common. Other causes of coma (e.g. bacterial meningitis, hypoglycemia) must be excluded. Management of convulsions with diazepam/midazolam and avoidance of harmful ancillary treatment like corticosteroids, mannitol, adrenaline and phenobarbitone is needed.

Severe Anemia

Packed red cell transfusion should be given slowly and cautiously when packed cell volume (PCV) is 12% or less, or hemoglobin is below 4 g/dL. Transfusion should also be considered in patients with less severe anemia in the presence of respiratory distress (acidosis), impaired consciousness or hyperparasitemia.

Lactic Acidosis

Indrawing of lower chest wall and deep sign respiration without any localizing chest signs suggest lactic acidosis. It is mostly seen in patients with cerebral malaria, anemia or dehydration. Correct hypovolemia, anemia and prevention of seizures are needed. Monitoring acid-base status with blood glucose, urea, and electrolyte level are also important.

Hypoglycemia

Patients with hyperparasitemia, children below 3 years or with convulsion and particularly those treated with quinine are prone to hypoglycemia. Manifestations are similar to cerebral malaria so it can be easily missed unless looked for carefully. Monitoring of blood sugar every 4–6 hourly is needed. Correct hypoglycemia with IV dextrose and it should be followed by slow infusion of 5% dextrose containing fluid to prevent recurrence.

Hyperpyrexia

Common in children and may lead to convulsion and altered consciousness. Tepid sponging, fanning and paracetamol 15 mg/kg should be given for hyperpyrexia.

Hyperparasitemia

High parasite density above 5% RBC infected is especially seen in nonimmune children associated with severe disease. Exchange transfusion/cytapheresis to be considered if greater than 20% of RBCs are parasitized.

Circulatory Collapse (Algid Malaria)

Resuscitation to be done with adequate use of fluids. Gram-negative septicemia should always be suspected. Blood sample for culture should be drawn before starting antibiotics.

Spontaneous Bleeding and Coagulopathy (DIC)

Mostly present in no immune children which should be managed with vitamin K, blood or blood products as required.

■ PREVENTION OF MALARIA

Prevention of malaria includes vector control and along with it personal protective measures taken both by the individual or community.

Chemical Control

Indoor residual spraying has been the backbone of mosquitoes control but they develop resistance to it with time.

Dichlorodiphenyltrichloroethane is the insecticide of choice for residual spray and if found to be resistance then malathion is the alternative choice. Resistance to both DDT and malathion requires synthetic pyrethroids.

Biological Control

Biological control is done with mosquito larvivorous fishes in tanks and other water bodies where they breed.

Personal Protection

Simple measures like screenings of house with wire mesh are ways of personal protection. Use of mosquito repellent creams, coils, mats and liquids and wearing long sleeve clothes are also effective. Sleeping under bednets impregnated with pyrethroid insecticide (permethrin, deltamethrin) is very effective.

Environmental Management

It includes reduction of breeding places, proper storage of water and reduction of unplanned construction.

■ SUGGESTED READING

1. Country profile: India. World Malaria Report 2018. World Health Organisation. Available from: <https://www.who.int/malaria/publications/country-profiles/en/>
2. Kundu R. Malaria. In: Gupta P, Menon PSN, Ramji S, Lodha R (Eds). PG Textbook of Pediatrics, 2nd edition. New Delhi: Jaypee Brothers Medical Publishers (P) Ltd.; 2018. pp. 1232-7.
3. Marx A, Pewsner D, Egger M, et al. Meta-analysis: accuracy of rapid tests for malaria in travelers returning from endemic areas. Ann Intern Med. 2005;142(10):836-46.
4. Moody A. Rapid diagnostic tests for malaria parasites. Clin Microbiol Rev. 2002;15(1):66-78.
5. National Strategic Plan for Malaria Elimination (2017-22). Directorate of National Vector Borne Disease Control Program. Directorate General of Health Services. New Delhi: Ministry of Health and Family Welfare, Govt. Of India; 2017. Available from: <http://www.indiaenvironmentportal.org.in/content/445149/national-strategic-plan-for-malaria-elimination-2017-22/>
6. White NJ. Malaria. In: Cook GC, Zumla A (Eds). Manson's Tropical Diseases. 21st edition. London: Saunders; 2003. pp. 1205-95.
7. World Health Organisation (WHO). Guidelines for the treatment of Malaria. 3rd edition. Geneva: World Health Organisation; 2015;23-5.

Leishmaniasis (Kala-azar)

Nigam Prakash Narain, Rajesh Kumar

INTRODUCTION

Leishmaniases are tropical and subtropical vector-borne intracellular protozoan diseases[1] caused by the flagellated parasites of genus *Leishmania* from family *Trypanosomatidae*.[2] Leishmaniasis in Indian subcontinent, Middle East and Africa is mainly caused by *Leishmania donovani* whereas *Leishmania infantum* is mostly responsible for disease along the Mediterranean coast, Middle East, Central Asia and in China.[3] *Leishmania* completes its life cycle in two hosts viz. definitive vertebrate host (man, dog, rodents, etc.) and insect vector, a female sandfly of *Phlebotomus* species. Leishmaniasis broadly presents as three main forms viz. (1) visceral leishmaniasis (VL) or kala-azar, (2) cutaneous leishmaniasis (CL) and (3) mucocutaneous leishmaniasis (MCL).[4]

EPIDEMIOLOGY

Worldwide annual incidence of VL is around 0.5 million whereas that of CL is around 1–1.5 million,[4] with VL and CL being endemic in 75 and 87 countries, respectively. Ninety percent of new cases of VL are contributed by 7 countries (Brazil, Ethiopia, India, Kenya, Somalia, South Sudan and Sudan).[5] In the WHO South-East Asia Region (SEAR) countries, VL mostly occurs in India, Bangladesh and Nepal. In India, VL is endemic in 54 districts in 4 states (Bihar, West Bengal, Jharkhand and eastern Uttar Pradesh)[6] which contributes for >70% cases. Sporadic cases are reported from Assam, Himachal Pradesh, Kerala, Madhya Pradesh, Sikkim and Uttarakhand. Approximately 50% of these new cases are of pediatric age group. The incidence of VL has decreased worldwide in last 5 years from 0.2–0.4 million new cases in 2012 to 50–90 thousands in 2017.[7]

TRANSMISSION

Leishmaniasis in humans is transmitted by female *Phlebotomus* sandflies in the Asia, Africa and Europe and by *Lutzomyia* sandflies in America.[2] These phlebotomine sandflies have varied hosts ranging from canids, rodents, marsupials, hyraxes to humans. Human leishmaniasis could have either zoonotic transmission, where from an animal reservoir; the disease is transmitted to humans or anthroponotic transmission patterns where disease is transmitted between humans to humans by a vector. Transmission by needles among intravenous (IV) drug abusers[8] and in utero transmission to fetus may also occur.

Morphology

Leishmania donovani exists in two forms: (1) amastigote (aflagellar) form and (2) promastigote (flagellar or leptomonad) form. *Amastigote* form is found in reticuloendothelial cells like macrophages, neutrophils, endothelial cells of liver, spleen and bone marrow of vertebrate hosts like man, dog, rodents, etc. It is an obligate intracellular form and is the infective stage to the vector, sandfly. Amastigotes are round to oval, 3–5 μm in size, having <1 μm, oval to round nucleus located in center or side of the cell. It has kinetoplast which lies at right angle to the nucleus and consists of copies of mitochondrial DNA. Axoneme represents the root of flagellum with no external flagellum and extends from blepharoplast. Adjacent to axoneme there is vacuole. *Promastigote* form is an extracellular form found in sandfly and in cultures. This stage is infective to humans. It is motile and contains single anterior flagellum. It is pear-shaped and measures 8–15 μm length. Nucleus is centrally placed and kinetoplast lies transversely near the anterior end and consists of parabasal body and blepharoplast. Axoneme represents the intracellular portion of flagellum, which projects from the front and may be of the same length as the body of parasite. Undulating membrane is absent.[3,9,10]

Life Cycle

Leishmania completes its life cycle in two hosts: (1) *vertebrate host* (man, dog, rodents, etc.) and (2) *insect vector* (female sandfly). In India, there is only one sandfly vector of kala-azar, i.e. *Phlebotomus argentipes*.[11] Sandflies are small insects, measuring only 1.5–3.5 mm. Adult sandfly is a small and fuzzy, having large wings with long hairs covering the whole body including the wings. Life cycle of sandflies consists of four stages viz. (1) egg, (2) four instars of larvae, (3) pupa and (4) adult form.[10] Female sandfly during its blood meal from infected person ingests amastigotes, which then transforms into promastigote forms in the insect's midgut. Promastigotes multiply by longitudinal fission and pass through various stages to form metacyclic promastigotes. The metacyclic promastigotes after multiplying in the midgut by binary fission, ascend to the foregut (proboscis) of the vector. These promastigote forms blocks the buccal cavity of *Phlebotomus,* which is forced to release them during the next blood meal, into the bite wound caused by its proboscis. Life cycle of *Leishmania* in sandflies varies from 4 days to 18 days. Fruit juice feed is required before the female sandfly becomes infective after blood meal from infected human. Promastigotes are phagocytosed by the skin macrophages and within next 12–24 hours are transformed into amastigote forms. The amastigote forms multiply inside the macrophages causing them to rupture and are then released into the circulation. Through circulation they are carried to various organs like liver, spleen and bone marrow and invade the reticuloendothelial cells like macrophages, endothelial cells, etc.

Host Factors

Children between ages 5 years and 9 years are most commonly affected pediatric population,[12] although any age group including infants could be affected. Males are infected more commonly in comparison to females, in ratio of 2:1,[12] probably due to more outside activities. Migrants, laborers, tourists, etc. moving from an endemic to a nonendemic area are often responsible for further propagating the disease. It commonly affects people of low socioeconomic status. Those in farming, forestry, mining and fishing are at increased risk.

Environmental Factors

Kala-azar is mostly confined to alluvial plains of river Ganges where there is enough monsoon rains with temperature ranging between 15°C and 38°C along with high humidity, rich vegetations and subsoil water,[7] and is unusual at altitude over 2,000 feet. During past epidemics, peaks were seen in March-April and in November. In the 1977 Bihar epidemic, it was observed that most cases occurred between April and September.[13] Prevalence usually increases during and after monsoon. Sandflies (*P. argentipes*) mostly lay eggs in cracks and crevices of various structures. Overcrowding, poor ventilatory conditions and organic wastes facilitate their transmission. Only female sandflies bite and they do so mostly at night.

■ CLINICAL FEATURES

Acute Onset

This rare presentation of VL is seen in the visitors or inhabitants of nonendemic areas. High grade intermittent or remittent fever is most common presentation and fever lasts for 2–6 weeks or longer. In these cases, there is rapid enlargement of spleen, which becomes palpable even in few days.

Chronic Onset

Chronic onset is the most common presentation of VL in endemic areas. The onset is insidious with incubation period ranging from 2 weeks to 32 weeks. Without appropriate treatment, patients with VL usually die within 2 years from secondary bacterial infection, severe anemia or hemorrhage due to thrombocytopenia. However, some of the infected cases might develop overt symptoms only after years, when they become immunocompromised. Infection in the reticuloendothelial system might have a subclinical course and patients may be mildly or overtly symptomatic. The typical manifestation of kala-azar consists of high fever, abdominal discomfort, emaciation and pallor. Fever is generally high grade and intermittent with a double rise of temperature in a day (double quotidian), the characteristic finding not commonly seen nowadays. Splenic enlargement is seen in nearly all cases, which becomes palpable by the first month of illness and thereafter enlarges at the rate of about 1 inch per month. It is huge, smooth, firm and nontender unless there has been a recent infarct. Marked splenomegaly and moderate hepatomegaly generally appear approximately 6 months after the onset of illness. Liver is usually enlarged but not to such an extent as the spleen. Hepatic functions remain unaltered. Jaundice with evidence of gross hepatocellular dysfunction is unusual and carries a grave prognosis. Other manifestations include pallor, lymphadenopathy, anemia, leukopenia, thrombocytopenia, night sweats, weakness, anorexia, asthenia, cutaneous pigmentation, and weight loss. In spite of the high fever, the children remain remarkably well and ambulant with reasonably preserved appetite. It may also be associated with acute malnutrition or wasting. Cytokine induced enhanced production of adrenocorticotropic hormone (ACTH) leads to hyperpigmentation of the skin, which gives VL, its Hindi name is *kala-azar*, meaning black fever.[7] However, nowadays this feature is not commonly seen in children.

The at-risk population includes preschool children, immunocompromised and undernourished individuals. Recently, leishmaniasis has been seen with increasing frequency in patients who have acquired immunodeficiency syndrome (AIDS) or who are IV drug users or both, suggesting a potential transmission mechanism through contaminated syringes.[8]

Those who present late might have hypergammaglobulinemia, which includes (nonprotective) antileishmanial antibodies. These children present characteristically with chronic diarrhea and growth retardation.

Cachexia and multisystem failure occurs if the disease progresses in the absence of treatment. A decrease in the number or function of CD4 cells may cause recurrence, as in the case of patients receiving corticosteroids or chemotherapy, in transplant recipients, or in association with infection with human immunodeficiency virus (HIV).

Features of Pancytopenia

Severe anemia, usually normocytic and normochromic, could be seen in VL as a result of multiple factors viz. autoimmune hemolysis, replacement of bone marrow with *Leishmania*-laden macrophages, hemorrhage, sequestration of erythrocytes in spleen, hemodilution, suppressive effects of cytokines on bone marrow and nutritional deficiencies.

Leukopenia is also seen in most patients, with total white blood cell (WBC) count being as low as 1,000/mm^3 in few patient. It is due to many factors like increased margination, splenic sequestration or an autoimmune process. Secondary infection is a common complication; most common association being tuberculosis. Other infections, which are commonly seen, are pneumonia, measles, otitis media, and cancrum oris. Cough and diarrhea are also common.

Eosinopenia, or absence of eosinophils, is frequently observed. Usually thrombocytopenia and hypergammaglobulinemia are also seen. Although bleeding manifestations could be seen presenting as epistaxis, hematemesis, petechiae and purpura due to severe thrombocytopenia, this is not a common presentation in endemic areas of Bihar.[14]

■ DIAGNOSIS

Clinical description: It is described as an illness with prolonged irregular fever, splenomegaly and weight loss as its main symptoms. In malaria endemic areas, VL should be suspected when fever lasts >2 weeks and no response has been achieved with antimalarial medicines (assuming drug-resistant malaria has also been considered).[6]

Case Classification (by WHO Operational Definition)[6,15]

1. *A kala-azar suspect case*: History of fever of >2 weeks with enlarged spleen and liver not responding to antimalarial in patient from an endemic area.
2. *A case of kala-azar*: A person from endemic area with fever of >2 weeks duration and with splenomegaly, who is confirmed by a rapid diagnostic test (RDT) or a biopsy.

Laboratory Diagnosis

Visceral leishmaniasis: Laboratory diagnosis of VL includes nonspecific tests along with direct and indirect evidences of *Leishmania*.

Nonspecific Tests

Complete blood count (CBC): It shows normocytic normochromic anemia, thrombocytopenia and leukopenia. Differential count shows neutropenia with relative lymphocytosis and monocytosis. The ratio of leukocyte to erythrocyte is greatly altered and may be about 1:2,000 (normal: 1:750). There is *hypergammaglobulinemia* with reversal of the albumin-to-globulin ratio. This hypergammaglobulinemia was the basis for *Napier's aldehyde or formogel test* and Chopra's *antimony test,* which are no longer used now. Liver function tests may be deranged with mild elevations of liver enzymes. Erythrocyte sedimentation rate (ESR) is usually increased.

Leishmanin skin test: It is, also known as *Montenegro test,* a delayed hypersensitivity test in which 0.1 mL of killed promastigote suspension (10%) is injected intradermally on the dorsoventral aspect of forearm. Induration of 5 mm or more after 48–72 hours suggests a positive result. Positive result is reflective of prior exposure to leishmanial parasite. In active kala-azar, this test is negative and becomes positive usually 6–8 weeks after cure from the disease.

Direct Evidence

Microscopy: *Gold standard* for diagnosis of VL is demonstrating amastigotes in smears of tissue aspirates. Sample could be obtained from bone marrow, splenic aspirate or very rarely from enlarged lymph node. The smears are stained by Leishman, Giemsa, or Wright's stains and examined under oil immersion microscope, which shows amastigote parasite within the macrophages, often in large numbers.

Culture: Aspirate from spleen, bone marrow or other tissues is inoculated and then incubated in special media like Novy-McNeal-Nicolle medium (NNN medium), Schneider's liquid medium with 20% calf serum, Bacto-agar biphasic medium, etc. Both microscopic examination as well as culture has a sensitivity of 85%.[16]

Animal inoculation: Animal inoculation is not used for routine diagnosis.

Indirect Evidence

Serodiagnosis:

- *Detection of antigen*: The concentration of antigen in the serum or other body fluids is very low. Enzyme-linked immunosorbent assay (ELISA) and polymerase chain reaction (PCR) have been developed for detection of leishmanial antigen. *KAtex test* is latex agglutination test which detects leishmanial antigen in urine and has high specificities (80%–100%) with moderate sensitivity (40%–95%).[17] It is especially useful in diagnosing case of VL-HIV coinfection and could help assess response to therapy. However, it is still in field trial but could be a promising bedside test in future.
- *Detection of antibodies:* Patients with VL show high parasite-specific antibody titers. Most of these serological tests have high sensitivity but lack adequate specificity. Thus, these tests alone cannot definitively confirm or exclude VL. Furthermore, antibody estimation fails to effectively differentiate current from past infection and could remain positive for long time in patients from endemic areas. Serological tests could be done through various methods like ELISA, complement fixation test, indirect immunofluorescence assay (IFA), and direct agglutination test (DAT).
- *rK39 rapid test for VL*: Due to simplicity and easy availability, it has become the method of choice for diagnosis of kala-azar and is often used as a bedside test for VL. Though, it has become the mainstay of serological diagnosis, its drawback is that it cannot predict response to therapy. It is a specific rapid immunochromatographic dipstick test developed using a recombinant leishmanial antigen *rK39,* consisting of 39 amino acids conserved in kinesin region of *Leishmania chagasi*.[18] The sensitivity of the test is 100% and specificity is 97%.[19] False-positive results could be seen in hepatitis and tuberculosis cases. In patients who do not fulfill the clinical case definition, positive result should be interpreted with caution. Results could be falsely negatives in HIV patients with depressed immune response. The RDTs could not be used to diagnose relapse cases as they remain positive for months to years after treatment of VL. In cases of suspected post-kala-azar dermal leishmaniasis (PKDL), negative RDT results rule out the disease. Confirmation of PKDL could only be done through parasitological diagnosis by bone aspirate or splenic aspirate.
- *Polymerase chain reaction*: It is a DNA detection method which recognizes parasite DNA and is highly sensitive as well as specific, and could detect even a single parasite in specimen.

TREATMENT

- *Antimony compounds*: Two compounds namely sodium stibogluconate (SSG) and meglumine antimoniate have been used for treating VL since 1930s. But since early eighties there has been emergence of large scale SSG resistance in North Bihar with only 35–38% patients responding to SSG and thus it has gone out of favor. In sensitive cases, SSG may be used in dose of 20 mg/kg body weight either by intramuscular (IM) injection or IV infusion, over the course of 28–30 days. Aside from IM injections being painful, major adverse effects of these compounds are arthralgia, myalgia, metallic taste and cardiotoxicity.
- *Oral miltefosine*: It is one of the most important developments in the treatment of VL for adults, as it eliminated the need for parenteral therapy and hospitalization. It was registered in India in 2002 and Asian elimination initiative adopted it as the first-line regimen in 2005. Miltefosine is the first oral drug that has proven to be effective against leishmaniasis, having cure rate of 95–100%. It is used in doses as followed; for children aged 2–11 years—2.5 mg/kg once daily after meals × 28 days, children > 12 years and weight < 25 kg—only one capsule of 50 mg daily × 28 days, children > 12 years and weight 25-50 kg—100 mg daily in two

doses of 50 mg each after meals for 28 days and for >50 kg body weight—150 mg/day orally for 28 days in divided doses.[6] Side effects of miltefosine include vomiting, diarrhea, asymptomatic transient elevation of hepatic enzymes and rarely nephrotoxicity. Because of its teratogenic effects, it should not be used in pregnant ladies and in females of childbearing age. It is presently being given as first-line drug in North Bihar at the primary health center (PHC) level to affected adults on outdoor basis, however, is not very successful in children due to gastrointestinal (GI) intolerance.

- *Amphotericin B*: This antifungal drug has excellent antileishmanial activity and is 400 times more potent than SSG. Amphotericin B deoxycholate is given at dose of 0.75–1 mg/kg slow IV infusion for 15–20 doses on alternate days. Total dose of 15 mg/kg achieves nearly 100% cure without any organ toxicity. Major side effects are infusion related, occasionally serious renal toxicity and electrolyte imbalance may occur.

- *Lipid formulations of amphotericin B*: They are the most important development in chemotherapy of VL. These are available in various forms like liposomal amphotericin B (LAmB; Ambisome), amphotericin B lipid complex (Abelect) and amphotericin B colloidal suspension (Amphomul/Amphocil). Conventional amphotericin B requires prolonged hospitalization along with renal monitoring whereas lipid formulations require much shorter stay and are relatively free from side effects with almost equal efficacy achieving cure rate of around 94% in VL.
    - *Liposomal amphotericin B*: It is recommended by WHO and included as the first-line treatment of VL by the National Vector Borne Disease Control Programme (NVBDCP) in Accelerated Plan for Kala-azar Elimination-2017 due to its ease of use, effectiveness and assured compliance. It is much safer than conventional amphotericin B; however, high cost is a limiting factor to its use. It is given as a single dose of 10 mg/kg IV (for all age groups), dissolved in 5% dextrose and is administered over 2 hours.

- *Injectable paromomycin (aminosidine)*: It is an aminoglycoside antibiotic marketed globally for >20 years. Its clinical efficacy in VL is established by clinical trials (Phase I/II) in Africa and India. It has high overall cure rates (final cure: 94.6%) and is also effective in patients failing previous treatment. It is very affordable and safe to use. Resistant cases of VL in North Bihar have been treated effectively by paromomycin.

- *Combination therapy*: Various combination therapies are recommended for treatment of kala-azar, like *antimonial with interferon-gamma, Ambisome with paromomycin, Ambisome with miltefosine, miltefosine with paromomycin and SSG with paromomycin.*

Treatment Outcomes in Kala-azar[6,15]

Treatment outcomes in kala-azar have to be assessed *twice*: (1) initial outcome is assessed at the last day of drug treatment whereas the (2) final outcome is assessed 6 months after the last drug intake.

Four main outcomes are identified in kala-azar elimination strategy:

1. *Cure*: A patient is considered clinically cured if he/she has completed full treatment and there are no signs and symptoms of kala-azar.
2. *Nonresponse*: Signs and symptoms persist or recur despite satisfactory treatment for more than 2 weeks.
3. *Relapse*: Any reappearance of kala-azar signs and symptoms within a period of 6 months after the end of treatment.
4. *Treatment failure*: Nonresponse or relapse.

◼ POST-KALA-AZAR DERMAL LEISHMANIASIS

About 3–10% cases of patients of VL in endemic areas develop PKDL, about 1 year or 2 years after recovery from the systemic illness.[3] It is seen mainly in India and East Africa and not seen elsewhere. PKDL is a nonulcerative lesion of skin. These lesions are of three types:

1. *Depigmented or hypopigmented macules*: These commonly appear on the face, trunk and extremities and resemble tuberculoid leprosy.
2. *Erythematous patches*: These are distributed on the face in a "butterfly distribution".
3. *Nodular lesion*: Both of the earlier mentioned lesions may develop into painless yellowish pink, nonulcerating, granulomatous nodules.

Diagnosis of Post-Kala-azar Dermal Leishmaniasis

The nodular lesions are biopsied and amastigote forms are demonstrated in stained sections. The biopsy material can be cultured or animal inoculation can be done. Immunodiagnosis has no role in the diagnosing PKDL.

Case Definitions[6]

- *Probable PKDL*: A patient from a kala-azar endemic area with multiple hypopigmented macules, papules, plaques or nodules, who is RDT positive.

- *Confirmed PKDL*: A patient from a kala-azar endemic area with multiple hypopigmented macules, papules, plaques or nodules, who is parasite positive in slit-skin smear (SSS) or biopsy.

Treatment of Post-Kala-azar Dermal Leishmaniasis

- First drug of choice is *miltefosine* orally for 12 weeks.
- *Sodium stibogluconate* may be given as 20 mg/kg/day for 40–60 days.
- *Amphotericin B deoxycholate* injection by IV infusion could be used in dose of 1 mg/kg/day for up to 60–80 doses over 4 months.
- *Liposomal amphotericin B* (Ambisome) is used as 2.5 mg/kg/day for 20 days.

Treatment Outcomes in Post-Kala-azar Dermal Leishmaniasis[6]

- *Initial cure*: Clinical improvement at the end of treatment is defined as a considerable reduction in the number and size of skin lesions.
- *Final cure*: Clinical cure 12 months after the end of treatment is defined as a complete resolution of macules, papules, plaques and nodules.

Coinfection with HIV: Visceral leishmaniasis is mostly an opportunistic infection in HIV patients. Atypical clinical presentations of these patients pose a diagnostic challenge. Nearly 2,000 cases of coinfection with HIV and VL are reported from 35 countries.[20] In these patients, hepatosplenomegaly may be absent. Diagnosis is usually made by bone marrow examination as sensitivity of antibodies based immunodiagnostic test is low. Amastigotes demonstration in buffy coat smear or PCR analysis of whole blood or its buffy coat could be used for screening and diagnosis in these patients.

HIV/VL coinfected patients are treated with LAmB, used in dose of 3–5 mg/kg daily or intermittently for 10 doses, days 1–5, 10, 17, 24, 31, and 38, total cumulative dose of 40 mg/kg.

Prevention: Due to sylvatic and rural nature of the disease, control is often difficult. Early detection and treatment of all cases are of utmost importance. Integrated insecticidal spraying could be considered to reduce sandfly population. Forest workers should use protective clothing and other protective measures. Although several trials for both killed and live-attenuated vaccines are going on but there are no vaccines currently available in market for prevention of leishmaniasis. A recently developed polyvalent vaccine using five *Leishmania* strains has been reported to be successful in reducing the incidence of CL in Brazil.

■ REFERENCES

1. Torres-Guerrero E, Quintanilla-Cedillo MR, Ruiz-Esmenjaud J, et al. Leishmaniasis: a review. F1000Res. 2017;6:750.
2. Karimi A, Alborzi A, Amanati A. Visceral leishmaniasis: an update and literature review. Arch Pediatr Infect Dis. 2016; 4(3):e31612.
3. Paniker's Textbook of Medical Parasitology, 8th edition, pp. 52-65.
4. Regional Strategic Framework for Elimination of Kala-azar from the South-East Asia Region 2011-2015.
5. Alvar J, Yactayo S, Bern C. Leishmaniasis and poverty. Trends Parasitol. 2006;22(12):552-7.
6. Hyperlink "https://www.nvbdcp.gov.in/WriteReadData/l892s/Accelerated-Plan-Kala-azar1-Feb2017.pdf" Accelerated Plan for Kala-azar Elimination 2017 - NVBDCP
7. Burza S, Croft SL, Boelaert M. Leishmaniasis. Lancet. 2018;392(10151):951-70.
8. Alvar J, Cañavate C, Gutiérrez-Solar B, et al. Leishmania and human immunodeficiency virus coinfection: the first 10 years. Clin Microbiol Rev. 1997;10(2):298–319.
9. Sastry AS, Bhat KS. Essentials of Medical Parasitology. 1st edition. Jaypee Brothers Medical Publishers; 2014. pp. 64-79.
10. Gupte S. The short textbook of medical microbiology; (Including Parasitology), 10th edition. pp. 367-71.
11. Guidelines on Vector Control in kala-azar Elimination, National Vector Borne Disease Control Progamme, Govt. of India.
12. Operational guidelines on kala-azar (visceral leishmaniasis) elimination in India – 2015, National Vector Borne Disease Control Programme.
13. Naraian NP, Kumar R. Textbook of Pediatric Infectious Diseases, 2nd edition. pp. 386-92.
14. Naraian NP. Partha's fundamentals of Pediatrics, 2nd edition. p. 153.
15. Indicators for monitoring and evaluation of the kala-azar elimination programme, August 2010, Bangladesh, India and Nepal, WHO.
16. Torres-Guerrero E, Quintanilla-Cedillo MR, Ruiz-Esmenjaud J, et al. Leishmaniasis: a review. F1000Res. 2017;6:750.
17. Sarkari B, Rezaei Z, Mohebali M. Immunodiagnosis of visceral leishmaniasis: current status and challenges: a review article. Iran J Parasitol. 2018;13(3):331-41.
18. Braz RF, Nascimento ET, Martins DR, et al. The sensitivity and specificity of Leishmania chagasi recombinant K39 antigen in the diagnosis of American visceral leishmaniasis and in differentiating active from subclinical infection, Am J Trop Med Hyg. 2002;67(4):344-8.
19. Guidelines on use of Rk39, National Vector Borne Disease Control Progamme, Government of India.
20. World Health Organization; 2019. [online] Available from: https://www.who.int/leishmaniasis/burden/hiv_coinfection/burden_hiv_coinfection/en/

Amebiasis, Cryptosporidiosis, and Giardiasis

Kiranpreet Kaur, Piyush Gupta

AMEBIASIS

INTRODUCTION

Entamoeba histolytica causes intestinal amebiasis as well as extraintestinal manifestations like liver, lung, and brain abscesses. It is a pseudopod forming nonflagellate protozoan. There are four species of intestinal amebae: *E. histolytica, E. dispar, E. moshkovskii,* and *E. bangladeshi. E. histolytica* causes symptomatic disease whereas *E. dispar* is nonpathogenic. *E. moshkovskii* is emerging as an important pathogenic organism. However, status of *E. bangladeshi* is still unclear.

EPIDEMIOLOGY

Amebiasis is a leading cause of diarrhea worldwide. The prevalence of amebiasis is disproportionately higher in developing countries as compared to developed nations because of poor hygiene and sanitation. In developed nations, prevalence is high in returning travelers or immigrants from endemic countries. Around 50 million people are affected annually and 100,000 people die making it the third leading cause of parasitic death in humans worldwide.[1] Prevalence in most of developing countries is 10–15% though estimates are as high as 40% in some populations. However, limited availability of methods to diagnose the infection pose a challenge to estimate the true prevalence in developing countries. According to Global Enteric Multicentric Study (GEMS), *E. histolytica* was one of the leading 10 causes of diarrhea in two of the seven study regions—sub-Saharan Africa and South Asia. Also, the recent reanalysis of GEMS using pathogen-specific polymerase chain reaction (PCR) analysis found that *E. histolytica* is the seventh most common cause of dysentery.

TRANSMISSION AND PATHOGENESIS

Transmission occurs primarily through fecal-oral route. There are two forms of the parasite: cyst and trophozoite. Cyst is the infective form whereas trophozoite is responsible for causing the invasive disease. Infection is acquired through ingestion of amebic cysts which are usually present in contaminated food or water. Viability of the cysts in the environment varies from weeks to months, and ingestion of a single cyst is enough to cause infection. Cysts excyst in the intestine to form trophozoites which invade the colonic mucosa to cause bloody diarrhea. Trophozoites kill both the epithelial cells and inflammatory cells by a variety of mechanisms:[2]

- Release of proteinases
- Cell lysis via a contact-dependent mechanism
- Apoptosis
- Formation of pores in the wall of cells known as ameba pores
- Alteration of tight junctions leading to increased permeability.

Trophozoites adhere to colonic epithelium via specific lectin, the galactose-N-acetylgalactosamine lectin. Cells which lack this lectin molecule are resistant to invasion by trophozoites. Other amebic molecules such as lipophosphopeptidoglycan, peroxiredoxin, arginase and lysine, and glutamic acid-rich proteins are also implicated in the pathogenesis of amebiasis.

Recently, it has been found that *E. histolytica* secretes a protein homolog of the proinflammatory cytokine; macrophage migration inhibitory factor (EhMIF). The inflammation produced by EhMIF leads to increased production of matrix metalloproteinases which breaks down extracellular matrix and helps in the invasion of the parasite. Interferon-gamma and acquired antibodies to EhMIF and Gal/GalNAc lectin have a protective role against the infection.

Due to its properties of chlorine resistance, environmental stability, and high transmission, the National Institute of Allergy and Infectious Diseases (NIAID) classified *E. histolytica* as a category B priority biodefense pathogen.

CLINICAL FEATURES

The infection is asymptomatic in 90% of the cases. Asymptomatic infection is known as intraluminal amebiasis. Factors that influence whether infection leads to asymptomatic or invasive disease include the *E. histolytica* strain and host factors such as genetic susceptibility, age and immune status. Risk factors for severe disease and increased mortality include young age, corticosteroid treatment, and malnutrition. Clinical amebiasis generally has a subacute onset, usually over 1–3 weeks. Clinical spectrum varies from mild diarrhea to severe dysentery, producing abdominal pain (12–80%), diarrhea (94–100%), and bloody stools (94–100%), to fulminant amebic colitis (0.5%). Fever occurs in around 40% of the cases. Fulminant colitis can occur in the form of bowel necrosis leading to perforation followed by peritonitis. Toxic megacolon has also been reported.

Localized colonic infection can result in mass of granulation tissue known as ameboma which can grow into lumen to cause pain, obstruction or intussusception. Rarely, intestinal amebiasis may manifest as a chronic syndrome of diarrhea, weight loss, and abdominal pain without dysentery. The chronic form lasts for years and mimics inflammatory bowel disease.

DIAGNOSIS

Polymerase chain reaction is the best diagnostic tool if available due to its high sensitivity. Other methods include stool microscopy, antigen detection, and serology. Newer commercially available antigen detection kits are increasingly becoming popular due to their sensitivity close to the PCR.[3]

Stool Microscopy

It is used to detect cysts or trophozoites either on wet mount or stained preparations. Cysts are small with four nuclei (size: 12–15 µm). Trophozoites are large and have a single nucleus (size: 15–20 µm). Trophozoites and cysts are shown in **Figures 1 and 2**, respectively. Stool microscopy cannot differentiate between different species of *Entamoeba* and is labor intensive.[4] A minimum of three

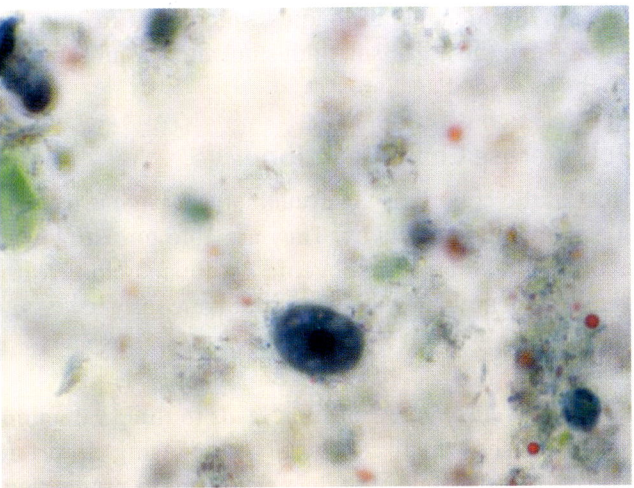

Fig. 1: This trichrome-stained photomicrograph revealed a parasitic *Entamoeba histolytica* trophozoite that contained a single round nucleus within which you can see peripherally situated chromatin, and a centrally located karyosome. Also, note the presence of numbers of vacuoles within the organism's cytoplasm.
Source: PHIL, CDC.

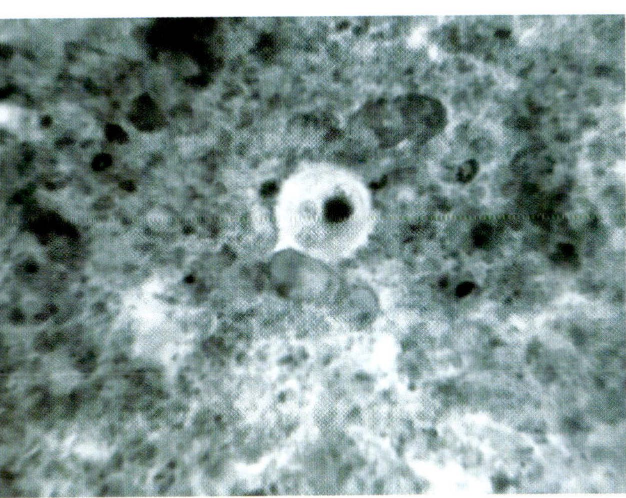

Fig. 2: Under a magnification of 900×, this photomicrograph of a chlorazol black-stained specimen revealed the presence of a cyst of the parasitic organism, *Entamoeba histolytica*. Though mature *E. histolytica* cysts contain four nuclei, in this particular view, you are only able to see three nuclei due in the focal plane presented, as well as a darkly staining chromatoid body.
Source: PHIL, CDC.

specimens sent on consecutive days are able to detect 85–95% of infections. In addition, stool may be positive for blood. However, fecal leukocytes may be absent due to destruction of the leukocytes by the organism.

Antigen Detection

Antigen detection is a very fast, sensitive, and specific method and gaining popularity in the recent years. It can differentiate between *E. histolytica* and *E. dispar*. They use specific monoclonal antibodies which bind to specific epitopes on the organism. Both stool and serum samples can be used for detection.

Polymerase Chain Reaction

Most of the commercially available PCR kits have 100% specificity and sensitivity. They are able to distinguish pathogenic and nonpathogenic organisms along with detection of multiple pathogens simultaneously.

Serology

Entamoeba histolytica infection leads to the production of antibodies which can be detected using different assays; *E. dispar* infection does not result in production of antibodies being nonpathogenic. Indirect hemagglutination is the most sensitive serologic assay; it is positive in approximately 90% of patients with symptomatic intestinal infection. It is not able to differentiate between acute and recent infection. In endemic areas, antibodies can be present in 10–30% of the population due to previous infection. Hence, serological tests have high negative predictive value.

Sigmoidoscopy or Colonoscopy

Its routine use is not advocated as it has risk of perforation. Amebic dysentery can show nonspecific mucosal thickening as well as flask-shaped ulcers in the colon. Cysts or trophozoites can be demonstrated on microscopy in biopsy samples taken from the edge of the ulcer. Antigen testing from the biopsy specimen may also show positive results.

■ DIFFERENTIAL DIAGNOSIS

Other causes of bloody diarrhea include *Shigella, Escherichia coli, Salmonella, Campylobacter, Clostridioides* (formerly *Clostridium*) *difficile,* and some *Vibrio* species. Noninfectious etiologies include ischemic bowel disease and inflammatory bowel disease.

■ TREATMENT

All *E. histolytica* infections should be treated, irrespective of symptoms because the infection carries a high risk of transmission and has the propensity to cause invasive disease.[5] The aims of antiparasitic therapy of intestinal amebiasis are to eliminate the invading trophozoites and to eradicate the cyst form seen in intestinal carriers.

Invasive colitis is generally managed with a tissue amebicide and an intraluminal agent. Tissue amebicides include:

- Metronidazole: 35–50 mg/kg/day in three divided doses for 7–10 days
- Tinidazole: 50 mg/kg once daily for 3–5 days
- Ornidazole: 40 mg/kg once daily for 3 days.

Second-line agents include nitazoxanide, dehydroemetine, and chloroquine.

Metronidazole and tinidazole are the most effective and first-line agents against amebiasis. Metronidazole causes side effects like nausea, headache, anorexia, and peripheral neuropathy. Tinidazole has shorter duration of therapy and once daily dosing. Also, tinidazole is better tolerated and has lesser side effects. However, it is uncertain whether tinidazole is superior to metronidazole for stool eradication of *E. histolytica*. Also, metronidazole alone may eliminate the intraluminal forms with its 10 day course; still we need to give the second drug which acts intraluminally. The intraluminal agents include:

- *Paromomycin*: 25–35 mg/kg/day in three divided doses for 7 day
- *Diloxanide furoate*: 20 mg/kg/day in three divided doses
- *Iodoquinol*: 30–40 mg/kg/day in three divided doses.

Asymptomatic carriers can be treated only with intraluminal agent. Surgical intervention is warranted in cases of bowel perforation, abscess, and toxic megacolon.

■ EXTRAINTESTINAL MANIFESTATIONS

The most common extraintestinal manifestation of amebiasis is liver abscess followed by involvement of pleura, heart, and brain.

Amebic liver abscess occurs as an ascending infection of trophozoites from the portal vein and involves the posterior segment of the liver. It presents with fever, right upper quadrant pain which is dull aching, anorexia, vomiting, cough, and weight loss. Concurrent diarrhea is present in one-third of the cases only. Physical examination reveals hepatomegaly and point tenderness over the liver in 50% cases whereas jaundice occurs in 10% cases only. Rupture of liver abscess can occur in pleural space four times more commonly than peritoneal space. Liver abscess rupture into the pleural space results in an amebic empyema; rupture into the lung can lead to consolidation, abscess formation, or a hepatobronchial fistula. Pleural involvement can also occur by hematogenous or lymphatic route. Rupture of left lobe abscess can result in cardiac involvement in the form of pericarditis, pericardial effusion, cardiac tamponade or constrictive pericarditis. Hepatic vein and inferior vena cava thrombosis secondary to amebic liver abscess have also been described. Uncommonly, patients with amebic hepatic abscesses may also have localized colonic infection resulting in a mass of granulation tissue forming an ameboma, which may mimic colon cancer.

Amebic liver abscesses contain acellular, protein-aceous debris, and a brown "anchovy sauce", consisting predominantly of necrotic hepatocytes. Trophozoites can be seen in the peripheral parts of the abscess in 20% of the cases on microscopy. Amebic liver abscess is generally diagnosed ultrasonographically. Amebic serology only has negative predictive value since positive serology can be due to past amebic intestinal infection. Aspiration of liver abscess is not routinely recommended until there is increased risk of rupture especially left lobe abscess and no clinical response with antimicrobial therapy after 5 days and in case of diagnostic dilemma. Pleural effusion due to ameba should always be aspirated. Antiparasitic therapy includes metronidazole or tinidazole for a duration of 7–10 days. This is followed by a luminal agent such as paromomycin even if the stool microscopy is negative.

Brain abscess can rarely occur due to hematogenous spread. If present, they are characterized by abrupt onset and rapid progression to death. Other rare presentation is cutaneous amebiasis which may manifest as painful perianal or perineal ulceration.[6]

■ FREE-LIVING AMEBAE

They are environmental protozoan parasites without any host and they do not require vector for transmission. Four genera of amebas are known to be pathogenic in humans: *Naegleria* (*N. fowleri* species), *Balamuthia* (*B. mandrillaris*), and *Sappinia* (*S. pedata*). All of these organisms primarily cause central nervous system (CNS) infections except *Acanthamoeba* which also causes extra-CNS infections. Free-living amebae are known for two clinical syndromes: primary amebic meningoencephalitis (PAM) and granulomatous amebic encephalitis (GAE).

Primary Amebic Meningoencephalitis

Naegleria fowleri is known to cause an acute hemorrhagic meningoencephalitis known as PAM. The life cycle of *N. fowleri* is completed in three stages: the infective trophozoite, a transient nondividing flagellate stage, and the cystic stage. Transmission to humans occurs through inhalation of water infested with *N. fowleri*. Trophozoites present in the water penetrate the cribriform plate to reach the olfactory bulb and cause PAM. Water exposure in children with ruptured tympanic membrane may also lead to PAM. Many fresh and warm water sources excluding sea water can lead to this devastating disease in humans. Thus, history of recreational activities in the water is the most important risk factor for acquiring PAM.

Primary amebic meningoencephalitis presents as an acute meningoencephalitis with rapid course progressing to death in few days due to raised intracranial tension. Mortality is more than 90%. Cranial nerves like olfactory and auditory nerves are most commonly affected indi-cating the pathway of spread of infection. Diagnosis is suspected on the basis of cerebrospinal fluid (CSF) picture with cell count ranging from 300 to 26,000 cells per mm^3 with marked polymorphonuclear predominance; presence of RBCs, 250–24,600 cells per mm^3, glucose is reduced and protein is elevated. Typically bacterial cultures and viral serology is negative and trophozoites of *N. fowleri* can be demonstrated in a fresh specimen. The wet mount preparation is used to immobilize the trophozoite and it is visualized using a phase contrast microscope. Giemsa or trichome stains can be used. PCR can usually diagnose the DNA of free-living ameba in 6 hours but they are not widely available. Serology is of no use because many asymptomatic children might harbor ameba in the nasal mucosa leading to false positive serology. Neuroimaging reveals nonspecific findings of meningoencephalitis. Lesions in the brain tend to be located in the orbitofrontal and temporal lobes, base of the brain, cerebellum, and upper spinal cord.[7]

Primary amebic meningoencephalitis should be differentiated from acute bacterial meningitis. History of exposure to water as well as negative bacterial cultures is an important indicator. However, most of the PAM cases have already received antibacterial therapy before they are diagnosed. There is lack of enough clinical data for guiding therapy against PAM due to low prevalence, delay in diagnosis, rapid progression, and high mortality of the disease. However, the available studies recommend the use of following drugs for a duration of 10–30 days:

- Conventional amphotericin B [1.5 mg/kg/day intravenously (IV) ± intrathecally]
- Rifampin (10 mg/kg/day orally in three divided doses or every 24 hours)
- Fluconazole (10 mg/kg/day IV or orally)
- Miltefosine (<45 kg: 50 mg orally twice daily; ≥45 kg: 50 mg orally three times daily)
- Azithromycin (10 mg/kg IV or orally).

In addition, steroids are recommended to reduce cerebral edema.

Granulomatous Amebic Encephalitis

Granulomatous amebic encephalitis is a rare subacute-chronic infection of the CNS caused by *Acanthamoeba* species, *B. mandrillaris,* and *S. pedata. Acanthamoeba* is the most common ameba found in the nature and it can be present in soil, air or water environments with a biofilm (brackish water, sewage, humidifiers, heating hospital environments, dental and dialysis units, and contact lenses). The *Acanthamoeba* life cycle includes two stages: a vegetative trophozoite and a cyst. Transmission occurs through inhalation of trophozoite/cyst or direct contact with the skin. *Acanthamoeba* is known to cause infection in immunocompromised hosts. GAE has a prolonged clinical course characterized by weeks or months of worsening headache, low-grade fever, visual disturbances, behavioral abnormalities, and focal neurologic deficits depending on the topographic location of lesions. As the disease progresses, signs of raised intracranial tension, cranial nerve palsies, altered sensorium, and death may occur.[8]

Lumbar puncture is generally contraindicated for patients who present with a focal lesion associated with elevated intracranial pressure. For patients in whom the CSF can be obtained, nonspecific findings are observed, including mild pleocytosis with lymphocytic predominance, high protein concentration, and low or normal glucose concentration. Trophozoites of *Acanthamoeba* can be seen with Giemsa stain. Brain tissue is needed to confirm the diagnosis. Staining with hematoxylin and eosin demonstrates both trophozoites and cysts. In patients with concomitant skin or pulmonary lesions, tissue samples from these organs may also demonstrate trophozoites. PCR provides a rapid diagnosis but it is not widely available. Brain CT scans and MRI show single or multiple space-occupying lesions with ring enhancement mainly in temporal and parietal lobes. Postmortem examination of the brain demonstrates extensive necrosis and the presence of multinucleated giant cells. Granulomas can be seen in immunocompetent patients, and an abundance of both trophozoites and cysts located in perivascular areas is characteristic finding.

Differential diagnosis includes tuberculosis, cysticercosis, toxoplasmosis, histoplasmosis, bacterial brain abscess, nocardiosis, cryptococcosis, aspergillosis, and primary CNS lymphoma.

Treatment

Regime includes empiric treatment with a combination of miltefosine, fluconazole, and pentamidine isethionate. Trimethoprim-sulfamethoxazole, metronidazole, and a macrolide (azithromycin or clarithromycin) can be added to this regimen as well.

Extra-CNS Manifestations of Acanthamoeba

Acanthamoeba can cause infection outside of the CNS; these include localized infections involving the skin, the nasopharyngeal area, keratitis, and disseminated infections.[9]

Cutaneous Manifestations

These are rare and seen primarily in immunocompromised hosts. Infection begins as papule which progresses to necrotic ulcers or may present as infiltrative plaques or cellulitis. The optimal approach to treatment of localized cutaneous infections is uncertain. Regimens that have been tried with success include twice-daily applications of topical chlorhexidine gluconate and 2% ketoconazole cream, combined with systemic therapy including intravenous pentamidine isethionate, an azole (itraconazole or ketoconazole), and flucytosine.

Nasopharyngeal Infection

Infection of the nasal mucosa and paranasal sinuses is a very rare condition and occurs in immunocompromised individuals only. The disease is characterized by a chronic course with nasal discharge and sinusitis unresponsive to antimicrobials. Findings on the physical examination include purulent nasal secretion, hard brown crusts, and erosion of the nasal septum. The diagnosis is established by a tissue biopsy which demonstrates a large number of trophozoites. Management consists primarily of surgical excision with medical treatment.

Keratitis

Acanthamoeba keratitis occurs in contact lens wearers who do not comply to the recommended cleaning procedures or following trauma. Clinical manifestations include conjunctival hyperemia, tearing, foreign body sensation, pain, and photophobia. Usually a single eye is affected, but bilateral involvement has been observed. Ring-shaped stromal infiltrates are characteristic late-stage lesions of *Acanthamoeba* keratitis. Trophozoites can be visualized via staining of cornea scrapings with fluorescent dye calcofluor. Cornea scrapings can be cultured and molecular methods can be applied to differentiate species and quantify the amebic load. In general, PCR methods are more sensitive than special stains and cultures. Combination therapy should be administered, including polyhexamethylene biguanide (0.02% PHMB) or biguanide-chlorhexidine in combination with propamidine (0.1%) or hexamidine (0.1%). Debridement may also be required.

Disseminated Infection

It occurs in immunocompromised hosts only. The skin and lungs are most frequently affected, with or without

CNS involvement. The condition is usually diagnosed postmortem.

CRYPTOSPORIDIOSIS

INTRODUCTION

Cryptosporidium is an intracellular protozoan responsible for causing diarrhea and biliary tract disease predominantly. There are about 20 species of *Cryptosporidium; Cryptosporidium parvum* is the main species responsible for human infections. *C. parvum* can be further divided into two species: *C. parvum* genotype 1 also known as *C. hominis* and *C. parvum* genotype 2 also known as *C. parvum.* The important difference between the two is that both infect humans but *C. parvum* infects animals as well. *C. hominis* has got the potential to cause more severe acute disease, more chances of recurrent infection as well as extraintestinal manifestations.

EPIDEMIOLOGY

Cryptosporidium mainly causes infection in developing countries with poor sanitation and hygiene. It is the leading cause of diarrhea caused by a parasite. The largest study ever conducted on diarrhea in children, Global Enteric Multicenter Study (GEMS), suggests that 2.9 and 4.7 million *Cryptosporidium*-attributable cases occur annually in children aged <24 months in sub-Saharan Africa and South Asia, respectively, with a total of approximately 202,000 *Cryptosporidium*-attributable deaths.[10] GEMS study also highlighted *Cryptosporidium* as one of the most common causes of moderate to severe diarrhea in under-5 children along with three other pathogens—rotavirus, *Escherichia coli* and *Shigella.*[11] *Cryptosporidium* is known to cause diarrhea in 1–3% of immunocompetent children in developed nations vs. 7–10% in developing countries.[12] Its incidence is high in immunocompromised patients especially HIV (human immunodeficiency virus)-infected children and children who are severely malnourished.[13] In recent years, due to newer diagnostic methods, incidence of diarrhea due to *Cryptosporidium* has increased in immunocompetent children as well.

LIFE CYCLE

Cryptosporidium completes its life cycle in a single host only **(Fig. 3)**. Oocyst is the infectious form which gets excysted in the small intestine of humans to release sporozoites. Sporozoites transform into meront which releases merozoites. These can either reinvade the intestinal wall leading to autoinfection or can undergo sexual maturation to release oocysts. The oocysts are excreted in the stool and remain viable in the environment for months.

TRANSMISSION

Transmission of cryptosporidiosis occurs primarily through fecal-oral route. Respiratory transmission has also been reported. Ingestion of only a few oocysts (10–50) can lead to severe disease and persistent infection, particularly in immunodeficient children. Since oocysts are resistant to many disinfectants (e.g. chlorine, iodine), they are able to escape the filtration systems and have a prolonged survival in the environment lasting for months. The risk of severe and/or prolonged disease is higher in children with both cellular and humoral immune deficiencies [e.g. HIV infection (particularly when the CD4 count is <100 cells/ μL)], post solid organ transplantation, immunoglobulin A deficiency, hypogammaglobulinemia, and recipients of immunosuppressive therapy.

PATHOGENESIS

Cryptosporidium alters the intestinal permeability and results in secretory diarrhea with low fecal osmotic gap. It also causes malabsorption. The organism does not remain confined to the gut and can spread from the intestinal lumen to the bile duct where it causes cholangitis and stricturing. *Cryptosporidia* being intracellular organism are found within epithelial cells and cause distortion of the villus architecture **(Fig. 4)**. Both humoral and cellular immunity are activated in response to the infection by the parasite. In cellular immunity, T-cell response is particularly important in combating the infection as evidenced by presence of severe disease in HIV children with CD4 count less than 100 μL.

CLINICAL FEATURES

Clinical spectrum of *Cryptosporidium* varies from asymptomatic infection, mild diarrhea, to severe diarrhea with malabsorption and biliary tract involvement. Pulmonary involvement has also been described. Incubation period is 7–10 days and it causes secretory diarrhea. The diarrhea usually resolves in 10–14 days in immunocompetent children. In immunocompromised children, cryptosporidiosis presents as chronic debilitating illness with persistent diarrhea and severe wasting. Other clinical manifestations include cholecystitis, cholangitis, hepatitis, and pancreatitis. Biliary tract involvement has been reported to affect 10–30% of patients with AIDS (acquired immunodeficiency syndrome).

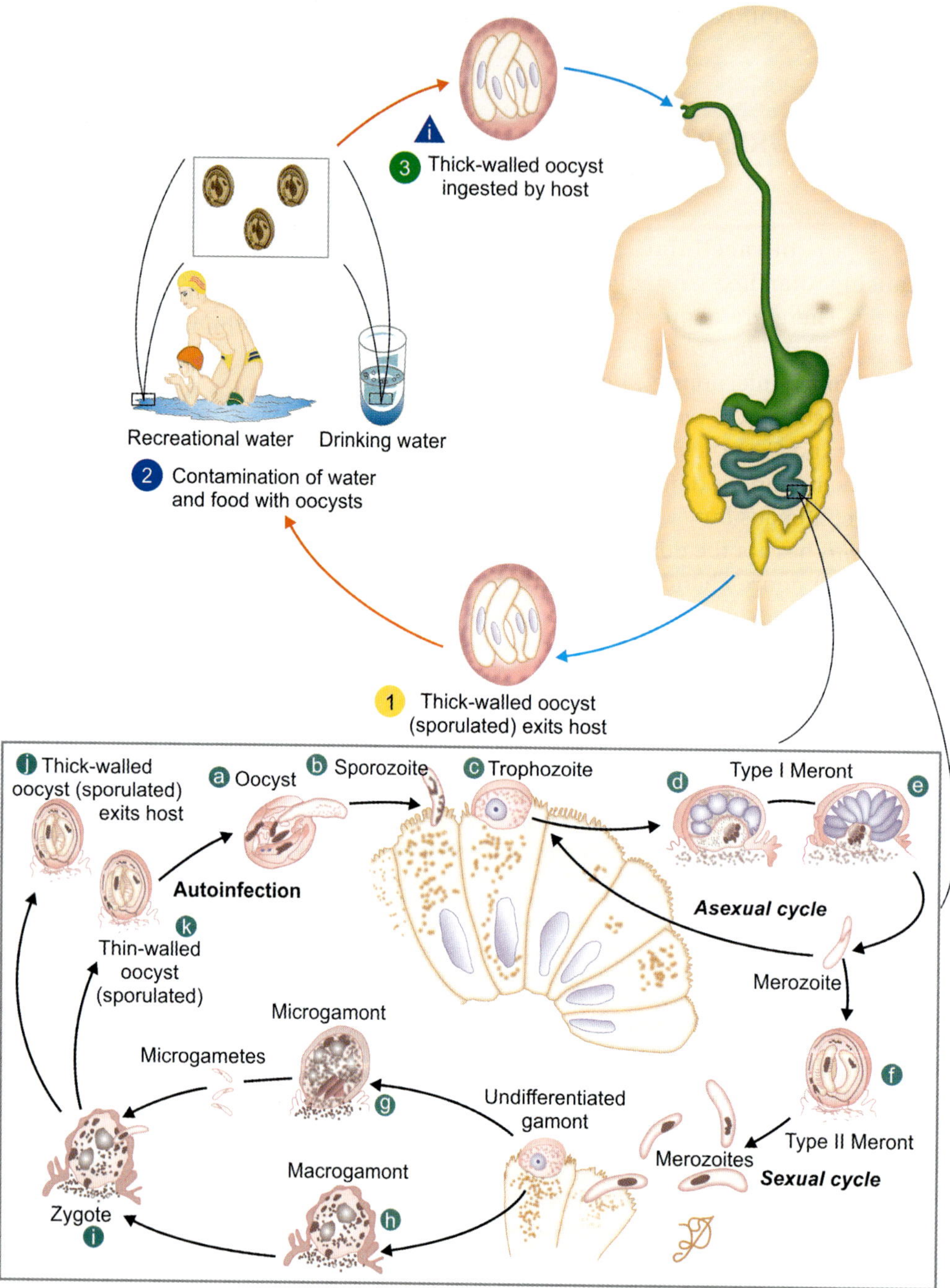

Fig. 3: The life cycle of different species of *Cryptosporidium* parasites, the causal agents of the disease cryptosporidiosis. *Source*: PHIL, CDC.

■ DIAGNOSIS

Stool Microscopy

The oocysts in the stool can be demonstrated by modified Ziehl-Neelsen (ZN) staining or immunofluorescent assays. Oocysts stain pink on modified ZN staining **(Fig. 5)**. Other stains like hematoxylin and eosin, Giemsa, or malachite green stains can also be used. Laboratories should be alerted to the potential diagnosis of *Cryptosporidium*, and specific stains for the organisms should be requested.

Immunofluorescent Assays

Cryptosporidium can be detected in fecal and tissue specimens with the help of immunofluorescent assays

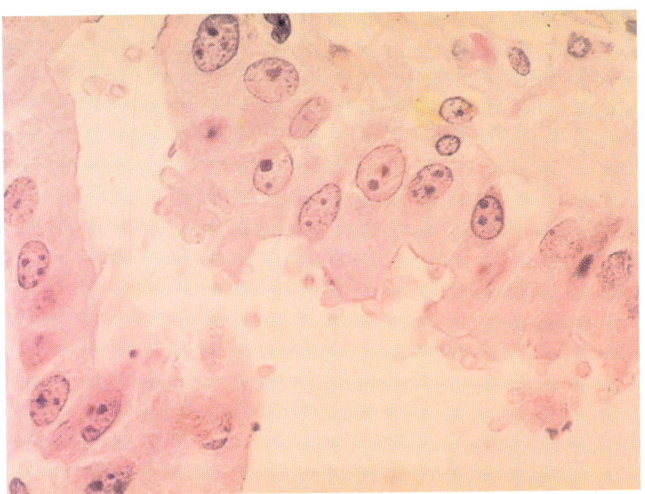

Fig. 4: This photomicrograph reveals some of the histopathology of a section of gallbladder tissue in a case of cryptosporidiosis. The paraffin-embedded tissue shows numerous *Cryptosporidium* spp. parasitic organisms lining the luminal surface of the epithelial cells. In this particular case, this patient had acquired immunodeficiency syndrome.
Source: PHIL, CDC.

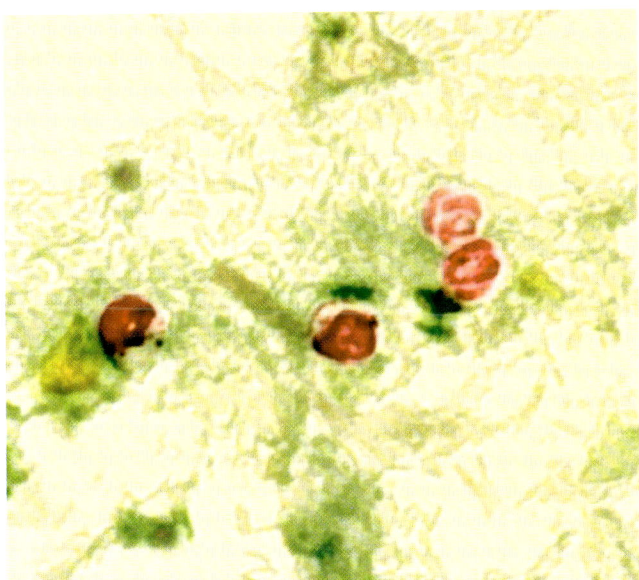

Fig. 5: This photomicrograph revealed the morphologic details of *Cryptosporidium parvum* oocysts, which had been stained using the modified acid-fast method. These oocysts exhibit a bright red coloration when using this staining technique, and in this case, you will note the sporozoites that were made visible inside the two oocysts on the right.
Source: PHIL, CDC.

which are based on monoclonal antibodies against the wall of oocyst.

Polymerase Chain Reaction

Polymerase chain reaction is increasingly being used as tool to diagnose cryptosporidiosis. It has the ability to distinguish between the different genotypes of *Cryptosporidium*. However, it is not able to distinguish between killed and live protozoan.[14]

Serology

Detection of antibodies using enzyme-linked immunosorbent assays/immunofluorescence assays (ELISA/IFA) is not recommended because it is not able to distinguish between recent and past infection.

Histopathology

Biopsy specimens are less sensitive than stool microscopy because of the patchy involvement of the organism.

■ TREATMENT

Most of the illness are self-limiting and may resolve with supportive care only. In case of severe and persistent diarrhea (>14 days), antimicrobial therapy may be required. Nitazoxanide is the preferred agent for all children more than 1 years of age. Its efficacy ranges from 56% to 86%. It has poor efficacy in immunocompromised children. Dose of nitazoxanide is as follows:

- *For children 1–3 years*: 100 mg twice daily for 3 days
- *For children 4–11 years*: 200 mg twice daily for 3 days
- *For patients 12 years and older*: 500 mg twice daily for 3 days.

In case it is not available, paromomycin can be used. Although its efficacy is less than nitazoxanide but studies have found that giving antiparasitic therapy has better outcome than giving placebo.

Antiretroviral therapy should be initiated as soon as possible. Retrospective analyses and case series have found that immune restoration with a CD4 count greater than 100 cells/μL is associated with resolution of symptoms.[15] If CD4 recovery is slow and diarrheal symptoms are persistent and severe, nitazoxanide is recommended.

In case of immunocompromised children other than those infected with HIV, refractory cryptosporidiosis is reported. Although there are no guidelines for management in such cases, one case series supports the use of nitazoxanide for a duration of at least 2 weeks. It evaluated six children who developed cryptosporidiosis following solid organ transplantation. All the patients eventually recovered; however, the two patients who received a short course (5 days) of therapy had an initial recurrence of symptoms when treatment was discontinued.[16]

■ PROGNOSIS

In patients with cryptosporidiosis and HIV infection, the prognosis without immune restoration is generally poor.

They are prone to develop fulminant disease in about 10% of cases characterized by passage of more than 21 stools per day from the time of presentation. In immunocompetent hosts, gastrointestinal and joint symptoms (e.g. painful and inflamed joints involving the knees, ankles, and feet) can persist for many months after the initial infection.

PREVENTION

Oocysts are resistant to most standard purification techniques, including chlorination. However, spores can be eliminated with freezing, boiling, and/or by filtration or using high concentrations of ammonia or formalin. Following preventive measures can be taken:

- Good hygiene.
- People with cryptosporidiosis should avoid swimming pools for at least 2 weeks after the diarrhea has resolved in order to prevent transmission.
- Children at high risk of severe disease, i.e. immuno-compromised children should avoid exposure to contaminated food and water (lakes, rivers, springs, etc.).
- For HIV-infected children, the best prophylaxis is early initiation of antiretroviral therapy. Antimicrobial prophylaxis for *Cryptosporidium* is not routinely recommended. However, clarithromycin or rifabutin (but not azithromycin) given for prophylaxis of *Mycobacterium avium* complex infection may be protective.[15]
- There is no therapy for asymptomatic family members although they may be shedding oocysts and must take care of their personal hygiene.

GIARDIASIS

EPIDEMIOLOGY

Giardia duodenalis (also known as *G. lamblia* or *G. intestinalis*) is a flagellated protozoan parasite known to cause diarrheal illnesses in humans worldwide.[17] There are five other species of *Giardia* but they do not affect humans. In resource-limited settings, the prevalence of giardiasis has been reported to be as high as 20–40% mainly in children <5 years of age.[18] Worldwide, *G. lamblia* is the third most common agent of diarrheal disease in children <5 years of age (after rotavirus and *Cryptosporidium* spp.). Apart from diarrhea, giardia infection may remain asymptomatic in significant number of cases.

LIFE CYCLE AND TRANSMISSION

There are two morphological forms: cysts and trophozoites. Trophozoites are pear-shaped, binucleate, multiflagellated

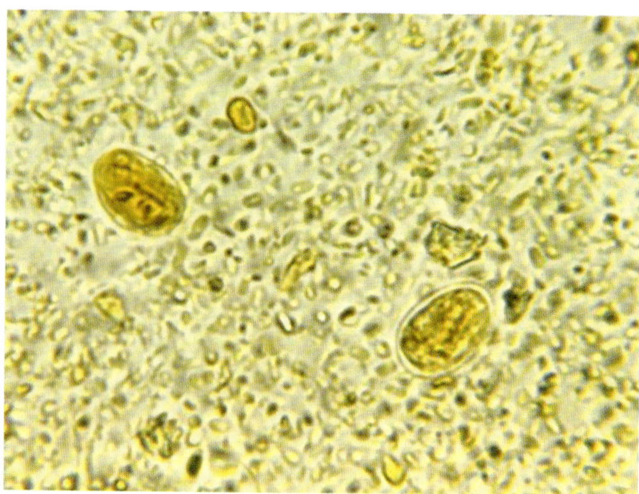

Fig. 6: Under a magnification of 900×, this photomicrograph of a fecal sample reveals the presence of two oblong-shaped, *Giardia lamblia*, intestinal protozoan cysts. *G. lamblia* is also known as *G. duodenalis* and *G. intestinalis*.
Source: PHIL, CDC.

parasite forms capable of division by binary fission. Cysts are the infectious form of the parasite; they are excreted in stool **(Fig. 6)**. Following cyst ingestion, excystation occurs in the proximal small bowel with release of trophozoites. Trophozoites bind to the mucosa of jejunum and duodenum with the help of adhesive disks on their surface but they do not invade the mucosa. Trophozoites which do not attach to small bowel mucosa reach the large intestine where they revert back to the infectious cyst form which appears in the stool. However, during acute diarrhea trophozoite may also appear in the stool.

Transmission of infectious cysts occurs via three routes: waterborne, foodborne, or fecal-oral transmission. Deep well water, in contrast with surface well water, is usually safe because filtration of water through soil removes *Giardia* cysts. *Giardia* cysts are resistant to chlorination; therefore, bacterial coliform counts are not a reliable measure of *Giardia* contamination in chlorinated water sources.

PATHOGENESIS

The species *Giardia duodenalis* consists of eight genetic groups (or assemblages); two assemblages are found in both humans and animals (A and B), and the remaining six are specific to nonhuman hosts, including canines, felines, rodents, and seals (assemblages C to H). The relative roles of *Giardia* assemblages and the human host responses that contribute to asymptomatic and symptomatic infections are relatively unclear. Infants, young children, immunocompromised children especially, travelers and those with cystic fibrosis are at increased risk of developing giardiasis.

■ CLINICAL MANIFESTATIONS

The severity of clinical manifestations associated with giardiasis is variable. In general, about half of exposed individuals clear the infection in the absence of clinical symptoms, approximately 15% of children shed cysts asymptomatically, and the remaining 35–45% of individuals have symptomatic infection. The nature of clinical manifestations in an individual likely depends on a number of factors including the virulence of the isolate, the parasite load, and the host immune response.

Asymptomatic Infection

Asymptomatic cyst shedding can occur up to 6 months. It is the most common presentation of *Giardia*.

Acute Infection

Symptoms usually develop after an incubation period of 7–14 days. Onset of acute gastrointestinal symptoms within 1 week of exposure is not likely attributable to infection with *Giardia*. Symptoms may last 2–4 weeks. Acute infection will present as diarrhea, steatorrhea, flatulence, fever, abdominal pain, and constipation.

Chronic Infection

It may follow acute illness or may occur without the acute phase. Chronic symptoms may occur in up to half of the symptomatic children. Symptoms of chronic giardiasis include persistent diarrhea, malabsorption, weight loss, lactose intolerance, dyspepsia, and stunted growth.

■ COMPLICATIONS

The common complications include weight loss, stunted growth, and malabsorption.[19] Hypersensitivity phenomena such as rash, urticaria, aphthous ulceration, and reactive arthritis or synovitis have also been described. Rarely, *Giardia* can spread from the duodenum to the biliary and pancreatic ducts, leading to cholecystitis, cholangitis, or granulomatous hepatitis. Certain studies have also found that giardiasis led to the development of irritable bowel syndrome subsequently.[20] Ocular manifestations like iridocyclitis, choroiditis, and retinal hemorrhages have also been reported.

■ DIAGNOSIS

Antigen Detection Assays

A number of immunoassays against antigens of trophozoites and cysts of giardia are available which have sensitivity and specificity comparable to conventional stool microscopy. Many of the commercially available assays can detect both *Giardia* and *Cryptosporidium* simultaneously.[21] One study of 325 stool specimens demonstrated that an enzyme-linked immunosorbent assay against a specific *Giardia* antigen (antigen 65) detected 30% more cases of *Giardia* than stool microscopy.[22] Another study that compared stool microscopy, DFA, and three immunodiagnostic techniques for diagnosis of *Giardia* found that there was agreement among the methods in 76% of cases and immunologic methods detected more positive results than stool microscopy in 12% of cases.[23] These immunoassays have limited utility following treatment as they may be falsely positive due to shedding of killed parasites.

Nucleic Acid Amplification Assays

Its utility following treatment is unclear as some studies reveal clearing of giardia DNA following treatment while some say persistence of DNA of killed parasite.

Stool Microscopy

This conventional method of detection is very specific and can detect multiple organisms simultaneously. However, sensitivity is low due to intermittent shedding and depends upon technical expertise. Stool microscopy should be done for 3 consecutive days to enhance sensitivity. Loose, watery stool is more likely to contain trophozoites whereas formed stools contain cysts.

Other Tests

There is no leukocytosis and eosinophilia. Fecal leukocytes are also absent but tests for malabsorption can be positive.

■ DIFFERENTIAL DIAGNOSIS

Giardia needs to be distinguished from other causes of diarrhea. Traveler's diarrhea is caused by enterotoxigenic *Escherichia coli* and *Campylobacter* spp. Onset of traveler's diarrhea caused by *Escherichia coli is* usually within days, whereas symptomatic giardiasis develops only after a week or more after infection. Presentation of cryptosporidium is also similar and hence can be distinguished by microscopy and immunoassays. Apart from it, we need to rule out other causes of malabsorption.

■ TREATMENT

All symptomatic children should receive appropriate therapy.[24] Among asymptomatic children, treatment is indicated in the following conditions in order to prevent transmission:

- Individuals in settings with risk for transmission to others (such as a child in a daycare setting)
- Household contacts of immunocompromised children (especially hypogammaglobulinemia or cystic fibrosis)
- Household contacts of pregnant women
- Food handlers.

For treatment of patients ≥3 years of age, tinidazole is better since it has a longer half-life than nitazoxanide and may be administered as a single dose with high efficacy (>90%). For treatment of patients 12–36 months of age, nitazoxanide is preferred. Given limited data regarding use of tinidazole and nitazoxanide for patients <12 months of age, metronidazole is used. Dosing of first line as well as alternative agents is given in the **Table 1**.

After appropriate treatment, clinical resolution as well as parasitological clearance from the stool occurs within 5–7 days. There is no need to repeat stool examination after the child becomes asymptomatic to check for parasite clearance.

Antimicrobial resistance has been observed in up to 20% of *Giardia* isolates, and cross-resistance between tinidazole and metronidazole (both are nitroimidazoles) has been observed. Antimicrobial resistance testing is not routinely done in giardiasis. If there is persistence or recurrence of symptoms, antimicrobial resistance should be suspected.

Persistent or Recurrent Symptoms

Persistent symptoms may be attributable to drug resistance, inadequate adherence, or immunosuppression. Recurrent symptoms after initial response to therapy may be due to persistent infection or reinfection. More often, however, persistent or recurrent symptoms occur as a result of noninfectious causes; these include postinfectious lactose intolerance, other absorptive deficiencies, and irritable bowel syndrome.

Table 1: Drugs used to treat *Giardiasis*.[25]

First-line agents	Dose
Tinidazole	50 mg/kg single dose
Nitazoxanide	Age 1–3 years: 100 mg bd for 3 days Age 4–11years: 200 mg bd for 3 days Age 12 years or more: 500 mg bd for 3 days
Second-line agents	
Metronidazole	15 mg/kg/day in three divided doses for 5–7 days
Albendazole	10–15 mg/kg/day od for 5 days
Paromomycin	10 mg/kg tds for 5–10 days
Furazolidone	2 mg/kg qid for 7–10 days
Quinacrine	2 mg/kg tds for 5 days

Patients with recurrent or persistent symptoms should have repeat stool examination for detection of giardiasis. Attempts should be made to know the source of infection and eliminate it. These patients should also be evaluated for any underlying immunodeficiency disorders.

Children who are confirmed to have persistent or recurrent giardiasis should receive a repeat course of antimicrobial. In case of recurrence, same antimicrobial agent is used but for longer duration. If there is persistence of infection, then antimicrobial agent from a different class is preferred. If there is refractory infection with repeated failures to monotherapy then a combination therapy may be warranted. Data on combination regimes are limited. Among the regimens studied, it is advisable to use albendazole (15 mg/kg/day orally, maximum dose 400 mg) plus metronidazole (15 mg/kg orally per day divided in three doses, with a maximum dose of 250 mg per dose) for 5 days. Other combinations include metronidazole/tinidazole plus quinacrine for 14–21 days.

■ PREVENTION

Infection Control

Proper hygiene is essential to prevent person to person transmission. Strict handwashing, care with diaper disposal, and treatment of symptomatic children can prevent the spread of giardiasis in daycare centers. Hand hygiene with soap and water is preferred over hand hygiene with alcohol-based hand disinfection (AHD). AHD is effective against trophozoites passed in the stool but is not effective against the cyst form that survives in the environment.

Water and Food Transmission

Giardia cysts are eliminated by boiling tap water at least 1 minute. Further, iodine-based treatments are better than chlorine.

Breastfeeding is protective against giardiasis in nursing infants in endemic areas since it may contain high levels of secretory immunoglobulin A. Zinc and vitamin A have been associated with a protective effect against giardiasis among children in resource-limited settings.

■ REFERENCES

1. Shirley DT, Farr L, Watanabe K, et al. A review of the global burden, new diagnostics, and current therapeutics for amebiasis. Open Forum Infect Dis. 2018; 5:ofy161.
2. Peterson KM, Singh U, Petri WA Jr. Enteric Amebiasis. In: Guerrant R, Walker DH, Weller PF (Eds). Tropical Infectious Diseases: Principles, Pathogens and Practice, 3rd edition, Saunders Elsevier, Philadelphia. 2011. p. 614.
3. Saidin S, Othman N, Noordin R. Update on laboratory diagnosis of amoebiasis. Eur J Clin Microbiol Infect Dis. 2019;38(1):15-38.

4. Parija SC, Mandal J, Ponnambath DK. Laboratory methods of identification of Entamoeba histolytica and its differentiation from look-alike Entamoeba spp. Trop Parasitol. 2014;4(2):90-5.

5. Gonzales MLM, Dans LF, Sio-Aguilar J. Antiamoebic drugs for treating amoebic colitis. Cochrane Database Syst Rev. 2019; 1:CD006085.

6. Salles JM, Salles MJ, Moraes LA, et al. Invasive amebiasis: an update on diagnosis and management. Expert Rev Anti Infect Ther. 2007;5(5):893-901.

7. Capewell LG, Harris AM, Yoder JS, et al. Diagnosis, clinical course, and treatment of primary amoebic meningo-encephalitis in the United States, 1937-2013. J Pediatric Infect Dis Soc. 2015;4:e68.

8. Marciano-Cabral F, Cabral G. Acanthamoeba spp. as agents of disease in humans. Clin Microbiol Rev. 2003;16(2):273-307.

9. Khan NA. Acanthamoeba: biology and increasing importance in human health. FEMS Microbiol Rev. 2006;30(4):564-95.

10. Sow SO, Muhsen K, Nasrin D, et al. The Burden of Cryptosporidium Diarrheal Disease among Children < 24 Months of Age in Moderate/High Mortality Regions of Sub-Saharan Africa and South Asia, Utilizing Data from the Global Enteric Multicenter Study (GEMS). PLoS Negl Trop Dis. 2016;10:e0004729.

11. Kotloff KL, Nataro JP, Blackwelder WC, et al. Burden and aetiology of diarrheal disease in infants and young children in developing countries (the Global Enteric Multicenter, Study, GEMS): a prospective, case-control study. Lancet. 2013;382:209.

12. Dabas A, Shah D, Bhatnagar S, et al. Epidemiology of Cryptosporidium in pediatric diarrheal illnesses. Indian Pediatr. 2017;54:299-309.

13. Bouzid M, Kintz E, Hunter PR. Risk factors for Cryptosporidium infection in low and middle income countries: A systematic review and meta-analysis. PLoS Negl Trop Dis. 2018;12:e0006553.

14. Aghamolaie S, Rostami A, Fallahi Sh, et al. Evaluation of modified Ziehl-Neelsen, direct fluorescent-antibody and PCR assay for detection of Cryptosporidium spp. in children faecal specimens. J Parasit Dis. 2016;40:958.

15. Panel on Opportunistic Infections in HIV-Infected Adults and Adolescents. Guidelines for the prevention and treatment of opportunistic infections in HIV-infected adults and adolescents: Recommendations from the Centers for Disease Control and Prevention, the National Institutes of Health, and the HIV Medicine Association of the Infectious Diseases Society of America. http://aidsinfo.nih.gov/contentfiles/lvguidelines/adult_oi.pdf [Last accessed on August 8, 2019].

16. Krause I, Amir J, Cleper R, et al. Cryptosporidiosis in children following solid organ transplantation. Pediatr Infect Dis J. 2012;31:1135.

17. Minetti C, Chalmers RM, Beeching NJ, et al. Giardiasis. BMJ 2016;355:i5369.

18. Laishram S, Kang G, Ajjampur SS. Giardiasis: a review on assemblage distribution and epidemiology in India. Indian J Gastroenterol. 2012;31(1):3-12.

19. Donowitz JR, Alam M, Kabir M, et al. A prospective longitudinal cohort to investigate the effects of early life giardiasis on growth and all cause diarrhea. Clin Infect Dis. 2016;63:792.

20. Nakao JH, Collier SA, Gargano JW. Giardiasis and Subsequent Irritable Bowel Syndrome: A Longitudinal Cohort Study Using Health Insurance Data. J Infect Dis. 2017;215:798.

21. Claas EC, Burnham CA, Mazzulli T, et al. Performance of the xTAG® gastrointestinal pathogen panel, a multiplex molecular assay for simultaneous detection of bacterial, viral, and parasitic causes of infectious gastroenteritis. J Microbiol Biotechnol. 2013;23:1041.

22. Rosoff JD, Sanders CA, Sonnad SS, et al. Stool diagnosis of giardiasis using a commercially available enzyme immunoassay to detect Giardia-specific antigen 65 (GSA 65). J Clin Microbiol. 1989;27:1997.

23. Aziz H, Beck CE, Lux MF, et al. A comparison study of different methods used in the detection of Giardia lamblia. Clin Lab Sci. 2001;14:150.

24. Shane AL, Mody RK, Crump JA, et al. 2017 Infectious Diseases Society of America Clinical Practice Guidelines for the Diagnosis and Management of Infectious Diarrhea. Clin Infect Dis. 2017;65:e45.

25. Granados CE, Reveiz L, Uribe LG, et al. Drugs for treating giardiasis. Cochrane Database Syst Rev. 2012;12:CD007787.

K Dhanalakshmi, Lakshan Raj

■ INTRODUCTION

Infections which are caused by the opportunistic free-living amebae such as *Acanthamoeba* species (spp.), *Balamuthia mandrillaris*, *Naegleria fowleri*, and *Sappinia* have been documented from all parts of the world, including the tropics.

Although these organisms share structural and pathogenic similarities, the infections they cause have distinctive epidemiology, clinical course, neuroimaging, and pathology.

Primary amebic meningoencephalitis (PAM) caused by *N. fowleri* is an acute fulminant disease that affects previously healthy children and youngsters and usually results in death within a week of presentation.[1] Almost invariably the patient has a recent history of swimming in bodies of warm fresh water, although there are recent reports of acquiring the infection through nasal irrigation using a Neti pot sinus rinse.

In contrast, granulomatous amebic encephalitis caused by *Acanthamoeba* spp. or *B. mandrillaris* is an insidious and protracted illness that affects primarily immunocompromised or debilitated patients and leads to death in weeks to months. Typically, the patient has no history of recent exposure to fresh water.

One other species of ameba belonging to the genus *Sappinia* has also been identified as a cause of severe encephalitis.[1]

Despite these differences, the prognosis of central nervous system (CNS) infection caused by

N. fowleri, *Acanthamoeba* spp., and *B. mandrillaris* is similarly dismal with few reports of survival.

■ EPIDEMIOLOGY

Pathogenic and opportunistic free-living amebae are ubiquitous in their distribution, living not only primarily in soil, but also in sea water, drinking water, swimming pools, sewage, eyewash solutions, contact lenses, dialysis units, dental treatment units, in dust, inside vertebrates, on plants, and in the air.[2-4]

As of 2015, well over 200 cases of primary amebic encephalitis have been documented worldwide, with approximately half occurring in the United States. 25,130 cases were reported in the United States between 1962 and 2008, 135 fatal cases of PAM were reported to the Centers for Disease Control and Prevention (CDC).[5]

Infections occur more frequently in previously healthy children, presumably because youngsters are most likely to remain in water for prolonged periods and they tend to disturb the sediment-containing amebae by diving and swimming underwater. Although it is most common in areas where water temperatures are higher, *N. fowleri* has the ability of overwintering, in cyst form, in sediment at the bottom of lakes.[3]

Though many were exposed to water containing *Naegleria*, why only few individuals got infected remains unknown. Many factors other than the presence of amebae, such as host susceptibility, size of inoculum, and time of exposure, have been considered to be taken into account.[4]

Acanthamoeba spp. are considered important components of the food chain and promote plant growth by predation on soil bacteria. *Acanthamoeba* spp. are prevalent in natural and artificial habitats that include fresh, brackish sea; in sewage; in improperly treated swimming pools; and in taps, dialysis units, dental units, ventilators, and ventilation units in homes and hospitals, sinks, hot tubs, and air-conditioning units.[6,7]

■ ORGANISMS

Naegleria spp. can exist in three forms—(1) an active feeding trophozoite, (2) a rarely seen dormant cyst, and (3) a flagellate form.

Only the trophozoite form is found in tissue or cerebrospinal fluid (CSF). The trophozoite of *N. fowleri* is a small measure of about 8–15 μm in diameter, with a conspicuous nucleus containing a large, dense central karyosome without peripheral chromatin lining the membrane.[8,9]

Naegleria trophozoites move slowly by extension of broad, rounded anterior pseudopodia (lobopodia). This feature may be noted on a warm saline preparation or in CSF specimens. *Naegleria* cysts are spherical, measure 7–12 μm in diameter, and have a single-layered outer membrane.

The life cycle of *Acanthamoeba* spp. consists of two stages—(1) an actively feeding and dividing trophozoite and (2) a dormant cyst stage.[8]

The trophozoite is 15–40 μm. The nucleus is vesicular; has a large, "targetoid" nucleolus; and is surrounded by vacuolated cytoplasm.

Locomotion typically is sluggish by extrusion of multiple fine spiny acanthopodia. *Acanthamoeba* trophozoites feed on bacteria, yeasts, and algae. *Acanthamoeba* cysts are smaller, 15–20 μm, with a wrinkled, thick double wall. Encystation occurs if environmental conditions are not favorable, such as desiccation, scarcity of food, and changes in pH or temperature. *Acanthamoeba* cysts are particularly hardy; they are intrinsically resistant to chlorination and sterilization of potable water and to biocides used for disinfecting bronchoscopes and contact lenses.[6,7] *Acanthamoeba* is the only pathogenic free-living species isolated from marine water. *Naegleria* spp. do not tolerate sea water.

■ CLINICAL MANIFESTATIONS

Naegleria Fowleri

Primary amebic meningoencephalitis caused by *N. fowleri* is an acute, rapidly progressive illness occurring principally in healthy young children that is almost uniformly fatal. Patients have an abrupt onset of severe bifrontal headache, high-grade fever, nausea and vomiting, nuchal rigidity, neurologic abnormalities, irritability, and other changes in mental status in 1–15 days after exposure (typically 5–8 days), most frequently after swimming or bathing in warm contaminated fresh water.[10,11]

Progression from fever to signs of meningitis and encephalitis is unrelenting and rapid. Seizures are common. Coma is present at or develops soon after hospital admission. In the absence of early diagnosis and appropriate treatment, the illness characteristically progresses rapidly to death within 1 week of the onset of symptoms (median, 72 hours).[11] The cause of death is usually from increased intracranial pressure with brain herniation, leading to cardiopulmonary arrest and pulmonary edema.

Apart from the clue of a recent history of exposure to warm fresh water, there is little to distinguish PAM from fulminant bacterial meningitis. CSF findings are similarly nonspecific, with increased pressure, elevated protein level (ranging from 100 mg/100 mL to 1,000 mg/100 mL), a normal-to-low glucose value, and modest polymorphonuclear (PMN) pleocytosis (ranging from 300 cells/mm^3 to as high as 26,000 cells/mm^3), but no bacteria, mycobacteria, or fungi are identified on culture.[10]

Smear of the CSF should be stained with Giemsa or Wright stains to identify the trophozoite, if present.

Acanthamoeba Species

Acanthamoeba cause granulomatous amebic encephalitis. The course is typically prolonged, with progression from focal neurologic signs to diffuse meningoencephalitis over weeks to months after exposure.[12] Patients most susceptible to contracting this disease include very young, old, debilitated, immunosuppressed, and chronically ill patients.

The clinical picture resembles that of a Space Occupying Lesion (SOL) with insidious onset of headache, intermittent low-grade fever, nausea, vomiting, lethargy, stiff neck, and symptoms of increased intracranial pressure. Altered mental status is particularly prominent.

As the infection progresses, depending on the area of the brain affected, hemiparesis, aphasia, ataxia, cranial nerve palsies, behavioral changes, and seizures develop. The incubation period after exposure to onset of CNS disease is unknown but is of the order of several weeks to months.

Routine CSF findings frequently are abnormal but nonspecific, with elevated protein level, low glucose value, and typically a mononuclear pleocytosis.[12]

Cutaneous *Acanthamoeba* infection is characterized by pustules, papules, skin ulceration which develop into nonhealing indurated draining ulcers or subcutaneous abscesses.[12-14] The most common sites where lesions occur are the face, trunk, and extremities. Disseminated disease without CNS involvement has a slightly better prognosis. In patients with AIDS (acquired immunodeficiency syndrome), mortality rates of 70% and 100% are reported for *Acanthamoeba* skin disease alone and in association with CNS disease, respectively.

Acanthamoeba **Keratitis**

Most cases of *Acanthamoeba* keratitis occur in otherwise healthy individuals who wear contact lenses or who have a history of corneal trauma. All soft contact lenses contain 50–75% water.[13] These lenses can absorb pathogens from contaminated cleaning solutions, carrying cases, and hands. When the lens comes into contact with the contaminated fluid, *Acanthamoeba* in the trophozoite stage bind to human corneal epithelial cells. If corneal trauma is present, they invade the corneal tissue and cause cytolysis of the cornea with formation of descemetocele and perforation. The nidus for infection most likely is trauma to the cornea or pre-existing herpes viral or bacterial conjunctivitis **(Fig. 1)**.

Amebic keratitis is characteristically painful and sight-threatening which fails to respond to conventional antibacterial or antiviral treatment. *Acanthamoeba* keratitis is frequently misdiagnosed, initially, as herpetic, bacterial, or fungal infection. Periods of temporary remission delay establishing the diagnosis further.

Recurrent corneal epithelial breakdown with dendritic infiltrates progresses to nonsuppurative keratitis, which waxes and wanes over several months and ends in a characteristic ring-shaped stromal abscess with secondary uveitis leading to loss of the cornea.[13,14]

Complications of infection include iritis, cataracts, corneal epithelial ulceration, hypopyon, glaucoma, scleritis, loss of visual acuity, and penetrating keratitis.

■ PATHOGENESIS

Naegleria trophozoites or cysts enter the body by aspiration of water or inhalation of soil. The trophozoites penetrate the olfactory mucosa and, after active phagocytosis by sustentacular neuroepithelial cells of the olfactory nerve, migrate along the nerve, pass through the cribriform plate, and gain entry to the CNS at the level of the olfactory bulbs.[10] From the olfactory bulb, which is bathed in CSF and lies in the highly vascularized subarachnoid space, *N. fowleri* gets disseminated throughout the CSF and CNS producing an intense inflammatory response associated with lytic necrosis hemorrhage surrounded by purulent exudates. Only trophozoites are found in the CNS lesions.

Macroscopically, *N. fowleri* produces diffuse meningoencephalitis, most severely affecting the cortical gray matter characterized by marked cerebral edema and purulent leptomeninges, particularly adjacent to the olfactory bulbs and base of the frontal and temporal lobes. Microscopically, an acute PMN fibrinopurulent leptomeningeal inflammatory infiltrate is seen throughout

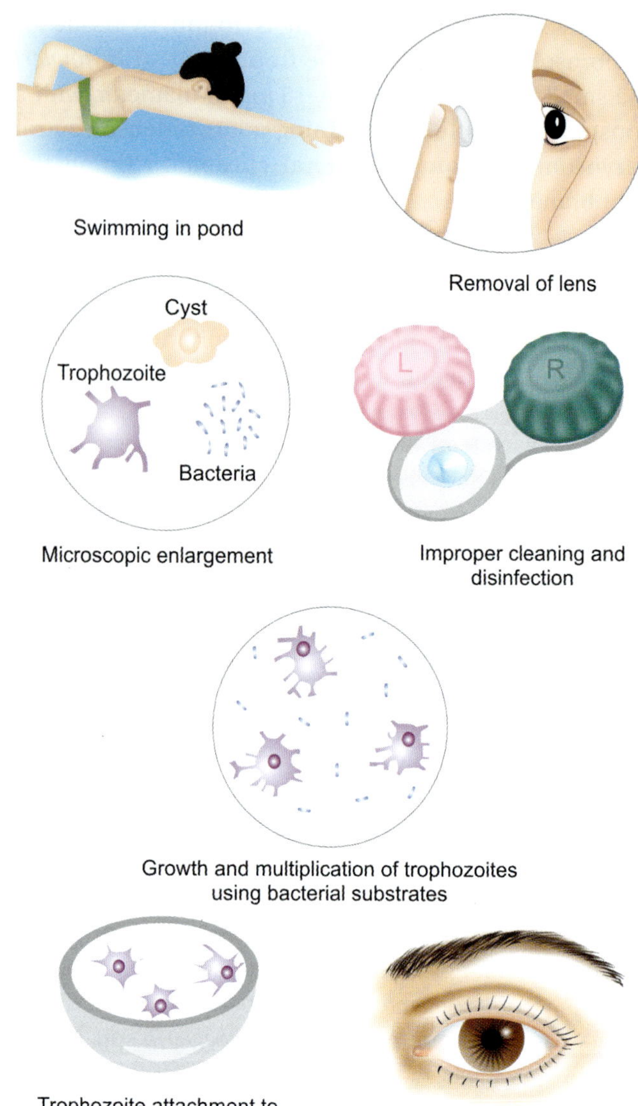

Fig. 1: Proposed mechanism for *Acanthamoeba* keratitis. Bacterial contaminants in the water on the lens support the growth of amebae, which lead to an increased number of invading organisms. The organisms adhere to the contact lens and enter tissue through the damaged cornea, with the subsequent development of keratitis.

the cerebrum, brain stem, and cerebellum and the upper spinal cord.

In contrast, most *Acanthamoeba* spp. infections seem to follow hematogenous dissemination from a primary lower respiratory or cutaneous focus. They are inhaled or inoculated through skin in the cyst phase. *Acanthamoeba* most likely enters the CNS through the blood–brain barrier, through the endothelial lining of cerebral capillaries.[5-7,10] Less commonly, *Acanthamoeba* is capable of causing CNS infection directly via the olfactory neuroepithelium. CNS infections caused by *Acanthamoeba* spp. are characterized macroscopically by diffuse cerebral edema and hemorrhage, with areas of softening and abscess formation. The meninges are spared except for areas overlying involved cerebrum. Microscopically, subacute or chronic necrotizing granulomatous infiltrates and multinucleate giant cells are scattered throughout the CNS, particularly in the cerebral hemispheres, basal ganglia, midbrain, and brain stem.

DIAGNOSIS

Previously, most cases of amebic meningoencephalitis were diagnosed with certainty only at autopsy or by brain biopsy.

Direct Microscopic Identification

If amebic infection of the CNS is suspected, a wet-mount preparation of fresh CSF should be examined for the presence of motile amebae. Ideally, the CSF specimen should be kept at room temperature and examined soon after collection. Although the specimen may be kept at 4°C for short periods, it never should be frozen.[15-17] If present, amebae tend to attach to the test tube wall or surface of the container, so gentle shaking and low centrifugation are recommended to dislodge the amebae. The supernatant should be placed gently on a slide.

Naegleria trophozoites move in a characteristic "slug-like" fashion by extrusion lobopodia anteriorly.

Naegleria, *Acanthamoeba*, and *Balamuthia* may be shown in fixed sections of brain tissue biopsy or autopsy specimens.

Reliably differentiating *Acanthamoeba* and *Balamuthia* by histology alone is difficult. Immunofluorescent stains using monoclonal and polyclonal anti-*Acanthamoeba* (available at the CDC), immunoperoxidase staining, and electron microscopy of tissue sections have been used to confirm the diagnosis. Amebic keratitis may be diagnosed by direct detection of trophozoites or cysts in smears of deep corneal scraping or biopsy.

Culture

Culture is useful for confirmation, speciation, and antimicrobial susceptibility testing. *N. fowleri* and *Acanthamoeba* spp. can be cultivated using bacteria as a food source or without bacteria, in an enriched cell-free nutrient medium that contains antimicrobial agents to inhibit growth of contaminating bacteria. Culture plates are incubated at 37°C and examined under low power daily for 10 days.

Both *N. fowleri* and *Acanthamoeba* spp. grow vigorously and produce detectable cytopathic effects in mammalian cell cultures.

Serology

Although specific *N. fowleri* antibody has been documented in survivors of primary encephalitis, serologic tests are of no use diagnostically.[17-19] The onset of PAM is rapid, and almost all patients die before significant antibody production can occur. In contrast, because the clinical courses of *Acanthamoeba* spp. are usually chronic, antibody responses have time to develop. Detection of serum or CSF antibody against *Acanthamoeba* spp. by indirect immunofluorescence staining has helped establish the diagnosis in many cases.

Detection of antibodies to *N. fowleri* and *Acanthamoeba* spp. in asymptomatic adult and pediatric populations presumably reflects unavoidable environmental contact with these ubiquitous organisms. Whether neutralizing antibodies play a role in the very low incidence of infections in healthy individuals, despite seemingly frequent environmental exposure, is unknown.

Immunofluorescent-antibody staining of serum for antibodies against *Acanthamoeba* spp. has proved to be a rapid noninvasive diagnostic test in many clinical cases. Potentially, this test is useful for establishing an earlier definitive diagnosis and initiation of therapy.

Molecular Diagnostics

Polymerase chain reaction (PCR) of DNA (deoxyribonucleic acid) extracted from frozen brain tissue has been used to confirm *N. fowleri* infection which has been diagnosed by histopathology and immunofluorescent staining.

Similarly, real-time PCR provides rapid, sensitive, and specific screening of environmental and recreational water sources for the presence of *N. fowleri*. The development of a multiplex real-time PCR assay for simultaneous detection of *N. fowleri* and *Acanthamoeba* spp. in clinical specimens of CSF and brain tissue obtained from primary amebic encephalitis patients antemortem offers the possibility of highly sensitive and specific rapid confirmatory diagnosis of CNS infection by free-living amebae and the chance of initiating earlier, more effective treatment.[19]

TREATMENT

Mortality among patients with primary and granulomatous amebic encephalitis is greater than 95%. The high fatality rate is undoubtedly due partly to late diagnosis or misdiagnosis and late initiation of potentially effective treatment.

Amebic Meningoencephalitis

Naegleria fowleri is exquisitely susceptible *in vitro* to amphotericin B, which remains the treatment of choice for PAM. All successfully treated cases have included amphotericin B in the treatment regimen. *Naegleria* is also susceptible *in vitro* to azithromycin and miconazole, with synergism *in vitro*.

Treatment regimens in cases with successful outcomes have included intravenous amphotericin, high-dose intravenous and intrathecal amphotericin and miconazole, oral rifampin, intravenous sulfisoxazole, and intravenous and intrathecal amphotericin in combination with oral rifampin.[20,21]

Liposomal amphotericin B seems less effective *in vitro* and in the animal model than conventional amphotericin (10-fold higher minimum inhibitory concentration) and is not recommended.[20]

Naegleria fowleri remains a trophozoite and does not encyst in tissues, so after it is destroyed by antimicrobial therapy, infection with *N. fowleri* should not recur.

The optimal treatment for CNS disease caused by *Acanthamoeba* spp. has not been established, and the prognosis remains grim, with few reports of survivors. Most cases are diagnosed at autopsy or a few days before death, leaving little time to evaluate treatment.

Combination treatment is favored because no single drug is active against trophozoites and cysts, and many drugs are amebistatic rather than amebicidal.[20-23] Among the few reports of successful treatment, orally administered trimethoprim-sulfamethoxazole, ketoconazole, and rifampin were associated with a favorable outcome in two apparently immunocompetent children with CNS disease.

Pentamidine is considered the most suitable treatment before CNS invasion has occurred because of its low penetration into the CNS. Because of its low penetration across the blood–brain barrier and nephrotoxicity, 5-fluorocytosine was preferred to pentamidine for CNS infection and in renal transplant recipients. Still, other regimens have included pentamidine isethionate, 5-fluorocytosine, and itraconazole.[23]

Similarly, Slater et al. reported successful treatment of disseminated cutaneous acanthamebiasis in a renal transplant recipient using 4 weeks of intravenous pentamidine, topical chlorhexidine, and 2% ketoconazole followed by maintenance oral itraconazole.

The anti-Leishmania drug miltefosine has been found to be useful both for systemic infections and for amebic keratitis.[22] Use of corticosteroids to treat cerebral edema and inflammation seems to exacerbate *Acanthamoeba* infection. At present, the risk of corticosteroid treatment probably outweighs any potential benefit and is best avoided.[23]

Amebic Keratitis

If not treated, amebic keratitis progresses to visual loss and enucleation. The presence of *Acanthamoeba* cysts in deeper corneal layers renders exposure to adequate drug levels problematic, making treatment difficult. In addition, *Acanthamoeba* cysts are resistant to most antibacterial agents at concentrations that are achievable but nontoxic to the cornea. In the early stages of infection, prolonged frequent application of drug is recommended. Combination treatment is preferred during prolonged treatment because of concerns for development of resistance. A variety of topical agents—the cationic antiseptic chlorhexidine gluconate and 0.02% polyhexamethylene biguanide (PHMB), a swimming pool disinfectant, alone or in combination with propamidine—are among the drugs of choice for amebic keratitis.[22,23] Both drugs are effective against trophozoites and are well-tolerated in the eye. Alternatively, two diamidines, propamidine isethionate and hexamidine, can be used, or chlorhexidine can be used along with diamidine. They should be used hourly as drops day and night for 48 hours initially, followed by hourly drops by day only for another 72 hours and, then, because of epithelial toxicity, tapered to 2 hours by day 5 for 3–4 weeks.

Newer agents, such as myristamidopropyl dimethylamine and miltefosine, are effective *Acanthamoeba* cysticidal agents, possess excellent antifungal and antibacterial activity, and show promise in treating recalcitrant keratitis.[20-23]

If medical treatment alone fails, keratoplasty and corneal grafting are required. In these cases, prolonged medical treatment aims to cure or control disease to allow for successful transplantation. The timing of surgery is controversial. Antiamebic drugs are usually continued for months after surgery to prevent late excystation of residual dormant cysts. Use of topical or systemic corticosteroid to treat severe pain or inflammation is controversial.

■ PREVENTION

Infections caused by free-living amebae are reported to be characterized by an absence of distinguishing symptoms, delayed diagnosis or misdiagnosis, and an almost uniformly poor prognosis without early appropriate treatment. Prevention of infection is of paramount importance. Strategies to prevent *Naegleria* infection exist; *N. fowleri* is susceptible to 1 µg/mL or less of chlorine, and adequate chlorination of water in swimming pools or hot tubs is a simple and sensible preventive measure. If water temperatures are higher, use of increased concentrations of chlorine (>2 to 3 mg/L) is recommended.

In certain parts of the world, environmental levels of *N. fowleri* are monitored to ensure that it is safe to swim and that the probability of acquiring an infection is low.[15]

Prevention of infection caused by *Acanthamoeba* spp. involves regular inspections of hot-water tanks, plumbing, and eyewash stations. Contact lens wearers should be aware of the importance of proper care of the lenses. Lenses should be cleansed in sterile benzalkonium-preserved saline or disinfected by heat. Use of homemade cleansing solutions and wearing lenses while swimming is contraindicated.

■ REFERENCES

1. Trabelsi H, Dendana F, Sellami A, et al. Pathogenic free-living amoebae: epidemiology and clinical review. Pathol Biol (Paris). 2012;60:399-405.
2. Dendena F, Sellami H, Jarraya F, et al. Free-living amoebae (FLA): detection, morphological and molecular identification of Acanthamoeba genus in the hydraulic system of a haemodialysis unit in Tunisia. Parasite. 2008;15:137-42.
3. Mergeryan H. The prevalence of Acanthamoeba in the human environment. Rev Infect Dis. 1991;13(Suppl 5):S390-1.
4. Shoff ME, Rogerson K, Kessler K, et al. Prevalence of Acanthamoeba and other naked amoebae in South Florida domestic water. J Water Health. 2008;6:99-104.
5. Centers for Disease Control and Prevention. Investigational drug available directly from CDC for the treatment of infections with free-living amebae. MMWR Morb Mortal Wkly Rep. 2013; 62(33):666.
6. Cope JR, Ratard RC, Hill VR, et al. The first association of a primary amebic meningoencephalitis death with culturable Naegleria fowleri in tap water from a US treated public drinking water system. Clin Infect Dis. 2015;60(8):e36-42.
7. Martinez AJ. Infection of the central nervous system due to Acanthamoeba. Rev Infect Dis. 1991;13:S399-402.
8. Shuster FL, Visvesvara GS. Free-living amoebae as opportunistic and non-opportunistic pathogens of humans and animals. Int J Parasitol. 2004;34:1001-7.
9. De Jonckheere JF. Molecular definition and the ubiquity of species in the genus Naegleria. Protist. 2004;155:89-103.
10. Baig AM. Pathogenesis of amoebic encephalitis: Are the amoebae being credited to an 'inside job' done by the host immune response? Acta Trop. 2015;148:72-6.
11. Kemble SK, Lynfield R, DeVries AS, et al. Fatal Naegleria fowleri infection acquired in Minnesota: possible expanded range of a deadly thermophilic organism. Clin Infect Dis. 2012;54:805-9.
12. Khan NA. Acanthamoeba and the blood-brain barrier: the breakthrough. J Med Microbiol. 2008;57:1051-7.
13. Lorenzo-Morales J, Khan NA, Walochnik J. An update on Acanthamoeba keratitis: diagnosis, pathogenesis and treatment. Parasite. 2015;22(10):1-20.
14. Visvesvara GS, Moura H, Schuster FL. Pathogenic and opportunistic free-living amoebae: Acanthamoeba spp., Balamuthia mandrillaris, Naegleria fowleri, and Sappinia diploidea. FEMS Immunol Med Microbiol. 2007;50:1-26.
15. Yoder JS, Eddy BA, Visvesvara GS, et al. The epidemiology of primary amoebic meningoencephalitis in the USA, 1962-2008. Epidemiol Infect. 2010;138:968-75.
16. Radford CF, Minassian DC, Dart J. Acanthamoeba keratitis in England and Wales: incidence, outcome, and risk factors. Br J Ophthalmol. 2002;86:536-42.
17. Schuster FL, Visvesvara GS. Free-living amoebae as opportunistic and nonopportunistic pathogens of humans and animals. Int J Parasitol. 2004;34:1001-27.
18. Qvarnstrom Y, da Silva AJ, Schuster FL, et al. Molecular confirmation of Sappinia pedata as a causative agent of amoebic encephalitis. J Infect Dis. 2009;199:1139-42.
19. Qvarnstrom Y, Visvesvara GS, Sriram R, et al. Multiplex real-time PCR assay for simultaneous detection of Acanthamoeba spp., Balamuthia mandrillaris and Naegleria fowleri. J Clin Microbiol. 2006;44:3589-95.
20. Schuster FL, Visvesvara GS. Opportunistic amoebae: challenges in prophylaxis and treatment. Drug Resist Updat. 2004;7:41-51.
21. Vargas-Zepeda J, Gómez-Alcalá AV, Vásquez-Morales JA, et al. Successful treatment of Naegleria fowleri meningoencephalitis by using intravenous amphotericin B, fluconazole and rifampicin. Arch Med Res. 2005;36:83-6.
22. Yoder JS, Straif-Bourgeois S, Roy SL, et al. Primary amebic meningoencephalitis deaths associated with sinus irrigation using contaminated tap water. Clin Infect Dis. 2012;55:e79-85.
23. Kato H, Mitake S, Yuasa H, et al. Successful treatment of granulomatous amoebic encephalitis with combination antimicrobial therapy. Intern Med. 2013;52:1977-81.

7.7 CHAPTER

Schistosomiasis, Flukes, and Filariasis

Rajesh Kumar Meena, Piyush Gupta

INTRODUCTION

Helminths are large, multicellular organisms which can be either free-living or parasitic in nature. The three main groups of helminths which are human parasites include flatworms (platyhelminthes), thorny-headed worms (acanthocephalins), and roundworms (nematodes). Platyhelminthes also include trematodes (flukes) and cestodes (tapeworms).[1]

In 2003, the World Health Organization (WHO) started focusing on the control and elimination of diseases which are endemic in tropical countries. These are closely associated with poverty and unhygienic lifestyle practices, causing approximately 1 billion cases globally. Schistosomiasis, visceral flukes, and filariasis are included in the "Neglected Tropical Diseases" by WHO.[2]

SCHISTOSOMIASIS

Schistosomes are the trematodes which parasitize humans. Five species of the genus *Schistosoma* which infect humans are *Schistosoma haematobium, S. mansoni, S. japonicum, S. intercalatum,* and *S. mekongi* among which the first three are the major causes of infection.

Human infection with *Schistosoma* species (spp.) parasites is known as schistosomiasis (bilharzia). Schistosomiasis has been reported from 78 countries across the globe; only 52 countries have moderate-to-high transmission rates requiring large-scale treatment. It infects almost 300 million people in developing countries of Africa, South America, Caribbean, Middle East, and countries such as Cambodia and Laos in Asia.[3] Though *Schistosoma* is not endemic in the Indian subcontinent, few case reports have been published about the existence of the disease. Seven new species of *Schistosoma* infecting animals have been found in India.[4,5]

Lifecycle

Schistosoma spp. have a complex lifecycle involving animals or human as the definitive host and freshwater snail as the intermediate host. **Figure 1** depicts the life cycle of *Schistosoma* spp. In the contaminated water source hatched eggs release miracidia, which infect the specific snail species. After release from snails, free-living cercariae penetrate human skin and develop into schistosomulae, which migrate via venous circulation to heart and then to various organs. Adult worms reside in either the mesenteric venous plexus or the vesicular venous plexus depending on the species of the parasite.

Clinical Features

Clinical features depend on the site affected and are due to local and systemic effects of the parasite and also due to the inflammation triggered by the host's immune response. Infected individuals can present acutely within a few weeks or can present months or years after the infection as a chronic form.

Acute Schistosomiasis (Katayama Syndrome)

Katayama syndrome is an early manifestation of schistosomiasis. It occurs 2–12 weeks after the first exposure in a nonimmune individual or heavy reinfection. Katayama syndrome is a cell-mediated inflammation related to migrating schistosomula and egg deposits in host presenting as a serum sickness-like syndrome. Clinical features include malaise, fever, abdominal pain, blood in the stools, cough, and erythematous maculopapular rash. Due to the long gap between exposure and clinical presentation with nonspecific manifestations, it often leads to misdiagnosis in nonendemic countries. Treatment

Schistosomiasis
(Schistosoma haematobium, S. intercalatum, S. japonicum, S. mansoni, S. mekongi)

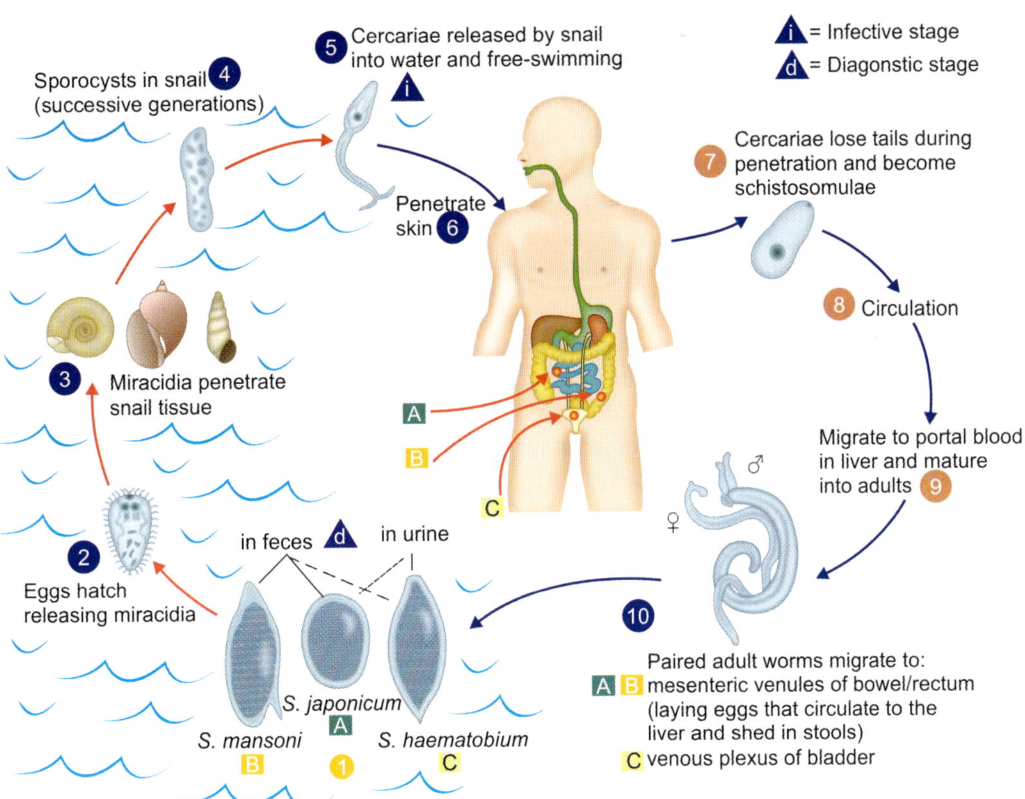

Fig. 1: Life cycle of flatworms of *Schistosoma*.
Source: Public Health Image Library (PHIL), Centers for Disease Control and Prevention (CDC), United States (US).

at this stage generates faster and more effective protection and reduces the rates of reinfection.[6,7]

Chronic Schistosomiasis

Chronic schistosomiasis occurs due to the immune response generated against the parasite eggs lodged in various organs such as liver, spleen, intestinal and urinary bladder wall. This leads to the granulomatous reaction resulting in organ injury and fibrosis. Clinical presentation depends on the site infected.

Table 1 describes the system-wise manifestations of chronic schistosomiasis.[8-10]

Neuroschistosomiasis is a rare manifestation which occurs due to a granulomatous reaction against the parasite eggs in the brain, appearing as lesions on neuroimaging.[11-13] Infection in children is associated with growth stunting and intellectual disability, and in adults with a reduced ability to work.[14]

Table 1: System-wise manifestations of chronic schistosomiasis.

System involved	Manifestations
Gastrointestinal	Abdominal pain, prominent vessels, dysentery, hepatomegaly, splenomegaly, ascites, esophageal varices, and portal hypertension
Urogenital	Dysuria, cystitis and hematuria, bladder fibrosis, bladder carcinoma*, infertility
Central nervous system	Headache, dizziness, and convulsions
Heart and lung	Persistent cough

Schistosoma haematobium is the cause.

Diagnosis

Diagnostic tests for schistosomiasis include coproparasitological examination (CopE), immunological, and molecular methods. CopE includes Kato-Katz (KK) thick smear technique, FLOTAC, etc. which detect the parasite eggs in stool or urine of the host. Demonstration of eggs in stool or urine is the gold standard for the diagnosis of schistosomiasis. Due to the need of less expertise and low cost, KK thick smear procedure is used in disease control programs. CopE methods lack sensitivity in nonendemic and low transmission areas, as eggs are shed in small quantities and intermittently depend on the host's parasite burden.[15]

An immunological method detects the circulating parasite antigen or antibodies generated by the host's immune system by ELISA (enzyme-linked immunosorbent assay). Serological tests are more relevant in low disease burden areas, but they do not distinguish between past and current infections. After confirmation of infection, microscopy is required for species identification and for estimating the disease burden. Tissue biopsy may demonstrate eggs embedded in the mucosa with granulomas in the surrounding tissue.

Molecular methods detect the presence of parasite DNA (deoxyribonucleic acid) by polymerase chain reaction (PCR), real-time PCR, and loop-mediated isothermal amplification (LAMP) in stool. Other samples which can be used are urine, blood, and saliva.[16]

Treatment

Praziquantel is the drug of choice for treatment of schistosomiasis. It is a highly efficacious and safe drug, which is active against all *Schistosome* spp. (20 mg/kg/dose PO TDS for *S. japonicum* and *S. mekongi*; 20 mg/kg/dose PO BD for *S. haematobium*, *S. mansoni*, and *S. intercalatum* for 1–2 days). But it is less active against juvenile schistosomula.

Combination therapy of praziquantel with artemisinin derivatives (artemether and artesunate) acts against all stages of the parasite, thus providing greater protection against schistosomiasis. But caution has to be taken about the use of this combination in areas where malaria is endemic.[17-19]

Prevention

Schistosomiasis infection can be prevented by avoiding swimming or playing in fresh water in endemic areas.

■ VISCERAL FLUKES

Trematodes are one of the classes under phylum platyhelminthes. Though trematode infections are uncommon in humans, foodborne trematodiases are zoonotic infections transmitted to humans through the vertebrate animal host. The parasite becomes infective after completing the life cycle in intermediate nonhuman hosts. The first intermediate host in all species is freshwater snail, while the second intermediate host varies as per the species; the host is always a mammal. Humans get the infection on consumption of raw or undercooked food (fish, crustaceans, and vegetables) that is infected with larval stages of the parasite. The main species which cause severe disease in humans are *Clonorchis*, *Opisthorchis*, *Fasciola*, and *Paragonimus*.[20]

The true global burden of foodborne trematodiasis is unknown, but as per the estimates by WHO Foodborne Disease Burden Epidemiology Reference Group (FERG) 2015, these four species cause approximately 200,000 illnesses and more than 7,000 deaths annually all over the world.[21] Countries in Asia and Latin America are the most affected, though cases about foodborne trematodes infections have been reported from more than 70 countries around the world.

Lung Flukes

Paragonimiasis is a foodborne zoonosis caused by *Paragonimus* spp. (*P. westermani*, *P. heterotremus*, *P. africanus*, *P. kellicotti*). *P. westermani* is the most common causative agent, and less frequently other species of *Paragonimus* cause human infection. This disease is endemic in Asia (China, Philippines, South Korea, Japan, Thailand, Vietnam, India), parts of West Africa (Eastern Nigeria and southwestern Cameroon), and several parts of Central and South America.[22]

In India, paragonimiasis is endemic in northeastern states. Multiple cases have been reported from Manipur, Arunachal Pradesh, and Nagaland, where interestingly *P. heterotremus* has been detected as the causative agent of paragonimiasis against the widely believed *P. westermani*.[23] Due to the lack of knowledge amongst healthcare providers and poor diagnostic facilities, this condition is underreported in our country, often misdiagnosed, and treated as tuberculosis.

Life Cycle

Human infection is relatively rare and associated with dietary habits such as eating raw crabs or crayfish (second intermediate crustacean host), which contains the infective metacercariae in their tissues **(Fig. 2)**. In humans metacercariae excyst in the duodenum, penetrate through the intestinal wall into the abdomen, and migrate to their final habitat in the lungs. Adult worms (5–10 mm) encapsulate within the lung parenchyma and deposit brown operculated eggs (60–100 μm). Inflammatory rupture

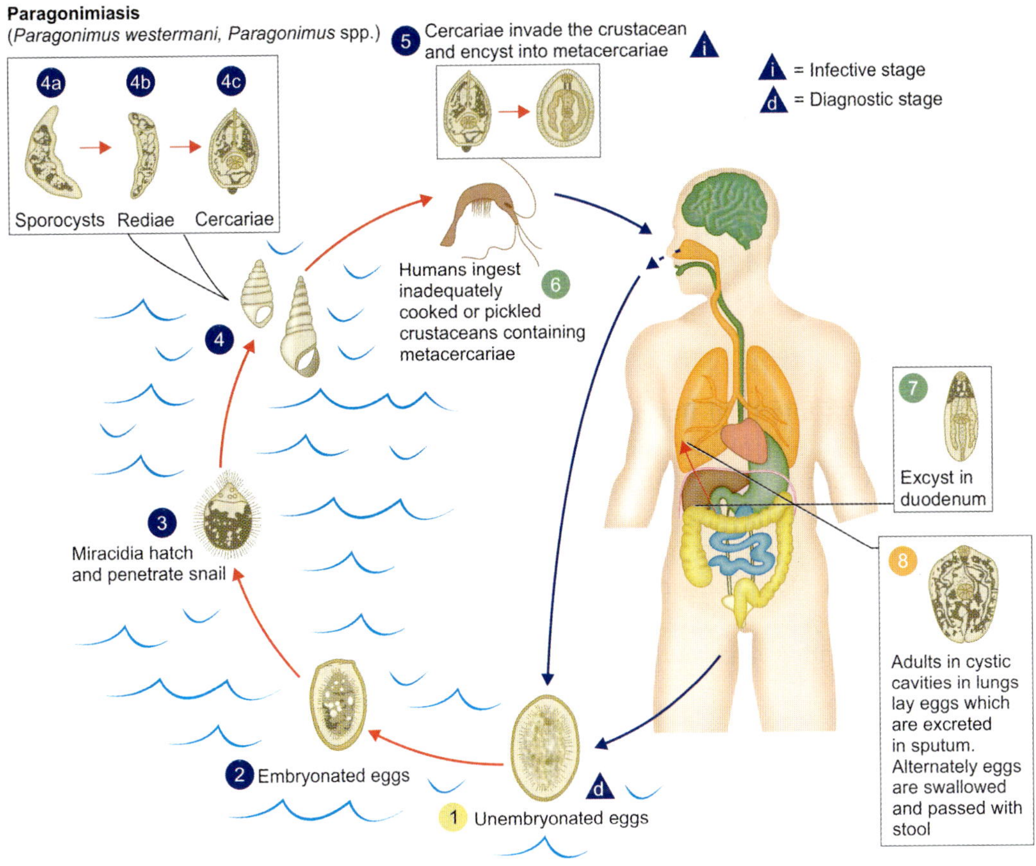

Fig. 2: Life cycle of flatworms of *Paragonimus* species (lung fluke).
Source: Public Health Image Library (PHIL), Centers for Disease Control and Prevention (CDC), United States (US).

of bronchioles leads to the release of eggs and necrotic material in lumen which is expectorated by coughing. Lung flukes lead to the development of parenchyma inflammation, hemorrhage, necrosis, and lung fibrosis.

Clinical Presentation

Most individuals are asymptomatic as they have low or moderate worm load. In humans, the highest incidence of paragonimiasis is found in 11–15-year-old children. *Paragonimus* infection leads to the development of respiratory symptoms such as cough, bloody sputum, and chest pain in majority of children apart from general features such as fever, loss of appetite, headache, and night sweats, mimicking pulmonary tuberculosis. Occasionally, the lung flukes migrate to other systems such as the central nervous system (CNS), liver, eye, skin, peritoneum, and pericardium.[24,25] CNS involvement occurs in individuals living in highly endemic regions and those who have a very high parasite burden. CNS infestation accounts for 50% of cases having extrathoracic disease. Presentations include headache, grand mal seizures, blindness, sensorimotor disturbances, etc.[26]

Diagnosis

In the absence of characteristic physical findings, laboratory examination plays an important role in diagnosing paragonimiasis. Complete blood count shows the presence of marked eosinophilia. For definitive diagnosis of paragonimiasis, sputum examination is the method of choice. Rust-colored sputum because of the presence of brown eggs and hemosiderin released from RBCs is the characteristic finding. This method has a low sensitivity, 30–40% for a single sputum sample, which improves to 54–89% on multiple examinations. Sensitivity for the demonstration of parasite eggs in stool samples is even less. Serologic tests are useful in the diagnosis of cerebral paragonimiasis in the initial course as antibodies decline with time.[27]

On radiological imaging, chest X-ray shows presence of small patchy infiltrates in middle lung fields; rarely features suggestive of lung abscess, pleural, or pericardial effusion or bronchiectasis may develop. In approximately 20% cases, radiological findings may be normal. Computed tomography (CT) shows the presence of clustered ring-enhancing lesions in the brain. The presence of multiple conglomerated lesions with irregular hemorrhage on MRI of brain is the characteristic finding very suggestive of cerebral paragonimiasis in children. Tunnel sign on MR images may be a specific indicator of the active cerebral disease.[28]

Treatment

Praziquantel (25 mg/kg TDS PO for 2 days) is the drug of choice. Triclabendazole (5 mg/kg PO daily for 3 days) can also be given.

■ INTESTINAL FLUKES

Among the several species of intestinal flukes known to cause human infection, the clinically important ones are *Fasciolopsis buski*, *Echinostoma*, *Heterophyes*, *Metagonimus*, and *Gastrodiscoides*. *F. buski* is endemic in Southeast Asian countries (China, Korea, India, Bangladesh, Thailand, Malaysia, Myanmar, Vietnam) and South and Central America. Cases due to the other species are also found in Russia along with Asian countries.[29]

Life Cycle

Human gets the infection by eating uncooked or undercooked infected freshwater fish, frogs, molluscs (clams, oysters, snails), crustaceans (crabs, shrimps), freshwater plants, watercress, water lily, and caltrop. Ingested metacercariae encyst in stomach and develop into flukes which inhabit the intestines, mainly duodenum and jejunum (**Fig. 3**). These adult flukes get attached to the duodenal or jejunal wall by the suckers causing mechanical damage and inflammation, leading to the formation of ulcers which can bleed and develop into intestinal abscesses. Adult intestinal flukes may develop up to 5 cm in length and these can live up to 25 years in human hosts. Mature *F. buski* can produce up to 16,000 eggs/day, which are released into feces, and it completes the life cycle through snail which acts as an intermediate host.

Clinical Presentation

The morbidity due to infestation depends on the parasite load. Mild infection with few flukes is usually asymptomatic, while high parasite burden presents with severe symptoms. In an acute stage, the presenting complaints include diarrhea, abdominal pain, flatulence, constipation, headache, and fever. Chronic cases present with features such as anemia, edema, anorexia, and prostration suggestive of malabsorption.[30] Rarely,

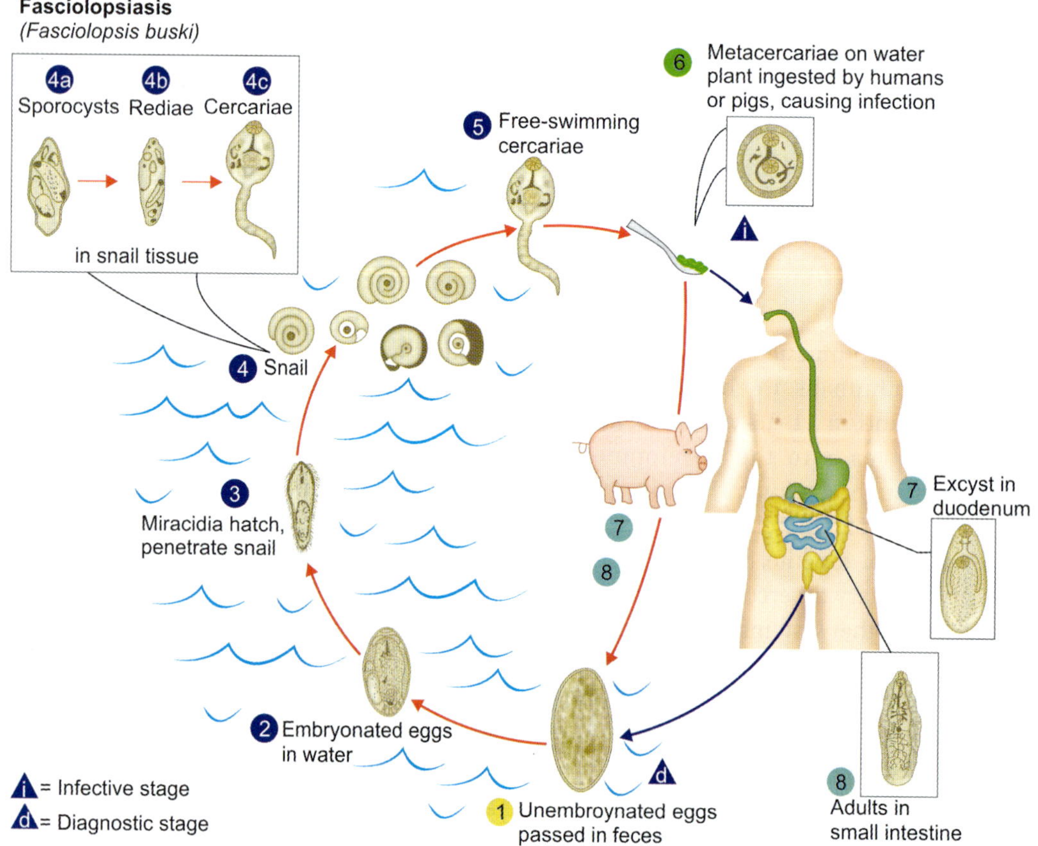

Fig. 3: Life cycle of *Fasciolopsis buski* (intestinal fluke).
Source: Public Health Image Library (PHIL), Centers for Disease Control and Prevention (CDC), United States (US).

intestinal perforation and upper gastrointestinal bleeding may occur.[31]

Diagnosis

The gold standard for the diagnosis of intestinal fluke infections is demonstration of eggs by fecal examination and identification of the species as the eggs of flukes like heterophyes and echinostomes are indistinguishable.

Treatment

Praziquantel (25 mg/kg/dose TDS PO for 2 days) is the drug of choice.

■ LIVER FLUKES

The most important species of foodborne trematodes which infect liver are *Clonorchis sinensis*, *Opisthorchis viverrini*, *Opisthorchis feline*, and *Fasciola hepatica*. Globally *C. sinensis* (Chinese liver fluke) causes approximately 35 million infections of which around half of the cases are reported from China, along with Taiwan, Northern Vietnam, and Korea. *O. viverrini* (Thai liver fluke) causes 10 million infections, endemic in Southeast Asian countries including Thailand, Cambodia, Laos,

and Central Vietnam. *F. hepatica* (sheep liver fluke) affects 2.4–17 million people worldwide, predominantly in Vietnam, Cuba, Egypt, South America, and Western European countries.[32] In the Indian subcontinent, fascioliasis has been from Bihar, Maharashtra, Assam, and Uttar Pradesh along with northeastern states.[33]

Life Cycle

Human gets infected after eating small freshwater fish or freshwater vegetation like wild watercress, lettuce, and alfalfa, which contains the metacercariae of *C. sinensis*, *O. viverrini*, and *F. hepatica* respectively. The life cycle of liver fluke is depicted in **Figure 4**. The ingested metacercariae excyst in human duodenum, cross the intestinal wall into the abdominal cavity, and enters liver parenchyma after penetrating the liver capsule. After entering the bile ducts, they mature into adult worms and produce eggs, which pass to intestines with bile and are finally excreted in feces.

Clinical Manifestations

Presentation of liver fluke infection varies from completely asymptomatic infection to severe manifestations depending on the phase of infection and parasitic load.

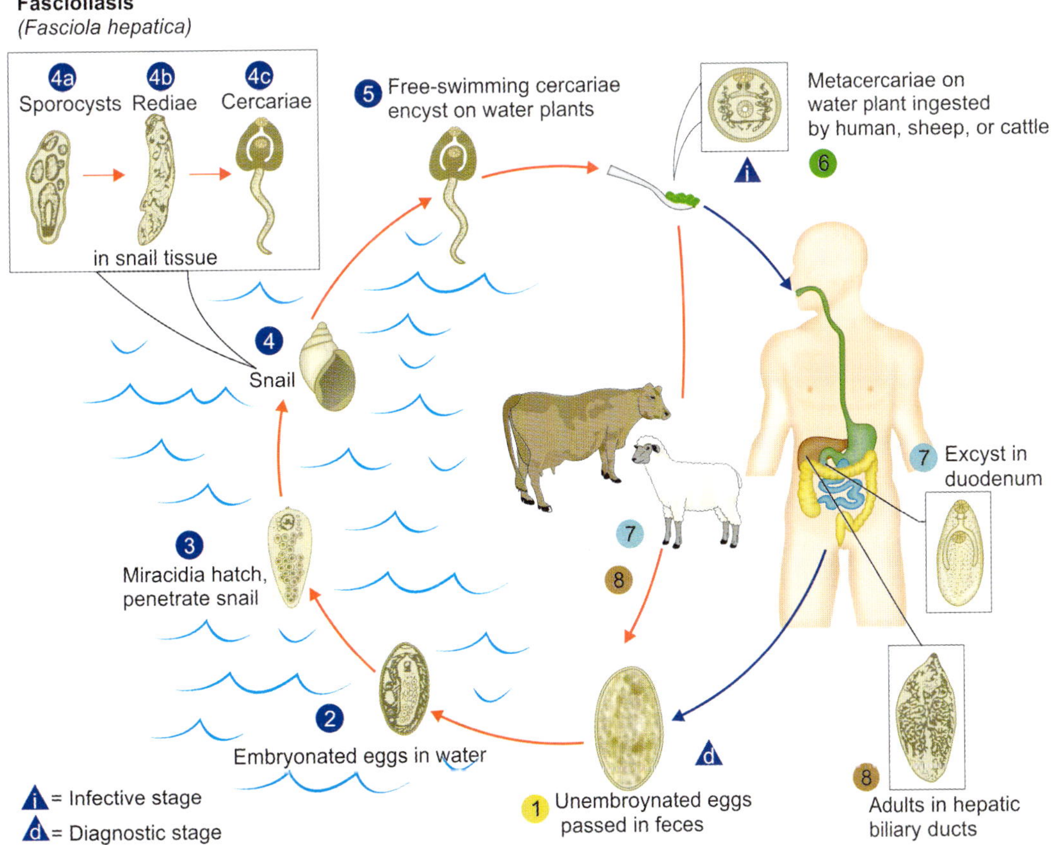

Fig. 4: Life cycle of *Fasciola hepatica* (liver fluke).
Source: Public Health Image Library (PHIL), Centers for Disease Control and Prevention (CDC), United States (US).

Manifestations commonly occur during the liver migratory phase (acute hepatic phase) or during the final lodging of the parasite in the bile ducts (chronic biliary phase).

Acute hepatic phase: Right hypochondriac pain, fever, urticaria, and loss of appetite which occur during the migration of larva in the liver parenchyma. This phase starts 6–12 weeks after ingestion of the infecting organism and the duration of this phase varies from weeks to months.

Chronic biliary phase: Features suggestive of ascending cholangitis, cholecystitis, cholelithiasis, and biliary abscesses occur due to the fluke-induced biliary epithelial hyperplasia and biliary duct fibrosis. Occasionally, invasion of the parenchyma results in liver abscess. *O. viverrini* infection is associated with cholangiocarcinoma in adults having very poor prognosis.

Diagnosis

Clinical diagnosis is presumptive while definitive diagnosis requires demonstration of parasite eggs in feces. Blood examination reveals presence of anemia and leukocytosis with eosinophilia. Liver function tests may show conjugated hyperbilirubinemia with elevated alkaline phosphatase and gamma-glutamyltranspeptidase (GGT) levels.

Stool examination shows unembryonated, ovoid, operculated eggs, the size of which varies as per the species. Eggs can also be demonstrated in biliary or duodenal aspirates and tissue biopsy. Microscopy has low sensitivity in mild infections and low specificity due to similar morphology of eggs of many species.

Serological tests include antibody or antigen detection by ELISA such as Fas2-ELISA which detects immunoglobulin G (IgG) against Fas2 antigen and Fasciola Circulating Antigens (CAs) or coproantigens in serum or feces respectively. Antibody-based kits lack the ability to differentiate between current and past infections. ELISA-based *Fasciola* antigen detection kits are more helpful in diagnosing current infections with 100% sensitivity and specificity.[34] Molecular methods such as PCR-restriction fragment length polymorphism (PCR-RFLP) based methods have high sensitivity and specificity, but due to the high cost and expertise requirements it cannot be used in routine practice.

Radiological imaging techniques such as ultrasound may reveal the presence of focal lesions in liver parenchyma, dilatation and thickening of intrahepatic bile ducts, and increased periductal echogenicity.[35] Abdominal CT may show multiple small hypodensities in the liver parenchyma during the acute phase and during chronic phase it reveals the thickening of liver capsule and hyperintense lesions within bile ducts suggestive of calcified dead flukes. Endoscopic retrograde cholangiopancreatography (ERCP) can be used for the diagnosis and therapeutic intervention in selected cases.

Treatment

The drug of choice for treatment of fascioliasis is triclabendazole (10 mg/kg single dose) but it has side effects such as abdominal pain, fever, pruritus, and vomiting. Oral bithionol (30–50 mg/kg/day on alternate days for a total of 10–15 doses) is another recommended drug, but these drugs are available in few countries only. Praziquantel (75 mg/kg in divided TID PO for 2 days) is another drug with a better safety profile.

Prevention

Foodborne trematode infections can be prevented by educating people about avoiding the consumption of raw crustaceans, molluscs, small freshwater fish, or freshwater vegetation. Other measures include the mass use of antihelminthics, proper disposal of human excreta, restraining pigs from having access to ponds and canals, etc.

■ FILARIASIS

Filariasis is caused by nematodes from the family Filarioidea. Almost 90% of infections are caused by *Wuchereria bancrofti* whereas few are caused by *Brugia* species. Humans are the exclusive host of *W. bancrofti*. Adult worms lodge in the lymphatic vessels and impair the drainage causing abnormal enlargement of the affected body parts leading to pain, severe disability, and social stigma.

Globally, around 120 million people living in tropical and subtropical countries are infected with lymphatic filariasis. Out of the total susceptible population, 57% live in the South-East Asia Region (SEAR). A recent estimation by WHO showed that in the last 13 years, more than 96.71 million cases were prevented or cured as a result of mass drug administration (MDA). In 2017, Thailand became the third country in SEAR to have achieved the criteria for elimination of lymphatic filariasis after Maldives and Sri Lanka.[36]

In the Indian subcontinent, lymphatic filariasis is still widely prevalent in 18 states and Union Territories. Brugian filariasis caused by *Brugia malayi* is mostly found in six states—Uttar Pradesh, Bihar, Andhra Pradesh, Orissa, Tamil Nadu, Kerala, and Gujarat, while Bancroftian filariasis is widely distributed. The National Filaria Control Programme was first launched in 1955. The activities were mainly confined to urban areas while in 1994 they were further extended to include the rural areas. In 2004, the elimination program was launched by the Government of India for lymphatic filariasis in 255 endemic districts of 16 States and five Union Territories of India. Initially, diethylcarbamazine (DEC) was given as MDA program and later on in the year 2006, albendazole was also added with DEC. Subsequently in 2015, 222 districts had a microfilaria rate of less than 1% whereas in 53 districts, MDA was stopped as the transmission cycle of the filaria was stopped successfully.[37,38]

Life Cycle

Adult filarial worms can live for almost 6–8 years and produce millions of larvae known as microfilariae that circulate in the blood of the infected host. On biting the infected humans, mosquito vector ingests the microfilariae, which subsequently undergo maturation in the mosquito. The mosquitoes can then spread infective larvae to susceptible hosts **(Fig. 5)**. The principal vector of *W. bancrofti* is the mosquito of the *Culex* genus (*culex quinquefasciatus*) while *Anopheles* and *Aedes* spp. are also known vectors in some parts of the world. *B. malayi* parasites are confined to some areas of Southeast Asia

including India and its principal vector is *Mansonia annulifera* and *Mansonia uniformis*. Factors such as the prevalence of the disease, density of vector, and density of microfilaria in the blood of the infected individual affect the disease transmission in an area.

Clinical Features

Filaria has a predilection of involving the lymphatic system of the body. Adult worm dwells in lymphatic vessels leading to lymphatic dilatation and lymphedema. Prevalence of lymphedema is significantly more in females, who can have all manifestations of the disease except hydrocele. Hydrocele as a result of scrotal lymphatic dilatation is the most common amongst all the presentations.

The disease rate is age dependent and it increases steadily after 10 years of age. Clinical presentation can be divided into acute or chronic. Acute presentation includes fever with chills and rigors, epididymo-orchitis, lymphangitis, and painful lymphadenopathy (cervical, axillary, inguinal and generalized). Chronic disease includes hydrocele, lymphedema which can be reversible initially on elevation or specific exercise of the limb, and elephantiasis (which is irreversible edema of the limb with

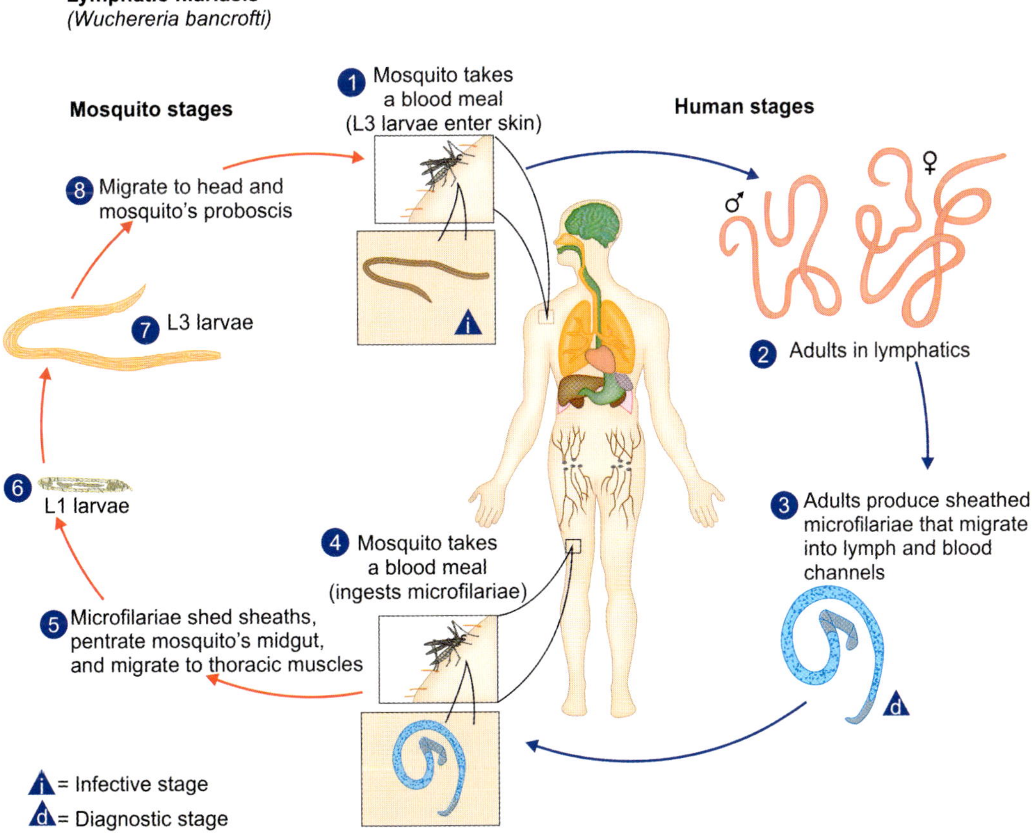

Fig. 5: Life cycle of *Wuchereria bancrofti*.
Source: Public Health Image Library (PHIL), Centers for Disease Control and Prevention (CDC), United States (US).

skin thickening, papillary, and nodular growth). Though lymphedema mostly affects the lower limbs, it can also involve the arms, breasts, and genitalia. Body deformities are mostly associated with social stigma, depression, and loss of occupation and thus increase the overall social burden.[39,40]

Tropical Pulmonary Eosinophilia

Microfilaria is mostly asymptomatic but can result in tropical pulmonary eosinophilia syndrome due to hyperresponsiveness of the host's immune system. This manifestation is typically found in Asian inhabitants. Symptoms typically include nocturnal cough, shortness of breath, and episodes of wheezing. Blood examination shows presence of eosinophilic leukocytosis [absolute eosinophil count (AEC) >3,000 cells/mm^3] with highly elevated levels of immunoglobulin E (IgE) and antifilarial antibodies.

Diagnosis

Diagnostic methods can be divided into nonspecific and specific. Nonspecific tests include presence of eosinophilia, elevated IgE levels, and dilated lymph channels on lymphoscintigraphy, but these tests have a low specificity. Tests such as the detection of microfilaria on blood smears, positive serology, and presence of DNA by PCR are the specific methods. Demonstration of microfilariae on the blood smear examination is considered as the gold standard for diagnosing the active infection. For examination, thick smear should be made from the blood collected between 10 pm and 2 am and stained with Giemsa or hematoxylin and eosin. Concentration techniques can be used to enhance the sensitivity.

Serological tests are the alternatives to microscopic diagnosis. Patients with active filarial infection generally have increased filarial antigen levels which lead to the easily detectable levels of Ig in the blood. These antibodies can be detected using ELISA and immunochromatographic methods. The advantage of the serological tests is that nocturnal sampling is not needed and have high sensitivity (96%). PCR-based assays have come up now which are even 10 times more sensitive than microscopy in detecting microfilaria. Antibody detection by measuring IgG4 has poor specificity (40%) as old infections also give positive results.

Treatment

Treatment of the affected person destroys microfilaria and adult parasites thus interrupts the transmission of *W. bancrofti*. Management includes drug therapy, limb positioning in early stages as drugs are not useful in chronic and advanced cases of lymphedema and surgical management of condition like hydrocoele. Early treatment prevents further deterioration and recurrence of lymphangitis. DEC is the drug of choice for more than 50 years; a single oral dose of 6 mg/kg is as effective as the 12-day regimen. The drug kills the microfilariae and few adult worms too. The most common side effects are dizziness, fever, headache, nausea, muscles, and joint pain. But people having chronic manifestations of disease like lymphedema and elephantiasis are unlikely to get any benefit from DEC treatment. In such cases simple measures such as maintaining proper hygiene, correct skin care regime, selective exercises, and elevation of the affected limbs are important for long-term outcome.

Preventive Strategies

Protection against the mosquito bites is the most effective way of prevention against lymphatic filariasis. Common measures such as use of mosquito nets while sleeping, wearing long-sleeve dresses, and use of mosquito repellent on exposed skin are quite effective. Another strategy includes MDA that will kill the microscopic worms. Annual mass treatment decreases the disease transmission rates by reducing the level of microfilariae in the blood and thus forms the basis of the Global Programme to Eliminate Lymphatic Filariasis which is still now considered as a neglected tropical disease. MDA regimens containing two drugs have interrupted the filaria transmission cycle when conducted annually for 4–6 years with effective coverage of the total population at risk. WHO recommended MDA regimens that include use of albendazole (400 mg) twice a year for areas coendemic with loiasis, while ivermectin (200 µg/kg) with albendazole (400 mg) is used in countries endemic with onchocerciasis. In countries without onchocerciasis like in India, DEC citrate (6 mg/kg) and albendazole (400 mg) are recommended. Successful campaigns to eliminate lymphatic filariasis have taken place in China and a few other countries.

In 2017, a new three-drug regimen consisting of ivermectin, DEC, and albendazole (IDA) is recommended by WHO. Annual use of IDA is recommended to accelerate the elimination of lymphatic filariasis as a public health problem.[41]

■ REFERENCES

1. US Centers for Disease Control and Prevention. About parasites; 2019. [online] Available from: https://www.cdc.gov/parasites/about.html. [Last accessed on August, 2019].

2. US Centers for Disease Control and Prevention. Diseases: Neglected tropical diseases; 2019. [online] Available from: https://www.cdc.gov/globalhealth/ntd/diseases/index.html. [Last accessed on August, 2019].

3. World Health Organization. Schistosomiasis; 2019. [online] Available from: https://www.who.int/news-room/fact-sheets/detail/schistosomiasis. [Last accessed on August, 2019].

4. Agrawal MC, Rao VG. Indian schistosomes: a need for further investigations. J Parasitol Res. 2011;2011:250868.

5. Kali A. Schistosome infections: an Indian perspective. J Clin Diagn Res. 2015;9(2):DE01-4.

6. Ross AG, Vickers D, Olds GR, et al. Katayama syndrome. Lancet Infect Dis. 2007;7(3):218-24.

7. Gordon CA, Kurscheid J, Williams GM, et al. Asian Schistosomiasis: Current Status and Prospects for Control Leading to Elimination. Trop Med Infect Dis. 2019;4(1):e40.

8. Karunamoorthi K, Almalki MJ, Ghailan KY. Schistosomiasis: a neglected tropical disease of poverty: a call for intersectoral mitigation strategies for better health. J Health Res Rev. 2018;5(1):1-12.

9. Gray DJ, McManus DP, Li Y, et al. Schistosomiasis elimination: lessons from the past guide the future. Lancet Infect Dis. 2010;10(10):733-6.

10. Ndhlovu PD, Mduluza T, Kjetland EF, et al. Prevalence of urinary schistosomiasis and HIV in females living in a rural community of Zimbabwe: does age matter? Trans R Soc Trop Med Hyg. 2007;101(5):433-8.

11. Li Y, Ross AG, Hou X, et al. Oriental schistosomiasis with neurological complications: case report. Ann Clin Microbiol Antimicrob. 2011;10:5.

12. Ferrari TC, Moreira PR. Neuroschistosomiasis: clinical symptoms and pathogenesis. Lancet Neurol. 2011;10(9):853-64.

13. Liu H, Lim CC, Feng X, et al. MRI in cerebral schistosomiasis: characteristic nodular enhancement in 33 patients. Am J Roentgenol. 2008;191(2):582-8.

14. Stecher CW, Sacko M, Madsen H, et al. Anemia and growth retardation associated with Schistosoma haematobium infection in Mali: a possible subtle impact of a neglected tropical disease. Trans R Soc Trop Med Hyg. 2017;111(4):144-53.

15. Habtamu K, Degarege A, Ye-Ebiyo Y, et al. Comparison of the Kato-Katz and FLOTAC techniques for the diagnosis of soil-transmitted helminth infections. Parasitol Int. 2011;60(4):398-402.

16. Utzinger J, Becker SL, van Lieshout L, et al. New diagnostic tools in schistosomiasis. Clin Microbiol Infect. 2015;21(6):529-42.

17. Utzinger J, Keiser J. Schistosomiasis and soil-transmitted helminthiasis: common drugs for treatment and control. Expert Opin Pharmacother. 2004;5(2):263-85.

18. Vale N, Gouveia MJ, Rinaldi G, et al. Praziquantel for Schistosomiasis: Single-drug Metabolism Revisited, Mode of Action, and Resistance. Antimicrob Agents Chemother. 2017;61(5):e02582-16.

19. Utzinger J, Keiser J, Shuhua X, et al. Combination chemotherapy of schistosomiasis in laboratory studies and clinical trials. Antimicrob Agents Chemother. 2003;47(5):1487-95.

20. Fürst T, Sayasone S, Odermatt P, et al. Manifestation, diagnosis, and management of foodborne trematodiasis. BMJ. 2012;344:e4093.

21. World Health Organization. Foodborne trematodiases; 2019. [online] Available from: https://www.who.int/news-room/fact-sheets/detail/foodborne-trematodiases. [Last accessed on August, 2019].

22. Procop GW. North American paragonimiasis (Caused by *Paragonimus kellicotti*) in the Context of Global Praragonimiasis. Clin Microbiol Rev. 2009;22(3):415-46.

23. Singh TS, Sugiyama H, Umehara A, et al. Paragonimus heterotremus infection in Nagaland: A new focus of Paragonimiasis in India. Indian J Med Microbiol. 2009;27(2):123-7.

24. Gadkowski LB, Stout JE. Cavitary pulmonary disease. Clin Microbiol Rev. 2008;21(2):305-33.

25. Keiser J, Utzinger J. Food-borne trematodiases. Clin Microbiol Rev. 2009;22(3):466-83.

26. Chen J, Chen Z, Lin J, et al. Cerebral paragonimiasis: a retrospective analysis of 89 cases. Clin Neurol Neurosurg. 2013;115(5):546-51.

27. Nakamura-Uchiyama F, Mukae H, Nawa Y. Paragonimiasis: a Japanese perspective. Clin Chest Med. 2002;23(2):409-20.

28. Zhang JS, Huan Y, Sun LJ, et al. MRI features of pediatric cerebral paragonimiasis in the active stage. J Magn Reson Imaging. 2006;23(4):569-73.

29. Chai JY, Shin EH, Lee SH, et al. Foodborne intestinal flukes in Southeast Asia. Korean J Parasitol. 2009;47(Suppl):S69-102.

30. Robinson MW, Dalton JP. Zoonotic helminth infections with particular emphasis on fasciolosis and other trematodiases. Philos Trans R Soc Lond B Biol Sci. 2009;364(1530):2763-76.

31. Sen Sarma M, Yachha SK, Srivastava A, et al. Endoscopic extraction of Fasciolopsis buski presenting as acute upper GI bleeding in a child. Gastrointest Endosc. 2015;82(4):743.

32. Khurana S, Malla N. Water- and food-borne Trematodiases in humans. In: Singh P, Sharma V (Eds). Water and Health. New Delhi: Springer; 2014.

33. Ramachandran J, Ajjampur SS, Chandramohan A, et al. Cases of human fascioliasis in India: tip of the iceberg. J Postgrad Med. 2012;58:150-2.

34. Ubeira FM, Muiño L, Valero MA, et al. MM3-ELISA detection of Fasciola hepatica coproantigens in preserved human stool samples. Am J Trop Med Hyg. 2009;81(1):156-62.

35. Choi D, Hong ST, Lim JH, et al. Sonographic findings of active Clonorchis sinensis infection. J Clin Ultrasound. 2004;32(1):17-23.

36. World Health Organization. Lymphatic filariasis; 2019. [online] Available from: https://www.who.int/news-room/fact-sheets/detail/lymphatic-filariasis. [Last accessed on August, 2019].

37. Directorate of National Vector Borne Disease Control Programme (NVBDCP). Ministry of Health and Family Welfare, Mass Drug Administration, Government of India. [online] Available from http://nvbdcp.gov.in/mda.html. [Last accessed on August 2019].

38. Dhariwal AC, Srivastava PK, Bhattacharjee J. Elimination of lymphatic filariasis in India: An update. J Indian Med Assoc (Vector Borne Dis Spec). 2015;113:189-90.

39. Raju K, Jambulingam P, Sabesan S, et al. Lymphatic filariasis in India: epidemiology and control measures. J Postgrad Med. 2010;56(3):232-8.

40. Shenoy RK, Bockarie MJ. Lymphatic filariasis in children: clinical features, infection burdens and future prospects for elimination. Parasitology. 2011;138(12):1559-68.

41. Khan AM. Lymphatic filariasis elimination programme in Assam, India, needs change in mass drug administration strategy to target the focus of infection. Indian J Med Res. 2018;147(1):7-10.

Soil-transmitted Helminths

Shalu Jain, Dheeraj Shah

INTRODUCTION

Soil-transmitted helminths (STH) refer to the intestinal worms, which are transmitted through contaminated soil. These infections are found mainly in areas where sanitation and hygiene are poor. These are included under the category of Neglected Tropical Diseases (NTD) because they inflict substantial illness and disability affecting approximately 1.5 billion people worldwide.

EPIDEMIOLOGY

More than 1.5 billion people worldwide are estimated to be infected with STH infections.[1] Infections are distributed in tropical and subtropical areas, majority in sub-Saharan Africa, America, China, and East Asia. Globally, India bears the highest burden of STH infections. In a study from 130 schools in Uttar Pradesh, the prevalence of STH infections was 75.6% among primary school children.[2] *Ascaris lumbricoides* was the most prevalent STH (69.6%), followed by hookworm (22.6%) and *Trichuris trichiura* (4.6%). In another study, children between 6 years and 14 years from 20 schools of Bihar were screened for STH infections. The overall prevalence of STH was 68%; ascariasis, hookworm, and trichuriasis were prevalent in 52%, 42%, and 5%, respectively.[3] In both of these studies, open defecation and absence of hand washing were the most important risk factors for STH.

COMMON SOIL-TRANSMITTED HELMINTHS

Intestinal worms vary in size ranging from 1 cm (*Enterobius*) to 10 m (*Taenia solium*) in length. Mature worms produce eggs or larvae that are responsible for transmission of infection outside the human host. The main species infecting people are the roundworm (*A. lumbricoides*), the whipworm (*T. trichiura*), and the hookworms (*Necator americanus* and *Ancylostoma duodenale*).

Helminths cause disease by the following mechanisms:

- Depriving the hosts of the nutrients (e.g. roundworm and tapeworm)
- Sucking blood (e.g. hookworm)
- Intestinal obstruction (e.g. roundworm)
- *Local effects*:
  - Abdominal pain and discomfort (e.g. roundworm, hookworm, and tapeworm)
  - Itching in the perianal area (e.g. pinworm)
- Abnormal migration (e.g. roundworms)
- Larval forms invading tissues (e.g. neurocysticercosis).

Table 1 lists the common worm infestations and their route of transmission in humans, whereas **Table 2** presents the salient features of their lifecycle.

Enterobiasis (Threadworm and Pinworm)

This is an infection due to an intestinal nematode, *E. vermicularis*. It is the most widespread of the helminths, but commonly escapes diagnosis due to absence of eggs in stools.

Epidemiology

Man is the only reservoir. Pinworm is easily transmitted from one child or person to a new host. The infection is common in lower socioeconomic families where personal hygiene is poor. Ova usually contaminate the area beneath the fingernails, and lack of proper hygiene favors the transmission. The eggs remain viable in linens and cloths for several days; hence, other family members can be rapidly infected. Infection occurs by oral ingestion of viable larvae or eggs by any of the following methods:

- Most commonly from perianal region to the mouth
- By ingestion of viable eggs present in soiled bed linen and other contaminated objects
- Via mouth or nose from eggs present in soil

Table 1: Major intestinal worm infestations.

Group or class	Infection	Organism	Mode of transmission to humans
Nematodes (roundworms)	Trichuriasis (whipworm)	Trichuris trichiura	Ingestion of embryonated eggs
	Enterobiasis (pinworm)	Enterobius vermicularis	Ingestion of eggs
	Ascariasis (roundworm)	Ascaris lumbricoides	Ingestion of embryonated eggs
	Hookworm	Ancylostoma duodenale, Necator americanus	Skin penetration by larvae
	Strongyloidiasis	Strongyloides stercoralis	Larva penetration of skin or colon
Cestodes (tapeworms)	Taeniasis saginata	Taenia saginata	Ingestion of cysticerci in beef
	Taeniasis solium	Taenia solium	Ingestion of cysticerci in pork
	Cysticercosis	Taenia solium	Ingestion of eggs
	Diphyllobothriasis	Diphyllobothrium latum	Ingestion of cysts in freshwater fish

Table 2: Life cycle of soil-transmitted helminths.

Parasite	Route of infection	Migration in body	Diagnostic form
Enterobius vermicularis	Mouth	Intestinal	Egg
Trichuris trichiura	Mouth	Intestinal	Egg
Ascaris lumbricoides	Mouth	Pulmonary	Egg
Ancylostoma duodenale	Skin	Pulmonary	Egg
Strongyloides stercoralis	Skin	Pulmonary	Rhabditiform larva

- Retroinfection, i.e. eggs hatch near anus and larvae migrate up the bowel.

Life Cycle

After being ingested, ova take about 35–60 days to develop into adults. The adult worm lies in the cecum and lays eggs in the perianal region.[4]

Clinical Features

Itching around the anus is the main symptom and occurs mainly at night. Excoriation and secondary infection can occur due to scratching. Itching also leads to restless sleep, irritability, and enuresis.

Diagnosis

Eosinophilia is usually absent. The diagnosis is made by the demonstration of characteristic eggs in feces, perianal swabs, and cellotape swabs from the perianal region. Eggs are present in only 5% of infected individuals. Cellotape swab is obtained by scraping of perianal region or a Scotch tape is touched lightly to the perianal region and examined for ova.

Treatment

The whole family of an infected person has to be treated to avoid reinfection. This should be combined with education and personal hygiene to prevent autoinfection. Albendazole is the drug of choice and is given as a single dose of 400 mg for adults and children. Alternatively, mebendazole (100 mg twice a day for 3 days) and pyrantel pamoate (10 mg/kg single oral dose) can also be used. The treatment should be repeated after 2 weeks to achieve a cure rate of 90–100%.

Trichuriasis (Whipworm)

This is an infection of the large intestine due to the nematode, *T. trichiura*. The prevalence of the infection in India varies from 0.1% in Delhi to as high as 95% in Tamil Nadu.

Epidemiology

Trichuris trichiura is a grayish white worm. It lives in the cecum and appendix.

Man is the major reservoir. Transmission occurs directly by mature eggs, which are ingested via contaminated fingers (contaminated from soil). Ova are excreted in feces and contaminate soil from where they are ingested by new hosts.

The infection is common in areas with high humidity, high rainfall, dense shade, and poor sanitation and in persons who have poor personal hygiene.

Life Cycle

Humans are infected by ingesting eggs, which migrate to the cecum and develop into mature worms.

Clinical Manifestations

The incubation period is usually 60 days. Light infections are asymptomatic or associated with abdominal pain, vomiting, distension, and flatulence. Heavy infections may present with severe dysentery. Hypoproteinemia, anemia, and growth retardation can occur in severe infection.

Diagnosis

Diagnosis can be made by identification of the characteristic ova in fecal samples. Egg counts can indicate the worm burden. Moderate eosinophilia is present.

Treatment

Asymptomatic infections need not be treated. Mebendazole (100 mg twice a day for 3 days) is the drug of choice. Albendazole can also be given as a single dose of 400 mg.

Ascariasis (Roundworm)

This is one of the most common and widespread human infections, infecting one in four of the world's population.

Epidemiology

Man is the only reservoir of infection. Infection is acquired by the ingestion of eggs in contaminated soil. This is usual in children while playing in soil. Infection is more common during rainy season.[5]

Life Cycle

The causative agent is *A. lumbricoides.* It is a comparatively large worm inhabiting the small intestine. Ova are passed in the feces, which develop in the soil (minimum 3 weeks) to become infective. These are ingested and hatch in the intestine, penetrate mucous membrane of the intestine, reach circulation from where they go to the lungs, passing up the respiratory tract to reach esophagus and thence the small intestine where they become the adult worms.

It takes 60–70 days after infection for the development of adult worms and excretion of eggs. Symptoms due to larval stages occur after 4–16 days of infection.

Larval ascariasis: Symptoms and signs caused by larval stages are as follows:

- *Ascaris* pneumonia after 4–16 days of infection due to migratory larvae. There is fever, cough, sputum, and radiological abnormalities. Pneumonitis lasts for about 3 weeks. Death from respiratory failure is also noted.
- General symptoms such as convulsions, meningism, epilepsy, palpebral edema, insomnia, and tooth grinding.

Adult ascariasis: Infection can lead to small bowel obstruction, especially with heavy infections in children. Colic, abdominal pain, and vomiting are quite common. The adult worms may migrate to various sites such as bile duct, ampulla of Vater, appendix, and perianal sinuses. Complications include intestinal perforation, peritonitis, liver abscess, cholangitis, etc.

Diagnosis

Diagnosis is made by demonstration of ova in fecal samples.

Treatment

All available anthelmintics are effective only against the adult worms. *Albendazole*: Children 2–5 years—200 mg single dose; older children and adults—400 mg single dose. *Mebendazole*: 100 mg twice daily for 3 days. *Levamisole*: Single dose, 5 mg/kg body weight. *Pyrantel pamoate*: 10 mg/kg single dose.

Ancylostomiasis (Hookworm)

Hookworm disease is due to two species of the parasite—*A. duodenale* and *N. americanus.* These inhabit the small intestine from where they suck blood and protein leading to the characteristic manifestations of hookworm anemia/disease. The two species of hookworms infect about 900 million persons in the world.

Epidemiology

Man is the only reservoir. Transmission peaks during the rainy season. Lack of wearing footwears predisposes to hookworm infection.

Life Cycle

The eggs are passed in feces which develop into rhabditiform larva, which gets double in size to develop into infective filariform larva. They pierce the skin and reach the lymphohematogenous system from where they go to lungs and like *Ascaris*, reach the esophagus and then to the small intestine where they become adult worms.

Infection is acquired through the penetration of the skin by the larvae present in the soil due to contamination with human feces.

Symptoms due to larvae appear 1–2 weeks after infection and ova appear after 42–45 days of infection.

Symptoms due to larvae: Itching occurs at the site of entry of larvae (ground itch), and after 1–2 weeks of this pulmonary symptoms in the form of dry cough and asthmatic wheeze, along with fever and eosinophilia, appear.

Adult worms: Light infection (up to 100 worms) does not cause symptoms. With worm loads of 500–1,000 worms, there is significant blood loss with iron deficiency anemia, and protein loss.

Management

Diagnosis: Diagnosis is made by examination of fecal samples for characteristic ova.

Treatment: Severe anemia may require blood transfusion, in addition to administration of iron. Adult worms can be eliminated by the use of anthelmintics as follows: *Albendazole*: Children 2–5 years: 200 mg single dose; older children and adults: 400 mg single dose. *Mebendazole*: 100 mg twice daily × 3 days. *Pyrantel pamoate*: A single dose of 10 mg/kg.

Prevention: Provision of proper sanitation facilities and prevention of contamination of soil are important preventive measures. Wearing shoes or sandals can prevent infection, as the larvae will not come in contact with skin.

Strongyloidiasis

It is caused by *Strongyloides stercoralis* which is the smallest of the intestinal worm. Like hookworm infections, it is also acquired by skin penetration; however, autoinfection can also occur by ingestion of filariform larva-contaminated food. They can be transmitted by direct physical contact as well.

Epidemiology

It is not as prevalent as other helminthic infections. The disease is more common in tropical climatic conditions.

Clinical Features

Ground itch is usually absent. *Intestinal* infections are usually asymptomatic but can cause epigastric pain, vomiting, diarrhea, and malabsorption. Autoinfection causes lesions over buttocks signifying larvae invasion of perianal area.

Management

Diagnosis is made by finding the larvae in the stool. Drugs of choice are ivermectin and thiabendazole. Health personnel should wear protective gear to prevent infection with larvae.

Taeniasis (Tapeworm)

These tapeworms are also known as beef tapeworm (*T. saginata*) and pork tapeworm (*T. solium*) reflecting the principle intermediate host for each of them. Man is the only definitive host for both the parasites. Pork tapeworm consists of a scolex with suckers and hooks, by means of which they attach to the intestinal wall. Hooks are absent in *T. saginata*.

Life Cycle

Adult worms reside in the small intestine of man. The eggs are passed in feces. Pig swallows these eggs and is infected. Larvae of tapeworm penetrate the intestinal wall of the pig and get encysted in the muscles and other tissues. Man is infected when he eats improperly cooked pork.

Clinical Features

Consumption of undercooked beef, pork, or unwashed raw vegetables infested with larvae or contaminated with eggs of *Taenia* results in human infection. Most infections are asymptomatic. Carriers have an increased risk of developing cysticercosis by repeated autoinfection.

Cysticercosis: Infection with larvae of *T. solium* result in cysticercosis. Ingested *Taenia* eggs develop into larvae in the small intestine. Larvae migrate across the intestinal wall and are carried to the target organ by bloodstream. The common target organs for cysticerci are brain, muscle, and subcutaneous tissue. In about 2 months' time, the larvae mature into cysticerci. The size of cysticerci varies from 2 mm to 2 cm. Only brain cysticerci are symptomatic, common presentation being a partial seizure. Active neurocysticercosis may manifest as raised intracranial tension, focal neurological deficits, or disturbances in consciousness.

Diagnosis

Diagnosis is established by the examination of the eggs in the stools or gross examination of proglottids or segments passed in the stools. Patients may pass motile segments of worms through anus. Diagnosis of neurocysticercosis is made by CT scan or MRI of brain.

Treatment

Treatment is similar for both infestations. Praziquantel in a single dose of 10 mg/kg is the drug of choice. Purgation is not essential.

Symptomatic active neurocysticercosis is treated with albendazole, in a dose of 15 mg/kg/day for 1–4 weeks along with steroids for initial 5–7 days.

CONTROL MEASURES OF INTESTINAL INFESTATIONS

The WHO (World Health Organization) (strategic plan 2011–2020) recommends deworming with anthelmintic medicines (albendazole 400 mg or 200 mg for children 1–2 years or mebendazole 500 mg) to all at-risk people living in endemic regions.[6] The at-risk population includes: Children > 1 year of age, nonpregnant adolescent girls (10–19 years), non-pregnant women of reproductive age group (15–49 years), and pregnant women in second or third trimester. Once-a-year treatment is recommended when the baseline prevalence of STH infections in the community is over 20% and twice-a-year treatment when it is 50%. In India, the National Deworming Day program was initiated in February 2015 achieving 85% coverage. Since then, only Madhya Pradesh and Rajasthan have continuing annual deworming programs. Schools are good targets for deworming activities because of accessibility, cost-efficacy, and provisions for health education. The global target is to eliminate morbidity due to STH in children by 2020. It is estimated that this can be obtained if at least 75% of the children are regularly treated in endemic areas.[6]

Most of the worm infestations are essentially preventable through good personal hygiene, improved environmental sanitation, and effective public health measures.

Proper Disposal of Feces

Borehole latrines should be constructed in the rural areas and the people should be encouraged to use these instead of defecating in the open fields.

Food

Ground or root vegetables used for making salads should be thoroughly cleaned and preferably peeled before use. Pork, beef, and fish should be well cooked to destroy the infective forms of the parasites embedded in the flesh.

Water

The drinking water should be boiled or filtered to prevent infection.

Skin

Children should be encouraged to wear shoes while playing in the fields to avoid penetration of feet by the larvae in soil contaminated with infected feces.

Health Education

- The habit of washing hands after defecation and before taking food should be encouraged.
- Nails should be cut and cleaned daily with soap and brush.
- Daily bath and scrupulous personal cleanliness should be advised. The underclothes should not be dirty.
- The children should be prevented from scratching of the perianal region. Irritation and itching should be relieved by the use of antipruritic creams containing crotamiton.
- Information about the mode of infection with the helminths, methods of prevention, and treatment should be widely disseminated.

REFERENCES

1. World Health Organization. Soil-transmitted Helminth Infections: Key Facts; 2019. [online] Available from: https://www.who.int/news-room/fact-sheets/detail/soil-transmitted-helminth-infections. [Last accessed on December, 2019].
2. Ganguly S, Barkataki S, Karmakar S, et al. High prevalence of soil-transmitted helminth infections among primary school children, Uttar Pradesh, India, 2015. Infect Dis Poverty. 2017;6(1):139.
3. Greenland K, Dixon R, Khan SA, et al. The epidemiology of soil-transmitted helminths in Bihar State, India. PLoS Negl Trop Dis. 2015;9(5):e0003790.
4. Ryan KJ, Ray GC. Parasites and Diseases. Sherris Medical Microbiology, 4th edition. New York: McGraw Hill; 2003.
5. Barabara JH. Lumen-Dwelling Helminths. Clinical and Pathogenic Microbiology, 2nd edition. US: Mosby; 1994.
6. Abraham D, Kaliappan S, Walson JL, et al. Intervention strategies to reduce the burden of soil-transmitted helminths in India. Indian J Med Res. 2018;147(6):533-44.

Echinococcosis (Hydatid Disease)

Baldev S Prajapati, Rajal B Prajapati

■ INTRODUCTION

Echinococcosis (hydatid disease) is a widespread parasitic infestation caused most commonly by *Echinococcus granulosus*, cestode (tapeworm). The parasites were, until recently, thought to be a single species, but recent molecular data have shown that there are a number of different species and genotypes, what was formally considered to be a single species. The other species are *Echinococcus multilocularis* (*E. multilocularis*) and *Echinococcus vogeli*. The disease is endemic in many sheep- and cattle-raising countries such as Australia, Africa, Middle East, and Latin America. However, the disease has spread to other parts of the world and it has become a global health problem. Man is an accidental host and dead end of the parasite.

■ LIFE CYCLE

The worm passes its life cycle **(Fig. 1)** in two hosts:

1. *Definitive hosts*: Dog, wolf, fox, and jackal. The adult worm lives in the intestine of these animals who

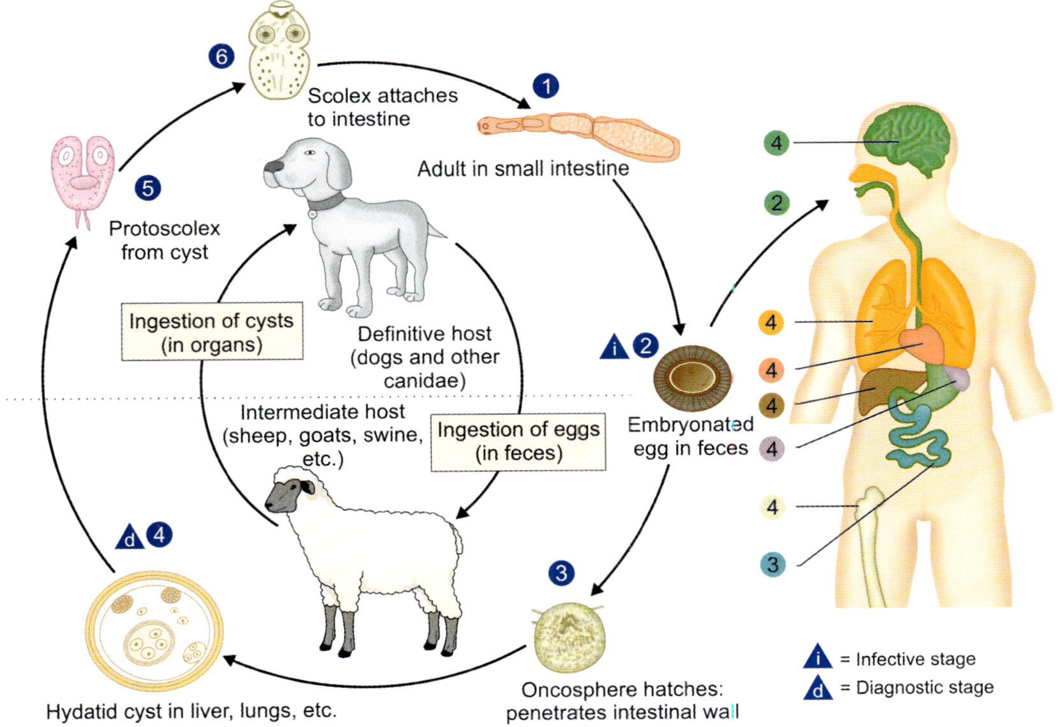

Fig. 1: Life cycle of *Echinococcus granulosus*.
Source: http://www.cdc.gov.

discharge a large number of eggs in their feces. The dog is the main definitive host.

2. *Intermediate hosts*: Sheep, pig, cattle, horse, goat, and man. The larval stage is passed in these animals and man, giving rise to hydatid cyst.

The eggs are excreted with feces of the definitive hosts, mainly dogs. These are swallowed by the intermediate hosts, sheep and other domestic animals, while grazing in the field and also by man, especially children, due to intimate contacts with infected dogs. In the duodenum, the embryos are hatched out. About 8 hours after ingestion of eggs, the embryos bore their way through the intestinal wall and enter the radicles of the portal vein. The embroys are carried to the liver and taken up in the sinusoidal capillaries. Thus, the liver acts as the first filter. Some of the embroys may pass through the liver and enter the pulmonary circulation and filter out in the lungs. The lungs act as the second filter. A few of them may pass the lung and enter the systemic blood circulation and lodge in the various organs. Practically, all the organs may be invaded, but they are commonly found in the liver and lungs.

Wherever the embryo settles, it forms a hydatid cyst. From the inner side of the cyst, brood capsules with a number of scolices are developed. A hydatid cyst developing from a single egg may contain thousands of scolices. A fully developed scolex is an end product and its presence inside the hydatid cyst is a sign of complete biological development. These fertile hydatids, when ingested by the dog, are capable of growing into adult worms in about 6–7 weeks' time in the intestine.

As the dogs have no access to the hydatid cyst developed in the viscera of a man, the life cycle of the worm comes to a dead end. Thus, the natural cycle is maintained by dogs and sheeps.

Human beings are an accidental host and a dead end for the parasite. They get infected by coming into contact with infected dogs, the mode of transmission being through the fecal-oral route. *E. multilocularis* has a similar life cycle with the difference that definitive hosts are fox and to some extent dogs and wolves and the intermediate hosts are small rodents.

PATHOGENESIS

Echinococcus granulosus parasites are commonly acquired in childhood, but the development of hydatid cysts requires several years to become large enough to detect or cause symptoms. In children, the lung is a common site for the development of hydatid cyst, but in adults 70% of hydatid cysts develop in the liver. The other organs to develop hydatid cysts are spleen, genitourinary system, bone, brain, and subcutaneous tissues. The host surrounds the primary cyst with a tough, fibrous capsule. Inside this capsule, the parasite produces a thick lamellar layer with the consistency of a soft-boiled egg white. Inside of this lamellar layer is the thin germinal layer of cells responsible for thousands of protoscoleces, remaining attached to the wall or floating free in the cyst fluid. Smaller internal daughter cysts may develop within the primary cyst capsule. The fluid in the cyst is clear, colorless, and watery. Rupture of the cyst can occur due to trauma or during surgery and can cause anaphylactic reaction. Protoscoleces released into the tissue can also develop into new cysts. *E. multilocularis* almost always involves the liver; the cysts develop very slowly and are rarely seen in children.

CLINICAL MANIFESTATIONS

- In the liver, hydatid cysts may remain asymptomatic.
- They may regress spontaneously or may produce nonspecific symptoms.
- Enlargement of the abdomen, hepatomegaly, a palpable mass, pain in the abdomen, and vomiting are common symptoms.
- They may cause compression effect on various organs.
- Mass effects can be noted in brain and bone.
- Anaphylaxis can develop with cyst rupture or spontaneous spillage from trauma or during surgery.
- Jaundice in a case of hydatid cyst is rare.
- The hydatid cyst in the lung commonly presents with cough, chest pain, or hemophysis.
- Cerebral and ocular hydatid cysts can become symptomatic even when they are small in size. Therefore, many a times, cerebral and ocular hydatid cysts are diagnosed in children.
- They can affect almost any organ including brain, eyes, heart, kidneys, spleen, pancreas, breast, bone, and muscles.

INVESTIGATIONS

The diagnosis of hydatid disease is commonly established by radiological imaging such as ultrasound or CT scan. Immunodiagnostic tests can also be used. Eosinophilia may be associated, but in less than 25% of cases.

Radioimaging

The most useful radioimaging modality for the diagnosis of hydatid cyst of the liver is abdominal ultrasonography. The presence of internal membranes or echogenic cyst material (hydatid sand) can be observed to aid the

Table 1: Hydatid cyst staging and treatment according to WHO.

WHO staging	Ultrasound picture	Treatment
CE$_1$	• Uniformly anechoic cyst with fine echoes • Settled representing hydatid sand	• <5 cm: Albendazole alone • >5 cm: Albendazole + PAIR
CE$_2$	Multiseptate honeycomb cyst	Surgery + albendazole
CE$_3$	Cyst with detached membranes	• <5 cm: Albendazole alone • >5 cm: Albendazole + PAIR
CE$_4$	Cysts with heterogeneous hypo/hyperechoic contents and no daughter cysts	Wait and watch
CE$_5$	Solid and calcified walls	Wait and watch

(PAIR: puncture, aspiration, injection, and reaspiration)

diagnosis. The World Health Organization (WHO) has developed a classification system for staging of hydatid cyst and its optimal therapy **(Table 1)**.

Computed tomography scan is the modality of choice for lung and brain hydatidosis. MRI is preferred for hydatid cyst involving muscles, salivary glands, and retroperitoneum.

Serology

Amongst the various immunological tests, Casoni's test is more popular. It is an immediate hypersensitive reaction-type test. It is positive in only 60% of cases. It can also be false positive in other parasitic infections. The indirect hemagglutination test is sensitive, but ELISA (enzyme-linked immunosorbent assay) is more accurate and is preferred for initial screening.

Aspiration

Percutaneous aspiration of the cyst under ultrasonographic guidance and demonstration of protoscoleces or hydatid membranes are confirmatory. This test is associated with a small risk of anaphylaxis. It is also advisable to start anthelmintic treatment before performing the aspiration. In patients with pulmonary hydatid cysts, protoscoleces can be demonstrated in sputum or bronchial lavage.

■ TREATMENT

Till the 1980s, surgery was considered to be the only modality for treatment of hydatid cysts. However, with the availability of more efficacious anthelmintic treatment, medical therapy has supplemented and in some cases replaced surgical treatment. Recently, treatment with percutaneous cyst aspiration, followed by injection of scolicidal agents, and then reaspiration [PAIR (puncture, aspiration, injection, reaspiration)] has been introduced with success. The various treatment options have been reviewed by WHO and recommended **(Table 1)**.

Surgery

Complete surgical removal of the intact hydatid cyst is the definitive treatment with complete cure. It should be completely removed without spilling the cyst contents and is best achieved by pericystectomy. Whenever lesser surgical procedures are being used, adjunctive anthelmintic treatment should always be given. Surgery is the treatment of choice for large liver cysts (>10 cm), cysts with secondary infection, cyst located in the lung, kidney, brain, etc. There is a definite risk of anaphylaxis during surgical intervention and can be minimized by instilling scolicidal agents in the cyst cavity during surgery. These agents include 10% formaldehyde, 3% hypertonic saline and 10% povidone-iodine. Formaldehyde is not preferred nowadays because of the risk of severe sclerosing cholangitis if cyst biliary communications are present. It is also important to pack the abdominal contents by pads soaked in 10% povidone-iodine to prevent dissemination of the protoscoleces.

Chemotherapy

Anthelmintic agents (albendazole and mebendazole) can be used as the sole modality of treatment in simple hydatid cysts less than 1 cm in diameter or as an adjunct to surgery. Albendazole is given in the dose of 15 mg/kg/day and mebendazole in 40–50 mg/kg/day. Albendazole is preferred to mebendazole because of its better absorption from the intestine and penetration into the cyst cavity. The minimum duration of treatment is 3 months. The adverse reactions in the form of hepatotoxicity, neutropenia, alopecia, etc. are known but they are reversible. Pregnancy, chronic liver disease, and bone marrow suppression are contraindications for medical therapy. Praziquantel has also been used in a dose of 50 mg/kg/day. A combination of praziquantel and albendazole is considered superior to albendazole alone. About one-third of patients treated with chemotherapy show a complete and permanent disappearance of the cyst while nearly 50% show a significant reduction in the cyst size. Still, about 20–40% of patients do not show a favorable response. Medical therapy is not useful in complicated, multiseptated cysts or in cysts with a thick and calcified cyst wall.

PAIR

It consists of percutaneous puncture (under sonographic guidance), aspiration of cyst contents, injection of the scolicidal agent (95% ethanol or hypertonic saline) for at least 15 minutes, and reaspiration. This method is useful for patients with smaller cysts and for those who cannot undergo surgery or refuse for surgery. PAIR is contraindicated for inaccessible or superficially located liver cysts and for inactive or calcified cysts. It is the best method for single or multiple cysts in the liver, spleen, kidney, and abdominal cavity. PAIR should not be used in liver cysts with cyst-biliary communication due to risk or sclerosing cholangitis. It is advisable to perform PAIR under anthelmintic coverage which should be continued for at least 1 month after the procedure. Recent studies indicate that PAIR combined with anthelmintic treatment has shown better clinical efficacy, lower morbidity, mortality, and shorter hospital stay than surgery.

◼ FOLLOW-UP

The response to treatment is best assessed by ultrasonography, CT scan, or MRI. It should be performed at an interval of 3 months and should be continued for at least 3 years.

◼ PREVENTION

Important measures to interrupt transmission include thorough handwashing, avoiding contacts with dogs, boiling or filtering water when camping, proper disposal of animal carcasses, and proper meat inspection. Strict procedures for proper disposal of refuse from slaughter houses must be instituted. Other useful measures are control or treatment of the dog population and regular praziquantel treatment of pets. Vaccines have been developed to prevent infection in grazing animals but are not used.

◼ SUGGESTED READING

1. Chatterjee KD. Parasitology; 12th edition. Kolkata: Chatterjee Medical Publishers; 1979. pp. 121-28.
2. Gupta S. Hydatid disease: Echinococcosis. In: Gupta P, Menon PSN, Ramji S, Lodha R (Eds). PG Textbook of Pediatrics, 1st edition. New Delhi: Jaypee Brothers Medical Publishers (P) Ltd; 2015. pp. 1274-77.
3. Kayal A, Hussan A. (2014). A Comprehensive Prospective Clinical Study of Hydatid Disease. [online] Available from: http://dx.doi.org/10.1155/2014/514757. [Last accessed on November, 2019].
4. Moro PL, Schantz PM. Echinococcus species (agents of cystic, alveolar & polycystic Echinococcosis). In: Long SS, Pickering, LK, Prober CG (Eds). 3rd edition. New York: Churchill Livingstone Elsevier; 2008. pp. 1327-31.
5. Rao SS, Mehra B, Narang R. The spectrum of hydatid disease in rural central India: an 11-year experience. Ann Trop Med Public Health. 2012;5:225-30.
6. WHO Informal Working Group. International classification of ultrasound images in cystic echinococcosis for application in clinical and field epidemiological setting. Acta Trop. 2003;85: 253-61.
7. World Health Organization. Guidelines for treatment of cystic and alveolar echinococcosis in humans. WHO Informal Working Group on Echinococcosis. Bull World Health Organ. 1996;74:231-42.

Tapeworms and Cysticercosis

Narayanappa D, Rajani HS

INTRODUCTION

Tapeworms are multicellular platyhelminthic parasites that belongs to a class of Cestodes.[1] The four clinically important cestodes are *Taenia solium, Taenia saginata, Diphyllobothrium latum* and *Echinococcus granulosus.* The clinical manifestations caused by *T. solium* are divided as either cysticercosis (cysts in various tissues including the brain) or taeniasis (intestinal tapeworm infection).[4] Cysticercosis is one of the most common parasitic disease of the human brain and also a neglected tropical disease.

TAPEWORMS

Tapeworms are multicellular platyhelminthic parasites that belong to a class of Cestodes.[1] The four clinically important cestodes are *Taenia solium, T. saginata, Diphyllobothrium latum,* and *Echinococcus granulosus.* Other cestodes of less importance are *E. multilocolosus, Hymenolepis nana,* and *Dipylidium caninum.*[3]

They live in human intestines and usually cause non-life-threatening diseases. Usually, infections result when humans ingest undercooked meat or fish contaminated with larvae which are invasive.

In two important human diseases, cysticercosis and hydatid disease, infection occurs by ingestion of eggs which hatch into larvae, resulting in disease.[3]

The adult worms are flat (platyhelminthes) and multisegmented with length varying from 8 mm to 10 m. They lack digestive tract and absorb nutrients directly from small intestine of definitive host.

Tapeworms have two main parts **(Figs. 1A to D)**:

1. The rounded head (scolex) which functions as an anchoring organ with suckers, hooks, or sucking grooves and gets attached to intestinal mucosa.
2. The flat body with numerous segments and each segment is called proglottid.

The neck next to scolex, an unsegmented region, is the germinal center with high regenerative capacity. Proglottids closest to the neck are new and undifferentiated. As proglottids move caudally, they develop hermaphroditic sex organs. Distal proglottids, the oldest, are gravid and produce eggs which are excreted in feces to infect intermediate hosts.

If treatment does not eliminate the neck and scolex of tapeworm, the entire worm may regenerate.

All tapeworms (cestodes) have a life cycle of three stages—eggs, larvae, and adults.

Adults inhabit guts of definitive hosts. Some tapeworms that infect humans are named after their intermediate host: Fish tapeworm (*D. latum*), beef tapeworm (*T. saginata*), and pork tapeworm (*T. solium*).[1]

Taenia asiatica (Asian tapeworm), similar to *T. saginata,* is acquired by eating pork and is more prevalent in Asia.[1]

Adult tapeworms living in the intestines of definitive hosts lay eggs which are excreted in the stools and are ingested by an intermediate host (typically another species). Intermediate hosts such as pigs and cattle can get infected when they ingest either egg or proglottids excreted in human feces. Larvae develop from ingested eggs in the intermediate host, enter the circulation, and may encyst in the musculature or other organs. When the intermediate host is consumed by definitive hosts, the larvae (cysticerci) are released from the ingested cysts in the intestines and develop into adult tapeworms thereby restarting the cycle.

Important features of adult tape worms that affect children are given in **Table 1**.[3]

Taeniasis and Cysticercosis

The clinical manifestations caused by *T. solium* are divided into either cysticercosis (cysts in various tissues including the brain) or taeniasis (intestinal tapeworm infection).[4]

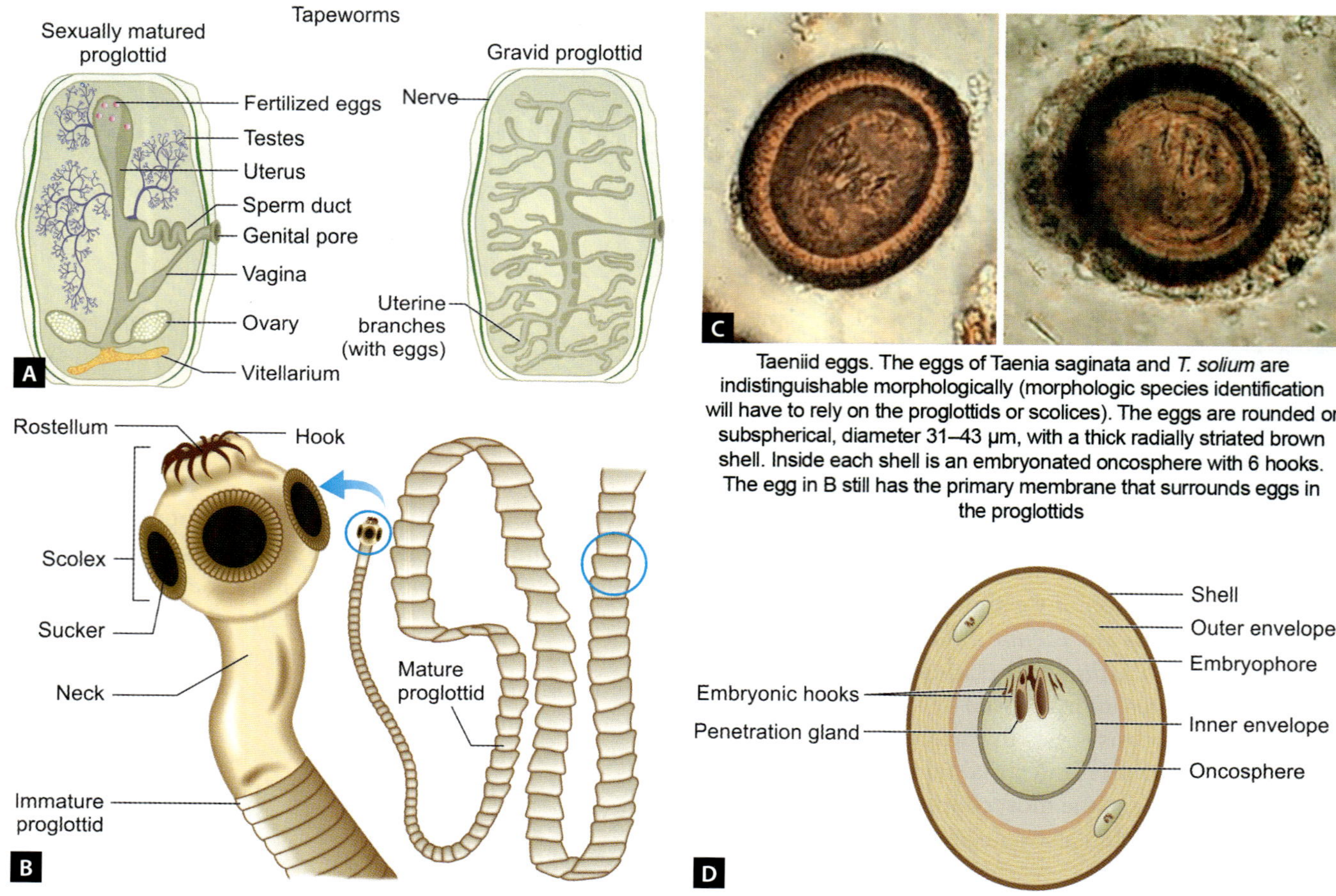

Taeniid eggs. The eggs of Taenia saginata and *T. solium* are indistinguishable morphologically (morphologic species identification will have to rely on the proglottids or scolices). The eggs are rounded or subspherical, diameter 31–43 μm, with a thick radially striated brown shell. Inside each shell is an embryonated oncosphere with 6 hooks. The egg in B still has the primary membrane that surrounds eggs in the proglottids

Figs. 1A to D: Structure of tapeworm.

Parasite species	Mode of transmission	Intermediate host	Main site affected in human body	Treatment
Taenia saginata	Ingesting larvae in undercooked beef	Cattle	*Intestine*: Abdominal discomfort, and passing proglottids in stool	Praziquantel or niclosamide, possibly nitazoxanide
Taenia solium	• Ingestion of larvae in undercooked pork • Ingestion of eggs in water or food contaminated with human stools	Pigs	*Intestine*: • Minimal abdominal discomfort, proglottids in stool • Brain and eyes (cysticercosis)	• Praziquantel or niclosamide, possibly nitazoxanide • Albendazole and praziquantel
Taenia asiatica	Ingestion of larvae in undercooked pork	Pigs	*Intestine*: Minimal abdominal discomfort	Praziquantel or niclosamide, possibly nitazoxanide
Diphyllobothrium spp.	Ingestion of larvae in undercooked freshwater fish	Copepods and fish	Intestine usually minimal; with prolonged or heavy infection with *Diphyllobothrium latum*, vitamin B12 deficiency	Praziquantel or Niclosamide
Echinococcus granulosus	Ingestion of eggs contaminated with dogs feces	Sheep	Liver, lungs, and brain	Albendazole and surgical removal

Table 1: Important features of adult tapeworms that affect children.

Source: Nelson textbook of pediatrics.

Taeniasis occurs when humans are infected by consuming raw or undercooked pork containing the larvae (cysticerci). A cysticercus is a pea-sized, fluid-filled bladder with an invaginated scolex. In the small gut, larvae get attached to the wall and take around 3 months to become an adult tapeworm. The terminal gravid proglottids with many eggs get detached and are excreted in human feces to be accidentally consumed by pigs. Pigs are infected by eggs which release a six-hooked embryo or oncosphere in the pig's intestine. This burrows through gut wall into a blood vessel and is carried to skeletal muscle, where it develops into a cysticercus and remains as cysticercus until consumed by human. Hence, humans are the definitive hosts and pigs are the intermediate hosts.[4]

Cysticercosis: Cysticercosis is different from "taeniasis" which is caused by adult tapeworm infection. Cysticercosis is a tissue infection with larval stage of *T. solium* or cysticercus due to ingestion of *T. solium* eggs. With species such as *T. solium*, the definitive host can act as an intermediate host; that is, if eggs in food or water contaminated with human stools are ingested, the eggs hatch into larvae in the small intestine, burrow through the wall, enter the circulation, and disseminate into many organs such as eyes, brain, skeletal muscle, and subcutaneous tissue, and encyst to form cysticerci. But larvae have high affinity for central nervous system (CNS), resulting in neurocysticercosis (NCC), a most common parasitic infection of CNS. In cysticercosis, humans get infected by eggs excreted in human stools and not due to ingestion of undercooked pork. Hence, NCC is seen in vegetarians as frequently as it is seen in nonvegetarians.[4]

Life Cycle of Taenia Solium (Fig. 2)

The lifecycle of *T. solium* is complex. The only definitive host in which pork tapeworm can complete its lifecycle and exists in adult form is humans. Both humans and pigs are intermediate hosts, where the tapeworm eggs develop to the metacestodes (larval) stage. In Asia, dogs have been identified as intermediate hosts.[1]

Cysticercosis results most commonly by ingestion of food or water contaminated with human feces containing eggs of *T. solium*. In the gut of host, eggs get uncoated liberating enclosed larvae (oncospheres) which penetrate gut wall to enter bloodstream and are transported and deposited in various tissues of the body such as brain, eyes, skin, and muscles. Oncospheres differentiate and develop into metacestodes, and passes through multiple stages of development to form established cysticerci.[1]

In "viable or vesicular stage," a first pathological stage, vesicle containing clear fluid with the head or scolex of a parasite with a membrane around each oncosphere is formed. These cysts remain dormant for several months or years depending on the nature of the immune response of the host.

"Colloidal stage" is the next stage in which scolex degenerates and vesicular fluid becomes turbid.

In granular nodular stage, the vesicular fluid becomes gradually more opaque and in calcified stage, the cyst calcifies to form a nonviable calcified nodule, eventually completing its evolution.

When a man ingests undercooked pork containing viable cysticerci, the life cycle is completed. Digestive enzymes in the small gut cause the scolices to evaginate from the cyst vesicle and with the help of powerful suckers and hooks, get attached to intestine wall and mature to adulthood, in which the terminal egg-containing sections of the tapeworm body, called "gravid proglottids," are excreted in feces.[1]

EPIDEMIOLOGY

Cysticercosis is one of the most common parasitic diseases of the human brain and also a neglected tropical disease. In 2010, the World Health Organization (WHO) recognized this disease due to its significant global impact, in terms of both disease and financial burden. Very limited data on prevalence, distribution, and transmission of NCC is available. Now steps for the control of both taeniasis and cysticercosis are being taken by the WHO.[2]

Neurocysticercosis is also the common cause of new-onset seizures in many regions of the world including India. In one of the community-based surveys involving over 50,000 individuals in Tamil Nadu district of south India, NCC was found to be the cause of active epilepsy in at least one-third of the patients and the prevalence of NCC as a cause of active epilepsy in India was calculated to be 1 per 1,000 population. That is, at least 1.2 million persons in India are suffering from active epilepsy due to NCC. The most common form of the disease in India was the solitary cysticercus granuloma (SCG) (first identified in 1989) which was seen in up to 60% of patients with NCC.[2]

Cysticercosis is associated with lack of sanitation, poor hygiene, and free-roaming pigs. Local transmission of the disease is, however, only possible in the presence of an adult *Taenia* carrier in the gut. Taeniasis is caused only by the consumption of pork infected with cysticercosis, but cysticercosis can also occur in vegetarians and non-pork eaters.

Although the disease can potentially be controlled if not eliminated, there are several socioeconomic and healthcare-related issues that constitute barriers to this goal.[2]

CLINICAL PRESENTATION[1,4]

The clinical presentation of NCC is pleomorphic and depends on parasite load, size and number of cysticerci, location of cyst, and immune responses and interactions.

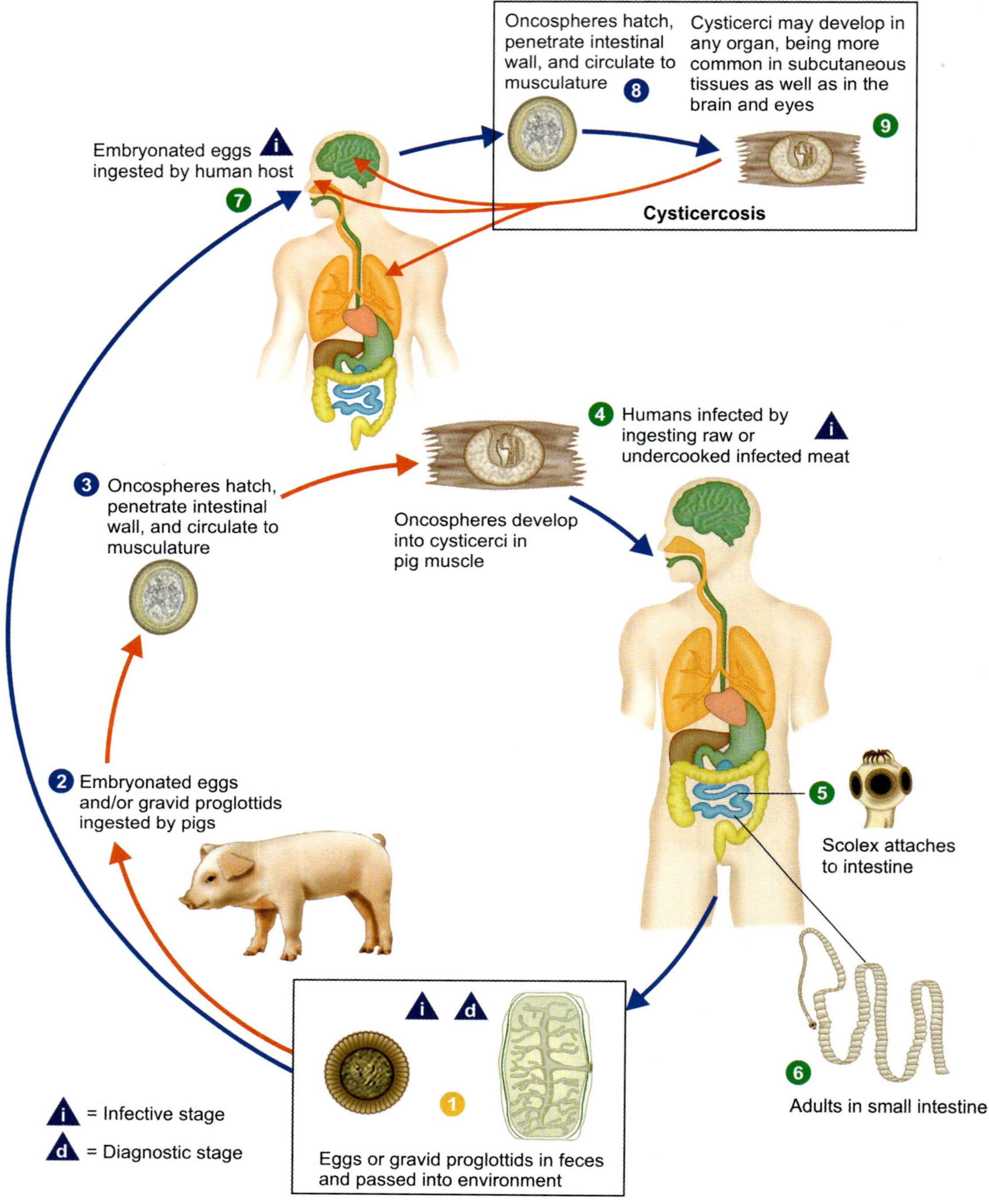

Fig. 2: Life cycle of *Taenia solium*.

Neurocysticercosis is classified on the basis of location as:

- *Parenchymal*: Cysticerci within the functional tissues of brain
- *Extraparenchymal*: Cysticerci in intraventricular, subarachnoid, spinal, or ocular.

Location of NCC is important because clinical presentation, radiologic appearance, prognosis, and management depend on the location.

The most common presentation of parenchymal NCC in majority of children is seizures. Other manifestations may be headache and vomiting due to raised intracranial tension (ICT), hydrocephalus, diffuse cerebral edema, or focal neurologic findings.

The seizures are usually focal but may be generalized also. Children may present with a single seizure or recurrent epilepsy. A fulminant encephalitis-like presentation is rare but may occur with massive initial infection associated with cerebral edema due to heavy parasite load.

Clinical manifestations of extraparenchymal NCC are more diverse depending on the location of lesion. It has poorer prognosis with higher rates of morbidity and mortality compared to parenchymal due to higher parasite, less restricted growth, and more irregularity of individual cysticerci.

Obstructive hydrocephalus is the most common presentation of intraventricular NCC (which is up to 20% of cases) associated with acute, subacute, or intermittent signs of increased intracranial pressure, usually without focal signs.

Subarachnoid NCC, rare in children, presents with signs of meningeal irritation, communicating hydrocephalus due to basilar arachnoiditis, cerebral infarction, or spinal disease with radiculitis or transverse myelitis.

Ocular NCC presents as iridocyclitis or decreased visual acuity because of cysticerci in the retina or vitreous resulting in retinal detachment.

Cysticerci in the tissues present with mass and focal findings from mass effect.

■ DIAGNOSIS[1,2,4-8]

Accurate diagnosis of NCC is difficult. A set of diagnostic criteria comprising clinical history, neuroimaging and immunological evidence and epidemiological factors proposed by Del Brutto et al. (2001)[5] may guide in diagnosis of NCC **(Table 2)**.

Investigations

Neuroimaging[1,2,4-8]

Neuroimaging is the most useful diagnostic study for NCC.

Magnetic resonance imaging (MRI) head provides information about location of cyst, cyst viability, and associated inflammation. The protoscolex, if visible within the cyst, is a pathognomonic sign for cysticercosis **(Fig. 3)**. A classical description in NCC is the "starry sky" appearance due to the presence of multiple cysts

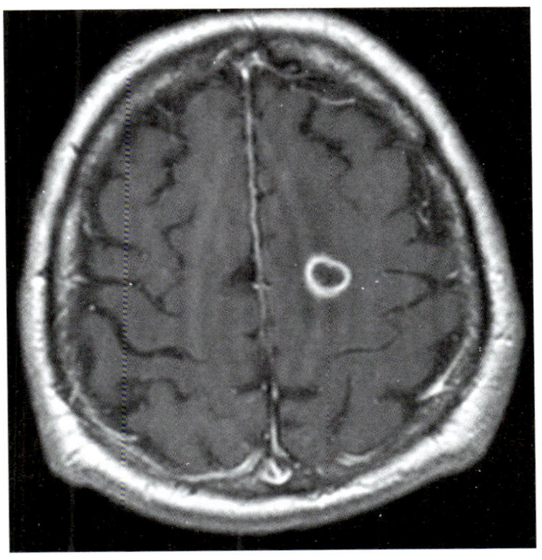

Figs. 3: Cerebral ring enhancing lesion.

Table 2: The "Del Brutto Criteria" for diagnosis of NCC.

Absolute criteria	Major criteria	Minor criteria	Epidemiological criteria
Histology: Visualization of parasite from biopsy of brain or spinal cord lesion	*Neuroimaging*: Lesions highly suggestive of NCC	*Neuroimaging*: Lesions suggestive of NCC	Patient country of origin endemic for NCC
Neuroimaging: Scolex visible within cystic lesion	*EITB assay*: Positive result for detection of *T. solium* antibodies	*Clinical manifestations*: Symptoms suggestive of NCC	Patient currently resides in NCC endemic area
Fundoscopy: Evidence of subretinal parasites	*Cysticidal drug therapy*: Lesion resolution following treatment with albendazole or praziquantel	*CSF ELISA*: Positive detection for detection of *T. solium* antibodies or antigens	Patient frequently travels to areas where NCC is endemic
		Evidence of cysticercosis outside the CNS	There is evidence that patient household has had contact with *T. solium* infection

Note: Diagnosis:
Definitive: 1 absolute OR 2 major plus 1 minor/1 epidemiological. *Probable*: 1 major plus 2 minor OR 1 major plus 1 minor plus 1 epidemiological OR 3 minor plus 1 epidemiological
Source: Del Brutto et al. (2001).
(CNS: central nervous system; CSF: cerebrospinal fluid; EITB: enzyme-linked immunoelectrotransfer blot technique; NCC: neurocysticercosis; ELISA: enzyme-linked immunosorbent assay)

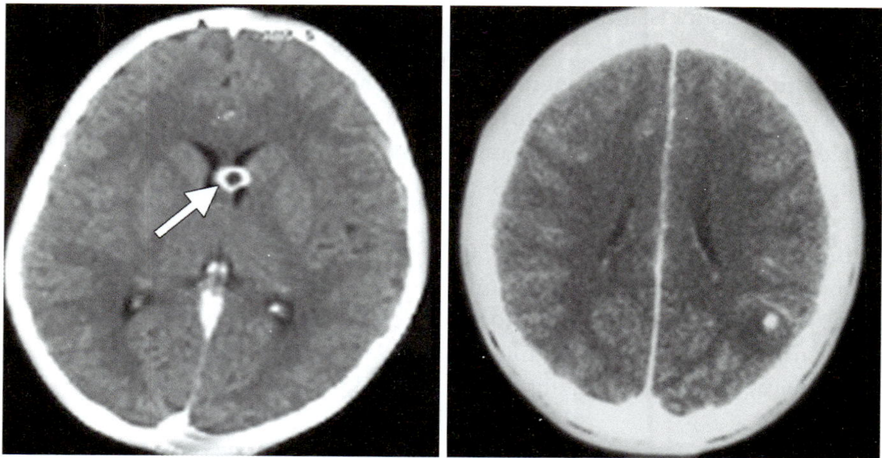

Fig. 4A: Intraventricular neurocysticercosis

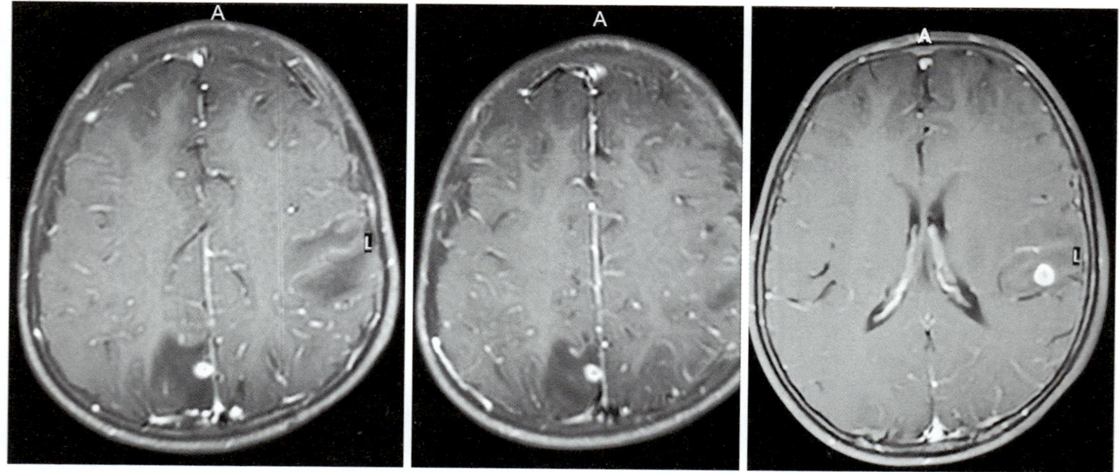

Fig. 4B: Well defined thick walled enhancing lesions in left frontal and right parietal lobe in subcortical and cortical areas: colloid vesicular stage of neurocysticercosis.

at different evolutionary stages **(Figs. 4A and B)**. The MRI is also a modality to detect basilar arachnoiditis, intraventricular cysts, and cysts in the spinal cord.

Computed tomography scans, which are cheaper and easily available, have higher sensitivity for detection of calcifications which occurs in around 50% of patients.

The most common finding in children is a solitary parenchymal cyst, with or without contrast enhancement, or CNS calcification.

In children from endemic areas, presentation with a single enhancing round lesion less than 2 cm in diameter without any evidence of other diseases (e.g. no fever or lymph nodes), with no focal findings or increased intracranial pressure, is highly specific for NCC.

Immunological Assays[1]

A reliable serological test will be useful in diagnosis as neuroimaging is expensive and requires expertise and infrastructure that are not easily available. New assays are under study that will show promising results.

- The lentil lectin purified glycoprotein (LLGP) enzyme-linked immunoelectrotransfer blot (EITB) assay uses targeted antigens to detect antibodies to *T. solium* in patient serum. This diagnostic test is reported to have a specificity of 100% and sensitivity of 98%.
- ELISA (Enzyme-linked immunosorbent assay)-based assay to detect *T. solium* antigens using monoclonal antibodies prepared from *T. saginata* indicates established infection.
- A lateral flow assay (LFA) based on the se of monoclonal antibody has been developed recently for diagnosis and monitoring of extraparenchymal NCC.

Stool Microscopy

Stool microscopy for the presence of *T. solium* eggs in the stool does not indicate an NCC infection but helps

Table 3: The main differences in the presentation of NCC and CNS tuberculomas in contrast MRI and CECT.

Neurocysticercosis	Tuberculoma
Lesions are smaller, <20 mm and may be single or multiple	Often multiple and larger, >20 mm because of conglomeration
Cystic	Solid
Less perilesional edema	More perilesional edema
Smooth margins	Irregular margin
Present at gray-white matter junction	More common in posterior fossa
Other involvements like eyes, muscles, or subcutaneous tissues	Spread is mostly secondary to infection somewhere else
T2W shows hyper intensity with hypointense scolex in it with no midline shift and Ring enhancement depends upon the staging	Hypointensity seen in T2W and midline shift may be present
MR spectroscopy shows multiple amino acid peaks	MR spectroscopy shows lipid peak
Meningitis feature is not there	Meningitis is usually associated

(CECT: contrast-enhanced computed tomography; CNS: central nervous system; MRI: magnetic resonance imaging; NCC: neurocysticercosis)

in detection of carriers and may help in disruption of cycle of transmission. PCR (polymerase chain reaction) and ELISA of stool samples may improve detection rates but impractical in many endemic settings due to lack of equipment and trained personnel.

Differential Diagnosis

Neurocysticercosis is often confused clinically with other seizure disorders. Clinical suspicion is based on travel history to an endemic region or from an endemic area, a history of contact with an individual who might carry an adult tapeworm, or suggestive imaging studies. The classical imaging appearance, ring-enhancing lesion, may be seen in other conditions such as brain abscess, granulomas (including tuberculomas) **(Table 3)**, fungal infections, Langerhans histiocytosis, and toxoplasmosis, demyelination, tumors, metastases, and subacute infarcts.

Recommendations to Diagnose Neurocysticercosis[1]

- Clinical manifestations of NCC are diverse. The two most common clinical presentations are seizures and headache and vomiting due to increased intracranial pressure.
- Initial evaluation should consider a detailed history, clinical examination, and neuroimaging studies.
- In inconclusive cases of suspected NCC, serologic testing with EITB for confirmation is recommended. ELISA using crude antigen has poor sensitivity and specificity and is not recommended for diagnosis.

■ TREATMENT (TABLES 4 AND 5)[1,2,4-8]

Because of the heterogeneity of clinical manifestations of NCC, diagnosis is difficult and also, there is no consensus on a single, standard therapeutic approach. There are different views about the use of anti-inflammatory drugs, cysticidal drugs, and anticonvulsants. Before treating, detailed evaluation is of utmost importance. The number, location, and viability of cysts; severity of the disease; and presence of raised ICT will determine the management of each case individually.

Cysticidal Drugs

The controversy regarding use of cysticidal drugs is that the destruction of cysts may result in paradoxical rapid increase in ICT due to extensive inflammatory response from the host and also the fact that parenchymal cysts may resolve naturally with benign asymptomatic course. Some experts opine that cysticidal drugs are unnecessary. However, several studies have proved the efficacy of cysticidal drugs in alleviating symptoms such as seizures and headaches, and hasten recovery of parenchymal lesions and also apprehensions regarding a live parasite in the brain being untreated, most clinicians support use of cysticidal drugs after thorough characterization of cyst by neuroimaging with the assumption that once inactive, they will cause fewer symptoms.

Antiparasitic treatment is important, but never an emergency.

The two most widely used cysticidal drugs are:

1. Albendazole, an imidazole, which impairs glucose uptake and metabolism in the parasite.
2. Praziquantel, an isoquinolone, which causes parasite paralysis by disrupting calcium pathways and homeostasis.

However, these cysticidal drugs are used only in the treatment of viable cysts in the vesicular or early colloidal stages of development and are not recommended for

Table 4: Treatment of extraparenchymal neurocysticercosis form.

Extraparenchymal form	Recommended treatment
Intraventricular (lateral or third ventricle)	Removal of the cysticerci by minimally invasive neuroendoscopy, when feasible Do not require antiparasitic drugs or shunt therapy, if all cysticerci are removed
Intraventricular (fourth ventricle)	Either endoscopic or microsurgical cystectomy
Intraventricular—when surgical removal not feasible (e.g. adherent cyst)	CSF shunting by ventriculoperitoneal shunt Adjuvant antiparasitic and anti-inflammatory therapy A CSF diversion (shunt) should always be performed prior to chemotherapy
Subarachnoid	*Surgical management of hydrocephalus*: Ventriculoperitoneal shunt *Antiparasitic therapy*: Albendazole or in combination with praziquantel *Anti-inflammatory therapy*: Corticosteroids

(CSF: cerebrospinal fluid)

Table 5: Treatment for different forms of parenchymal neurocysticercosis (NCC) form.

Form	Treatment	
Viable parenchymal Single	Antiparasitic therapy	Antiparasitic drugs should be used in all patients with viable parenchymal NCC unless there is increased intracranial pressure
	1–2 viable cysts	Monotherapy with albendazole (15 mg/kg/d in 2 daily doses up to 1,200 mg/d) with food for 10 days
	>2 viable cysts	Albendazole (15 mg/kg/d in 2 daily doses up to 1,200 mg/d) combined with praziquantel (15 mg/kg/d in 3 daily doses) for 10 days
	Anti-inflammatory therapy	Corticosteroids should be used whenever antiparasitic drugs are used
	Antiepileptic therapy	Antiepileptic drugs should be used in all patients with seizures
• Single enhancing lesion due to neurocysticercosis • Calcified	Antiparasitic therapy	Albendazole (15 mg/kg/d in 2 daily doses up to 800 mg/d) for 1–2 weeks
	Anti-inflammatory therapy	Corticosteroids should be given concomitantly with antiparasitic agents
	Antiepileptic therapy	Antiepileptic drugs should be used in all patients with seizures
Calcified parenchymal neurocysticercosis with or without perilesional edema	Antiparasitic therapy	Antiparasitic treatment not recommended Antiepileptic
	Anti-inflammatory therapy	Treatment with antiepileptic drugs
	Antiepileptic therapy	Corticosteroids should not be routinely used
Cysticercal encephalitis (with diffuse cerebral edema)		Avoid antiparasitic drugs, treat diffuse cerebral edema with corticosteroids

calcified cysts, as cysticidal drugs are ineffective as parasites are already dead in calcified cysts.

Albendazole is the drug of choice because of its efficacy as antiparasitic drug compared to praziquantel, better cerebrospinal fluid (CSF) penetration, less interaction with co-administered anti-inflammatory drugs such as corticosteroids, easily available, well tolerated, and cost-effective.

The usual regimen of albendazole is 15 mg/kg/day in two divided doses for 7–28 days. Both short- and long-duration therapies were found to be equally effective for parenchymal NCC.

Subarachnoid NCC does not respond well to single antiparasitic drug at doses and durations used for parenchymal NCC. Optimal management may require chronic anti-inflammatory therapy, intensive antiparasitic therapy, that is, high doses of albendazole for longer duration, and surgical therapy.

Contraindications for Cysticidal Drugs

Cysticidal drugs are generally contraindicated in a markedly raised ICT, in cases with pre-existing risk of developing hydrocephalus, such as in subarachnoid NCC and encephalitic NCC, heavy parasite load and disseminated infection due to paradoxical response of sudden raise in ICT due to degradation of viable cysts and flared-up host immune response and may even result in death. Inappropriate use of cysticidal drugs in calcified NCC should be avoided.

Antiepileptics

Seizures are the most common clinical presentation of parenchymal NCC. In cases presenting with convulsions and multiple viable cysts, antiepileptic treatment may be considered. Carbamazepine or phenytoin are the preferred antiepileptics in NCC. Carbamazepine is preferred over phenytoin due to its associated side effects. A shorter duration of antiepileptics for 1 year may be considered till the neuroimaging abnormalities disappear.

Steroids

Steroid administration before use of cysticidal drugs is important to regulate the flared-up inflammatory response which might be due to degradation of viable cysts and also due to decreased perilesional edema. Usually, oral prednisolone or intravenous dexamethasone in children with raised ICT is used as an adjunct to cysticidal therapy. They are administered around 3 days prior to starting cysticidal drugs and continued for approximately a week till the end of the cysticidal course treatment. In children with a markedly raised ICT, heavy parasite load, and disseminated infection, the use of cysticidal therapy is contraindicated as sudden raise in ICT can occur due to host immune responses and steroids may be used alone.

Surgery

Surgery was once considered the primary modality of treatment for NCC; with recent development of pharmacological therapies, the role of surgery has decreased and is now restricted only for very severe diseases with significant risk of complications if left untreated, such as extraparenchymal NCC and racemose NCC, or due to risk of inflammatory response that may be associated with cysticidal drugs. Surgical cyst extirpation may be considered.

For subarachnoid NCC, surgical intervention may include CSF shunting for hydrocephalus or minimally invasive surgical debulking.

Ventricular NCC of the third and lateral ventricles should be treated with minimally invasive surgery when possible.

Open craniotomy or CSF diversion along with antiparasitic drugs are optimal in selected cases. Antiparasitic therapy should be deferred until after surgical therapy.

The common surgical intervention considered is shunt insertion in severe cases with hydrocephalus.

■ CONCLUSION

Neurocysticercosis, a leading cause of epilepsy in the developing world. Thorough understanding of pathogenesis of neurocysticercosis and the life cycle of *T. solium* is necessary to develop appropriate intervention and prevention programs. Development and enforcement of Global strategies for prevention and control is the need of the hour.

■ REFERENCES

1. Gripper LB, Welburn SC. Neurocysticercosis infection and disease–A review. Acta Trop. 2017;166:218-24.
2. Rajshekhar V. Neurocysticercosis: Diagnostic problems & current therapeutic strategies. Indian J Med Res. 2016;144(3): 319-26.
3. Fischer PR, White AC Jr. Adult tapeworm infections. In: Kliegman R, Stanton B, Geme J St, Schor N (Eds). Nelson's textbook of pediatrics. First South Asian 2nd edition. Elsevier, Philadelphia; 2016;3:1749-52.
4. White AC Jr, Fischer PR. Cysticercosis. In: Kliegman R, Stanton B, Geme J St, Schor N (Eds). Nelson's textbook of pediatrics. First South Asian, 2nd edition. Elsevier, Philadelphia; 2016;3: 1749-52.
5. Del Brutto OH, Rajshekhar V, White AC Jr, et al. Proposed diagnostic criteria for neurocysticercosis. Neurology. 2001;57:177–83.
6. White AC Jr, Coyle CM, Rajshekhar V, et al. Diagnosis and treatment of neurocysticercosis: 2017 clinical practice guidelines by the Infectious Diseases Society of America (IDSA) and the American Society of Tropical Medicine and Hygiene (ASTMH). Am J Trop Med Hyg. 2018;98(4):945–66.
7. World Health Organization (WHO). Taeniasis/cysticerosis; 2019. [online] Available from: www.who.int/mediacentre/factsheets/fs376/en/] [Last accessed on August, 2019].
8. Sharma BB, Sharma S. Neurocysticercosis (NCC) vs Central Nervous System (CNS) Tuberculoma in Children—Dilemma over Clinico-Radiological Diagnosis? Open Journal of Pediatrics. 2016;6(3):245-51.

8

Fungal Infections

Jaydeep Choudhury

Superficial Cutaneous and Subcutaneous Fungal Infections

Sandipan Dhar, Sahana M Srinivas

INTRODUCTION

Fungal infections in children which were once thought to be uncommon in the past few decades have been increasing recently due to the changing scenarios. Fungal infections of skin and nails affect 13–25% of the world's population and pose a major health problem in school children and cause significant morbidity. The epidemiology of fungal infections in children has greatly changed in the last few years. There has been an increasing incidence not only in immunocompromised children but also in an immunocompetent child. Factors such as widespread use and misuse of corticosteroids, broad-spectrum antibiotics and cytotoxic agents have contributed to the increased incidence of both superficial and deep fungal infections. Modifiable environmental and host factors also contribute to the rising pediatric cases. Fungal infections are widely prevalent in this part of the globe due to the tropical environment with high temperature and humidity.

There is increased epidemic of steroid-induced and resistant tinea in India, especially in adults, which has become a major source of infection in children. Use of over-the-counter (OTC) and fixed-drug combination (FDC) medications by parents and lack of knowledge of giving timely healthcare facilities, resistance to antifungal agents has led to increased and recurrent fungal infections in children. This chapter will discuss superficial and subcutaneous fungal infections in children.

CLASSIFICATION

Fungi are a large, diverse group of eukaryotic aerobic organisms and exist as parasites, saprophytes, or commensal. They can occur as yeast, mold, and dimorphs. Yeasts are unicellular, round to oval, and reproduce through budding and molds occur as hyphae, which are long tubular structures and reproduce by forming spores (conidia) that occur at the end of hyphae. Dimorphs grow as both yeast (humans) and mold form (environment). Fungi can evoke allergic reactions or inflammatory response in the host by direct tissue invasion or through their products.

Fungal infections in children are classified into three types as described in **Table 1**.

Superficial Cutaneous Fungal Infections

Superficial infections are the most common type of fungal infection seen in both younger and older children. Superficial fungal infections are dermatophytosis, tinea versicolor, tinea nigra, piedra, and candidiasis. The causative agents of these superficial fungal infections are described in **Table 2**. Few Indian studies have documented the prevalence of superficial fungal infections from 19% to 32%. Majority of the cases were seen in the age group of 10–15 years with a male preponderance. Published literature has shown that 83% of children affected with superficial fungal infections had contact with an affected family member. The most common family source was the mother followed by siblings. Other predisposing factors included rural background, low socioeconomic status,

Table 1: Classification of fungal infections in children.	
Type of fungal infection	*Features*
Superficial/cutaneous	Affects skin, hair, nails, mucous membranes
Subcutaneous	Affects subcutaneous tissue
Systemic/opportunistic	• *True pathogen*: Affects healthy children • *Opportunistic*: Affects immunocompromised children

Table 2: Superficial fungal infections and their causative agents.

Superficial fungal infections	Causative agents
Dermatophytosis	Dermatophytes: *Trichophyton, Microsporum, Epidermophyton*
Tinea versicolor	*Malassezia* species
Candidiasis	*Candida*
Tinea nigra	*Hortaea werneckii*
Piedra	*Trichosporon, Piedraia hortae*

Table 3: Classification of dermatophytes based on natural habitat.

Anthropophilic	Geophilic	Zoophilic
• *E. floccosum* • *M. audouinii* • *M. ferrugineum* • *T. rubrum* • *T. tonsurans* • *T. violaceum* • *T. schoenleinii* • *T. concentricum* • *T. mentagrophytes*	• *M. gypseum* • *M. flavum*	• *M. canis* • *M. equinum* • *T. verrucosum* • *T. mentagrophytes*

Table 4: Classification of dermatophytosis based on the location.

Tinea infection	Site
Tinea capitis	Scalp
Tinea corporis	Trunk, flexures, extremities except palms, soles, scalp
Tinea cruris	Groins, inner thigh, buttocks, perianal region
Tinea barbae	Beard area
Tinea pedis	Foot and toe web spaces
Tinea manuum	Palms and interdigital web spaces
Tinea faciei	Face
Tinea imbricata	Anywhere on the body
Tinea unguium	Nail plate
Tinea incognito	Anywhere on the body
Onychomycosis	Nails

joint family setup, hostel setup, poor personal hygiene, direct skin-to-skin contact with an infected person, sharing of clothes, toys, combs, damp clothes and history of atopy.

Dermatophytosis (Tinea Infections)

Etiopathogenesis

Dermatophytosis, also called as tinea, is a superficial fungal infection affecting the keratinized tissue like skin, hair, and nail and is caused by dermatophytes. They invade the keratinized tissue by digesting them and cause different clinical reactions. These dermatophytes belong to the family Arthrodermataceae. Depending on the natural habitat, dermatophytes are of three groups: anthropophilic which affect only humans, zoophilic whose normal hosts are animals but can infect humans, and geophilic which are found in soil and rarely pathogenic to humans **(Table 3)**. Factors such as trauma, abrasion of the skin, moisture, and warmth help penetration of fungal spores with desquamation of stratum corneum. Unsaturated fatty acids and transferrin in sebum and serum act as inhibitory factors preventing dermatophyte infections. Th1 cell-mediated immunity plays an important role in the pathogenesis of fungal infections by activation of T lymphocytes and production of chemotactic factors and cytokines resulting in inflammation.

Based on the sites affected, dermatophytosis are classified into various types as described in **Table 4**.

■ CLINICAL FEATURES

Tinea Capitis

Tinea capitis is the common type of dermatophyte infection seen in children affecting the hair shaft of scalp. It is seen more commonly in prepubertal children in the age group of 3–7 years. Rarely it is seen in infants. Past studies have shown the prevalence of tine capitis from 26.9% to 64.9%. Boys are affected more than girls in the ratio of 5:1. Predisposing factors include poverty, overcrowding, low socioeconomic status, hygiene status, protein deficiency, and vitamin A deficiency. Based on the hair invasion, dermatophytes can be classified into endothrix, ectothrix, and favus. In endothrix, the fungus grows completely within the hair shaft. The hyphae are converted to arthroconidia (spores) within the hair without destruction of the hair shaft. In ectothrix, the hyphae grow outside the hair shaft and destroy the cuticle. Arthroconidia may develop both within and outside the hair shaft. In favus, the hyphae is seen parallel to the long axis of hair shaft and leave long tunnels in the hair shaft after degeneration. It is caused by various microsporum and *Trichophyton* species but more commonly affected by *Trichophyton tonsurans* and *Microsporum canis*. It is transmitted by close contact with affected children, shared brushes, combs, clothing, bed linen, used hats, and fomites. The reservoir of infection has been demonstrated in asymptomatic children contributing to the epidemiological factors. The pathogenesis of tinea capitis is described in **Box 1**.

Clinically, tinea capitis is classified into two types: noninflammatory and inflammatory. The noninflammatory

> **Box 1:** Pathogenesis of tinea capitis.
>
> *Trauma/abrasion*
> - Invasion of hyphae, grows down between the space between hair shaft and follicle wall
> - Hyphae spreads into and around hair shaft
> - Intrapilary hyphae grows down towards the hair bulb, stops at the upper limit of keratogenous zone

type includes grey patch, seborrheic dermatitis, and black dot. The inflammatory type is of two types: kerion and favus. Noninflammatory is the most common type of tinea capitis seen in children. Easy pluckability of hair is a common feature of tinea capitis.

Noninflammatory Type

Grey patch: It clinically presents as asymptomatic, well-defined patches with slight hyperkeratosis on scalp with loss of hair presenting as broken stumps of gray lusterless hair and minimal scaling **(Fig. 1)**. It is often the cause of epidemics in school.

Seborrheic dermatitis type: It is characterized diffuse scaling all over the scalp with no evident hair loss.

Black dot: It clinically manifests as multiple, ill-defined patchy alopecia with black dots and diffuse scaling **(Fig. 2)**. The appearance of black dots is due to breakage of hair at the level of scalp.

Inflammatory Type

Kerion: It is a distinct type of inflammatory tinea capitis presenting as boggy indurated swelling studded with vesicles, pustules, and crusting along with broken hairs leading to scarring alopecia **(Figs. 3 and 4)**. There may be multiple discharging sinuses with matting of hair. It is associated with posterior cervical, retroauricular, and occipital lymphadenopathy.

Favus: Favus in Latin word means "honeycomb." It is characterized by the formation of cup-shaped yellow crusts called "scutula" with protruding hairs. It is often associated with mousy odor and scarring alopecia.

Tinea capitis should be differentiated from alopecia areata, seborrheic dermatitis, atopic dermatitis, psoriasis, trichotillomania, and bacterial folliculitis. Diagnosis is mainly based on clinical features. Potassium hydroxide (KOH) examination may be useful. Wood's lamp examination may be useful in ectothrix organisms. Fungal culture is the gold standard investigation in tinea capitis.

Tinea Corporis

Tine corporis, also called "ringworm of the body," is the most common superficial fungal infection seen in

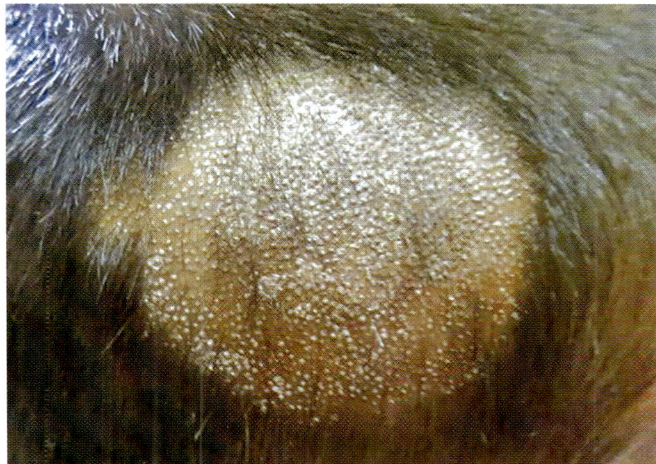

Fig. 1: Grey patch type tinea capitis showing broken stumps of grey hairs with scaling.

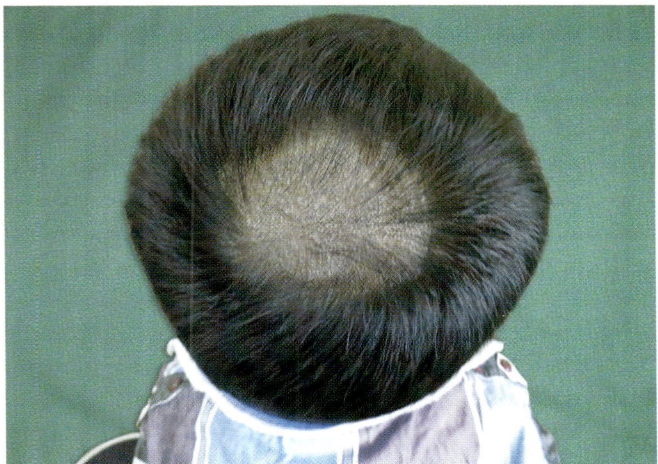

Fig. 2: Patchy alopecia with black dots and scaling on scalp.

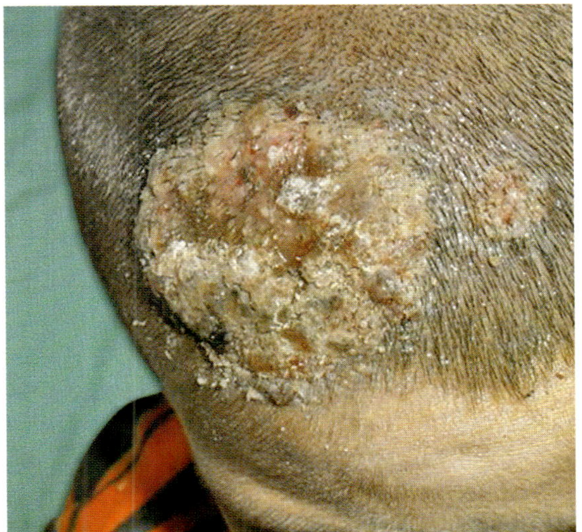

Fig. 3: Kerion showing boggy indurated swelling studded with pustules, crusting and broken hairs.

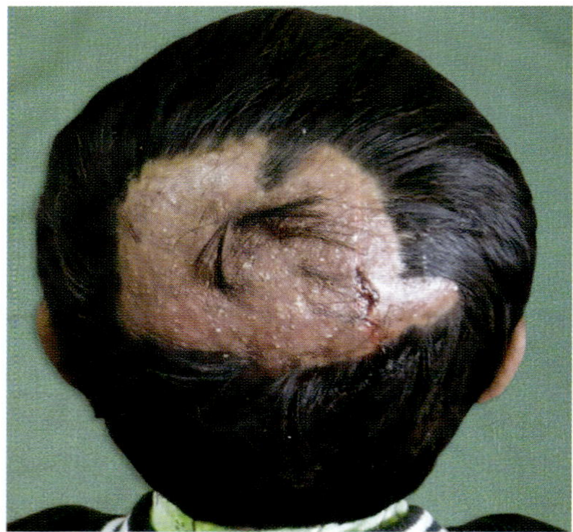

Fig. 4: Scarring alopecia in kerion after treatment.

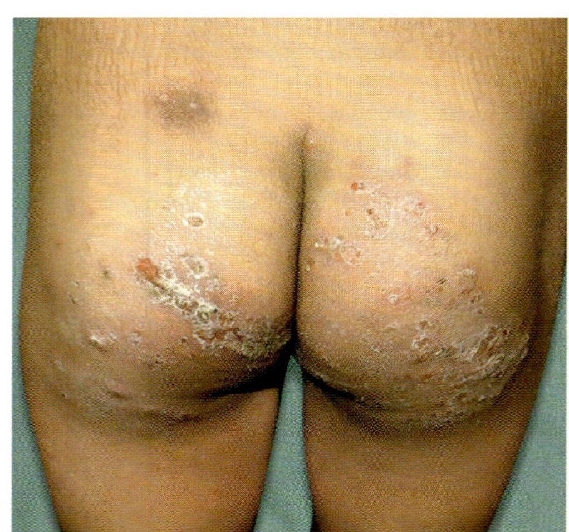

Fig. 5: Well-defined erythematous scaly annular plaque in tinea corporis on the gluteal region.

children. Studies have shown the prevalence of tinea corporis in children ranging from 45% to 47%. It affects mainly the nonhairy areas of the body such as face, trunk, and extremities with exclusion of palms, soles, and groins. The causative organism in young children is usually *M. canis* and in older children it is *T. rubrum*, *T. verrucosum*, *T. mentagrophytes*, *T. tonsurans*, or *Epidermophyton floccosum*. Transmission is by direct contact with infected peer groups and contact with pets such as puppies and kitten. The source of infection in children could be affected parents with tinea pedis, tinea unguium, or onychomycosis. Other predisposing factors include warm, humid climate, diabetes, leukemia, and immunodeficiency. It is clinically characterized by pruritic, single to multiple annular to polycyclic erythematous to hyperpigmented scaly plaques with central clearing and raised peripheral border **(Fig. 5)**. Other morphological variants include vesicular, pustular, and eczematous types. Complications include secondary infections. It usually resolves with postinflammatory hyperpigmentation. Rarely it becomes generalized.

Diagnosis of tinea corporis is mainly on clinical presentation. Diagnostic tests include KOH examination of skin scrapings and fungal culture. Differential diagnosis includes granuloma annulare, psoriasis, pityriasis rosea, contact dermatitis, nummular eczema, seborrheic dermatitis, and annular erythema.

Tinea Cruris

Tinea cruris, also called "jock itch," affecting the groins and upper thighs is commonly seen in adolescents and adults. In the past few years, it has been increasingly seen in children. Indian studies have shown the prevalence of tinea cruris from 28% to 50%. The causative organism includes *E. floccosum*, *T. rubrum*, and *T. mentagrophytes*.

Predisposing factors include hot humid climate, tight clothes, obesity, and physical activity. Clinically, it presents as pruritic, well-defined, sharply marginated, not always symmetrical erythematous to hyperpigmented scaly plaques with central clearing located on the intertriginous folds, inner thighs, perianal region, buttocks, and lower abdomen **(Figs. 6 and 7)**. Scrotum, penis, and labia majora are usually spared, but if involved the diagnosis of candidiasis should be considered. Long-standing, not treated tinea cruris may become lichenified. Differential diagnosis includes erythrasma, intertrigo, psoriasis, and seborrheic dermatitis. Wood's light examination shows coral-red fluorescence.

Tinea Barbae

Tinea barbae is an uncommon infection affecting the beard area seen in adolescents and adults. The causative organism is mainly *T. mentagrophytes*, *T. verrucosum* and rarely by *T. violaceum* and *T. rubrum*. It usually affects one side of the face and involves hair follicles resulting in inflammatory papules, pustules, crusting, and rarely kerion-like nodules. Lesions can persist for months resulting in scarring alopecia. Differential diagnosis includes bacterial folliculitis, herpes simplex, and contact dermatitis.

Tinea Pedis

Tinea pedis though common in adolescents and adults can be seen in children. Use of occlusive footwear for a prolonged period, increased sweating, and source of infection in the family can be predisposing factors in children. *T. tonsurans* is commonly associated with tinea pedis in children. There are four clinical types of tinea

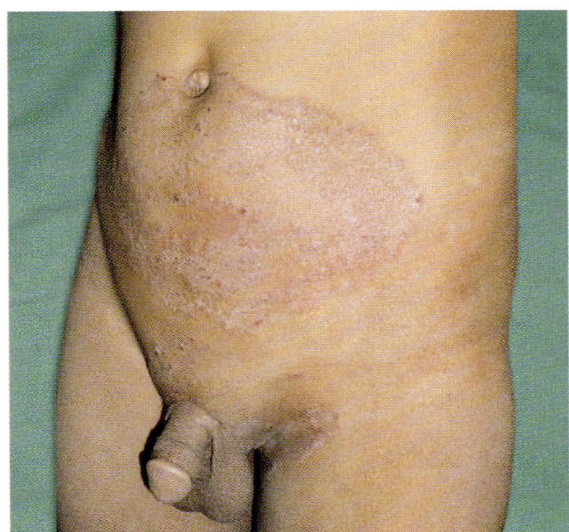

Fig. 6: Tinea corporis and tinea cruris showing well-defined hyperpigmented scaly plaque on abdomen and inner aspect of thighs.

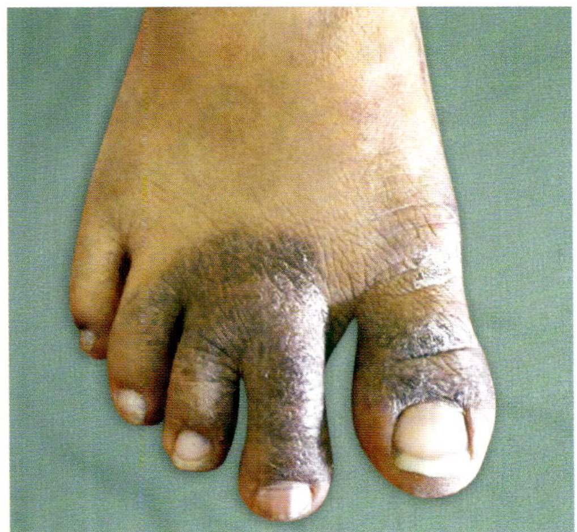

Fig. 8: Tinea pedis with annular scaly plaque on the dorsum of feet and web spaces.

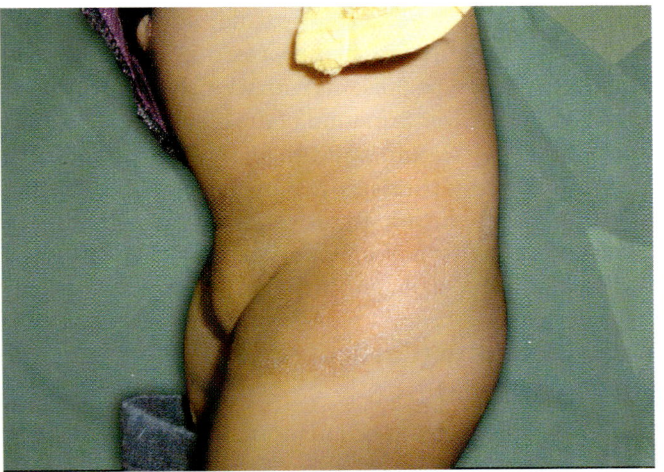

Fig. 7: Tinea cruris extending to inner aspect of thigh, and lower abdomen.

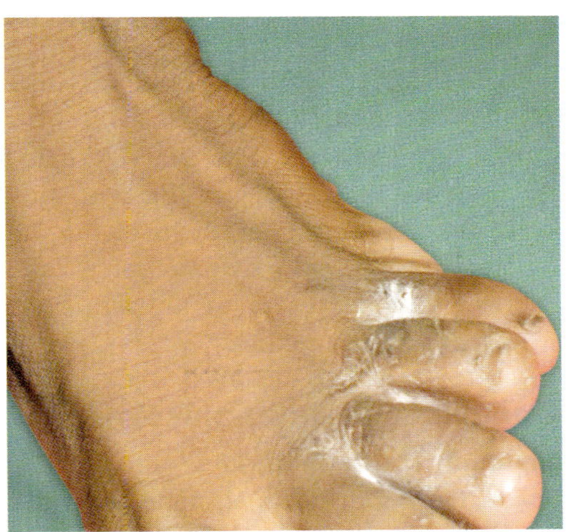

Fig. 9: Maceration in web spaces in chronic intertriginous type of tinea pedis.

pedis: (1) chronic intertriginous type, (2) vesicular type, (3) moccasin type, and (4) ulcerative type. The chronic intertriginous type is the most common type characterized by erythema, scaling, and maceration in the toe web spaces **(Figs. 8 and 9)**. The vesicular type manifests as vesicles and bullae along with erythema in the foot. There is diffuse erythema with scaling and hyperkeratosis in the moccasin type. Ulcerative form is rarely seen in children and it is a severe form of tinea pedis manifesting with bullous and ulcerative lesions. Differential diagnosis includes psoriasis and contact dermatitis.

Tinea Manuum

Tinea manuum affects palms and web spaces of hands. The causative organism is *T. tonsurans*. It is clinically characterized by pruritic, well-defined erythematous to hyperpigmented, hyperkeratotic scaly plaques on the palms and web spaces. It is mostly unilateral but can become bilateral. Rarely, tinea manuum manifests with vesicular lesions similar to dyshidrotic eczema. Tinea manuum of one hand with tinea pedis of both feet is termed as "two feet one hand syndrome." Differential diagnosis of psoriasis, contact dermatitis, pompholyx, and id reaction should be considered.

Tinea Faciei

Tinea faciei is a subtype of tinea corporis occurring on face. It presents as erythematous annular scaly plaque with central clearing **(Fig. 10)**. Tinea faciei should be differentiated from psoriasis, seborrheic dermatitis, granuloma annulare, polymorphic light eruption, and lupus erythematosus.

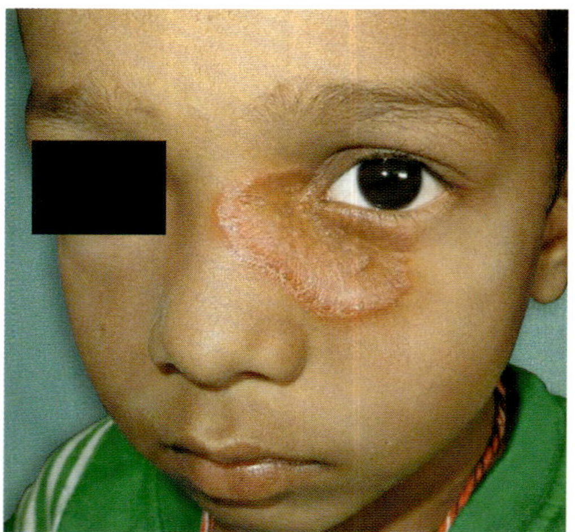

Fig. 10: Tinea faciei showing erythematous scaly plaque on the medial aspect of left eye extending to lower eyelid and nose.

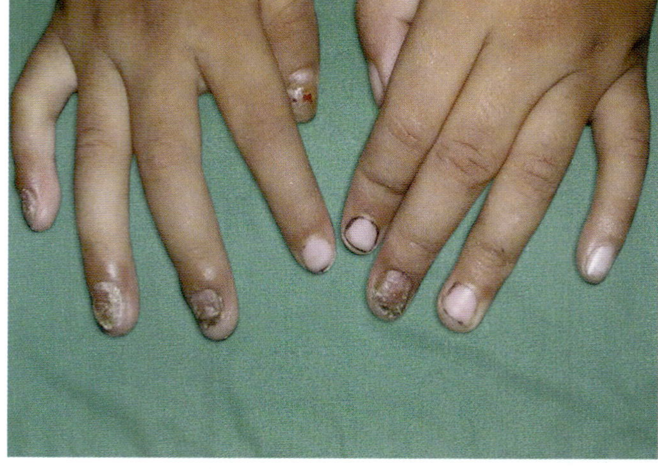

Fig. 11: Onychomycosis of fingernails with total nail dystrophy.

Tinea Imbricata

Tinea imbricata is a distinct type of superficial dermatophyte infection caused by *T. concentricum*. It involves only skin and nails. The characteristic feature includes concentric rings of scaling with polycyclic borders. It can spread peripherally involving the entire skin often sparing the scalp, axillae, palms, and soles. Application of topical steroid to tinea infection may present with similar presentation.

Tinea Unguium and Onychomycosis

Tinea unguium is a dermatophyte infection affecting the nail plate. Onychomycosis, also affecting the nails, is caused by both dermatophytes and nondermatophytes and yeasts. They are often associated with tinea manuum and tinea pedis. Tinea unguium and onychomycosis are uncommon in children as compared to adults due to faster nail growth, less trauma, smaller surface area, and lower incidence of tinea manuum and pedis. The worldwide prevalence of onychomycosis is 0–2.6%. Tinea unguium is caused by *T. rubrum*, *T. mentagrophytes var interdigitale*, and *E. floccosum*. Onychomycosis is caused by the *Trichophyton* species along with *Candida albicans*, *Candida parapsilosis*, and molds. *Candida* causes periungual infection. Nail changes in tinea unguium include onycholysis, subungual hyperkeratosis, and total dystrophy.

Onychomycosis is classified into distal subungual, proximal subungual, and white superficial types. Distal subungual is the most common type affecting nail bed and distal part of nail plate. It presents as onycholysis, subungual hyperkeratosis, and yellowish discoloration of the nail plate **(Fig. 11)**. Proximal subungual is an uncommon type affecting the proximal nail fold. The white superficial type presents with whitish plaques on the dorsal nail plate. Confirmation of the diagnosis is by KOH wet mount preparation and fungal culture. Differential diagnosis includes psoriasis, lichen planus, traumatic nail dystrophy, and chronic paronychia. Asymmetrical nail involvement with tinea infection elsewhere in the body can provide a clue to diagnose fungal infection of the nail.

Tinea Incognito (Corticosteroid Modified Tinea)

Steroid-modified tinea infections are termed tinea incognito. Recently, there has been a tremendous increase in the use of OTC and FDC (fixed drug combination) products containing steroids. Misuse of topical corticosteroids by caregivers has led to increased incidence of tinea incognito. In an Indian study of dermatophytosis in children, 94% had applied topical steroid/steroid antifungal combination before presentation to a dermatologist. The typical presentation of annular scaly plaque is not present in tinea incognito. Well-defined border, no scaling, hypopigmentation, and appearance of lesions after stopping creams, concentric rings of erythema, atrophy, and telangiectasia aid to the diagnosis of tinea incognito **(Figs. 12 and 13)**.

Dermatophytid

Dermatophytid is a delayed type of hypersensitivity reaction to the fungal antigens and manifests at a site distant from the primary source of fungal infection. This "id" reaction is seen during active infection or during initiation of systemic antifungal therapy. It is associated with kerion

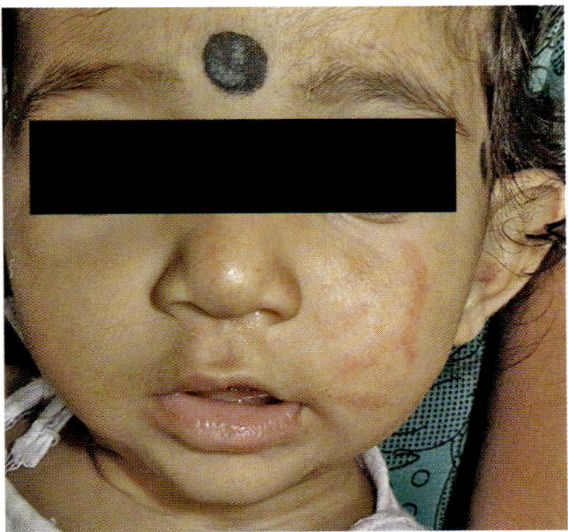

Fig. 12: Tinea incognito with ill-defined border and no scaling.

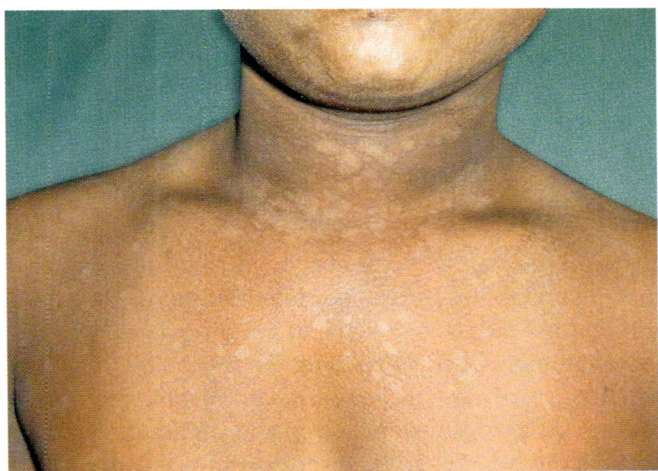

Fig. 14: Multiple, well-defined hypopigmented mild scaly macules on the neck and chest in tinea versicolor.

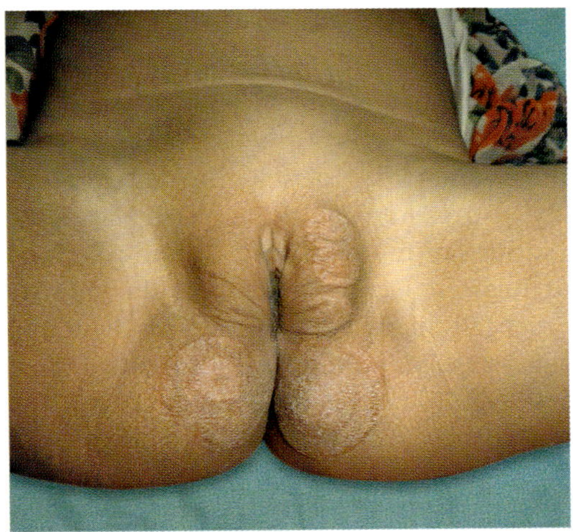

Fig. 13: Tinea incognito showing hyperpigmented plaques with concentric layers on genitalia.

and acutely inflamed tinea pedis. It clinically manifests as symmetrical, pruritic, papules, and papulovesicles on the face, trunk, and extremities. Other types of "id" reaction associated are pompholyx type, urticaria, erythema nodosum, erysipelas, and pityriasis rosea-like reaction. Dermatophytid should be differentiated from drug reactions. Management includes treatment of the primary source with antifungals and topical steroids.

Tinea Versicolor

Tinea versicolor is a common superficial fungal infection caused by yeast forms of dimorphic fungus *Malassezia furfur* (*Pityrosporum orbiculare/Pityrosporum ovale*). It is seen in humid and tropical climate. It affects both children and adolescents. It is rarely seen in neonates. It is characterized by asymptomatic, well-defined

hypopigmented to hyperpigmented macules with mild scaling distributed over the face, upper chest, back, and proximal arms **(Fig. 14)**. The face and periocular region are often affected in neonates due to close contact with the mother during feeding, thus increasing the humidity. Sometimes, scaling is very mild and not visible. Scales can be visible on stretching of skin often termed a "coup'de onglee" sign. Diagnosis is mainly clinically and by KOH examination of the scales. Tinea versicolor is differentiated from pityriasis alba, vitiligo, pityriasis rosea, psoriasis, and postinflammatory hypopigmentation.

Tinea Nigra

Tinea nigra is a superficial fungal infection of the stratum corneum caused by *Phaeoannellomyces* or *Hortaea werneckii*. It is a misnomer as it is not caused by dermatophyte infection. It is seen more in the costal and marine climate. Clinically, it presents as well-defined light to dark brown or black macules involving the palms and soles. KOH examination of skin scrapings for hyphae and budding yeast cells and fungal culture is confirmatory. Differential diagnosis includes postinflammatory hyperpigmentation, contact dermatitis, chemical stain, and fixed drug eruption. It is often misdiagnosed as malignant melanoma. Topical antifungals are the treatment of choice **(Table 5)**.

Piedra

Piedra is a superficial fungal infection of the hair shaft. It is of two types: black piedra caused by *Piedraia hortae* and white piedra caused by *Trichosporon beigelii*. The clinical features of both white and black piedra are given in **Table 6**. KOH showing septate hyphae and spores and fungal culture confirms the diagnosis. Clipping or shaving the hairs is curative. Topical antifungal creams or ketoconazole shampoo can be given as an adjuvant therapy.

Candidal Infections (Moniliasis)

Candidiasis is an acute or chronic infection of skin and mucous membrane. It can affect internal organs. It is caused by yeast-like fungus belonging to the genus *Candida*. The most common organism causing candidiasis is *C. albicans* which exists as normal commensal in the microflora of the oral cavity, gastrointestinal tract, and vagina. It becomes pathogenic due to various predisposing factors such as genetic disorders (chronic mucocutaneous candidiasis), endocrine disorders (diabetes mellitus, Addison's disease, hypothyroidism, Cushing's syndrome), immunological factors (HIV, leukemia, lymphoma), drugs (antibiotics, systemic corticosteroids, immunosuppressive drugs), low birth weight children, prematurity, and candidal vaginitis in mother.

Oral Candidiasis (Thrush)

Oral candidiasis, also called as thrush, is most commonly caused by *C. albicans*. Newborns and infants, immunocompromised children, use of antibiotics, and steroids are susceptible to oral candidiasis. Oral thrush can be acquired in neonates at the time of delivery during passage through an infected birth canal. It is characterized by white to gray pseudomembranous plaques resembling milk curds present on the dorsal aspect of tongue and buccal mucosa. It can be differentiated form milk curds by gentle scrapping of the whitish plaque with a cotton applicator or tongue blade. In oral candidiasis, the whitish plaque adheres to the oral mucosa with an underlying eroded mucosa. KOH wet-mount preparation shows budding yeast cells and fungal culture can identify the type of *Candida* infection. Different morphological patterns of oral candidiasis are described in **Table 7**.

Perleche (Angular Cheilitis)

Perleche is characterized by fissuring and inflammation at the corners of the mouth along with maceration and oozing. Predisposing factors in children include dental malocclusion or lip-licking behavior. It is not associated with nutritional or vitamin deficiency.

Candida Diaper Rash

Diaper dermatitis can be secondarily infected with candidiasis. Diaper dermatitis is an irritant contact dermatitis caused by excessive wetness, friction, high pH, and high enzymatic activity due to feces and urine. Clinically, it presents as erythema and scaling on the convex surface of the pubic area, buttocks, and medial aspect of thighs, reflecting the areas of the body in contact with the diaper. It spares the inguinal folds. Candidal diaper rash involves the deep inguinal folds with maceration, peripheral scaling, and satellite pustules **(Fig. 15)**.

Table 5: Common topical and systemic fungal agents for superficial fungal infections in children.

Topical antifungal agents	Systemic antifungal agents
• *Imidazole group*—clotrimazole 1%, miconazole 2%, ketoconazole 2%, oxiconazole, sertaconazole 2%, econazole 1% • *Allylamines*—terbinafine hydrochloride 1%, ciclopirox 0.77%	• Griseofulvin • Fluconazole 3–6 mg/kg • Terbinafine 3–6 mg/kg • Itraconazole 3–5 mg/kg

Table 7: Different clinical patterns of oral candidiasis.

Clinical type	Features
Acute or chronic pseudomembranous	Whitish membrane that is easily removable, present on the buccal mucosa, gums, palate, dorsum of tongue, and rarely esophagus
Acute or chronic erythematous	Mucosa appears red and glazed
Hyperplastic	Thick, adherent, whitish plaques on tongue and buccal mucosa
Median rhomboid glossitis	Diamond-shaped plaque on the tongue with loss of papillae

Table 6: Clinical features of white and black piedra.

Features	White piedra	Black piedra
Climate	Temperate/subtropical	Tropical
Sites	Hairs of scalp, eyebrows, eyelashes, axillae, pubic region	Hairs of scalp, eyebrows, eyelashes, axillae, pubic region
Clinical features	Asymptomatic, soft white elongated nodules on hair shafts	Small, hard, adherent, brown-black nodules on the hair shafts
Differential diagnosis	Nits (pediculosis), hair casts, scales, monilethrix, trichorrhexis nodosa	Pediculosis, trichorrhexis nodosa, scales

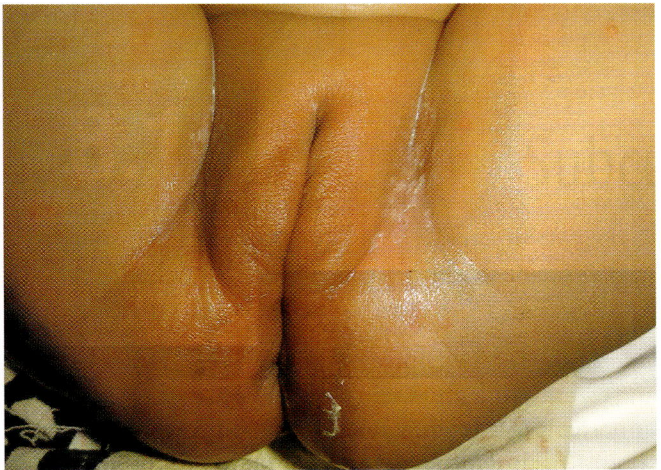

Fig. 15: Ill-defined erythema with scaling and pustules in the inguinal folds in candidal diaper rash.

Intertrigo

Intertrigo is characterized by intense bright red erythema, maceration, papulovesicles, and satellite pustules in the skin folds seen in infants and children. It is commonly associated with *C. albicans* and sometimes secondarily infected with *Staphylococcus aureus*. Predisposing factors include warm and humid environment, friction, sweat, moisture, and overdressed and chubby children.

Candidal Vulvovaginitis

Candidal vulvovaginitis is common in adults and rarely seen in prepubertal children. Symptoms include itching, burning, and dysuria. There is erythema, edema of the labia, and vaginal mucosa along with whitish plaques. Curdy white discharge is a classical feature of candidal vulvovaginitis. Differential diagnoses that is considered are psoriasis, atopic dermatitis, bacterial infection, contact dermatitis, poor hygiene, and lichen sclerosus. Candidal vulvovaginitis in prepubertal children should raise the suspicion of child abuse and investigated. Demonstration of budding yeast cells in KOH examination and fungal culture confirms the diagnosis.

Chronic Paronychia

Inflammation of the nail folds is termed paronychia. Chronic paronychia is commonly caused by *C. albicans* and presents as loss of cuticle, transverse ridging, erythema, and edema of nail folds. Finger sucking in children can lead to chronic paronychia. It should be differentiated from acute paronychia which is caused by bacterial infection. Acute paronychia is acute in nature and presents with pain, edema, and pustule.

Neonatal Cutaneous Candidiasis

Candidal infection in neonates can occur vertically by an infected mother or horizontally by nosocomial infection. About 75% of neonatal candidiasis is caused by *C. albicans*. Other candida species implicated in neonatal candidiasis include *C. tropicalis*, *C. parapsilosis*, *C. lusitaniae*, and *C. glabrata*. Neonatal cutaneous candidiasis is of two types: congenital form which occurs at birth and neonatal type which is seen after 1 week of life.

Congenital cutaneous candidiasis is a benign infection presenting at birth or within 1 week of life in neonates exposed to *Candida* infection in utero. About 20–25% of pregnant women develop candidal vulvovaginitis, but only few neonates born to infected mothers develop congenital candidiasis. Risk factors include prolonged rupture of the membrane, chorioamnionitis, and foreign body in uterus. Clinically, it presents with erythematous macules which evolve into vesicles, pustules, or bullae on an erythematous base distributed on trunk, extremities, and flexures including palms and soles **(Fig. 16)**. It resolves within 1–2 weeks. It is differentiated from neonatal candidiasis where it presents after 1 week of life and acquired through an infected birth canal or through the skin of affected caregivers. Clinically, it presents with similar features of congenital candidiasis but associated with oral thrush. KOH smear shows budding yeast cells. The presence of white microabscesses on the surface of placenta and umbilical cord is pathognomonic of congenital cutaneous candidiasis.

Chronic Mucocutaneous Candidiasis

Chronic mucocutaneous candidiasis is characterized by recurrent and refractory infections of the skin, hair and nails, and mucosa. It often presents in infancy and can occur as an autosomal-dominant or autosomal-recessive form. It is also associated with immunological defects such as severe combined immunodeficiency, dedicator of cytokines 8 (DOCK 8) deficiency and signal transducer and activator of transcription (STAT) 3 deficiency and polyendocrinopathy like hypothyroidism, hypoparathyroidism, hypoadrenocorticalism, and gonadal failure. Chronic mucocutaneous candidiasis presents as recurrent or persistent oral thrush, esophageal candidiasis, candidal diaper dermatitis, intertrigo, or paronychia.

■ LABORATORY DIAGNOSIS

- *Specimen collection:* Skin scrapings for KOH examination are taken from the blunt edge of the scalpel blade or by scrapping the lesions by a glass

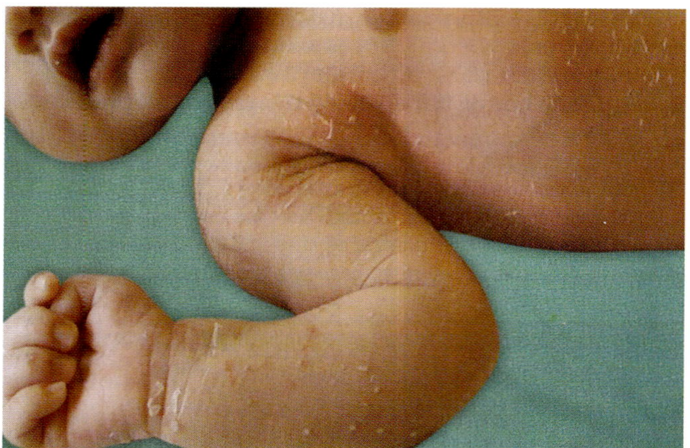

Fig. 16: Multiple pustules and exfoliation present on the trunk and extremities in neonatal candidiasis.

slide. For scalp lesion scrapping as well as plucked hairs is necessary for KOH examination and fungal culture. For nail examination, nail clippings should be obtained from the proximal part of nail plate as well as from the undersurface of the nail plate. For intertriginous lesions, moistened swab can be used for collection of the sample.

- *Wood's lamp examination:* Wood's lamp examination is a very useful and noninvasive screening method for the diagnosis of tinea infections as well as control of epidemics in school. Some of the dermatophyte species produce characteristic fluorescence when exposed to ultraviolet rays (320–400 nm). It is mainly used to diagnose tinea capitis caused by *Microsporum* **(Table 8)**.
- *KOH wet mount preparation:* KOH examination is used for identification of fungal hyphae and spores in skin, hair, and nails. About 10% to 20% KOH examination is added to the specimen and then the slide is examined under the microscope after 5–10 minute. For hair specimen, 30 minutes is necessary to examine the slide under a microscope. Dermatophytes appear as uniformly refractile, septate branching filaments. Candidiasis is seen as budding oval yeast cells (pseudohyphae).
- *Fungal culture:* Fungal culture is the gold standard for diagnosis of fungal infections. The specimen collected is grown on Sabouraud Dextrose Agar media or Dermatophyte Test Medium.

MANAGEMENT OF SUPERFICIAL FUNGAL INFECTIONS

There are various topical and systemic antifungals for the treatment of superficial fungal infections in children

Table 8: Characteristic florescent features of organisms causing tinea capitis.

Organism	Fluorescent color
Microsporum canis	Blue-green
Microsporum audouinii	Blue-green
Microsporum gypseum	Blue-green
Trichophyton schoenleinii	Dull-blue
Trichophyton tonsurans	No fluorescence

(*see* **Table 5**). The choice of therapy depends on age, site, and extent of infection, causative organism, and associated underlying systemic disorders. The source of the infection should be treated while managing fungal infections in children to prevent recurrent and persistent infections. Management of various superficial fungal infections is described in **Table 9**. General management includes good hygiene, wearing loose cotton clothes, washing clothes separately, and drying them in sunlight. Sharing of clothes, hats, jackets, hairbrushes, and toys should be discouraged in children. Treatment of the affected family members and close contacts is necessary. Education of parents and school staff is necessary in children. Another important aspect of treatment is that both topical and systemic antifungals should be given 2 weeks beyond symptom resolution.

SUBCUTANEOUS MYCOSES

Subcutaneous fungal infection affects skin and subcutaneous tissue and rarely presents with systemic involvement. They are uncommon in children. They are acquired through direct inoculation of the causative agent through the skin. Deep dermatophytosis is associated with primary immunodeficiency, HIV, or immunosuppressive therapy. Studies have shown CARD9 deficiency in developing idiopathic deep dermatophytosis. There is evidence that there is role of CARD9 in antifungal defense against dermatophytes. Some of the subcutaneous mycoses seen in children are discussed in the following text.

Mycetoma (Madura Foot/Maduromycosis)

Mycetoma is a chronic granulomatous subcutaneous infection caused by fungi and anaerobic bacteria. Though mycetoma occurs worldwide, it is more common in tropical and subtropical regions. Children in rural areas are more susceptible to mycetoma infection. The causative organisms are "eumycetoma" (fungi) and "actinomycetoma" (bacteria) causing eumycotic

Table 9: Management of dermatophyte and non-dermatophyte infections in children.

Fungal infection	Topical treatment	Systemic treatment
Dermatophyte infections		
Tinea capitis	Ketoconazole shampoo (reduce fungal shedding)	• Griseofulvin micronized 20–25 mg/kg/day: 6–12 weeks (given along with fatty food) • Griseofulvin ultramicronized 10–15 mg/kg/day: 6–12 weeks • Terbinafine 3–6 mg/kg/day: 4–6 weeks • Fluconazole 3–6 mg/kg/day: 4–8 weeks • Itraconazole 5 mg/kg/day: 4–6 weeks • Systemic antibiotics (secondary infection) • Systemic corticosteroids 0.5–1 mg/kg body weight for 2 weeks (kerion to prevent scarring)
Tinea corporis/tinea cruris/ tinea faciei/tinea imbricate/ tinea incognito	All azoles and allylamines: Twice/day for 2 weeks	Terbinafine/itraconazole/griseofulvin/fluconazole for 2–4 weeks (dose similar to tinea capitis)
Tinea pedis/tinea manuum	• Topical antifungals similar to above	• Systemic antifungals similar to tinea capitis
Tinea unguium/ onychomycosis	• Ciclopirox nail lacquer (once/week)	• Antifungals similar to above • *Finger nails*: 6 weeks • *Toe nails*: 12 weeks
Tinea versicolor	• Both azoles and allylamines twice/day for 2–3 weeks	• Itraconazole 200 mg once/day for 3–7 days (recurrent lesions) • Fluconazole 400 mg (one dose)
Candidiasis	Topical imidazoles (clotrimazole cream/paint, miconazole, ketoconazole, econazole)	• Treatment of underlying predisposing factors • Fluconazole single dose for oral thrush and vulvovaginitis • Intravenous fluconazole for neonatal candidiasis • Itraconazole • IV amphotericin B (neonatal candidiasis)

mycetoma and actinomycotic mycetoma. They gain entry through skin trauma. Eumycetoma fungi include *Madurella mycetomatis*, *Pseudallescheria boydii*, and *Acremonium* species. Actinomycotic mycetoma is caused by genus *Nocardia*, *Streptomyces*, and *Actinomadura*. Actinomycotic mycetoma is more commonly encountered in India.

Clinically, it presents as three characteristic features of nodules, tumefaction, and sinuses discharging grains. Initially, it starts as a small, firm, painless subcutaneous nodule at the site of injury that gradually increases in size with edema and multiple discharging sinuses. The discharge contains grains. The color of the grain helps in identification of the causative agent. The sites involved are extremities more commonly on feet and hands. Other sites such as trunk, chest wall, abdomen, perineum, buttocks, and thighs can be rarely involved. Infection can spread to deeper planes involving muscles, ligaments, and bones. Differential diagnosis includes chromoblastomycosis, cutaneous tuberculosis, chronic osteomyelitis, and sporotrichosis.

Eumycetoma produces black to whitish to yellow grains and actinomycetoma produces white grains. Microscopy for KOH examination and culture of the grains aids to the diagnosis. Tissue culture is confirmatory. Histopathological examination from the skin tissue shows a suppurative inflammatory and granulomatous reaction in dermis consisting of epithelioid cells, plasma cells, lymphocytes, neutrophils, and giant cells. Actinomycetoma responds to antibiotics such as sulfonamides, cotrimoxazole, streptomycin, cephalosporins, amikacin, tetracyclines, rifampicin, minocycline, and dapsone. Eumycetoma is unresponsive to treatment and requires radical surgical excision. Medical therapies include ketoconazole, itraconazole, and amphotericin B for prolonged periods. Newer antifungals such as voriconazole 400–600 mg daily and posaconazole 800 mg daily is highly effective.

Chromoblastomycosis

Chromoblastomycosis is rarely seen in children and caused by several pigmented fungi such as *Phialophora verrucosa*, *Fonsecaea pedrosi*, *Cladosporium carrionii*, and *Wangiella dermatitidis*. It is seen in rural children, especially in the endemic region. The youngest age reported is 2 years. Literature review has shown genetic susceptibility to develop chromoblastomycosis in children.

Clinically, it starts as small warty papule, gradually increases, and becomes verrucous plaque. It heals with central atrophy and scarring (**Fig. 17**). Rarely it can manifest as an ulcerative or sporotrichoid form. The sites

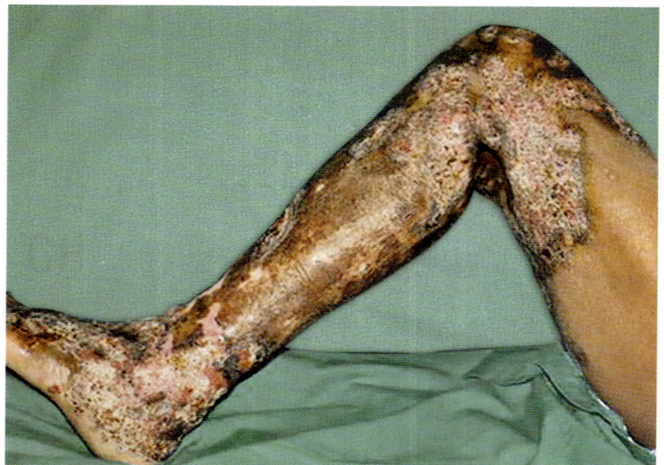

Fig. 17: Chromoblastomycosis showing well-defined hyperkeratotic, verrucous plaque with dyspigmentation on the lower limb.

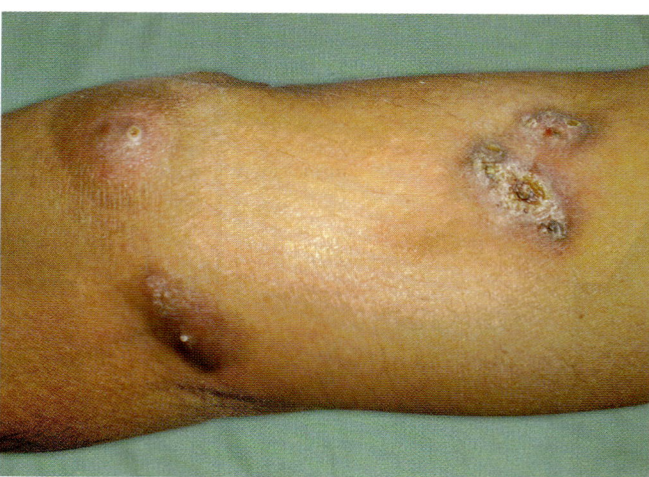

Fig. 18: Sporotrichosis showing multiple, well ill-defined erythematous nodules to crusted plaque on the lower leg with lymphatic spread.

involved are usually trauma-prone areas like extremities. Systemic involvement such as the bone and nervous system can be rarely involved. KOH examination shows septate hyphae and sclerotic bodies. Skin biopsy from the tissue shows pseudoepitheliomatous hyperplasia with granulomatous inflammation and presence of characteristic bodies called sclerotic bodies (Medlar bodies or copper pennies). Sclerotic bodies are thick-walled spherical bodies with thick, planate septal calls and are the hallmark of chromoblastomycosis. For a small, localized lesion, surgical excision is the treatment of choice. Systemic antifungals such as terbinafine and itraconazole for prolonged periods of 6 months to 1 year is effective. Newer antifungals such as voriconazole and posaconazole are also effective, especially when associated with systemic involvement.

Sporotrichosis

Sporotrichosis is a granulomatous fungal disorder caused by saprophytic dimorphic fungi *Sporothrix schenckii*. The disease is prevalent in tropical and subtropical regions. In India, it is more reported from the sub-Himalayan belt. In a study conducted in the region of Peru, children were affected more commonly than adults and they were aged less than 15 years. The main route of entry to skin is through minor trauma or abrasion. Possible modes of exposure in children are playing in the fields, pets, dirty floors in house, and raw wood ceiling. After inoculation, it spreads through lymphatics.

The different clinical types of sporotrichosis are lymphocutaneous form, fixed cutaneous form, disseminated form, and extracutaneous form. Clinically,

it starts as a small nodule at the site of trauma, ulcerates, and spreads through lymphatics. The fixed cutaneous form is common in children. It can present as papule, verrucous, or ulcerated plaques **(Fig. 18)**. About 40–60% affects face in children. The disseminated form is seen in immunodeficiency. The extracutaneous form involving lungs, bones, joints, and central nervous system is rarely seen in children. Differential diagnosis includes sarcoidosis, nocardiosis, mycetoma, chromoblastomycosis, cutaneous anthrax, and atypical mycobacterial infection. Histopathology shows granulomatous inflammation with asteroid bodies that appear as thick, radiating eosinophilic material surrounding fungal elements termed as Splendore–Hoeppli phenomenon. The treatment of choice is saturated solution of potassium iodide (KI). It is given in the dose of 1–3 g/day (one to two drops three times daily). Itraconazole, terbinafine, and fluconazole are also effective. Amphotericin B is effective for disseminated disease.

Rhinosporidiosis

Rhinosporidiosis is a chronic granulomatous infection caused by fungus *Rhinosporidium seeberi* seen more commonly in India and Sri Lanka. It affects mucosal surfaces such as nose, eyes, and sinuses. It affects older children and adults. Clinically, it presents with papules, nodules, and pedunculated vascular polypoid or sessile growths in the nasal mucosa, naspharynx, soft palate, and conjunctiva. Rarely it involves larynx, genitalia, and rectum. Differential diagnosis includes rhinoscleroma, mucoromycosis, and nasal polyps. Fine Needle Aspiration Cytology (FNAC) shows sporangia and spores. Skin biopsy shows granulomatous reaction with pseudoabscess and

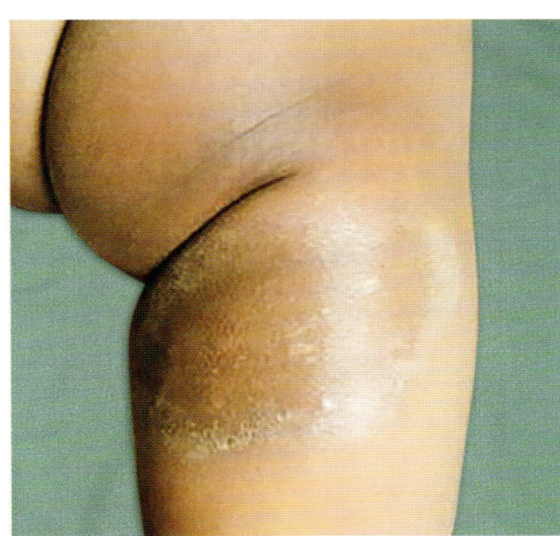

Fig. 19: Well ill-defined hyperpigmented, indurated subcutaneous swelling in zygomycosis.

fibrosis. Excision is the treatment of choice. Dapsone and antifungals such as ketoconazole and clotrimazole are effective in management.

SUBCUTANEOUS ZYGOMYCOSIS

Zygomycosis is an acute or chronic subcutaneous fungal infection caused by saprophytic fungi belonging to class zygomycetes with two fungal orders: Mucorales and Entomophthorales. Mucorales is seen in immuno-compromised children. Entomophthorales include two types *Basidiobolus* and *Conidiobolus* and affects immunocompetent children. The disease is most common in South India. *B. ranarum* affects the subcutaneous tissue of arms, trunk, thighs, and buttocks and is mostly seen in children. The mode of transmission is through minor trauma or insect bite.

Clinically it starts as a hard nodule, slowly progresses to form subcutaneous mass, and spreads locally. The overlying skin is tense, hyperpigmented, or edematous **(Fig. 19)**. There is nonpitting edema of the extremity. It can extend to the underlying muscle and viscera. KOH mount shows broad, pauciseptate, branching hyphae. Histopathological examination shows granulomatous inflammation with the Splendore–Hoeppli phenomenon. Differential diagnosis includes lymphatic edema, soft-tissue sarcoma, and lymphoma. KI and itraconazole is the first line of treatment in subcutaneous zygomycosis. Other treatment modalities include miconazole, cotrimoxazole, ketoconazole, itraconazole, terbinafine, and amphotericin B.

SUGGESTED READING

1. Chakrabarti A, Roy SK, Dhar S, et al. Sporotrichosis in north-west India. Indian J Med Res. 1994;100:62-5.
2. Dash M, Panda M, Patro N, et al. Sociodemographic profile and pattern of superficial dermatophytic infections among pediatric population in a tertiary care teaching hospital in Odisha. Indian J Paediatr Dermatol. 2017;18(3):191.
3. Gandhi S, Patil S, Patil S, et al. Clinicoepidemiological study of dermatophyte infections in pediatric age group at a tertiary hospital in Karnataka. Indian J Paediatr Dermatol. 2019; 20(1):52.
4. Groll AH, Tragiannidis A. Update on antifungal agents for paediatric patients. Clin Microbiol Infect. 2010;16(9):1343-53.
5. Jain A, Jain S, Rawat S. Emerging fungal infections among children: A review on its clinical manifestations, diagnosis, and prevention. J Pharm Bioallied Sci. 2010;2(4):314.
6. Kaufman DA, Coggins SA, Zanelli SA, et al. Congenital Cutaneous Candidiasis: Prompt Systemic Treatment is Associated with Improved Outcomes in Neonates. Clin Infect Dis. 2017;64(10):1387-95.
7. Lanternier F, Cypowyj S, Picard C, et al. Primary immuno-deficiencies underlying fungal infections. Current Opin Pediatr. 2013;25(6):736-47.
8. Mishra N, Rastogi MK, Gahalaut P, et al. Clinicomycological study of dermatophytoses in children: Presenting at a tertiary care center. Indian J Paediatr Dermatol. 2018;19(4):326.
9. Oke OO, Onayemi O, Olasode OA, et al. The prevalence and pattern of superficial fungal infections among school children in Ile-Ife, South-Western Nigeria. Dermatol Res Pract. 2014; 2014:842917.
10. Srinivas SM, Gowda VK, Mahantesh S, et al. Chromo-blastomycosis associated with bone and central nervous involvement system in an immunocompetent child caused by Exophiala Spinifera. Indian J Dermatol. 2016;61(3):324-8.
11. Verma S, Heffernan MP. Superficial fungal infection: Dermatophytosis, onychomycosis, tinea nigra, piedra. In: Wolff K, Goldsmith LA, Katz SI, Gilchrest BA, Paller AS, Leffell DJ (Eds). Fitzpatrick's Dermatology in General Medicine, 7th edition, Vol. 2. USA: McGraw Hill Professional; 2008. pp. 1807-31.

Systemic Mycoses

Kheya Ghosh Uttam

■ INTRODUCTION

Fungus constitutes approximately 7% (611,000 species) of all eukaryotic species on earth. Six-hundred fungal species can act as human pathogens.

A million of people die every year from fungal infections, and invasive fungal infection is recognized as a major cause of worldwide morbidity and mortality. Invasive fungal infection is a very serious challenge in the developing world where both diagnostic and therapeutic facilities are limited. A major contributor to this widespread emergence of fungal infection is increasing number of immunocompromised individuals, more availability of intensive care facilities, and use of broad-spectrum antimicrobial therapy.

■ SYSTEMIC FUNGAL INFECTIONS

Systemic fungal infection is synonymous with invasive fungal infection (IFI). The standard definition of IFI was developed by members of the European Organization for Research and Treatment of Cancer (EORTC), Invasive Fungal Infection Cooperative Group (IFICG) and Mycology Study group (MSG) of National Institute of Allergy and Infectious disease (NIAID). According to them, the presence of fungal elements either as mold or as yeast in deep tissues of biopsy or needle aspirates that is confirmed on culture and histopathological examination can be described as an IFI. Systemic illnesses are caused by many fungal agents of which *Candida, Cryptococcus,* and *Aspergillus* species are important. Epidemiologically fungal infection may be classified into opportunistic and endemic mycoses. Endemic mycoses are infections caused by fungi that are not part of normal human flora and are acquired from environment almost exclusively by inhalation. The common agents are dimorphic fungus (histoplasmosis, blastomycosis, coccidioidomycosis, and paracoccidioidomycosis). Opportunistic mycoses are caused by fungus that are frequently components of normal human flora like yeast (*Candida* and *Cryptococcus spp.*) and mold (*Aspergillus* and *Mucor spp.*).

Opportunistic Systemic Fungal Infection

Systemic Candidiasis

Invasive candidiasis is the most common invasive mycotic infection across the world. Incidence varies from 1 to 12 per 1,000 admissions in different hospitals across India. All intensive care units report high incidence of invasive candidiasis. Prolonged hospitalization, central venous access, total parenteral nutrition, use of broad-spectrum antibiotics for prolonged duration, mechanical ventilation, major abdominal surgery, and immune suppression (corticosteroid or other immunosuppressive therapy, neutropenic patients, children with endocrine disorders, HIV, burn and malignancy, and neonates) are risk factors for candidemia. *Candida albicans* is the most common cause of invasive candidiasis among immunocompromised children and has a higher rate of mortality and morbidity than non-*albicans* species. Systemic candidiasis usually result from hematogenous spread. But it may result from contiguous spread from skin as in superficial erosions, deep wounds, catheter related or from alimentary tract to other abdominal organs during perforation of gastrointestinal (GI) tract.

Enteric infection: Esophageal involvement is common in HIV-infected children. It manifests as substernal pain, dysphagia, painful swallowing, and anorexia. Nausea and vomiting are common in young children. Most patients do not have thrush. Stomach or intestinal ulcers also occur. Oral involvement mainly manifest as thrush. Beside thrush, three types of oral candida infection occur in HIV-infected children—atrophic candidiasis characterized by erythematous mucosa or loss of papillae of tongue, chronic hyperplastic candidiasis characterized by oral symmetric white plaques, and angular cheilitis. A syndrome of mild diarrhea in normal individuals who shows predominant *Candida* on stool culture has also been described, although *Candida* is not considered a true enteric pathogen. Its presence more often reflects recent antimicrobial therapy.

Pulmonary infection: Because the organism frequently colonizes the respiratory tract, it is commonly isolated from respiratory secretions. Thus, demonstration of tissue invasion is needed to diagnose *Candida* pneumonia or tracheitis. It is rare, being seen in immunosuppressed patients and patients intubated for long periods, usually while taking antibiotics. The infection may cause fever, cough, abscesses, nodular infiltrates, and effusion.

Urinary tract infection: Candiduria may be the only manifestation of disseminated disease. More often, candiduria is associated with instrumentation, an indwelling catheter, anatomic abnormality of the urinary tract, or immunosuppressed host especially in diabetics. It is usually asymptomatic but symptoms of cystitis may be present. Masses of *Candida* (fungal balls) may obstruct ureters and cause obstructive nephropathy. Candida casts in the urine suggest renal tissue infection.

Other infections: Endocarditis, myocarditis, meningitis, and osteomyelitis may occur in immunocompromised patients or neonates.

Disseminated Candidiasis

This occurs in neonates, especially in premature infants, in an intensive care setting, and is recognized when the infant fails to respond to antibiotics or when candidemia is documented. These infants have unexplained feeding intolerance, cardiovascular instability, apnea, new or worsening respiratory failure, glucose intolerance, thrombocytopenia, or hyperbilirubinemia. Treatment for presumptive infection is often undertaken because candidemia is not identified in many such patients.

Hepatosplenic candidiasis occurs in immuno-suppressed, severely neutropenic patients with chronic fever, variable abdominal pain, and abnormal liver function tests. Symptoms persist even when neutrophils return. It may occur with or without fungemia. Ultrasound or CT scan of the liver and spleen demonstrates multiple round lesions. Biopsy is confirmative.

Diagnosis

A definitive diagnosis of systemic candidiasis requires isolation of organism from a sterile body site or demonstration of organism in a tissue biopsy specimen. Diagnosis is often presumptive in neutropenic and immunocompromised patients with prolonged fever or failure of clinical improvement in spite of sensitive antibiotic therapy. Endoscopy is useful for diagnosis of esophagitis. Ultrasonography, CT scan, or MRI can detect lesions in brain, heart, kidney, liver, and spleen, but these lesions are not typically detected by imaging until late in the course of diseases or after neutropenia has resolved. In high-risk patients, serial serum level of $(1,3)$-β-D-glucan may be helpful in the diagnosis, but it has low sensitivity and specificity.

Treatment

Fungal prophylaxis: High-risk oncology patients and bone marrow and solid organ transplant recipients need fungal prophylaxis. In oncology patients, both fluconazole and echinocandins are used as prophylaxis at a lower dose than the therapeutic dose. In bone marrow transplant recipients, voriconazole is preferred for prophylaxis as it gives an additional mold prophylaxis. Solid organ transplant recipients similarly benefit from antifungal prophylaxis by fluconazole, voriconazole, or caspofungin.

Antifungal therapy: Selection of the initial antifungal therapy depends upon previous use of azole either as prophylaxis or therapy, severity of the disease, organ involvement, immune status of the patient, common isolates of that unit and their sensitivity pattern. Moderate-to-severely ill children require empirical therapy with echinocandins or Amphotericin B. Fluconazole may be started for those who are less critically ill. Though studies has failed to show any statistically significant difference in outcome in patients with candidemia who were treated with fluconazole, from that of patients who were treated with conventional Amphotericin B. Definitive therapy should be made based on susceptibility testing result. Renal function should be monitored closely in patients who receive Amphotericin B. In addition to antifungal drugs, the indwelling catheter, infected valve or prosthesis should be removed. Presently, majority of *C. albicans* are sensitive to fluconazole. *C. glabrata*, *C. parapsilosis*, and *C. krusei* are less sensitive to fluconazole and more sensitive to polyenes and echinocandins. *C. auris* new species causing nosocomial infection across world is resistant to most antifungals.

ASPERGILLOSIS

The genus *Aspergillus* has 250 species, but most human diseases are caused by *A. fumigatus, A. flavus, A. niger, A. terreus,* and *A. nidulans.* Invasive disease is most commonly caused by *A. fumigatus.* Aspergillosis may present differently depending upon the host. Invasive aspergillosis is common in immunodeficient hosts, whereas immuno-competent atopic hosts tend to develop allergic disease. Nonallergic colonization leading to noninvasive syndromes, such as pulmonary aspergilloma, occurs in immunocompetent or mild-degree immunosuppressive patients.

Systemic or Invasive Aspergillosis

Systemic or invasive aspergillosis (IA) is the second most common invasive fungal infection in immunocompromised children. Children at highest risk include those with new-onset acute myelogenous leukemia, relapse of hematologic malignancy, recipients of allogenic hematopoietic stem cells, and solid organ transplantation. It may also occur in children with neutrophil or macrophage dysfunction, as in severe combined immunodeficiency or chronic granulomatous disease, prolonged steroid use, and HIV. Hallmark of invasive disease is angioinvasion and necrotizing bronchopneumonia with invasion of the pulmonary vessels. This may result in widespread fungal embolization to heart, GI tract, skin, kidney, liver, bone, and central nervous system (CNS) and occasionally erosion of blood vessel wall with catastrophic hemorrhage.

Invasive pulmonary aspergillosis: It is the most common form of aspergillosis. Clinical features are persistent fever, in spite of broad-spectrum antibiotic, cough, chest pain, hemoptysis, and pulmonary infiltrates. Patients with CGD (chronic granulomatous disease) are at particular risk for pulmonary aspergillosis. In CGD, local invasion to pleura, ribs, and vertebrae is seen.

Diagnosis

Chest X-ray may show multiple ill-defined nodules, lobar or diffuse consolidation or may be normal. CT scan shows halo sign, cavitary lesion, or lesions with an air crescent sign, though the last two are less commonly seen in children than in adults. MRI shows target sign, a nodule with low signal centrally with peripheral ring enhancement. Isolation of *Aspergillus* from blood culture is uncommon, as fungemia is of low level and intermittent. Conclusive diagnosis requires either culture positivity from sterile site or histologic identification of tissue invasion by fungal hyphae but obtaining tissue specimen is often impractical. Unlike aspergilloma and allergic aspergillosis, serology is of low yield for invasive disease. ELISA-based test for galactomannan in serum, bronchoalveolar lavage (BAL) fluid, and cerebrospinal fluid (CSF) is of choice for IA. It has a high rate of false negativity in patients with CGD. Beta-glucan assay is a nonspecific fungal assay and cannot discriminate different fungal infections.

Treatment

Voriconazole is the treatment of choice as primary therapy for pulmonary IA. Multiples studies has shown improved response rates and survivals and better tolerability in patients receiving voriconazole than patients receiving Amphotericin B. The dose required is higher than in adults. The other triazoles (itraconazole, and posaconazole) can also be used for first-line therapy of IA. The echinocandins are generally considered second-line treatment for IA.

Invasive sinonasal disease: It is difficult to diagnose as presentation vary widely. Clinically, it may present with congestion, rhinorrhea, headache, facial pain or swelling, orbital swelling, fever or abnormal appearance of nasal turbinates. Diagnosis depends on direct visualization via endoscopy and biopsy, as imaging is often normal. Treatment is voriconazole, but mucormycosis must be ruled out as voriconazole does not act on it.

Central nervous system: CNS involvement occurs due to secondary involvement due to bloodstream dissemination or via local extension of sinus disease. Clinical presentation includes change in mental status, seizures, coma, ophthalmoplegia, and paralysis. The hyphae invades CNS vasculature, causing hemorrhagic infarcts leading to abscess. Prognosis is extremely poor. Neuroimaging helps in diagnosis. Galactomannan assay testing of CSF may be future methodology to confirm diagnosis. Surgical resection and high-dose voriconazole are the best treatment options.

Cutaneous aspergillosis: Primary cutaneous disease occurs at the site of skin disruption, especially in premature infants. Secondary cutaneous disease occurs due to hematogenous spread in transplant recipients. Lesions are erythematous indurated papular lesion that progress to painful, ulcerated and necrotic lesion. Treatment comprises surgical debride-ment and systemic voriconazole.

Eye: Endophthalmitis and keratitis may be seen in disseminated aspergillosis. Clinically, it present with pain, photophobia, and decreased visual acuity. Endophthalmitis is treated with intravitreal injection of either Amphotericin B or voriconazole, surgical intervention, and systemic antifungal therapy with voriconazole. Keratitis is treated with topical and systemic antifungals.

Other sites: Aspergillus can infect the bone and the heart. The most commonly involved bones are vertebrae and ribs. Cardiac involvement presents with endocarditis, myocarditis, and pericarditis. Treatment depends on combination of surgical debridement and systemic fungal therapy.

Noninvasive Syndromes

In immunocompetent children, pulmonary aspergillomas, otomycosis, and sinus aspergillosis are manifestations of nonallergic colonization or noninvasive syndromes of *Aspergillus* species. Aspergilloma grows in pre-existing pulmonary cavities and almost all patients have underlying lung disease, such as cystic fibrosis or tuberculosis.

Allergic Diseases

Allergic bronchopulmonary aspergillosis (ABPA) is a hypersensitivity lung disease that manifests as episodic wheezing, low-grade fever, eosinophilia, and transient pulmonary infiltrates often with expectoration of brown mucus plug. It is primarily seen in patients with asthma and cystic fibrosis. There are eight primary diagnostic criteria for ABPA: Episodic bronchial obstruction, peripheral eosinophilia, immediate cutaneous reaction to *Aspergillus* antigens, precipitating IgE antibodies to *Aspergillus* antigen, elevated total IgE, serum precipitin (specific IgG) antibodies to *A. fumigatus*, pulmonary infiltrates, and central bronchiectasis. Secondary diagnostic criteria include repeated detection of *Aspergillus* from sputum, coughing brown plugs or specks. Radiological characteristics are bronchial wall thickening, pulmonary infiltrates, and central bronchiectasis.

Allergic *Aspergillus* sinusitis, though less common, occurs as an allergic response in children with nasal polyps, previous sinusitis, or after a sinus surgery. They present with symptoms of chronic sinusitis or recurrent acute sinusitis, such as congestion, headache, and rhinitis. Laboratory findings include elevated IgE levels, precipitating antibodies to *Aspergillus* antigen, and immediate cutaneous reaction to *Aspergillus* antigens. Sinus tissue specimen may contain eosinophils, Charcot–Leyden crystals, and fungal elements.

Diagnosis

The diagnosis is made by culture from lung, sinus, and skin biopsy specimen. The organism is usually not recoverable from blood. Microscopic examination of potassium hydroxide (KOH) wet mount of tissue or BAL specimens also helps in diagnosis. An enzyme immunosorbent assay serological test for detection of galactomannan from serum or BAL is useful in both children and adults. A positive results indicates invasive aspergillosis whereas a negative does not rule out. So, galactomannan test is of greater utility in monitoring response to treatment rather than diagnostic marker. In allergic aspergillosis, typical clinical symptoms and elevated total concentration of IgE (>1,000 ng/mL), *Aspergillus*-specific serum IgE, eosinophilia, and a positive result from a skin test for *Aspergillus* antigen clinch the diagnosis.

Treatment

Voriconazole is the drug of choice for invasive aspergillosis, except in neonates where Amphotericin B is recommended. Voriconazole therapy is continued for at least 12 weeks, but treatment duration should be individualized. Monitoring of serum galactomannan level in those with significant elevation at the onset, on a twice weekly basis may be useful to assess response to therapy along with clinical and radiological evaluation. Surgical excision of a localized lesion (pulmonary lesion and sinus debris) is usually required.

■ CRYPTOCOCCOSIS

Out of the 30 cryptococcal species, two species (*Cryptococcus neoformans* and *C. gattii*) are mainly responsible for majority of cryptococcosis.

Cryptococcus, which can cause disease in the immunocompetent host, is more likely to be clinically apparent and severe in immunocompromised patients with T-cell immune defect such as those seen in HIV infection or with leukemia or lymphoma or those taking prolonged corticosteroids or those who have undergone solid organ transplantation. Other risk factors include immunosuppression associated with diabetes mellitus, renal failure, cirrhosis, rheumatological conditions, and patient receiving monoclonal antibodies. Overall, cryptococcosis is significantly less common in children than in adults. The agent may disseminate hematogenously to any organ system. Sites of infection include lung, CNS, blood, skin, bone, eyes, and lymph nodes.

Central nervous system: The CNS is the most common site of infection and is the most serious form of cryptococcal disease. It presents with features of meningitis, meningo-encephalitis, or space-occupying lesion but sometime may have subtle nonspecific features like fever, headache, and behavioral changes. Despite antifungal therapy, the mortality rate is high. Factors associated with poor prognosis are high CSF fungal burden, low CSF white blood cell (WBC) count (<10 cells/mm^3), failure to rapidly sterilize the CSF, and increased intracranial pressure (ICP).

Lungs: After CNS infection, pneumonia is the most common form of cryptococcosis which may present as acute respiratory distress syndrome and may mimic pneumocystis pneumonia (alveolar and interstitial infiltrates) or it may be asymptomatic and detected radiographically (chest X-ray shows pulmonary nodules). Others may present with cough, fever, pleuritic chest pain, and weight loss. Chest X-ray may reveal solitary or multiple masses, patchy or lobar consolidation, or nodular or reticulonodular interstitial changes.

Skin: Cutaneous disease is usually due to disseminated cryptococcosis and rarely due to local inoculation. Early lesions are erythematous, variably indurated, and tender. They may be ulcerated with central necrosis and raised border.

Bone: About 5% patients with disseminated disease have bone involvement. Vertebrae are the most common site followed by tibia, ileum, rib, femur, and humerus. Arthritis may also occur.

Sepsis syndrome: It occurs almost exclusively in HIV-infected patients. It is characterized by fever, followed by respiratory distress and multi-organ involvement, and the disease is often fatal. Cryptococcal-associated immune reconstitution inflammatory syndrome (C-IRIS) occurs in HIV patients treated with antiretroviral therapy due to improvement of immune function. IRIS is particularly problematic in CNS cryptococcosis and leads to worsening of increased ICP.

Diagnosis

Definitive diagnosis is done by culture of the organism from body fluid or tissue specimen, or demonstration of the fungus in histologic section of infected tissue or body fluids by Indian Ink staining. Cryptococci grow easily on standard culture media. Rapid detection test for detection of cryptococcal capsular polysaccharide antigen in serum or CSF specimen is very useful. Antigen is detected from serum or CSF in more than 98% of patients with cryptococcal meningitis. Antigen titers of >1:4 in body fluids strongly suggest infection. Patients with pneumonia typically do not have elevated serum antigen level. The result may be falsely negative when antigen concentration is very low or very high (prozone effect), if infection is caused by unencapsulated strain. As the antigen persists for prolonged period, serial measurement for disease monitoring is not useful.

Treatment

The choice of antifungal therapy depends on the sites of involvement and the host immune status. Amphotericin B (1 mg/kg/day) or lipid-complex Amphotericin–B (3–6 mg/kg/day) in combination with flucytosine (100–150 mg/kg/day) is indicated as initial therapy for patients with meningeal and other serious cryptococcal infections. In meningitis, the combination therapy (induction therapy) should be for at least 2 weeks followed by consolidation therapy with fluconazole (10–12 mg/kg/day) for a minimum of 8 weeks or until CSF culture is sterile. Longer periods of induction (4–6 weeks) is needed in meningitis secondary to *C. gattii*, with neurological complications, absence of flucytosine in the induction regimen and in immunocompetent patients. For mild disease limited to lungs in absence of dissemination or CNS disease, oral fluconazole (6–12 mg/kg/day) is given for 6–12 months to prevent disseminated disease. Alternative treatment includes itraconazole (5–10 mg/kg/day), voriconazole, and posaconazole.

■ MUCORMYCOSIS

Mucormycosis is a group of disorder caused by opportunistic fungal infection of the order Mucorales. The most common disease-causing genera are *Rhizopus, Mucor,* and *Lichtheimia*. It is uncommon in children and occurs in hematological malignancy patients, patients with renal failure and diabetes and receiving iron chelation therapy. It is characterized by rapidly evolving course, tissue necrosis, and blood vessel invasion. It can occur as any of several clinical syndromes, including sinus/rhinocerebral, pulmonary, GI disseminated or cutaneous or subcutaneous disease.

Diagnosis

Imaging procedures may suggest the etiology, but they are best diagnosed by culture or histopathological examination of aspirated or biopsy of infected tissues. Mucorales can be cultured on standard culture media from different specimens.

Treatment

Except for localized cutaneous disease, all forms of mucormycosis is difficult to treat. It requires early diagnosis, prompt institution of medical therapy, and extensive surgical debridement of all devitalized tissue. Amphotericin B is the mainstay of therapy. Voriconazole is not active against mucormycosis. Posaconazole, though active against mucormycosis, is not recommended for primary therapy but often used as salvage therapy.

■ MALASSEZIA FURFUR

Members of the genus *Malassezia* usually cause different dermatological conditions. *Malassezia furfur* is the most common species to cause fungemia and *M. pachydermatis* causes several outbreak in neonatal intensive care unit (NICU), especially in preterm babies and in those associated with prolonged parenteral nutrition that includes fat emulsion. The yeast, which requires skin lipids for its growth, can infect lines when lipids are present in the infusate. Some species will grow in the absence of lipids. The use of lipid emulsion containing medium-chain triglycerides inhibits the growth of the species and can prevent infection. Unexplained fever and thrombocytopenia are common. Pulmonary infiltrates may be present.

Diagnosis

The diagnosis is done by culture of blood, catheter tip, or tissue specimen facilitated by alerting the bacteriology laboratory to add olive oil to culture media, as the fungus does not grow readily on standard fungal media.

Treatment

Treatment involves removal of the involved catheter and discontinuing the lipid infusion. Persistent or invasive infection requires Amphotericin B. Fluconazole and itraconazole are also effective. Flucytosine has no activity against *Malassezia*.

■ ENDEMIC MYCOSES

Endemic mycoses are caused by dimorphic fungus. Histoplasmosis, blastomycosis, coccidioidomycosis, and paracoccidioidomycosis are the four important endemic mycoses affecting humans.

Histoplasmosis

Exposure to *Histoplasma* is common in endemic areas; majority of infections are subclinical. Less than 1% of infected patients shows clinical symptoms and mostly presents with pulmonary histoplasmosis. Acute pulmonary histoplasmosis presents with flu-like symptoms and progresses to significant respiratory distress and hypoxia. Hepatosplenomegaly may also be there. It may also present with prolonged illness of weight loss, dyspnea, high fever, asthenia, and fatigue. In disseminated disease, extrapulmonary manifestations are destructive bony lesions, Addison's disease, meningitis, multifocal chorioretinitis, and endocarditis. Disseminated histoplasmosis can either be self-limited or progressive.

Diagnosis

Culture is the definitive method of diagnosis. Culture sensitivity of tissue or body fluid is highest for children with progressive disseminated histoplasmosis due (PDH) to large inoculum of organisms. The yeast can be recovered from blood or bone marrow in >90% of patients with PDH. Histological examination can identify yeast forms in different tissue specimens. Antigen detection is the most widely available diagnostic study. *H. capsulatum* polysaccharide antigen can be detected in urine, blood, BAL fluid, and CSF. Antigenuria has been shown to correlate with severity of disseminated histoplasmosis. False-positive result is common. Testing both the urine and the serum samples for *Histoplasma* antigen increases the sensitivity compared with testing only urine or serum alone.

Treatment

Acute pulmonary histoplasmosis does not require treatment, unless it fails to improve clinically within 1 month; in that case it requires treatment with oral itraconazole for 6–12 weeks. Patients with pulmonary histoplasmosis who become hypoxemic or require ventilatory support, who has obstructive symptoms caused by granulomatous mediastinal disease and patients with PDH requires initial treatment with Amphotericin B for 2–4 weeks or until improvement followed by oral itraconazole as maintenance therapy for 3–6 months.

Other Endemic Mycoses

Blastomycosis, coccidioidomycosis, and paracocci-dioidomycosis are quite rare and are restricted to certain geographical areas of the world.

Blastomycosis remains asymptomatic or subclinical in 50% of infected people. Only 2–13% of blastomycosis cases occur in the pediatric population. The most common manifestation in children is pneumonia, which may be acute or chronic. Extrapulmonary blastomycosis most commonly affects skin and then bone. CNS blastomycosis occurs in less than 10% of immunocompetent patient but may be 40% in patients with HIV infection. Diagnosis is by demonstration of species in histopathological specimen or by culture as clinical and radiological features mimic other diseases. Mild-to-moderate infections can be treated with itraconazole for 6–12 months. Severe infections require initial therapy with Amphotericin B followed by itraconazole.

Paracoccidioidomycosis occurs primarily in adult; children represents only 5–10% of all cases. There are two clinical forms—acute and chronic. The acute form (juvenile paracoccidioidomycosis) is rare and occurs exclusively in children and targets the reticuloendothelial system. Pulmonary symptoms may be absent. Patients typically present with fever, malaise, wasting, lymphadenopathy, and hepatosplenomegaly. Adults develop chronic progressive illness. Itraconazole orally for 6 months is the treatment of choice. Fluconazole may be used but it requires higher dose and longer duration. Amphotericin B is recommended in disseminated disease where other therapy has failed.

Coccidioidomycosis is asymptomatic or self-limited in 60% of infected children. It can present clinically as pulmonary and extrapulmonary diseases (5–10%). Pulmonary infection occurs in 95% of cases and can be divided into primary, complicated, and residual infections. Treatment depends upon the clinical spectrum of the disease. Acute mild pneumonia usually does not require treatment (spontaneous recovery in 75–85% of cases) but require follow-up every 1–3 months for 2 years. If there are constitutional symptoms (weight loss and night sweats) or in special circumstances (immunosuppression or late pregnancy), treatment with azole daily for 3–6 months with follow-up every 1–3 months for 2 years is required. Chronic pneumonia and disseminated, non-meningeal disease require treatment with an azole for ≥1 year. Diffuse pneumonia, reticulonodular or military infiltrates suggest underlying immunodeficiency and possible fungemia and require initial treatment with Amphotericin B, followed by an azole for ≥1 year.

CONCLUSION

Systemic mycoses or invasive fungal infections are significant health problem in certain group of pediatric population. Awareness of the treating clinician is essential for early diagnosis and treatment of this group.

SUGGESTED READING

1. Chakrabarti A, Chatterjee SS, Shivaprakash MR. Overview of opportunistic fungal infections in India. Nihon Ishinkin Gakkai Zasshi. 2008;49:165-72.
2. Chakrabarti C, Sood SK, Parnell V, et al. Prolonged candidemia in infants following surgery for congenital heart disease. Infect Control Hosp Epidemiol. 2003;24:753-7.
3. Chakrabarty A, Das A. Emergence of non-albicans Candida species. J Int Med Sci Acad. 2004;17:186-9.
4. Chander J. Candidiasis. In: Chander J (Ed). Textbook of Medical Mycology. 3rd edition. New Delhi: Mehta Publishers; 2009. pp. 266-83.
5. Edwards JE. Candidiasis. In: Fauci AS, Braunwald E, Kasper DL (Eds). Harrison's Principles of Internal Medicine. 17th edition. USA: McGraw-Hill; 2008. pp. 1254-6.
6. Sievert DM, Ricks P, Edwards JR, et al; National Healthcare Safety Network (NHSN) Team and Participating NHSN Facilities. Antimicrobial-resistant pathogens associated with healthcare-associated infections: summary of data reported to the National Healthcare Safety Network at the Centers for Disease Control and Prevention, 2009–2010. Infect Control Hosp Epidemiol. 2013;34(1):1-14.

Pneumocystis Jirovecii (Previously Classified as Pneumocystis Carinii)

Ira Shah, Himali Meshram

INTRODUCTION

Pneumocystis jirovecii (Pneumocystis carinii), previously considered as a protozoa, is an opportunistic fungus that resides in the human and other mammalian bronchoalveolar lumen.[1] *Pneumocystis* species infection is host specific. *P. jirovecii* infection is characteristic for humans.[1] *P. jirovecii* cysts are transmitted by the airborne route and lungs are the most commonly affected organs. This microorganism replicates under immunosuppressive conditions, ultimately resulting in interstitial pneumonia called *Pneumocystis* pneumonia (PCP), which is generally lethal if left untreated. Patients with decreased immunity and CD4+ T-cell count less than 200/μL have a higher risk to develop PCP. Information on prevalence of PCP in immunocompromised children with pneumonia in Southeast Asia is limited. The occurrence of PCP is global and most of the children are exposed to this organism by 3–4 years of age.

PATHOPHYSIOLOGY

The life cycle of the *Pneumocystis* species can be divided into two phases and it has two morphological forms. The proliferative phase has the haploid trophozoites and cysts represent the reproductive stage.[1] The cyst is 5–7 mm in size and contains up to eight sporozoites. Once these sporozoites are excysted, they become trophic forms called trophozoites. These different forms of *Pneumocystis* when inhaled reside in the alveoli of lungs. The trophic form attaches to the lung alveoli. Host immunity, importantly, CD4+ T-cells and macrophages, hinder the multiplication and spread of *Pneumocystis* and subsequent formation of disease in immunocompetent hosts. In immunocompromised hosts, where alveolar macrophages and CD4+ T-cells are not able to remove *Pneumocystis*

organisms, pneumonia and other manifestations of the disease ensue. The lung injury is related to the inflammatory response against the *P. jirovecii* organism as compared to the organism itself. Thus, there seems to be a role of steroids to control the inflammation and hypoxia in these patients.

Children with primary immunodeficiencies, e.g. hypogammaglobulinemia, severe combined immunodeficiency (SCID), HIV infection with low CD4+ T levels, malignancies, and those on immunosuppressive therapy, are at increased risk of acquiring PCP.

CLINICAL FEATURES

Pneumocystis pneumonia presents with nonspecific respiratory symptoms, including tachypnea, increasing dyspnea, dry cough, fever, and hypoxia (PaO$_2$ <65 mm Hg). PCP in non-HIV patients has rapid onset, with more severity of disease, and progresses at a faster rate as compared to HIV-infected individuals. A greater neutrophil count which is seen in non-HIV patients is thought to cause more lung injury than in HIV patients.[1] The fatality in non-HIV patients is higher (35–55%) as compared to HIV-positive patients (10–20%).[2,3] The classification to determine severity of PCP is depicted in **Table 1**.

The clinical presentations of the PCP disease have been observed to occur in two different patterns. The infantile form has led to outbreaks in infants in nursing homes in Europe. Infants present with interstitial pneumonia with tachypnea and dyspnea and no fever. They have severe intercostal retractions and as the disease progresses, nasal alae flaring and cyanosis can also be seen. Bilateral crepitations can also be heard. There may be nonspecific symptoms such as anorexia, diarrhea, vomiting, and listlessness. Left untreated, the disease course is over several weeks and at least 50% of these patients die. PCP

Table 1: Classification to determine severity of *Pneumocystis* pneumonia.[4]

Clinical factor	Disease severity		
	Mild	*Moderate*	*Severe*
Dyspnea	On exertion	On minimal exertion or at rest	Even at rest
Resting arterial tension (PaO$_2$)	More than 11.0 kPa	Between 8.1 kPA and 11.0 kPa	Less than 8.0 kPa
Oxygen saturation (SaO$_2$)	More than 96%	Between 91% and 96%	Less than 91%
Radiological changes in chest (CXR)	Normal or minimal changes	Diffuse changes in interstitium	Severe interstitial changes with diffuse alveolar shadowing

(CXR: chest X-ray; PaO$_2$: partial pressure of oxygen in blood; SaO$_2$: oxygen saturation)

disease in older children and adults presents as acute presentation with fever, cough, and progressive tachypnea. Nasal alae flaring and intercostal retractions may occur. The disease is progressive, and all untreated patients die. An occasional older child may have complaints of substernal pain.

Pneumocystis pneumonia needs to be differentiated from similar conditions such as CMV (*Cytomegalovirus*) pneumonia, acute respiratory distress syndrome (ARDS), lymphocytic interstitial pneumonia (LIP), *Mycoplasma* infections, legionellosis, tuberculosis, and *Mycobacterium avium* complex (MAC) infection.

■ APPROACH TO DIAGNOSIS

Since the initial symptoms are nonspecific, always suspect PCP in those at risk. Suspect PCP in a clinical setting of immunosuppression (primary or secondary) with signs of respiratory distress and hypoxemia. Chest X-rays (CXR) and CT scan of the chest show interstitial shadows with a ground-glass pattern[1] **(Fig. 1)**. CT chest should be considered even when CXR are normal as seen during the early stages of the disease. A normal CT is useful to exclude PCP.[4]

Isolation of *P. jirovecii* on microscopy and indirect immunofluorescence with monoclonal antibodies staining against *P. jirovecii* cysts are useful.[1,4] Cytochemical staining with toluidine blue or Giemsa and Wright stains on samples such as bronchoalveolar lavage (BAL) and lung biopsies are conventional methods.[2] Polymerase chain reaction (PCR) assays that amplify various genetic fragments have been used on the BAL or biopsy samples. PCP PCR has a high sensitivity of ≥97% and a high negative predictive value (NPV) ≥99%.[4]

Lactate dehydrogenase (LDH) level greater than 500 mg/dL is associated with lung damage and high levels indicate severe disease. It can be used as an added test in the HIV-infected patient. The utility of LDH levels in

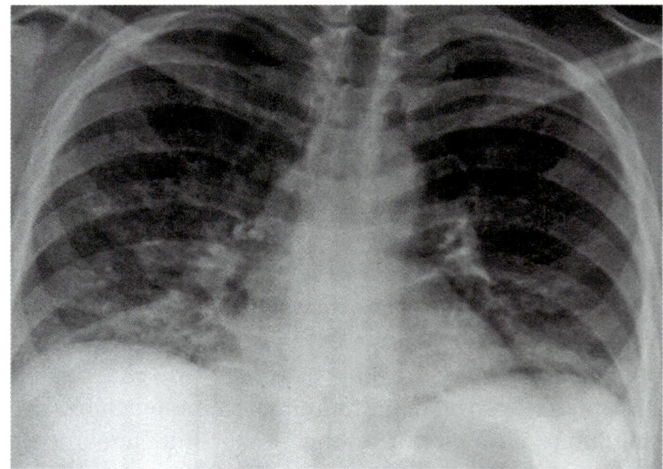

Fig. 1: Chest X-ray showing *Pneumocystis* pneumonia with basal and perihilar haziness.

the HIV-negative patients is limited, with poor sensitivity and specificity.[4]

■ MANAGEMENT

It is difficult to treat PCP infection with typical drugs which are used for the treatment of fungal infections. The therapeutic agents aim at disrupting the folic acid pathway required for proper organism functioning in pneumocystis organisms. Prophylaxis includes combination of trimethoprim (TMP) and a sulfa drug, sulfamethoxazole (SMX).[1] Addition of caspofungin, which is an inhibitor of the (1→3)-B-D-glucan synthase, to TMP-SMX enhances the inhibition effect.[1] The drugs used for the treatment of PCP are depicted in **Table 2**. Patients with severe illness and those with gastrointestinal side effects can be given treatment with the parenteral route. In patients with PaO$_2$ less than 70 mm Hg, or A-a gradient of 35 mm Hg and more, corticosteroids are used as adjunctive initial therapy. Methylprednisolone (2 mg/kg/day) can be tried. Corticosteroids should be tapered and stopped as

Table 2: Drugs used in the treatment of PCP.[4]

HIV infected	Patients with hematological manifestations	SOT
• *First line:* TMP/SMX (15–20 mg/kg/day of TMP) IV/PO in four divided doses for 21 days. Convert to oral therapy as soon as patient tolerates • Corticosteroids can be used if there is hypoxia	*First line:* TMP/SMX (15–20 mg/kg/day of TMP) IV/PO in four divided doses for 21 days. Convert to oral therapy as soon as patient tolerates	• *First line:* TMP/SMX (15–20 mg/kg/day of TMP) IV/PO in four divided doses for 21 days. Convert to oral therapy as soon as patient tolerates • Corticosteroids can be used if there is hypoxia
Second line (for mild/moderate disease): • Dapsone—2 mg/kg/day OD PO + trimethoprim 15 mg/kg/day in three divided doses PO for 21 days • Atovaquone *Second line (for severe disease):* • Primaquine base 0.3 mg/kg OD PO (max—30 mg/day) + clindamycin 10 mg/kg IV or PO every 6 hours (max—600 mg IV, 300–450 mg PO) for 21 days • IV pentamidine (4 mg/kg) OD IV for 14–21 days	*Second line:* • Primaquine base 0.3 mg/kg OD PO (max —30 mg/day) + clindamycin 10 mg/kg IV or PO every 6 hours (max—600 mg IV, 300–450 mg PO) for 21 days • IV Pentamidine (4 mg/kg) OD IV for 14–21 days • Atovaquone	*Second line:* IV pentamidine (4 mg/kg) OD IV for 14–21 days

(HIV: human immunodeficiency virus; SOT: solid organ transplantation; TMP/SMX: trimethoprim/sulfamethoxazole)

soon as recovery from pneumonia occurs. As dictated by the clinical condition, supportive care must aim to achieve adequate oxygenation and hydration. Mechanical ventilation may be required in 5–10% of patients with AIDS and 50–60% of patients without AIDS.

■ PROPHYLAXIS IN *PNEUMOCYSTIS* PNEUMONIA[4]

For prevention of PCP, chemoprophylaxis is advisable for HIV-positive children <6 years of age with severe immunosuppression (CD4 cell counts <500 cells/mm^3 or CD4 percentage <15%). It is also recommended in all HIV-infected infants irrespective of CD4 count. All HIV-exposed infants should be on prophylaxis from 1½ months of age, till proved negative. Patients with hematological conditions such as acute lymphoid leukemia (ALL), bone marrow transplant recipients, patients on treatment with immunosuppressive agents, and patients with primary immune deficiencies should receive chemoprophylaxis for PCP.[3] Due to ease of administration, relative lack of toxicity, and established role against PCP, TMP-SMX (5 mg/kg TMP and 25 mg/kg SMX) given orally in one to two divided doses daily or on alternate days is the most commonly used drug for primary and secondary prophylaxis in immunocompromised children. For those intolerant to TMP-SMX, aerosolized pentamidine, atovaquone, or dapsone may be used. Dapsone is given in the dose of 2 mg/kg/day or 4 mg/kg once weekly PO (max—100 mg/day or 200 mg per dose weekly).

■ PROGNOSIS

Without treatment, PCP is universally fatal, within 3–4 weeks of onset. The mortality depends on the inflammatory response against the *P. jirovecii* organism as compared to the organism itself. Patients requiring mechanical ventilation have a higher mortality rate. Immunosuppressed patients are at a risk for PCP, and hence chemoprophylaxis is warranted in these patients.

■ REFERENCES

1. Sokulska M, Kicia M, Wesołowska M, et al. Pneumocystis jirovecii—from a commensal to pathogen: clinical and diagnostic review. Parasitol Res. 2015;114(10):3577-85.
2. Zajac-Spychała O, Gowin E, Fichna P, et al. Pneumocystis pneumonia in children—the relevance of chemoprophylaxis in different groups of immunocompromised and immuno-competent paediatric patients. Cent Eur J Immunol. 2015; 40(1):91-5.
3. Liu Y, Su L, Jiang SJ, et al. Risk factors for mortality from pneumocystis carinii pneumonia (PCP) in non-HIV patients: a meta-analysis. Oncotarget. 2017 4;8(35):59729-39.
4. White PL, Price JS, Backx M. Therapy and management of Pneumocystis jirovecii infection. J Fungi (Basel). 2018; 4(4):pii:E127.

Noncommunicable Diseases in Children: Burden, Action, and Targets

Rekha Harish, Deepak Pande

INTRODUCTION[1-4]

The term *noncommunicable diseases (NCDs)* refer to those conditions that are not infectious (hence nontransmissible among people). Typically, they are chronic, evolve slowly, and are likely to continue progressively unless intervened. Though NCDs are a large group of diseases, cardiovascular diseases (CVDs), cancers, diabetes, and chronic respiratory diseases are the most prominent among them. NCDs are the result of a combination of genetic, physiological, environmental, and behavioral factors. The importance of NCDs stems from the fact that currently most of the deaths worldwide are resulting from direct or indirect consequences of NCDs and the proportion of such deaths is rising rapidly in many regions of the world, most notably, in the tropical countries. On account of their enormous burden of morbidity and mortality on healthcare systems across the world, huge impact on individual productivity and national economies, rising prevalence, and severe long-term consequences, the prevention of NCDs has become a public health priority globally, and more so, in the low- and middle-income tropical countries. Children and youth have commonly been becoming victims of NCDs on account of air pollution and unhealthy lifestyle and behaviors, such as tobacco and alcohol use, physical inactivity, and unhealthy diets. Overweight and poor social and economic conditions combine with such risk factors to create a potent setting for genesis of NCDs. Though many NCDs take decades to develop overt signs of disease, their predisposing risk factors are known to start early in life, calling for a life-course approach to their prevention and control. NCDs often result from modifiable lifestyle factors, and this fact needs to be utilized aggressively to devise effective intervention strategies. Various such strategies, including those targeting children, are being developed internationally to combat the present scourge of NCDs. Early detection, screening, treatment, palliative care, a comprehensive primary healthcare approach, effective monitoring, surveillance, strong leadership, and accountability are all key components of programs designed to prevent NCDs.

BURDEN[3]

Noncommunicable diseases are usually perceived as ailments of older age groups, but it is now well known that children, adults as well as the elderly, i.e. all age groups, are vulnerable to each of the major risk factors contributing to NCDs. Like all age groups, all regions and countries are affected by NCDs, though in varying proportions. Unplanned urbanization, rising income levels, unhealthy lifestyles including unhealthy diets, insufficient physical activity, tobacco addiction, and alcoholism are the sociodemographic and metabolic factors that are the major driving forces behind the rise in prevalence of NCDs. Poverty, a common problem in most of the tropical countries, has been closely associated with NCDs, and is predicted to impede poverty eradication measures in low-income countries, by increasing costs of health care. The poor, vulnerable, and socially disadvantaged individuals get sicker and die sooner than others, as they face greater risk of exposure to major risk factors like tobacco and unhealthy dietary practices, and have less access to quality healthcare. Exorbitant costs of lengthy treatment and loss of breadwinners force millions of people into poverty annually, and stifle development of their respective nations and society.

Obesity and overweight among children have well-known associations with several NCDs. The World Health Organization (WHO) Commission on Childhood Obesity has revealed obesity to be increasing at alarming rates, by 10 times in the past 4 decades. The majority of this increase is in developing countries, where the rate of rise is more than 30%. Prevalence of overweight/obesity in very young children (between 0 year and 5 years) was a total of 131 million in 1990, which rose to 41 million in 2016, and is projected to rise to 70 million by 2025. Overall among children and adolescents, prevalence of obesity is about 124 million. Without intervention, these children face a high risk of becoming obese adolescents and obese adults.

Lifestyle-related diseases among adolescents have also emerged as a major challenge to public health. Unhealthy lifestyles are well known to lead to NCDs.

■ GLOBAL SCENARIO[3-7]

It is widely acknowledged that the burden of NCDs constitutes one of the major challenges for global development in the 21st century **(Fig. 1)**. The WHO (2018) has reported NCD to be contributing to 41 million deaths annually, which amounts to about 71% of all deaths globally. About 15 million of these deaths are "premature". NCDs disproportionately affect people in low- and middle-income countries (like almost all of the tropical countries), with over 85% of the NCD-related deaths occurring in such countries. Four groups of diseases account for most (over 80%) of these deaths—CVDs account for most (17.9 million) of the deaths, followed by cancers (9 million), respiratory diseases (3.9 million), and diabetes (1.6 million). India is among the tropical low- and middle-income countries, in which the majority of "premature" NCD deaths have been occurring, and are undergoing an

Table 1: Annual global burden of mortality attributable to major risk factors for noncommunicable diseases.[3]	
Risk factor for NCDs	*Annual global burden of mortality*
Tobacco	7.2 million
Excess salt intake	4.1 million
Use of alcohol	3.3 million
Insufficient physical activity	1.6 million

epidemiological health transition, due to rapid unplanned urbanization, globalization of unhealthy lifestyles, and technological changes, leading to economic betterment, but at the cost of addition of serious risks to health.

Table 1 highlights some of the leading risk factors of causes of deaths due to NCDs, and the magnitude of burden of mortality caused by them. Additionally, several metabolic risk factors contributing to the risk of NCDs are hypertension (19% of global deaths attributed), overweight/obesity, hyperglycemia, and hyperlipidemia.

■ INDIAN SCENARIO[1,5,8-10]

As per the recently published (2019) Comprehensive National Nutrition Survey (CNNS) (2016–2018) National Report of Government of India, United Nations Children's Fund (UNICEF), and Population Council, there is a growing risk of NCDs among children aged 5–9 years, and adolescents aged 10–19 years in India. Diabetes is being increasingly diagnosed in children and adolescents, and is no longer considered a disease associated with affluence. According to the CNNS report, one in 10 school-aged children and adolescents have been found to be prediabetic with fasting plasma glucose of 101–125 mg/dL or glycosylated hemoglobin (HbA1c) of 5.7-6.4% and 1% has been found to be diabetic, with fasting plasma glucose of >126 mg/dL. Moreover, 3% of school-aged children and 4% of adolescents had high total cholesterol (≥200 mg/dL) and high low-density lipoprotein (LDL) (≥130 mg/dL). About 26% of school-aged children and 28% of adolescents had low high-density lipoprotein (HDL) (<40 mg/dL). 34% of school-aged children and 16% of adolescents had high serum triglycerides. About 7% of school-aged children and adolescents were at-risk for chronic kidney disease. About 5% of adolescents were found to be hypertensive. Wide variations in prevalence have been noted across various states of India.

Goa and Nagaland are identified as the states with the highest prevalence of overweight in children 5–9 years of age. In addition to these two states, the highest prevalence of abdominal obesity has been observed in Arunachal

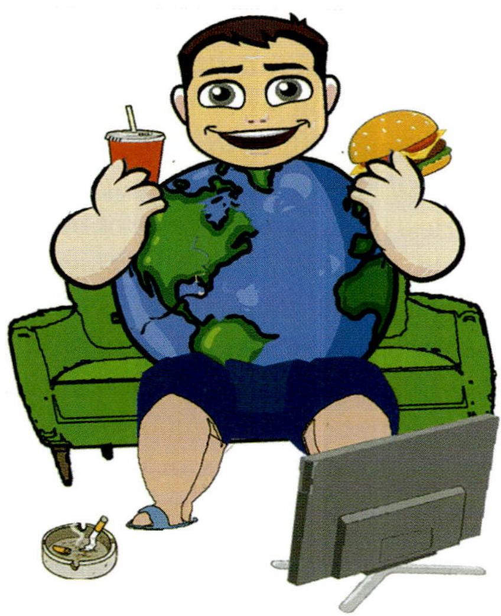

Fig. 1: Combating noncommunicable diseases (NCDs) and their risk factors—a major challenge for global health.

Pradesh. For adolescents, highest prevalence of abdominal obesity has been found in Delhi and Tamil Nadu. In the states of Sikkim and West Bengal, more than 20% of school-aged children and adolescents have been found to have high total cholesterol. More than 30% prevalence of low HDL cholesterol have been found in Arunachal Pradesh, Chhattisgarh, Uttar Pradesh, Bihar, and Meghalaya in both age groups, and in Karnataka among adolescents; a higher prevalence of low HDL cholesterol was found in rural areas and poorest health quintile. Among school-aged children and adolescents, respectively, 67% and 43% prevalence of high serum triglyceride have been noted in West Bengal. Highest prevalence of at-risk for chronic kidney disease among school-aged children and adolescents has been found in the states of Andhra Pradesh, Sikkim, Nagaland, Telangana, and West Bengal. States with highest recorded prevalence of hypertension among adolescents are Delhi, Uttar Pradesh, and Manipur.

Noncommunicable diseases contribute to over 60% of the mortality in India. In year 2016, leading CVD (ischemic heart disease and stroke) was the largest contributors to the total burden of mortality in India, at 28.1%, with their contribution to mortality increasing by 34.3% from 1990 to 2016. This can be attributed to rapid population aging and significantly increasing levels of the main risk factors for CVD—high systolic blood pressure, air pollution, high cholesterol, high fasting plasma glucose, and high body mass index—during that period. The prevalence of CVD and their share of mortality are higher in the states of Andhra Pradesh, Goa, Himachal Pradesh, Kerala, Maharashtra, Tamil Nadu, and West Bengal.

Chronic respiratory diseases, mainly chronic obstructive pulmonary disease (COPD) and Asthma, at 10.9%, make the second largest contribution to the mortality burden in India, with the prevalence of both reported to have increased by 29.2% and 8.6%, respectively. Higher crude COPD prevalence was reported in the states of Jammu and Kashmir, Himachal Pradesh, Uttarakhand, and Haryana.

Diabetes has been shown to contribute 3.1% of the total mortality burden, with slight preponderance in women, and a rise in disease burden of 29.7% between 1990 and 2016. Diabetes has been found to be especially prevalent in the southern states.

India houses almost a fifth of the world's population, and the emergence of obesity and NCDs associated with it, in the background of widespread undernutrition, has come at a significant cost to population health, well-being, and the already overburdened health systems. To gauge the economic impact of NCDs in India (2012–2030), the estimated cumulative cost associated with the common NCDs was about ₹38,302,200 crores (US\$ 6.15 trillion) in 2010.[5] Up to 80% of Indians incur huge out-of-pocket expenses on medical care, resulting in debt and devastation; 39 million Indians are pushed into poverty annually, due to diagnostic and treatment costs. The Government of India and UNICEF apprehend that if overweight and obesity are not aggressively addressed, the burden of NCDs will exact a terrible cost on the development of India and reduce its contribution to global health and economic progress.

■ DOUBLE WHAMMY OF MALNUTRITION IN LOW- AND MIDDLE-INCOME COUNTRIES[1,11]

The coexistence of undernutrition and overweight/obesity, or diet-related NCDs constitutes a double whammy of malnutrition and diet-related NCDs, within individuals, households, and populations. In low- and middle-income countries, with undernutrition continuing to cause nearly half of the deaths in children under 5 years, now concurrently overweight and obesity in children are increasing at a rate 30% faster than in rich nations. Now India, undergoing a nutrition transition from an underweight to an overweight population during recent decades has also taken serious cognizance of the rapidly growing epidemic of overweight and obesity in the country, identified onset of overweight and obesity at an early age as a public health concern, and felt the urgent need to aggressively address overweight and obesity, concurrently with undernutrition **(Fig. 2)**.

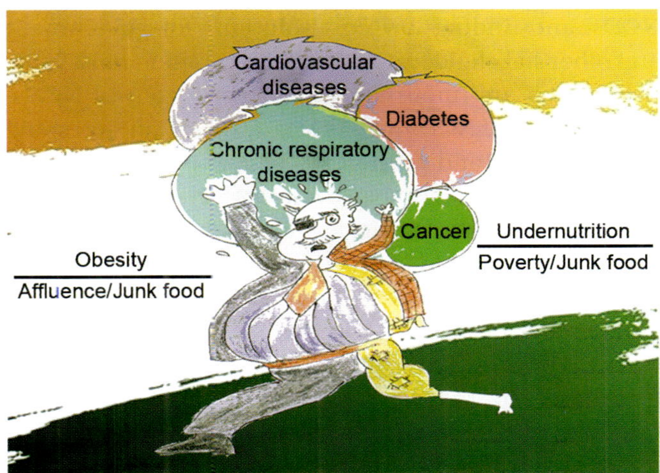

Fig. 2: India, like most other tropical countries, reeling under a double whammy of undernutrition in one section of its population and overweight/obesity in another section, each crippling it under an unbeatable and mounting burden of major noncommunicable diseases.
Source: Inspired by the *"Common Man"* character created by the legendary Indian cartoonist late Shri RK Laxman.

Such a double whammy of malnutrition can be seen at various levels, for instance:

- *At individual level*: Nutritional anemia in an obese adolescent.
- *At household level*: An overweight mother with an underweight child.
- *At population level*: A large proportions of the population afflicted by undernutrition and another large proportion of the population suffering from overweight/obesity. This may be seen within the same community, nation, or region.

Moreover, undernutrition early in life (even *in utero*) may predispose to overweight and NCDs such as diabetes and heart disease in later life. Also, overweight in mothers can predispose to overweight and obesity in her child. The biological, environmental, and social influences thus exemplified, being important drivers in the burden of malnutrition across the life course, obviously complicate the burden of NCDs and development of effective strategies to control them.

However, this double whammy also presents an important opportunity for comprehensive and integrated action against all forms of malnutrition. Effective tackling of this double whammy of malnutrition, particularly by the low- and middle-income countries, will be the key to achieving the Sustainable Development Goals (SDGs) (Goal 2 and Target 3.4) of the WHO.

Action[1,3,5,10,12,13]

A focus on reducing the risk factors associated with NCDs, and finding low-cost solutions for government and other stakeholders to reduce the common modifiable risk factors are important strategies to control NCDs. Management of NCDs includes early detection, screening and treatment, and providing access to palliative care to those in need. A comprehensive approach is multisectoral, involving collaboration between health, finance, transport, education, agriculture, planning, and others, to reduce the risks associated with NCDs, and promote interventions to prevent and control them. High impact essential interventions can be delivered through a primary healthcare approach focused on early detection and timely treatment. Such interventions are cost-effective too, as they reduce the need for more expensive treatment. Effective monitoring and accountability frameworks are also necessary, inter alia, to meet the time-bound goals and targets.

The WHO has assumed a leadership and coordination role, to control the epidemic of NCDs. The 2030 Agenda for Sustainable Development has recognized NCDs as a major challenge for sustainable development. As part of the Agenda, Heads of State and Governments have committed to develop ambitions national responses, to meet the SDG target 3.4, of reducing premature mortality from NCDs by one-third by 2030. To support countries in their national efforts, the WHO has developed a *global action plan for the prevention and control of NCDs 2013–2020*, which includes nine global targets that have the greatest impact on global NCD mortality. The targets address prevention and management of NCDs.

The Government of India is implementing a National Program for Prevention and Control of Cancer, Diabetes, CVD and stroke (NPCDCS), with objectives including increasing awareness of risk factors, to setup infrastructure such as NCD clinics, cardiac care units, and to carry out opportunistic screening. With reference to the *Global Action Plan and monitoring framework to prevent and control NCDs* of the WHO (2013), India was the first country to adopt the National Action Plan, with 10 targets and 21 indicators. Accordingly, the Government of India has taken the initiative to prepare and disseminate guidelines for mass screening for hypertension, diabetes, and common cancer, with the objective of early detection of common NCDs. Inspired by an SDG vision, tackling NCDs will require a comprehensive approach based on preventive, curative, and rehabilitative services. India has gained some early momentum in this regard by addressing the challenges of leadership and intersectoral coherence, and prioritizing prevention. New guidelines addressing comprehensive primary healthcare propose, a community outreach, and preventive approach to NCDs. For the first time in India, the CNNS has provided a comprehensive set of biomarkers for NCDs in children and adolescents, at the national and state level **(Table 2)**.

Surveillance and collection of data concerning risk factors are critical for monitoring, policy planning, and implementation, particularly in countries like India with a rapidly increasing burden of NCDs. A recent systematic review[5] concluded that India has a much delayed response on NCD risk factors surveillance and information of the same are sporadic and incomplete. The situation may not be very different in most other tropical countries. So, development of cost and time effective NCD surveillance system is emphasized.

Targets[1,6]

The 2030 Agenda for Sustainable Development, adopted at the United Nations Summit on sustainable development in September 2015, recognizes NCDs as a major challenge for sustainable development, and as part of its agenda,

Table 2: Biomarkers of noncommunicable diseases for Indian children and adolescents.[1]

1. *Fasting plasma glucose and glycosylated hemoglobin*		
Age	*Fasting plasma glucose*	*HbA1c*
5–9 years	Prediabetic: >100 mg/dL and ≤126 mg/dL Diabetic: >126 mg/dL	Prediabetic: >5.6% and ≤6.4% Diabetic: >6.4%
10–19 years	Prediabetic: >100 mg/dL and ≤126 mg/dL Diabetic: >126 mg/dL	Prediabetic: >5.6% and ≤6.4% Diabetic: >6.4%
2. *Lipid profile*		
Age	*Plasma lipid and lipoprotein concentrations*	
Children (5–9 years) And Adolescents (10–19 years)	• High total cholesterol ≥200 mg/dL • High LDL ≥130 mg/dL • Low HDL <40 mg/dL • High serum triglycerides: For 5–9 years ≥100 mg/dL, for 10–19 years ≥130 mg/dL	
3. *Serum creatinine*		
5–12 years	Serum creatinine >0.7 mg/dL	
>12 years	Serum creatinine >1.0 mg/dL	
4. *Blood pressure*		
10–19 years	• Systolic blood pressure level ≥140 mm Hg, or • Diastolic blood pressure level ≥90 mm Hg	

(HDL: high-density lipoprotein; LDL: low-density lipoprotein; HbA1c: glycosylated hemoglobin)

heads of states and governments committed inter alia to reduce by one-third premature mortality from NCDs. Globally, by year 2025, a 25% relative reduction in risk of premature mortality from NCDs is targeted. The 2030 Agenda for Sustainable Development (WHO) includes a target for reducing premature deaths from NCDs by one-third, by year 2030.

WHO, in its World Health Assembly in May, 2008, put forth an Action Plan of Global Strategy for the Prevention and Control of NCDs. India, being a WHO member state, is committed for implementing the same and has been taking the required steps and initiative to meet the objectives, and was the first to adapt the Global Monitoring Framework for NCDs, and to develop specific national targets and indicators aimed at reducing the number of premature deaths from NCDs by 25% by 2025. As a part of this plan, India has developed a long-term National Action Plan and Monitoring Framework with 10 targets **(Table 3)** to prevent NCDs, and is continuing to develop several national public health programs. In recognition of the current challenges in nutrition and health, the government of India has recently launched the POSHAN Abhiyaan (National Nutrition Mission), and to provide robust data on the shifting conditions of under nutrition and obesity, the ministry of health conducted the Comprehensive National Nutrition Survey to collect comprehensive data on nutritional status of Indian children 0–19 years of age by using gold standard biomarkers of NCDs for the first time in India. Also, the National Health Mission (NHM) includes programmatic components for prevention and treatment of NCDs.

■ FOUR MAJOR NCDS AND FOUR MAJOR RISK FACTORS[1,5,8]

Though the list of medical conditions qualifying as NCDs is very long, as only four of those conditions account for most of the premature mortality due to NCDs, WHO has identified those four major NCDs—(1) CVDs such as heart attacks and stroke, (2) diabetes, (3) chronic respiratory diseases (chronic obstructive pulmonary diseases and asthma), and (4) cancer. In India too, these four conditions account for a high proportion of (over 60%) premature deaths, placing them ahead of injuries, communicable diseases, maternal, prenatal, and nutritional conditions. In 2016, ischemic heart disease, chronic obstructive pulmonary disease, and cerebrovascular disease were noted among the top five causes of disability-adjusted life years; and malnutrition, air pollution, dietary factors, high blood pressure, and high blood glucose were noted among the top risk factors for the same. However, data from community-based NCD programs in India suggest that NCDs other than the said four also contribute a significant proportion of morbidity.

A risk factor is defined as "*An aspect of personal behavior or lifestyle, an environmental exposure, or a hereditary*

Table 3: Targets for noncommunicable diseases (NCDs) prevention and control in India.[15]

Framework element	Outcome	Targets 2020	Targets 2025
Premature mortality from NCDs	Relative reduction in cardiovascular disease, cancer, diabetes, or chronic respiratory disease	10%	25%
Alcohol use	Relative reduction in alcohol use	5%	10%
Obesity and diabetes	Halt the rise in obesity and diabetes prevalence	No mid target set	Halt the rise in obesity and diabetes prevalence
Physical inactivity	Relative reduction in prevalence of insufficient physical activity	5%	10%
Raised blood pressure	Relative reduction in prevalence of raised blood pressure	10%	25%
Salt/sodium intake	Relative reduction in mean population intake of salt with the aim of achieving recommended levels of less than 5 g/day	20%	30%
Tobacco use	Relative reduction in prevalence of current tobacco use	15%	30%
Drug therapy to prevent heart attacks and stroke	Eligible people receiving drug therapy and counseling (including glycemic control) to prevent heart attacks and strokes	30%	50%
Essential NCD medicines and basic technologies to treat NCDs	Availability and affordability of quality, safe, and efficacious essential NCD medicines including generics and basic technologies in both public and private facilities	60%	80%
Household indoor air pollutions	Relative reduction in households, of solid fuels as a primary source of energy for cooking	25%	50%

characteristic that is associated with an increase in the occurrence of a particular disease, injury, or other health condition" (Centers for Disease Control and Prevention, 2006). These behavioral and biological risk factors, with a predisposition to the development of NCDs, are insufficient physical activity, use of tobacco and alcohol, overweight and obesity, increased fat and sodium intake, low fruit and vegetable intake, and raised levels of blood pressure, blood glucose, and cholesterol (WHO, 2013). In respect of the aforementioned four major NCDs, WHO has identified four major modifiable risk factors—insufficient physical activity, unhealthy diet, tobacco and alcohol use, and air pollution[2] **(Fig. 3)**. To curb the growing burden of NCDs, the Government of India has also initiated prompt action by targeting these four major risk factors.

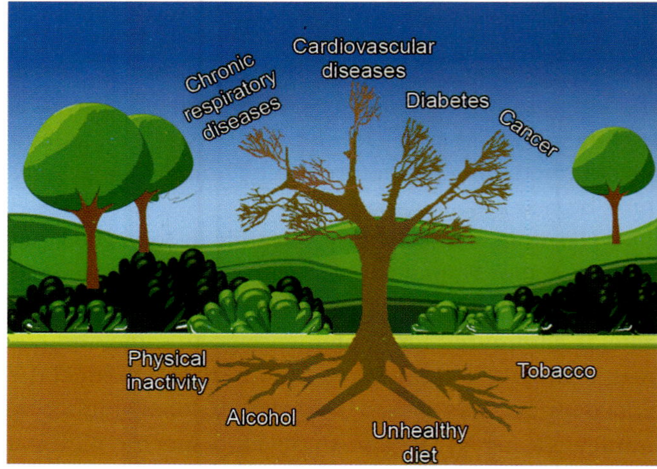

Fig. 3: The noncommunicable disease (NCD) tree—four major NCDs and four main modifiable risk factors.

RELEVANCE FOR CHILDREN AND YOUTH, THE ROLE OF IAP

With the above background, there is an obvious felt need for prevention of NCDs to begin early through public health campaigns directed toward lifestyle changes in the family. It is now well known that many of the NCDs actually begin in childhood (and even earlier, in fetal life) and manifest later, in childhood or adulthood, due to accumulations of various risk factors and interactions between them, throughout the life course. Lifestyle-related diseases among adolescents are becoming a major challenge to public health globally. Pediatricians, therefore, have a central role in the prevention and control of the NCD epidemic.

In the private sector, the IAP, being the second largest academic body in the world and the largest and most representative association of pediatricians in India, has been at the forefront in matters of child advocacy and in leading such campaigns for children. For over five decades, IAP has been committed to the well-being of children of India, not only for curative but also for preventive and promotive healthcare. IAP has also been standing for professional and academic improvement, building awareness, and partnering with the Government and non-government bodies. Therefore, IAP shares a moral as well as professional responsibility for contributing significantly to the task of tackling the growing menace of NCDs in the country, and is ideally placed to utilize its huge and nationwide network of very capable experts for primary prevention of NCDs and to inculcate healthy behaviors across schools for the estimated 200 million school-going children in the country with the aim of bringing about the necessary lifestyle changes to reduce the alarming burden of NCDs in future generations.

KEY LEARNING POINTS

- The prevalence of NCDs is rising globally and low-income societies are getting affected disproportionately.
- India, facing a double whammy of undernutrition and overweight/obesity, is already well into the rising epidemic of NCDs, a large number of its children and adolescents are already affected by, else at-risk for development of NCDs, and interventions to curb the epidemic are urgently required in the private sector as well.
- There are wide, regional variations in prevalence of NCDs and their risk factors.
- The foundations of most NCDs are laid down in childhood and adolescence. So, they are the ideal age for targeting preventive strategies.
- WHO has identified four major NCDs and four main modifiable risk factors for NCDs, which can become the priority areas for preventive action.
- IAP is very well-positioned to play a major role in NCD prevention in India, and to show the way to other tropical countries of the world, and has initiated fresh action in this regard.

CONCLUSION

The burden of NCDs and their risk factors should be viewed broadly for their impact on life expectancy, quality of life, and social and economic implications. The NCD threat can be overcome by using existing knowledge and highly cost-effective solutions are available. Comprehensive and well-integrated actions at national levels, led by the respective governments, are the key to success.[14] In line with the Global Action Plan for the prevention and control of NCDs 2013–2020 of WHO, India was the first country to develop specific national targets and indicators aimed at reducing the number of global premature deaths from NCDs by 25% by 2025. India has

to achieve the Sustainable Development Goal 3 to ensure healthy life and promote well-being at all ages as well as Target 3.4 to reduce by one-third the premature mortality from NCDs through interventions prominently including primary prevention.[4] The Indian Academy of Pediatrics (IAP) has decided to rise to the occasion to meet the challenges by contributing in a big way to prevent and control NCDs through interventions directed at children and adolescents through a multi-pronged strategy including advocacy, behavior change communication, capacity building, health promotion, mass awareness, and creation of healthy environments in schools.

REFERENCES

1. Ministry of Health and Family Welfare (MOHFW), Government of India, UNICEF, Population Council (2019). Comprehensive National Nutrition Survey (CNNS) National Report, New Delhi. [online] Available from: https://www.popcouncil.org/uploads/pdfs/2019RH_CNNSreport.pdf. [Last accessed on December, 2019].
2. Proimos J, Klein JD. Noncommunicable diseases in Children and Adolescents. Pediatrics. 2012;130:379-81.
3. Noncommunicable Diseases. World Health Organization (2018). Noncommunicable diseases: Key Facts. [online] Available from: https://www.who.int/news-room/fact-sheets/detail/noncommunicable-diseases accessed 08-08-2019. [Last accessed on December, 2019].
4. World Health Organization (2017). Noncommunicable diseases: the slow motion disaster. [online] Available from: http://www.who.int/publications/10-year-review/ncd/en/index2.html accessed 08-09-2019. [Last accessed on December, 2019].
5. Nethan S, Sinha D, Mehrotra R. Noncommunicable disease risk factors and their trends in India. Asian Pac J Cancer Prev. 2017;18(7):2005-10.
6. Ministry of Health and Family Welfare, Government of India (2012-13). National Action Plan and Monitoring Framework for prevention and control of Noncommunicable diseases (NCDs) in India. [online] Available from: https://mohfw.gov.in/sites/default/files/9967643039National_Action_Plan_and_Monitoring_Framework.pdf. [Last accessed on December, 2019].
7. World Health Organization (2015). India: first to adapt the Global Monitoring Framework on non-communicable diseases. [online] Available from: https://www.who.int/features/2015/ncd-india/en/. [Last accessed on December, 2019].
8. National Health Mission. Ministry of Health & Family Welfare, Government of India (2016). Prevention, Screening and Control of Common Non-Communicable Diseases. [online] Available from: https://mohfw.gov.in/sites/default/files/Module%20for%20Multi-Purpose%20Workers%20-%20Prevention%2C%20Screening%20and%20Control%20of%20Common%20NCDS.pdf. [Last accessed on December, 2019].
9. Arokiasamy P. India's escalating burden of non-communicable diseases. Lancet Glob Health. 2018; 6(12):e1262-3.
10. Harvard Initiative for Global Health Quality (2013). The economic impact of non-communicable diseases in China and India: Estimates, projections and comparisons. [online] Available from: https://www.google.com/url?sa=t&source=

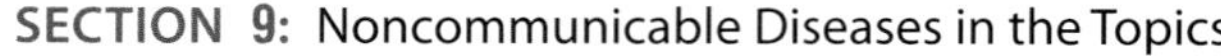

web&rct=j&url=http://www.isec.ac.in/WP%2520300%2520-2520David %2520E%2520Bloom%2520et %2520al. pdf&ved=2ahUKEwj7jdSHia7mAhXRg UsFHcrtCu8QFj AKegQIBhAC&usg=AOvVaw0WBSUR 5vhn 8dReKHtJewdk [Last accessed on December, 2019].

11. World Health Organization. Double burden of malnutrition. [online] Available from: https://www.who.int/nutrition/double-burden-malnutrition/en/ [Last accessed on December, 2019].

12. Bachani D. Need for strategic revamping to prevent and control non-communicable diseases in India. Indian J Community Med. 2017;42(1):1-3.

13. Mondal S, Belle SV. India's NCD strategy in the SDG era: are there early signs of a paradigm shift? Global Health. 2018; 14(1):39.

14. World Health Organization. Global Health Observatory (GHO) Data. [online] Available from: http://www.who.int/gho/ncd/en/ [Last accessed on December, 2019].

15. National Centre for Disease Informatics and Research. Indian Council of Medical Research (2017). National Stroke Registry Program. [online] Available from: http://ncdirindia.org/stroke/BS_FactSheet_MonitoringFramework.aspx [Last accessed on December, 2019].

"It is a matter of great concern that India is witnessing an epidemiological transition. Noncommunicable diseases are on the increase."
Shri M Venkaiah Naidu, Honorable Vice President of India, addressing the National Interventional Council of the Cardiological Society of India at the Sanjay Gandhi Postgraduate Institute of Medical Sciences, Lucknow, April 5, 2019, while urging doctors to educate people on dangers of lifestyle diseases.

Genetic Disorders in Tropics

Kausik Mandal

BURDEN OF GENETIC DISORDERS

Genetic disorders are as prevalent in Southeast Asia as in any other part of the world. Though the burden of genetic disorders is still not recognized as agonizing as the infectious diseases in India, this group of disorders is gradually going to be the foremost public health problem few years down the line.

Genetic contribution to various human diseases can vary from subtle genetic predisposition, like that in bronchial asthma, to specific inherited genetic disorders such as sickle cell disease (SCD). Moreover, cancers are essentially genetic disorders; for many of them, there can be inherited mutations and in many others there can be only mutations in the somatic cells leading to clonal proliferation. Many congenital anomalies can be due to genetic and nongenetic disruptions (e.g. congenital rubella, amniotic band disruption sequence, or fetal valproate syndrome), which occur during the period of embryogenesis. In view of lack of a clear-cut delineation and definition of genetic disorders, it is difficult to estimate its incidence and prevalence in a population. We, however, will stick to congenital anomalies and inherited childhood genetic disorders, which is common in the southeast Asia/India.

Worldwide, around 3%–5% of all live born infants have a major congenital anomaly. A single minor anomaly is found in around 14% newborns. About 4–5% of all babies born have a genetic disorder. A chromosomal abnormality is detected in 0.5% of all newborn babies and 7% of all stillborns. Around 15% of all pediatric admissions have underlying genetic defects and around 20–30% of all infant deaths are due to genetic disorders. About 50% of individuals found to have mental retardation have a genetic basis for their disability.

In India and southeast Asia, the estimated incidence genetic disorders are similar to the world, except for the striking preponderance of β-thalassemia and related disorders such as SCD [hemoglobin (Hb)S] and HbE, HbC (hemoglobin C), and HbD with various combinations, all arising from beta-globin gene mutations. Due to endogamy in certain populations, some very common mutations are observed for a distinctive phenotype; e.g. homozygous MLC1:c.320insC (homozygous insertion of a cytosine in exon 2 in *MLC1* gene), leading to megalencephalic leukoencephalopathy with subcortical cysts (MLC), is observed in Indian Agarwals.[1]

Considering an extremely expanding population, the numbers must have increased exponentially now; but estimation done a decade back had shown that about 495,000 infants with congenital malformations, 390,000 with G6PD deficiency, 21,400 with Down syndrome, 9,000 with β-thalassemia, 5,200 with SCD, and 9,760 with amino acid disorders are born every year in India. If we consider the common malformations, the highest is neural tube defects (NTDs) with an estimated birth of 36.3 cases in 10,000 live births, leading to around 88,532 cases in a year in India.[2]

CLASSIFICATION OF GENETIC DISORDERS

As stated earlier, due to genetic contributions to various childhood illnesses, a clear-cut classification is sometimes difficult. The various disorders as per their etiology and importance are described in **Table 1**.

Down Syndrome

Down syndrome is the most common genetic cause of mental retardation, accounting for around 20–30% of children with mental retardation. The physical characters

Table 1: Classification of genetic disorders.

Classification		Common examples	Important Indian/Southeast Asian disorders*
Chromosomal	Defects in chromosome number	Down syndrome Turner syndrome Klinefelter syndrome	
	Defects in chromosome structure	Chromosomal large deletions, duplications, and translocations	
	Submicroscopic copy number variations (microdeletion syndromes)	Williams syndrome Velocardiofacial syndrome Prader–Willi and Angelman syndromes	
Single gene disorders	Autosomal dominant disorders	Achondroplasia Tuberous sclerosis Neurofibromatosis type 1 and type 2	
	Autosomal recessive disorders	Phenylketonuria Gaucher's disease Mucopolysaccharidosis type 1 Cystic fibrosis	β-thalassemia and sickle cell disease Spinal muscular atrophy
	X-linked recessive disorder	G6PD deficiency Mucopolysaccharidosis type 2 (Hunter syndrome)	Hemophilia A and B Duchenne muscular dystrophy
	X-linked dominant disorder	Rett syndrome	
Non-Mendelian disorders	Polygenic and multifactorial	Nonsyndromic cleft lip	Neural tube defect
	Oligogenic	Hirschsprung disease	
	Mitochondrial (Mitochondrial mutations)†	Leigh disease Leber hereditary optic neuropathy (LHON)	
	Imprinting disorders	Beckwith–Wiedemann syndrome Albright hereditary osteodystrophy	

*Importance is related to prevalence and/or public awareness and government policies.
†Mitochondrial disorders can be due to mutation in nuclear genes or mitochondrial genes. Those due to mutation in nuclear genome follow Mendelian inheritance. The same phenotype, like Leigh disease, can be due to mutation in either genome.

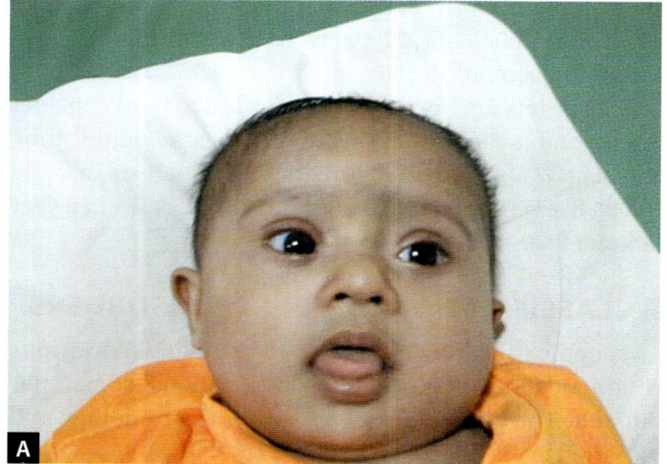

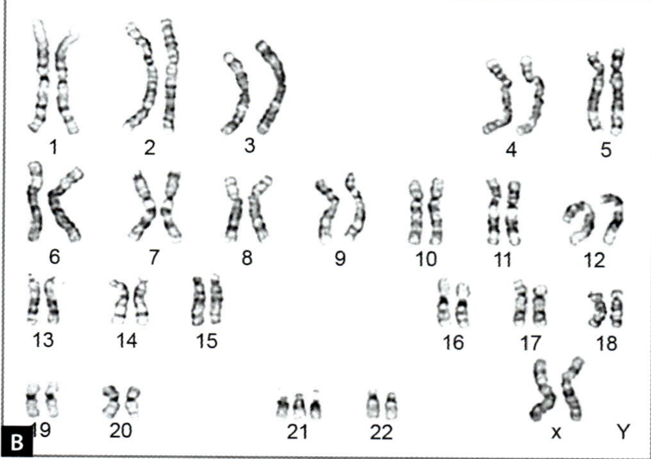

Figs. 1A and B: *Down syndrome*: Flat facial profile, depressed nasal bridge, epicanthic folds, hypertelorism, upslant of eyes, protruding tongue, brachycephaly, and karyotype showing trisomy 21.

are easily recognized by trained eyes (**Figs. 1A and B**). Chromosome analysis is indicated in all children with Down syndrome not only because there are other known genetic disorders with similar features, but also to know the exact chromosomal constitution giving rise to Down syndrome. Children with Down syndrome might have

Table 2: Frequency and recurrence risk associated with different translocations in Down syndrome.

Chromosomes involved in translocation	Relative frequency among translocation	Prevalence of de novo translocation*	Prevalence of inherited translocation	Carrier mother	Carrier father
21 with D group (14,13,15)	54.2%	55%	45%	10–15%	1–5%
21 with G group (21,22)	40.9%	96%	4%		
			t21;21	100%	100%
			t21;22	10–15%	1–5%
21 with chromosomes other than D or G	4.9%	Few	Most	10–15%	1–5%

*For de novo translocations, the risk of recurrence of Down syndrome in siblings is 1%.

different chromosomal constitutions; 95% of such children have 47 chromosomes with an extra 21, 4% have translocation involving chromosome 21, and around 1% are mosaic for two cell lines. All have near similar phenotypes.

The risk of recurrence in case of a free trisomy 21 (having 47 chromosomes) and that of mosaic Down syndrome is 1%. The risk of recurrence however differs in a child with Down syndrome due to translocation involving chromosome 21 and has either of the parents as a carrier of the translocation as stated in **Table 2**.

The following points need to be remembered before ordering a chromosome analysis:

- A pretest counseling needs to be offered to all families before the analysis.
- Chromosome analysis should be done from a reliable laboratory. A good chromosome analysis from a reliable laboratory has the following attributes:
  - The report is accompanied by a picture with depiction of the anomaly (if any) in the picture. Information about number of metaphases analyzed is stated.
  - In case of chromosomal analysis for prenatal diagnosis, the regulations of PNDT Act (Prenatal diagnostic techniques Act) are strictly followed.
  - Chromosome analysis of parents is required only if the child has Down syndrome due to translocation. Chromosomal analysis also may be needed if the child with Down syndrome is not alive and his/her karyotype was not done.

Breaking the News

Diagnosis of Down syndrome is obvious at birth to the doctor but not to the family unless the child has some major malformation. Disclosing the news that the child has a disorder associated with mental handicap is a challenging talk and needs to be done by an expert clinician with knowledge of Down syndrome. The diagnosis should be disclosed to the parents within first few days after birth. It should be done with great care and preferably to both the parents together. Information about major problems should be provided in a balanced manner. Positive aspects, such as ability to achieve self-care, some education, and ability to lead happy and useful life, need to be stated. Detailed counseling may follow after the karyotype report is available.

Investigations and surveillance plan of a case with Down syndrome:

- Clinical evaluation and investigations to look for associated cardiac and gastrointestinal malformations need to be done immediately after birth.
- *Chromosome analysis*: Once at the onset.
- *Complete hemogram [Hb, TLC (total leukocytes count), DLC (differential leukocytes count), ESR (erythrocyte sedimentation rate), and RBC (red blood cell) indices]*: At the onset and yearly (more frequently if any abnormality is detected). It is not necessary to tell parents about less frequent associations such as leukemias to the parents.
- *Thyroid profile [Free T4 (Free thyroxine), TSH (thyroid-stimulating hormone)]*: At the onset and yearly if normal. Treating all children with Down syndrome with thyroxine supplementation is not recommended. Thyroxine supplementation is done for children with confirmed hypothyroidism.
- *Pediatric cardiology evaluation*: Echocardiography and treatment as per requirement.
- Ophthalmological examination for squint and cataract.
- Audiometry.

Management Issues

- *Hypotonia and motor delay*: Physiotherapy
- Infant stimulation program
- *Eye and vision*: It is important to detect ocular problems such as refractive errors, cataract, glaucoma,

nasolacrimal outflow obstruction, and keratoconus, and treat accordingly.

- *ENT and hearing*: Conductive deafness is common; 90% are due to otitis media. Such children need to be periodically evaluated for obstructive sleep apnea.
- *Neurology and seizure*: Epilepsy and dementia are more common in such children.
- *Gastrointestinal*: Frequency of duodenal atresia and Hirschsprung disease is more common in Down syndrome.
- *Immune system complications*: These children are more prone to autoimmune disorders and infections.
- Education and vocational training as per IQ assessment.

Counseling Issues

The following points need to be remembered during counseling a family with Down syndrome:

- Mental retardation is a lifelong problem. Breaking such news should be done in an ideal genetic counseling session and not casually in a crowded OPD setting. Such children require social and family support and need special education.
- Increased maternal age increases the risk of Down syndrome; however, most Down syndrome children are born to women less than 35 years of age. Women with increased maternal age should not feel stigmatized.
- Aneuploidy screening during pregnancy needs to be explained so that other family members and friends plan and act accordingly.
- Prenatal testing in next pregnancy should be offered to every couple with a child with Down syndrome. Recurrence risk is according to the chromosomal constitution and can vary from 1% to 100% as depicted in the preceding text.
- A female child with trisomy 21 when grows old and gets married is likely to transmit the same to around 30–50% of her offspring. Males with Down syndrome are usually infertile.

Turner Syndrome

Turner syndrome (TS) is present in 1 in 2,500 to 1 in 3,000 live born females. It is more frequently found in pregnancy losses. More than 99% of conceptuses with 45,X are spontaneously aborted, accounting for around 20% of all spontaneous abortions. Clinical features vary from *in utero* lymphedema **(Figs. 2A to C)** to infertility in females of reproductive age group. The typical dysmorphic features are as follows:

- *Eyes*: Epicanthic folds, squint, nystagmus, ptosis, hypermetropia, cataracts, amblyopia.

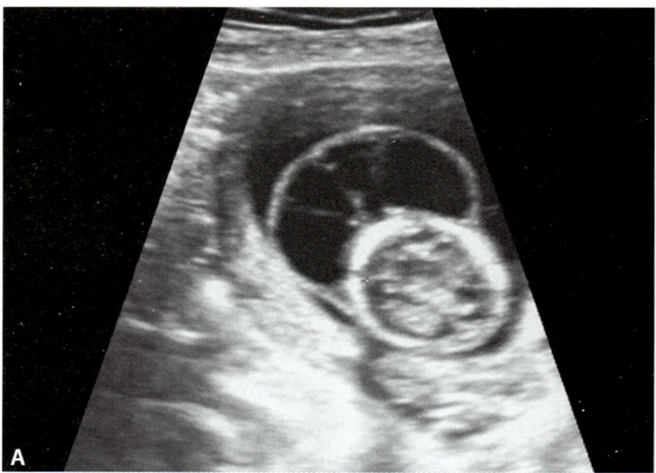

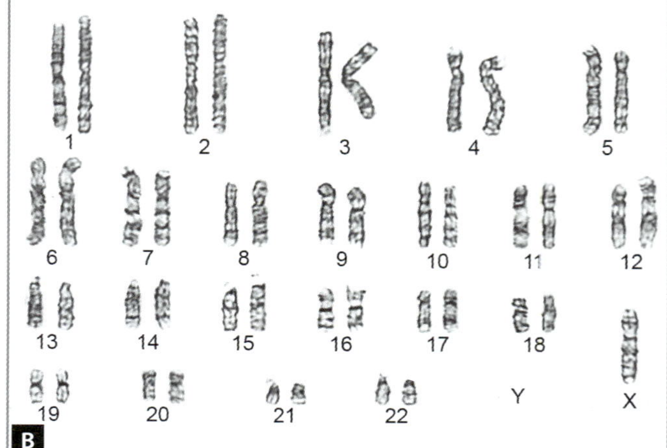

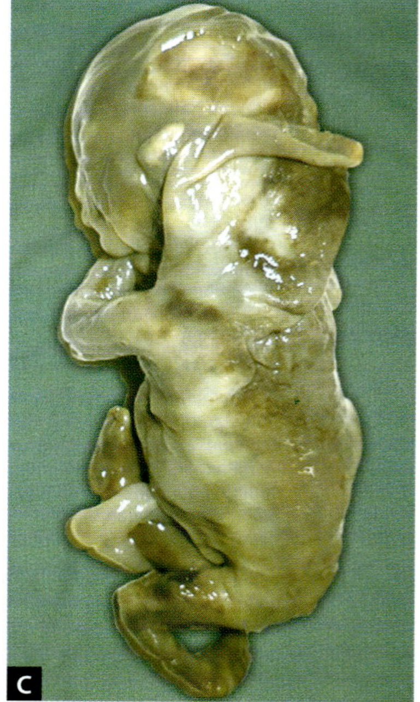

Figs. 2A to C: *Turner syndrome*: Ultrasonography showing cystic hygroma, antenatal karyotype showing 45,X and the same fetus at autopsy showing skin edema and cystic hygroma.

- *Ears*: Posteriorly rotated low-set ears. Chronic otitis media may lead to deafness, or there can be associated sensorineural deafness.
- *Mouth*: Crowding of teeth and malocclusion, and micrognathia.
- *Neck*: Low hairline, short, and webbed neck.
- *Chest*: Widely spaced nipples, pectus excavatum.
- *Upper limbs*: Cubitus valgus.
- *Hands*: Short 4th/5th metacarpals, short fingers, nail hypoplasia, and hyperconvex nail.
- *Lower limbs*: Congenital hip dislocation.

A significant number of cases may not have any Turner stigmata and may present only as short stature or delayed puberty. Hence, karyotype of all prepubertal girls with short stature needs to be done. It is to be remembered that TS is not synonymous with 45,X karyotype; other chromosomal abnormalities leading to a hypofunctioning or inactive X can also lead to similar phenotype. The various chromosomal constitutions associated with TS are described in **Table 3**.

Though there is no definite genotype–phenotype correlation in case of TS, certain features have been described with specific chromosomal constitutions, e.g. congenital lymphedema for 45,X and mental retardation and more severe phenotype for ring chromosome X. Presence of Y confers risk of gonadoblastoma of 7–30%.

During routine karyotyping, where 20 cells are counted, mosaicism of 5% may be detected. However, if 46,XX karyotype is found in a clinically suspected Turner individual, counting 100 or more metaphases or assaying a second tissue-like skin fibroblast is necessary to look for mosaicism for an abnormal cell line (for attributes of a good chromosome analysis, see Down syndrome).

Table 3: Various chromosomal constitutions associated with Turner syndrome.

Chromosomal constitution	Remarks	Percentage of Turner syndrome
45,X	Monosomy of X in all cells	40–60%
46,X,i(Xq)	Isochromosome of long arm of X (duplication of long arm with loss of short arm)	5–10%
Other structural defects involving X chromosome	Ring X, partial deletion of p or q arms, isochromosome of p arm, X-autosome or X-Y translocations	Rest
45,X/46XX; 45,X/47,XXX; rarely 45,X/46,XY	Mosaicism of 45,X with various other cell lines	Rest

Management Issues

The major issues in TS are short stature and hypogonadism.

Short stature and growth hormone (GH): Growth velocity is reduced even in infancy; however, the overt sign of short stature is often delayed till 5–10 years of age.

- Females with TS produce sufficient GH; still it has been seen that GH therapy has been the beneficial effect of final adult height.
- Provocative GH testing should not be routinely done, except in those with abnormal growth than expected for TS, determined on TS-specific growth curves.
- Growth hormone therapy is generally initiated at a dose of 0.375 mg/kg/wk (0.054 mg/kg/d or 0.162 IU/kg/d or 4.8 IU/m^2/d). This is most effective when given daily and as a custom, it is administered in the evening.
- Follow-up should include regular monitoring of growth velocity at 3–6-month intervals to assess the efficacy of GH treatment and also monitoring of thyroid function, serum glucose, and side effects such as orthopedic problems, especially scoliosis.
- Growth hormone dose adjustments should be according to the patient's growth response and IGF-I (insulin-like growth factor I) levels.
- Development of scoliosis or kyphosis is a side effect of GH therapy; however, it should not prevent the use of GH. Therapy is generally stopped when expected height has been attained or there remains very little further growth potential (bone age >14 years and growth velocity <2 cm/yr).
- The optimum age of starting GH has not been established; for practical purpose, it is 4 years or as soon as diagnosed at a later age.
- Escalation of GH dosing beyond approved 0.375 mg/kg/wk appears unwarranted as it has produced small gains in adult height. Elevated IGF-I levels, idiopathic intracranial hypertension, and slipped capital femoral epiphysis are often associated with high doses of GH.
- For girls above 9 years of age, especially with extreme short stature, one may consider adding a non-aromatizable anabolic steroid, such as oxandrolone (0.05 mg/kg/d or less); one needs to monitor liver enzymes and virilization.
- All families need to be counseled about the modest increase in height with GH, which needs to be balanced against injections, cost, monitoring, and potential risks such as increased insulin level and blood pressure.

Gonadal function

- Absent pubertal development is a common problem of TS. Some spontaneous pubertal development is seen in up to 30% children with TS. Practically, in the long run, over 90% of TS will have gonadal failure.

- Before initiation of estrogen therapy, determine serum gonadotropin to exclude delayed spontaneous puberty.
- Low-dose estrogen therapy starting at 12 years of age helps in normalized development of secondary sexual characteristics, a normal pace of puberty, uterine and bone mineral development. It also probably improves cognitive and hepatic functions. Overall, it improves quality of life without interfering with the effect of GH on final adult height.
- It is better to avoid oral contraceptive pill (OCP) for pubertal development as the synthetic estrogen doses in most preparations are too high and the synthetic progestin may interfere with optimal breast and uterine development.
- Replacement with estrogen (E2) is usually begun at one tenth to one eighth of the adult replacement dose and then gradually, it is increased over a period of 2–4 years.

- Equivalent initial E2 doses are: Depot (intramuscular) E2, 0.2–0.4 mg/mon; transdermal E2, 6.25 µg/d; micronized E2, 0.25 mg/d.

Other concomitant associations which need to be looked for and managed accordingly are:

- *Cardiovascular*: Bicuspid aortic valve with or without coarctation of aorta
- *Renal*:
  - Structural anomalies are present in up to 40%
  - Renal agenesis, horseshoe kidney, duplicated collecting system, obstructed outflow, and aberrant vasculature
- *Hypothyroidism* occurs in 5–10% in mid or late childhood
- *Diabetes* in adulthood, especially in obese.

Williams Syndrome

Williams syndrome (WS) is often first suspected following an echocardiography detecting a supravalvular aortic stenosis or distinct facial features **(Fig. 3)** and characteristic behavior phenotype (overfriendly behavior). Prevalence is

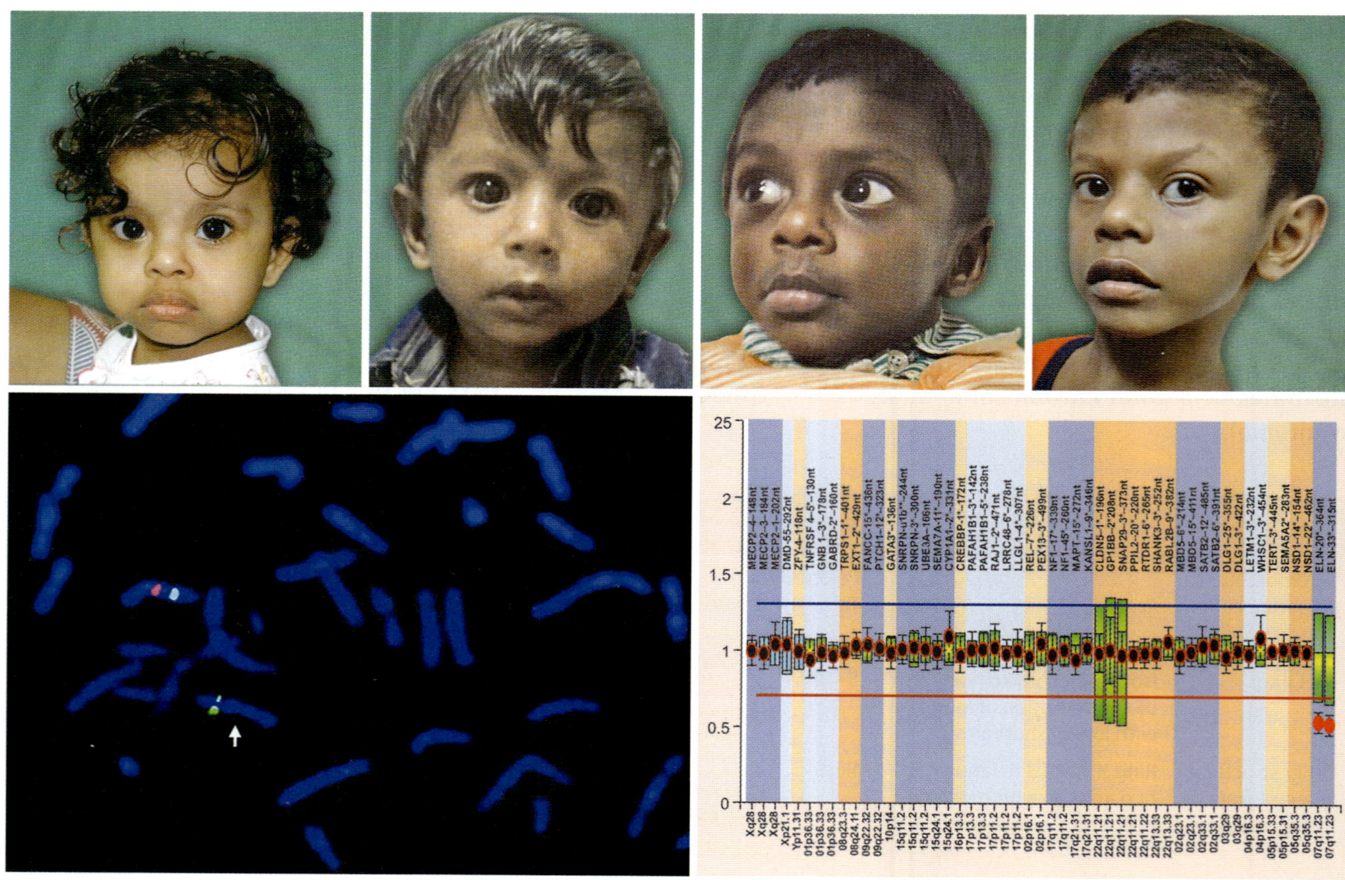

Fig. 3: *Williams syndrome (WS):* Facial features of WS include small upturned nose, long philtrum, wide mouth, full lips, small chin, and puffiness around the eyes. FISH showing deletion (lack of magenta color probe, shown by arrow) at 7q11.23 locus, in one of the chromosome 7 (marked with green colored control probe). MLPA (for common microdeletion syndromes) showing heterozygous deletion (probe ratio near 0.5) at 7q11.23. (FISH: fluorescent in-situ hybridization; MLPA: multiplex ligation-dependent probe amplification)

estimated to be 1 in 20,000 to 1 in 50,000 live births. It is a microdeletion syndrome diagnosed by FISH (fluorescent in-situ hybridization) using a probe complementary to the region 7q11.23, containing the elastin gene. These days, FISH is replaced by MLPA (multiplex ligation-dependent probe amplification), the diagnostic modality. MLPA is cheaper, easy to perform, and looks for more disorders at a time.

Preliminary evaluation once WS is diagnosed:
- Growth monitoring (preferably on WS growth charts)
- Ultrasound examination of the bladder and kidneys
- *Cardiology evaluation*:
  - Evaluation by a pediatric cardiologist
  - Blood pressure in all four limbs
  - Echocardiogram, including Doppler flow studies
- Serum calcium or ionized calcium, blood urea nitrogen (BUN), and creatinine
- Calcium/creatinine determination on a spot urine sample
- *Thyroid function*: Free T4, TSH
- Ophthalmologic evaluation
- Baseline hearing evaluation.

Agents to Avoid

It is a common practice to give multivitamins to all children with poor growth. Though they have poor growth, *multivitamins are contraindicated in children with WS*. Most pediatric multivitamin preparations contain vitamin D, which might aggravate nephrocalcinosis.

Medical Management

- Developmental disabilities need to be addressed by early intervention and special education programs.
- Psychological and psychiatric interventions.
- Monitoring and treatment of hypertension.
- Management of hypercalcemia.
- *Diet*: The dietary calcium intake should not be more than the recommended daily allowance (RDA). If the serum concentration of calcium is found to be elevated, dietary calcium should be reduced according to the serum concentration, which needs to be periodically monitored.
- Refractory hypercalcemia may be treated with oral steroids.
- Intravenous pamidronate, at times, has been used to treat infants with severe symptomatic hypercalcemia.
- Treatment of nephrocalcinosis may need input from nephrologists.

Surgical Management Issues

- Around 30% children require surgical correction of supravalvular aortic stenosis. Some might require surgical correction for mitral valve insufficiency as well.
- Renal artery stenosis may require surgical intervention.
- Refractive error strabismus is treated with corrective lenses and various other interventions, including surgery.
- Recurrent otitis media may need tympanostomy tubes.
- There is risk of myocardial insufficiency during surgery. A well-equipped center is necessary for any surgical procedure.

Follow-up

The following are recommended for monitoring at specified time interval:

Time interval	Evaluations
Every year	• Vision for refractive errors and strabismus • Blood pressure in both arms • Calcium/creatine ratio in a random spot urine and urine routine
Every 2 years	Serum concentration of calcium
Every 3 years	Thyroid function
Every 5 years	Hearing assessment
Every 10 years	Renal and bladder ultrasound
In adults	• Glucose tolerance test (GTT) starting at age 30 years for diabetes mellitus (repeat every 5 years if normal) • Cardiac evaluation for mitral valve prolapse, aortic insufficiency, and arterial stenoses • Evaluation for cataracts

Counseling Issues

Almost all microdeletions in WS are de novo in origin (sporadic) although in some patients, parent-to-child transmission has been reported. When parents are normal, the recurrence risk is negligible in siblings; in such a situation, prenatal testing is rarely sought for, though clinically readily available.

Achondroplasia

Achondroplasia is the most common cause of disproportionate short stature. Such individuals are easily recognizable because of their large head with frontal bossing, midface hypoplasia, and short arms and legs **(Fig. 4)**.

Intelligence and overall life span are usually normal. However, craniocervical junction compression predisposes to a risk of death in infancy.

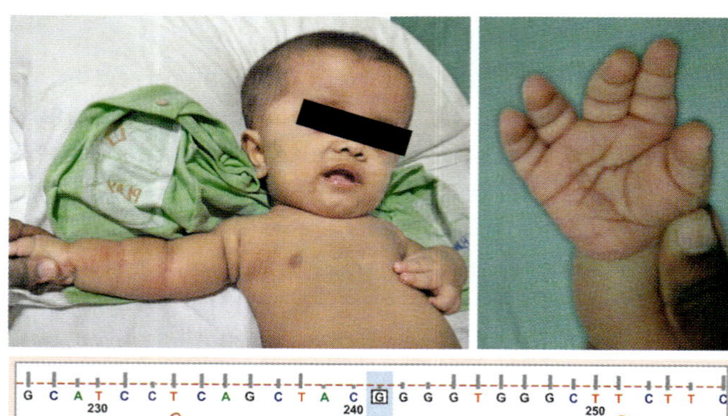

Fig. 4: *Achondroplasia*: Prominent forehead, rhizomelia, trident hand in a child with achondroplasia. Common sequence variation: NM_000142: Heterozygous *FGFR3:c.1138G > A (G380R)*.

There are several skeletal dysplasias which cause short stature. Conditions that may be confused with achondroplasia are hypochondroplasia, cartilage–hair hypoplasia, and other metaphyseal dysplasias. A definitive diagnosis by X-ray and mutation testing should be done for proper genetic counseling.

Evaluations Following Initial Diagnosis

- Genetics consultation and consultation with a pediatric orthopedic surgeon dealing with bone dysplasia are advisable
- Achondroplasia-specific growth charts should be used for documentation of length, weight, and head circumference
- Baseline CT or MRI of the brain
- Craniocervical junction assessment includes history and neurological examination, CT or MRI of the craniocervical junction, and polysomnography.

Treatment of Manifestations

Short stature:
- Growth hormone therapy shows initial acceleration of growth, but with lessening effect over time. It has got very little effect on adult stature.
- *Limb-lengthening surgeries*:
  - Increase in height of up to 12–14 inches
  - Age of surgery is debatable. It can commence as early as 6–8 years of age according to one group; the other group prefers postponing surgery until the affected individual is able to make an informed decision.

Obesity: Early interventions are required to control obesity.

Neurosurgical intervention may be required for:
- *Hydrocephalus*: Ventriculoperitoneal shunting, rather than third ventriculostomy, is preferable.
- *Spinal stenosis*: May require urgent extended and wide laminectomies
- *Craniocervical junction constriction*: Predictors are:
  - Increased deep tendon reflexes or clonus affecting lower limbs
  - Polysomnography detecting central hypopnea
  - Reduced foramen magnum size as determined by CT of the craniocervical junction. Comparison should be made with norms for individuals with achondroplasia.

ENT evaluation and interventions are required for:
- Obstructive sleep apnea
- Middle ear dysfunction.
  Orthopedic interventions may be required in conditions other than correction of short stature, for varus deformity and kyphosis.

Socialization: Support groups and social awareness programs.

Agents/circumstances to avoid:
- Collision sports
- Gymnastics
- Diving from height during swimming.

Genetic Counseling

Achondroplasia is inherited in an autosomal dominant manner. Most such individuals have de novo mutation in the *FGFR3* gene. Two common mutations account for almost all individuals (the first in 98% and the second in 1%). About 80% of children with achondroplasia have parents with average stature. The risk of having another child with achondroplasia, in normal parents, is negligible; however, in view of possibility of germ line mosaicism, prenatal testing in next pregnancy is advisable. An individual with achondroplasia, when grows up and marries a person of normal stature, has a 50% risk in each pregnancy of having a child with achondroplasia; prenatal testing can be done by mutation testing in such a situation.

β-thalassemia

β-thalassemia, also called Cooley's anemia or Mediterranean anemia, is a genetic disorder, prevalent in the southeast Asia. It is characterized by reduced or defective synthesis of beta-chain of hemoglobin leading to microcytic hypochromic anemia and in severe cases requiring transfusion of blood or packed RBC to sustain life.

Prevalence

Approximately 1.5% of the world population are supposed to be carriers (trait/heterozygous) of the β-thalassemia. The trade along the great Silk Road, which extends from China through the Indian subcontinent to Iran and the Eastern Mediterranean, and the invasion of the Mongols (1,220 AD) and the Tatars (1,380–87 AD) probably explain the high incidence and distribution of the disease in populations from the Mediterranean basin, throughout the Middle East, the Indian subcontinent, southeast Asia, and Melanesia to the Pacific Islands.

India has a large population which is ethnically diverse. The frequency of β-thalassemia trait/carrier status has been reported from <1% to 17% and an average of 3–4% throughout India. There is also a regional distribution of the beta-chain-related hemoglobinopathies throughout the country.[3] A high frequency of HbD in the Northern Punjabi population, HbE in the eastern region (West Bengal), and HbS (sickle cell) from populations of tribal origin in central India has been reported. Considering the prevalence of β-thalassemia in India, around 10,000–12,000 children are born with β-thalassemia major every year.

Molecular Pathology

Human hemoglobin is a tetramer of globin polypeptide chains, with a pair of α-like chains and a pair of β-like chains. The major portion, adult hemoglobin A (HbA), consists of two α and two β chains $(\alpha_2\beta_2)$; the next in proportion, minor adult hemoglobin (HbA2), has two α and two δ chains $(\alpha_2\delta_2)$; and fetal hemoglobin is made up of two α and two γ chains $(\alpha_2\gamma_2)$.

The beta-chains are transcribed from two alleles of the beta-globin genes (*HBB* gene) and the alpha-chains from four alleles of alpha-globin genes (a pair of *HBA1* and a pair if *HBA2* genes). Unpaired polypeptide chains of hemoglobin are insoluble and tend to precipitate, form inclusions, and damage RBCs. β-thalassemia essentially occurs due to defective beta-globin synthesis, thus producing a relative excess to alpha-globin chains, triggering inclusions and red cell damage. Associated defect/deletion of alpha-chains causes amelioration of symptoms and alpha triplication, leading to excess alpha chains, causes more severe disease (e.g. transforming a carrier to thalassemia intermedia phenotype). Thus, alpha-genes are considered as modifier genes for beta-gene phenotypes.

According to severity, beta-globin mutations can be β^0 (where no beta-chain is produced) and β^+ (in which beta-globin protein is produced but at a reduced level).

Genetics

HBB gene is a small gene located at 11p15.4. It has got 3 exons **(Fig. 5)**. Like most protein-coding genes, the coding sequence starts with the "ATG" codon which codes for methionine. While giving nomenclature about any sequence change/mutation, the c. number starts from the "A" of "ATG" (e.g. c.20 means 20th nucleotide from the first nucleotide and c.20A > T means at the 20th nucleotide A is replaced by T). The common mutations found in India are c.92 + 5G > C [IVS (IVS stands for intervening sequence) 1-5 G > C], c.92 + 1G > T, and c.92 + 1G > C at splice sites following exon 1; c.51delC, c.26_27insG, and c.92G > C in exon 1; C.126_129delCTTT in exon 2, etc. The old nomenclature used was not standardized and was either using codon number in various ways or using positions in the introns; for example, IVS 1-5 G > C denotes the sequence change in 5th nucleotide in intron 1. Most of the literatures still use the old nomenclature due to its familiarity among physicians and scientists. Previous ARMS-PCR (amplification-refractory mutation system-polymerase chain reaction) was done to look for targeted mutations. Nowadays, Sanger sequencing of coding exons, 5'UTR (untranslated regions, containing the cap site mutations) and conserved splice sites are done to look for all point mutations and small deletions and duplications. There is a common 619bp (base pair) deletion mutation involving the exon 3; for this mutation PCR amplification of two fragments, one amplifying the flanking regions and one amplifying the area of suspected deletion, is being done to detect homozygous or heterozygous mutation.

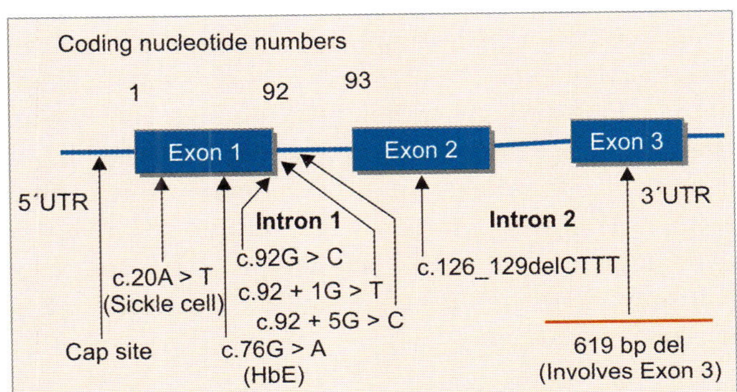

Fig. 5: *HBB* gene: It contains 3 exons. The various common mutations and their positions are marked. The most common mutation, c.92 + 5G > C is located in intron 1, 5 nucleotide downstream of the last nucleotide (c.92) of exon 1. The 619bp deletion involves exon 3.

It is important to note that HbS (sickle cell), HbC, HbD, and HbE (HBB:c.76G > A) are abnormal hemoglobins due to mutation in the beta-chain (*HBB* gene). Homozygous HbS is SCD and is discussed later. Homozygous HbE has very mild symptoms and may not get detected, except during investigations for any major associated illness. However, HbE along with another pathogenic β^0 or β^+ mutation is likely to cause thalassemia intermedia, many a times becoming transfusion dependent with time. HbC is a structural variant caused by an amino acid substitution of lysine for glutamic acid at the same codon of HbS (position six after initiation codon) of the beta-hemoglobin chain. Persons with hemoglobin C trait (HbAC) are phenotypically normal. Individuals with hemoglobin C disease (HbCC) may have a mild degree of hemolytic anemia and, splenomegaly. Although the clinical complications of hemoglobin C disease are not very severe, inheritance with other hemoglobinopathies such as hemoglobin S may lead to appreciable consequences. Hemoglobin D carriers (HbAD) and homozygous HbD disease (HbDD) have no or mild phenotypes, and at times remain nonrecognizable even when they co-occur with another beta-mutation. HbD can be due to various mutations; HbD Punjab is a very specific mutation in exon 3. Otherwise, exon 3 mutations are very rare.

Modifier genes: As stated earlier, alpha-genes modify the phenotype of β-thalassemia; alpha deletions make the phenotype milder and duplication/triplication makes it more severe.

Activating mutations in the promoter region of gamma-globin genes causes increased gamma chain formation thus raising the fetal hemoglobin, HbF ($\alpha_2\gamma_2$). This condition is designated as HPFH (hereditary persistence of fetal hemoglobin), which though being a benign condition, at HPLC (high-performance liquid chromatography) for Hb variant, will show very high fetal hemoglobin, like thalassemia major. It, however, needs to be remembered that when there is heterozygous deletion of the whole *HBB* gene, there is again high HbF, which is also called "deletional form of HPFH." This condition is actually carrier status of β-thalassemia, which when compounded with another beta-mutation will give rise to thalassemia major-like phenotype; the sequencing will show homozygous beta-mutation, due to complete absence of one allele.

Inheritance: The disease is inherited as autosomal recessive disorder, which means that both the alleles of the gene are mutated to cause the disease. Father and mother are generally asymptomatic carriers. When both the mutations are same, the affected child's genetic status is designated as "homozygous" and when the two mutations are different, it is "compound heterozygous."

Symptoms

According to manifestations, β-thalassemia is divided into:
- Thalassemia major
- Thalassemia intermedia
- Thalassemia minor.

β-*thalassemia major (mutation in both alleles of the HBB gene) is generally suspected in the following condition*:
- An infant or child younger than age 2 years
- Severe anemia (microcytic)
- Hepatosplenomegaly
- Evidence of hemolysis.

These children cannot sustain life without regular blood transfusion. Untreated, there is expansion of the bone marrow due to ineffective erythropoiesis. These children develop hemolytic facies, if not adequately treated. Later in life, they may have areas of extramedullary hematopoiesis. Poorly treated children may have typing "hair-on-end" appearance in skull X-ray.

Thalassemia intermedia (mutation in both alleles of the HBB gene) should be suspected:
- Children who present at a later age
- Milder clinical findings.

Children with thalassemia intermedia do not require regular treatment with blood transfusion to sustain life; however, in view of ineffective erythropoiesis and chronic anemia, they may develop facial changes and short stature **(Fig. 6)**.

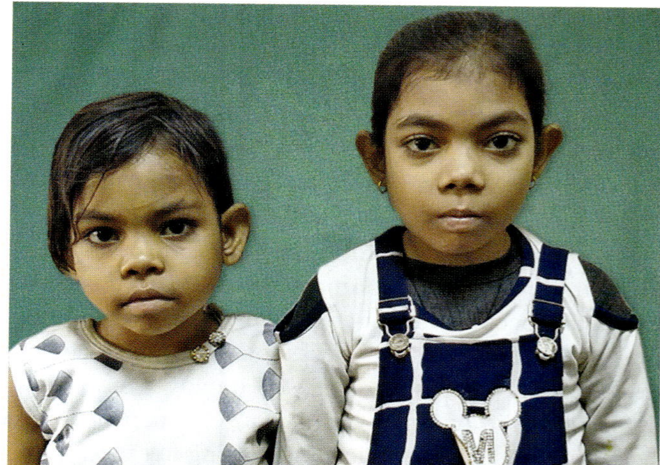

Fig. 6: *Thalassemia*: Facial features of two siblings with thalassemia intermedia. They are having hemolytic facies characterized by frontal bossing, depressed nasal bridge, prominent malar bones, and malocclusion of teeth.

Thalassemia minor (mutation in one allele of the HBB gene):

- They are carriers.
- They are usually clinically asymptomatic, but sometimes a mild anemia is present along with microcytosis.

Laboratory Diagnosis

Hematological parameters, peripheral smear examination, RBC indices, and Hb variant analysis by HPLC give near-accurate diagnosis for β-thalassemia. These tests should be carried on before doing a molecular testing. Previously done Hb electrophoresis is no longer used for diagnosis though sometimes, Hb variant analysis by HPLC is often termed Hb electrophoresis by some.

Hematological parameters show low Hb. Peripheral smear shows microcytosis, hypochromia, anisocytosis, poikilocytosis (spiculated teardrop and elongated cells), and nucleated RBCs (erythroblasts). The nucleated red cells are often mistaken as lymphocytes and the total leucocyte count (TLC) is seen elevated. It is markedly increased following splenectomy.

The other different parameters used to diagnose β-thalassemia and distinguish each variety are depicted in **Tables 4 and 5**.[4,5]

In affected children lower than 12 months, the HbF remains elevated and sometimes it becomes difficult to diagnose thalassemia in them. The diagnosis of β-thalassemia below 1 year of age and during newborn screening is sometimes aided by the following:

- *Complete absence of HbA*: Generally seen, when both alleles have severe mutations.
- When one or both alleles have a less severe mutation, Hb variant analysis is not helpful, especially in the newborn period, because the diminished amount of hemoglobin A overlaps the range for normal babies.
- Microcytic hypochromic anemia with anisopoikilocytosis and nucleated RBCs on peripheral blood smear
- Molecular testing detecting biallelic pathogenic variants in *HBB* gene.

Molecular testing: It is the gold standard and is essential for prenatal testing. It is important to note that the proband needs to be tested and at times the carrier parents need to be screened for mutations before prenatal testing is offered. The various mutations and methods have been discussed in the preceding text under genetics.

Management

It is important to distinguish between children having thalassemia intermedia (requiring intermittent transfusions on an as-needed basis) and those with thalassemia major (who need a regular transfusion or hypertransfusion program).[6,7] For practical management guidelines, refer to chapter of hematology.

Table 4: RBC indices for diagnosis of β-thalassemia.

	Normal	Normal	Affected	Carrier
	Male	Female	β-thal major	β-thal minor
Mean corpuscular volume (MCV fl)	89.1±5.01	87.6±5.5	50–70	<79
Mean corpuscular hemoglobin (MCH pg)	30.9±1.9	30.2±2.1	12–20	<27
Hemoglobin (Hb g/dL)	15.9±1.0	14.0±0.9	<7	*Males*: 11.5–15.3 *Females*: 9.1–14

Source: Galanello R, Melis MA, Ruggeri R, et al. Beta 0 thalassemia trait in Sardinia. Hemoglobin. 1979;3(1):33-46.

Table 5: HPLC for Hb variant for diagnosis of β-thalassemia after 1 year of age.

	Normal	Affected (thalassemia major or intermedia)		Thalassemia minor/carrier
		* β^0/β^0	† β^+/β^+ or β^0/β^+	
HbA	96–98%	0	10–30%	92–95%
HbF	<1%	95–98%	70–90%	0.5–4%
HbA$_2$	2–3%	2–5%	2–5%	>3.5%

(HPLC: high-performance liquid chromatography)
*Both alleles with severe mutations.
†Both alleles with less severe or at least one allele with less severe mutation.
Source: Telen MJ, Kaufman RE. The mature erythrocyte. In: Lee GR, Paraskevas F, Foerster J, Lukens J (Eds). Wintrobe's Clinical Hematology, 10th edition. Baltimore, MD: Lippincott Williams & Wilkins; 1999. p. 207.

Genetic Counseling and Prenatal Testing

β-thalassemia is an autosomal recessive genetic disorder. The parents of an affected child are asymptomatic carriers. When parents are carriers, the risk of having an affected child is 25%. Carrier testing by RBC indices and Hb variant by HPLC is indicated in all couples from southeast Asia, especially in communities where the disease is prevalent and in at-risk family members of an affected child. When both the spouses are found to be carriers, mutation testing is indicated to identify the putative mutations. Prenatal testing during pregnancy is being offered to know the status of the baby. When there is an affected child with homozygous or compound heterozygous mutations, prenatal testing is being provided in every subsequent pregnancy. Prenatal testing is done from DNA extracted from samples obtained by CVS (chorionic villous sampling) in earlier weeks (around 12 weeks) or amniocentesis in later part (16–20 weeks) of pregnancy. CVS is preferred, since it provides better DNA and has an advantage of earlier detection. It is important to note that detection of mutation in the proband is essential before offering prenatal testing.

Sickle Cell Disease

Sickle cell disease is a hemoglobinopathy which occurs due to mutation in the beta-globin gene and is characterized by intermittent vaso-occlusive events and chronic hemolytic anemia.

Prevalence

Sickle cell disease, in India, was first described in 1952 from the Nilgiri Hills of northern Tamil Nadu. At present, it is widespread among people of the central India, in the Deccan plateau, with a smaller focus in the north of Kerala and Tamil Nadu, and this region is commonly known as "sickle cell belt".[8] There is a large tribal population in this region, and so it is assumed that HbS is more prevalent among the tribal population. However, it is now clear that HbS is prevalent among both tribal and nontribal people. At times, differences in phenotype have been reported between different populations; a tribal population in Valsad has a milder disease than a non-tribal population in Nagpur and this difference is attributed to extremely high frequencies of alpha thalassemia in the tribal group. The frequency of the sickle cell trait is very varied; it is found to be as high as 35% in some communities.

Pathophysiology

Sickle cell mutation occurs in *HBB* gene at the 20th nucleotide from the starting of exon 1, where A is changed to T, designated as *HBB*:c.20A > T. There is a change in 6th codon from the initiation codon and the glutamic acid codon (GAG) is changed to a valine codon (GTG). This change forms an abnormal hemoglobin called HbS. When people with HbS are exposed to extreme conditions such as hypoxia or dehydration, the sickle hemoglobin (HbS) can polymerize, and the RBC reversibly assumes a sickled shape. These RBCs, whether sickled or unsickled, can adhere to vascular endothelium, resulting in acute and chronic vaso-occlusion, vascular injury, and organ damage.

Clinical Features

Though the mutation in SCD is in beta-globin gene, the main manifestation in this disorder is due to vaso-occlusive events rather than chronic hemolytic anemia like β-thalassemia. Homozygotes (HbS/S) are generally symptomatic, though heterozygotes (HbS) may sometimes have symptoms, albeit milder than that of homozygotes. Due to tissue ischemia, there is acute and chronic pain as well as organ damage. It can affect any organ system, including the bones, joints, liver, spleen, lungs, kidneys, and brain.

The following manifestations:

- *Dactylitis* (pain and/or swelling of the hands or feet): The spleen can become engorged with blood cells in a "splenic sequestration," and the child presents with splenic crisis with severe anemia. The spleen is particularly vulnerable to infarction. Individuals with SCD who are not on hydroxyurea or transfusion therapy virtually become functionally asplenic with time, thus increasing their risk for certain types of infections with capsulated organisms.
- Acute chest syndrome.
- Chronic hemolysis can result in anemia, jaundice, cholelithiasis, and delayed growth and sexual maturation. Individuals with the highest rates of hemolysis are predisposed to pulmonary artery hypertension, priapism, and leg ulcers but may be relatively protected from vaso-occlusive pain.

Other forms of SCD result from coinheritance of HbS with other abnormal β-globin chain variants, the most common form in India being sickle β-thalassemia (HbS/β⁺-thalassemia and HbS/β⁰-thalassemia). Others are sickle E, sickle D-Punjab, sickle HbC, sickle O-Arab, etc.

Diagnosis

The diagnosis of SCD is established by identification of HbS in significant quantities. Mutation testing confirms the diagnosis.

Newborn screening programs perform isoelectric focusing sometimes with HPLC of an eluate of dried blood spots. It is always prudent to confirm results with molecular testing.

Management: Refer to chapter of hematology.

Genetic Counseling and Prenatal Testing

As girls grow up, the family should be aware about pregnancy management. Pregnant women with SCD require close follow-up and monitoring. There is an increased risk for preterm labor, thrombosis, infectious complications, and acute painful episodes during pregnancy. Hydroxyurea should be discontinued during pregnancy.

Sickle cell disease (homozygous) is an autosomal recessive condition. The risk of recurrence in siblings is 25%. When a person with homozygous SCD marries a person who is a carrier (heterozygous/trait) of sickle cell, the risk of recurrence in offspring is 50%. This phenomenon is called "pseudo-dominance."

Prenatal testing in sickle cell is debatable, since the disease even in homozygous form has mild manifestations in many individuals and has various treatment options. Though not as frequent as for β-thalassemia, many couples do opt for prenatal testing, especially those who have experienced severe morbidity and mortality in the family.

Neural Tube Defect

Neural tube defect is one of the most common major malformations found in a fetus or a neonate. An analysis of around 515,500 births from various parts of India revealed the frequency of anencephaly as 2.5 per 1,000 and that of spina bifida as 1.5 per 1,000. The overall prevalence was extremely high in north India, especially in the state of Punjab (more than 4 per 1,000 births).[9]

Neural tube defects can result from alterations in any of the processes that are involved in the formation of the primary neural tube. Though the underlying causes of neural tube closure defects are likely to be quite heterogeneous, periconceptional folic acid supplementation has been found to reduce the risk by around 70%. The process of neurulation occurs at the 4th week of human gestation. This gives the idea about the requirement of folic acid much early in the development even before the woman has learned that she is pregnant as she misses a period. It is recommended that a woman should start taking folic acid as soon as she plans a pregnancy (at least 3 months prior to pregnancy) to prevent NTDs in the fetus. The common practice of starting folic acid after a positive pregnancy test offers limited protection.

Classification

The failure of neural tube closure is associated with defects in the overlying bony structures (i.e. cranial vault and neural arches) resulting in exposure of the underlying neural tissue. As a result, defects of primary neural tube closure are often referred to as "open" NTDs. Further classifications of the NTDs are based on the location and extent of the defect.

Anencephaly: In this condition, there is absence of the cranial vault along with markedly diminished cerebral hemispheres. The cerebellum might also be absent and the brain stem hypoplastic. As per severity, anencephaly is classified as holocrania and mesocrania:

- *Holocrania*: When the defect involves the foramen magnum
- *Merocrania*: When the foramen magnum is not involved.

Folic acid deficiency in the mother is still considered to be the most common cause of anencephaly. Sometimes, genetic or chromosomal disorders are also implicated. Rarely anencephaly is seen as a disruption sequence following amniotic band entanglement of the fetus *in utero*.

Most fetuses with anencephaly are either aborted spontaneously or undergo medical termination following detection of the defect by prenatal ultrasonography. On rare occasions, anencephalic infants are live born and can survive for short periods without significant medical support. This disorder is considered universally as a lethal disorder.

Acalvaria: Acalvaria is a condition often diagnosed as anencephaly. Unlike in anencephaly, there is not much diminution of brain size. The cranial contents in acalvaria are generally complete, though there can be associated pathologies in the brain. It consists of absence of the calvarial bones, dura mater, and associated muscles in the presence of a normal skull base and normal facial bones. It is considered to be a postneurulation defect. The likely pathogenesis of acalvaria is faulty migration of the membranous neurocranium. The normal placement of the embryonic ectoderm results in an intact layer of skin over the brain parenchyma. Some children are reported to live for some time in case studies.

Encephaloceles: They are characterized by protrusion of intracranial contents through a congenital defect in the dura and skull. They are usually midline defects and based on the anatomical locations they are named as:

- Occipital
- Parietal
- Temporal
- Frontal or frontoethmoidal (sincipital)
- Transsphenoidal
- Nasal.

As per the contents, pathologically they are sometimes classified as meningocele (leptomeninges and CSF), meningoencephalocele (leptomeninges, CSF, and brain), meningoencephalocystocele (leptomeninges, CSF, brain, and ventricles), atretic cephalocele (small nodule of fibrous fatty tissue), or gliocele (CSF lined by glial tissue).

Sometimes occipital encephaloceles are associated with known single gene defects, e.g. Meckel–Gruber syndrome, where there is occipital encephalocele associated with enlarged polycystic kidneys with or without polydactyly.

Iniencephaly: It is a rare NTD that combines extreme retroflexion (backward bending) of the head associated with occipital bone defects and defects in the cervicothoracic spine.

Craniorachischisis: Craniorachischisis, also called craniospinal rachischisis, is failure of neural tube closure over the entire body axis **(Fig. 7)**. It is a lethal condition.

Spina bifida: Neural tube closure defects that are restricted to the caudal portion of the neural tube are referred to generally as spina bifida or sometimes as meningomyeloceles.

This condition is associated with bony defects in the overlying neural arches, through which the meninges and spinal cord tissue are exposed to the body surface.

Most lumbosacral meningomyeloceles are associated with Chiari II (Arnold Chiari) malformation and ventricular dilatation **(Fig. 8)**.

The majority of babies with meningomyeloceles are live born. These babies need to be evaluated for associated ventricular dilatation and other neurological functioning like lower limb movements soon after birth. With proper neurosurgical intervention and medical treatment, survival into the adulthood is common. Neurosurgical interventions mainly comprise repair of the defect and ventriculoperitoneal shunt for associated hydrocephalus. However, many such babies might have residual neurodeficit such as bladder incontinence and lower limb weakness, even after successful surgical correction.

Occult spinal dysraphisms: Occult spinal dysraphism includes meningocele (that may be partially skin

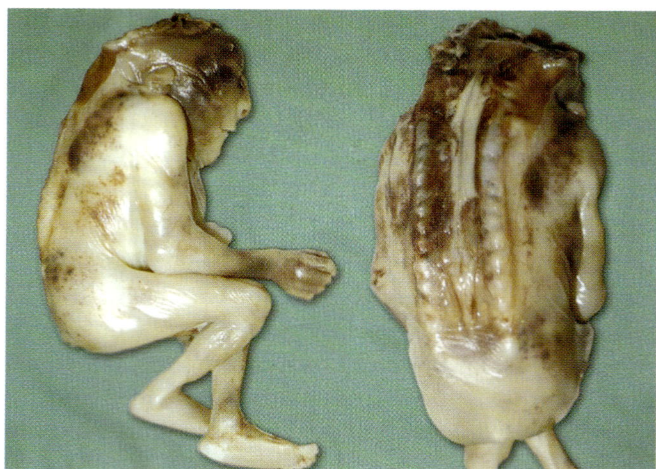

Fig. 7: *Craniorachischisis*: Fetus with craniorachischisis showing failure of neural tube closure over the entire body axis.

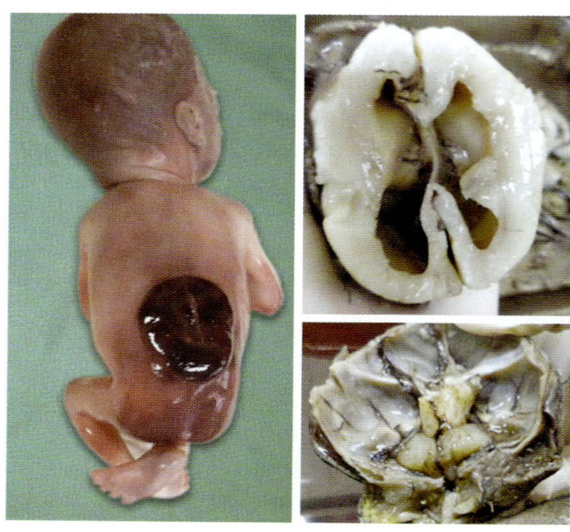

Fig. 8: *Lumbosacral meningomyelocele*: Typical lumbosacral meningomyelocele with Arnold–Chiari malformation (caudally displaced cerebellar vermis) with lateral ventricular dilatation in brain. Such displaced and compressed cerebellum is described as "banana sign" in antenatal ultrasonography.

covered), spinal lipomas (lipomyelomeningocele or lipomeningocele), myelocystocele, split cord malformations, and various forms of sacral agenesis. A number of closed or skin-covered conditions such as encephalocele, iniencephaly along with occult spinal dysraphisms are sometimes referred to as closed NTDs as opposed to the open NTDs (anencephaly, meningomyelocele or spina bifida, and craniorachischisis). In general, the occult spinal dysraphisms are conditions, thought not to result from defects in primary neural tube closure but may arise due to defects in secondary neural tube development.

Risk Factors for Neural Tube Defects

The open NTDs, which are relatively common, are recognized as being etiologically heterogeneous.

Folic acid deficiency: Folic acid deficiency in the mother has been implicated as the single most important risk factor for NTDs. It has been shown that the incidence decreases by 50–70% by folic acid supplementation in women in childbearing age, in various studies.

Though found in a small number of individuals, the following are other risk factors for NTDs:
- *Maternal use of medications*: Valproic acid, carbamazepine (CBZ), etc. or other antifolate drugs.
- *Family history*: Risk in siblings of affected individuals is 3–8%.
- Maternal insulin-dependent diabetes.
- *Obesity*: The risk of having a child with an NTD increases with increasing maternal body mass index (BMI).
- *Hyperthermia*: There is an increased risk for NTDs, in particular anencephaly, in infants whose mothers were exposed to hyperthermia during the first trimester of pregnancy.
- *Reproductive technologies*: There is an association between assisted reproductive technologies and the risk of congenital malformations, including NTDs.
- Autoantibodies to folate receptors.
- Environmental occupational hazards.
- *Chromosomal and genetic disorders*: Though rare, some chromosomal and Mendelian disorders have been associated with NTD.

Prevention Strategies

Neural tube defects as a group are amenable to prevention at different stages.

Primary prevention: Use of periconceptional folic acid (starting 3 months prior to conception as a common practice) is being universally accepted as the best prevention strategy. The recommended dose is 0.5 mg daily; however, the preparation available in the market contains 5 mg of folic acid per tablet. Folic acid is a water-soluble vitamin and the extra is supposed to be excreted in urine without any side effects.

Fortification of food with folic acid has been tried by some countries.

Secondary prevention: Screening to identify pregnant women, who are at an increased risk of carrying an NTD-affected fetus, can be achieved by the evaluation of maternal serum alpha-fetoprotein levels as a part of biochemical screening for aneuploidies (such as triple test). However, a more practical approach is a careful ultrasonography, as a part of anomaly scan. It is likely to pick up a high percentage of all NTDs before 20 weeks of gestation (legal gestational age for termination of the affected pregnancy). When a diagnosis of spina bifida is confirmed by ultrasound before 20 weeks of gestation, the couple needs to be counseled about the advantages of detection of the anomaly before the legal gestational age of termination of pregnancy. Ultrasonography and sometimes fetal MRI are used to identify spontaneous leg movements, spine deformities, and the presence of associated Chiari II malformation. The couple can take decisions of termination of pregnancy or continuation of the same according to the associated complications, probable outcome after surgery, and social and religious beliefs.

Management and Outcome

Although anencephaly and craniorachischisis are lethal conditions, individuals with spina bifida can survive with appropriate medical and surgical treatment. Those babies who are live born with a spina bifida are likely to get their spinal lesion closed postnatally early in the neonatal period, usually within 3 days after birth. In advanced centers, a small proportion of fetuses undergo surgeries *in utero*. Literature depicts better outcome in babies who undergo surgeries *in utero*; however, the expertise required for such procedures is high. Whether treated *in utero* or postnatally, children with spina bifida are at risk of hydrocephalus, complications of Chiari II malformations, lower limb paralysis, sensory loss, bowel and bladder dysfunction, spinal deformities, and club foot. Though most children treated adequately have normal intelligence, some cognitive and learning problems are common in such children. The most important determinant of neurological outcome is the level of the lesion—the more proximal the lesion, the poorer the outcome. Postsurgery, 1-year survival among individuals with spina bifida is around 85–90%; however, many of these individuals have significant comorbidities and increased mortality, sometimes presenting as sudden death.

Genetic Counseling

Apart from the issues for counseling mentioned in the preceding text, the couple must be counseled about the chance of chromosomal abnormality, single gene disorder, or teratogenic exposure in a small percentage of such babies. Prenatal testing for chromosomes and probable single gene disorders should be offered to all couples.

Those who opt for termination with or without prenatal testing should be offered postmortem examination. Such testing and examination are essential for effective genetic counseling which helps couples to take future reproductive decisions. Recurrence risk depends on the underlying cause, if any. When a chromosomal and single gene disorder is not identified, the empiric recurrence risk is around 3–5%. Special care should be taken during counseling of women, where there is a probable teratogenic cause. Women on antiepileptic drugs need to be counseled about possible teratogenic effects including NTD. As a rule, possible monotherapy at possible lowest dose for effective control of seizures needs to be adjusted prepregnancy. Valproate use should be preferably avoided in pregnant women by all possible means.

Congenital Heart Disease

Heart malformation is one of the most common birth defects, affecting about 7 in 10,000 newborns. Despite the high prevalence of the disease, the role of genetics was not recognized in the past. Children with heart defects are now surviving till adulthood, thanks to surgical advances; this bring families and their treating physicians to think about recurrences and possible methods to prevent recurrences. With increasing awareness about genetics and availability of cytogenetic and molecular genetic testing facilities, pediatric cardiologists and surgeons have started taking interest in genetic workup and prenatal testing facilities.

As with most congenital and genetic disorders, all children with congenital heart defects need clinical genetic evaluation. This includes a detailed history taking, dysmorphology evaluation by a trained geneticist, and relevant tests related to the possible etiology. A detailed family history might give a clue toward a known form of familial heart defect, and antenatal history might identify a known teratogen. This brief overview will focus on various disorders in major groups.

Chromosomal Defects

Children with congenital cardiac disorders require a routine chromosomal analysis whether or not a child has clinical features of a known chromosomal disorder. The common chromosomal disorders are listed in **Table 6**.

Microdeletion Syndromes

It is to be remembered that the large telomeric deletions or duplications may be detected by routine karyotype; however small deletions or duplications, also called CNVs (copy number variations), may be missed and might require other modalities such as FISH, MLPA, or cytogenetic microarray for confirmation. Some common microdeletion syndromes are easily recognizable and are listed in **Table 7**.

Table 6: Chromosomal disorders associated with congenital heart disease (CHD).

Chromosomal disorder	Percent with CHD	Main features	Heart anomaly
Trisomy 21 (Down syndrome)	40–50	Hypotonia, mental retardation epicanthal fold transverse palmar crease, brachydactyly	AVSD, VSD, ASD, TOF
Trisomy 13 (Patau syndrome)	80	Polydactyly, cleft lip and palate, holoprosencephaly, profound mental retardation, omphalocele, 80% die in first year	ASD, VSD, PDA, HLHS, laterality defects, atrial isomerism
Trisomy 18 (Edwards syndrome)	90–100	IUGR, rocker-bottom feet, overlapping fingers and toes, profound mental retardation; 90% die in first year	ASD, VSD, PDA, TOF, DORV, D-TGA, CoA
Monosomy X (Turner syndrome, 45,X)	25–35	Lymphedema of hands and feet, widely spaced hypoplastic nipples, webbed neck, primary amenorrhea, short stature	CoA, BAV, valvar AS, HLHS, aortic dissection
Klinefelter syndrome (47,XXY)	50	Usually normal appearing, tall stature, small testes, delayed puberty, variable mental retardation	MVP, venous thromboembolic disease, PDA, ASD
Deletion 4p (Wolf–Hirschhorn syndrome)	50–65	Pronounced microcephaly, widely spaced eyes, Greek helmet appearance of nose, severe mental retardation and seizures	ASD, VSD, PDA
Deletion 5p (cri du chat)	30–60	Cat-like cry, prenatal and postnatal growth retardation, round face, widely spaced eyes, epicanthal fold, simian crease, severe mental retardation	VSD, ASD, PDA

(ASD: atrial septal defect; AS: aortic stenosis; AVSD: atrioventricular septal defect; BAV: bicuspid aortic valve; CoA: coarctation of the aorta; DORV: double outlet right ventricle; D-TGA: D-transposition of great arteries; HLHS: hypoplastic left heart syndrome; IUGR: intrauterine growth retardation; MVP: mitral valve prolapse; PDA: patent ductus artery; TOF: tetralogy of Fallot; VSD: ventricular septal defect)

Table 7: Recognizable microdeletion syndromes associated with congenital heart disease (CHD).

Microdeletion (interstitial)	Percent with CHD	Main features	Heart anomaly
Deletion 22q11 (DiGeorge, velocardiofacial syndrome)	75	Prominent nose, thymic and parathyroid hypoplasia, hypocalcemia, feeding/speech/learning/behavioral disorders, immunodeficiency, palate/skeletal/renal anomalies	IAA-B, truncus arteriosus, isolated aortic arch anomalies, VSD
Deletion 7q11.23 (Williams–Beuren syndrome)	53–85	Infantile hypercalcemia, skeletal and renal anomalies, cognitive deficits, "social" personality, elfin facies	Supravalvar AS and PS, PPS

(AS: aortic stenosis; IAA-B: interrupted aortic arch type B; PS: pulmonary stenosis; PPS: peripheral pulmonary stenosis; VSD: ventricular septal defect)

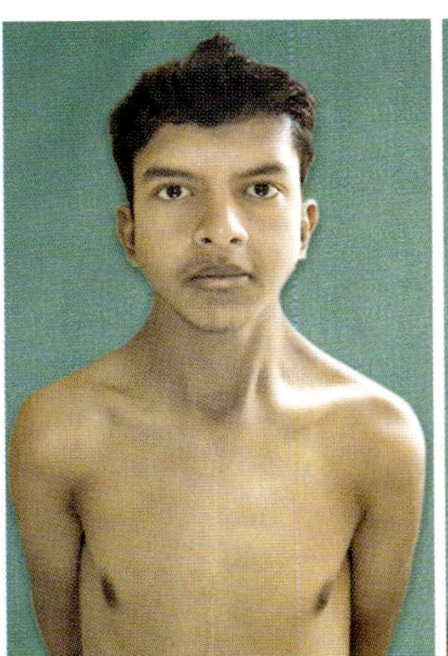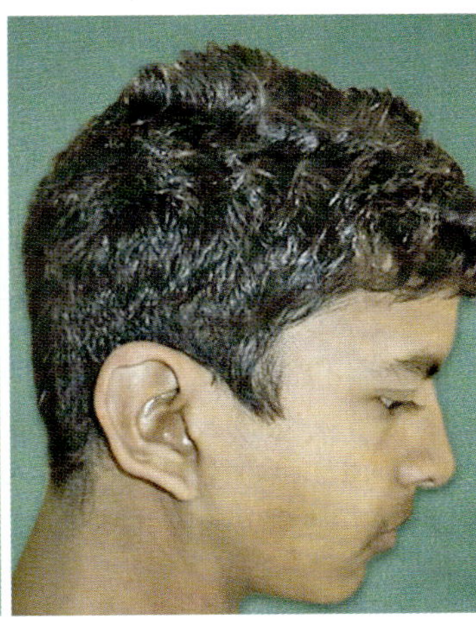

Fig. 9: *Noonan syndrome*: Typical recognizable features of Noonan syndrome includes eyes that are wide-spaced, downslanted, with epicanthal folds and ptosis; ears that are low-set, posteriorly rotated with fleshy helices; broad or webbed neck; superior pectus carinatum, widely set nipples.

Single Gene Disorders

Many congenital cardiac disorders are due to defect in genes which have been recognized to have a specific phenotype. Knowing the gene and the pattern of inheritance, genetic counseling and prenatal testing have become feasible. Mutation testing in most such cases are done by molecular methods involving PCR and sequencing techniques. The list of single gene disorder is large, notable are Noonan syndrome (*PTPN11* and other genes),[10] Holt–Oram syndrome (*TBX 5* gene), etc. Noonan syndrome is a fairly common, autosomal dominant disorder, which is clinically recognizable by the facial features **(Fig. 9)**.

Teratogens

A teratogen is an agent that can produce a permanent alteration of structure or function in an organism exposed during embryonic or fetal life. An important example is congenital rubella, which presents with the triad of sensorineural deafness, eye abnormalities (retinopathy, cataract, glaucoma, or microphthalmia), and congenital heart disease (pulmonary artery stenosis or patent ductus arteriosus), present in around 50% of patients.

Nonsyndromic Isolated Heart Malformations

Nonsyndromic isolated heart malformations are usually sporadic; particular defects such as atrial septal defect (ASD) can be inherited. Many genes are found to be involved in the development of heart. The possibility that several genes might act additively for a defect is being suggested.[11] Empirical risk for siblings for isolated heart malformations is 2–5% and empirical risk for offspring 3–5%. Various risk assessment models are being tried to assess risk in future pregnancies; however, careful evaluation is required in each case.

■ REFERENCES

1. Gorospe JR, Singhal BS, Kainu T, et al. Indian Agarwal megalencephalic leukodystrophy with cysts is caused by a common MLC1 mutation. Neurology. 2004;62(6):878-82.
2. Verma IC, Bijarnia S. The burden of genetic disorders in India and a framework for community control. Community Genet. 2002;5(3):192-6.
3. Nadkarni AH, Gorakshakar AC, Sawant PM, et al. The phenotypic and molecular diversity of hemoglobinopathies in India: A review of 15 years at a referral center. Int J Lab Hematol. 2019;41(2):218-26.
4. Galanello R, Melis MA, Ruggeri R, et al. Beta 0 thalassemia trait in Sardinia. Hemoglobin. 1979;3(1):33-46.
5. Telen MJ, Kaufman RE. The mature erythrocyte. In: Lee GR, Paraskevas F, Foerster J, Lukens J (Eds). Wintrobe's Clinical Hematology, 10th edition. Baltimore, MD: Lippincott Williams & Wilkins; 1999. p. 207.
6. Taher A, Vichinsky E, Musallam K, et al. Guidelines for the Management of Non Transfusion Dependent Thalassaemia (NTDT) [Internet]. Nicosia, Cyprus: Thalassemia International Foundation; 2013.
7. Cappellini MD, Cohen A, Porter J, et al. Guidelines for the Management of Transfusion Dependent Thalassaemia (TDT), 3rd edition. Nicosia, Cyprus: Thalassemia International Foundation; 2014.
8. Serjeant GR, Ghosh K, Patel J. Sickle cell disease in India: A perspective. Indian J Med Res. 2016;143(1):21-4.
9. Verma IC. High frequency of neural-tube defects in North India. Lancet. 1978;1(8069):879-80.
10. Narayanan DL, Pandey H, Moirangthem A, et al. Hotspots in PTPN11 gene among Indian children with Noonan syndrome. Indian Pediatr. 2017;54(8):638-43.
11. Hirayama-Yamada K, Kamisago M, Akimoto K, et al. Phenotypes with GATA4 or NKX2.5 mutations in familial atrial septal defect. Am J Med Genet A. 2005;135(1):47-52.

Hematological Disorders in the Tropics

Maharshi Trivedi, Pooja Dewan

Disorders of blood or reticuloendothelial system are fairly common in tropics and subtropics. These include infectious causes (like malaria, dengue, leishmaniasis, etc.) or noninfectious conditions including nutritional anemias. In this chapter, we will cover mainly the noninfectious hematological conditions prevalent in tropics.

■ THALASSEMIA

Thalassemia is a genetic disorder characterized by reduction in globin chain synthesis. Depending on whether there is a decreased production of α or β globin chain, thalassemia may be labeled as α- or β-thalassemia, respectively.

Gene for β globin chain is located on chromosome 11, one gene on each chromosome. β-thalassemia syndromes are a result of genetic mutations in both these genes. In β^0-thalassemia, there will be complete absence of the β-globin, while β^+ and β^- thalassemia denotes decreased amounts of normal β-globin. β-thalassemia major is used to describe the most severe form of transfusion dependent β-thalassemia with a presentation in early age. β-thalassemia intermedia is the term used for thalassemia that generally is asymptomatic in childhood and these patients begin to require blood transfusion in adolescence. Thalassemia carriers or traits or minor, with a single β-globin mutation, are usually asymptomatic but are found to have microcytosis on peripheral smear and mild anemia.[1] Based on the clinical severity, β-thalassemia is categorized as *β-thalassemia major, minor,* and *intermedia.*

Chromosome 16 carries the gene for α globin. Normal individuals have four α globin genes. An α^0 or α^- mutation indicates absence of α-chain production, and α^+ mutation results in decreased amount of α-globin chain. Mutation of one α gene causes carrier state, mutation of two genes produces α-thalassemia minor, mutation of three genes results in hemoglobin H (HbH) disease, and mutation of all four genes produces fatal Bart's hydrops fetalis.[2]

In India nearly 4% of the population has thalassemia minor while annually 12,000 new children of thalassemia major are added to the normal population.[3] More than 200 different mutations could lead to thalassemia. Of these, the 20 most common mutations are responsible for 80% of the known thalassemias worldwide. Thalassemia is more common in North-West India. The case rate can be as high as 5–15% in some ethnic groups of North India (*Punjabis* and *Sindhis*).

Pathophysiology

Basic pathophysiology in β-thalassemia constitutes: (1) inadequate β-globin gene production which results in inadequate amount of HbA and (2) imbalance between α and β globin chain production. Alpha globin chains are in excess to non-α globin chains, and α globin tetramers ($\alpha4$) are formed, which get precipitated in red cell precursors, damaging the red cell membrane and causing early red cell death. There is compensatory erythroid hyperplasia and bone marrow (BW) expansion. In β-thalassemias, the excess of α chains combine with γ chains, resulting in increased fetal hemoglobin (HbF$\alpha_2\gamma_2$), and δ-chain producing relative or absolute increase in HbA$_2$ production ($\alpha_2\delta_2$).[4]

In the α-thalassemia syndromes, an excess of β and γ globin chains is produced which form Bart hemoglobin (γ_4) in fetal life and HbH (β_4) after birth, which have a very high oxygen affinity, and result in extravascular hemolysis. Most severe form of α-thalassemia (hydrops fetalis) results *in utero* anemia and fetal loss.[2] As β-thalassemia is more prevalent in India, focus of our discussion is mainly on features and management of β-thalassemia.

Clinical Presentation

The clinical manifestation of thalassemia is as a result of reduced normal hemoglobin in erythrocytes which leads to increased hemolysis and ineffective red cell production.[3] Infants become anemic between 3 months and 18 months of age and require regular blood transfusions. As these children grow, they develop thalassemic facies characterized by malar prominence due to flattened facial bones. Hepatosplenomegaly develops due to extramedullary hematopoiesis. Chronically transfused children will have features of iron overload. Hemosiderosis affects the cardiac, hepatic, endocrinal glandular, and skin tissues. Patients with β-thalassemia intermedia can present in later half of first decade with mild-to-moderate anemia and variable transfusion requirements.[1]

Management

Transfusion Therapy

Packed red cell transfusion therapy should be started once diagnosis is established and at hemoglobin cut-off of <7 g/dL documented on at least two occasions.[5] Children are transfused every 3–4 weeks with the aim to maintain a pretransfusion hemoglobin level of 9.5–10.5 g/dL (also known as moderate transfusion). A pretransfusion hemoglobin level of 11–12 g/dL (hematocrit level >27%) is recommended for patients with cardiac comorbidity or other medical conditions and for those patients with evidence of extramedullary hematopoiesis (known as hypertransfusion regimen).[5] While in case of supertransfusion regimens hemoglobin is never allowed to fall below 13 g/dL (hematocrit >35%).[6]

Before starting transfusion therapy child's extensive red cell phenotype and/or genotype should be done. Also, genetic counseling followed by human leukocyte antigen (HLA) typing of sibling and parents can help ascertain the possibility of finding a suitable donor for hematopoietic stem cell transplantation (HSCT). Hepatitis B vaccination should be offered at the earliest.[3]

It is preferable to transfuse irradiated or washed packed cells, because it reduces the risk of transfusion transmitted of infection and also protects against the development of antibodies against leukocyte or platelet antigens (alloimmunization), respectively. Leukocytes can also be filtered out at the time of transfusion by using microfilters (leukodepletion). Cytomegalovirus-negative red cell units are indicated in stem cell transplantation candidates.

In patients with nontransfusion dependent thalassemia (NTDT), worse outcome has been seen at hemoglobin less than 10 g/L.[7]

Iron Overload Monitoring

Conventional tests to measure iron level are serum ferritin and liver biopsies. Invention of super conducting quantum interference device (SQUID) and magnetic resonance imaging (MRI) T2 FerriScan has replaced invasive procedure of liver biopsy nowadays and it is useful for quantifying liver and cardiac iron load. Serum ferritin concentrations should be measured every 3–6 months.[8,9] Serum ferritin concentrations consistently higher than 2,500 µg/L indicate a need for optimization of iron-chelation therapy.[8,10,11] In patients with NTDT, chelation should be initiated if ferritin concentrations exceed 800 µg/L. Once ferritin concentration is less than 300 µg/L, chelation therapy may be discontinued.[9] Other tests for measuring iron load depends upon target organ to be evaluated like such as ECHO for cardiac function, thyroid stimulating hormone (TSH), T3 and T4 levels to assess effect of iron overload over thyroid, and similarly estimation of growth hormone levels, serum testosterone, gonadotropins, venous blood sugars (fasting, postprandial or random), hemoglobin A1C (HbA1C), dual-energy X-ray absorptiometry (DEXA) scans, etc. to evaluate other hormone deficiencies.[10,11]

Chelation Therapy

Currently approved iron chelators are: (1) desferrioxamine, (2) deferasirox, and (3) deferiprone. Indication for starting chelation therapy are: (1) serum ferritin is >1,000 µg/L or (2) the child has received 15–20 units of transfusion; usually this occurs after 1 year of transfusion therapy.[3,8]

Desferrioxamine has half-life of less than 30 minutes necessitating subcutaneous or intravenous administration. It should be administered over 8–10 hour daily, 5–7 days/week. Dose is 20–40 mg/kg. Problems with desferrioxamine are noncompliance because of the route of administration, bradycardia and hypotension on intravenous administration, local reaction, allergy on subcutaneous administration, ototoxicity, retinal changes, and bone dysplasia with truncal shortening.[3,8]

Deferasirox requires once-a-day administration because of long half-life of 16 hours. Dose is 20–40 mg/kg. Common adverse effects are gastrointestinal symptoms, increase in creatinine and increase in liver enzymes. It causes excretion of iron through fecal route.[3,8]

Deferiprone has a half-life of approximately 3 hours and given in doses of 75–100 mg/kg/day in three divided doses. It reduces cardiac iron load effectively. Side effects of deferiprone include transient agranulocytosis, gastrointestinal side effects, and arthralgia.[3,8]

Combination therapy is advised in case of high serum ferritin despite compliance to a single chelating agent, or evidence of cardiac, hepatic, and endocrine dysfunctions due to hemosiderosis.[3,8,12]

Hydroxyurea

Hydroxyurea (HU) is used in persons with thalassemia intermedia to reduce extramedullary hematopoiesis, increase the hemoglobin levels, and, in some cases, to improve leg ulcers, decrease the vascular disease, and pulmonary hypertension. It is usually started at a dose of 10 mg/kg.[4]

Bone Marrow Transplant

This option should be offered in case of availability of HLA-matched sibling. The most important factors affecting the survival after HSCT are: (1) presence of hepatomegaly, (2) portal fibrosis, and (3) serum ferritin >1,000 µg/L. Transplant conditioning, graft-versus-host disease, and graft failure together may account for 5–10% mortality and this could be a major deterrent to HSCT.[1,3]

Splenectomy

Patients developing splenomegaly, features of hypersplenism, or with annual packed red cell transfusion requirement in excess of 200 cc/kg may warrant a splenectomy.[8,9] There is increased risk of venous thrombosis, pulmonary hypertension after splenectomy. They are also predisposed to increased occurrence of leg ulcers and silent cerebral infarctions post splenectomy.[13,14] It should be undertaken only after 6 years of age, after vaccination against diseases due to *Streptococcus pneumoniae*, *Haemophilus influenzae*, and *Neisseria meningitidis* at least 3–4 weeks before the surgery. Prophylactic penicillin therapy must be continued life-long after splenectomy.

Preventive Monitoring

Serial echocardiograms are needed to monitor the cardiac function and pulmonary artery pressure. After 8 years of chronic transfusion therapy, cardiac T2* MRI studies are recommended.[8,15] Children older than 5 years or those having at least 3-year duration of chronic transfusions should be monitored for endocrine dysfunction.[8,15] Height, weight, and sitting height and nutritional assessments should be monitored.

■ SICKLE CELL DISEASE

Sickle cell disease (SCD) is a group of inherited disorders that is defined by the presence of atypical hemoglobin molecules called "hemoglobin S". The red blood cells (RBCs) with hemoglobin S are prone to distortion into a sickle, or crescent shape, in the presence of hypoxia, high altitude, dehydration, change in temperature, or stress. SCD is the most common monogenic disorder.[16] Tribals in India have a very high prevalence of SCD.[17]

Pathophysiology

Sickle cell disease is a result of single gene mutation of β globin chain where glutamine is replaced by valine at 6th position (i.e. *HBB* Glu6Val, rs334). Most severe of the SCD spectrum is homozygous HbSS (sickle cell anemia) which results due to inheritance of βS from both parents. Other forms include compound heterozygous conditions, HbSC, HbS/β⁰-thalassemia or HbS/β⁺ or HbS/β⁻ thalassemia, HbSD, HbSE or HbSO Arab. Coinheritance of HbA and HbS (HbAS) results in sickle cell trait which might also be mildly symptomatic.[18] With the exception of HbS–β⁰-thalassemia, other compound heterozygous genotypes have milder form of disease.[18,19]

Sickle cell disease is characterized by abnormal erythrocytes damaged by HbS. HbS polymerizes in conditions of hypoxia or dehydration. This in turn can damage the erythrocyte membranes leading to hemolysis and vaso-occlusion. HbS polymerization, vaso-occlusion, and hemolytic anemia precipitate a cascade of pathologic events, which include vascular-endothelial dysfunction, nitric oxide deficiency, inflammation, oxidative stress, hypercoagulability, increased neutrophil adhesiveness, and platelet activation.[18]

Clinical Features and Complications[18,19]

Clinical features and complications of SCD are mentioned in **Table 1**. Chronic complications may be attributed to either large vessel vasculopathy or progressive ischemic organ damage.

Diagnosis

Anemia with reticulocytosis, presence of target cell and Howell-Jolly bodies, are seen on peripheral smear. Sickling of the RBCs can be induced by the addition of sodium

Table 1: Clinical features and complications of sickle cell disease.	
Acute complications[18,19]	
Painful event	Dactylitis, pain in ribs, sternum, long bones, and priapism
Infection	Bacteremia, sepsis, meningitis, osteomyelitis, pneumonia especially from encapsulated organisms such as *Streptococcus pneumoniae* and *Haemophilus influenzae* type B; malaria
Anemia	Due to splenic sequestration (sequestration crisis), transient aplastic crisis, transfusion reaction or papillary necrosis, and acute hemolytic crisis with coexistent G6PD deficiency
Other organ damage	Ischemic stroke, acute chest syndrome*, papillary necrosis, and splenic infarct
Chronic organ damage[18,19]	
Kidney	Hyposthenuria, glomerular hyperfiltration, glomerulosclerosis, hematuria, albuminuria, end-stage renal disease, and nocturnal enuresis
Heart/lung	Restrictive lung disease, elevated tricuspid jet velocity, pulmonary hypertension, restrictive cardiomyopathy, dysrhythmias, and sudden death
Central nervous system	Acute ischemic stroke, hemorrhagic stroke, venous sinus thrombosis, silent cerebral infarction, chronic pain, and cognitive impairment
Liver/gastrointestinal system	Jaundice, cholelithiasis, cholangiopathy, hepatopathy, and mesenteric vaso-occlusion
Spleen	Infarction and hyposplenism
Musculoskeletal system/skin	Avascular necrosis and leg ulcers
Eyes	Proliferative retinopathy and orbital infarction
Genital	Impotence and infertility

*Acute chest syndrome is characterized by fever, respiratory symptoms (cough) with new pulmonary infiltrates and hypoxemia; and can range in severity from mild respiratory distress to acute lung disease.

metabisulfite which may then be seen on a peripheral blood smear. "Sickle solubility test" is a useful test to detect the presence of hemoglobin S. Diagnosis is established by hemoglobin electrophoresis, using standard alkaline gel, isoelectric focusing (IEF), capillary zone electrophoresis (CZE), or high performance liquid chromatography (HPLC). Recent advances include diagnosis based on deoxyribonucleic acid (DNA) microarrays.[18]

Management

Supportive Management

Appropriate analgesia using nonsteroidal anti-inflammatory drugs (NSAIDs) and opioid agents should be provided.[20] For children presenting with acute chest syndrome, antibiotics covering microorganisms including pneumococcus, chlamydia, and mycoplasma, oxygen therapy and blood transfusion are recommended. Respiratory deterioration with worsening hypoxemia and acute stroke necessitates urgent exchange transfusion.[18] Sequestration crisis may be managed by good supportive care including blood transfusion and is a medical emergency.

Prevention of Infection

Penicillin V at a dose of 62.5–250 mg per day at least until 5 years of age should be given. Children should be vaccinated with pneumococcal vaccines beginning at the age of 2 years and followed by a booster shot every 5 years. Malarial prophylaxis should be given when appropriate. Parents should be educated to consult a healthcare professional for fever.[20]

Blood Transfusion

Red cell transfusion constitutes the most important component of treatment for SCD. There are two types of transfusion: (1) simple transfusion and (2) chronic transfusion.

Indications for simple transfusion are: (1) acute splenic sequestration, (2) transient aplastic crisis, (3) symptomatic severe anemia, (4) severe acute chest syndrome, and (5) preoperative preparation. This is aimed at reducing the proportion of sickle hemoglobin to improve oxygenation and to prevent acute vaso-occlusion with target hemoglobin level ≥10 g/dL.

Child should be put on chronic transfusion therapy in events of clinical stroke, transcranial Doppler (TCD) showing high time average mean velocity of ≥200 cm/sec, and multisystem organ dysfunction. Pregnancy, hepatic sequestration, and recurrent splenic sequestration are other indications for transfusion.[18]

For primary stroke prevention or prevention of additional silent cerebral infarctions HbS should be kept,

<30% by frequent transfusions (every 3–6 weeks). In case of secondary stroke prevention target, HbS should be kept <30% or <50% with transfusions every 3–6 weeks.[18,19]

Hydroxyurea

Hydroxyurea is a powerful inducer of HbF production. HbF inhibits intracellular HbS polymerization, and in turn reduces the morbidity and mortality. The dose for HU is 10–20 mg/kg/day which helps in preventing acute pain, acute chest syndrome, and primary stroke.[19]

Transplant

Transplant using stem cells harvested from BW or umbilical cord has shown an overall survival and event-free survival of 90%. Transplantations are effective in preventing future clinical complications associated with vaso-occlusion due to sickled hemoglobin.[18,21,22] However, the nonavailability of unaffected MSDs and the high mortality and morbidity following HSCT are the major obstacles.

Universal Transcranial-Doppler Screening

Children with maximum time-averaged mean velocity (TAMV) of blood flow in the intracranial arteries ≥200 cm/sec are at highest risk of developing stroke. Evidence suggests that TCD screening can be a major weapon to tackle primary stroke in SCD. Additionally, it can be used to monitor the response to treatment.[18,23]

Prevention of Cerebrovascular Disease

The need for prophylactic transfusions must be justified as there would be issues like iron overload, increased costs, and availability of phenotype-matched blood supply. As per the recommendations of National Institutes of Health (NIH), infants ≥9 months of age should be prescribed hydroxycarbamide. However, its use may be deferred as it may be toxic and adversely affect the fertility. Early HSCT, before developing stroke, seems promising.[18,24]

Early screening of neonates and comprehensive care can curb the morbidity and mortality of SCD patients in the first decade of life.[17]

■ APLASTIC ANEMIA

Aplastic anemia (AA) is a serious and potentially life-threatening BW failure disorder. It can occur across all ages but it typically has two peak ages viz. mid to late childhood and another peak in the geriatric age group. Incidence is 2–3 per million in developed countries whereas Asian studies from India, Thailand, and China have showed 2–3 times higher incidence.[25,26] Etiology of AA can be inherited or acquired (**Table 2**).

Clinical Features

Anemia leads to fatigue, headaches, breathlessness, palpitations, and rarely chest pain in severe anemia. Leukopenia, especially neutropenia, can predispose the patient to infections. Thrombocytopenia leads to increased tendency for bruising and bleeding. Inherited marrow failure syndromes present with characteristic facies, short stature, other congenital anomalies, and features specific to syndrome. **Table 3**, depicts classification of AA on the basis of severity.[27]

Diagnostic Workup

Careful history including family and drug history must be taken. Laboratory tests to be done should include a complete hemogram with reticulocyte count and absolute

---

Table 2: Etiology of aplastic anemia.

Inherited aplastic anemia:
- Fanconi anemia
- Shwachman-Diamond syndrome
- Dyskeratosis congenita
- Congenital amegakaryocytic thrombocytopenia
- Reticular dysgenesis
- Unclassified inherited bone marrow failure syndromes
- Other genetic syndromes: *Down syndrome, Dubowitz syndrome, Seckel syndrome, Schimke immune-osseous dysplasia, Cartilage-hair hypoplasia, and Noonan syndrome*

Acquired aplastic anemia:
- Radiation, drugs, and chemicals: *Predictable—chemotherapy, benzene; Idiosyncratic—chloramphenicol, antiepileptics, and gold 3,4-methylenedioxymethamphetamine*
- Viruses: *Cytomegalovirus, Epstein-Barr, Hepatitis B, Hepatitis C, Hepatitis non-A, non-B, non-C (seronegative hepatitis), HIV*
- Immune diseases: *Eosinophilic fasciitis, hypoimmunoglobulinemia, and thymoma*
- Paroxysmal nocturnal hemoglobinuria
- Marrow replacement: *Leukemia, myelodysplasia, and myelofibrosis*
- Autoimmune

Table 3: Classification of aplastic anemia (Camitta criteria).[27]
Severe: Bone marrow cells <25%, or 25–50% with less than 30% of stem cells in BM and two of the following: • Neutrophils <0.5×10^9/L   • Platelets <20×10^9/L   • Reticulocyte <20×10^9/L
Very severe: As for severe but neutrophils <0.2×10^9/L
Nonsevere: Values not meeting above criteria for severe/very severe

(BM: bone marrow)

neutrophil count, peripheral blood smear, serum vitamin B_{12} and serum folate levels, liver function test, and tests to determine any possible viral etiology, autoantibody screen, and test for paroxysmal nocturnal hemoglobinuria (Ham's test, complement lysis sensitivity test, and flow cytometry). BM aspiration and biopsy are needed to diagnose and check for abnormal chromosomes. Following tests are mandatory for initiating definitive therapy:[28,29]

- Chromosomal breakage test (diepoxybutane/ mitomycin-C stress test—Fanconi anemia)
- Telomere length
- Fluorescence in situ hybridization (flow-FISH)— dyskeratosis congenita
- Lymphocyte subset testing (to look for B cell lymphopenia).

Treatment

Supportive therapy including blood component therapy and antibiotics to treat infections is needed. Nonsevere AA (sometimes referred to as "mild" AA) may not need any blood or platelet transfusions.[30]

Definitive treatment in inherited AA is stem cell transplantation. Treatment options in acquired AA aim to restore BM to normal cell production by use of immunosuppressants or curative treatment by using a HSCT.[29,30]

In case of severe or very severe AA, first choice of treatment is HSCT where a matched sibling donor (MSD) is available.[29,30] If MSD is not available, then next line of treatment is immunosuppressive therapy (IST) with antithymocyte globulin (equine ATG in a dose of 20 mg/ kg/day for 5 days) and cyclosporine (5 mg/kg/day for 6–12 months followed by slow tapering). Equine ATG has been results compared to rabbit ATG for the treatment of idiopathic severe AA. As ATG can lead to serum sickness, steroids should be given along with ATG. Poor results with IST have been observed if it has not been started within 6 weeks of diagnosis. IST takes average of 3–4 months to produce response, so second course of IST has been recommended no earlier than 4–6 months.[29,30] Matched

unrelated donor (MUD) HSCT within initial 3 months of diagnosis is another option in the absence of MSD HSCT.[31] MUD is favored over IST in presence of life-threatening infections. In the presence of cytogenetically abnormalities or if the age of donor is <45 years (and preferably <30 years) or the donor is not a multiparous female, a MUD would be preferable.[29-31]

In case of unavailability of MUD and after failure of IST, mismatched unrelated donor (9/10) (MMUD) HSCT can be considered at 3–4 months after IST. In case of unavailability of any donor, other available options are 2nd course of IST (rabbit ATG following horse ATG failure), androgens, alemtuzumab, eltrombopag or haploidentical donor transplant, according to availability of trial or therapy. In the absence of a matched BM donor, there is a scope for transplant using cord blood stem cells, or BM stem cells from a half matched family member. Survival benefit has not been found in AA with use of erythropoietin ("Epo") and granulocyte colony-stimulating factor (G-CSF) therefore they are usually not preferred.[28,29,32]

■ HEMOPHILIA

Hemophilia A and B are X-linked inherited clotting disorders due to deficiencies of the clotting factors VIII and IX, respectively. Male individuals are affected while the females are asymptomatic or mildly affected carriers.[33,34]

Diagnosis

A prolonged activated partial thromboplastin time (aPTT) with a normal prothrombin time (PT) is suggestive of hemophilia. Estimation of activity of factor VIII or IX clotting factors confirms the diagnosis. It also aids the grading of severity of hemophilia. Hemophilia is classified into three main forms: severe (<1% of normal activity), moderate (1–5% of normal activity), and mild (5–40% of normal activity). Affected females may very rarely manifest with bleeding when factor activity is <40%.[34-36]

Prenatal diagnosis can be done by mutational analysis of fetal DNA obtained by chorionic villus sampling in the first trimester or amniocentesis in the second trimester.

Preimplantation genetic diagnosis (PGD) of hemophilia is also available.

Clinical Manifestations

The clotting factor activity and the age of the patient will determine the risk for hemorrhage. Neonates can present with intracranial hemorrhage (1–4% of cases) or extracranial hemorrhage, including both subgaleal bleeding and cephalohematoma. Other presentations are bleeding from circumcision, spontaneous muscle hemorrhage in the weight bearing parts of body, and spontaneous intra-articular bleeding (hemarthrosis). Recurrent hemorrhages in the same joint (i.e. a target joint) can lead to hemophilic arthropathy. In patients with moderate hemophilia; hemorrhages tend to occur after injury or surgery. In mild hemophilia, nearly all incidents are triggered by trauma or surgery. Female carriers of hemophilia may present with menorrhagia, bruising, postsurgical or peripartum hemorrhage.[37,38]

Treatment

Contact sports are contraindicated, however, some form of regular physical activity (noncontact sports) can foster strengthening of the musculoskeletal system. Use of NSAIDs is not recommended. Paracetamol may be taken. Maintaining oral and dental hygiene is recommended. Vaccines should be given subcutaneously instead of intramuscular route, using a thin needle (25–27 G), and firm pressure should be applied for 5–10 minutes.[35]

Factor Replacement Therapy

On-demand treatment, i.e. replacing the deficient factor during the bleeding episode is usually the prevalent mode of treatment in resource-constrained settings. Prophylactic treatment involves routine injection of factor concentrates even in the absence of any overt bleeding episode. This helps to prevent bleeding and thereby the development of hemophilic arthropathy. It may be classified as:

- Episodic (given only during evident bleeding), or continuous (children receive replacement of factor at least >85% of the year).
- Primary (initiated just after the first joint bleed but before another episode), secondary (after ≥2 joint bleeds but before developing hemophilic arthropathy), or tertiary (after the onset of joint disease).
- Various protocols recommend different doses of factor for prophylaxis:
  - Malmo protocol (25–40 IU/kg/dose)
  - Utrecht protocol (15–30 IU/kg/dose).

Data suggests that prophylactic administration of low doses of factor VIII (10–20 IU/kg twice or thrice per week) can also limit the number of acute bleeds.[34,35,39,40]

Treatment of Acute Bleeding

Following a bleeding in the joint, management needs to be comprehensive which is represented by the pneumonic RICE (Rest, Ice, Compression, and Elevation) and replacement therapy. The site and severity of bleed are the determinants of dosage. In case of epistaxis, the patient is made to sit in erect position while breathing through the mouth and pinching the nose for 10–15 minutes. Local antifibrinolytics are also useful.[35]

Calculation of Dose of Factors

Factor VIII (IU per dose) = U/dL desired rise (%) × Body weight (kg) × 0.5

(1 U/kg of factor VIII increases the body level by 2%, half-life of factor VIII is 8–12 hours, given 12 hourly)

Factor IX (IU per dose) = U/dL desired rise (%) × Body weight (kg)

(1 U/kg of factor IX increases the body level by 1%; half-life of factor IX is 18–24 hours, given 24 hourly).

Recombinant factor IX should be given 1.2–1.5 times the dose of plasma derived factor IX, as its activity is less than that of plasma-derived factor IX.[35]

Desmopressin Acetate

Desmopressin acts by increasing the plasma concentrations of factor VIII and von Willebrand factor and can be used in patients with mild hemophilia A.[34] It may be administered intravenously or subcutaneously in a dose of 0.3 µg/kg body weight.[41]

Antifibrinolytics

Tranexamic acid can be used at a dose of 25 mg/kg oral or 10 mg/kg IV given at 6–8 hourly interval. In case of oral bleeds, swish and swallow technique can be applied. Antifibrinolytics are contraindicated in hematuria and those receiving activated prothrombin complex concentrates (PCCs) as it increases the risk of thrombosis.[35]

Inhibitor

Inhibitors are neutralizing alloantibodies which are targeted against factor VIII or IX. Nijmegen-Bethesda assay is useful to quantify the inhibitors. Repeated administration of factor concentrates leads to immune tolerance induction (ITI) where over a period of time body stops reacting to the treatment product. ITI is a useful treatment strategy to tackle inhibitors. In case of failure of ITI, trial of intravenous immunoglobulin (IVIG) or immunosuppressants like rituximab and cyclophosphamide can be given along with ITI.[42,43]

Depending on the titers, patients may be categorized as low titer (<5 BU) or high titer (≥5 BU). Standard replacement therapy with increased doses is adequate to handle low titer inhibitors. For patients with a high titer or high-responding inhibitors, bypassing agents like activated PCC and recombinant activated factor VII are used.[44]

IMMUNE THROMBOCYTOPENIC PURPURA

Immune (or idiopathic) thrombocytopenic purpura (ITP) is characterized by isolated thrombocytopenia (<100,000 platelets/mL) without any conditions known to reduce platelet count. ITP may be further described as "newly diagnosed" (from diagnosis until 3 months), "persistent ITP" (3–12 months' duration) and "chronic ITP" (>12 months' duration).[45] ITP may follow a viral infection or immunization. It is possible that ITP may be triggered by an autoimmune dysfunction in response to infection. The usual age at the time of diagnosis is 2–6 years of life.[46,47]

Presentation and Workup

Usual presentation is normal looking child presenting with petechiae and purpura. Oral or nasal bleeding, or overt bleeding manifests in less than a third of patients.[48,49] ITP is a clinical diagnosis without a specific confirmatory test. It is usually diagnosed after excluding other conditions which are associated with thrombocytopenia. A meticulous history and detailed physical examination should be done to look for constitutional symptoms, which suggest diagnoses other than ITP. Complete blood count reveals thrombocytopenia without affecting other cell lines. BM examination may be deferred in children with classical features of ITP. BM examination should be done to exclude other diagnoses (particularly leukemia and AA), in patients with unusual features or those refractory to treatment and before starting glucocorticoids.[50,51]

Pathophysiology

Immunoglobulin G (IgG) directed against platelet antigens binds platelets followed by their destruction in the reticuloendothelial system primarily the spleen. Megakaryocytes in the marrow may also be targeted by autoantibodies. Impaired hepatic production of thrombopoietin may also be contributory.[48]

Management

First line treatment of ITP has been outlined in **Table 4**.[48-50,52] The preferred initial approach is IVIg or anti-D therapy as glucocorticoids may be toxic and there may be a concern over partially treating an unrecognized acute lymphoblastic leukemia.

If there is no improvement after 3–6 months of therapy, child must undergo BM aspiration and in newly diagnosed children tests to identify underlying infection (HIV/HCV/*Helicobacter pylori*), testing for antinuclear antibody, testing for antiphospholipid antibody, lupus anticoagulant, and serum immunoglobulins (IgG, IgA, and IgM) must be done. Additionally, review the compliance and medication dosage.[52]

The American Society of Hematology (ASH) recommends using rituximab or high-dose dexamethasone as a second-line pharmacotherapy.[50]

MEGALOBLASTIC ANEMIA

Megaloblastic anemia (MA) is a group of disorders wherein the BW produces abnormally large and immature red cells due to impaired DNA synthesis. Most cases of childhood MA are the result of folic acid or vitamin B_{12} deficiencies. We discuss here about vitamin B_{12} and folic acid deficiency anemia. Vitamin B_{12} and folate deficiency can be due to decreased intake, decreased absorption or increased demand from various causes. Drugs and inborn error of metabolism also can cause vitamin B_{12} or folate deficiency. Deficiency in mothers is the usual cause of deficiency in infants and young children.[53,54]

Clinical Features

Anemia, anorexia, irritability, and easy fatigability are common clinical features. Clinical features typical of MA include hyperpigmented knuckles and terminal phalanges, hepatosplenomegaly (30–40%), and petechiae and other bleeding manifestations (25%). Cases may mimic AA or acute leukemia.[55,56] Cases of MA may also exhibit tremors—known as infantile tremors syndrome, developmental retardation/regression and microcephaly, hypotonia, developmental delay, listlessness, and failure to thrive. Neuroimaging may reveal diffuse frontotemporoparietal cortical atrophy.[53,57]

Diagnosis

Megaloblastic anemia is suspected based on clinical features coexisting with laboratory features like the presence of macrocytes on peripheral smear [increased

Table 4: Treatment options in ITP.

Treatment options[48–50,52]	Dose	Comments
Front line therapy		
Observation alone	Patients with skin manifestations (bruising and petechiae) only and no other bleeding	Symptoms resolves and platelet counts typically improves within weeks to months
IVIg	0.8–1 g/kg, IV over 4–6 hours, may repeat dose if no response	Platelet count typically begins to rise in 24 hours, Effect typically lasts roughly 3 weeks
Anti-D therapy	250 U/kg (50–75 mg/kg), IV over 30 minutes	Platelet count typically rise in 24–48 hours, effect typically lasts roughly 3 weeks
Steroids	Prednisone 1–2 mg/kg/d divided into bid dosing for at least 1–2 weeks, followed by slow tapering	Duration is often determined by platelet response If steroids must be used chronically, then should be given at lowest therapeutic dose to minimize toxicity
Second line therapy		
Rituximab	Weekly infusion (375 mg/m^2) for 4 consecutive weeks	31–70% response
Dapsone	1–2 mg/kg/day (max 100 mg) for 3 weeks	Response rate 50–60%
High-dose dexamethasone	20 mg/m^2 for 4 sequential days every 28 days	Up to 80% response
Methyl prednisolone	30 mg/kg IV × 3 days then causes 20 mg/kg IV × 4 days	60–100% response may be more useful as a front-line agent for ITP May be worth trying before splenectomy in severe symptomatic chronic ITP
Immunosuppressive agents	Cyclosporine 5 mg/kg/day in two divided doses for 3 weeks Tacrolimus and sirolimus Mycophenolate mofetil 10 mg/kg BD for 4–6 weeks	Response rate 40–55% Variable responses Response rate 60%
Chemotherapy	Cyclophosphamide 500–1,000 mg/m^2 IV every 4 weeks Azathioprine 1–2 mg/kg/d PO for 2–3 months Vincristine 1.5 mg/m^2/week for 4–6 weeks, others	Variable response, insufficient data in children Response rate 40% Variable response, insufficient data in children
Thrombopoietin agonists	Eltrombopag and romiplostim	Being tested in children

(ITP: immune thrombocytopenic purpura; IVIg: intravenous immunoglobulin; IV: intravenous)

red cell mean corpuscular volume (MCV)] accompanied by anisopoikilocytosis and hypersegmented neutrophils. Neutropenia (17–49%) and thrombocytopenia (44–80%) may also be present.[53,54,56] The RBC precursors exhibit disparity in nuclear-cytoplasmic maturation. B_{12} levels of <200 pg/mL are indicative of vitamin B_{12} deficiency. Plasma or serum folate level of <4 mg/L indicates folate deficiency. Increased methylmalonic acid (MMA) levels are considered to be a highly sensitive and specific test for identifying B_{12} deficiency. Hyper homocysteinemia is seen in both B_{12} and folate deficiency.[54,58,59] Reduced red cell folate level is seen not only in folate deficiency but also known to coexist with B_{12} deficiency. RBC folate estimation reflects average folate status of the individual during the preceding 3–4 months and is not affected by recent dietary intake of folate.[54,58,59] MA is also characterized by raised serum bilirubin and lactate dehydrogenase (LDH) levels.[60]

Treatment

Replacement therapy is required. Conventionally, oral folic acid 5 mg/day has been used.[53] For B_{12} deficiency, parenteral or oral administration of B_{12} may be used, the former being preferred in pernicious anemia. The duration of treatment is not as standardized. Patients may be given frequent doses of 1 mg of B_{12} on alternate days for the initial 1–2 weeks, followed by weekly supplementation for a few weeks, and then monthly supplementation for 3–4 months after clinical improvement.[54,61] BW abnormalities have been shown to normalize with disappearance of megaloblastic erythroid changes as early as within 36–48 hours of treatment. By the end of first week there would be reticulocytosis.

High-dose oral (2 mg of B_{12} daily) and parenteral therapy have been proven to be equally effective.[54,61] Treatment of pernicious anemia, or any B_{12} deficiency that is caused by malabsorption/post-total gastrectomy, requires lifelong supplementation with parenteral vitamin B_{12}. Vitamin B_{12} deficiency due to secondary causes requires treatment of underlying cause along with supplementation.[54]

GLUCOSE-6-PHOSPHATE DEHYDROGENASE DEFICIENCY

Glucose-6-phosphate dehydrogenase (G6PD) deficiency is the most common human enzyme defect, affecting more than 400 million people worldwide. It is an X-linked, hereditary genetic defect caused by mutations in the *G6PD* gene.[62]

Diagnosis

The definitive diagnosis of G6PD deficiency is by estimation of enzyme activity. G6PD activity can be measured qualitatively or, preferably by quantitative spectrophotometric analysis of the rate of reduced nicotinamide adenine dinucleotide phosphate (NADPH) production from NADP. It should not be measured during the acute hemolytic event, in young neonates, or in the presence of any condition associated with reticulocytosis, because G6PD activity is higher in young erythrocytes leading to false negative results. Molecular tests is the only method for definitive diagnosis in heterozygous females.[63]

Variants of G6PD deficiency[64]

- *Class I*: Severely deficient, associated with chronic nonspherocytic hemolytic anemia (<10% normal activity).
- *Class II*: Severely deficient (<10% normal activity), associated with acute hemolytic anemia.
- *Class III*: Moderately/mildly deficient (10–60% of normal activity).
- *Class IV*: Very mild or no enzyme deficiency (60–150% of normal activity).
- *Class V*: Increased activity (>150% normal activity).

Clinical Manifestations

Glucose-6-phosphate dehydrogenase deficiency usually presents as acute hemolytic anemia, neonatal jaundice, or chronic nonspherocytic hemolytic anemia. Acute hemolytic anemia, is usually precipitated by an extraneous agent, such as drugs (quinolones, sulfa drugs, nalidixic acid, aspirin, nitrofurantoin, etc.), infection (viral infections), or eating fava beans.[62] G6PD deficient individuals have a normal life expectancy and quality-of-life.[65] Clinically,

patient presents with fatigue, back pain, pallor, dark urine, abdominal pain, and jaundice. Neonates could present with prolonged and severe jaundice. Hyperbilirubinemia (indirect type), raised serum LDH, and reticulocytosis are suggestive of the disorder.[62]

Management

Most patients would recover spontaneously but there is a risk for recurrent episodes, hence, prevention is of utmost importance. Oxidative stressors must be avoided. Acute hemolysis usually does not need specific treatment and may require transfusions of RBCs.[62] Neonatal jaundice caused by G6PD deficiency should be managed as other causes of neonatal jaundice.[66]

Individuals with congenital nonspherocytic hemolytic anemia may have a well-compensated anemia and may not require any transfusion. However, the degree of anemia can severely be worsen by any exacerbating event. So they should be monitored for development of severe anemia especially in presence of precipitating factors. Very rarely, congenital nonspherocytic hemolytic anemia may require regular transfusions.[62] Antioxidant agents like vitamin E and selenium could be beneficial in patients with chronic hemolysis.[67] Patients with congenital nonspherocytic hemolytic anemia are at risk of developing splenomegaly and gallstones.[62]

VITAMIN K DEFICIENCY BLEEDING

Vitamin K deficiency bleeding (VKDB) is a rare bleeding disorder due to vitamin K (VK) deficiency seen more commonly in early infancy. VK is needed for the synthesis in the liver of certain clotting factors namely factors, VII, IX, and X wherein gamma-carboxylation of these factors occurs.[68] Unlike in disseminated intravascular coagulation, these infants are relatively well appearing and not sick. The condition is also referred to as hemorrhagic disease of the newborn (HDN).[69]

Classification

Depending upon the age of onset VKDB may be classified as early, classic, and late **(Table 5)**.[70,71] Early onset VKDB presents with bleeding within 1 day of birth or may even be *in utero* or during delivery due to intake of medicines like phenytoin, isoniazid or rifampicin by mother during pregnancy. Classical form is seen in neonates 2–7 days old and occurs due to physiological deficiency of VK leading to deficiency of factors II, VII, IX, and X. Neonates are also have poor placental transfer of VK,

Table 5: Classification of vitamin K bleeding disorder.

Type of vitamin K deficiency syndrome[70,71]	Timing of presentation and features	Bleeding sites	Causative factors
Early	0–24 hours	Scalp subperiosteal, intracranial, intrathoracic, and intra-abdominal	Maternal drugs interfering with vitamin K metabolism or vitamin K dependent coagulation factors (i.e. warfarin, anticonvulsants)
Classical	Days 2–7	Gastrointestinal (most common), skin, nose, umbilical, circumcision	Mainly idiopathic, breastfeeding (low milk intakes)
Late	Day 8 to 6 months (peak 3–8 weeks) More common in males (2:1)	Intracranial (much higher prevalence), skin, gastrointestinal	Idiopathic, secondary to breastfeeding, cholestasis, long-term antibiotics, secondary causes of malabsorption, chronic diarrhea

poor hepatic storage of VK and also may have a delayed colonization of the gut. Breastfed neonates are also prone to VKDB as the breast milk is relatively deficient in VK. Affected infants are normal at birth but subsequently develop bleeding manifestations like ecchymoses, gastrointestinal bleeding, nasal bleeding, bleeding after circumcision or bleeding from umbilical stump or rarely cephalohematoma. Classical HDN can be treated by intravenous VK, Also, babies receiving prophylactic VK at birth are usually protected.[72] Late VKDB is seen between 4 weeks and 8 weeks in healthy breastfed infants with risk factors like underlying disorders with malabsorption, prolonged therapy with antibiotics, cholestasis, and biliary atresia.

Assessment of Vitamin K Status

Coagulation assays such as PT and aPTT are recommended to screen for VKDB. PT becomes prolonged only when the prothrombin concentration drops below about 50% of normal.[73] Thus, it may not be useful for detecting subclinical deficiency. In the presence of VK deficiency, functionally defective molecules of VK-coagulation factors are released into the bloodstream known as proteins induced by VK absence or antagonism (PIVKA). Enzyme immunoassay (EIA) for PIVKA-II is an useful functional marker of subclinical VK deficiency.[73-75]

Diagnostic criteria of VKDB include prothrombin time (PT) ≥4s above control and additionally have at least one of the following:

- Normal or elevated platelet count, normal fibrinogen, and absent fibrin degradation products.
- Prothrombin time normalizing following VK administration.
- Proteins induced by VK absence or antagonism (usually that of factor II) level exceeding normal controls.

A probable case of VKDB is defined as presence of one in which the PT and aPTT are deranged along with one of the three criteria listed above.[76] Long half-life of clearance of PIVKA-II enables diagnosis of VKDB to be made even days after the original bleeding event.[77]

Treatment

Infants who present with a nonlife threatening bleed should be treated with phylloquinone (VK1; phytomenadione; phytonadione) given slowly by intravenous or subcutaneous injection. The dose range of 1–2 mg is more than sufficient to fully correct VK deficiency in infants aged up to 6 months. Fresh frozen plasma (FFP), or PCC can be given in cases of massive bleeding.[71] If a child is suspected to have VKDB, VK may be given intravenously while we await the blood product.[71] Intramuscular administration may lead to a painful hematoma. However, if venous access cannot be established, subcutaneous route could be used.[71] In case of severe intracranial hemorrhage recombinant factor VIIa (rFVIIa) has also been tried.[72]

Prevention

Single parenteral dose of 0.5–1.0 mg IM VK should be given to all newborn infants within 6 hours of life.[73,75]

■ REFERENCES

1. Taher AT, Weatherall DJ, Cappellini MD. Thalassaemia. Lancet. 2018;391:155-67.
2. Piel FB, Weatherall DJ. The α-thalassemias. N Engl J Med. 2014;371:1908-16.
3. Choudhry VP. Thalassemia minor and major: current management. Indian J Pediatr. 2017;84:607-11.
4. Origa R. β-thalassemia. Genet Med. 2017;19:609-19.
5. Sara T, Alan C. Blood transfusion. In: Domenica M, Cappellini Alan C, John P, Ali T, Vip V (Eds). Guidelines for the Management of Transfusion Dependent Thalassaemia (TDT),

3rd edition. Cyprus: Thalassaemia International Federation; 2014. pp. 28-41.

6. Propper RD, Button LN, Nathan DG. New approaches to the transfusion management of thalassemia. Blood. 1980;55:55-60.

7. Taher AT, Musallam KM, Saliba AN, et al. Hemoglobin level and morbidity in non-transfusion-dependent thalassemia. Blood Cells, Mol Dis. 2015;55:108-9.

8. Cappellini MD, Cohen A, Porter J, et al. Guidelines for the Management of Transfusion Dependent Thalassaemia (TDT), 3rd edition. Cyprus: Thalassaemia International Federation; 2014.

9. Taher A, Vichinsky E, Musallam K, et al. Guidelines for the Management of Non Transfusion Dependent Thalassaemia (NTDT). Cyprus: Thalassaemia International Federation; 2013.

10. Belhoul KM, Bakir ML, Saned M-S, et al. Serum ferritin levels and endocrinopathy in medically treated patients with β thalassemia major. Ann Hematol. 2012;91:1107-14.

11. Olivieri NF, Nathan DG, MacMillan JH, et al. Survival in Medically Treated Patients with Homozygous β-thalassemia. N Engl J Med. 1994;331:574-8.

12. Taher AT, Musallam KM, Cappellini MD, et al. Optimal management of β thalassaemia intermedia. Br J Haematol. 2011;152:512-23.

13. Musallam KM, Taher AT, Karimi M, et al. Cerebral infarction in β-thalassemia intermedia: Breaking the silence. Thromb Res. 2012;130:695-702.

14. Taher AT, Musallam KM, Karimi M, et al. Overview on practices in thalassemia intermedia management aiming for lowering complication rates across a region of endemicity: the OPTIMAL CARE study. Blood. 2010;115:1886-92.

15. Taher AT, Saliba AN. Iron overload in thalassemia: different organs at different rates. Hematology. 2017;265-71.

16. Piel FB, Hay SI, Gupta S, et al. Global Burden of Sickle Cell Anaemia in Children under Five, 2010–2050: Modelling Based on Demographics, Excess Mortality, and Interventions. PLoS Med. 2013;10:e1001484.

17. Colah R, Mukherjee M, Ghosh K. Sickle cell disease in India. Curr Opin Hematol. 2014;21:215-23.

18. Ware RE, de Montalembert M, Tshilolo L, et al. Sickle cell disease. Lancet. 2017;390:311-23.

19. Piel FB, Steinberg MH, Rees DC. Sickle cell disease. N Engl J Med. 2017;376:1561-73.

20. Yawn BP, Buchanan GR, Afenyi-Annan AN, et al. Management of Sickle cell disease. JAMA. 2014;312:1033.

21. Dallas MH, Triplett B, Shook DR, et al. Long-term outcome and evaluation of organ function in pediatric patients undergoing haploidentical and matched related hematopoietic cell transplantation for sickle cell disease. Biol Blood Marrow Transplant. 2013;19:820-30.

22. Walters MC, De Castro LM, Sullivan KM, et al. Indications and results of HLA-identical sibling hematopoietic cell transplantation for sickle cell disease. Biol Blood Marrow Transplant. 2016;22:207-11.

23. Hankins JS, McCarville MB, Rankine-Mullings A, et al. Prevention of conversion to abnormal transcranial Doppler with hydroxyurea in sickle cell anemia: A Phase III international randomized clinical trial. Am J Hematol. 2015;90:1099-105.

24. Nickel RS, Hendrickson JE, Haight AE. The ethics of a proposed study of hematopoietic stem cell transplant for children with less severe sickle cell disease. Blood. 2014;124:861-6.

25. Gupta V, Pratap R, Kumar A, et al. Epidemiological features of aplastic anemia in Indian children. Indian J Pediatr. 2014;81:257-9.

26. Young NS, Kaufman DW. The epidemiology of acquired aplastic anemia. Haematologica. 2008;93:489-92.

27. Camitta BM. Pathogenesis and treatment of aplastic anemia. Rinsho Ketsueki. 1984;25:459-69.

28. Benson-Quarm N, Gandhi S, Kulasekararaj A, et al. Aplastic anaemia. Hematology. 2014;19:60-1.

29. Samarasinghe S, Veys P, Vora A, et al. Paediatric amendment to adult BSH guidelines for aplastic anaemia. Br J Haematol. 2018;180:201-5.

30. Barone A, Lucarelli A, Onofrillo D, et al. Diagnosis and management of acquired aplastic anemia in childhood. Guidelines from the Marrow Failure Study Group of the Pediatric Haemato-Oncology Italian Association (AIEOP). Blood Cells, Mol Dis. 2015;55:40-7.

31. Samarasinghe S, Steward C, Hiwarkar P, et al. Excellent outcome of matched unrelated donor transplantation in paediatric aplastic anaemia following failure with immunosuppressive therapy: a United Kingdom multicentre retrospective experience. Br J Haematol. 2012;157:339-46.

32. Killick SB, Bown N, Cavenagh J, et al. Guidelines for the diagnosis and management of adult aplastic anaemia. Br J Haematol. 2016;172:187-207.

33. Mannucci PM, Tuddenham EGD. The Hemophilias—From Royal Genes to Gene Therapy. N Engl J Med. 2001;344:1773-9.

34. Peyvandi F, Garagiola I, Young G. The past and future of haemophilia: diagnosis, treatments, and its complications. Lancet. 2016;388:187-97.

35. Sachdeva A, Gunasekaran V, Ramya HN, et al. Consensus Statement of the Indian Academy of Pediatrics in Diagnosis and Management of Hemophilia. Indian Pediatr. 2018;55:582-90.

36. White GC, Rosendaal F, Aledort LM, et al. Definitions in hemophilia. Recommendation of the scientific subcommittee on factor VIII and factor IX of the scientific and standardization committee of the International Society on Thrombosis and Haemostasis. Thromb Haemost. 2001;85:560.

37. Paroskie A, Gailani D, DeBaun MR, et al. A cross-sectional study of bleeding phenotype in haemophilia A carriers. Br J Haematol. 2015;170:223-8.

38. Luck JV, Silva M, Rodriguez-Merchan EC, et al. Hemophilic arthropathy. J Am Acad Orthop Surg. 2004;12(4):234-45.

39. Gouider E, Jouini L, Achour M, et al. Low dose prophylaxis in Tunisian children with haemophilia. Haemophilia. 2017;23:77-81.

40. Verma SP, Dutta TK, Mahadevan S, et al. A randomized study of very low-dose factor VIII prophylaxis in severe haemophilia: a success story from a resource limited country. Haemophilia. 2016;22:342-8.

41. Mannucci PM, Pareti FI, Ruggeri ZM, et al. 1-Deamino-8-D-Aarginine vasopressin: a new pharmacologica approach to the management of haemophilia and von Willebrand's disease. Lancet. 1977;309:869-72.

42. Oldenburg J, Jiménez-Yuste V, Peiró-Jordán R, et al. Primary and rescue immune tolerance induction in children and adults: a multicentre international study with a VWF-containing plasma-derived FVIII concentrate. Haemophilia. 2014;20:83-91.

43. Franchini M, Mannucci PM. Inhibitor eradication with rituximab in haemophilia: where do we stand? Br J Haematol. 2014;165:600-8.

44. Kempton CL, White GC. How we treat a hemophilia A patient with a factor VIII inhibitor. Blood. 2009;113:11-7.

45. Rodeghiero F, Stasi R, Gernsheimer T, et al. Standardization of terminology, definitions and outcome criteria in immune thrombocytopenic purpura of adults and children: report from an international working group. Blood. 2009;113:2386-93.

46. Terrell DR, Beebe LA, Vesely SK, et al. The incidence of immune thrombocytopenic purpura in children and adults: a critical review of published reports. Am J Hematol. 2010;85:174-80.

47. Yong M, Schoonen WM, Li L, et al. Epidemiology of paediatric immune thrombocytopenia in the General Practice Research Database. Br J Haematol. 2010;149:855-64.

48. D'Orazio JA, Neely J, Farhoudi N. ITP in children. J Pediatr Hematol Oncol. 2013;35:1-13.

49. Anoop P. Immune thrombocytopenic purpura: historical perspective, current status, recent advances and future directions. Indian Pediatr. 2012;49:811-8.

50. Neunert C, Lim W, Crowther M, et al. The American Society of Hematology 2011 evidence-based practice guideline for immune thrombocytopenia. Blood. 2011;117:4190-207.

51. Naithani R, Kumar R, Mahapatra M, et al. Is it safe to avoid bone marrow examination in suspected ITP? Pediatr Hematol Oncol. 2007;24:205-7.

52. Provan D, Stasi R, Newland AC, et al. International consensus report on the investigation and management of primary immune thrombocytopenia. Blood. 2010;115:168-86.

53. Chandra J. Megaloblastic anemia: back in focus. Indian J Pediatr. 2010;77:795-9.

54. Green R, Datta Mitra A. Megaloblastic anemias. Med Clin North Am. 2017;101:297-317.

55. Marwaha RK, Singh S, Garewal G, et al. Bleeding manifestations in megaloblastic anemia. Indian J Pediatr. 1989;56:243-7.

56. Gomber S, Kela K, Dhingra N. Clinico-hematological profile of megaloblastic anemia. Indian Pediatr. 1998;35:55-8.

57. Grattan-Smith PJ, Wilcken B, Procopis PG, et al. The neurological syndrome of infantile cobalamin deficiency: developmental regression and involuntary movements. Mov Disord. 1997;12:39-46.

58. Green R. Metabolite assays in cobalamin and folate deficiency. Baillieres Clin Haematol. 1995;8:533-66.

59. Green R. Indicators for assessing folate and vitamin B12 status and for monitoring the efficacy of intervention strategies. Food Nutr Bull. 2008;29:S52-63.

60. Green R, Dwyre DM. Evaluation of macrocytic anemias. Semin Hematol. 2015;52:279-86.

61. Stabler SP. Vitamin B12 deficiency. N Engl J Med. 2013;368:149-60.

62. Cappellini M, Fiorelli G. Glucose-6-phosphate dehydrogenase deficiency. Lancet. 2008;371:64-74.

63. Minucci A, Giardina B, Zuppi C, et al. Glucose-6-phosphate dehydrogenase laboratory assay: how, when, and why? IUBMB Life. 2009;61:27-34.

64. Glucose-6-phosphate dehydrogenase deficiency. WHO Working Group. Bull World Health Organ. 1989;67:601-11.

65. Cocco P, Todde P, Fornera S, et al. Mortality in a cohort of men expressing the glucose-6-phosphate dehydrogenase deficiency. Blood. 1998;91:706-9.

66. Newman TB, Maisels MJ. Evaluation and treatment of jaundice in the term newborn: a kinder, gentler approach. Pediatrics. 1992;89:809-18.

67. Hafez M, Amar ES, Zedan M, et al. Improved erythrocyte survival with combined vitamin E and selenium therapy in children with glucose-6-phosphate dehydrogenase deficiency and mild chronic hemolysis. J Pediatr. 1986;108:558-61.

68. Newman P, Shearer MJ. Vitamin K metabolism. Subcell Biochem. 1998;30:455-88.

69. Suttie JW. Vitamin K and human nutrition. J Am Diet Assoc. 1992;92:585-90.

70. Shearer MJ. Vitamin K deficiency bleeding (VKDB) in early infancy. Blood Rev. 2009;23:49-59.

71. Williams MD, Chalmers EA. Gibson BES, Haemostasis and Thrombosis Task Force BC for S in H. The investigation and management of neonatal haemostasis and thrombosis. Br J Haematol. 2002;119:295-309.

72. Flood VH, Galderisi FC, Lowas SR, et al. Hemorrhagic disease of the newborn despite vitamin K prophylaxis at birth. Pediatr Blood Cancer. 2008;50:1075-7.

73. Ng E, Loewy AD. Position Statement: Guidelines for vitamin K prophylaxis in newborns: A joint statement of the Canadian Paediatric Society and the College of Family Physicians of Canada. Can Fam Physician. 2018;64:736-9.

74. Widdershoven J, van Munster P, De Abreu R, et al. Four methods compared for measuring des-carboxy-prothrombin (PIVKA-II). Clin Chem. 1987;33:2074-8.

75. American Academy of Pediatrics. Committee statement, Committee on Nutrition. Vitamin K supplementation for infants receiving milk substitute infant formulas and for those with fat malabsorption. Pediatrics. 1971;48:483-7.

76. Cornelissen M, von Kries R, Loughnan P, et al. Prevention of vitamin K deficiency bleeding: efficacy of different multiple oral dose schedules of vitamin K. Eur J Pediatr. 1997;156:126-30.

77. Humpl T, Brühl K, Brzezinska R, et al. Fatal late vitamin K-deficiency bleeding after oral vitamin K prophylaxis secondary to unrecognized bile duct paucity. J Pediatr Gastroenterol Nutr. 1999;29:594-7.

Noncommunicable Respiratory Disorders in the Tropics

Hema Gupta Mittal, Sarika Gupta

INTRODUCTION

Currently, major respiratory burden in Indian children includes asthma, recurrent infections, and bronchiectasis unlike in adults where chronic obstructive pulmonary diseases (COPD) and lung cancers are the main causes of morbidity and mortality. Recent trends have shown changes in etiologies from infectious to noninfectious diseases and emerging noninfective etiologies such as genetic disorders including cystic fibrosis (CF) and primary ciliary dyskinesias (PCDs), bronchopulmonary dysplasia, interstitial lung diseases (ILDs), gastroesophageal reflux diseases (GERD), neuromuscular illnesses, sleep disorders, and lung malformations.

BURDEN AND CLASSIFICATION

Cystic fibrosis is reported with low prevalence in Asia (1:10,000 to 1:40,750) with mainly in Caucasians (1 in 2,500). Recent reviews have concluded high underreporting in India and other tropical countries such as Sri Lanka and China.[1-3] With availability of genetic testing and screening by reduced fraction of exhaled nitric oxide (FENO), ciliary dyskinesias are being increasingly recognized in children. Besides these, other major diseases in children include asthma, bronchiectasis, lung malformations, immunodeficiency disorders, rheumatological disorders, and environmental disorders, such as hypersensitivity pneumonitis and lung pollution, etc.

Noninfective respiratory diseases in children may be broadly classified as shown in **Box 1**. Some common disorders are discussed in detail in the following text.

TROPICAL PULMONARY EOSINOPHILIA

It is endemic in the tropical and subtropical regions of the India, southeast Asia, South America, south Pacific islands, and Africa and manifests as a triad of wheezing, fever, and eosinophilia in less than 1% of filarial infections. In India, it is mostly found around the coastal regions from Maharashtra to Kerala and West Bengal to Tamil Nadu (prevalence of 0.5–9.9%).[4]

Etiopathogenesis

The pathogenesis is due to an exaggerated as a hypersensitivity reaction (type I, type III, and type IV reactions) to the microfilariae of *Wuchereria bancrofti* and *Brugia malayi*. Mature gravid human filarial parasites, living in the lymphatics, periodically release microfilaria which are trapped within the pulmonary microcirculation and hence microfilaremia is rarely observed in tropical pulmonary eosinophilia (TPE). The degenerating microfilaria releases antigenic constituents which trigger interleukin-4-mediated immune response and airway hyperreactivity. An IgE-inducing antigen of *B. malayi* known as Bm23-25 has been detected in bronchoalveolar lavage (BAL) studies patients with TPE. Molecular mimicry between Bm23-25 and gamma-glutamyltranspeptidase present on the human pulmonary epithelium surface is well known. The pathology may vary from time to time with predominant acute eosinophilic infiltration, eosinophilic bronchopneumonia, and eosinophilic abscesses in first 6 months followed by mixed cell type of infiltrate (i.e. eosinophils and histiocytes) with generally well-marked fibrous tissue formation till 2 years and histiocytic infiltration and fibrosis beyond 2 years. In advanced stage lung scarring, restrictive lung and progression to ILD is known.

Clinical Features

Tropical pulmonary eosinophilia is commonly seen in adolescents and young males (15–40 years) but has been

Box 1: Common etiologies of noninfective respiratory diseases in children.

- *Inflammatory and immune-mediated disorders*: Asthma, sarcoidosis, systemic lupus erythematosus (SLE), rheumatoid arthritis, dermatomyositis, scleroderma, Wegener's granulomatosis, etc.
- *Metabolic and genetic disorders*: Cystic fibrosis, α-1 antitrypsin deficiency, primary ciliary dyskinesias (PCDs)
- *Immunodeficiency disorders* including *primary immunodeficiency* disease such as T cell and B cell or combined defects, chronic granulomatous diseases, etc. and *secondary disorders* such as human immunodeficiency virus (HIV), post-transplants or chemotherapy, etc.
- *Interstitial and diffuse lung diseases,* e.g. developmental anomalies—alveolar capillary dysplasia and malalignment of pulmonary veins, neuroendocrinal cell hyperplasia, pulmonary interstitial glycogenosis, surfactant dysfunction mutations, immune-mediated collagen vascular disorders, etc.
- *Bronchiectasis and chronic suppurative lung disease* due to immune disorders, ciliary dyskinesias, cystic fibrosis, congenital tracheobronchomegaly syndromes, aspirations, allergic bronchopulmonary aspergillosis (ABPA), autoimmune disorders, etc. hypersensitivity pneumonitis
- *Environmental exposures* disorders such as hypersensitivity pneumonitis secondary to molds, pigeon breeders lung, malt, maple bark, house dust, etc. and pollution
- *Pulmonary hypertension*—idiopathic or secondary to hereditary, drug or toxins; connective tissue disorders, developmental anomalies, persistent pulmonary hypertension of newborn, altitude sickness, etc.
- *Congenital lung malformations* including *airway malformations,* e.g. web, cysts, hemangioma, malacia, stenosis, bronchial atresia, *parenchymal malformations,* e.g. congenital thoracic malformations (CTM), agenesis, hypoplasia or sequestrations of lung, bronchogenic or duplication cysts, congenital large hyperlucent lobe (CLHL) and *vascular malformations,* e.g. aberrant subclavian or pulmonary arteries, arch anomalies such as double aortic arch and right-sided arch, *chest wall and respiratory muscle disorders* such as muscular dystrophies, and neuromuscular disorders
- *Aspiration syndromes* such as gastroesophageal reflux disease (GERD), swallowing defects, foreign bodies, and trachea esophageal fistulas
- *Sleep disorders* including *central* causes such as congenital hypoventilation syndromes, hypothalamic dysfunction *OR peripheral* etiologies such as obstructive disorders secondary to craniofacial syndromes, adenoid hypertrophy
- *Tumors* like hamartomas, mesodermal and tracheal tumors, mediastinal and metastatic tumors
- *Miscellaneous* such as drowning, pulmonary hemosiderosis, traumatic pneumothorax, and sudden infant death syndrome (SIDS)

well reported in children also. The respiratory symptom manifestations include predominantly nocturnal and are cough with scanty mucus, wheezing, breathlessness, and chest pain. On chest examination, in three-fourth children, wheezes and crackles may be found. Rare presentations include consolidation, cavitation, pneumothorax, and bronchiectasis. Systemic symptoms include fever, weight loss, fatigue, and malaise. Extrapulmonary systemic manifestations include lymphadenopathy and hepatosplenomegaly.

■ DIAGNOSIS

Peripheral blood eosinophilia is the hallmark of disease with levels greater than 3,000/μL being common. Diurnal variations in eosinophil count with paradoxical increase at night and during worsening of symptoms possibly due to pulmonary eosinphillic sequestration. Raised erythrocyte sedimentation rate (ESR) with sputum and BAL eosinophilia is often present. Increased levels of total serum IgE, filarial-specific IgE and IgG, complement fixation test to *Dirofilaria immitis* antigen, and presence of microfilaria in lungs are other tests. Patients with a TPE-like syndrome due to other helminthes may have serological tests which cross-react with filarial antigens. ELISA (enzyme-linked immunosorbent assay) test for Og4C3 antigen is sensitive and specific for *Wuchereria bancrofti* infections whereas sandwich ELISA estimating antibodies to Bm-SXP-1 antigen may be useful for *B. malayi*

infection. Chest X-ray may show reticulonodular shadows and miliary mottling similar to miliary tuberculosis. Computed tomography (CT) chest may show miliary mottling, interstitial shadows, bronchiectasis, air trapping, lymphadenopathy, cavitations, consolidation, or pleural effusions, etc. Spirometry may show mixed restrictive and obstructive findings and reduced diffusion capacity.

Differential diagnosis of eosinophilia may include other parasite infestations (*Ascaris, Toxocara,* Strongyloides, hookworm, lung flukes, *Schistosoma, Trichinella,* etc.), asthma, allergic bronchopulmonary aspergillosis (ABPA), acute or chronic eosinophilic pneumonia, Churg-Strauss syndrome, idiopathic hypereosinophilic syndrome, drug reactions, etc. Filarial TPE may be differentiated from nonfilarial TPE by nocturnal symptoms, pulmonary infiltrates on chest X-ray, leukocytosis with peripheral eosinophilia > 3,000/μm, increased serum IgE and filarial specific IgG and IgE, and improvement with diethylcarbamazine (DEC) therapy.

Treatment

Diethylcarbamazine for 3 weeks (6 mg/kg/day) is treatment of choice. Relapses may be seen in one-fourth patients. Repeated monthly courses of DEC at 2–3 monthly intervals for up to 2 years may be useful in patients with relapse and persistent mild ILD. Steroids may be beneficial by reducing inflammation and release of oxidants but the exact dose and duration is not established.

CYSTIC FIBROSIS

It is an autosomal recessive disorder caused by mutations in gene, encoding a protein called cystic fibrosis transmembrane conductance regulator (CFTR) in chromosome 7. The abnormality of cAMP (cyclic adenosine monophosphate)-regulated chloride conductance by epithelial cells on various mucosal surfaces leads to dehydration of secretions that are too viscid and difficult to clear. Till date, more than 2,500 variants in *CFTR* gene are identified, but not all of them may cause the disease.

Clinical Features

Besides respiratory involvement, other systems affected include exocrine pancreas, gastrointestinal and hepatobiliary system, male genitourinary tract, and exocrine sweat glands. Characteristic clinical features include chronic sinopulmonary disease, pancreatic insufficiency and recurrent pancreatitis, neonatal bowel obstruction, rectal prolapse, focal biliary cirrhosis, failure to thrive (FTT), Pseudo-Bartter syndrome, and male infertility (obstructive azoospermia).

Diagnosis

Cystic fibrosis is diagnosed if a patient has characteristic phenotypic features *OR* history of CF in sibling *OR* positive newborn screening (NBS) test result *AND* any one of the following: (1) Increased sweat chloride concentration, (2) two CF mutations, and (3) demonstration of abnormal nasal epithelial ion transport.

In developed countries, CF is diagnosed by NBS programs using immunoreactive trypsin assay. Beyond neonatal period, quantitative pilocarpine iontophoresis sweat chloride test remains the gold standard. Availability of *CFTR*-modulating therapies specific to certain mutations may benefit patients with positive sweat chloride criteria. Patients with intermediate sweat test results may benefit from *CFTR* genotyping for confirmation of diagnosis.

Different regions across globe have shown variations in CF mutations. ΔF508 is highest in Caucasian population and common in Sri Lankan patients as compared to Indian subcontinent and similar ethnicity-specific variant distribution was also observed in China with p.Gly970Asp as the most common mutation and p.Phe508del, rare in comparison to Caucasians.

Treatment

Specific pancreatic enzyme replacement, supplementation of fat-soluble vitamins, salt supplementation, airway clearance, and antibiotics form the mainstay of treatment. Supportive care with a multidisciplinary team of physician, physiotherapist, dietician, psychologist, and social scientist is required. Gene therapy using a viral or liposomal vector does not appear to be a therapeutic option for the near future. CFTR modulators such as ivacaftor and lumacaftor are very costly and unaffordable in developing countries.

Tropical countries share common problems such as lack of neonatal screening programs, reduced life expectancy, poor availability of necessary drugs, and a lack of CF services. Socioeconomic factors along with rare genotypes may contribute to worse disease outcome in tropical children. Increasing awareness of CF and availability of diagnostic tests will lead to the early identification and reduce morbidity and mortality.

ALLERGIC BRONCHOPULMONARY ASPERGILLOSIS

It is a respiratory illness attributed to establishment of the fungus in the airways and the development of hypersensitivity to its antigens. It is a well-documented phenomenon in adults with increasing significance in children recently. It usually occurs in immunocompetent but susceptible children with bronchial asthma and CF. *Aspergillus* spores are entangled in the viscid sputum generating a cascade of inflammatory reactions resulting in ABPA. ABPA is mostly attributed to be caused by *Aspergillus fumigatus*. Other species *A. niger, A. flavus,* and other fungi—*Stemphylium lanuginosum, Helminthosporium* species; *Candida* species have been also reported in association with ABPA.

Epidemiology

In the pediatric population, ABPA has mostly been observed in children with CF with a reported prevalence of 2–15% with multiple reports from the Indian subcontinent. In a study from AIIMS, Delhi, proportion of ABPA with CF was reported to be around 18%. Predisposing factors included low CF score, age >12 years, airway reversibility, atopy, and eosinophilia.[5] Other risk factors for ABPA in CF include poor nutritional status, use of inhaled antibiotics, inhaled corticosteroid, long-term azithromycin consumption, rhDNase (recombinant human DNase) therapy, and *Pseudomonas* infection. Similarly, studies have shown occurrence of ABPA in children with poorly controlled asthma leading to significant morbidity. A recent Indian study reported ABPA in 26% of children with poorly controlled asthma.[6] Another similar study reported ABPA in 15% of children with asthma and in 6.5% of total asthmatic children screened.[7] Undiagnosed and untreated

ABPA may lead to parenchymal and airway damage sacking in respiratory failure and secondary heart failure.

Pathogenesis

Allergic bronchopulmonary aspergillosis is characterized pathologically by mucoid impaction of the bronchi, eosinophilic pneumonia, and bronchocentric granulomatosis. Important role of T cells with increase in Th2 CD4+ cell responses to *Aspergillus* antigens has been observed in ABPA. Aspergillus-responsive T cells generate interleukin (IL)-4, IL-5, and IL-13, which in turn account for the increase in blood and airway eosinophils and IgE in ABPA. *Aspergillus* spores adhere to preactivated epithelium in genetically susceptible patients with asthma or CF and grow into hyphae. After bronchial penetration, *Aspergillus* antigens activate immune response resulting in bronchial/bronchiolar inflammation and destruction. A number of genetic factors are associated with ABPA including *HLA-DR2, HLA-DR5, HLA-DQ2, CFTR* gene mutations, *surfactant protein-A2, IL-4 alpha-chain receptor* polymorphisms, *IL-10* polymorphisms, *toll-like receptor* polymorphisms, etc.

Clinical Features and Staging

Allergic bronchopulmonary aspergillosis may be suspected in difficult-to-control asthma despite good compliance to therapy. The points for suspicion in children with CF include wheezing, transient pulmonary infiltrates, and exacerbations responding inadequately to antibiotics. The clinical picture of ABPA is dominated by asthma/CF and recurrent exacerbations. Episodes of exacerbation present with episodes of bronchial obstruction, fever, malaise, expectoration of brownish mucus plugs, and hemoptysis. Patients with fibrotic stage present with severe dyspnea and cyanosis, and there is extensive bronchiectasis, cavitary lesions, and fibrosis in lungs.

The conventional five stages of ABPA progression include: (1) Acute, (2) remission, (3) exacerbation, (4) corticosteroid-dependent asthma, and (5) fibrosis (end stage). Recently, Agarwal et al. suggested the seven stages of ABPA: *Stage 0* (asymptomatic—ABPA criteria are fulfilled in a patient of controlled asthma), *Stage 1* (acute—ABPA criteria positive along with uncontrolled symptoms), *Stage 2* (response—clinically better with total IgE decreased by >25% from baseline), *Stage 3* (exacerbation—clinically worsened with total IgE increased >50% from baseline), *Stage 4* (remission-clinically improved with total IgE at baseline or increase is <50%), *Stage 5* (treatment dependent—≥2 exacerbations in 6 months or worsening

Box 2: Diagnostic criteria for ABPA.

Predisposing conditions (one must be present): Asthma *OR* cystic fibrosis
Obligatory criteria (both must be present):
- *Aspergillus* skin test positivity or elevated IgE levels against *Aspergillus fumigatus*
- Elevated total IgE concentration (typically > 1,000 IU/mL, but if the patient meets all other criteria, an IgE value < 1,000 IU/mL may be acceptable)

Other criteria (at least two must be present):
- Precipitating serum antibodies to *A. fumigatus* or elevated serum *Aspergillus* IgG by immunoassay
- Radiographic pulmonary opacities consistent with ABPA
- Total eosinophil count >500 cells/μL in glucocorticoid-naïve patients (may be historical)

(ABPA: allergic bronchopulmonary aspergillosis)

on tapering steroids), and *Stage 6* (advanced—extensive bronchiectasis and cor pulmonale).[8]

Diagnosis and Treatment

The diagnosis of ABPA may be made as per criteria in **Box 2**.[8] The mainstay of treatment aims to control episodes of acute inflammation and to limit progressive lung injury. Glucocorticoids are considered the mainstay of treatment of acute ABPA and antifungal therapy may help to decrease exacerbations, reduction in sputum eosinophilic count, IgE levels, and eosinophilic cationic proteins. Inhaled glucocorticoids may help control symptoms of asthma but do not have documented efficacy in preventing acute episodes of ABPA. In asthmatic patients with ABPA, the recommended dosage of prednisolone is 0.5 mg/kg/day for the first 2 weeks, and further tapering and discontinuation at 3 months. For ABPA in CF patients, recommended dose of prednisolone is 0.5–2.0 mg/kg/day (maximum 60 mg) for 1–2 weeks, then 0.5–2.0 mg/kg/day every other day for 1–2 weeks, and then taper in next 2–3 months. There is lack of studies evaluating the efficacy of itraconazole for ABPA in asthmatic children. The dose of itraconazole recommended for children is 5 mg/kg/day (maximum dose: 400 mg/day). The total duration of therapy should be 3–6 months.

◼ FOREIGN BODIES IN AIRWAY

Foreign body aspiration constitutes a significant cause of morbidity and mortality, in children between age of 6 months and 5 years. The anatomical position of the larynx, episodes of shouting, crying and playing while eating, and lack of parental supervision while eating and playing contribute to it. Since it is an emergency and if not managed appropriately, it may contribute to chronic lung injury and cause chronic pulmonary infections, bronchiectasis, and lung abscess. It is misdiagnosed most commonly as asthma or pneumonia. Timely diagnosis and management of an inhaled foreign body offer a diagnostic challenge to the physician.

Classification

The most common site for foreign body aspiration is the right lower bronchus or bronchus intermedius as it is more vertical, shorter, and wider. Foreign bodies may be classified as follows:

- On the basis of grade of foreign body airway obstruction, foreign body aspiration causes *partial* OR *complete* obstruction. The partial obstruction causes mild-to-moderate effects contrary to magnitudes of complete occlusion.
- On the basis of origin, foreign bodies may be either *internal or external.* Examples of internal or endogenous sources include mucus masses—mucocele. External or exogenous bodies include food particles (in 40% of cases) such as peanuts, pulses, seeds, and almonds. Nonorganic materials include toys, pen caps, stone, marbles, and balloons. Vegetative foreign body predominates in rural areas and in winter season (peanut), whereas nonorganic materials predominate in urban areas. In India, peanuts account as the most common foreign body.

Clinical Features

Classically, the onset of symptoms is sudden. A study from Delhi reported common clinical features of choking (90%), paroxysmal cough, and fast breathing followed by stridor and decreased air entry, as most common features of foreign bodies in airways. The triad of wheezing, paroxysmal cough, and decreased air entry is documented in about 35–39% of patients. Another study documented triad of cough, dyspnea, and wheezing as more common and seen in 60–70% of presentations.[9,10] A significant proportion of children come to the hospital after few weeks of aspiration. It may be attributed to parental inattention and wrong diagnosis, absence of classical symptoms, after the acute initial phase of symptoms, and diverse clinical features due to inhalation of foreign body.

Diagnosis and Treatment

A typical history of sudden onset of symptoms such as choking and respiratory distress after eating is quite suggestive of foreign body. Chest X-ray is not a fairly acceptable investigation as most of the foreign bodies are radiolucent, which are missed on chest X-ray. However, focal hyperinflation and lung collapse may be suggestive based on the background of suggestive history of foreign body aspiration. Rigid bronchoscopy is the treatment of choice for removal of tracheobronchial foreign body. Rigid bronchoscopy should be considered the definitive diagnostic and therapeutic intervention in all cases where history and physical examination are suggestive or suspicious of airway foreign body.

■ INTERSTITIAL LUNG DISEASE

Interstitial lung disease or diffuse lung disease (DLD) consists of a diverse group of disorders which share the common characteristics of involvement of pulmonary parenchyma and interference with gas exchange. These disorders are classified together because of similar clinical, radiographic, physiologic, or pathologic manifestations. Underlying pathology includes extensive alteration of alveolar and airway architecture, and changes in the interstitial compartment. The term ILD is less precise because the interstitium is not involved in some of the conditions, such as neuroendocrine cell hyperplasia of infancy. Another term used in the literature is "diffuse parenchymal lung disease." This may be classified in **Table 1**.[11,12]

Clinical Features

The clinical features of ILD include symptoms such as cough, rapid and/or difficult breathing, exercise intolerance and signs of resting tachypnea, adventitious sounds, retractions, digital clubbing, failure to thrive, hypoxemia or respiratory failure. These are nonspecific and thus the first step in diagnostic evaluation is to exclude more common causes including immunodeficiency, infections, congenital heart disease, recurrent aspiration, cystic fibrosis, and PCD. Extrapulmonary invovlement including skin, eye and nail changes, anemia or pancytopenia, lymphadenopathy, arthritis, hepatosplenomegaly, etc; are helpful in differentiating ILD, especially in older children.

■ DIAGNOSIS AND TREATMENT

The first step in diagnostic evaluation is to exclude more common causes of DLD including HIV and other immunodeficiency disorders, testing for infectious etiologies, barium swallow esophageal pH/impedance probe, echocardiogram, bronchoscopy (infection, aspiration, pulmonary hemorrhage, etc.), and sweat chloride testing. Lung function status to know the severity and extent of disease includes radiological tests (X-ray chest, chest CT, electrocardiogram for secondary pulmonary hypertension), pulmonary function tests (spirometry, plethysmography, 6-minute walk test and

Table 1: Classification of interstitial lung diseases (ILD) in children.

Diseases specific to infancy	Disorders with primary pulmonary involvement
Acinar/alveolar dysgenesis	Alveolar hemorrhage syndromes (idiopathic pulmonary capillaritis)
Congenital alveolar dysplasia	Genetic disorders of surfactant production and metabolism
Alveolar capillary dysplasia with misalignment of pulmonary veins (ACD-MPV)	Pulmonary vascular disorders
Pulmonary hypoplasia (oligohydramnios, congenital diaphragmatic hernia)	Pulmonary interstitial glycogenosis
Bronchopulmonary dysplasia	Chronic eosinophilic pneumonia
Neuroendocrine cell hyperplasia of infancy (NEHI)	Pulmonary alveolar proteinosis (PAP)
Pulmonary interstitial glycogenosis	NEHI
Surfactant dysfunction disorders	Infectious or post-infectious chronic lung disease
Diseases nonspecific to infancy	Hypersensitivity pneumonitis
Hypersensitivity pneumonitis or toxic inhalation	Drug or radiation induced lung disease
Aspiration syndromes	Aspiration syndromes
Eosinophilic pneumonia	Disorders of lung growth and development
Acute interstitial pneumonia (AIP)	Systemic disorders with associated pulmonary involvement
Nonspecific interstitial pneumonia (NSIP)	Connective tissue disease [e.g. systemic lupus erythematosus (SLE) polymyositis/dermatomyositis, systemic sclerosis, mixed connective tissue disease, or systemic juvenile idiopathic arthritis (JIA)]
Idiopathic pulmonary hemosiderosis	Dyskeratosis congenita (bone marrow hypoplasia, often with skin, nail and mucosal changes)
Immunodeficiency and lymphoproliferative disorders	Storage diseases
Storage diseases	Neurocutaneous syndromes
Sarcoidosis	Immunodeficiency and lymphoproliferative disorders
Langerhans cell histiocytosis	Langerhans cell histiocytosis
	Lymphatic disorders
	Malignancies

infant pulmonary function testing, diffusion studies, pulse oximetry and arterial blood gases). Other investigations for systemic illness disorders including immune studies, connective tissue disorders, hypersensitivity pneumonitis, etc. are also suggested. Lung biopsy may be required in many DLD. Largely, the assessment ensues from least-to-most invasive procedures, but it can vary depending on the context, acuity, and severity of the patient's condition.

Management is mostly supportive, which comprises supplemental oxygen and ventilator support, nutritional support, proper immunizations including annual influenza vaccinations, supervised exercise (for older children), bronchodilators for reversible airway obstruction, vigorous treatment of superimposed infections, and avoidance of harmful environmental exposures (cigarette smoke and other inhaled irritants). Conditions that may respond to glucocorticoids include ILD associated with connective tissue disorders, hypersensitivity pneumonitis, lymphocytic interstitial pneumonia, and cryptogenic organizing pneumonia. Connective tissue disorders respond well to immunosuppressive medications, but there is no clear evidence of efficacy of systemic corticosteroids or hydroxychloroquine in most other forms of childhood DLD. Pulse therapy with intravenous methylprednisolone (10–30 mg/kg per day), for 3 consecutive days each month or a single dose weekly is often preferred in comparison to daily oral therapy with 1–2 mg/kg of prednisolone.

Other specific treatments include antimicrobials for certain infections, management of swallowing dysfunction and/or reflux in patients with chronic aspiration, avoidance of the offending antigen in hypersensitivity pneumonitis, and whole lung lavage for older children with pulmonary alveolar proteinosis. Granulocyte-macrophage colony-stimulating factor may be tried as an alternative to lung lavage in acquired pulmonary alveolar proteinosis. Glucocorticoids are not beneficial for neuroendocrine cell hyperplasia of infancy, alveolar capillary dysplasia with misalignment of the pulmonary veins, and pulmonary hypoplasia. Lung transplantation is an option for children with end-stage lung disease. Genetic counseling and family support are also important components of care.

AIR POLLUTION AND LUNG HEALTH

It is obvious that the quality of air that we breathe determines the health of our lungs as well as of other organs. With increasing urbanization, industrialization, deforestation, etc. the quality of air is deteriorating rapidly. An article published in Lancet reports that DALY due to chronic respiratory disease in India has increased from 4.5% to 6.4% over a period of 20 years, and 53.7% of it is attributed to air pollution.[13] Major components of air pollutants include carbon monoxide, nitrogen oxide, sulfur oxide, particulate matters, volatile organic compounds, diesel exhaust particles, and ozone. It is surprising that exposure to air pollutants starts before the birth. Placenta, assumed to be an efficient barrier, allows passage of several air pollutants into the fetal circulation. Such exposure creates impact on cognitive function as well as on the immune system. Mothers exposed to higher level of particulate matter give birth to child with decreased telomere length symbolizing lesser quantity of buffer for postnatal influence of factors, thereby promoting biological aging. This may be compounded by exposure during neonatal period and early childhood which is another critical period of growth of lungs and immune system.

The hypothesis of an early origin of chronic respiratory diseases supports the theory that noxious agents acting during periods crucial to lung development may give rise to permanent structural or functional changes in the lung, with potential lifelong consequences. Air pollutants trigger a series of biological processes including innate immunity inflammation, oxidative stress, apoptosis and autophagy, and an imbalance of T helper cells, all of which are associated with pathological changes in allergic respiratory diseases. There is increase in the risk of respiratory tract infection by direct toxic effects on the mucosa, impaired ciliary function, and impaired local immune defenses resulting in prolonged inflammation, congestion, or predisposition to infection. Air pollution is also associated with reduced lung function and enhanced airway reactivity in children with asthma. On the top of it, air pollutants induce epigenetic changes too, which is passed across the generation. Preventive measures include reduced exposure, strengthening of antioxidant defense and enforcing strict legislative norms to reduce air pollution.

ALLERGIES IN TROPICS

There is progressive increase in the prevalence of allergic diseases globally and in India. Presently, about one-fourth of Indians are sensitized to a varied number of allergens.[14] Allergic disorders include both IgE-mediated and non-IgE-mediated reactions. Data document a sharp increase in the prevalence rate of IgE-mediated atopic diseases. Spectrum of allergic disorders includes bronchial asthma, atopic rhinitis, dermatitis, allergic conjunctivitis, urticaria, food allergy, insect allergy, and anaphylaxis. Allergic rhinitis (AR) and asthma are chronic in nature, while anaphylaxis, and food, drug, and insect allergies are often acute. Major sources of allergen in India include pollen grains, fungal spores, foods, insects, and dust mites. With mélange of climate, vegetation, and food habits, India has a varied range of allergens. Eliminating the modifiable risk factors could help reduce huge amount of allergy disorders, for example by providing education, cessation of smoking, reduction of air pollution, and providing clean fuel (LPG) to poor and vulnerable households.

BRONCHIECTASIS AND ASTHMA

Most common etiologies for bronchiectasis remain cystic fibrosis and noncystic types including ABPA and immunodeficiency disorders in the west. In Indian children, the profile of bronchiectasis remain same, however postinfectious bronchiectasis secondary to tuberculosis, measles, HIV, bacterial infections, and foreign body also contribute significantly.

Asthma remains a global burden. In India and other tropical countries, the incidence continues to rise as per latest reports. The acceptability of disease, treatment adherence, and financial implication and support in tropical countries still remain a challenge.

CHALLENGES OF DIAGNOSIS AND TREATMENT OF NONINFECTIVE RESPIRATORY DISORDERS IN TROPICS

The hurdles in diagnosis of chronic lung diseases are multiple, especially in tropical countries. Specialized techniques, such as pediatric bronchoscopy and endobronchial ultrasound (EBUS)-guided biopsy, which are helpful in direct visualization and samples for cytopathological evaluation are not widely available. Neonatal screening program (NBS) for CF is not available in most of the tropical countries as compared to west and sweat testing chloride remains the gold standard, however, with limited availability. The mutation analysis has limited role due to multiple mutations identified and only few having therapeutic implications. Limited availability of electron microscopy for diagnosis of PCDs, polysomnography for evaluation of sleep disorders, estimation of exhaled nitric oxide levels (FeNO and Nasal

NO), and nonstandardization of allergy testing panels for hypersensitivity pneumonitis and asthma exist. Most helpful and widely used tests include radiological evaluation [high-resolution CT (HRCT)/contrast-enhanced CT (CECT)] which provides information about disease localization, pattern and extent and clue to underlying etiology. Though lung function tests including spirometry are available for older children, for infants and toddlers, newer techniques such as impulse oscillometry rapid thoracic compression (RTC) or raised volume rapid thoracic compression (RVRTC) or whole body plethysmography are limited to specialized centers only. Similarly, treatment of most of noninfective diseases has financial constraints such as enzyme supplementation and CFTR modulators in cystic fibrosis, immunodeficiency disorders requiring immunoglobulin replacements or transplantation or practical limitations in environmental exposures. Home oxygen and ventilation are very poorly developed in India and elsewhere.

Hence, there is a need to develop more centers to enhance services including (a) assessment of pulmonary physiology by performing pulmonary function testing in all age groups, (b) improving diagnostic and therapeutic role of bronchoscopy and BAL (c) sweat testing, (d) molecular diagnostics for various respiratory illnesses, and (e) utilizing advanced imaging and minimally invasive technologies for diagnosis and treatment of respiratory illnesses.

KEY MESSAGES

- After acute respiratory tract infections and tuberculosis, noninfective causes remain important cause of mortality and morbidity in children.
- Noninfective diseases such as asthma, tropical pulmonary eosinophilia, immunodeficiency and connective tissue disorders are common in pediatric population from tropical countries.
- Cystic fibrosis is not rare in India and other tropical countries and should be highly suspected in young children with wet cough and failure to thrive.
- Children with eosinophilia from endemic areas should be evaluated for tropical pulmonary eosinophilia.
- Allergic bronchopulmonary aspergillosis should be highly suspected in children with poorly controlled asthma and exacerbations of cystic fibrosis; and not uncommon.
- A previously well child with sudden onset of choking, cyanosis, and distress should be evaluated always for foreign body.

- Interstitial lung disease though rare, but not uncommon in children, may be suspected as underlying chronic respiratory settings.
- Environmental factors such as exposure to pets, fungi, plantations, pigeons, and factories are important in chronic respiratory diseases.
- Asthma and other allergic disorders are on increasing trends in tropics and west and cause of global concern.
- Environmental pollution and its ill effects affect both adult and pediatric lung health.

REFERENCES

1. Kabra SK, Lodha R, Mehta P. 50 years of pediatric pulmonology: progress and future. Indian Pediatr. 2013;50:99-103.
2. Indika NLR, Vidanapathirana DM, Dilanthi HW, et al. Phenotypic spectrum and genetic heterogeneity of cystic fibrosis in Sri Lanka. BMC Medical Genet. 2019;20(1):89.
3. Guo X, Liu K, Liu Y, et al. Clinical and genetic characteristics of cystic fibrosis in CHINESE patients: a systemic review of reported cases. Orphanet J Rare Dis. 2018;13(1):224.
4. Mullerpattan JB, Udwadia ZF, Udwadia FE. Tropical pulmonary eosinophilia: a review. Indian J Med Res. 2013;138(3):295-302.
5. Sharma VK, Raj D, Xess I, et al. Prevalence and risk factors for allergic bronchopulmonary aspergillosis in Indian children with cystic fibrosis. Indian Pediatr. 2014;51(4):295-7.
6. Singh M, Das S, Chauhan A, et al. The diagnostic criteria for allergic bronchopulmonary aspergillosis in children with poorly controlled asthma need to be re-evaluated. Acta Paediatr. 2015;104(5):e206-9.
7. Chetty A, Bhargava S, Jain RK. Allergic bronchopulmonary aspergillosis in Indian children with bronchial asthma. Ann Allergy. 1985;54(1):46-9.
8. Agarwal R, Chakrabarti A, Shah A, et al. Allergic broncho-pulmonary aspergillosis: review of literature and proposal of new diagnostic and classification criteria. Clin Exp Allergy. 2013;43(8):850-73.
9. Salih AM, Alfaki M, Alam-Elhuda DM. Airway foreign bodies: A critical review for a common pediatric emergency. World J Emerg Med. 2016;7(1):5-12.
10. Sehgal A, Singh V, Chandra J, et al. Foreign body aspiration. Indian Pediatr. 2002;39(11):1006-10.
11. Deutsch GH, Young LR, Deterding RR, et al. Diffuse lung disease in young children: application of a novel classification scheme. Am J Respir Crit Care Med. 2007;176(11):1120-8.
12. Kurland G, Deterding RR, Hagood JS, et al. An official American Thoracic Society clinical practice guideline: classification, evaluation, and management of childhood interstitial lung disease in infancy. Am J Respir Crit Care Med. 2013;188(3):376-94.
13. India State-Level Disease Burden Initiative CRD Collaborators. The burden of chronic respiratory diseases and their heterogeneity across the states of India: the Global Burden of Disease Study 1990–2016. Lancet Glob Health. 2018;6(12):e1363-74.
14. Bhattacharya K, Sircar G, Dasgupta A, et al. Spectrum of Allergens and Allergen Biology in India. Int Arch Allergy Immunol. 2018;177:219-37.

Noncommunicable Tropical Gastrointestinal and Pancreatobiliary Diseases

Moinak Sen Sarma

INTRODUCTION

Communicable diseases are mostly infectious and commonly found in tropical settings. This chapter focuses on some of the noncommunicable, gastrointestinal, and pancreatobiliary diseases that are predominantly found in tropical developing countries. They may be seen sporadically occurring in the West, especially in the migrant population. Though some of the disorders are still prevalent, others are on a declining trend possibly due to better hygiene standards or shift in etiopathophysiology in tropical countries. Due to lack of resources for workup, in developing countries, noncommunicable diseases may remain undiagnosed, despite strong clinical suspicion.

EXTRAHEPATIC PORTAL VENOUS OBSTRUCTION

This is a disorder of occurring in childhood with a manifestation continuum into adulthood. The major bulk of portal hypertension (PHT) in Indian and Asian children is due to extrahepatic portal venous obstruction (EHPVO) in contrast to cirrhosis in the developed countries. Disease burden in Indian children is mostly reported from Northern (sub-Himalayan) and Eastern (draining areas of the Gangetic-Yamuna belt) states, lesser from Western and Southern parts (author's observation). EHPVO is the consequence of portal vein thrombosis (PVT) of an unknown etiology just outside the liver. It may have variable extension proximally into the intrahepatic radicles, distally into its confluence, tributaries (splenic and superior mesenteric vein) or entire splanchnic system. Isolated involvement of the splenic, superior mesenteric, or inferior mesenteric vein is not included under the definition of EHPVO. For the working definition of EHPVO, it is mandatory to document a "portal cavernoma" (portal vein replaced by a web of collaterals) on imaging.

Etiopathogenesis

Since PVT may be a subacute process, it is often clinically missed at the time of onset. Hence what exactly causes PVT is largely known. It is known to occur predominantly in the lower socioeconomic strata. Hence with the hygiene hypothesis, the most popular putative mechanism is an occult intra-abdominal infection to incite the process. Bacteria and endotoxins draining from the superior mesenteric vein relatively decrease the blood flow at the portal vein confluence before entering the liver. This results in portal vein phlebosclerosis, thrombosis, and subsequent cavernoma formation in approximately 3–8 weeks. Various studies have shown that umbilical sepsis, umbilical catheterization, and *Bacteroides* bacteremia are the causative agents of portal phlebitis. Infections and inflammation in the hepato-pancreato-biliary system due to anatomical (e.g. choledochal cyst, Caroli disease) or acquired (e.g. liver abscess, acute pancreatitis) factors are known causes of secondary portal vein thrombosis. Studies have failed to show any preexisting hypercoagulable states responsible for this condition. Rarely, congenital anomalies of the portal vein and iatrogenic trauma during surgery have been reported to cause EHPVO.[1]

Clinical Presentation

Eighty-five percent of children, mostly in the first decade present with single or multiple bouts of variceal hemorrhage (hematemesis and melena). The rest 15% are nonbleeders presenting with incidentally detected isolated splenomegaly. Antecedent febrile illness and respiratory tract infection (Valsalva maneuver) tend to rupture the varices. Bleeding is worsened by ingestion of nonsteroidal anti-inflammatory drugs (e.g. ibuprofen and diclofenac) used for fever. They cause gastric erosions and worsens the pre-existing portal hypertensive gastropathy. Variceal bleeding is characteristically painless, large volume, and well tolerated necessitating the requirement of packed cell transfusion. Presence of postural signs (dizziness, syncope, and prostration) and hypotension indicates significant blood loss. Presence of gastrointestinal (GI) bleeding and the absence of jaundice are 97.5% accurate in predicting the diagnosis of EHPVO as compared to cirrhosis.[2] Clinical examination reveals isolated splenomegaly without any stigmata of chronic liver disease. Liver may be palpable if the patient is in cardiac failure due to anemia (postbleeding). Splenic size may acutely decrease just after a massive hemorrhage (to compensate for the volume loss) and resume prebleeding size after blood transfusion. Massive splenomegaly may be accompanied by dragging sensation, left upper quadrant pain, splenic infarction **(Fig. 1)**, mild unconjugated hyperbilirubinemia and poor quality of life. Though hypersplenism is common, symptoms related to the same (symptomatic anemia and spontaneous skin bleeds) are rare (5%). Chronic dragging sensation and apprehensions of rupture of a massive spleen may preclude them from contact sports. Massive bleeding may be accompanied by diuretic-responsive transient transudative ascites (13–18%). Jaundice is seen in advanced EHPVO due to symptomatic portal cholangiopathy (7–10%) resulting from obstruction of extrahepatic bile ducts (compression by collaterals or ischemic biliary strictures). Unscreened blood transfusion in the past may cause chronic hepatitis B or C infection manifesting later with frank liver disease.

Growth retardation (stunting and wasting) occurs in up to 33–54% of children.[3] Portal colopathy is a complication which presents with bleeding per rectum from anorectal varices and mucosal changes in the colon.

INVESTIGATIONS

Hemogram detects hypersplenism (decrease of any two cell lines assessed in a nonbled state, 12 weeks after last blood transfusion). Liver functions tests are usually preserved, except hypoproteinemia–hypoalbuminemia postbleeding. Baseline hepatitis B, hepatitis C, and human immunodeficiency virus (HIV) status (12 weeks after last blood transfusion) is required as most patients are multitransfused. Doppler ultrasonography (DUS) is sensitive (94–100%) and specific (96%) to confirm portal cavernoma. A dominant collateral (irregular walls with the sluggish flow) along the sclerosed portal vein may rarely be mistaken as a patent portal vein leading to confusion in diagnosis. DUS gives additional information about the degree of splenomegaly, presence of splenic infarction, patency of veins in portal circuit (splenic, superior mesenteric, inferior mesenteric), size of shuntable systemic veins (e.g. left renal vein), peribiliary collaterals, intrahepatic biliary dilatation (suggestive of portal cholangiopathy), and presence of ascites. Computed tomography (CT) angiography **(Fig. 2)** or MR portovenogram is indicated in cases where DUS has been inconclusive and as a definitive road map before contemplating shunt surgery. Magnetic resonance (MR) cholangiography delineates the degree of portal cholangiopathy **(Fig. 3)**.[4] Liver biopsy and hepatic wedge venous pressures are not routinely required.

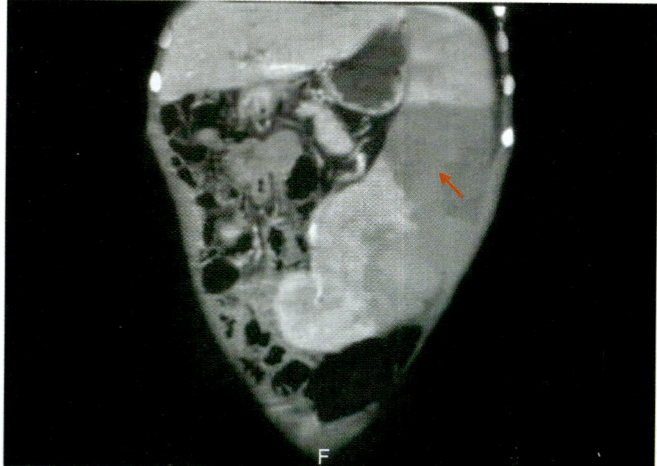

Fig. 1: Computed tomography abdomen showing massively enlarged spleen with splenic infarct (arrow) in extrahepatic portal venous obstruction (EHPVO).

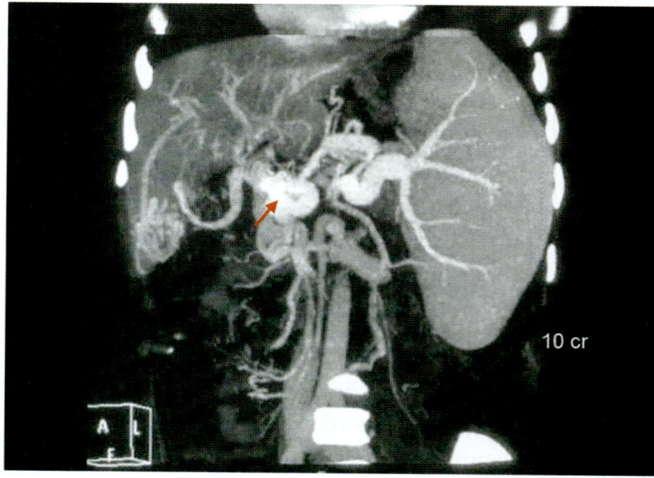

Fig. 2: Computed tomography portovenogram showing portal cavernoma (arrow).

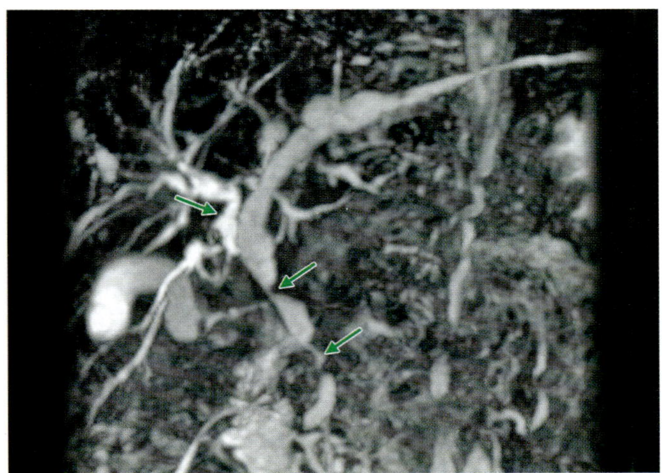

Fig. 3: Magnetic resonance cholangiogram showing intrahepatic and extrahepatic strictures (arrows) in extrahepatic portal venous obstruction (EHPVO) suggestive of portal cholangiopathy.

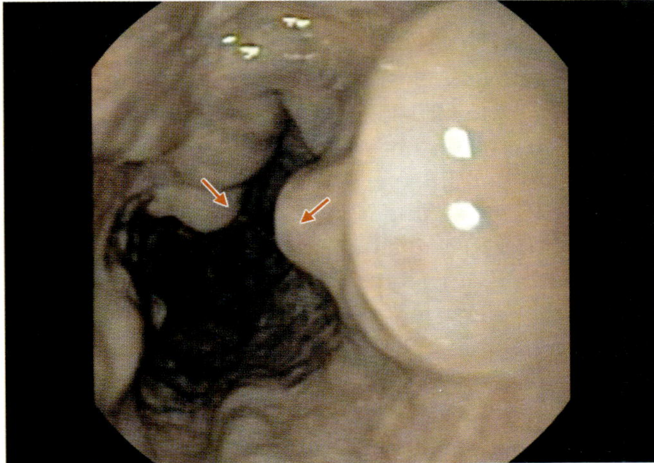

Fig. 4: Upper gastrointestinal endoscopy showing large esophageal varices (arrows).

Management

Acute Variceal Bleed

Acute variceal bleeding occurs due to rupture of large esophageal varices in 97% of first-time bleeders **(Fig. 4)**. Gastric variceal bleeding is less frequent. Ongoing bleed is assessed by tachycardia, hypotension, or postural hemodynamics and saline lavages. Packed red cell transfusion should target to maintain hemoglobin at 8 mg/dL. Hypertransfusion may increase portal pressure and aggravate further bleeding from varices. In today's era, the pediatric Sengstaken–Blakemore tube is used only in settings of uncontrolled variceal bleeding when medical and endoscopic therapy have failed or when endoscopic facilities are not available in remote areas. Octreotide is a somatostatin analog that decreases the splanchnic and azygos blood flow, thus reducing the pressure in the varices. It is infused as 1 mcg/kg bolus followed by 1–5 mcg/kg/hour gradual escalation till hemostasis is achieved and maintained for 3–5 days after endoscopic therapy before tapering. Overall this therapy is well tolerated, with mild reversible side effects like hyperglycemia, abdominal discomfort, nausea, and diarrhea. Beta-blockers (propranolol 0.5–2.0 mg/kg/day or carvedilol) may be initiated in those without medical contraindications (asthma and heart block) after control of the bleeding episode or as prophylaxis in nonbleeders. Hemodynamic resuscitation with packed cell transfusion and octreotide should be followed by endoscopic therapy.

Endoscopic Therapy

Details of endoscopic therapy are beyond the purview of this chapter. The goal of endoscopic management in bleeders is to find the cause, localize the site of bleeding, and control acute variceal bleeding. During endoscopy, one should look for the presence of esophageal varices, gastric varices, portal hypertensive gastropathy, and for any other cause of bleeding like duodenal or gastric ulcers. Endoscopic procedures are performed at intervals of 2–3 weeks till the esophageal varices are eradicated, primarily by two modalities of therapy—endoscopic variceal ligation and/or endoscopic sclerotherapy. Nonbleeders with large esophageal varices (who are not on beta-blockers) are prophylactically tackled endoscopically before they rupture. Bleeding gastric varices are managed with glue injection (N-butyl 2-cyanoacrylate or isobutyl 2-cyanoacrylate). Balloon deployed self-expandable metallic stents and endosonography-deployed microcoils in gastric varices have been used successfully in adults with torrential variceal bleeding but are not yet recommended in children. Hemospray has been used in limited settings with success in children until definitive therapy is offered. Esophageal stents have been used in uncontrolled variceal bleeding in adults with 80% success.

Surgery

It is advisable for all EHPVO patients to undergo an elective portosystemic shunt surgery soon after control of acute variceal bleeding. An ideal physiological shunt is a mesoportal Rex bypass (MPRB) where a graft is placed between the superior mesenteric vein and a patent left branch of PV through the Rex venous recessus, thereby restoring normal hepatopetal blood flow. This procedure is technically demanding and needs favorable anatomy, which is rarely encountered (patent left branch and communication with right branch of PV) with high rates of shunt block (40%). In poor socioeconomic countries, where referral is delayed, disease is longstanding and resources are limited, this procedure is rarely performed. In those where anatomy is not favorable and issues related to large spleen, central end-to-side splenorenal with splenectomy and end-to-side mesocaval shunts are performed, especially in developing countries. Due to relative deprivation of portal blood supply to the liver, mild liver ischemia and transient hepatic encephalopathy (3–5%) are known to occur. In trained surgical hands, rates of shunt blocks may be as low as 8–10%. Gastric devascularization for treatment of bleeding gastric varices is performed where there are no suitable shuntable veins. Symptomatic portal cholangiopathy that does not respond to portosystemic shunt surgery may require resection of bile duct stricture with bilioenteric anastomosis.[5]

◼ NONCIRRHOTIC PORTAL FIBROSIS

Noncirrhotic portal fibrosis (NCPF) is a condition where there is neither cirrhosis nor extrahepatic portal obstruction, but phlebosclerosis of the intrahepatic portal radicles. Though reported from all over the world, maximum cluster of pediatric cases is reported from lower socio-economic strata of the Indian subcontinent. In Japan, the terminology to describe this condition is "idiopathic portal hypertension" with preponderance in females in the fourth and fifth decades. The etiology is unclear but chronic exposure to vinyl chloride, copper sulfate or arsenic poisoning (West Bengal) have been postulated. *Escherichia coli* gastrointestinal infections in early life, prothrombotic states, primary immunodeficiencies, HIV, immunological disorders (celiac disease, autoimmune thyroiditis, and scleroderma) and exposure to thiopurines have been associated. In rare scenarios, there may be familial clustering (HLA DR3) and link with certain genetic conditions [Noonan, Turner, Adams–Oliver and POEMS (Polyneuropathy, Organomegaly, Endocrinopathy, Monoclonal protein, Skin changes) syndromes]. NCPF accounts of 4–5% of all pediatric portal hypertension. The condition presents just like EHPVO but predominantly in the second decade (adolescent or young adult) as well tolerated variceal bleeding or massive splenomegaly (nonbleeders). Issues related to large spleen (similar to EHPVO) are seen in the majority. Liver may be mildly enlarged or normal in the span. A small proportion (10–20%) may progress to behave like cryptogenic (nodular) cirrhosis with the shrunken liver, ascites, jaundice, hepatic

encephalopathy, or hepatopulmonary syndrome.[6] In contrast to EHPVO, portal vein is patent and dilated on imaging. The splenic vein is often more dilated than the portal vein. Liver functions are preserved except in advanced disease. For confirmation of diagnosis, liver biopsy, and hepatic venous pressure gradient (HVPG) are recommended. Characteristic obliterative portal venopathy in liver histology is seen in 40–60%. Rest may show aberrant portal vessels, sinusoidal dilatation, or even normal parenchyma. Most importantly liver histology is required to show the absence of cirrhosis. HVPG is normal (<5 mm Hg) or near normal (7–8 mm Hg) suggestive of a presinusoidal block. Management of acute variceal bleeding, endoscopic and pharmacotherapy are similar to EHPVO. Portosystemic shunt is controversial as it may ameliorate all symptoms but risk hepatic decompensation, especially in those where the disease may be progressive. Hence 20–30% may ultimately require liver transplantation.

◼ BUDD–CHIARI SYNDROME

Budd–Chiari syndrome (BCS) is a hepatic venous outflow obstruction at the level of all hepatic veins (HV), inferior vena cava (IVC), or both. This entity accounts for 3–7% of pediatric portal hypertension. In adults, the disease occurs due to an underlying prothrombotic state or myeloproliferative disorder and is reported from all over the world. In contrast, pediatric series of idiopathic etiology has been reported predominantly from India and China. Chronic BCS is most commonly caused due to thrombosis, phlebitis or web in the all three HV or IVC. Rarely, it may be caused from a secondary underlying cause (benign or malignant tumor, abscess, cyst, etc.) causing compression or invasion of HV and IVC. The antecedent thrombotic event that results in hepatic venous outflow obstruction is often innocuous and unidentified in children. If the obstruction is left untreated, chronicity ensues and the disease progresses to fibrosis and cirrhosis. In advanced stages, chronic BCS is indistinguishable from sinusoidal causes of portal hypertension. In Indian children, outflow obstructions are isolated IVC (2–9%), isolated HV (74–100%), and combined HV–IVC (23–25%). Though thrombophilia is an important etiology in BCS, the search for a causative prothrombotic workup is often unyielding, inconclusive, or ambiguous in children. Clinical settings to suspect thrombophilia are associated portal or mesenteric vein thrombosis, family history, thrombotic event in past (deep vein thrombosis), associated systemic diseases (inflammatory bowel disease, systemic lupus erythematosus, Behçet's disease, etc.) and recurrent stent block (after intervention).

Although an abnormal thrombophilia profile may be seen in 68–75% of children, the establishment of cause and effect is not straightforward. Low quantitative levels of protein C, protein S, homocysteine, and antithrombin III may reflect poor synthetic functions of the liver rather than thrombophilia state. Documentation of genetic mutation of the particular thrombophilia in a child and parents is confirmatory. Implications of thrombophilic state in children would mean imperative life-long anticoagulation. They would be at a lifetime risk of venous thrombosis elsewhere (abdominal, systemic) and increased comorbidities (hematological, cardiac).

CLINICAL MANIFESTATIONS

The usual age of presentation is 10 (1.5–17) years but children as young as 4–5 months have been reported. Chronic BCS is the most common presentation in children which is most often symptomatic. Hallmark feature is a tense intractable ascites (83–96%) that rapidly accumulates despite repeated large-volume paracentesis and is poorly controlled even with optimal diuretics. Often dilated tortuous veins (60–70%) with cephalad flow (above and below umbilicus) are seen over abdomen and flanks **(Fig. 5)**. Similar collaterals over back with flow upward is the hallmark of an intrahepatic IVC obstruction. As BCS is considered a "good cirrhotic", synthetic functions are relatively preserved at a presentation. At the onset, the child is usually anicteric with firm hepatomegaly, near-normal liver enzymes, low-to-normal albumin and normal

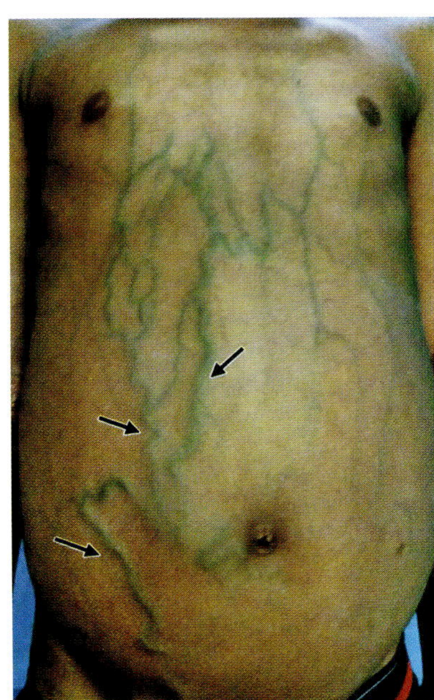

Fig. 5: Dilated tortuous abdominal veins with collateralization (arrows) in Budd–Chiari syndrome.

coagulation. Variceal bleeding (8–25%), overt jaundice (13–24%), hepatic hydrothorax (20–36%) and growth failure (28–36%) are relatively uncommon features. The end-stage disease manifests just like any other cirrhotic with jaundice, shrunken liver, encephalopathy, and coagulopathy. About 10% of chronic BCS are clinically asymptomatic but have features of portal hypertension (varices on endoscopy and splenomegaly ± hypersplenism). Tender hepatomegaly with minimal jaundice and ascites indicate acute or subacute presentation. Of the known causes of pediatric acute liver failures, BCS as a fulminant presentation is rare (1%).[7]

Diagnosis

Invasive venography ± cavography is the gold standard for diagnosis of BCS. In children, this procedure is deferred till the time of endovascular intervention. Hence, DUS, which is radiation-free assumes prime importance in the confirmation of diagnosis (60–96%). Narrowed, fibrotic, cord-like or thrombus-filled HV with loss of normal flow pattern is the usual finding. In IVC obstruction, a membrane, stenosis, and proximal prestenotic dilatation are found. Intrahepatic venovenous collaterals, caudate lobe hypertrophy and dilated caudate vein indicate the chronic process. Noninvasive angiography (CT or MR) is required when there is a diagnostic ambiguity. DUS not only diagnoses the condition, but also assesses the "health of the hepatic vein" as well as flow. Length of block, presence of hepatic vein "stump", dominant accessible collaterals, and orientation of the hepatic vein help in deciding the modality of endovascular management.

Management

Severe tense ascites that causes abdomino-respiratory discomfort and difficulty in ambulation needs immediate attention in the form of large-volume paracentesis (LVP). In a single-time LVP, it is advisable to drain <200 mL/kg ascitic fluid under albumin infusion (0.5–1 g/kg) to prevent postparacentesis circulatory dysfunction.[8] Multiple LVP and diuretics (furosemide and spironolactone in ratio of 2.5:1) are required till definitive intervention. Hepatic hydrothorax is also relieved with LVP but may occasionally require thoracocentesis in case of severe respiratory compromise. Varices need to be downgraded endoscopically 2–3 weeks before endovascular intervention and initiation of anticoagulation after the intervention. Between stabilization of the above issues and early recurrence of symptoms, an optimal therapeutic window is sought for definitive intervention in children. The aim of endovascular management is to relieve hepatic

Table 1: Management of Budd–Chiari syndrome.

Presentation	Site of block	Preferred technique	Route	Comments
Fulminant	Usually HV	None	Not applicable	LT only option
Acute	HV	TIPS	Transjugular	LT if TIPS fails
Chronic	HV (short segment <5 cm occlusion)	• Angioplasty only (infants) • Angioplasty preferably with stenting (older children)	• Transjugular preferred • Percutaneous transabdominal approach if transjugular fails	LT if radiological techniques fail or presentation as advanced liver disease
	HV long segment (>5 cm) or no HV stump	Direct intrahepatic portocaval shunt (DIPS) also known as modified TIPS	Transjugular	
	IVC web/segmental occlusion	IVC balloon angioplasty preferably with stenting (if placement of stent is appropriate for age)	Transfemoral	

(HV: hepatic vein; IVC: inferior vena cava; LT: liver transplantation; TIPS: transjugular intrahepatic portosystemic shunt)

congestion either through correction of obstruction or creation of a bypass radiologically. Most physiological intervention is restoration of flow within one HV and/or the occluded IVC. The definite therapies for the management of BCS are summarized in **Table 1**. Post procedure the patients are maintained on lifelong anticoagulation (warfarin) with target International Normalised Ratio 2 to 3. Pre-intervention pediatric end-stage liver disease (PELD) score <4 determines the favorable outcome of radiological intervention. The overall vascular patency rates are 87%, 82%, and 62% at 1, 5, and 10 years of follow-up.[7] Restenosis and repeat intervention is required in 30%. Liver transplantation is indicated in fulminant BCS, failure of endovascular intervention, advanced liver disease, genetically proven protein C, protein S, or antithrombin III deficiencies.

Hepatic Vena Cava Syndrome

Classified under BCS, hepatic vena cava syndrome (HVCS) is a primary obliterative disease of the hepatic portion of IVC characterized by a localized stenosis **(Fig. 6)**, long segment stenosis or web. For reasons unknown, the disease has shown a paradigm shift from Europe and North America to Afro-Asian countries including Japan. Presently, the disease is endemic in Nepal. Malnourished children and pregnant women with pelvic infections are most prone. Postulations include congenital "coarctation" of IVC and infections. Translocation of Gram-negative bacteremia from gut results in thrombophlebitis typically of the posterior wall of hepatic IVC. This area is in constant motion with the movement of the diaphragm making the blood flow turbulent and prone for endothelial damage. In time, the thrombophlebitis causes fibrosis, shrinkage, and complete circumferential stenosis of the IVC. In acute stages, HVCS presents as high fever and abdominal pain with neutrophilic leukocytosis

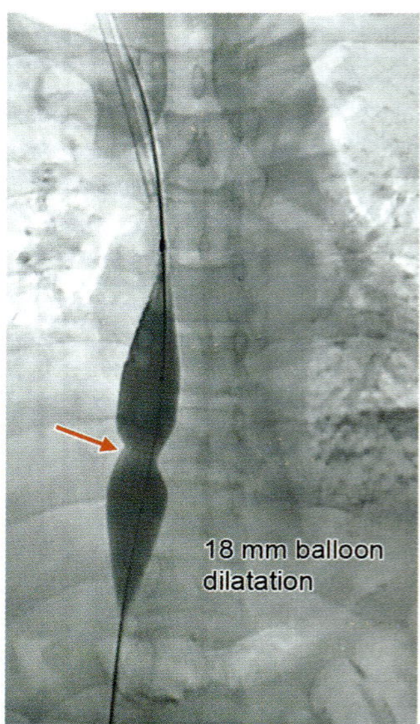

Fig. 6: Balloon angioplasty of localized inferior vena cava stenosis (arrow showing waist of stenosis).

followed by rapid progression to tender hepatomegaly, ascites, pedal edema, and mild jaundice. Blood culture may yield an organism in 40–60%. Acute thrombus with IVC narrowing is seen on DUS. Mainstay of therapy is long-term antibiotics, diuretics, and anticoagulation. Once chronicity ensues, the clinical manifestation and management is akin to chronic BCS described above. In HVCS, liver cirrhosis is known to occur in 3–8 months with a higher predisposition to hepatocellular carcinoma as compared to BCS. Acute clinical exacerbations (due to formation of new thrombi) on underlying chronic HVCS is known.[9]

ORIENTAL CHOLANGIOHEPATITIS

Oriental cholangiohepatitis (OCH) is a disease predominantly seen in East Asia with declining incidence, earlier seen in elderly but now reported in young adults too. It is characterized by intrahepatic bile duct strictures with stones causing recurrent bacterial cholangitis and predisposition to cholangiocarcinoma. Differential diagnosis include primary sclerosing cholangitis, Caroli disease, portal cholangiopathy, and low-phospholipid-associated cholelithiasis. Although the etiology remains unknown, *Clonorchis sinensis* or *Ascaris lumbricoides* infections are thought to be initiating factors of the disease. Smoldering bacterial infection leading to portal bacteremia, intraductal inflammation, and hepatic stone formation is a suggested potential cause. MR cholangiography is the preferred modality of investigation. Predominant involvement of central and left hepatic ducts are seen. Abrupt tapering of the peripheral bile ducts with mural irregularity is frequently encountered (arrowhead sign). Gall bladder stones may be seen in 70%. It is doubtful whether routine screening for parasitic infections should be practiced as there is no firm evidence for the same. Initial management includes treatment of cholangitis with antibiotics and biliary drainage. Endoscopic retrograde cholangiopancreatography (ERCP) is usually the preferred interventional procedure. Percutaneous transhepatic cholangiography may be helpful in cases of failed ERCP. Those with localized or unilateral involvement may require segmental resection or hemihepatectomy with or without hepaticojejunostomy. Recurring symptoms and residual stones are seen in 30% after ERCP.[10]

JODHPUR DISEASE

This is a rare condition which is also known as acquired, late-onset gastric outlet obstruction, or pyloric achalasia. In contrast to congenital hypertrophic pyloric stenosis (CHPS), in this condition there is a pyloric narrowing without muscular hypertrophy. Clustering of cases have been encountered in Jodhpur, India and neighboring areas of Sindh, Pakistan. It has been sporadically reported also from other Indian states, Turkey, and Mexico. Age range varies from newborns to 17 years, but most commonly encountered in the preschool years. Patients present with a long-standing history of recurrent, nonbilious stale food vomiting and progressive weight loss. Visible gastric peristalsis is noted. Unlike CHPS, ultrasonography does not show pyloric thickening and barium series do not show windsock deformity. Dilated stomach is noted on imaging. Pylorus is non-negotiable on endoscopy. *Helicobacter pylori* tests are negative. Therapy is initiated with hydration, correction of dyselectrolytemia, and alkalosis. Though most cases have been treated in the past with pyloroplasty,

there is evidence that endoscopic pyloric dilatation may be an alternative and effective therapy.[11]

CAUSTIC INJURIES AND BATTERY INGESTION

In the Indian subcontinent and other developing countries, corrosive and button/disc battery ingestion is a major problem. Caustic agents are not kept out of reach of children and irresponsibly stored in empty beverage bottles to which children are lured. Additionally there is a lack of strict implementation of childproof packing, biohazard labeling, and unrestricted open availability in the market. Accidental ingestion in younger children (<10 years of age) and suicidal intention in socially stressed adolescents are the most common reasons. Various agents and their characteristics are summarized in **Table 2**. Larynx, mouth, esophagus, and stomach may be injured. It is uncommon to see effects of corrosive intake in the bowel. Clinical manifestations of acute ingestion are shown in **Table 3**. Management is shown in **Tables 4 and 5**. Chronic sequelae are gastrointestinal strictures in 20–30% of corrosive ingestions **(Fig. 7)**. Button battery is a unique foreign body that has intensely alkaline and electrical properties. It causes rapid progressive necrosis of gut wall and surrounding structures **(Fig. 8)**. Persistent tissue necrosis is seen even after endoscopic

Table 2: Corrosive ingestion: Difference between acid and alkali ingestion.

	Alkali	Acid
Examples	• Drain cleaners • Oven cleaners • Dishwasher detergents • Bleach	• Toilet bowel cleaners • Battery liquid • Aqua regia (goldsmith) • Rust removers
Characteristics	• Available as solid or liquid • Odorless, colorless (consumed in large quantities)	• Available as liquid • Pungent, noxious (consumed in small quantities)
Site of injury	• Mouth and laryngeal (common) • Esophageal > Gastric (increased viscosity, contact time, and volume)	Gastric > esophageal (less viscous and runs downs the esophagus and lesser curvature quickly)
Type of necrosis	Liquefactive	Coagulative
Extent of injury	Deep and circumferential	Superficial and patchy (protective eschar prevents deeper extension)
Systemic complications	Less	More (induces disseminated intravascular coagulation and organ dysfunction)

Table 3: Clinical manifestations of corrosive injury.

Site of injury	Clinical manifestations	
	Immediate	*Delayed*
Lips, oral cavity	Drooling, spitting, incessant crying, burns and mucosal ulcers	Submucosal fibrosis, scars, yperpigmentation
Larynx, pharynx	Upper airway obstruction (stridor and suprasternal retractions)	Hoarseness of voice
Esophagus	Odynophagia, hematemesis, and chest discomfort	Dysphagia to solids and liquids (stricture formation)
Stomach	Epigastric pain	• Early satiety (reduced stomach capacity) • Stale food vomiting (gastric outlet obstruction due to antropyloric structure)

Complications:
- Esophageal perforation and mediastinitis (persistent chest and back pain, fever, toxic appearance)
- Gastroesophageal reflux disease (due to shortening of esophageal length)
- Tracheoesophageal fistula
- Gastric perforation (acute abdomen, guarding, and rigidity)

or surgical removal. They are found in toys, watches, and other electronic goods. Toy safety is a major concern in the West where other than material quality and toxicity, it is mandatory to screw or fasten the battery compartments. Changing of batteries is hence responsibly performed by the guardian. In developing countries, cheaper toys

Table 5: Zargar classification and management of corrosive injury.

Grade	Appearance	Management	Follow-up
0	Normal	Oral feeding	Not mandatory
1	Edema and hyperemia		
2a	Superficial ulcers	Oral feeding, antibiotics, PPI	
2b	Deep circumferential ulcers	• Nil orally initially followed by TPN/NG feeds, Antibiotics, PPI • Steroids only in 2b	• Barium swallow followed by serial endoscopic dilatations (esophageal and/or gastric) till luminal patency is achieved • Surgery if nonresponsive to repeated dilatations
3a	Few scattered areas of necrosis (greyish-black discoloration)		
3b	Extensive or confluent areas of necrosis		

(PPI: proton pump inhibitors; TPN: total parenteral nutrition; NG: nasogastric)

Table 4: General principles in management of acute corrosive ingestion.

Steps	Components	Comments
Examination	Look for crepitus (pneumomediastinum) and signs of perforation in abdomen. Laryngoscopy if required	
Resuscitation	• Airway, breathing, circulation • Nil per oral	Intubation, inotropes (if required). Do not give gastric lavage, activated charcoal, emetics, neutralizing agents, and milk
Radiography	• Plain X-ray chest and abdomen • Contrast studies with thin soluble contrast (not mandatory)	For pneumomediastinum and perforation. To document sites of involvement and leaks
Endoscopy	• Minimal air insufflation • Grade the severity of injury (Zargar classification)	In asymptomatic or symptomatic, acid or alkali ingestion, accidental or suicidal. Preferably in first 12–24 hours, no later than 72 hours. Avoided between days 5–15 of ingestion due to (high chances of perforation)
Antibiotics	• Used in higher grades of injury • Gram-positive and negative cover • Anaerobic cover if leaks or perforation suspected	Use intravenous or suspension, not tablets or capsules
Nutrition	• Gradually progress from liquid diet to semisolids and then solids • Parenteral nutrition if perforation, delayed oral feeding • Jejunostomy feeds in gastric outlet obstruction	Placement of nasogastric tube is controversial due to risks of perforation and but preferred in many centers to keep lumen patent and allow feeding
Proton pump inhibitors	Used in higher grades of injury	May be given as intravenous initially followed by oral (sachet/powder) if lumen patency permits
Steroids	To be used only in Zargar grade 2B, not in other grades. 1 g/1.73 m^2/day dexamethasone for 3 days	Overall not practiced in most centers. May delay progression of strictures. Contraindicated in adults and those suspected of perforation

have accessible battery compartments which can be easily unlocked or broken. Discarded batteries are not properly disposed. Hence young children are prone to accidental ingestion of the battery. Ingestion of smaller batteries may not be witnessed always by caretakers. They may pass out of the gastrointestinal tract and yet have delayed presentation. Most of the damage occurs above the diaphragm. The simple rule of immediate and mandatory endoscopic removal is 4 A's: all ages, all sizes (big or small), anywhere in upper gastrointestinal tract (accessible by endoscope), anytime (irrespective of hours of ingestion). Contrary to guideline policy in the West for smaller batteries in stomach of older children, the wait-and-watch policy is not recommended in developing countries (personal opinion). This is due to a lack of general awareness and poor referral systems. After endoscopic removal, serial CT angiography or MRI of the upper GI tract is required to assess ongoing tissue necrosis for an impending vascular complication. The child should be

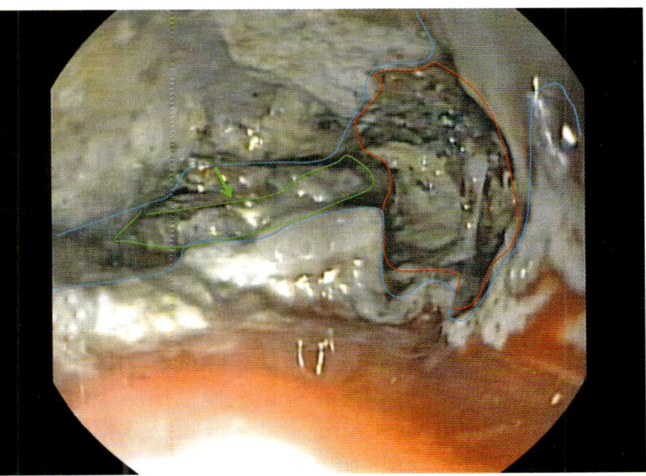

Fig. 8: Upper gastrointestinal endoscopy showing impacted button battery (green arrow and demarcated area) in esophagus with areas of eschar-necrosis (red demarcation), extensive ulceration (blue demarcation), and bleeding.

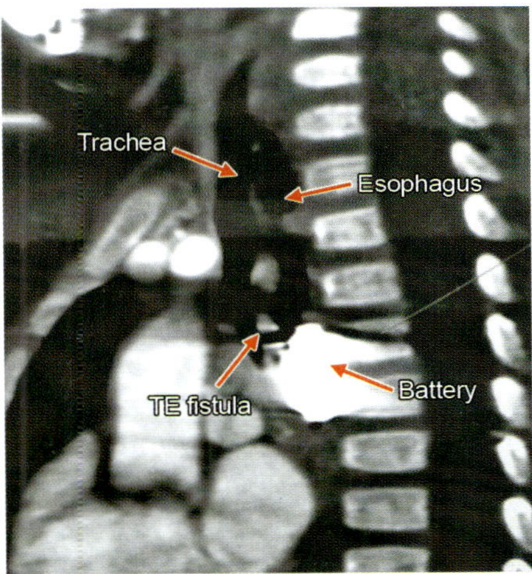

Fig. 9: Lateral X-ray chest showing impacted esophageal button battery causing tracheoesophageal (TE) fistula.

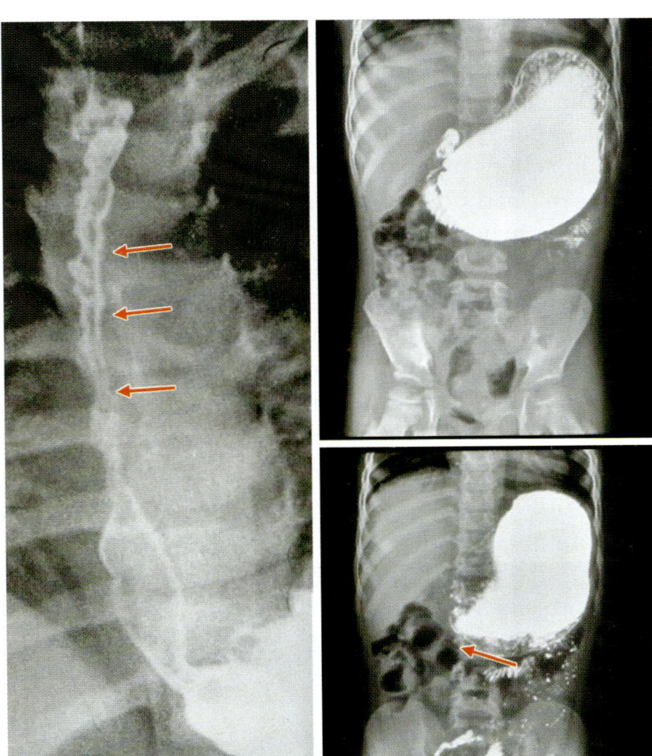

Fig. 7: Contrast esophagram showing postcorrosive long esophageal stricture (arrows) and barium meal retention of contrast in stomach (arrow) suggestive of gastric outlet obstruction.

kept nil per oral and preferably on parenteral nutrition till inflammation subsides. Empirical antibiotics and proton-pump inhibitors are recommended. Batteries that have advanced beyond the reach of endoscope into small bowel

do not require routine enteroscopy. Hastening small bowel transit by osmotic agents and laxatives has been tried with anedoctal success. Vascular catastrophes (aortoesophageal fistulae and arterial aneurysms), esophageal perforation, and tracheoesophageal fistulae **(Fig. 9)** are notorious complications. Registries in the United States of America report 46% short-term and 70% long-term case fatality.[12] Emergent surgical referral is considered in luminal perforation (frank or impending), pneumomediastinum or any other complication. Invariably the child will require multiple chest surgeries. The surgical planes of resection are challenging for even expert surgeons due to unhealthy friable tissue in the proximity of great vessels and nerves. Leaks, gaping wounds, suture line dehiscence, and restenosis of the lumen are the recurrent problems. Replacement grafts are expensive.

■ TROPICAL CALCIFIC PANCREATITIS

Tropical calcific pancreatitis (TCP) is a special type of chronic pancreatitis that affects children, adolescents, and young adults. The disease is characterized by large pancreatic duct calculi, pancreatic endocrine insufficiency, and aggressive course of the disease. The highest prevalence of 1/500 to 1/800 has been reported from India, especially from the state of Kerala. The disease has also been reported from Southern Africa and other Asia-Pacific countries (China, Indonesia, and Malaysia). The association in Southern India was initially linked with cassava (tapioca) ingestion which contains cyanogenic glycosides toxic to the pancreas. Later studies failed to show cassava ingestion as a risk factor in humans or animal models and growing prevalence in northern India (where cassava is not a staple diet). In recent studies, it has been noted that there is a shift of the disease to older age groups and lesser prevalence of diabetes. The same disease has now been associated with genetic mutations in *SPINK1, CFTR,* and *CTRC* suggesting that the erstwhile nomenclature of TCP may actually be a misnomer. Morphology of pancreas at the time of diagnosis is severe pancreatic parenchymal atrophy with marked main pancreatic duct (MPD) dilatation and large MPD calculi showing burnt out disease **(Fig. 10)**. Pancreatic symptoms include recurrent or chronic severe epigastric pain with radiation to back and hunched postures to relieve pain. Steatorrhea is present in 25% of patients. Weight loss precedes in 15–20% before disease onset and 50–67% after symptoms have commenced. Typically the body mass index is <18.5. Diabetes mellitus indicates that >90% of the parenchyma is lost. About 30–40% have presenting symptoms of diabetes before the pancreatic atrophy is detected.[13] Hence the term "fibrocalculous pancreatic diabetes" was once suggested. Increased morbidity results from malnutrition, recurrent infection, and poor control of hyperglycemia. Management includes limiting the ongoing oxidative stress by antioxidants, pain relief, pancreatic enzymes, and nutritional supplementation, preferably with medium-chain triglycerides. Extracorporeal shock wave lithotripsy and endoscopic pancreatic stenting are management modalities for the MPD stones and drainage. Surgery (Puestow operation and lateral pancreaticojejunostomy) is considered in case of failure of endoscopic therapy for pain or drainage.

■ TROPICAL SPRUE

Once thought to be a major cause of chronic diarrhea and malabsorption in tropical countries, this entity is now declining for reasons unknown. The disease has been reported from South and Southeast Asia, Central America, South America, the Caribbean islands, parts of Africa, and tropical Australia. Epidemics and war outbreaks in the yester years are now limited to local clustering and sporadic cases. Since expatriates visiting tropical areas are also affected, the disease is postulated to be incited by an infectious organism. However, no causative agents have been clearly identified. Postinfectious malabsorption is another hypothesis where an infectious diarrhea in the recent past activates innate immunity leading to villi damage and malabsorption. The disease is seen in older children, adolescents, and young adults. Tropical sprue (TS) is defined as an intestinal mucosal disease characterized by partial villous atrophy and malabsorption of 2 or more unrelated nutrient groups (e.g. fat, carbohydrate, and vitamins) for which other known causes of malabsorption have been excluded (e.g. celiac disease, parasitic infections,

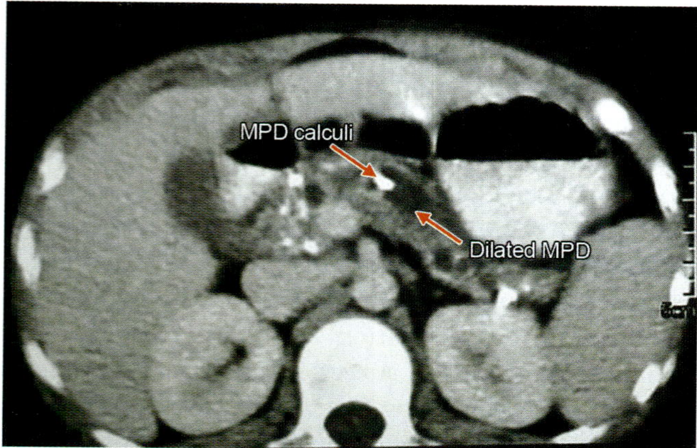

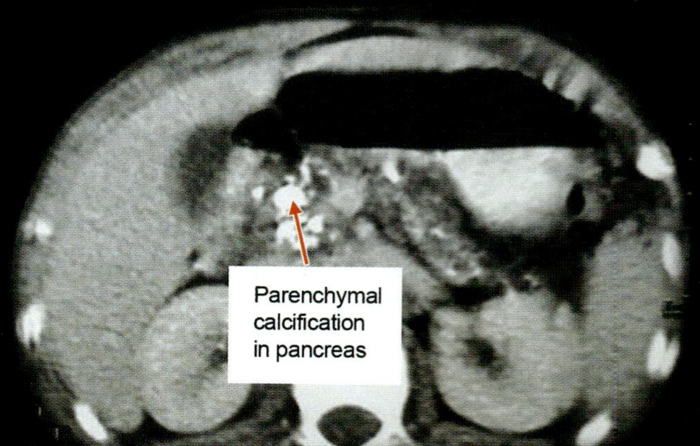

Fig. 10: CT abdomen in tropical calcific pancreatitis.
(MPD: main pancreatic duct)

immunodeficiencies, neoplasm, and chronic pancreatitis). The typical presentation is with chronic diarrhea and/or steatorrhea (pale, bulky, frothy, and foul-smelling stools) with weight loss. This results from carbohydrate, fat, protein, and bile acid malabsorption. Symptoms and signs are attributable to multivitamin (vitamins A, B, C, D, E, and K) deficiencies, loss of trace elements (iron and zinc), electrolyte losses (K, Ca, P, and Mg), and hypoproteinemia–hypoalbuminemia **(Fig. 11)**. Rarely patients may have colonic pseudo-obstruction (Ogilvie syndrome). Presence of clubbing and complete or subtotal villous atrophy suggests an alternative diagnosis. There is no single test to diagnose TS. Test of malabsorption, though recommended is not practically available in most centers. Hence the diagnosis is presumptive based on the clinical features and exclusion of other diseases. Malabsorption commonly is established by testing for fecal fat (72-hour fecal fat) and D-xylose absorption. Being a disease of distal small bowel and terminal ileum, TS has low vitamin B12 and normal folic acid levels. In contrast, celiac disease involves proximal small bowel and hence presents with low folic acid and normal vitamin B12 levels. A three-stage Schilling test may be required to rule out other causes of vitamin B12 deficiency. Fecal examination screening for parasites and abdominal imaging (for tuberculosis and neoplasm) is essential. Endoscopy shows scalloped folds similar to celiac disease. Deep duodenal (from the third and fourth parts of duodenum) and jejunal biopsies show partial villous atrophy. Small bowel aspiration culture >10[5] bacteria/mL and positive glucose hydrogen breath tests are suggestive of small bowel bacterial overgrowth syndrome.[14] Treatment consists of hydration and correction of all deficiencies, electrolytes, and trace elements. Tetracycline 250 mg 4 times daily (or doxycycline 100 mg once daily) for 3–6 months is prescribed as specific therapy for TS in adults and similarly extrapolated in children. There is anecdotal experience with other antibiotics, especially if the above drugs are contraindicated. A high-calorie, high-protein, medium chain triglyceride (MCT) enriched, and long chain fat-restricted diet is usually prescribed.

■ IMMUNOPROLIFERATIVE SMALL INTESTINAL DISEASE

Non-Hodgkin lymphoma can primarily involve the gastrointestinal tract. About 90% are B-cell lymphomas. One of the variants of B-cell lymphoma is immuno-proliferative small intestinal disease (IPSID). Earlier termed as Mediterranean lymphoma, this disorder is not uncommon in tropics and found in poor socioeconomic strata. The disease has been reported in Northern and Southern India, mainly in young adults. The disease has

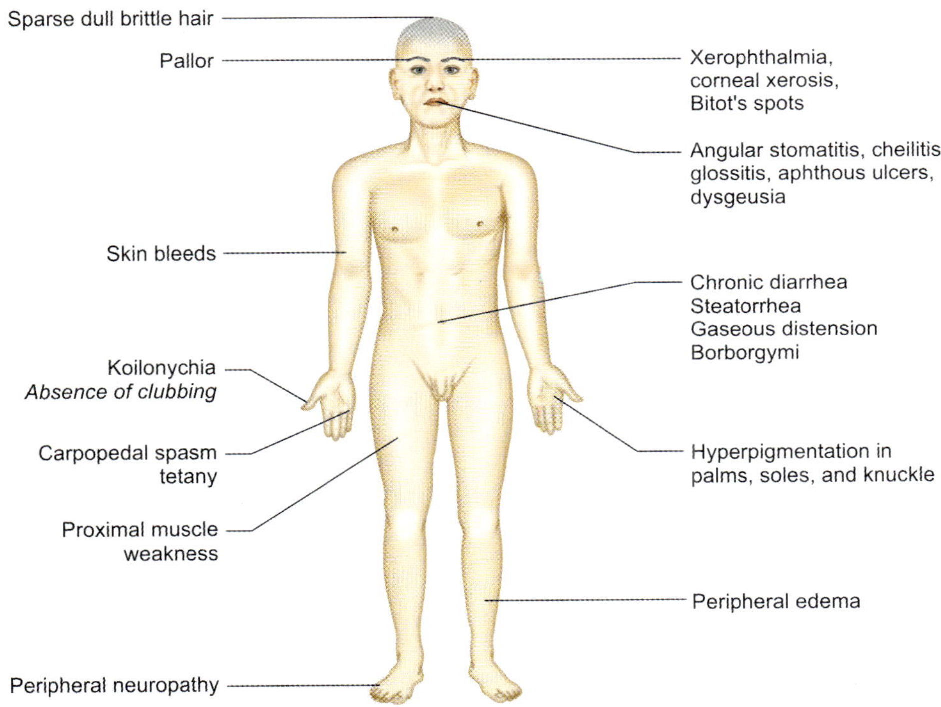

Fig. 11: Symptoms and signs in tropical sprue.

lack of association with *H. pylori* but close association with a past *Campylobacter jejuni* infection.[15] The infective pathophysiology is not fully understood. One of the postulations is a bacterial toxin-induced mutation in gut plasma cells that produce alpha-heavy chains instead of normal immunoglobulin A (IgA). This leads to diffuse clonal proliferation of abnormal plasma cells throughout the gut, heavy lymphoplasmacytic infiltrates in lamina propria and crypt effacement.[16] IPSID is a differential diagnosis of older children and adolescents presenting with chronic diarrhea. IPSID closely mimics celiac disease. However, unlike celiac disease which has short stature, children with IPSID have normal height indicating that the child had been growing well and disease-free in the past. The disease indolently progresses over months to produce symptoms of malabsorption, chronic diarrhea, abdominal pain, weight loss, anasarca, anemia, and clubbing. In advanced disease with adjacent lymph nodal involvement, abdominal masses are palpable, similar to abdominal lymphomas. Confirmation of the disease is cumbersome. Alpha-heavy chain assessment by routine immunoelectrophoresis is not available in most centers. Nodular thickened duodenal folds are seen on endoscopy. Mucosal biopsies are inadequate as deeper layers may show malignant cells. Hence full thickness small bowel biopsies with adjacent lymph nodes are required for staging. Early involvement is known to respond to antibiotics such as tetracycline 1 g/day for 6 months in adults. Success is seen in 30–70%. There is limited experience in children. An advanced disease which has poor prognosis must be treated as lymphoma with chemotherapy. Debulking surgery may be required.

CONCLUSION

- Noncommunicable GI and hepatobiliary disorders may be uncommon yet challenging to diagnose
- Most of the causes of pediatric portal hypertension in tropics are potentially salvageable
- Corrosive and button battery ingestion is unique to developing countries and is preventable if awareness is raised
- Advanced TCP and IPSID have a poor outcome.

REFERENCES

1. Yachha SK. Portal hypertension in children: an Indian perspective Journal of Gastroenterology and Hepatology. 2002; 17:S228-31.
2. Peter L, Dadhich SK, Yachha SK. Clinical and laboratory differentiation of cirrhosis and extrahepatic portal venous obstruction in children. Journal of Gastroenterology and Hepatology. 2003;18:185-9.
3. Krishna YR, Yachha SK, Srivastava A, et al. Quality of life in children managed for extrahepatic portal venous obstruction. J Pediatr Gastroenterol Nutr. 2010:50:531-6.
4. Sen Sarma M, Yachha SK, Rai P, et al. Cholangiopathy in children with extrahepatic portal venous obstruction. J Hepatobiliary Pancreat Sci. 2018;25:440-7.
5. Lal R, Sarma MS, Gupta MK. Extrahepatic portal venous obstruction: what should be the mainstay of treatment? Indian J Pediatr. 2017;84(9):691-9.
6. Prasad D, Sen Sarma M, Yachha SK, et al. Pediatric non-cirrhotic portal fibrosis: role of endoscopic management in determining long-term outcome. Hepatol Int. 2019.
7. Singh SK, Sen Sarma M, Yadav R, et al. Prognostic scoring systems and outcome of endovascular radiological intervention of chronic Budd-Chiari syndrome in children. Liver Int. 2018; 38:1308-15.
8. Sarma MS, Yachha SK, Bhatia V, et al. Safety, complications and outcome of large volume paracentesis with or without albumin therapy in children with severe ascites due to liver disease. J Hepatol. 2015;63:1126-32.
9. Shrestha SM, Kage M, Lee BB. Hepatic vena cava syndrome: new concept of pathogenesis. Hepatology Research. 2017;47: 603-15.
10. Verweij KE, van Buuren H. Oriental cholangiohepatitis (recurrent pyogenic cholangitis): a case series from the Netherlands and brief review of the literature. Neth J Med. 2016;74(9):401-5.
11. Sharma KK, Ranka P, Goyal P, et al. Gastric outlet obstruction in children: an overview with report of Jodhpur disease and Sharma's classification. J Pediatr Surg. 2008;43:1891-7.
12. Jatana KR, Litovitz T, Reilly JS, et al. Pediatric button battery injuries: 2013 task force update. Int J Pediatr Otorhinolaryngol. 2013;77(9):1392-9.
13. Garg PK. Chronic Pancreatitis in India and Asia. Curr Gastroenterol Rep. 2012;14:118-24.
14. Ghoshal UC, Srivastava D, Verma A, et al. Tropical sprue in 2014: the new face of an old disease. Curr Gastroenterol Rep. 2014;16(6):391.
15. Lecuit M, Abachin E, Martin A, et al. Immunoproliferative small intestinal disease associated with Campylobacter jejuni. N Engl J Med. 2004;350(3):239-48.
16. Al-Saleem T, Al-Mondhiry H. Immunoproliferative small intestinal disease (IPSID): a model for mature B-cell neoplasms. Blood. 2005;105(6):2274-80.

Swathi Kiran Shiri, Anil Vasudevan

9.6 CHAPTER

Renal Disease in Tropics

■ INTRODUCTION

The tropics can be defined either geographically or ecologically. Geographically, tropics can be defined as the regions around the equator where the sun is directed at least once during the solar year (Tropic of Cancer 23° north–Tropic of Capricorn 23° south latitude). Ecologically, the tropics are those areas where there are high year-round temperatures without winters or snow. Tropical regions include parts of Central America, South America, the Caribbean, Africa, the Middle East, and Southeast Asia. These regions are economically backward compared to other regions of the world and share common healthcare challenges. Among the various healthcare problems commonly encountered in the tropical regions is kidney disease which may due to infectious or noninfectious causes. An understanding of the common causes of tropical renal diseases, their epidemiology and clinical presentation along with early diagnosis and management, patient awareness and improvement in healthcare facilities will lead to a better outcome and lower mortality. This chapter provides an overview of acquired causes of renal injury in the tropics which includes infection, toxins, envenomation, medications and natural disasters.

■ RISK FACTORS FOR RENAL DISEASE IN TROPICS

Risk factors for renal diseases in tropics can be classified as environmental derived factors and socioeconomic factors.

Environmental Factors

- Poor sanitation, lack of access to clean drinking water and poor infection control.
- Due to higher temperatures and humidity, minerals and some organic compounds are leached which contaminate the flowing water resulting in pollution of the fields and water-borne diseases.
- Overcrowding and poor living conditions.
- Heat, humidity, and higher saline content in water provide a conducive environment for infectious agents to thrive. Water flooding of burrows in the rainy season forces the snakes out of their home and to the surface.

Socioeconomic Factors

- Poor and deprived population are exposed to various health hazards including environmental hazards and often have difficult access to health care.
- Large slum areas with congestion and overcrowding, poor sanitation, absence of basic amenities like piped water supply, closed drainage and sewerage and disposal of garbage.
- Increased risk of exposure to natural medicines and industrial toxins that can result in acute kidney injury (AKI).

■ CLINICAL SPECTRUM OF RENAL DISEASE

The spectrum of renal involvement includes asymptomatic proteinuria or pyuria, electrolyte abnormalities, nephritic or nephrotic syndrome, AKI, and chronic kidney disease.

■ MECHANISMS OF RENAL INJURY

Pathophysiology of renal involvement in tropical infections is due to multiple factors as mentioned above that results in glomerular, microvascular, or tubulointerstitial lesions.
- *Direct kidney damage*:
  - Infiltration of various cells and triggering of inflammation in kidney and lower urinary by direct invasion of the organism as seen in leptospirosis and schistosomiasis.

- Damage of glomerular endothelium (e.g. falciparum malaria) secondary to interaction between the infected and deformed red blood cells (RBCs) and the intact vascular endothelium. The infected RBCs adhere to these endothelial cells resulting in obstruction of the capillaries and also triggering the inflammatory cascade.
- *Indirect kidney damage*:
  - Indirect renal damage are a consequence of multiple factors such as rhabdomyolysis and hemolysis due to the release of myoglobin and hemoglobin respectively, increased level of bile acids in the body, generation of oxygen-free radicals and release of certain lytic enzymes like phospholipases. These changes are mainly seen in case of snakebite.
  - Activation of cell mediated as well as humoral immunity by bacterial antigens and endotoxins resulting in immune-mediated kidney damage.
  - Certain parasitic infections cause acute systemic toxicity because of decrease in systemic vascular resistance due to generalized vasodilatation. This is usually seen in patients with scrub typhus, malaria, leptospirosis, and rare infections like hanta virus. The generalized vasodilatation further lead to the activation of rennin aldosterone axis and sympathetic nervous system causing vasoconstriction of the intrarenal vessels which are end arteries causing irreversible ischemic injury resulting in AKI.

Acute Cortical Necrosis

The severity renal injury and outcome is determined by the extent of necrosis of the renal tissue which can be patchy or can be diffuse in nature. Acute cortical necrosis is commonly seen in children with hemolytic uremic syndrome and following snakebite.

ETIOLOGY OF RENAL DISEASE IN TROPICS

The tropical renal disease can be classified as infective, toxin mediated (animal, plant, medicines) or natural disasters **(Table 1)**. Among the various causes the most common cause of renal involvement in tropical areas are community acquired infections resulting in severe forms acute tubular necrosis (ATN). In a study from a tertiary care center in South India, 40% of adult patients with tropical infections had AKI. Malaria, scrub typhus, leptospirosis and dengue were the most common etiology that resulted in AKI in the study.

Infections

Infective causes are due to bacterial, viral, parasitic and fungi infections depending on the region. Most commonly tropical infection presents with high-grade fever with myalgia, severe pallor and jaundice. Laboratory evaluation shows evidence of intravascular hemolysis in the form of anemia and thrombocytopenia with occasional deranged coagulation profile. Acute gastroenteritis due to viral or bacterial etiology is one of the common causes of kidney disease in children. The severity of renal involvement is determined by underlying organism, severity of infection and susceptibility of the individual to infection **(Table 2)**. While AKI is the most common renal complication, certain infections like tuberculosis (TB) and leprosy follow a subacute or indolent long clinical course.

Malaria

The majority of AKI due to malaria are secondary to *Plasmodium falciparum* infection followed by

Table 1: Common causes of renal injury in tropics.				
Vector-borne infections	*Plant and fungal toxins*	*Chemical toxins*	*Environmental factors*	*Others*
• Malaria • Dengue fever • Scrub typhus • Hemorrhagic • Rift valley fever • Leptospirosis • Hantaviruses • Zygomycosis • Diarrheal diseases (*Escherichia coli, Entamoeba histolytica Shigella*) cholera and viral gastroenteritis • Melioidosis • Typhoid • *Chlamydia* • Legionellosis	• Herbal medicines • Impila food plants • Djenkol beans • Marking nut • Mushroom • Plant-derived toxins used as insecticides and to kill fish • Animal poisons • Snake bites • Wasp, hornet, and bee stings • Spider bite • Jellyfish sting • Scorpion sting • Carp gallbladder or bile	• Ethylene glycol • N,N'-dimethyl-4,4'-bipyridinium dichloride • Ethylene dibromide • Copper sulfate • Chromic acid	• Natural disasters • Heat stroke	Glucose 6 phosphate dehydrogenase (G6PD) deficiency

Table 2: Renal involvement in tropical bacterial and viral infections.

Infection	Pathogen	Abnormal urinary sediment	Proteinuria	AKI %	Renal pathology	Risk of CKD
Enteric fever	Salmonella typhi, paratyphi	++	++	0.2–1%	MPGN, AIN	NA
Leptospirosis	Leptospira spirochetes	++++	++++	40–87%	ATN, AIN, vasculitis	Present
Scrub typhus	Orientia tsutsugamushi	+	++	20–60%	ATN, AIN	Present
Tuberculosis	Mycobacterium tuberculosis	++	+	20–40%	AIN	Present
Dengue	Dengue virus	++	++	0.9–30%	MPGN, AIN, TMA	NA
Malaria	Plasmodium	+++	++	1–60%	ATN, CN, TMA, GN	Present

(AIN: acute interstitial nephritis; AKI: acute kidney injury; ATN: acute tubular necrosis; CN: cortical necrosis; GN: glomerulonephritis; MPGN: membranoproliferative glomerulonephritis; TMA: thrombotic microangiopathy; CKD: chronic kidney disease)
Source: Kamath N, Iyengar A. Infections and the kidney: a tale from the tropics. Pediatr Nephrol. 2018;33(8):1317-26.

Plasmodium vivax, *Plasmodium knowlesi*, and rarely *Plasmodium ovale*. AKI is diagnosed in 1–4% of affected patients, and in case of severe malarial disease incidence of AKI is up to 60%. Clinical manifestations can range from high-grade fever with chills to seizures, altered sensorium, and hemoglobinuria along with major organ dysfunction. Young children (<5 years of age), high parasitic load, children with suppressed immunity as seen in those with human immunodeficiency virus (HIV), severe sepsis with multiorgan dysfunction are some of the identified risk factors for AKI. Pathophysiology as described above is due endothelium damage due to attachment of parasitized RBCs to the intact glomerular capillaries which results in obstruction of small vessels, cellular infiltration, and cytokines causing damage of the glomerulus and tubules, renovascular hemodynamic instability due to inflammatory mediators like tumor necrosis factor (TNF) alpha and interleukin 10 (IL-10). Histopathological examination of renal tissue reveals changes of ATN and in very severe cases cortical necrosis as well. Certain other histological changes that have been observed in renal biopsy specimen include acute tubulointerstitial nephritis, mesangioproliferative and diffuse proliferative changes and thrombotic microangiopathy. Clinically falciparum malaria is known to present as acute glomerulonephritis or nephritic syndrome as well. Chronic malarial nephropathy is one of the rare manifestations seen in *Plasmodium malariae* infection and in endemic regions.

The treatment of choice for *P. falciparum* malaria is artemisinin-based combination therapy. Prompt treatment with antimalarial agents and timely initiation of dialysis in those with severe renal injury results in better survival rates and recovery from AKI due to malaria. Whereas in case of chronic malarial nephropathy it is usually unresponsive to the medical antimalarial management and invariably progresses to end-stage renal disease (ESRD).

Leptospirosis

Leptospirosis is one of the common infections encountered in tropical countries. It is primarily a zoonotic infection and humans are accidentally infected. It is usually due to consumption of water that is contaminated with the stool and urine of animals like rats, cats, dogs, and cattle. Renal injury often occurs in the immune phase by direct infiltration by spirochetes. The direct kidney damage can result in tubulointerstitial nephritis which is the most common form of renal involvement. The affected patients have nonoliguric AKI with dyselectrolytemia like hypokalemia and myoglobinuria. Sometimes, the reduced expression of aquaporin-2 channels resulting in impaired renal tubule concentrating ability resulting in polyuria, hypokalemia and hypomagnesemia. In severe cases there may be rhabdomyolysis and hemolysis causing anemia, and hyperbilirubinemia. The incidence of mortality due to the AKI is about 40–50% in the affected population. Management includes prompt administration of crystalline penicillin or doxycycline within 7 days of infection. This reduces the incidence and severity of AKI.

Dengue

Dengue is caused by arbovirus of genus *Flavivirus* which transmitted by female aedes mosquitoes, i.e. *Aedes aegypti* and *Aedes albopictus*. Renal involvement in dengue is a part of multiorgan dysfunction and constitutes severe dengue as per classification. The prevalence of AKI in dengue varies from 0.9% to 30.7%. Kidney involvement can range from isolated proteinuria, hematuria, AKI, infection-related glomerulonephritis (IRGN), hemolytic uremic syndrome or tubulointerstitial nephritis.

Acute kidney injury is often multifactorial resulting from direct effects of the virus on the kidneys or secondary to poor hemodynamic status and shock. The renal injury may be rarely due to rhabdomyolysis, acute hemolysis or secondary to infection related glomerulonephritis.

Histopathology show features of ATN, tubulointerstitial nephritis, thrombotic microangiopathy, and glomerular proliferative changes in case of IRGN. Presence of AKI increases the risk of mortality and morbidity. Management includes prevention of AKI by careful fluid therapy to maintain perfusion and supportive care. Once AKI sets in, the management depends on the underlying severity and type of renal involvement. Dialysis is often required in those with severe AKI.

Rickettsial Infections

Rickettsial infection is a zoonotic disease transmitted by ticks, fleas or mites. Scrub typhus which is caused by the bacterium *Orientia tsutsugamushi* is the most common rickettsial infection encountered in India. AKI secondary to scrub typhus is increasing being reported and was probably under reported due to lack of appropriate diagnostic facilities. Clinical manifestations can range from mild, asymptomatic disease at times to severe life-threatening illness. Severe disease is characterized by multiorgan involvement in the form of acute respiratory distress syndrome, bleeding, coagulation disorders, meningoencephalitis, and shock.

Renal involvement is more frequent with Rocky Mountain spotted fever, tick typhus and Q fever. Clinically, they either have AKI with features of fluid overload, gross hematuria and hypertension secondary to IRGN or nonoliguric AKI due to tubulointerstitial nephritis. Urine analysis reveals active urinary sediments with hematuria, proteinuria, pyuria, and presence of granular casts in up to 80% of patients. Abnormal renal function is seen in nearly half of the affected children. AKI may be seen in more than half of children with scrub typhus and is more common in children with hepatic and central nervous system (CNS) involvement. Histopathological lesions seen are ATN, interstitial nephritis, and feature of IRGN with mesangial and endocapillary proliferation. Presence of AKI and renal dysfunction is associated with higher mortality.

Acute Gastroenteritis

Diarrheal disease is the most common cause of renal injury in children. The underlying cause is infectious which could be viral most commonly followed by bacteria or parasitic. The damage to the kidneys is due to the hypoperfusion secondary to severe dehydration resulting in severe forms of ATN and AKI. Certain factors contribute to the AKI like ingestion of nephrotoxic medications like nonsteroidal anti-inflammatory drugs (NSAIDs), antibiotics like aminoglycosides and penicillin. In the case series from tertiary care centers in North India, diarrheal disease related AKI contribute up to 50% of all children undergoing dialysis. AKI can be prevented by preventing dehydration using oral rehydration solution and by early recognition and correction of dehydration using oral or parenteral fluid. The renal outcome is usually complete recovery from AKI. The complete recovery depends on the severity and duration of dehydration before correction.

Chronic Infections

Tuberculosis: TB, a major public health problem in India and other developing countries, is caused by *Mycobacterium tuberculosis*. One-third of extrarenal manifestations are caused by urogenital TB which is rare in children. Renal involvement in TB can be secondary to disseminated infection or due to localized genitourinary disease.

Kidneys are commonly affected in miliary TB due to hematogenous spread. The miliary lesions are usually seen in the cortical parenchyma of the kidneys. This contrasts with localization of tubercular infection in the medullary region in localized genitourinary disease wherein granulomas are formed with severe caseous necrosis. In case of extensive renal involvement, papillary necrosis with cavitary lesions replaces the functional renal parenchyma that may also extend into the collecting system. The lesions may also extend and infiltrate beyond the renal capsule leading to a significant mass lesion that may be palpable and at times closely mimic a malignant lesion. The involvement of the collecting ducts and the ureters can result in significant stenosis which is often segmental. The ureteric stenosis results in urinary obstruction and reflux. Lower urinary tract symptoms are observed with involvement of the bladder. On laboratory evaluation, proteinuria, sterile pyuria along with abnormal renal function is usually observed. Rarely, isolated hematuria can be the only presenting manifestation. Secondary amyloidosis, an important late complication of TB manifests as nephrotic range proteinuria. The management of urogenital TB is antitubercular therapy as per RNTCP guidelines. Surgical treatment will be required in those with obstructive lesions, infundibular and pelvic stenosis with severe bladder symptoms.

Other Infections

In children with HIV infection, renal involvement can range from AKI, HIV-associated nephropathy (HIVAN), HIV-related glomerular disease and renal injury secondary to antiretroviral therapy. It could also be secondary to infections, septic shock, dehydration, and use of nephrotoxic medications.

TOXINS

Snake Envenomation

Snakebite-related deaths are highly prevalent in India contributing to 45,000 deaths per year. AKI is observed in 12–30% of those bitten by poisonous snakes. The clinical manifestations depend on the species of snake and dose of the toxic venom. Clinical manifestations of viper snakebite are pain and swelling around bite site, excessive bleeding from the bite site, and tender and enlarged regional lymph nodes. Systemic manifestations include bleeding and hypotension. Renal involvement in the form of AKI occurs within 4–6 hours to 7 days after the bite. Grossly, the kidney will be swollen with flea bitten petechial hemorrhages. Histopathological lesions are ATN with pigment casts in the renal tubules which may be observed in up to 80% of the patients with snakebite and AKI. Other renal biopsy findings are changes of endocapillary proliferation, features of thrombotic microangiopathy, mesangiolysis, interstitial inflammation, vasculitis, renal infarcts, and acute cortical necrosis **(Table 3)**. Management of patients includes local wound care, compression dressing of the extremity and prompt administration of anti-snake venom. Early administration of antivenom is important to prevent the development of hematological abnormalities, rhabdomyolysis, and AKI. Coagulopathy is corrected by transfusion of fresh frozen plasma. Anti-tetanus toxoid should be administered to all patients with snakebite. Patients with myotoxic snakebite are at risk of myoglobinuria and subsequent AKI. Hence, aggressive fluid therapy along with forced alkaline diuresis helps prevent intratubular precipitation of myoglobin. The prognosis of AKI due to snakebite is good in patients who receive early supportive management and antivenom.

Scorpion Sting

Scorpions are among the most poisonous insects belonging to the family of arthropods. Scorpion envenomation has been recognized as a significant problem worldwide especially in areas of America, Africa, and Middle East countries. In India, *Mesobuthus* is most commonly encountered species of scorpion. The venom is made up of several toxins among which most relevant for clinical manifestations are A toxins (alpha-toxins) (polypeptide). These toxins cause prolonged depolarization at the voltage-gated sodium channels resulting in sympathetic and parasympathetic overactivity and massive release of vasoactive mediators and cytokines. The clinical picture is dominated by signs and symptoms due to autonomic activity, cardiac arrhythmias, myocardial dysfunction, and neurological manifestations. Severe multiorgan dysfunction can result in death. The venom rapidly concentrates in kidney resulting in interstitial damage. The most common histopathological changes are ATN, interstitial fibrosis, focal segmental glomerulosclerosis (FSGS), thrombotic microangiopathy, and cortical necrosis.

Native Medications

Native medications have been in use in worldwide for various indications based on local practices. Medicines are extracted from local flora and fauna and also derived from chemical sources. The composition of these medications depends on the prevalent practices and is usually not tested for efficacy and safety. Toxic chemicals are usually added to enhance the texture and potency of the medications. Kidneys are the main site of metabolism and excretion of these substances which are highly nephrotoxic. A high index of suspicion, along with careful history taking, and an awareness of local practices is important for proper diagnosis and management of renal injury caused by these toxins in the tropics. Clinical manifestations can range from isolated kidney involvement as AKI or multisystemic involvement of which hepatic involvement can usually be

Table 3: Envenomation and renal injury.			
Organism	*Russell's viper*	*Cobra*	*Scorpion*
Clinical features	*Local injury*: • Hemolysis • Rhabdomyolysis • Coagulopathy • Neurotoxicity	*Neurotoxicity*: Rhabdomyolysis	*Autonomic overactivity*: • Cardiac dysfunction • Pulmonary edema • Neuromuscular • Excitation
AKI (%)	18.7–45%	10–33%	Unknown
Histology	ATN, CN, AIN, GN	ATN	ATN, CN, TMA

(AIN: acute interstitial nephritis; AKI: acute kidney injury; ATN: acute tubular necrosis; CN: cortical necrosis; GN: glomerulonephritis; TMA: thrombotic microangiopathy)

severe leading to worsening of underlying renal injury. The most common histopathology lesions seen are ATN, interstitial nephritis, and acute cortical necrosis.

■ MISCELLANEOUS CAUSES

Disaster-related Acute Kidney Injury

Natural and manmade disasters like earthquakes, tsunami, hurricane, and war have significant impact on the kidneys causing various effects. The AKI can be classified into two categories:

1. *Traumatic causes*: Crush syndrome, hemorrhage causing ischemic ATN and trauma to urinary tract.
2. *Nontraumatic causes*: Nephrotoxicity due to antibiotics, contrast agents, NSAIDs and sepsis associated AKI.

Acute kidney injury due to crush syndrome is mainly due to the rhabdomyolysis causing severe ATN with pigment nephropathy. Clinically as early as 2–24 hours post the crush injury, patients are noted to develop oliguria with passing brownish-colored urine. AKI is more common in those patients who do not receive adequate intravenous fluids post injury. Confirmation of diagnosis is based on the clinical setting and urine positivity for myoglobin in the absence of RBCs. Renal biopsy shows features of ATN with pigment casts. Management is conservative. Hydration with intravenous fluids and diuretics to maintain good urine output are key interventions to prevent AKI. In the presence of oliguric AKI, renal replacement therapy (RRT) is the supportive modality of choice.

Glucose 6 Phosphate Dehydrogenase Deficiency and Intravascular Hemolysis

Deficiency caused by glucose 6 phosphate dehydrogenase (G6PD) deficiency causes intravascular hemolysis. Drugs (primaquine, nitrofurantoin, and NSAIDs), toxins or infections are the common triggers for hemolysis. AKI secondary to hemoglobinuria is seen in 5–10% of cases. The initial symptom is passage of dark colored urine followed by oliguria. In the presence of abnormal renal functions after an episode of hemolysis, AKI needs to be considered.

■ CONCLUSION

Renal disease in tropical countries is a major public health problem. Socioeconomic factors, climate and environmental conditions in tropical regions contribute to the high burden of renal disease in the tropics. Infection, which is the most common cause of renal involvement in the tropical countries, includes diarrheal diseases, malaria, leptospirosis and dengue. Envenomation, consumption of toxic herbs or chemicals and poisoning are other major causes of renal diseases in the tropics. Many causes of renal disease in tropical countries are preventable. The major barrier to prevention of kidney involvement is failure to recognize the risk factors and early signs of renal injury. Early identification and specific management of certain infections and envenomation could prevent the risk of subsequent renal injury and its sequelae. Once the AKI sets in, appropriate management and avoidance of nephrotoxic medications becomes important. RRT is indicated in those with severe renal failure.

■ SUGGESTED READING

1. Burdmann EA, Jha V. Acute kidney injury due to tropical infectious diseases and animal venoms: a tale of 2 continents. Kidney Int. 2017;91(5):1033-46.
2. Jha V, Parameswaran S. Community-acquired acute kidney injury in tropical countries. Nat Rev Nephrol. 2013;9(5): 278-90.
3. Jha V, Rathi M. Natural medicines causing acute kidney injury. Semin Nephrol. 2008;28(4):416-28.
4. Kamath N, Iyengar A. Infections and the kidney: a tale from the tropics. Pediatr Nephrol. 2018;33(8):1317-26.
5. Luyckx VA, Naicker S. Acute kidney injury associated with the use of traditional medicines. Nat Clin Pract Nephrol. 2008;4(12):664-71.

Allergic Disorders in the Tropics

Remesh Kumar R, Krishna Mohan R

INTRODUCTION

"Allergy" is an umbrella term, which includes a variety of disorders such as asthma, allergic rhinitis, food allergy, urticaria, atopic dermatitis (AD), contact dermatitis, drug allergy, allergic conjunctivitis, and anaphylaxis. The spectrum of allergic disorders in childhood is very wide and still expanding. Being an ecosystem determined disorder, the various risk factors and triggers of allergic diseases vary according to geographical, climatic, cultural, and socioeconomic conditions. A majority of the theoretical concepts of allergy are derived from studies in temperate zones. Compared with the temperate zones, prevalence of allergic diseases in the tropics is as high and in some regions even higher, though food allergy is comparatively less common.

FACTORS AFFECTING ALLERGY IN THE TROPICS

- The climatic conditions in the tropics with a mean annual temperature of 28°C and relative humidity 85% favor the existence of house dust mites (HDM) and intestinal helminth infections. The influence of perennial mite allergen exposure is one of the most important particularities of the tropics with regards to allergy. The high humidity also favors the cockroaches and molds and therefore a higher allergen load in homes and bedding materials. The climate also predisposes to insect bites that induce papular urticaria.
- Most allergic conditions are frequently underdiagnosed due to socioeconomic reasons, lack of health facilities as well as lack of awareness. For example, the use of inhaled corticosteroids (ICS) among patients with persistent asthma is often inadequate, which is related to the perception of disease as an acute condition only.

- Urbanization is a very important factor modifying allergic susceptibility, as evidenced by the fact that prevalence of allergic diseases in urban and suburban areas of the tropics is comparable to those found in affluent countries, but is comparatively low in rural communities. Air pollution is also an important factor influencing allergic susceptibility.
- Diverse viruses have been detected in children suffering from acute respiratory illnesses in the tropics. So there is high prevalence of virus-induced wheeze as well as asthma triggered by the viral infections in many of the tropical regions.
- The timeline in which immunoglobulin E (IgE) sensitization and symptoms evolve in the tropics differs to the atopic march that has been described. In the atopic march, the symptoms often appear in a particular sequence starting with AD as the first manifestation of allergy in an infant, followed by food allergy, seasonal, or perennial allergic rhinitis (PAR) and finally asthma at late childhood. But, at least in some tropical areas, the allergy symptoms debut with respiratory symptoms.

ALLERGENS IN PEDIATRIC ALLERGY

The term *allergen* refers to an antigen that can trigger an allergic reaction. Allergens can sensitize the immune system via respiratory tract (aeroallergens), gastrointestinal tract (food allergens), or skin (contact allergens) **(Box 1)**.

Food allergens usually play a major role in the first 2 years of life. As a fetus can produce IgE as early as 11 weeks of gestation and sensitization can occur with food antigens crossing placenta, food allergies can manifest even in the newborn period. Sensitization to inhalant allergens becomes evident later as it depends upon local

Box 1: Common allergens in children.		
Aeroallergens	*Food allergens*	*Contact allergens*
House dust mites, molds, cockroach, pollens, animal dander (cat, dog)	Milk, peanut, soy, egg, tree nut, fish, shellfish, wheat	Nickel, chromate, thiomersal, aluminium, rubber chemicals, cosmetics

Table 1: Pharmacotherapy of allergic rhinitis.	
Intranasal corticosteroids	• Most effective for all symptoms of allergic rhinitis • Also useful in associated allergic conjunctivitis
Oral antihistamines	• Effective in all symptoms of allergic rhinitis except nasal congestion • 2nd and 3rd generation antihistamines preferred
Decongestants	• Effective only for nasal congestion • Decongestant nasal drops should not be used continuously for more than 3 days to avoid rhinitis medicamentosa
Leukotriene receptor antagonists	Effective for most of the symptoms but less effective than intranasal corticosteroids
Ipratropium bromide nasal spray	Effective especially for watery rhinorrhea
Normal saline	Adjunctive role

aerobiology and child's environment and it takes a few seasons for seasonal allergens to sensitize the immune system.

PECULIARITIES OF ALLERGENS IN TROPICS

- Sensitization to pollens is less frequent and less intense than to mite allergens.
- Immunoglobulin E sensitization to food allergens is frequently detected without symptoms and aeroallergen sensitization is not usually preceded by food sensitization. The sources of food allergens are slightly different; for instance hypersensitivity to shellfish, fish, and fruits is more common than reactions to nuts, peanut, and wheat.
- Immunoglobulin E sensitization to aeroallergens occurs early in life and at higher frequencies compared to temperate areas.
- The main sensitizers in allergic patients living in tropical urban environments are HDM and cockroach.

THE SPECTRUM OF ALLERGY DISEASES IN THE TROPICS

Allergic Rhinitis

The International Study of Asthma and Allergies in Childhood (ISAAC) Phase I (conducted in the early 1990s) and Phase III (2001–2003) detected an overall increase in the prevalence of rhinoconjunctivitis which was more marked in older children.

In India, ISAAC study was conducted in 14 centers. Phase I included 30,879 children in the 6–7-year age group, while there were 37,171 children in the 13–14-year age group. Data from India revealed that nasal symptoms were present in 12.5% children in the 6–7-year age group and 18.6% in the 13–14-year age group. Allergic rhinoconjunctivitis was seen in 3.3% and 5.6%, respectively.

Allergic rhinitis should be suspected in patients with any two of the following: paroxysmal sneezing, rhinorrhea, nasal obstruction, and itching in nose. Itching in eyes, palate, throat, and ears may also be present.

Children with allergic rhinitis may have typical allergic facies, i.e. open mouth breathing, dark coloration under the eyes (allergic shiners), and a crease across the lower eyelid (Dennie's sign). There may be a transverse crease across the lower nose caused by chronic upward rubbing on the tip of the nose; a motion called the "allergic salute." Inspection of the nasal cavity may reveal pale, boggy, and sometimes bluish mucosa.

As per the ARIA (Allergic Rhinitis and its Impact on Asthma) guidelines, allergic rhinitis is classified based on the frequency of symptoms and the symptom severity into mild, moderate-severe, intermittent, and persistent.

Based on the frequency and duration of symptoms, allergic rhinitis can be of three types:
1. *Seasonal allergic rhinitis (SAR)*: Symptoms during specific season only; common allergens—pollens and outdoor mold spores
2. *Perennial allergic rhinitis*: Symptoms present almost throughout the year; common allergens—HDM, cockroaches, indoor molds, and animal danders
3. *Perennial allergic rhinitis with seasonal exacerbation*: Symptoms of both SAR and PAR.

Allergic rhinitis is diagnosed by combination of clinical features, examination of nose, and *in vivo* and *in vitro* allergy tests.

Management of allergic rhinitis includes allergen avoidance, pharmacotherapy **(Table 1)**, and allergen-specific immunotherapy.

Pediatric Asthma

Pediatric asthma is one among the most common chronic respiratory disease which affects children in all countries and ethnic groups. The prevalence of pediatric asthma is definitely on a rise in the tropical countries. Possible reasons include urbanization, changing dietary patterns, air pollution, etc. ISAAC Phase III showed a definite increase in the prevalence of pediatric asthma in many tropical regions compared with the phase I results.

Management of pediatric asthma has undergone drastic changes over the years. Gone are the days when asthma was considered only as a disease of bronchoconstriction. The present understanding of asthma as a chronic inflammatory disease with airway remodeling, emphasizes the key role of ICS in the management of asthma. But with the recent advances in the pathophysiology, it has been shown that ICS is most effective in eosinophilic inflammation. Other drugs like long-acting beta-2 agonists, long-acting antimuscarinic, and drugs which are effective against other mediators in airway inflammation like leukotrienes, IgE, interleukin-6 (IL-6), IL-4, and IL-5 may also have role in those with poor control of symptoms. The goals of the treatment are not only to reduce the airway inflammation and risk for acute exacerbations, but also to reduce the fatalities in asthma. Treating the comorbid conditions and trying to modify or reduce indoor air pollution wherever possible is equally important in the management.

The inhaled medications are of two types—controller and reliever. Beclomethasone, budesonide, and fluticasone are the controller drugs available in India. Among the controller medications, fluticasone has the least bioavailability of less than 1% due to its nearly complete first-pass mechanism.

Reliever medications are those that are used to relieve the bronchoconstriction. Short-acting beta-2 agonists (SABA) include salbutamol and levosalbutamol. Other drugs used as reliever medications along with SABA are systemic corticosteroids and ipratropium.

Atopic Dermatitis

Atopic dermatitis is a chronic inflammatory skin disorder which is widely distributed, particularly among children under 5 years. Although there are several population studies on AD, very little is known about the actual prevalence, especially outside Europe. As per ISAAC Phase I and Phase III, which had the participation of centers from several tropical countries too, the prevalence of AD was found higher than in other regions in some centers. AD is characterized by pruritus, chronic or relapsing course, and typical distribution involves face, scalp, and extensor surfaces in infants and children while flexural folds are involved in older children and adolescents. Xerosis, ichthyosis, pityriasis alba, palmar hyperlinearity, nonspecific hand or feet eczema, and facial erythema may also be seen. Lichenification is a feature of chronic AD. In tropical countries, especially in underdeveloped areas, the other causes of pruritus and lichenified lesions such as scabies, papular urticaria, seborrheic dermatitis, and miliaria are very common. This poses practical difficulty in the diagnosis of AD in tropics.

Diagnosis is mainly clinical. Personal or family history of allergic disorders, aeroallergen, or food allergen sensitization on allergy tests and elevated serum IgE levels may be present and are supportive to diagnosis.

Moisturizers and topical corticosteroids are mainstay of therapy. Twice-daily application of moisturizers after a 10-minute warm soaking bath is recommended. Low-potency steroids are recommended for the face or intertriginous areas. Low- to mid-potency steroids are suggested for the trunk, extremities, or scalp. Long-term application of high-potency steroids is often necessary for lichenification.

Topical calcineurin inhibitors (Tacrolimus ointment and Pimecrolimus cream) are frequently used nowadays as effective steroid-sparing agents for AD in children with age more than 2 years.

First-generation oral antihistamines (diphenhydramine or hydroxyzine) are preferred for children with significant nocturnal pruritus. Topical or systemic antistaphylococcal antibiotic may be required due to high colonization of *Staphylococcus aureus* in children with AD.

Identification and avoidance of food allergens is very important as IgE-mediated food allergy is present in 35% of children with moderate-to-severe AD. Irritants and emotional stressors should also be avoided.

Urticaria

Urticaria usually presents as pruritic generalized eruption with erythematous circumscribed borders and pale, slightly elevated centers. When the symptoms are present for less than 6 weeks, it is considered acute urticaria, otherwise it is termed chronic urticaria. Angioedema is usually a nonpruritic, asymmetric nondependent swelling which may involve subcutaneous tissues such as the eyelids, lips, tongue, genitals, and dorsum of the hands or feet. Urticaria is a common problem in the tropics and seems to be clinically similar to that in temperate zones.

Due to similar pathophysiology, approximately 50% of affected patients have both urticaria and angioedema together; urticaria and angioedema alone may be seen as 40% and 10% in patients, respectively. Although allergic reactions are a very common cause of acute urticaria

Table 2: Causes of acute urticaria/angioedema.	
Food allergens	Egg, milk, soy, peanut, tree nuts, wheat, fish, seafood, etc.
Infections	Viral infections, parasites, *Mycoplasma*, and others
Stings and bites	Honeybee, wasp, bedbugs, fleas, and mites
Medications	Penicillins, other antibiotics, opioids, volume expanders, etc.
Contact urticaria	Latex, pollen, nettle plants, industrial chemicals, etc.

(Table 2), allergy is an uncommon cause of chronic urticaria/angioedema. Common causes of chronic urticaria/angioedema are infections, physical urticaria, autoimmune urticaria, collagen vascular disorders, or idiopathic. In children with recurrent angioedema without urticaria, hereditary angioedema (HAE) should be suspected. In the tropics, various infections and parasitic infestations are comparatively more common and they should be considered as an important cause of both acute and chronic urticaria. There are reports of acute and chronic urticaria associated with giardia lamblia, fasciola hepatica, toxocara canis, echinococcus granulosus, strongyloides stercoralis, hymenolepis nana, blastocystis hominis, ascaris lumbricoides, etc.

Papular urticaria is an allergic, chronic skin disease caused by insect bites, especially with fleas and mosquitoes. It is a common manifestation in the tropics. It usually appears during the first year of life; normally, it improves by the age of 7 years, but there are exceptions that persist until adulthood. Although this is common in the tropics, it can be observed in any place where causal insects are present.

Second-generation H_1-antihistamines are drug of choice for management of acute urticaria/angioedema. Sedative H_1-antihistamines are also effective. Rarely, a severe episode may require a short course of systemic corticosteroids. Urticaria/angioedema as a part of anaphylaxis must be treated with intramuscular adrenaline. Identification and avoidance of the trigger is important for preventing recurrence of allergic urticaria/angioedema.

Food Allergy

Adverse reactions to foods can be a true (immunologically mediated) food allergy or nonimmunological adverse reactions to foods like food poisoning and food intolerance. A food allergy is an adverse health effect arising from a specific immune response that occurs reproducibly on exposure to a given food.

Though food allergy has been noted in the urbanized western world for some time, nowadays it is becoming common all round the world. Food allergy is estimated to affect more than 1–2% and less than 10% of the population. The overall prevalence of self-reported or questionnaire-based food allergy in Asia is reported to be 3.4–11%. Although more than 170 foods have been identified as triggers of food allergy, those causing most of the significant allergic reactions include milk, egg, peanut, tree nuts, fish, shellfish, wheat, soy, and seeds. The prevalence of peanut allergy is relatively low in the tropical region compared to temperate climates, though the prevalence of sensitization to peanut is relatively high. Genetic and ethnic factors, environmental immunomodulatory factors, exposure to aeroallergens, and age of introduction of foods are the probable reasons why peanut allergy is less common in some tropical populations. The high rates of asymptomatic sensitization may be due to cross-reactive allergens, which have poor correlation with clinical allergy.

Immunoglobulin E-mediated food allergies can affect a variety of target organs: the skin, manifested as urticaria and/or angioedema; the gastrointestinal tract, causing vomiting, abdominal pain, and/or diarrhea; the respiratory tract, as wheezing and/or allergic rhinitis; and the cardiovascular system resulting in hypotension and/or cardiac arrhythmias. An immediate, systemic IgE-mediated reaction is anaphylaxis and can develop into a potentially fatal allergic reaction. With non-IgE mediated (or T-cell mediated) food allergies, patients can have reactions to food, such as AD flare-ups or severe vomiting and diarrhea progressing to shock on ingestion/exposure to the offending food.

The only proven therapy for food allergy is strict elimination of the offending food. But complete elimination of common foods (milk, egg, soy, wheat, rice, chicken, fish, peanut, nuts) is very difficult because of their widespread use in a variety of processed foods. This requires extensive education and work on the part of the parents and any other caregiver, including babysitters, grandparents, etc. and includes reading all food labels as well as taking special care when ordering food in restaurants, notifying schools regarding snacks/meals, etc. Parents of younger children with food allergies should be trained to identify early allergic symptoms and should have antihistamines and epinephrine available at all times. Allergen-specific therapies such as oral, sublingual, and epicutaneous immunotherapy and allergen nonspecific therapies such as Chinese herbal formula Food Allergy Herbal Formula-2 (FAHF-2) and omalizumab are tried, but more data on efficacy and safety are needed before these therapies become mainstream.

CONCLUSION

Pediatric allergic diseases are as rampant in the tropics as in any part of the world. The various factors affecting the development and progression of allergy diseases in the tropics slightly vary, compared with the temperate regions. Adequate knowledge about this is essential while managing allergic diseases in tropics. High priority should be given to creating awareness among the general public about the allergic diseases and the importance of early diagnosis and treatment.

SUGGESTED READING

1. Andiappan AK, Puan KJ, Lee B, et al. Allergic airway diseases in a tropical urban environment are driven by dominant mono-specific sensitization against house dust mites. Allergy. 2014;69(4):501-9.
2. Björkstén B, Clayton T, Ellwood P, et al.; ISAAC Phase III Study Group. Worldwide time trends for symptoms of rhinitis and conjunctivitis: Phase III of the International Study of Asthma and Allergies in Childhood. Pediatr Allergy Immunol. 2008;19(2):110-24.
3. Budge PJ, Griffin MR, Edwards KM, et al. A household-based study of acute viral respiratory illnesses in Andean children. Pediatr Infect Dis J. 2014;33(5):443-7.
4. Demirci M, Yildirim M, Aridogan BC, et al. Tissue parasites in patients with chronic urticaria. J Dermatol. 2003;30(11): 777-81.
5. Dennis R, Caraballo L, Garcia E, et al. Asthma and other allergic conditions in Colombia: a study in 6 cities. Ann Allergy Asthma Immunol. 2004;93(6):568-74.
6. Dharmage SC, Lowe AJ, Matheson MC, et al. Atopic dermatitis and the atopic march revisited. Allergy. 2014;69(1):17-27.
7. Kidon MI, Chiang WC, Liew WK, et al. Mite component-specific IgE repertoire and phenotypes of allergic disease in childhood: the tropical perspective. Pediatr Allergy Immunol. 2011;22(2):202-10.
8. Larenas-Linnemann D, Michels A, Dinger H, et al. Allergen sensitization linked to climate and age, not to intermittent-persistent rhinitis in a cross-sectional cohort study in the (sub)-tropics. Clin Transl Allergy. 2014;4:20.
9. Lecha Estela LB. Biometeorological classification of daily weather types for the humid tropics. Int J Biometeorol. 1998; 42(2):77-83.
10. Lee AJ, Gerez I, Shek LP, et al. Shellfish allergy–an Asia-Pacific perspective. Asian Pac J Allergy Immunol. 2012;30(1):3-10.
11. Raj D, Lodha R, Pandey A, et al.; New Delhi Childhood Asthma Study Group. Aeroallergen sensitization in childhood asthmatics in northern India. Indian Pediatr. 2013;50(12): 1113-8.
12. Robinson CL, Baumann LM, Romero K, et al. Effect of urbanisation on asthma, allergy and airways inflammation in a developing country setting. Thorax. 2011;66(12):1051-7.
13. Shek LP, Lee BW. Food allergy in Asia. Curr Opin Allergy Clin Immunol. 2006;6(3):197-201.
14. Vedanthan PK, Mahesh PA, Vedanthan R, et al. Effect of animal contact and microbial exposures on the prevalence of atopy and asthma in urban vs rural children in India. Ann Allergy Asthma Immunol. 2006;96(4):571-8.

Vasculitis in Children

Purushothaman KK, Geetha P

INTRODUCTION

The term vasculitis indicates the presence of inflammation of the vessel wall leading to vascular stenosis, aneurysm, rupture or occlusion resulting in ischemia, necrosis or injury to tissues. Clinical features vary widely depending on the type and location of vessels involved and the extent of the pathological changes. Vasculitis can occur as a primary disorder or secondary to other disorders like infections, malignancies, autoimmune/autoinflammatory conditions. Primary vasculitis is rare in children. The incidence varies in different parts of the world. In tropical countries Henoch–Schönlein purpura (HSP) [immunoglobulin A (IgA) vasculitis as recent terminology] and Kawasaki disease (KD) are the most common. Generally, they are complex and challenging disorders and can involve multiple organs and systems. Presentation may be acute and self-limiting, waxing and waning or indolent. They may be associated with significant morbidity and mortality, particularly if the diagnosis is delayed. This chapter provides an overview on the epidemiology, classification and clinical approach of vasculitis in children. Clinical features and treatment of few of the common vasculitis are also included.

EPIDEMIOLOGY

There are striking geographic differences noted in the relative frequency of vasculitis. The incidence and prevalence of various vasculitis in children in India is unknown. Most common are HSP and KD and all the others are rare. KD and Takayasu arteritis are most prevalent in Japan. Polyarteritis nodosa and cutaneous polyarteritis are also more common in Japan and Turkey. The estimated incidence of new cases of pediatric vasculitis is approximately 50 cases per 10,000 children per year. Giant cell arteritis and essential cryoglobulinemic vasculitis are exclusively seen in adults. There is paucity of data about the disease prevalence in developing countries.

Kawasaki disease is showing a trend of increase in incidence over the last two decades in Asian countries compared to western countries. World over Kawasaki and HSP are reported in males more than females, the proportion varies in different countries.

CLASSIFICATION

In 1990, the American College of Rheumatology had proposed classification criteria for adult patients with vasculitis, but it was widely recognized that these criteria were not suitable for children. So at the international conference held at Vienna, in June 2005, the vasculitis working group of Pediatric Rheumatology European Society (PReS) with the endorsement of European Society of Pediatric Nephrology and European League against Rheumatism (EULAR) proposed a new classification criteria for childhood vasculitis. These criteria have been modified and validated using a large international web-based registry. The final Ankara 2008 classification criteria have high sensitivity and specificity and have been endorsed by EULAR, PReS, and the Pediatric Rheumatology International Trials Organization (PRINTO).

Later in 2012, the International Chapel Hill Consensus Conference updated the previous recommendations and the notable changes were the addition of new categories like single organ vasculitis (which includes isolated central vessel vasculitis), vasculitis associated with probable etiology (such as hepatitis or drug induced vasculitis) and vasculitis associated with systemic diseases (such as systemic lupus erythematosus). The presence or absence of antineutrophilic cytoplasmic antibody (ANCA) is also incorporated within in the classification framework and thus small vessel vasculitis is subcategorized into immune complex and ANCA-associated vasculitis. This classification currently followed is given in **Box 1**.

■ KAWASAKI DISEASE

Kawasaki disease is a medium vessel vasculitis predominantly affecting children less than 5 years. It is characterized by the development of coronary artery abnormalities (CAA) in 15–25% of the affected children which may lead to mortality and lifelong morbidity, if not diagnosed and treated early. It is the leading cause of acquired heart disease in developed countries. In the absence of pathognomonic tests, diagnosis rests on clinical findings and exclusion of other disease entities with known causes.

Epidemiology

First described in Japan, now KD is occurring worldwide with maximum cases reported in Japan. Recurrence rates and familial occurrences are also maximally reported from Japanese ancestry. Increase in incidence during the winter season is observed in US. But in India no seasonal variation is observed.

Etiology

Even after four decades of its description exact etiology of KD is not known. Present concept is an immune-mediated inflammation triggered by an infectious organism in a genetic susceptible person. Genetic factors seems to be responsible for the varying ethnic susceptibility. Asians are more susceptible with highest incidence in Japan. Incidence of cases in children of parents who had KD in their childhood, higher rates of KD in siblings of index cases and twins argue for a genetic susceptibility. Risk of concordance in identical twins is 13%. Many candidate genes are considered as "susceptible genes" or "genes increasing severity, susceptibility" for KD and disease outcome, including response to management. These polymorphisms vary across populations, and the important difference in allele frequency will explain the increased incidence of disease among Asian populations. Aneurysm formation and response to intravenous immunoglobulin (IVIG) are influenced by variants in several different genes and signaling pathways.

Many reasons to suspect a triggering infectious agent. Occurrence in clusters and epidemics, self-limited nature, occurrence in young, sparing of older population and very young all suggest this possibility. An unidentified cytoplasmic agent in the macrophages in the respiratory epithelium and coronaries reported in many cases. Earlier concept about the immune response was a superantigen. Current concept is immune response to a classic antigen which is protective against future exposure.

The self-limited nature and rarity of future recurrence suggest the possibility of immune memory which is protective against future encounters with an infectious agent.

Pathology

Although coronary artery involvement decides the long-term outcome, KD inflammation involves all the medium-sized arteries and organs during the acute febrile phase. Hepatitis, interstitial pneumonitis, aseptic meningitis, myocarditis, pericarditis, pancreatitis, and sterile pyuria may cause organ specific manifestations. Even though liver and kidney are involved hepatic failure and renal failure are rare. Pathological changes in arteries progresses in three phases. First phase of necrotizing arteritis occur within the first 2 weeks after fever onset. The second

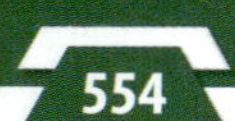

phase is subacute/chronic vasculitis due to infiltration of lymphocytes and plasma cells macrophages. The third stage is luminal myofibroblastic proliferation (LMP), which persists for months to years which may lead to vascular stenosis. Very mildly dilated vessels may return to normal, but the severely involved ones will lead to long-term sequelae like irreversible dilatation, stenosis, thrombosis which may predispose for later tissue ischemia. Large or giant coronary aneurysms >8 mm in diameter will not resolve. They may rupture and always contain thrombi. Predisposition to atherosclerosis is rare.

Clinical Features

Box 2 describe the criteria for diagnosis.

Patients who meet the criteria are said to have classic or typical KD. Patients who do not have sufficient criteria are labeled as atypical or incomplete. Classic KD is diagnosed when fever last 5 or more days with the presence of four of five principal clinical criteria. Typically all the clinical features may not be present at one point of time. Few of the principal features may be late to appear and some clinical features may disappear if the patient is seen late in the course of illness. Fever usually continues for 1–3 weeks if appropriate treatment is not given.

Fever lasting less than 5 days argues against KD but spontaneous resolution of fever after 7 days does not argue against the possibility of KD. Fever usually resolves within 36 hours after IVIG administration. Average duration of fever is 12 days. Duration of fever correlates with risk of coronary aneurysms.

Extremity changes. Erythema of palms and soles and painful induration of hands and feet occur in the acute phase. Desquamation of fingers and toes usually begin in the periungual region within 2–3 weeks after onset of

fever, and may extend to palms and soles. Deep transverse grooves across nails may occur after 1–2 months.

Diffuse maculopapular rash and rarely scarlet fever or erythema multiforme like rash appear within 5 days of beginning of fever. Urticarial or micropustular rashes are still rare. Primarily trunk is involved but accentuation at groin is characteristic. Bullous, vesicular and petechial rashes are very rare and suggests other possibilities.

Bilateral nonexudative bulbar conjunctival injection spares the limbus leaving an avascular zone around the iris. Anterior uveitis is common.

Changes of lips and oral cavity are: (1) erythema, dryness, fissuring, peeling, cracking, and bleeding of lips; (2) "strawberry tongue" with prominent fungiform papillae; (3) diffuse oropharyngeal mucosa. Ulcers and pharyngeal exudates will not occur and argues against KD.

Cervical lymph node is the least common of the principal clinical features. It is usually unilateral, >1.5 cm in diameter and occur in the anterior triangle. Rarely, lymph node enlargement may precede other clinical features leading to wrong diagnosis of other entities at the beginning. Diagnosis becoming obvious with typical features occurring later.

Rarer features:

- Transient unilateral or bilateral lower motor neuron (LMN) facial palsy and sensorineural hearing loss.
- Hepatitis, pancreatitis, gallbladder involvement occasionally may be severe.
- Arthritis of large joints may be severe in the second or third week of illness.
- Peripheral vessel involvement with aneurysm formation and ischemia severe enough to cause gangrene.
- X-ray findings may confuse with pneumonia especially in cases with respiratory symptoms.
- Erythema and induration at the site of Bacille Calmette Guérin (BCG) vaccination may occur.
- Rarely macrophage activation syndrome occur which may lead to a severe course not responding to IVIG.

Laboratory features typically shows high erythrocyte sedimentation rate (ESR) and C-reactive protein (CRP) and leukocytosis with neutrophilia. Low sodium and albumin levels, elevated transaminase and sterile pyuria may be present. Thrombocytosis is common in the second week of fever onset **(Figs. 1A to D)**.

Incomplete (Atypical) Kawasaki Disease

Small percentage of cases, especially infants less than 6 months of age may present with prolonged fever without

---

Box 2: Diagnosis of classic Kawasaki disease (KD).
Classic KD is diagnosed in the presence of fever for at least 5 day together with at least 4 of 5 following principal clinical features. In the presence of more than four principal features particularly when redness and swelling of the hands and feet are present, diagnosis of KD can be made with 4 days of fever
1. Erythema and cracking of the lips, strawberry tongue and/or erythema of oral and pharyngeal mucosa
2. Bilateral bulbar conjunctival injection without exudates
3. *Rash*: Maculopapular, diffuse erythroderma, or erythema multiforme like
4. Erythema and edema of hands and feet in acute phase and/or periungual desquamation in subacute phase
5. Cervical lymphadenopathy (>1.5 cm in diameter), usually unilateral

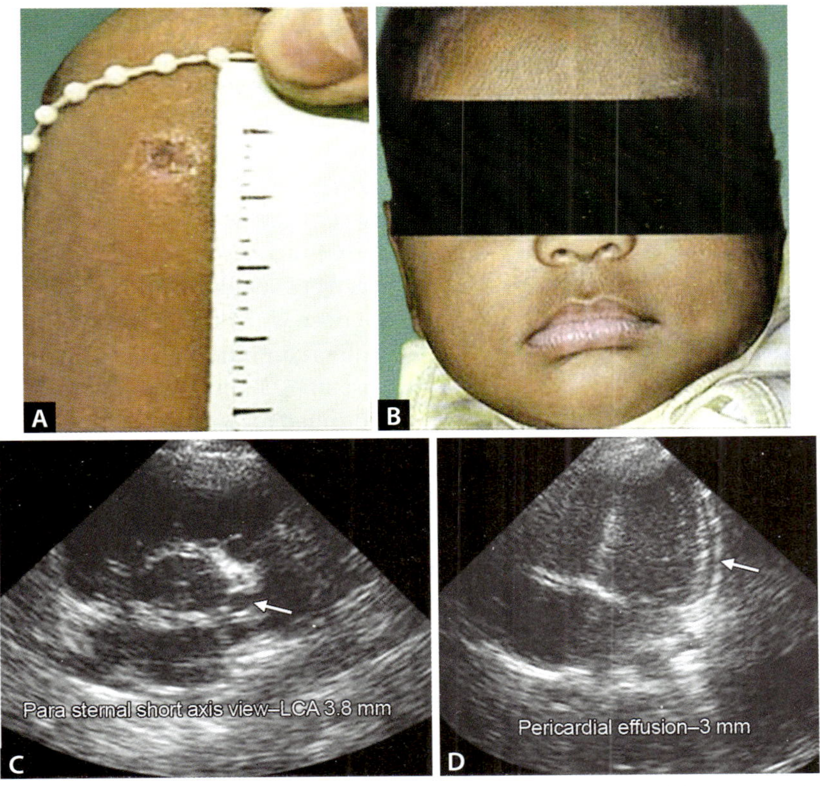

Figs. 1A to D: (A) BCG site induration; (B) Red lips; (C) Dilated coronary LCA; and (D) Pericardial effusion.
(BCG: Bacille Calmette Guérin; LCA: left coronary artery)

classical criteria where ECHO show coronary artery abnormalities. A high index of suspicion for the diagnosis and early ECHO is important in these cases. In these cases of incomplete KD diagnostic algorithm proposed in 2004 guidelines American Heart Association (AHA).

Differential Diagnosis

Exudative conjunctivitis and Koplik spots helps to differentiate KD from measles, supported by leukopenia in laboratory result which practically rules out KD. Absence of conjunctival involvement and response to antibiotics helps to differentiate from scarlet fever. Presence of bleeding manifestations, liver dysfunction renal dysfunction support the possibility of leptospirosis. Even though involvement of kidney and liver occur in KD features of failure of the systems very rare.

Common Pitfalls in Diagnosis

Babies less than 6 months may present with prolonged fever and unexplained irritability only without the classical features. Unless we keep this possibility in mind and do ECHO as a routine in all cases of prolonged fever in this age group with fewer than four principal criteria, many cases of KD are likely to be missed in this age group.

As the most common age group involved is less than 5 years we are likely to miss rare case of KD occurring in older age group especially adolescents. Both these age groups have a higher prevalence of coronary artery involvement.

High fever irritability and presence of cells in the cerebrospinal fluid in many cases are diagnosed as meningitis till the classical features evolve.

Prolonged fever with pus cell in urine wrong diagnosis of urinary tract infection is often made.

Prolonged fever with prominent cervical lymph node with throat congestion may be wrongly diagnosed as tonsillitis. Consider possibility of KD when expected response to antibiotics is not seen.

High-grade fever with rash presenting in shock is likely to be diagnosed as sepsis with myocardial involvement. This presentation is especially common with staphylococcal infections. Few cases of Kawasaki may present with predominant shock. Most of the markers of sepsis and KD are common except thrombocytosis which is less common in septic shock. This should be kept in mind in a case of suspected septic shock when blood culture negative.

Treatment

Mainstay of treatment in both complete and incomplete KD is a single high dose of IVIG with acetylsalicylic acid (ASA). Acute treatment should be started from the onset and to be continued until the resolution of acute systemic inflammation and coronary artery luminal dimensions has stabilized and no more expanding. Timely initiation of IVIG has reduced the incidence of coronary artery involvement from 25% to less than 5%.

Cases with typical features may be started on IVIG and ASA. An algorithm will be helpful in case of incomplete KD to decide in patients with fever and less than four classical diagnostic criteria.

Ideally IVIG should be started within the first 10 days. Those who are presenting after 10 days may also be treated if there is evidence of ongoing inflammation manifested as high ESR or CRP (more than 3 mg/dL) or persistent fever without other reasons or coronary artery dilatation or aneurysm (luminal dimension more than 2.5 Z score). Mechanism of action of IVIG is unknown. IVIG appears to have generalized anti-inflammatory effect. Possible mechanisms of action include modulation of cytokine production, neutralization of toxins augmentation of regulatory T-cell activity, suppression of antibody synthesis, and provision of anti-idiotype antibodies.

Single infusion of IVIG 2 g/kg given over 10–12 hours is shown to have superior efficiency than smaller repeated doses. About 20% of children treated as above still develop coronary artery dilatation in the proximal LAD or proximal right coronary artery (RCA) by Z-score criteria, 5% may develops coronary artery aneurysm (Z > 2.5) and 1% develops giant aneurysm according to Japanese Ministry Health Criteria. If cutoff point of dilatation is taken as >2, 30% of patients will have coronary artery dilatation.

Acetylsalicylic acid does not appear to lower the frequency of development of coronary abnormalities during the acute phase of disease. There is no consensus in the dose and duration of ASA during the acute phase of management. Dose used in the United States is 50–80 mg/kg and in Japan and Western Europe 30–50 mg/kg is used during the acute phase. There is no data to support the superiority of either dose. Practices regarding duration of high dose ASA also vary between different institutions. Many centers reduces the dose when the child is afebrile for 48–72 hours. Other centers continue high dose until the 14th day of illness or at least 48–72 hours of cessation of fever. Aspirin 3–5 mg/kg is continued for 6–8 weeks and no coronary changes persists. For children who develop coronary abnormalities ASA will be continued for long. Concomitant use of ibuprofen antagonizes the platelet inhibition by ASA and is should not be used along with ASA.

Long-term prognosis is determined by the coronary artery involvement. Long-term management of those patients rests on judicious use of thromboprophylaxis and vigilant follow up of pathological changes.

Intravenous Immunoglobulin Resistance

Approximately 10–20% of patients continue to have fever after 36 hours of IVIG infusion. Mechanism of nonresponse is unknown. They are at increased risk of coronary artery abnormalities. A scoring system developed in Japan to identify these high risk cases so that they may benefit from more aggressive therapy. This high risk prediction model is not applicable in other countries **(Table 1)**.

Adjunctive Therapies for Primary Treatment

In cases where chance of nonresponse to IVIG predictable by scoring system adjunctive therapies for primary

Table 1: Treatment options for IVIG resistant KD patients.	
Most frequently administered	
IVIG: Second infusion	2 g/kg IV
IVIG + steroid	IVIG 2 g/kg IV + methylprednisolone 2 mg/kg divided 8 hourly IV until fever subsides. Then continue orally till C-reactive protein (CRP) normalizes and then taper and stop
Infliximab	Single infusion 5 mg/kg IV given over 2 hours
Alternative agents	
Cyclosporine	3 mg/kg divided 12 hourly IV or 4–8 mg orally 12 hourly
Anakinra	2–6 mg/kg SC
Cyclophosphamide	2 mg/kg IV
Plasma exchange	

(IVIG: intravenous immunoglobulin; KD: Kawasaki disease)

resistance tried. With IVIG high administration of steroids high or low dose showed lesser incidence of coronary artery involvement.

Few studies where infliximab was used with IVIG showed lesser infusion reaction to IVIG, but no difference in coronary artery aneurysm.

Vaccination Following Treatment of Kawasaki Disease

Those who had high dose of IVIG better avoid live parenteral vaccines for 10–11 months. Those who are on low dose aspirin are more prone for Reye syndrome especially during infection with varicella and influenza viral infections. They may get vaccinated against these infections. Aspirin may be replaced with clopidogrel 3 days before and 3 months after vaccination.

■ HENOCH–SCHÖNLEIN PURPURA OR IMMUNOGLOBULIN A VASCULITIS

Henoch–Schönlein vasculitis is one of the most common primary vasculitides seen in children. William Heberden in 1802 first described this disease. Later in 1837, Shönlein from Germany proposed the diagnostic triad of purpuric rash, arthritis, and abnormalities of urinary sediment. In 1874, Henoch described the association of gastrointestinal symptoms and proteinuria with this triad. Hence it came to be known as HSP. The term anaphylactoid purpura was applied by Gairdner in 1948. The disease is now called as IgA vasculitis as it is characterized by deposition of IgA1 in the walls of the small vessels.

Epidemiology

Henoch–Schönlein purpura is predominantly a disease of childhood, although a similar syndrome can be seen in adults also though uncommon. It is rare in children less than 2 years. The peak age of onset is between 4 years and 6 years of age. In a study from the United Kingdom, wherein 1.1 million children <17 years were screened, the annual incidence was found to be around 20 per 100,000 and greater incidence was found in children from the Indian subcontinent (24 per 100,000). The mean incidence of HSP nephritis in Asian children has been reported to be 4.9 cases per 100,000 children. Males are affected more commonly than females.

Pathogenesis

Immunoglobulin A has a key role in the pathogenesis of this disease as there is almost universal deposition of IgA1 in the vascular tissue. It is reported that many infectious agents like group A β-hemolytic *Streptococcus* and allergy to insect bites, dietary allergens and even exposure to certain drugs can predispose to HSP. Although the pathogenesis of HSP still remains unknown, studies suggest that serum levels of poorly glycosylated IgA1 is increased in HSP especially in HSP nephritis and these are recognized by antiglycan IgG or IgA antibodies which are perhaps triggered off by some infection leading to the formation of circulating immune complexes, which get deposited in the mesangium and other tissues resulting in vasculitis. Disorders of coagulation and its activation are also associated with the occurrence of HSP. In patients with severe abdominal involvement, it is seen that there may be a rapid decline of factor VIII.

It is recognized that the genetic contribution to the pathogenesis of HSP is complex and possibly polygenic in nature. Familial clusters of the disease may occur with siblings affected simultaneously or sequentially.

Clinical Features

Skin

The characteristic skin manifestation is palpable purpura seen most prominently on the extensor surface of the dependent areas or pressure bearing surfaces especially on the lower extremities and buttocks but it may occur on other areas also including arms and ears. The abdomen, chest and face are relatively spared. It is the presenting manifestation in 50% of children. The rash is usually symmetrical, typically appears in crops and can persist for 3–10 days. The lesions can be induced by mild trauma. New crops may continue to develop for several months after the disease onset and gradually fade over time **(Figs. 2 to 5)**.

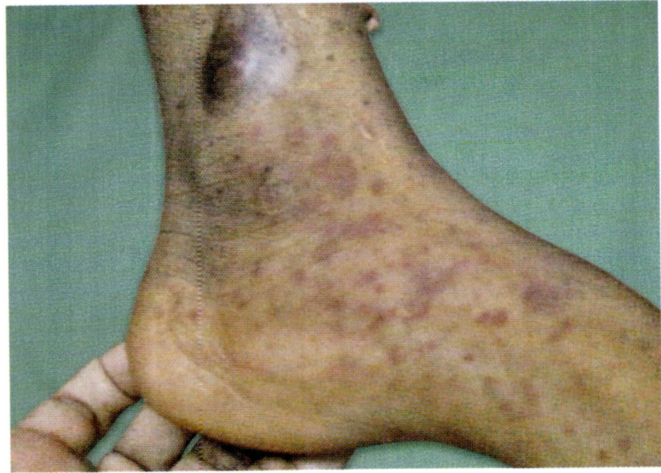

Fig. 2: Palpable purpura in Henoch–Schönlein purpura.

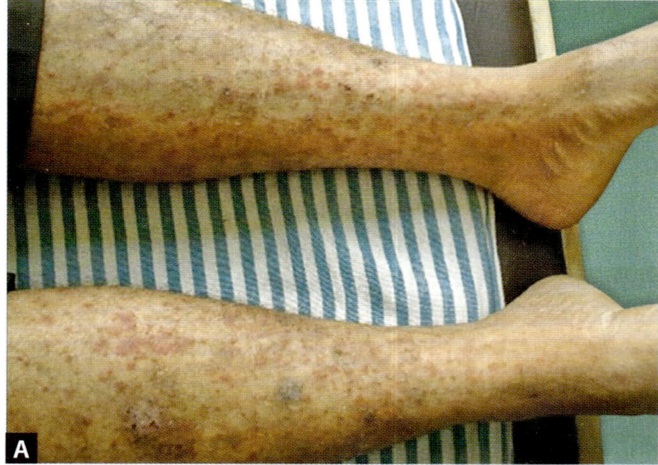

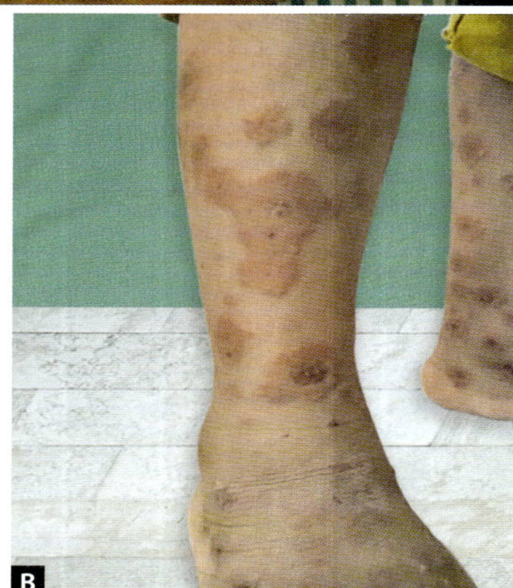

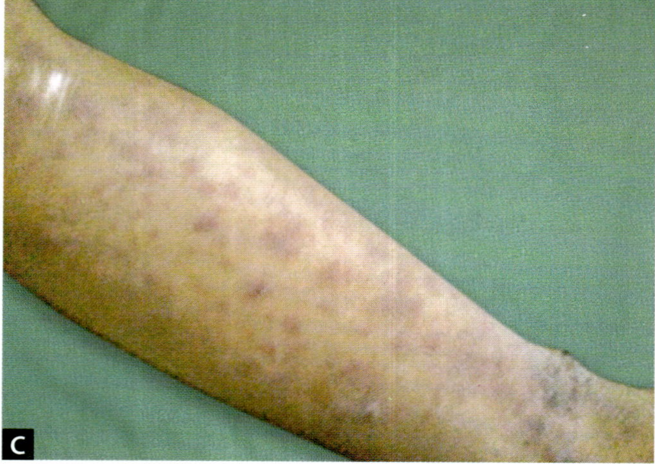

Figs. 3A to C: Skin lesions in Henoch–Schönlein purpura.

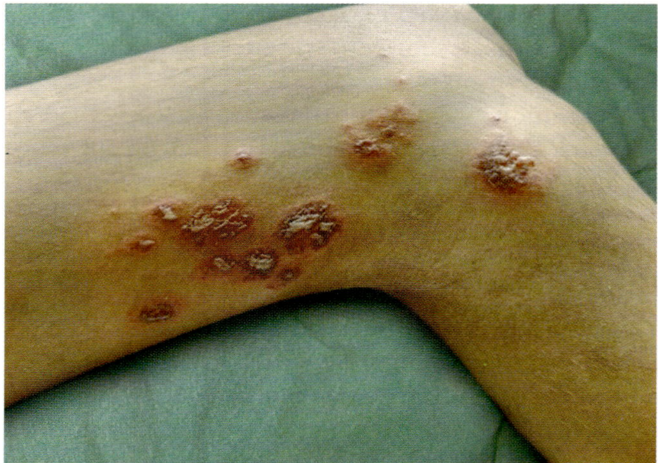

Fig. 4: Rare presentation of vesicular lesions in Henoch–Schönlein purpura.

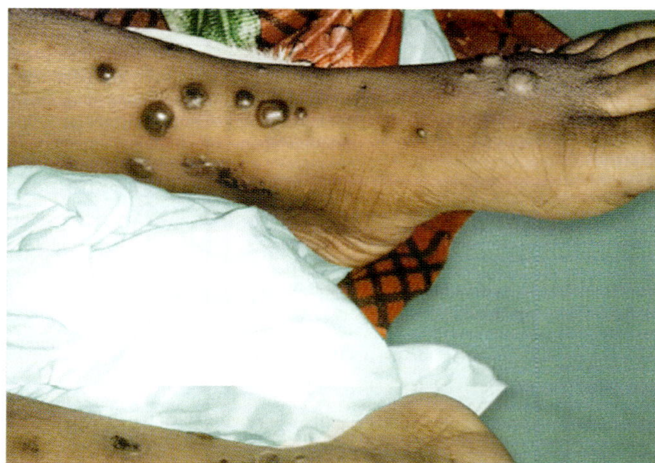

Fig. 5: Hemorrhagic bullae in Henoch–Schönlein purpura.

Other skin lesions like small petechiae, large ecchymosis, and rarely hemorrhagic bullae and skin ulcerations can occur. The rash is often preceded by maculopapular or urticarial lesions.

Subcutaneous edema over the dorsum of hands and feet and around the eyes, forehead, scalp and scrotum may occur especially in young children.

Musculoskeletal

Arthralgia or arthritis involving a few joints occur in 50–80% of children with HSP and are the presenting symptoms in about 15–25% of children. Large joints such as the knee and ankle are most commonly involved but other joints may also be involved. Characteristically, there is prominent periarticular swelling, limitation of movement and considerable pain without erythema, warmth or effusion in the joint. The arthritis is usually nonerosive and fleeting in nature. It may recur again during the disease course.

Table 2: 2010 classification criteria for Henoch–Schönlein purpura.

Criterion	Definition
Abdominal pain	*Diffuse, acute, colicky pain*: May include intussusception and gastrointestinal bleeding
Histopathology	Leukocytoclastic vasculitis with predominant Ig A deposits or proliferative glomerulonephritis with predominant IgA deposits
Arthritis, arthralgias	• *Arthritis*: Acute joint swelling or pain with limitation of motion • *Arthralgia*: Acute joint pain without joint swelling or limitation of motion
Renal involvement	• Proteinuria > 0.3 g/24 hrs; spot urine albumin to creatinine ratio > 30 mmol/mg; or ≥ 2+ on dipstick • *Hematuria*: Red ell casts; urine sediment showing > 5 red cells per high power field or red cell casts

Adapted from Ozen et al. EULAR/PRINTO/PRES criteria for Henoch–Schönlein purpura, childhood polyarteritis nodosa, childhood Wegener granulomatosis and childhood Takayasu arteritis; Ankara 2008. Part II: Final Classification Criteria, Ann Rheum Dis 69; 2010.

Gastrointestinal

More than 50% of children develop abdominal symptoms usually within a week after the onset of the first symptom and almost always within 30 days. The symptoms range from mild colicky abdominal pain, nausea, and vomiting to serious symptoms of bowel vasculitis like intestinal hemorrhage, ischemia, necrosis, intussusception, and bowel perforation. Vasculitis of the bowel wall causes edema and submucosal and intramural hemorrhage and this can occasionally lead to intussusception usually confined to small bowel. Intestinal bleeding presenting as gross or occult blood per rectum can occur in 30% of cases. Intussusception and massive intestinal hemorrhage are seen in less than 5% of children. Other rare manifestations are acute pancreatitis, hepatobiliary disease, ulcerative colitis, protein losing enteropathy, steatorrhea, etc.

Renal

Renal involvement is seen in 20–60% of children with HSP and usually manifests within a few days to a few weeks after the first clinical presentation but can occur 2 months or more from presentation but 97% of children will develop renal disease within 6 months. The most common presentation is microscopic hematuria with or without proteinuria. Renal involvement can be microscopic or macroscopic hematuria, proteinuria alone or associated with hematuria, acute nephritis, nephrotic syndrome or a mixed picture or even renal failure acute

or chronic. Renal disease may become serious in 10% of cases and is more prevalent in older children and adults.

Increased risk of nephritis is seen in the following situations:

- Age of onset >7 years
- Persistent purpuric rash
- Severe abdominal symptoms
- Decreased factor VIII.

Though renal involvement is typically early, end-stage disease may not be obvious for a number of years.

Other less common clinical features are:

- Central nervous system vasculitis
- Guillain–Barré syndrome
- Ocular involvement
- Orchitis
- Pulmonary hemorrhage, etc.

Scrotal pain and swelling can occur in 13% of boys and then torsion testis has to be ruled out.

Recurrence of symptoms can occur in around 30% of children and is more common in children with renal disease.

Investigations

Henoch–Schönlein purpura by and large is a diagnosis of exclusion. No specific diagnostic laboratory tests are available for confirming the diagnosis. Complete blood counts may be totally normal or there may be leukocytosis with shift to left and a mild increase in acute phase reactants. Normal or increased platelets help to rule out idiopathic thrombocytopenic purpura. Normochromic anemia is seen if there is gastrointestinal blood loss which can be confirmed by a positive stool guaiac test. Microscopic examination of urine to look for hematuria and estimating urinary protein are important investigations done to look for renal involvement. If there is renal involvement, blood urea, serum creatinine, and serum electrolytes may be deranged. Although levels of C1q, C3, and C4 are usually normal, low levels of total hemolytic complement and decreased levels of properdin and factor B are seen in 50% of affected children during the acute illness due to activation of the alternate complement pathway. Serum IgA and IgM concentrations are increased in half of the patients during the active phase of the disease ANCAs are typically absent. Antinuclear antibody and rheumatoid factor are usually absent. Antistreptolysin (ASO) may be elevated.

Imaging studies of abdomen are usually done in patients with significant gastrointestinal symptoms and imaging of other areas is done depending on the clinical presentation. Plain radiographs of the abdomen may demonstrate dilated loops of intestine denoting decreased intestinal motility. Ultrasound abdomen can demonstrate specific abnormalities like increased bowel wall thickness, fluid in the peritoneal cavity, hematomas, and intussusception. Ultrasonography is extremely useful in detecting intussusception. Ultrasound and color Doppler examination of the scrotum is indicated in scrotal pain and swelling to rule out torsion testis which is a known complication of HSP.

Tissue biopsy is not needed to diagnose HSP in most of the cases as the diagnosis is purely clinical. Skin biopsy is indicated in children with atypical skin findings and it shows leukocytoclastic vasculitis in postcapillary venules and dermal capillaries with perivascular accumulation of neutrophils and mononuclear cells. Immunofluorescence studies show IgA, complement component 3 (C3) and fibrin deposition in the walls of involved vessels. The biopsy should be taken from a fresh lesion as far as possible (within 24 hours of onset). Also IgA deposition may be absent if biopsy is taken from the center of the lesion as the presence of proteolytic enzymes can result in negative staining.

The indications of renal biopsy in children with HSP are:

- Nephritis or nephrotic presentation
- Raised creatinine, hypertension or oliguria
- Heavy proteinuria at 4 weeks
- Persistent proteinuria (not declining after 4 weeks)
- Impaired renal function.

The renal finding usually seen in HSP is a focal and segmental proliferative glomerulonephritis with IgA deposition. Severe and rapidly progressive cases can show glomerular necrotizing lesions and cellular crescents correlating with poor renal outcomes.

Treatment

Henoch–Schönlein purpura, mostly being a self-limiting disease, supportive treatment is advised which includes good hydration, nutrition and electrolyte balance, control of pain with simple analgesics like paracetamol and monitoring closely for development of abdominal and renal manifestations. Arthritis responds well to NSAIDs. Skin lesions do not require treatment except for severe cases which may require a short course of oral steroids. Severe gastrointestinal symptoms and orchitis need a short course of steroids. Steroids are indicated in severe abdominal pain, significant GI bleeding and intussusception which is the only condition in which surgery may be indicated. Initially, intravenous steroids and later oral steroids in

tapering doses may be given. Steroids are also indicated in neurological involvement, torsion testis, severe soft tissue or scrotal swelling, and pulmonary hemorrhage.

Recent studies suggest that steroids given prophylactically, do not prevent the onset of HSP nephritis but in those with severe renal involvement, early steroids could be helpful in treating the disease and thus altering the disease course. Children with mild renal disease like microscopic hematuria or mild proteinuria, watchful expectancy is what is needed. There is no need of any specific therapy. Children with more severe or persistent proteinuria or impaired renal function need to be seen by a nephrologist and renal biopsy is usually recommended. Steroids are needed for these patients, intravenous steroids to be given initially followed by oral. In more severe cases intravenous cyclophosphamide also may be required for control of symptoms. Other drugs like azathioprine or mycophenolate mofetil (MMF) may be considered as second line agents. In children with renal disease, nephrotic range proteinuria and crescents in more than 50% of glomeruli carry a uniformly poor prognosis.

Outcome

Henoch–Schönlein purpura is a benign and usually a self-limiting disease. The most important complications are gastrointestinal in the acute stage and renal in long-term. Prognosis is excellent in most children. Over all less than 5% of children progress to end-stage renal failure. Children with HSP should be followed up for development of renal manifestations for a minimum period of 6 months.

Infantile Acute Hemorrhagic Edema

This disorder in older children overlaps clinically with Henoch–Schönlein purpura syndrome affects infants between 4 months and 24 months of age (**Figs. 6A and B**). It usually begins acutely with fever, purpura, ecchymoses and inflammatory edema of the face, ears and limbs. It has a benign course and spontaneous remission is the rule, but attacks may recur. This disorder in older children overlaps with Henoch–Schönlein purpura. Histopathology shows leukocytoclastic vasculitis with occasional IgA deposits.

■ TAKAYASU ARTERITIS

Takayasu arteritis also known as "pulseless disease" is the only large vessel vasculitis which occurs in pediatric age group. Tricuspid atresia (TA) occurs throughout the world with the highest incidence in the East Asians. Pathological changes leading to "predominantly stenotic"

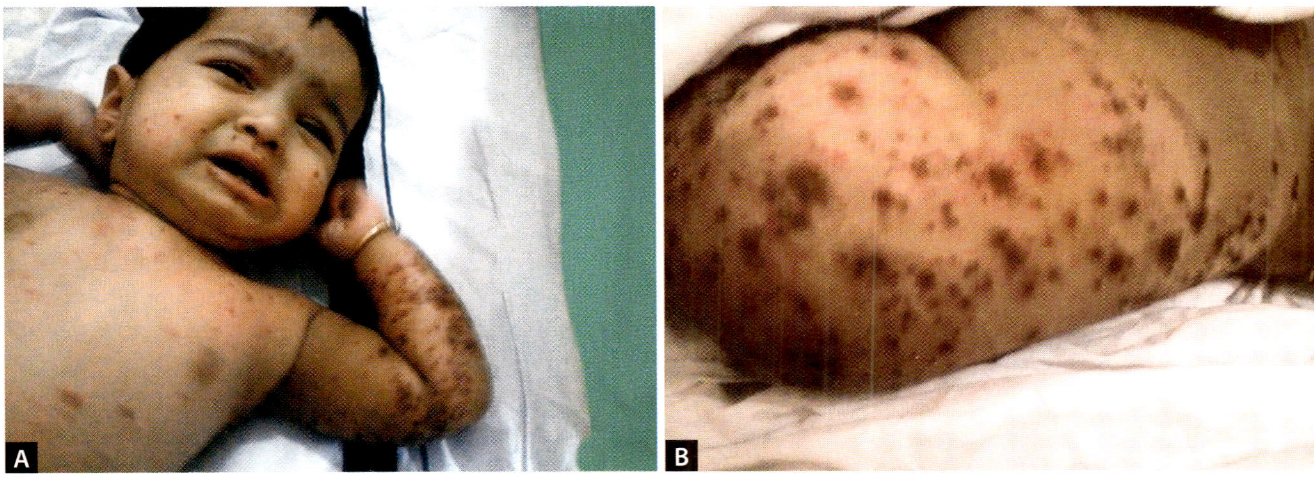

Figs. 6A and B: Infantile hemorrhagic edema.

or "predominantly aneurysmal" type with regional variation in occurrence, Asians have the predominant stenotic type. There are two types depending on the involvement of aorta, with predominant involvement of "supradiaphragmatic aorta and branches" or "middle aortic syndrome" where infradiaphragmatic aorta and its branches. Persistent chronic inflammation leads to blood vessel dilatation and aneurysm formation or intimal proliferation leading to scarring and progressive stenosis. Age of onset is between 10 years and 40 years but can occur in younger age group (20%), rare reports from infants also. Average age of onset is 13 years. Females are more commonly involved in all age groups, especially in adults.

Predilection of certain groups and occurrence in twins argue for a genetic basis for Takayasu arteritis. Pathological changes show more of lymphocytic inflammation in children compared to adults where granuloma formation is more common.

Clinical Features

Even though hypertension/or its sequelae is most common manifestations in all age groups overall clinical features differ from adult when it occurs in children. Early clinical manifestations are usually nonspecific. Most cases diagnosis is delayed as they present with vague complaints without symptoms or signs of vascular involvement.

Hypertension is the most frequent presentation (82%) followed by headache (31%), fever (29%), dyspnea (23), and weight loss (22%). Musculoskeletal symptoms are rare in all age groups, but it is more common when it occurs in children. Only after significant vessel wall injury, evidence of hypoperfusion becomes evident. These usually include low volume pulse, asymmetry in the blood pressure, claudication. Aortic valve damage may lead to regurgitation. Ocular manifestations are rare in children compared to adults. Takayasu was an ophthalmologist who reported retinal vascular changes in a Japanese girl.

Diagnosis

No specific laboratory diagnostic tests to confirm. ESR and CRP is elevated during activity. Autoantibodies including ANA, ANCA are done to rule out other autoimmune diseases.

Conventional catheter digital subtraction catheter arteriography is the most accepted method but it will not provide the pathological changes in the walls of the vessel. MRI, MRA, and CT angiography give details of vessel wall and are more helpful in monitoring the disease severity, but their sensitivity and specificity in children are not validated.

Treatment

Corticosteroids are the mainstay of treatment, but methotrexate, azathioprine, MMF, and cyclophosphamide are all used in children. Anti-tumor necrosis factor (anti-TNF) therapy and anti-interleukin-6 (anti-IL-6) were also tried rarely in children. Surgical intervention frequently indicated if the symptoms of stenosis of vessels in end-organ damage or severe symptoms. Outcomes of interventions are worse if they are done during activity of the disease.

Mortality is more common in children compared to adults suggesting more severe course when it occurs in children.

◼ POLYARTERITIS NODOSA

Polyarteritis nodosa is a form of primary systemic vasculitis characterized by necrotizing inflammatory changes with nodules along the walls of the medium and small muscular arteries, affecting multiple organ systems throughout the body. It was first described by Kussmaul and Maier in 1866. There is some overlap with smaller vessel disease but PAN is considered as a distinct entity. The disease spectrum varies from a relatively benign cutaneous form which may be self-limiting to a severe systemic variety that can be fatal.

Epidemiology

Polyarteritis nodosa is rare in the pediatric age group although it is considered to be the third most common systemic vasculitis seen in children. PAN in children seems to be worldwide in distribution with no sex predilection and majority present in midchildhood. Currently, there is lack of data regarding the epidemiology of childhood PAN (**Box 3**).

Etiopathogenesis

The immunopathogenesis causing vascular injury in PAN is unclear and probably heterogeneous. A number of infectious triggers like hepatitis B, parvovirus, cytomegalovirus, HIV, etc. and diseases like hematological malignancies have been reported to be associated. But such associations are rare in childhood PAN. There are reports of PAN in children linked to recent streptococcal infection and also immunization. There is some evidence suggesting the role of superantigens in the pathogenesis. There may be a genetic predisposition that makes an individual susceptible to PAN as evidenced by the occurrence in siblings and also the association of childhood PAN with

Box 3: The EULAR/PReS criteria for classifying polyarteritis nodosa (PAN).*
Essential: *Histologic evidence* of necrotizing vasculitis in medium- or small-sized artery or an angiographic abnormality showing aneurysm, stenosis, and occlusion. *Plus one of the following:* • Skin involvement • Myalgia or muscle tenderness • Hypertension • Peripheral neuropathy • Renal involvement

*(100% specific, 73% sensitive)
(EULAR: European League Against Rheumatism; PReS: Pediatric Rheumatology European Society)

mutations in the Familial Mediterranean gene (*MEFV* gene). Mutations in the *CERC1* gene encoding adenosine deaminase 2 have been recently reported in patients with symptoms suggestive of PAN.

Clinical Manifestations

The most common clinical features of this condition include fever, weight loss, malaise, and fatigue. There can also be myalgia, muscle tenderness, abdominal pain, arthralgia, and arthritis. Systemic involvement is variable but the skin, musculoskeletal system, kidneys, nervous system, and gastrointestinal tract are predominantly affected with cardiac and respiratory manifestations occurring less frequently.

The characteristic skin finding is livedo reticularis and occasionally, tender subcutaneous nodules overlying the affected arteries and also lesions resembling those of HSP are seen. The lesions can sometimes be necrotic and peripheral gangrene and skin infarction can occur.

Myalgias and arthralgias affecting large joints are seen.

Severe intestinal ischemia and associated abdominal pain and vomiting can be the presenting manifestation sometimes. Rarely, rupture of arterial aneurysms resulting in peritoneal bleeding and perirenal hematoma can occur. Widespread infarction can also occur in the affected viscera.

Neurologic involvement can affect both peripheral and central nervous system, the former being more common. Mononeuritis multiplex, polyneuropathy, focal deficits, hemiplegia, isolated cranial nerve palsy, encephalitis, visual loss, and rarely ischemic stroke, progressive encephalopathy and organic psychoses can occur.

Common renal manifestations are proteinuria and/or hematuria but sometimes anuric renal failure can occur. Renovascular involvement is also seen and can present as hypertensive emergency.

Laboratory Evaluation

There is usually anemia, leukocytosis, thrombocytosis, elevated ESR, and CRP showing systemic inflammation. Urinary abnormalities like proteinuria and hematuria may also be seen.

A high index of suspicion is usually needed for diagnosing PAN and the diagnosis is usually established by radiological investigations. Conventional angiography is the gold standard of diagnosis but recently magnetic resonance (MR) and especially computed tomography (CT) angiography have emerged as alternative noninvasive techniques to demonstrate vasculitis in PAN. Angiographic findings seen in PAN include aneurysms reflecting the necrotic vasculitis of renal, celiac, mesenteric, cranial or arteries in other parts of the body. Renal and mesenteric arteries are predominantly involved. There may also be microaneurysms, segmental narrowing, occlusion or beaded pattern of arteries. However, MRA may fail to demonstrate small or microaneurysms or may overestimate vascular stenotic lesions. Tc99m–dimercaptosuccinic acid (DMSA) scan of the kidneys demonstrating patchy areas of decreased isotope is an indirect evidence of medium vessel vasculitis of renal arteries.

The characteristic histopathologic lesions seen in PAN are fibrinoid necrotizing inflammation of the walls of medium or small arteries with marked inflammation of the vessel wall. However, if the biopsy specimen is not properly sampled, this finding may be absent. Immune deposition is not usually seen in immunofluorescence studies in PAN.

Treatment

The mainstay of treatment for remission of this disease is corticosteroids. For mild disease, oral steroids may be sufficient. For severe life-threatening or organ damaging disease, intravenous methylprednisolone in a dose of 20–30 mg/kg for 3–6 doses followed by oral steroids with subsequent tapering may be needed for 3–6 months. Additional cytotoxic agents such as cyclophosphamide to induce remission also will be needed in patients with severe systemic involvement. Intravenous cyclophosphamide is better than oral in view of low cumulative dose and similar efficacy.

Once remission is achieved, maintenance therapy with daily or alternate day prednisolone in a low dose and oral azathioprine are commonly used for an additional 12–18 months. Low dose aspirin is used as an antiplatelet agent by some methotrexate, cyclosporine, and MMF are also used for this condition by many physicians. Sometimes, plasma exchange may be needed in severe cases. IVIG has also been found to be useful in refractory cases.

Recently, biological agents such as infliximab (TNF inhibition) or rituximab (anti-CD20 blockade) have been successfully used in severe life-threatening or organ damaging disease not responding to steroids and other medications. Penicillin prophylaxis may be effective when streptococcal infection is implicated. Allogeneic hematopoietic stem cell transplantation has been found to be successful in a few patients and in the future gene therapy may be an option.

Outcome

Polyarteritis nodosa is usually a monophasic disease in children and relapses are much less common when compared to adults. However, life-threatening complications can occur if treatment is delayed or inadequate. Mortality has considerably reduced now when compared to pre-steroid era. But long-term follow-up of these children is necessary as late morbidity can occur due to chronic vascular injury leading to diffuse endothelial dysfunction and premature atherosclerosis.

Cutaneous Polyarteritis Nodosa

Cutaneous polyarteritis nodosa (cPAN) a form of vasculitis affecting small- and medium-sized vessels. It is characterized by the presence of fever, subcutaneous nodules, and painful nonpurpuric lesions with or without livedo reticularis occurring predominantly in the lower extremities and with no systemic involvement except for myalgia, arthralgia, and nonerosive arthritis. The condition is often associated with a preceding streptococcal infection. The age of onset is early, commonly in the first decade and the incidence of peripheral gangrene is seen to be more in Indian children **(Figs. 7 and 8)**.

The acute phase reactants are not as elevated as seen in systemic PAN. The skin lesions and histopathology are same in both cPAN and systemic PAN. Rarely this can evolve into full blown PAN. There may be periodic exacerbations and remissions and this may persist for a long time.

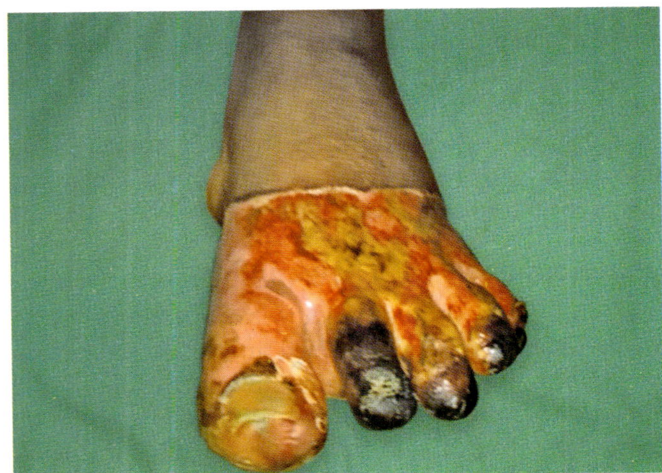

Fig. 7: A child with partially treated polyarteritis nodosa.

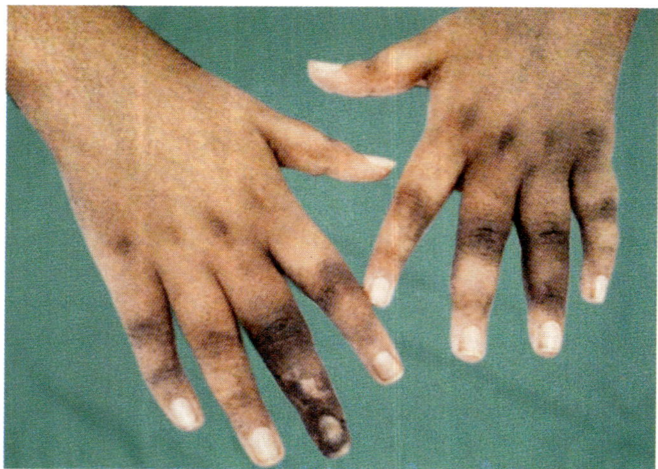

Fig. 8: Child with polyarteritis nodosa.

ANTINEUTROPHILIC CYTOPLASMIC ANTIBODY-ASSOCIATED VASCULITIS

Antineutrophilic cytoplasmic antibody-associated vasculitis (AAV) is a group of vasculitis characterized by small to medium sized blood vessel inflammation and the presence of ANCAs. The recent identification of ANCA has resulted in classifying small vessel vasculitis as immune complex small vessel vasculitis and ANCA-AAV. AAV include granulomatosis with polyangiitis (GPA) previously known as Wegner's granulomatosis, eosinophilic granulomatosis with polyangiitis (EPGA) previously known as Churg–Strauss syndrome, and microscopic polyangiitis (MPA).

Antineutrophilic cytoplasmic antibodies are detected by immunofluorescence microscopy and can be divided into predominantly cytoplasmic ANCA (c-ANCA), perinuclear ANCA (p-ANCA), indeterminate or atypical pattern. The target antigen of c-ANCA is PR3, a serine protease and the predominant target antigen of p-ANCA is myeloperoxidase (MPO) and antibodies to these target organs are called PR3 ANCA and MPO–ANCA, respectively.

Although AAV are rare in children, they can be associated with significant morbidity and mortality, especially if the diagnosis is delayed.

Granulomatosis with Polyangiitis

Granulomatosis with polyangiitis is a chronic vasculitis involving small to medium sized arteries characterized by granulomatous necrotizing inflammation of the upper and lower respiratory tracts, pauci-immune glomerulonephritis, and frequently vasculitis involving other organs.

The pediatric specific EULAR/PRINTO/PReS criteria for classification of GPA:
At least three out of six of the following:

1. Upper airway involvement
2. Pulmonary involvement
3. Subglottic, tracheal or bronchial stenosis
4. Renal involvement
5. Histopathology showing granulomatous inflammation
6. Antineutrophil cytoplasmic antibody positivity.

The cause of GPA is essentially unknown and it is likely to be multifactorial. It is probably the result of interactions between genetic factors and triggering environmental exposures.

Clinical Features

The most common clinical features are fatigue, weight loss, and fever followed by pulmonary, renal, and ear, nose, and throat (ENT) manifestations. The common pulmonary manifestations are shortness of breath, cough, hemoptysis or alveolar hemorrhage. There can also be nasal and sinus mucosal inflammation causing sinusitis, persistent otitis media, persistent rhinorrhea, purulent or bloody nasal discharge, epistaxis and oral or nasal ulcers.

Subglottic stenosis is a specific manifestation of GPA seen quite frequently and is included in the new classification criteria for GPA. In long standing disease, there can be cartilage ischemia with nasal cartilage perforation leading to saddle nose deformity. Renal involvement can be abnormal urine analysis and progressive renal failure. Other organs like skin, gastrointestinal tract, nervous system, and eyes can also be involved.

Diagnosis

The diagnosis of GPA can be made by the characteristic clinical features, the presence of serological markers specifically ANCA most commonly PR3–ANCA or c-ANCA, and the characteristic histopathologic findings. The pulmonary radiographic abnormalities seen in GPA are nodules, fixed infiltrates, cavities, and sometimes ground-glass appearance.

Treatment

Combined use of corticosteroids and cyclophosphamide for induction of remission has considerably improved the outcome of childhood GPA. Mortality has also been considerably reduced. Both oral and pulsed intravenous cyclophosphamide have been used with success. Rituximab is also an effective alternative for the initial treatment of GPA. The drugs that are commonly used for maintenance include azathioprine, methotrexate, and leflunomide.

Prognosis has improved considerably in recent years due to early diagnosis and aggressive immunosuppressive therapy.

Microscopic Polyangiitis

Microscopic polyangiitis is described as a small vessel vasculitis in both adults and children. It is defined as a necrotizing vasculitis with few or no immune deposits predominantly affecting small vessels. Necrotizing glomerulonephritis and pulmonary capillaritis are common and granulomatous inflammation is absent. Clinically, kidneys, lungs, skin, joints, and gastrointestinal tract can get involved. Mononeuritis multiplex, glomerulonephritis, pulmonary hemorrhage, and fever are important manifestations. The presence of p-ANCA in 75% of patients with MPA is useful in diagnosing this condition. The disease is rare in children.

Eosinophilic Granulomatosis with Polyangiitis

Eosinophilic granulomatosis with polyangiitis (EGPA), previously known as Churg–Strauss syndrome or allergic granulomatosis and angiitis is a rare necrotizing vasculitis involving predominantly small vessels. There are no pediatric classification criteria for EGPA. Clinically, EGPA is characterized by severe asthma or allergic rhinitis, skin disease, and vasculitis that commonly involves the cardiovascular system, kidneys, nervous system, and gastrointestinal tract. p-ANCA or MPO-ANCA is associated in high frequency in this condition. There can be presence of extravascular granulomas and eosinophilic infiltrates.

Behçet's Disease

Behçet's disease is a multisystem disease of unknown etiology described by the Turkish dermatologist Hulusi Behçet in 1937. The clinical triad of this disease is aphthous stomatitis, genital ulcerations, and uveitis. It is now classified under the category of variable vessel vasculitis as it can involve vessels of any size and can involve both arteries and veins.

Criteria of the International Study Group for the Diagnosis of Behçet's Disease

Recurrent oral ulcerations: Plus two of the following:

- Recurrent genital ulcers
- Eye lesions
- Skin lesions
- Pathergy.

There is no specific laboratory test that can diagnose Behçet's disease. Acute phase reactants may be increased in active disease. Direct angiography or magnetic resonance angiography can delineate the extent and character of the vascular lesions.

Corticosteroids, azathioprine, cyclosporine, thalidomide, cyclophosphamide, and anti-TNF drugs have been successfully used in managing Behçet's disease depending on the organ involved.

Noncommunicable Endocrinological Diseases in the Tropics

Pinky Meena, Piyush Gupta

■ INTRODUCTION

Endocrinological disorders pose significant burden in the developing world of tropics. Rapid urbanization and lifestyle changes are associated with disease burden similar to developed world while they still cope with the other spectrum of malnourishment. Spectrum is wide including pituitary dysfunction, growth hormone deficiencies (GHDs), hypo/hyperthyroidism, diabetes mellitus, puberty disorders, obesity, and adrenal dysfunctions. In this chapter, we will be dealing with hypopituitarism, hypothyroidism, and diabetes mellitus.

■ HYPOPITUITARISM

The prevalence of pituitary diseases in pediatric population in the tropical countries is lacking. An Indian study in adult population estimated 4% of the Indian population is affected by it.[1] It is estimated to affect 1 in 4,000 to 1 in 10,000 live births worldwide. The incidence increases with age.[2]

Etiology

In children, hypopituitarism can be congenital or acquired. There is a significant difference in the etiology of the disease in the west and tropical countries; however, most data in the tropics comes from adult studies. Tropical countries have higher burden from pituitary adenoma, infection, abscess, and pituitary hemorrhage due to snake bite, HIV infection, road traffic accidents, and iron overload states such as thalassemia.[3] Most cases are due to tubercular bacterial meningitis (TBM) causing pituitary involvement, especially in children.[4] Pituitary insufficiency have been reported after bacterial, viral, and fungal meningitis too.[5] Craniopharyngioma is the most common tumor associated with multiple pituitary deficiencies in children which usually manifest with GHD. Septo-optic dysplasia (SOD) is the most common congenital cause of hypopituitarism, with an incidence as high as 1 in 10,000. **Table 1** enumerates causes of neonatal hypopituitarism. **Box 1** enumerates cause of hypopituitarism in general.

Clinical Features

Neonates

All newborns with midline defects and micropenis should be evaluated for hypopituitarism. Assessment for other associated features such as optic nerve hypoplasia should be done. Suspicion should be strong in cases of refractory hypoglycemia, prolonged jaundice [indirect hyperbilirubinemia in TSH axis deficiency, or direct hyperbilirubinemia as in growth hormone (GH) or adrenocorticotropic hormone (ACTH) axis deficiencies]. The clinical manifestations vary from isolated growth hormone deficiency (IGHD) to multiple pituitary hormone deficiency (MPHD) causing thyroid hormone deficiency, diabetes insipidus, hyperprolactinemia, and secondary gonadal dysfunction.[6] IGHD presents with normal looking child at birth later lacking in growth rapidly during infancy, or with hypoglycemia in children. MPHD presents with various spectra of hormonal deficiency. Early transcription

Table 1: Causes of neonatal hypopituitarism.	
Time of onset	*Causes*
Congenital causes	Maternal hyperglycemia, congenital infections (syphilis, toxoplasmosis), hypothalamus–pituitary development defects, midline defects, cleft lip/palate, and genetic mutations
Perinatal–neonatal causes	Birth trauma-asphyxia (pituitary stalk junction), neonatal sepsis, and hemochromatosis (transient)

Box 1: Causes of hypopituitarism.

Primary hypopituitarism:
- Neoplasms leading to pituitary destruction
  - Intrasellar tumors (adenomas, craniopharyngiomas)
  - Parasellar tumors (meningiomas, optic nerve gliomas)
  - Metastatic tumors (breast, lung, melanoma, renal cell carcinoma)
- Ischemic necrosis of the pituitary
  - Postpartum (Sheehan's syndrome)
  - Diabetes mellitus
  - Other systemic disorders (sickle cell disease and traits, temporal arteritis, eclampsia, atherosclerotic disease, hemorrhagic fever with renal syndrome)
- Pituitary apoplexy (nearly always secondary to a pituitary tumor)
- Cavernous sinus thrombosis
- Aneurysms of intracranial internal carotid artery
- Infectious disease (tuberculous meningitis, fungal disease, malaria, HIV)
- Infiltrative disease (hemochromatosis, secondary amyloidosis)
- Immunological or inflammatory (lymphocytic or granulomatous hypophysitis, sarcoidosis)
- Primary empty sella syndrome
- Iatrogenic
  - Nasopharyngeal, pituitary, or brain irradiation
  - Surgical destruction
- Genetic (PIT-1, GH, β-LH, GHRH-R mutations or deletions)
- "Idiopathic" (GH, ACTH, TSH, others): Frequently monohormonal

Secondary hypopituitarism:
- Pituitary stalk, hypothalamus, or other central nervous system diseases
- Tumors (craniopharyngioma, germ cell tumor, metastasis, lymphoma, leukemia)
- Infiltrative (hemochromatosis, lipid storage disease)
- Traumatic brain injury
- Hormone-induced (glucocorticoids, gonadal steroids)
- Iatrogenic (surgical, irradiation)
- Infectious (HIV, tuberculosis)
- Nutritional (starvation, obesity)
- Anorexia nervosa
- Severe systemic illness (interleukin mediated)
- Psychoneuroendocrine (psychosocial dwarfism, stress-associated amenorrhea)
- Genetic (vasopressin-neurophysin gene, *KAL1* gene).

Table 2: Common signs and symptoms associated with hormone deficiencies.

Hormone deficiency	Signs and symptoms
Growth hormone	• Linear growth failure, increased adiposity, decreased muscle mass, fatigue • *If congenital*: Neonatal hypoglycemia, micropenis
Corticotropin	Nausea, vomiting, weight loss, prolonged duration of common illnesses, hypotension, fatigue
Thyrotropin	• Fatigue, dry hair, dry skin, linear growth failure, constipation, weight gain despite decreased intake, bradycardia • *If congenital and untreated*: Development delays, intellectual disability
Prolactin	Inability to lactate after pregnancy
Luteinizing hormone/follicle-stimulating hormone	• Delayed or absent pubertal development with lack of pubertal growth spurt, secondary amenorrhea, decreased libido, osteoporosis • *If congenital*: Micropenis, undescended testicles
Antidiuretic hormone	Polyuria, polydipsia, nocturia, dehydration, hypernatremia

Investigations

A brain magnetic resonance imaging (MRI) is the preferred imaging study for visualizing hypothalamic pituitary anatomy; it can also detect the midline malformations, absent corpus callosum, suprasellar associated.[7,8] GHD can be confirmed using GH levels, insulin-like growth factor-I (IGF-I), and insulin-like growth factor binding protein 3 (IGFBP-3) matched with normal levels for bone age. Corticotropin challenge test, ACTH stimulation test, and cortisol levels detect ACTH deficiency.[9]

Treatment

The principle of treatment is replacement of the deficient hormones. Recombinant human GH is used to treat growth failure and metabolic abnormalities related to GHD. Replacement doses range from 0.16 to 0.25 mg/kg per week. Growth velocity and IGF1 levels guide the GH therapy, which is continued until the desired height is achieved or if the growth velocity is <1 inch/year or till attainment of skeletal age >14 years in girls and >16 years in boys. Thyroid and adrenal hormones if deficient are supplemented before GH. Hydrocortisone and fludrocortisone are used to treat adrenal insufficiency resulting from ACTH deficiency or primary disorders of the adrenal gland. The maintenance replacement hydrocortisone dose is 7–9 mg/m^2 per day. In gonadotropin deficiency, replacement (estrogen or testosterone) is started when bone age reaches the age

factor gene mutations (*LHX3, LHX4, HESX1, SOX3,* and *PITX2*) are associated with anomalies in other organ systems. Mutation of genes expressed in late stages cause isolated pituitary involvement (*PIT1/POU1F1, PROP1*).

Older Infants and Children

Growth failure is the most common presentation in this age group; however, hypoglycemia can also be the presenting symptom in few cases. Disorders of pubertal development and diabetes insipidus are also common. In adolescents, acquired hypopituitarism may present with subtle fatigability symptoms which are often neglected. **Table 2** depicts various symptoms associated with hormone deficiency.

of puberty for the patient's sex (i.e. age 10 years for girls, age 11–12 years for boys). Vasopressin or desmopressin (DDAVP) may be required to treat diabetes insipidus.

■ HYPOTHYROIDISM

Hypothyroidism is among the most common endocrine diseases. It is one of the leading causes of preventable intellectual deficiency. Prevalence of congenital hypothyroidism (CH) in India is 1 in 2,640 neonates as compared to world average of 1 in 3,800.[10] Early diagnosis and treatment are pertinent to prevent neurodevelopmental impairment.

Acquired hypothyroidism is more common in older children, which is mainly due to autoimmune destruction (Hashimoto's thyroiditis). In India, the prevalence of hypothyroidism and subclinical hypothyroidism in adults are 3.9% and 9.4%, respectively.[11] Autoimmune thyroiditis is more common in girls, as high as 7.5% in India. It has emerged to be a common cause in areas of iodine sufficiency.[12]

Congenital Hypothyroidism[13]

Etiology

Thyroid dysgenesis is the most common cause of CH (85%). It is sporadic in most cases, but is occasionally familial due to mutation/deletion of gene) involved in fetal thyroid formation (*TSHR, PAX8, NKX2-1, FOXE1,* and *NKX2-5*). Thyroid tissue can be absent (agenesis), hypoplastic, or ectopic in site. Although low serum T4 level with high serum TSH level is present in all cases, the absence of serum thyroglobulin (Tg) differentiates thyroid agenesis from ectopic/hypoplastic thyroid. Ultrasound and radioscintigraphy aid in confirming the diagnosis of all three types.

Familial thyroid dyshormonogenesis: Patients have defect in hormone synthesis and release pathway. The following eight inborn errors have been identified: (1) TSH resistance [deactivating mutations of the thyroid receptor and cAMP (cyclic adenosine monophosphate) signal transduction pathway], (2) iodide trapping defect (Na-I symporter mutations), (3) iodide oxidation defects (thyroid peroxidase deficiency), (4) defective coupling of iodotyrosines, (5) deiodination defects, (6) defective thyroglobulin synthesis, (7) defective proteolysis of thyroglobulin, and (8) release of T3 and T4 into the circulation.

Other causes: Resistance to thyroid hormones in peripheral tissues, multiple pituitary hormone deficiency,

transplacental passage of maternal TSH-binding inhibitory antibodies, maternal radioiodine, and antithyroid drug exposure (propylthiouracil/methimazole).

Endemic goiter: Endemic goiter results from nutritional iodine deficiency. The Indian subcontinent has a high prevalence of endemic cretinism due to iodine deficiency. Iodine deficiency disorders (IDDs) are not limited to the Himalayan and Tarai region but are reported from all over the country. In national survey of districts, 263 of 325 districts were endemic for IDD making the prevalence of IDD > 10%.[14]

Clinical Features

At birth, hypothyroid neonates are asymptomatic due to effect of transplacental passage of T4, which fulfils about 30% of fetal T4 requirement. Thus, biochemical screening is pertinent for early diagnosis in most cases. Thus, CH has near-normal fetal growth and manifests in early infantile age. However, few cases can present with goiter at birth, especially those with maternal goitrogen exposure. It can present with delayed passage of meconium, constipation, prolonged neonatal jaundice, hypothermia, poor feeding, lethargy, hoarse cry, and hypotonia. On examination, neonates have coarse facies, myxedema of the eyelids, hands, and/or scrotum, wide open fontanelles, large protruding tongue, goiter, umbilical hernia, delayed relaxation of deep tendon reflexes, and mild pericardial effusion. Untreated CH in early infancy results in profound developmental delay, and impaired cognitive development (cretinism).[15]

Endemic cretinism: IDD has wide spectrum of presentation. It is the single largest cause of preventable intellectual disability worldwide. Antenatal iodine deficiency leads to abortions, stillbirths, congenital anomalies, increased perinatal mortality, and endemic cretinism. In childhood and adolescence, impaired learning and psychosocial functions, short stature, and goiter are some of the clinical features. Objective assessment reflected mean IQ loss of 13.5 points in children.[16] **Table 3** demonstrates the two types of presentation of endemic cretinism.

Acquired Hypothyroidism

Chronic lymphocytic thyroiditis (CLT)/autoimmune thyroiditis is the most common cause of acquired hypothyroidism and goiter in children living in iodine-sufficient areas. It has female preponderance (M:F ratio 2:1 in adolescence and 4:1 in childhood). CLT is associated with other autoimmune disorders, trisomy 21 syndrome, Turner syndrome, and Klinefelter syndrome. In children,

Table 3: Comparative clinical features in neurological and hypothyroid cretinism.[1]

Features	Neurological cretin	Hypothyroid cretin
Mental retardation	Present, often severe	Present, less severe
Deaf mutism	Usually present	Absent
Cerebral diplegia	Often present	Absent
Stature	Usually normal	Severe growth Retardation usual
General feature	No physical signs of hypothyroidism	Coarse dry skin Husky voice
Reflexes	Excessively brisk	Delayed relaxation
ECG X-ray limbs	Normal Normal	Small voltage QRS Complexes and other abnormalities of hypothyroidism Epiphyseal dysgenesis
X-ray limbs	Normal	Epiphyseal dysgenesis
Effect of thyroid hormones	No effect	Improvement

autoantibodies [antithyroglobulin antibody, antithyroid peroxidase antibody (TPO)] are detected in the serum in 95% cases.

Subacute thyroiditis due to viral illness, although rare in children, presents with painful goiter; initially it has thyrotoxic phase, followed by a euthyroid phase, and then a hypothyroid phase. Amiodarone, thioamides, lithium, and excess dietary iodine can cause hypothyroidism. Surgical removal/irradiation of thyroid can be other causes.

Clinical Features

Acquired hypothyroidism is typically insidious in onset usually with asymptomatic or symptomatic goiter, decrement of growth velocity, delayed bone age, and mild weight gain even with complaints of reduced diet, dull facial expression, lethargy, decreased energy, dry skin, puffiness, sleep disturbance, cold intolerance, and constipation, slowed metabolism, and impaired memory. Transient toxic thyroiditis can be the initial presentation in about 5–10% CLT cases preceding hypothyroidism. Hyperthyroidism present with heat intolerance, weight loss, tremors, and sexual pseudoprecocity, galactorrhea, and short stature.

Laboratory Studies

In primary hypothyroidism, serum thyrotropin (TSH) concentration increases due to low T4 levels. In patients with secondary or tertiary hypothyroidism, serum free T4 measurement by equilibrium dialysis is the gold standard.

The concentration of serum TSH is low. Serum antithyroid antibody test (anti TPO and Tg) are required to establish a diagnosis of CLT.

Newborn screening for CH, a combination of T4 and TSH, yields the best outcome. In infants, if the serum total T4 is less than 85 nmol/L (<7 µg/dL), with TSH more than 40 mIU/L, CH is likely. If total T4 is low, and serum TSH is not elevated, TBG deficiency, central hypothyroidism, or euthyroid sick syndrome should be considered.

Imaging Studies

Ultrasound is required to locate thyroid gland when suspecting agenesis. Thyroid scan with iodine-123 or technetium-99m, which concentrates in the thyroid gland, is useful to detect the absence or ectopic location of thyroid tissue. It is also helpful in differentiating hot and cold goiter and organification defects. X-ray helps in bone age calculation.

Treatment

Treatment of CH should be initiated as early as possible. In CH, treatment should be initiated as soon as the diagnosis is suggested preferably before 2 weeks of life. The outcome of cognitive development is directly related to time of initiation of hormone replacement. The recommended starting dose of levothyroxine for CH is 10–15 µg/kg/day. Newborns with elevated TSH should be treated empirically with thyroid hormone replacement until they are aged 2 years. When on thyroid hormone replacement therapy, serum TSH and T4 levels are followed to adjust the dose of levothyroxine, initially monthly until normalization of T4 levels, then 3 monthly till 3 years age, and further 6 monthly.

Children with CLT may require lifelong levothyroxine, as few as 20% show complete remission. The dose of levothyroxine at initiation is lower than in CH and titrated further as per serum TSH concentration. Trial of stopping hormone therapy should only be attempted once puberty and desired height is achieved.

In the case of hypopituitarism with concomitant thyroid and corticotropin/adrenal insufficiency, glucocorticoid should be replaced before thyroid hormone replacement to avoid risk of adrenal crisis due to increased demand from enhanced metabolism.

The management of IDD is dependent on primary prevention by ensuring adequate iodine intake and is implemented through food fortification with iodine (bread, milk, water, and salt). India adopted World Health Assembly-endorsed Universal Salt Iodization (USI) in 1990, post which significant legislative, manufacturing, and educational measures were taken to ensure the same. The WHO (World Health Organization) recommends to add 20–40 mg of iodine per kg of salt in order to meet iodine requirements assuming that the average consumption of salt per capita is 10 g per day. Household level iodized salt coverage in India is 91% with 71% households consuming adequately iodized salt.[17] The WHO recommends regular assessment of iodine status in the population. The two most common markers used for this purpose are *urinary iodine concentration* which indicates recent dietary iodine intake and *goiter prevalence* which reflects past iodine status.[18]

DIABETES MELLITUS

Diabetes mellitus (DM) poses significant health concern in tropical region, where most of the countries are in developing phase facing the double burden of undernutrition and obesity. Due to lack of diabetes registry in most countries, the prevalence of DM in southeast region is derived from India. Although there is no national directory for diabetes in India, regional data from the country is available. Two from urban Chennai (prevalence of 0.26 cases per 1,000 person years),[19,20] one from Karnataka (0.3 per 100,000 person years in the under-25 year age-group),[21] and from Haryana (0.18 per 1,000 person years).[22]

The prevalence of T1DM (type 1 diabetes mellitus) in children is 111,500 according to a WHO report of the International Diabetes Federation for the southeast Asian region. Although T1DM is more prevalent in children and its incidence is increasing by 3% per year, T2DM (type 2 diabetes mellitus) is strikingly becoming more common in children and adolescence. The age of onset of T2DM is declining with obesity being major risk factor.[23] This alarming trend has already set foot in countries such as Japan where 80% of childhood diabetes is T2DM.[24]

Etiology

Type 1 diabetes mellitus is characterized by the destruction of insulin-producing pancreatic β-cells during the prodromal period which is mainly implicate to autoimmune mechanisms. Most common antibodies associated with T1DM include islet-cell antibodies, insulin autoantibodies, autoantibodies to glutamic acid decarboxylase (GAD), the tyrosine phosphatase-related insulinoma-associated 2 molecule, and the zinc transporter. Presence of two or more of these antibodies forecasts increased risk of development of T1DM over the next 5–10 years. However, environmental triggers have significant role in modifying disease occurrence

even in predisposed person. T2DM results from complex interaction of genetic and environmental factors.[25]

Diabetes mellitus has been linked to both chronic undernutrition[26] and obesity.[27] Although its relationship with chronic undernutrition is controversial, the WHO earlier gave classification category of malnutrition-modulated diabetes mellitus (MMDM). MMDM is subdivided into protein-deficient diabetes mellitus (PDDM) and fibrocalculus pancreatic diabetes (FCPD). FCPD manifests as pancreatic calculus and is common in tropical regions. PDDM exhibits ketosis-resistant hyperglycemia. MMDM presentation is similar to T1DM in a background of chronic malnutrition; young age at onset requires insulin therapy for glycemic control but also exhibits insulin resistance and has less propensity to develop ketosis on insulin withdrawal.[26]

Obesity is the single major type 2 diabetes risk. Alarmingly the incidence of T2DM associated with obesity is increasing even in the tropical countries.[27] Obesity also predisposes to metabolic condition "prediabetes," which predisposes to future development of diabetes and is characterized by impaired fasting glucose and/or glucose tolerance.[28]

Clinical Features

Both types of DM are characterized by hyperglycemia and glycosuria. Insulin-dependent diabetes mellitus (IDDM) or T1DM usually present with diabetic ketoacidosis. Patients with T2DM or non-insulin-dependent diabetes mellitus (NIDDM) characteristically have insulin resistance, and are associated with other metabolic syndrome, obesity, and hypertension. T2DM presents with classical symptoms of polyuria, polyphagia, and polydipsia. Long-term complications of micro-macrovascular, neuropathy, leg ulcer, renal failure, and retinopathy are common and warrant screening for same.

Investigations

To designate diagnosis of diabetes, one of the following criteria should be fulfilled: (1) Fasting plasma glucose (PG) (>126 mg/dL), (2) 2-hour PG after 75-g oral glucose tolerance test (OGTT) (>200 mg/dL), (3) random PG (>200 mg/dL) with classic signs and symptoms of hyperglycemia, or (4) hemoglobin A1C level > 6.5%.[28]

Management

Type 1 diabetes mellitus: Insulin by injection or chronic-infusion pumps along with dietary management. Novel implanted chambers containing insulin-secreting cells may release insulin in a more natural way.

Type 2 diabetes mellitus: Main therapy is oral hypoglycemics (metformin) along with lifestyle modification (nutrition and physical activity). Insulin therapy is indicated if the child is in diabetic ketoacidosis or if classification into type 1 or 2 is difficult, and in cases who despite of being on oral hypoglycemics cannot maintain blood sugar levels [RBG (random blood glucose) ≥ 250 mg/dL; or HbA1c is >9%]. Apart from blood glucose levels, HbA1c concentrations (3 monthly) should be done to adjust the dose and assess compliance. Physical activity involving moderate-to-vigorous exercise for at least 1 hour daily is recommended, along with limitation of screen time to less than 2 hours a day.[29]

CONCLUSION

Most countries of tropical region face double burden of communicable and noncommunicable disease. Noncommunicable endocrinological diseases' mortality and morbidity can be combated by early diagnosis and management. Neonatal screening mechanisms need to be implemented stringently. Lifestyle modifications warrants another scope of improvement.

REFERENCES

1. Kochupillai N. Clinical endocrinology in India. Curr Sci. 2000;79:1062-7.
2. Pierce M, Madison L. Evaluation and initial management of hypopituitarism. Pediatrics in Review. 2016;37:370.
3. Chatterjee P, Mukhopadhyay P, Pandit K, et al. Profile of hypopituitarism in a tertiary care hospital of eastern India–is quality of life different in patients with growth hormone deficiency? J Indian Med Assoc. 2008;106(6):384-5,388.
4. Dhanwal DK, Vyas A, Sharma A, et al. Hypothalamic pituitary abnormalities in tubercular meningitis at the time of diagnosis. Pituitary. 2010;13(4):304-10.
5. Dhanwal DK, Kumar S, Vyas A, et al. Hypothalamic pituitary dysfunction in acute nonmycobacterial infections of central nervous system. Indian J Endocrinol Metab. 2011;15(Suppl 3):S233-7.
6. Kurtoğlu S, Özdemir A, Hatipoğlu N. Neonatal hypopituitarism: diagnosis and treatment approaches. J Clin Res Pediatr Endocrinol. 2019;11(1):4-12.
7. Prabhakar VK, Shalet SM. Aetiology, diagnosis, and management of hypopituitarism in adult life. Postgrad Med J. 2006; 82 (966):259-66.
8. Argyropoulou MI, Kiortsis DN. MRI of the hypothalamic-pituitary axis in children. Pediatr Radiol. 2005;35(11):1045-55.
9. Rosenfeld RG. Disorders of growth hormone and insulin-like growth factor secretion and action. Pediatr Endocrinol. 1996:117-69.
10. Desai PM. Disorders of the thyroid gland in India. Indian J Pediatr.1997;64:11-20.
11. Usha Menon V, Sundaram KR, Unnikrishnan AG, et al. High prevalence of undetected thyroid disorders in an iodine sufficient adult south Indian population. J Indian Med Assoc. 2009;107(2):72-7.
12. Marwaha RK, Tandon N, Karak AK, et al. Hashimoto's thyroiditis: countrywide screening of goitrous healthy young girls in postiodization phase in India. J Clin Endocrinol Metab. 2000;85(10):3798-802.
13. Agrawal P, Philip R, Saran S, et al. Congenital hypothyroidism. Indian J Endocrinol Metab. 2015;19(2):221-7.
14. Ministry of Health and Family Welfare, Government of India. (2011). Annual Report to the people on Health, 2010-2011. [online]. Available from: https://mohfw.gov.in/sites/default/files/6960144509.pdf. [Last accessed on December, 2019].
15. Cheetham T. Congenital Hypothyroidism: Screening, Early Management, and Outcome. Encyclopedia of Endocrine Diseases. 2019:285-95.
16. Hetzel BS. The story of iodine deficiency, an international challenge in nutrition. New Delhi: Oxford University Press; 1989. pp. 36-51.
17. World Health Organization. (1996). Recommended iodine levels in salt and guidelines for monitoring their adequacy and effectiveness. [online] Available from: https://apps.who.int/iris/bitstream/handle/10665/63322/WHO_NUT_96.13.pdf?ua=1. [Last accessed on December, 2019].
18. World Health Organization, United Nations Children's Fund, International Council for the Control of Iodine Deficiency Disorders. Assessment of the Iodine Deficiency Disorders and monitoring their elimination. Geneva: WHO; 2001.
19. Ramachandran A, Snehalatha C, Abdul Khader OM, et al. Prevalence of childhood diabetes in an urban population in south India. Diabetes Res Clin Pract. 1992;17(3):227-31.
20. Ramachandran A, Snehalatha C, Krishnaswamy CV. Incidence of IDDM in children in urban population in southern India. Madras IDDM Registry Group Madras, South India. Diabetes Res Clin Pract. 1996;34(2):79-82.
21. Kumar P, Krishna P, Reddy SC, et al. Incidence of type 1 diabetes mellitus and associated complications among children and young adults: results from Karnataka Diabetes Registry 1995–2008. J Indian Med Assoc. 2008;106(11):708-11.
22. Kalra S, Kalra B, Sharma A. Prevalence of type 1 diabetes mellitus in Karnal district, Haryana state, India. Diabetol Metab Syndr. 2010;2:14.
23. Alberti G, Zimmet P, Shaw J, et al. Type 2 diabetes in the young: the evolving epidemic: the international diabetes federation consensus workshop. Diabetes Care. 2004;27:1798-1811.
24. Kitagawa T, Owada M, Urakami T, et al. Increased incidence of non-insulin dependent diabetes mellitus among Japanese schoolchildren correlates with an increased intake of animal protein and fat. Clin Pediatr (Phila). 1998;37:111-5.
25. Atkinson MA, Eisenbarth GS. Type 1 diabetes: new perspectives on disease pathogenesis and treatment. Lancet. 2001;358:221-9.
26. Samal KC, Kanungo A, Sanjeevi CB. Clinicoepidemiological and biochemical profile of malnutrition-modulated diabetes mellitus. Ann NY Acad Sci. 2002;958:131-7.
27. Hu FB. Globalization of diabetes: the role of diet, lifestyle, and genes. Diabetes Care. 2011;34:1249-57.
28. American Diabetes Association. Diagnosis and classification of diabetes mellitus. Diabetes Care. 2014;37(Suppl 1):S80-90.
29. Copeland KC, Silverstein J, Moore KR, et al. Management of newly diagnosed type 2 Diabetes Mellitus (T2DM) in children and adolescents. Pediatrics. 2013;131(2):364-82.

Tropical Neurological Disorders

Lokesh Saini, Shivan Kesavan

INTRODUCTION

Tropical neurological disorders have been on the rise in recent years even in the Western world, thanks to global warming and increased human migration practices. Also, there is resurgence in these disorders in endemic countries such as India due to population explosion, depleting water resources, sanitation facilities, and urbanization; however, most of the tropical neurological disorders belong to infectious category, the most common example being neurocysticercosis. Noninfectious neurological disorders are rare. Two common tropical disorders (noninfectious) which affect the child's nervous system are infantile tremor syndrome (ITS) and rheumatic chorea (RC), and this chapter deals with both conditions.

INFANTILE TREMOR SYNDROME

Infantile tremor syndrome is a clinical entity which has been described as a syndrome characterized by anemia, hyperpigmentation of skin, hair changes, delayed developmental milestones, and tremors. This clinical syndrome of infants and young children with neurological manifestations has been reported in Indian children since the beginning of the second half of 20th century. From India, the first description of this entity was given by Dikshit who described it as "nutritional dystrophy and anemia."[1] A few years later, Pohowalla and colleagues discussed the condition as "infantile meningoencephalitic syndrome."[2] Jadhav and associates later brought about a publication describing it as "Vitamin-B12 deficiency in Indian infants—a clinical syndrome."[3]

Infantile tremor syndrome generally occurs in infants between the age of 6 months and 2 years and is characterized by developmental delay and tremors which are associated with listlessness, apathy, hypotonia, and hypokinesia. Other accompaniments of the syndrome are anemia, skin hyperpigmentation, and hair changes suggestive of micronutrient deficiencies.

In India, it is predominantly described in children who are exclusively breastfed by mothers who are predominantly vegetarians. Literature from the Western world describes this condition in infants born to vegan mothers or those with a disorder of vitamin B12 malabsorption, most notably pernicious anemia. They are either developmentally delayed or have developed normally, but have lost all or some of the gained milestones. Tremor is the defining criteria to label as ITS. Those without tremors but with the other features of this disorder are said to be in the "pre-ITS" phase. Other neurologic manifestations include myoclonic jerks, choreiform movements, brisk reflexes, and tone abnormalities. The children often have a chubby look, apathy, and listlessness and may have fever, cough, diarrhea, hepatomegaly, or edema. They may also have signs of other multinutrient deficiencies including rickets and angular cheilitis.

In our population (Northern India and some pockets in South India), where majority of people consume vegetarian diet, most of the women in the childbearing age group are depleted of vitamin B12 reserves in their body. These mothers, when they breastfeed their children, put them at risk of vitamin B12 deficiency. Prolonged exclusive breastfeeding as opposed to introduction of complementary feeds at 6 months of age also prevents accretion of vitamin B12 through complementary foods. Studies have shown that duration of exclusive breastfeeding is usually longer in B12-deficient infants. Children with this condition have a general unacceptance of solid food which can be attributed to anorexia, oro-lingual dyskinesias, and hypotonia, which leads to continuation of breastfeeding

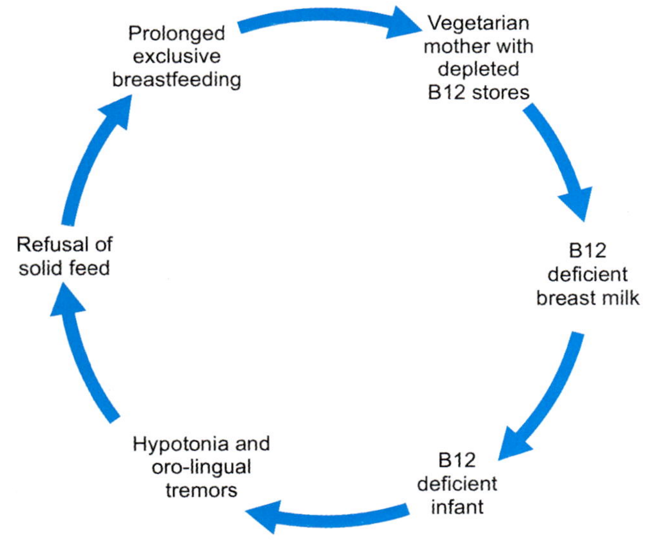

Fig. 1: Vicious cycle in the pathogenesis of the infantile tremor syndrome.

as the sole feeding modality, leading to a vicious cycle **(Fig. 1)**.

Jadhav et al. were the first to describe serum B12 deficiency as the putative cause in their six cases. Their cases showed remarkable improvement on daily oral administration of vitamin B12. They attributed the deficiency to B12 deficiency in mother, as the cause of the syndrome and also found low B12 levels in breast milk in addition to low maternal serum B12 levels. Five years later, Srikantia et al. reported similar results in their 30 infants whom they treated with vitamin B12 administration.[4] While this seems to be the case in most of the papers on this condition, other investigators have argued against a major role of vitamin B12, some even demonstrating normal B12 levels and no clinical response to B12 therapy. The definitive and singular role of vitamin B12 in this syndrome is yet to be proved, though isolated vitamin B12 deficiency appears to be causative of this syndrome. Despite the fact that more than five decades have passed since its first description, the optimal treatment regimen for this syndrome is not clear. The condition continues to plague children of our country and with possible long-term consequences on their intellect.

Etiology

A literature search regarding the possible etiologies for the "ITS" reveals a lack of consensus, and is therefore reflected in the variability of treatment regimens advocated. Of the postulated etiologic hypotheses, vitamin B12 deficiency seems to be most commonly incriminated cause.[5] Published literature from the past has mainly considered malnutrition, infection, and vitamin B12 deficiency as causative agents. The following factors have been discussed in the literature:

- *Infection*: Pohowalla et al. suggested that this condition may be a meningoencephalitic process of obscure origin. Some well-known epidemiologic features, e.g. seasonal incidence, association with fever, self-limiting course and abrupt onset, are favorable for this hypothesis. However, no conclusive evidence is forthcoming in this regard.
- *Protein–energy malnutrition*: Since there is some resemblance between ITS and nutritional recovery syndrome described by Kahn et al., malnutrition was postulated as an etiologic agent.[6] However, malnutrition and hypoproteinemia are not common features of ITS and vast majority of children have 75–100% of expected weight and tremors appear before the start of therapy in most patients, which clearly distinguishes ITS from "recovery syndrome."

Vitamin B12 Deficiency

Maternal vitamin B12 deficiency can be attributed to two main causes. First is due to the nutritional deficiency that can occur in exclusive vegetarians or if animal source food consumption is low. Maternal intake and absorption during pregnancy and lactation has a direct implication not only on her own health but also in preserving the neurological well-being of the child who is dependent on the mother for his/her nutrition in the early months of extrauterine life.

The other most important etiology of maternal vitamin B12 deficiency is malabsorption, which may be due to pernicious anemia, worm infestation, surgical resection of parts of the gut, recurrent gastrointestinal infections, or achlorhydria.

The least common group of disorders include those resulting in functional vitamin B12 deficiency in the child exemplified by inborn errors of cobalamin absorption and transport and cobalamin receptor defects.

Pregnant women who practice vegetarianism, including those who consume limited quantities of animal products, run a high risk of delivering an infant who may develop vitamin B12 deficiency, since breast milk has been shown to have low amounts of the vitamin. With prolonged breastfeeding, this deficiency state persists and leads to progressive neurological damage. Up to 50–60% of women in the childbearing age have been found to have subclinical vitamin B12 deficiencies, which might not become clinically significant in the mothers.[7] However, children born to these mothers have a high risk of poor neurodevelopmental outcome.

It has been estimated that approximately 25 µg of vitamin B12 is stored at birth in the body of an infant born to a vitamin B12 replete mother and about 0.1–0.4 µg per day of vitamin B12 is consumed in tissue synthesis by the baby. Healthy and vitamin B12 replete mothers, if they exclusively breastfeed their infants, need an average of 0.25 µg per day of the vitamin from breast milk to fulfill the infants' requirement during the first 6 months of life.[8]

People consuming a balanced vegetarian diet generally do not have nutritional deficits. Nevertheless, vitamin B12 deficiency has been seen in vegetarian people, particularly in impoverished locations, who consume very minimal food from animal source. Vitamin B12 is generally present in a very minimal amount in the available vegetarian food. Hence, food from animal sources such as milk, curd, meat, and fish have to be consumed in adequate amounts to have adequate vitamin B12 homeostasis. The public health implication of cobalamin insufficiency is not well acknowledged in spite of its high prevalence. Some recent studies have postulated that nearly one out of every three children have cobalamin deficiency with a wide range in severity.[9]

Peripheral blood films and marrows of patients with ITS have been studied; many studies showed a megaloblastic picture in blood and bone marrow. Keeping this in mind, vitamin B12 and folate estimation has also been done in a few studies. Quantitative measurements of vitamin B12 levels in the mother, in breast milk, and in infants have been done and have been found to be low to low-normal. Studies from the past which have refuted the causative role of vitamin B12 deficiency have relied of bone marrow megaloblastosis to define a vitamin B12 deficiency state. A comprehensive study was conducted by Garewal and Narang where they studied both vitamin B12 and folate levels in 23 children with ITS, 17 of them showed a vitamin B12 levels less than 100 pg/mL. Folate levels were also studied, out of the 23 children enrolled, 14 showed normal folate levels, and only 4 had a low folate levels in their blood.[10] In the context, it should be noted that serum vitamin B12 level is not a robust marker of cellular B12 deficiency status and requires other surrogate markers for a sensitive diagnosis (further detailed below in the investigations and differential diagnosis section) and neurological manifestations can occur in the complete absence of hematological manifestations of B12 deficiency.

Pathophysiology

Many theories have been laid down in an attempt to define the role of vitamin B12 in the neurodevelopment of children.

Defective Myelination or Demyelination

A prolonged deficiency of vitamin B12 causes impairment in myelination of the brain and spinal cord. Myelination of the brain is most dynamic in the first 6 months of life. Nerve cells are surrounded by myelin which protects the cell and facilitates communication. Hence, loss of myelin integrity alters the neuronal function. In addition, initial damage to the myelin sheath is followed by axonal degeneration. The two forms of vitamin B12, adenosylcobalamin and methylcobalamin, are cofactors in two enzymatic reactions which impact myelin formation. Adenosylcobalamin is the cofactor in the conversion of methylmalonyl CoA (coenzyme A) to succinyl CoA **(Fig. 2)**. A defect in this conversion results in an excess of the precursor propionyl CoA, which further leads to synthesis of odd-chain fatty acids. This leads to the integration of large amounts of abnormal C15 and C17 fatty acids into the nerve sheaths, which results in altered myelin which has reduced amounts of ethanolamine, sphingomyelin, and phospholipids.[11]

This is corroborated by neuroimaging abnormalities in children with ITS found in literature. Though these changes are nonspecific and have been reported to be seen in cases of malnutrition as well as any severe systemic illness. In a recent study, cranial neuroimaging of 10 cases of ITS was done. Most common findings noted were cerebral atrophy with ex-vacuo enlargement of ventricles and prominent subarachnoid spaces. Hyperintense signal in frontal and periventricular white matter on T2-weighted images in MRI scan may signify demyelination or edema. Three cases had thinning of corpus callosum, an association which had not been reported earlier; this provides support to the effect of B12 on myelin formation and maintenance, since the corpus callosum forms the major interhemispheric white matter tract rich in myelinated nerve fibers.[12]

ALTERATION IN SAM:SAH RATIO, HYPERHOMOCYSTINEMIA, AND ASSOCIATED NEUROTOXICITY

Homocysteine is converted to methionine using the enzyme methionine synthase. The reaction entails the transfer of a methyl group from 5-methyltetrahydro-folate to homocysteine hence forming tetrahydrofolate (THF) and methionine as a byproduct. In this reaction methylcobalamin acts as the cofactor. Methionine is converted to S-adenosylmethionine (SAM) and eventually to S-adenosylhomocysteine (SAH) upon donation of its methyl group. SAH is hydrolyzed to regenerate methionine. In vitamin B12 deficiency, there is a folate trap where

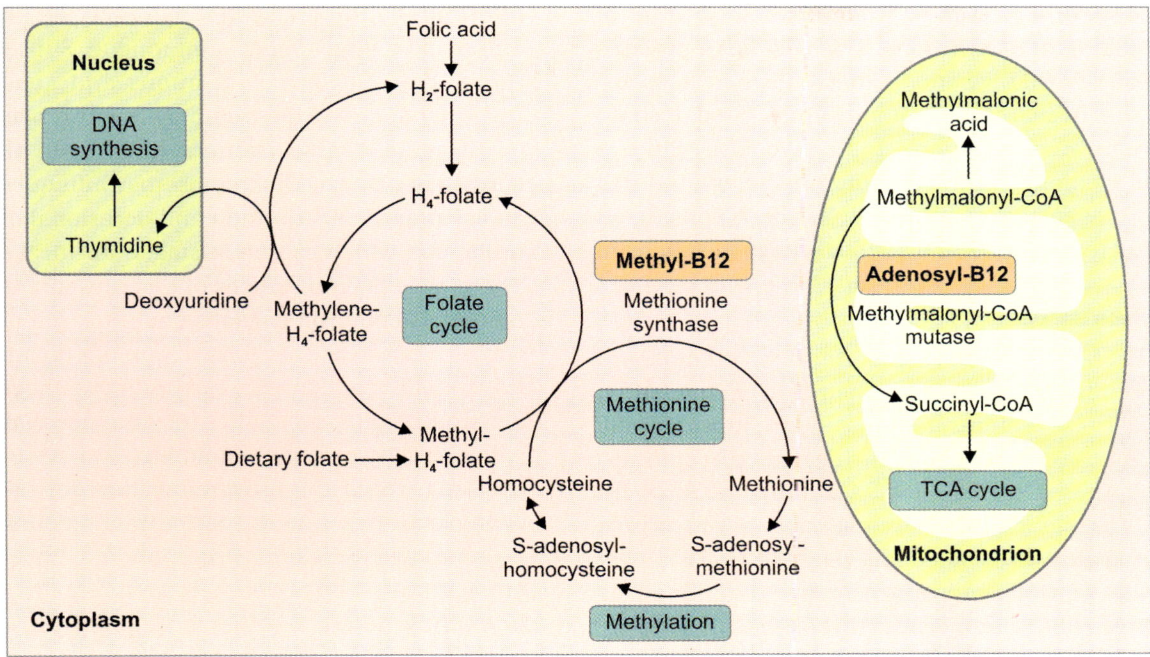

Fig. 2: The two biologically active forms of vitamin B12 (methylcobalamin and adenosylcobalamin) and their role in the two vital metabolic pathways is shown. The mechanism of elevation of homocysteine levels and methylmalonic acid levels resulting from metabolic block due to vitamin B12 deficiency is evident.
(DNA: deoxyribonucleic acid; TcA tricarboxylic acid; CoA: coenzyme A)
Source: Adapted from Green R, Allen LH, Bjørke-Monsen AL, et al. Vitamin B12 deficiency. Nat Rev Dis Primers. 2017;3:17040.

folate is ensnared as THF. Hence, SAH and homocysteine levels are elevated and SAM levels are depressed **(Fig. 2)**. This decreased SAM:SAH ratio messes up the methylation reactions which are essential for synthesis of lipids, proteins, and neurotransmitters in the central nervous system (CNS).

Hyperhomocysteinemia has been linked with many of the neurodegenerative diseases. There could also be a possible neurotoxic effect of homocysteine causing overstimulation of N-methyl-D-aspartate receptors. A decrease in the SAM:SAH ratio has been proposed to result in inhibition of DNA synthesis and cell division because the trapped folate cannot be recycled in the deficiency of cobalamin.

Tumor Necrosis Factor-α and Epidermal Growth Factor Imbalance

A novel theory has been put forward by Scalabrino regarding the pathophysiology of neurological damage associated with vitamin B12 deficiency. The CNS glial cells produce various growth factors and cytokines. Some cytokines such as tumor necrosis factor-α (TNF-α) serve as neurotoxins in CNS diseases, like the ones characterized by demyelination. Other cytokines such as epidermal growth

factor (EGF) are neurotrophic. These cytokines have been studied in the adult population with vitamin B12 deficiency presenting with subacute combined degeneration and it has been shown that the deficient individuals have higher serum concentrations of TNF-α and lower concentrations of EGF. It has also been shown that the imbalance can be rectified by vitamin B12 therapy.[13]

There is a study in which it has been postulated that SAM decreases the serum TNF-α in rats which had been stimulated with lipopolysaccharides and also lowers gene expression of TNF-α in lipopolysaccharide-treated murine macrophages. Till date no study has evaluated cytokine imbalance in vitamin B12-deficient infants and it has not been causally linked with the neurological derangements seen in ITS. Decreased EGF and increased TNF-α have been associated with the hematological and neurological manifestations of cobalamin deficiency, so they can have a role in the loss of neural integrity which can hamper the neural development of these children.[14]

Alteration of Oxidative Metabolism and Accumulation of Lactate

In a recent case study of a 6-month-old vitamin B12 deficient infant, proton MRS (magnetic resonance spectroscopy) of the brain showed an accumulation of lactate in the brain parenchyma. This signifies a possible interruption of oxidative energy metabolism in neurons. Although the mechanism is not fully understood, it could be due to an increase in anaerobic glycolysis. Since a rapid improvement in clinical symptoms of vitamin B12 deficiency is seen after treatment, it has been considered as a result of restored cerebral aerobic energy metabolism.

Clinical Features

The classic features of ITS are tremors, mental and physical retardation, light-colored hair, skin pigmentation, and pallor. These features are present in almost all fully manifesting cases. These babies are described as "plump" or "well contoured" or "chubby." Additional features are excessive skin pigmentation, excessive salivation, muscle flabbiness, apathy, and listlessness **(Figs. 3A to D)**.

Infantile tremor syndrome can be understood as a syndromic state comprising three phases, namely "pretremor," "tremor," and "post-tremor" phases.

- *Pretremor (prodromal) phase (pre-ITS)*: This phase is characterized by regression of milestones after a period of normalcy or after a delayed development, anemia, pigmentation, hair changes, plumpness despite existence of malnutrition, expressionless facies with open mouth, and drooling. Children may present with isolated developmental delay with the neurocutaneous features without regression in this phase.
- *Tremor (classical) phase*: Appearance of coarse rhythmic tremors on top of the clinical features of pretremor phase characterizes this phase. To begin, tremors are intermittent and are seen only on crying or feeding and involve fingers, face, and tongue. Subsequently, these often become continuous and generalized. Predominance of axial tremors have also been noted. Oro-lingual coarse tremors have been the most consistent pattern. The tremors may infrequently have an asymmetric distribution and occasional be strictly unilateral, which can be mistaken for focal seizures. There have been instances of this presentation being treated as epilepsia partialis continua, often without success. However, true seizures are not uncommon in this condition and the two can be differentiated only by electrophysiological studies (electroencephalography with electromyography). Children may have associated dystonia, when the movement disorder takes on a "wing-beating" quality. Since involvement of the oropharyngeal region is common and since tremors are aggravated by action, a bleating quality to cry is frequently noted. Another infrequent presentation in these children is in "metabolic crisis," with acute encephalopathy, metabolic acidosis, and acute severe worsening of the movement disorder. These infants are initially suspected to have an inborn error of metabolism and are later diagnosed to have vitamin B12 deficiency when the biochemical workup returns.
- *Post-tremor (recovery) phase*: Regression of tremors and other features of the syndrome takes place slowly, over a period of days to weeks. However, the earliest signs of improvement are noted in the form of increased alertness of the child and interactiveness with the environment and the appearance of a general

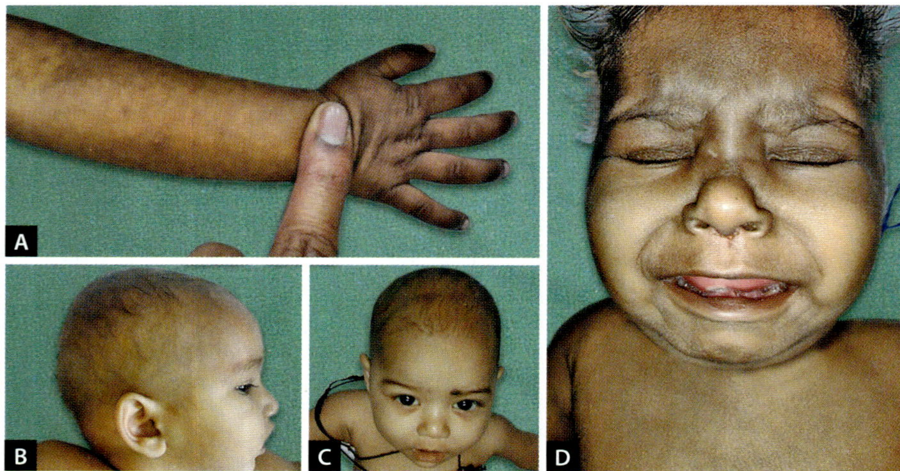

Figs. 3A to D: Clinical manifestations of infantile tremor syndrome. (A) Peripheral (knuckles and dorsum of the hands) hyperpigmentation with reticulate (lace-like or honeycomb) hyperpigmentation of the forearm is evident; (B) thin sparse hypopigmented hair; (C) severe pallor as a result of anemia; (D) angular cheilitis with a red tongue can be seen.

sense of well-being as reported by parents. This is evident as early as 48–72 hours after initiation of therapy. The other features of the syndrome gradually improve. It is to be noted that tremors may increase (or appear, in children who are started on treatment in the pretremor phase i.e. pre-ITS) for a brief period of time usually lasting less than a week during treatment.[5] The mechanism underlying this phenomenon is unclear, though a similar phenomenon of increasing paresthesias in adults with vitamin B12 deficiency on treatment has been attributed to disordered remyelination of the affected nerves. A similar central phenomenon may partly explain this feature.

Investigations and Differential Diagnoses

The complete blood count frequently reveals a macrocytic anemia with high mean corpuscular volume (MCV) and low to low-normal platelet counts. Pancytopenia can occasionally be a part of the presentation. Mild hyperbilirubinemia can be an accompaniment to this blood picture. The authors have seen referrals suspecting acute leukemia in view of hepatosplenomegaly and pancytopenia. Characteristically, the bone marrow examination shows a hypercellular marrow with megaloblastosis without blasts. As mentioned above, the blood picture can be normal ("hematological-neurological dissociation") due to unclear reasons, or can be altered due to blood transfusions.[5] A dimorphic picture can be seen in the hemoglobin indices resulting in an apparent normal or even low MCV as a result of coexistent iron deficiency. The peripheral smear may reflect a similar picture.

The diagnosis is usually easily made with a low serum vitamin B12 level which is low in the majority of the patients.

However, the level may be normal in a certain number of patients. This can be explained by the fact that serum vitamin B12 level is not a robust and sensitive measure of the intracellular vitamin B12 sufficiency status. This is because only 10–30% of the measured vitamin B12 level is bound to the cellular delivery protein, transcobalamin; the remainder is bound to haptocorrin, which is a protein of unknown function. Certain laboratories can measure transcobalamin levels which can make the assay more sensitive, but this is not universally available. Blood homocysteine levels and urine methylmalonic acid levels are more sensitive markers of vitamin B12 deficient status.[15] The mechanism of elevation of these compounds are evident from **Figure 2**.[11] In patients with a normal or low-normal serum vitamin B12 level, homocysteine levels are uniformly high, helping to make the diagnosis. Other micronutrients levels are not consistently deranged and their role in causation of the syndrome is unclear, but appears noncontributory.

Neuroimaging in these infants shows a global cerebral atrophy involving both the cortex and white matter and consequent ventriculomegaly (ex-vacuo). Dysmyelination is evident in the form of diffuse or patch white matter hyperintensities on T2/FLAIR (fluid-attenuated inversion recovery) sequences. Some or most of these changes are reversible on follow-up imaging after completion of treatment. Acute metabolic crisis-like presentations can be associated with bilateral basal ganglia changes simulating an inborn error of metabolism, and these changes are also frequently reversible **(Figs. 4A to D)**.

Certain inborn errors of metabolism, the most important of which are inherited defects of cobalamin metabolism, can be clinically and biochemically similar

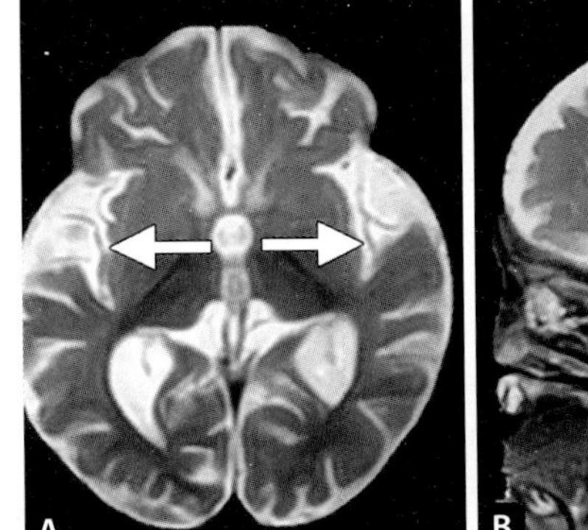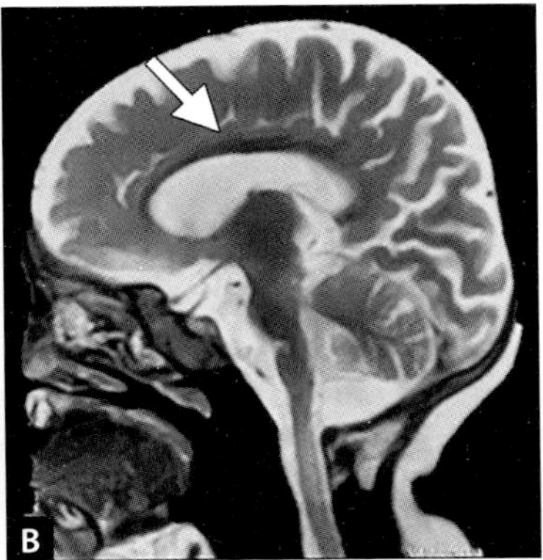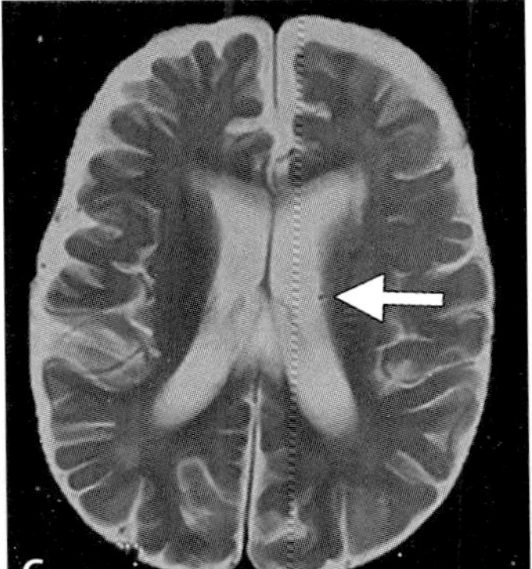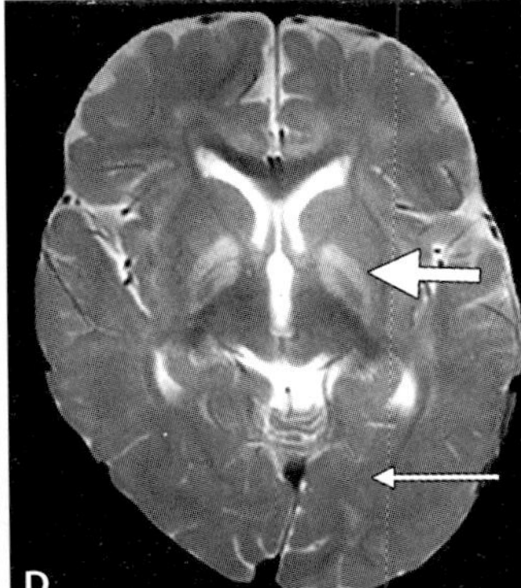

Figs. 4A to D: Neuroimaging (MRI) in infants with infantile tremor syndrome (ITS). (A) T2 axial section showing fronto-temporal predominant global cerebral atrophy leading to widening of the Sylvian fissure bilaterally (arrows); (B) T2 sagittal section showing thinned-out corpus callosum (arrow) demonstrating the severe white matter loss; (C) T2 axial section showing cortical atrophy, loss of cerebral white matter, and secondary ventricular dilation (arrow); (D) T2 axial image of an infant of ITS presenting in an acute metabolic crisis with dystonia and tremors, showing bilateral globus pallidus involvement (thick arrow) and dysmyelination (thin arrow).

and short of a genetic testing for variations associated with the specific disorder is done, a clear differentiation cannot be made. However, since these are genetic disorders, they tend to be life-long and less likely to be completely reversed by the proposed therapeutic regimen for ITS (discussed below). Homocystinuria due to methylenetetrahydrofolate reductase (MTHFR) deficiency, biotinidase deficiency, and glutaric aciduria type I and methylmalonic academia are differentiated easily by their characteristic clinical features and unique biochemical profile.

Management

As already mentioned above, there is a lack of consensus among clinicians regarding the optimal therapeutic regimen, mainly because of ongoing misconceptions about the etiology.[5] Though it is agreed that affected children may harbor deficiencies of other micronutrients (though unsubstantiated yet), it is certain that vitamin B12 deficiency plays a central role in the causation of this disorder. A majority of these patients appear to be well nourished, although children may also present with protein–energy malnutrition with dominant clinical features of tremors, hyperpigmentation, and hair changes, in which complete nutritional rehabilitation needs to be done. In others, vitamin B12 therapy remains the mainstay. Large doses are required to reverse the cellular deficiency and replenish stores. We suggest daily injections followed by gradually tapering doses **(Flowchart 1)**.

Evidence of iron deficiency is frequently found at diagnosis and may also develop in due course of therapy as a result of enhanced erythropoiesis after vitamin B12 therapy, in which cases it needs to be supplemented. The routine addition of other multivitamins and minerals seems unnecessary, except for calcium and vitamin D deficiency when clinical signs of rickets exist.

A parenteral route is preferred in the initial stages since infants are unable to feed well due to the hypotonia and movement disorder in addition to poor appetite. A parenteral route also circumvents concerns of poor absorption of oral drugs due to intestinal megaloblastosis in at least some of these children. After at least 14 doses of parenteral therapy, the rest of the regimen can be completed orally.

Profound feeding difficulties may require hospital admission and nasogastric feeding until the oro-lingual tremors subside. Tremors have been treated with a number of medications, the most popular of which is propranolol. However, other than the feeding difficulties mentioned above, tremors and dyskinesias do not limit functioning

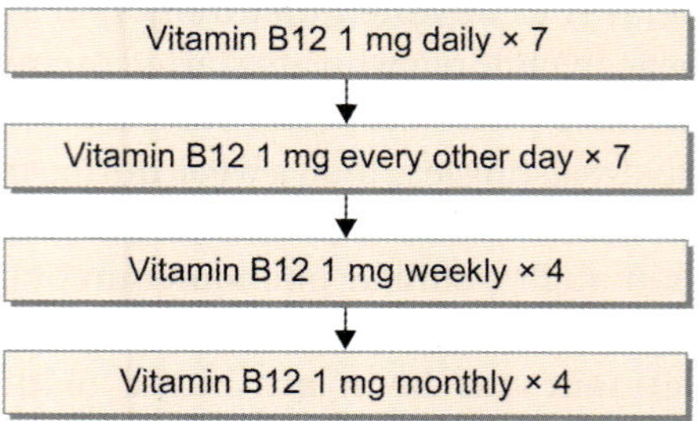

Flowchart 1: The proposed regimen for treatment of nutritional B12 deficiency in infants (ITS). Alternatively, after a total of 14 doses, the regimen can be completed with equivalent or higher (1,500–2,000 micrograms per day) doses of oral vitamin B12.

and subside during sleep. There is no evidence to support the efficacy of medications to control tremors, particularly the troublesome oro-lingual tremor, which the authors feel do not respond satisfactorily to any of the medications. The best therapy for tremors in this disorder appears to be vitamin B12, on which they subside in a variable period ranging from 3 days to 2 weeks.

Treatment Response and Short-term Outcome

A dramatic improvement in the general condition of the child comprising time spent awake, responsiveness, spontaneous limb movements, visual and auditory alertness, general cheerfulness and smiling, production of spontaneous sounds, and betterment of appetite are the earliest changes noted, usually within the first 3 days of initiation of therapy. Some children, as mentioned above, develop tremors or have a transient worsening in tremors. Treatment needs to be continued, and these tremors gradually subside with therapy (complete resolution in 1–4 weeks). This can be concerning to parents and may need reassurance from the treating pediatrician. Improvement in pallor and hematological parameters takes place within a week. Hyperpigmentation of the skin and hair changes are the last ones to resolve, taking one or more months to recover, with skin changes showing an earlier improvement **(Figs. 5A and B)**.[5]

Long-term Outcome

There have been reports depicting complete reversibility of the neurological effects in the short term after nutritional rehabilitation; however, the long-term sustenance of such a benefit is unclarified. It is commonly seen in practice that although the short-term improvement is substantial and appears rewarding, the long-term outcomes are variable. This has suggested that this disorder in not completely reversible and probably results in some

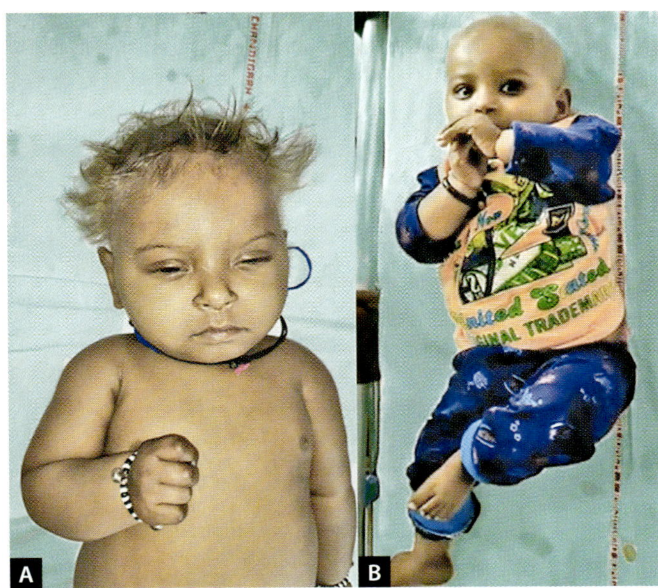

Figs. 5A and B: Pre- (A) and post-treatment (B) images. An apathetic, listless child can be seen before commencement of treatment (A). On day 30 of treatment (B), the same child was alert, playful, showed good visual tracking, and had a monosyllabic babble.

permanent damage to the developing brain. Most studies describing children with this disorder have not assessed development of these children on a standard development scale. In addition, what proportion of them have delayed development starting in early infancy and what proportion regress after a normal period of development is also not very clearly described. Being a potentially treatable and preventable disorder, the developmental features and long-term outcome need further clarification. It can be postulated that infants with tremors, those with a preexistent developmental delay before onset of regression and those infants presenting in an acute "metabolic crisis" may have a less than complete reversal of clinical features, and especially may be left with delay in development and intellectual disability.

RHEUMATIC (SYDENHAM'S) CHOREA

Rheumatic chorea or Sydenham's chorea (SC) is one of the major criteria for the diagnosis of rheumatic fever. The typical age of onset of SC is 5–15 years and there is a gender predilection as females are more affected than males in all the epidemiological studies.[16] Chorea tends to manifest later (usually beyond 6–8 weeks) than other manifestations of rheumatic fever, such as carditis or arthritis, which usually develop 2–3 weeks following an infection of group A beta hemolytic streptococcal (GABHS) infection (pharyngitis).[16-18]

Conventionally, chorea in SC is generalized; however, hemichorea can also occur in about one-fourth of children. Symptoms can be mild in form of just subtle difficulties in writing, combing, etc. to severe symptoms in form of interference with daily activities in school, leading to school absenteeism and frequent falls because of incoordination. Other infrequent manifestations in SC can include motor restlessness, hypotonia, clumsiness, speech disarticulation, tics, and weakness. The associated hypotonia can be completely disabling, a variant coined as chorea paralytica or chorea mollis. Neuropsychiatric symptoms, including obsessive compulsive behaviors and changes in personality and emotional lability, are common and used to predate the appearance of chorea. Neuropsychiatric symptoms are difficult to treat and tends to last even after complete resolution of chorea in most of the cases.[19-21]

Children initially presenting with isolated chorea, but no other symptoms of rheumatic fever may develop cardiac involvement during a recurrence. RC is expected to resolve in 1–6 months based on previously published cohort studies. Recurrences of chorea are not uncommon, occurring in 25% of patients. The most important trigger for relapse in children is poor prophylactic penicillin adherence. Elevated antistreptococcal [antistreptolysin O (ASO)] titers are present in about 10–20% and imaging is usually normal, except for possible acute phase T2 hyperintensities and swollen appearance of the caudate and putamen.[17,19]

Pathophysiologically, acute SC is believed to be associated with antibodies against GABHS that cross-react, through the process of molecular mimicry, with either neuronal extracellular surface and/or intracellular (cytoplasmic or cytoskeletal) antigens.[20-23]

Treatment

Proposed treatments of chorea in SC currently include penicillin therapy for acute phase as well as for prophylaxis, symptomatic medications, and possibly immunomodulatory therapy. The list of recommended symptomatic therapies is wide and consist of anticonvulsants (valproate and carbamazepine) and neuroleptics (haloperidol and risperidone). Once the patient becomes symptom free for at least 1 month, it is suggested that medications can be gradually tapered. In the case of uncontrolled or persisting chorea, recognizing the proposed autoimmune etiology for SC, reports have recommended the use of steroids, intravenous immunoglobulin (IVIg) or plasma exchange. Proposed treatment protocol is given in **Flowchart 2**.[16,21-23]

Flowchart 2: The proposed treatment protocol for children with Sydenham's chorea. Symptom severity is judged in terms of functional impairment (disruption of activities of daily living). Chorea paralytica denotes a rare and the most severe form with hypotonia resulting in severe disability.

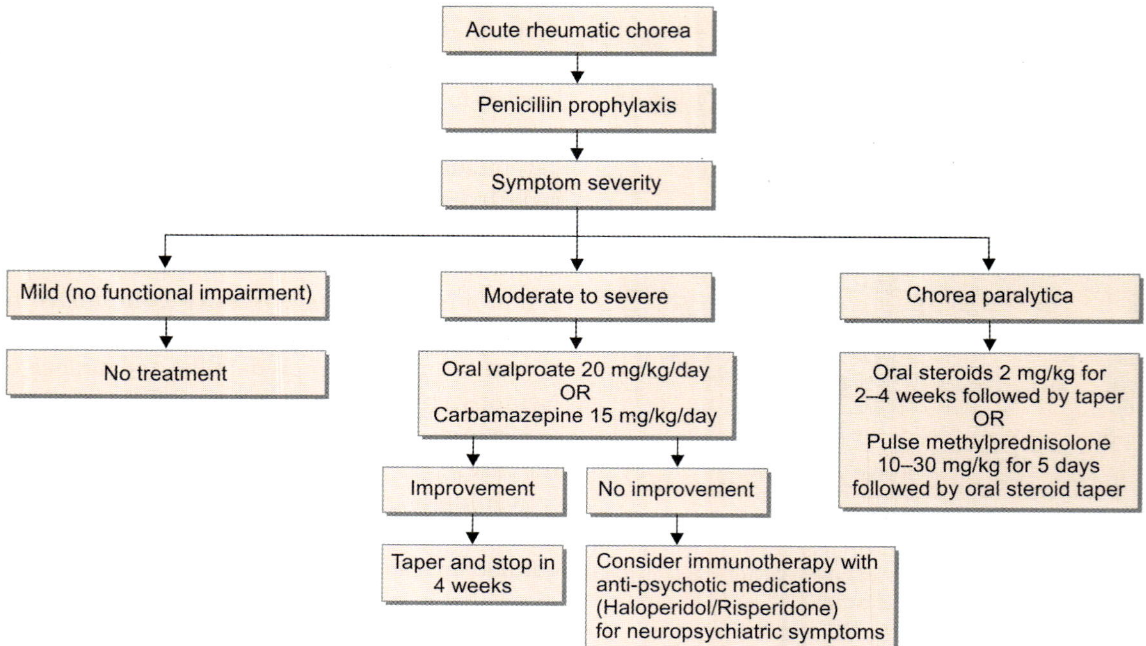

■ REFERENCES

1. Dikshit AK. Nutritional dystrophy with anemia. Indian J Child Health. 1957;6:132-6.
2. Pohowalla JN, Kaul KK, Bhandari NR, et al. Infantile "meningo-encephalitic" syndrome. Indian J Pediatr. 1960;27:49-54.
3. Jadhav M, Webb JK, Vaishnava S, et al. Vitamin B12 deficiency in Indian infants. A clinical syndrome. Lancet. 1962;2(7262):903-7.
4. Srikantia SG, Reddy V. Megaloblastic anaemia of infancy and vitamin B12. Br J Haematol. 1967;13(6):949-53.
5. Goraya JS, Kaur S. Infantile tremor syndrome: a review and critical appraisal of its etiology. J Pediatr Neurosci. 2016;11(4):298-304.
6. Kahn E. A neurological syndrome in infants recovering from malnutrition. Arch Dis Child. 1954;29(145):256-61.
7. Finkelstein JL, Kurpad AV, Thomas T, et al. Vitamin B12 status in pregnant women and their children in India. The FASEB journal. 2014;28:135.6.
8. McPhee AJ, Davidson GP, Leahy M, et al. Vitamin B12 deficiency in a breast fed infant. Arch Dis Child. 1988;63(8):921-3.
9. Taneja S, Bhandari N, Strand TA, et al. Cobalamin and folate status in infants and young children in a low-to-middle income community in India. Am J Clin Nutr. 2007;86(5):1302-9.
10. Garewal G, Narang A, Das KC. Infantile tremor syndrome: a vitamin B12 deficiency syndrome in infants. J Trop Pediatr. 1988;34(4):174-8.
11. Green R, Allen LH, Bjørke-Monsen AL, et al. Vitamin B12 deficiency. Nat Rev Dis Primers. 2017;3:17040.
12. Jamwal A, Sharma S, Saini G. Cranial neuroimaging in infantile tremor syndrome. J Evol Med Dent Sci. 2015;(44):7643-6.
13. Scalabrino G. Subacute combined degeneration one century later. The neurotrophic action of cobalamin (vitamin B12) revisited. J Neuropathol Exp Neurol. 2001;60(2):109-20.
14. Veal N, Hsieh CL, Xiong S, et al. Inhibition of lipopoly-saccharide-stimulated TNF-alpha promoter activity by S-adenosylmethionine and 5'-methylthioadeno-sine. Am J Physiol Gastrointest Liver Physiol. 2004;287(2):G352-62.
15. Stabler SP. Clinical practice. Vitamin B12 deficiency. N Engl J Med. 2013;368(2):149-60.
16. Dean SL, Singer HS. Treatment of Sydenham's chorea: a review of the current evidence. Tremor Other Hyperkinet Mov (N Y). 2017;7:456.
17. Punukollu M, Mushet N, Linney M, et al. Neuropsychiatric manifestations of Sydenham's chorea: a systematic review. Dev Med Child Neurol. 2016;58:16-28.
18. Panamonta M, Chaikitpinyo A, Auvichayapat N, et al. Evolution of valve damage in Sydenham's chorea during recurrence of rheumatic fever. Int J Cardiol. 2007;119:73-9.
19. Gurkas E, Karalok ZS, Taskin BD, et al. Predictors of recurrence in Sydenham's chorea: clinical observation from a single center. Brain Dev. 2016;38:827-34.
20. Peña J, Mora E, Cardozo J, et al. Comparison of the efficacy of carbamazepine, haloperidol and valproic acid in the treatment of children with Sydenham's chorea: clinical follow-up of 18 patients. Arq Neuropsiquiatr. 2002;60:374-7.
21. Genel F, Arslanoglu S, Uran N, et al. Sydenham's chorea: clinical findings and comparison of the efficacies of sodium valproate and carbamazepine regimens. Brain Dev. 2002;24:73-6.
22. Green LN. Corticosteroids in the treatment of Sydenham's chorea. Arch Neurol. 1978;35:53-4.
23. van Immerzeel TD, van Gilst RM, Hartwig NG. Beneficial use of immunoglobulins in the treatment of Sydenham chorea. Eur J Pediatr. 2010;169(9):1151-4.

10

Pediatric Subspecialties in Tropics

Raju C Shah

Tropical Childhood Ophthalmology

Meenakshi Swaminathan, Abhishek Paul

■ INTRODUCTION

Pediatric examination poses a unique challenge to the physician owing to the lack of communication, short attention span, and unreliability of the traditional subjective methods of visual assessment, especially in developmentally delayed or uncooperative children. These can be overcome by examining the child in a comfortable, playful, and friendly environment, crowded with ample toys and bright objects of interest.

Table 1 highlights the important visual milestones in development of pediatric eyes.

■ IDEAL TIMING OF VISION SCREENING

There is no definitive guideline regarding vision screening in preschool children. However, the All India Ophthalmological Society (AIOS) expert committee consensus suggests vision screening by an ophthalmologist at least once between birth and 3 years. The high-risk group comprising of low birth-weight, premature or syndromic babies needs screening at the time of discharge or within 1 month of age.

For children ages 3–5 years, the 2017 United States Preventive Services Task Force (USPSTF) report

Age (months)	Clinical function	Visual acuity
Birth	Blinks to torch light; Sluggish pupillary reflex (pupillary reflex present since 29–31 weeks of gestation)	6/360–6/120 (by OKN)
1	Small saccades develop; follows horizontal moving objects; fixation starts developing; normal OKN; pupillary reflex well-developed	6/480–6/120 (by preferential looking tests)
2–3	Fixation well-developed; larger saccades; pursuits and convergence movements starts developing; follows vertically moving objects	6/120–6/60 (by preferential looking tests)
3	Watches movements of own hands and reaches out toward interesting objects; prefers photographs to patterns	
4	Foveal differentiation complete; sensory fusion and accommodation begins to develop	6/120–6/30 (by preferential looking tests)
5	Blink response to visible threat (menace response); grasps and explores objects; stereopsis begins to develop	6/90–6/24 (by preferential looking tests)
6	Accommodation well-developed; fusional vergence well-developed	
9	Picks up small objects; responds (turns) on calling name	6/48–6/12
12	Hands over toy on request with accompanying hand-out gesture	
36	Visual acuity at adult levels on pediatric acuity charts; contrast sensitivity well developed	6/12–6/6 (Lea symbols, HOTV)
>60	Stereopsis fully developed; adult-type visual acuity testing possible	6/6

(OKN: optokinetic nystagmus)

recommends vision screening, to detect amblyopia or its risk factors.

Referral to an Ophthalmologist

The following children should be referred for comprehensive evaluation to a pediatric ophthalmologist:

- High-risk group as mentioned above.
- Parents providing history of delayed developmental milestones (avoidance of following light, or no eye contact).
- Structural abnormality (e.g. ptosis).
- Absent, white or asymmetric red reflex on distant direct ophthalmoscopy.
- Pupil abnormality (unequal size, shape, and sluggish reaction to light).
- Symptoms or signs suggestive of visual discomfort (squeezing, excessive eye rubbing, and avoidance of sunlight).

Refractive Errors

Refractive errors are the most commonly encountered clinical entity. Myopia, hypermetropia, and astigmatism comprise the refractive errors in decreasing order of prevalence. A recent research estimated global myopia prevalence to be 22.9%, which by 2050, will increase to an alarming figure of 49.7%!

Symptoms and Signs

Complaints of frequent squeezing or rubbing of eyes, bringing the object of interest closer, difficulty in copying from blackboard or eye strain on near work, should arouse the suspicion of a refractive error. Some refractive errors may also present as a squint (misalignment of eyes). Refractive errors are easily identified by use of screening methods such as school screening by trained teachers, volunteers or primary vision care professionals such as technicians and optometrist or photoscreening. Children who fail screening are referred for more detailed evaluation including a cycloplegic refraction.

Management

Spectacles are prescribed for correction of refractive error in children. Pathophysiology of myopia is multifactorial, with both genetic and environmental factors. More outdoor activities have been shown to be protective, while prolonged intense education, and increased near work may be associated with progression of myopia.

Recent focus on halting progression of myopia has involved use of progressive addition lens to minimize peripheral defocus [Correction of Myopia Evaluation Trial (COMET) study] in those who fulfill specific inclusion criteria, pharmacological agents {low dose atropine in concentrations ranging from 0.1% to 0.01% [Atropine in the Treatment of Myopia (ATOM) and Low-Concentration Atropine for Myopia Progression (LAMP) study], pirenzepine and tropicamide}, orthokeratology (involving temporary reshaping of cornea with contact lens), and lifestyle modifications (more outdoor activities and less near work).

AMBLYOPIA

Amblyopia (lazy eye) is a partial decrease of vision in the absence of any anatomical abnormality. It occurs when there is inadequate foveal stimulation or abnormal binocular interaction between the two eyes due to different visual input from the two foveae. The critical period of visual development and foveal maturation is during the first 5 years of life. When there is a difference in the quality of the images received by each eye, the brain disregards the blurred image from the amblyopic eye, resulting in the abnormal development of visual system for that eye.

Types

- *Strabismic*: The most common type and occurs due to presence of squint that results in an inability to fuse dissimilar images coming from two eyes.
- *Refractive*: It results from formation of a constant blurred image on the retina. It is of two types: *Anisometropic* amblyopia (dissimilar refractive errors of the two eyes) and *Isoametropic* amblyopia (large uncorrected similar refractive errors in both eyes).
- *Visual deprivation*: It is the least common, but most difficult to treat. It occurs due to media opacities that obstruct the visual axis; most common causes are congenital cataract, ptosis, and corneal opacities.

In preverbal children, suspect poor vision in one eye when the child protests covering of one eye (the eye with better vision), shows fixation preference for one eye, has unilateral squint or eccentric fixation.

Management

- *Optical*: Aim is to enable formation of a clear image on the fovea; obtained by correction of refractive error by spectacle or contact lens and treatment of the cause of visual deprivation (like media opacity such as cataract).
- *Occlusion*: Patching of the sound eye so that the weak amblyopic eye is forced to work (conventional occlusion). If children resist occlusion, topical atropine

maybe tried once or twice a week to blur vision in the normal eye (pharmacological penalization).

- *Orthoptics*: They include antisuppression and foveal stimulation exercises to facilitate the development of binocular vision.
- *Surgical correction*: The endpoint of the above mentioned conservative therapy is alternation of fixation or equal vision in the two eyes. At this point, strabismus is managed surgically, which yields favorable outcomes due to improved sensory status of the patient.

■ STRABISMUS (SQUINT)

Strabismus refers to misalignment of visual axes of the two eyes relative to each other. The misalignment can be horizontal (esotropia, in which one eye is nasally deviated inward or exotropia, in which one eye is temporally deviated outwards) or vertical (hypertropia in which one eye is directed upward relative to the other).

True squint must be differentiated from a false appearance of squint (pseudostrabismus), due to a broad nasal bridge, or epicanthal folds that makes the eyes appear esotropic.

Strabismus may be also be classified as concomitant or incomitant. Concomitant squint has equal angles of deviation in all gazes; the angles vary in incomitant squint; the common cause of which is paralytic.

Etiology

In most cases, the etiology is not known. In some cases, there is a strong family history (like in infantile esotropia). Squint may occur in uncorrected hypermetropia (excess accommodation to clear the image and hence excess convergence too); due to poor vision in one eye; or due to central nervous system (CNS) conditions such as cerebral palsy, hydrocephalus or brain injury.

Symptoms and Signs

In squint, the fovea of each eye is focusing on a different object; thus, two different images reach the brain leading to confusion. Also, the same object is imaged at two different places in retina, leading to diplopia. To eliminate the symptoms of confusion and diplopia, the brain ignores the image coming from the deviated eye, leading eventually to development of strabismic amblyopia in that eye. Furthermore, as binocular vision does not develop, the child lacks depth perception.

Most squints manifest in the initial 3–4 years of life. Newborn babies may squint occasionally, until their binocular reflexes develop; thus, any squint that presents or persists after the age of 3–4 months must be investigated.

Squint may be constant, being present throughout the day, or it may be intermittent and appears occasionally.

Management

Intermittent squint permits each fovea to receive adequate stimulation and allows partial development of stereopsis due to occasional binocular cooperation seen during the times when eyes are straight; hence treatment, though mandatory, is not an emergency. Constant squint needs early diagnosis and aggressive treatment. Children should wear the spectacles constantly for refractive errors. In many cases, no other treatment is required. As the child grows, spectacle power is adjusted appropriately. If any squint remains in spite of using spectacle, muscle surgery is the end treatment.

A small proportion of children require surgery on the eye muscles to straighten the eye alignment. After surgery, it is usually necessary to continue spectacles, occlusion, and exercise for managing amblyopia, as advised by the ophthalmologist.

■ EYELID INFECTIONS

The common acute infections are blepharitis, stye (hordeolum externum) and chalazion, and hordeolum internum.

Blepharitis

Blepharitis is a subacute or chronic inflammation of lid margins. Predisposing factors include lack of lid hygiene and low immunity, especially in persons living in crowded places.

Symptoms

These include irritation, watering, itching, and sticking of lashes along with occasional burning sensation.

Management

General treatment common to all forms of blepharitis includes maintenance of lid hygiene (warm compresses for 5 minutes and cleaning of lid margin with diluted baby shampoo), topical antibiotic eye drops 3–4 times in a day, and topical antibiotic ointment at bedtime.

Specific types of etiologically classified blepharitis are as follows:

- *Bacterial blepharitis*: It is caused by *Staphylococcus* and *Streptococcus*. Yellow crusts are seen at the root of lashes, which bleed when removed. Treatment includes the above with oral antibiotics in unresponsive cases.

- *Meibomitis (posterior blepharitis)*: It is caused by inflammation of meibomian glands. White foam-like secretions are seen on eyelid margins and canthi. Prominent meibomian gland openings and expression of thick secretions on applying pressure on the tarsus. Treatment includes the above with oral doxycycline (to inhibit staphylococcal lipase formation) in older children.
- *Seborrheic blepharitis*: It is caused due to seborrhea and may be associated with dandruff of scalp. Accumulation of white dandruff-like scales on the lid margin is seen. Treatment includes the above with use of antidandruff shampoo to treat the scalp seborrhea.
- *Parasitic blepharitis*: It is caused by lice; *Phthirus* or *Pediculus*. Lice anchoring the lashes are seen on slit-lamp examination. Treatment includes the above after mechanical removal of individual louse with forceps, and delousing of the patient and family members, clothing and bedding to prevent recurrence.

Hordeolum Externum (Stye)

It is a painful swelling caused by acute suppurative inflammation of lash follicle and its associated gland of Zeis or Moll. *Staphylococcus aureus* is the causative organism. Uncorrected refractive errors, chronic blepharitis, habitual eye rubbing, and reduced immunity may predispose to recurrent lid infections.

Management

Treatment of predisposing and hot fomentation with use of topical antibiotic eye drops and ointment. If a lid abscess forms, it must be drained under cover of systemic and topical antibiotics.

Chalazion (Tarsal or Meibomian Cyst)

A chronic nonsuppurative lipogranulomatous inflammation of meibomian gland that leads to a painless eyelid swelling. It may resolve on its own with frequent hot fomentation. If it is large or does not resolve, intralesional steroid (triamcinolone acetonide) injection is an alternative. Nonresponsive lesions may be incised and its contents curetted under regional anesthesia.

Hordeolum Internum

It is a suppurative inflammation of the meibomian gland associated with blockage of the duct. It may be caused by the primary infection by *S. aureus* or secondary infection in a chalazion. It causes a painful lid swelling. It can be differentiated from hordeolum externum by having the point of maximum tenderness and swelling, away from the lid margin. The pus usually points on the tarsal conjunctiva (seen as yellowish area on everting the lid) and not on the root of cilia.

Management is similar to that of external hordeolum, except that, when the pus forms, it should be drained by a vertical incision from the tarsal conjunctiva.

■ OPHTHALMIC NEONATORUM

Ophthalmia neonatorum, or neonatal conjunctivitis, refers to conjunctivitis occurring within the first month of life. It is important to diagnose and treat the cause as it can lead to certain systemic comorbidities. It is less common in developed countries due to prophylaxis, but it is still a significant cause of blindness in underprivileged tropical countries.

Etiology and Presentation

It has diverse etiology and the time of presentation helps point toward the causative factor. Spread is via direct contact during passage through the birth canal or via ascending route to the cervix in prolonged rupture of membranes. Bacterial (usually between 3 days and 7 days), viral (usually in the 2nd week), or chemical agents (within hours of instillation of prophylactic agent) can cause this condition.

In the first 24 hours, the cause most likely is due to chemical conjunctivitis (silver nitrate instilled for prevention and treatment of conjunctivitis). On presentation, there is serous discharge with conjunctival congestion.

In the first 3–7 days, the cause is commonly infectious and the causative organisms are *Neisseria gonorrhoeae, Neisseria meningitidis, Streptococcus pneumoniae, S. aureus, Haemophilus*, and *Pseudomonas* (rare). Gonorrhea presents with profuse discharge, chemosis and congestion and in severe cases can cause corneal ulceration and perforation. Hence, prompt diagnosis (culture aided) is important and treatment is necessary to prevent ocular complications. Systemic antibiotics also need to be started to prevent meningitis and sepsis.

In postpartum days 5–14, the organisms commonly causing infection are *Chlamydia trachomatis* (D-K) causing trachoma inclusion conjunctivitis (TRIC) and *Herpes simplex* virus.

Management

It is based on specific organism. Gonorrhea and Chlamydia respond to topical erythromycin and tetracycline eye ointments. Gonorrhea requires systemic ceftriaxone. For Chlamydia, the treatment of choice is systemic erythromycin. Chemical conjunctivitis can be prevented by using less toxic erythromycin eye drops and even topical povidone-iodine drops is helpful in low cost setup.

■ CONJUNCTIVITIS

It is caused by inflammation of the conjunctiva due to cellular infiltration and exudation and vascular dilation. Symptoms include eyelid fullness and swelling, chemosis, gritty foreign body sensation, discharge, stickiness and matting of lashes, follicles, papillae, membranes, and pseudomembranes. Acute conjunctivitis has duration of less than 3 weeks and chronic conjunctivitis is of a longer duration. Conjunctivitis can also be classified into infectious and noninfectious.

Infectious

Bacteria and viruses are common causes. Can present unilaterally or bilaterally. Purulent discharge is suggestive of bacterial infection; mucopurulent discharge of viral and chlamydial infection and serous or watery discharge of viral or allergic reaction. Membraneous or pseudomembraneous conjunctivitis is seen in severe viral or bacterial conjunctivitis. Membraneous conjunctivitis is commonly seen with infections such as beta-hemolytic streptococci, pneumococci, *Corynebacterium diphtheriae,* and *N. gonorrhoeae.*

Viral

This is one of the common causes of infective conjunctivitis in children and spread through contact. Adenovirus is the most common etiology. It can present throughout the year; more commonly seen in winter. Other causes of viral conjunctivitis are epidemic keratoconjunctivitis, herpes simplex, varicella, and Epstein-Barr virus among others.

Serous discharge with an admixture of blood, preauricular and/or submandibular lymphadenopathy, febrile illness, and follicular conjunctivitis are common features. Acute follicular conjunctivitis is seen in epidemic keratoconjunctivitis, herpes zoster keratoconjunctivitis, infectious mononucleosis, and Epstein-Barr virus infection. Chronic follicular reaction is seen in chronic chlamydial infections (trachoma and lymphogranuloma venereum).

Treatment

Supportive; over treatment with antibiotics should be avoided when etiology is viral. Corneal subepithelial infiltrates are seen in some cases of adenoviral and epidemic keratoconjunctivitis.

Bacterial

Common causes of conjunctivitis among children. Purulent and mucopurulent discharge is common along with other features of conjunctivitis. Can be acute, hyperacute, and chronic.

S. aureus, S. pneumoniae, Haemophilus influenzae, and *Moraxella* are common causes. Other causes are *C. diptheriae* and *N. gonorrhoeae.*

Treatment

Topical antibiotics (broad spectrum) and lubricants.

Chlamydial

Chlamydia trachomatis infection is seen commonly in children. Trachoma and inclusion conjunctivitis in adolescents.

Trachoma is commonly seen in developing countries with poor hygienic conditions. Clinical manifestation includes follicular conjunctivitis, papillary hypertrophy, corneal vascularization, cicatricial changes of conjunctiva (Arlt's line), and cornea leading to lid abnormalities and corneal scarring and blindness.

Treatment

Hygiene to control the spread of infection. Topical and systemic erythromycin and tetracycline (in children >8 years).

Adult Inclusion Conjunctivitis

Presentation with follicular conjunctivitis, mucopurulent discharge, and preauricular adenopathy.

Treatment

Tetracycline.

Noninfectious

Causes include allergic conjunctivitis, dry eye, trauma, foreign body, toxic or chemical agents, chemical injury, neoplasm, and factious and idiopathic causes.

Allergic Conjunctivitis

Allergic conjunctivitis consists of acute forms (seasonal allergic conjunctivitis and perennial allergic conjunctivitis) and chronic forms [vernal keratoconjunctivitis (VKC), atopic keratoconjunctivitis (AKC), and giant papillary conjunctivitis (GPC)]. All these are type 1 hypersensitivity reactions in which allergen causes mast cell degranulation causing release of histamine, among others, causing a cascade of reactions (vasodilatation, increased vascular permeability, and increased serous/mucoid discharge).

Seasonal allergy is the most common form and presents commonly with congestion, itching, ropy serous discharge, chemosis, etc. These patients often have associated systemic allergic reaction such as wheezing, eczema, and rhinoconjunctivitis.

Treatment

Avoidance of allergens and symptomatic treatment (antihistamines, mast cell stabilizers, nonsteroidal anti-inflammatory agents, and steroids).

Vernal Keratoconjunctivitis

It is a more severe and chronic form with seasonal exacerbations. It is caused by type 1 and type 4 hypersensitivity reactions. It tends to be bilateral and affects superior and limbal conjunctiva. Systemic eczema and asthma are seen in 75% cases with VKC.

Clinical presentation: All features of allergic conjunctivitis maybe seen along with Horner-Trantas dots (pathognomonic), giant cobble-stone papillae in upper tarsal conjunctiva, ropy discharge, and corneal shield (Togby's) ulcer.

Treatment: Symptomatic relief with cold compresses and controlling of hypersensitivity reaction with topical medications ranging from mast cell stabilizers combined with antihistamine and topical nonsteroidal agents.

Phlyctenular Keratoconjunctivitis

Inflammatory process secondary to an allergic hypersensitivity to bacterial antigens (commonly *S. aureus* but also with *Mycobacterium tuberculosis*, *Chlamydia*, *Candida albicans*, and parasites such as *Ascaris* and *Ancylostoma*). Elevated, hard, yellowish-white nodule is seen clinically near the limbus and is a delayed hypersensitivity reaction.

Treatment

Removal of offending agent and symptomatic treatment.

■ VITAMIN A DEFICIENCY

Malnutrition and infections such as measles are common causes of vitamin A deficiency in developing countries. 190 million children worldwide are vitamin A deficient; it is the second most common nutritional disorder after protein-energy malnutrition (PEM) and both can coexist together. It is one of the common causes of bilateral corneal ulcers in children.

Classification of Xerophthalmia [World Health Organization (WHO) Grading]

- XN night blindness
- X1A conjunctival xerosis
- X1B Bitot's spots
- X2 corneal xerosis
- X3A corneal ulceration/keratomalacia <1/3 of corneal surface
- X3B corneal ulceration/keratomalacia >1/3 of corneal surface
- XS corneal scar
- XF xerophthalmic fundus.

Treatment

Diagnosis of xerophthalmia is a medical emergency and prompts massive vitamin A supplementation.

World Health Organization recommended dose based on age is as follows:

- *Children above 12 months of age:* Orally 110 mg of retinol palmitate or 66 mg retinol acetate (*200,000 IU vitamin A*) immediately and again the following day. An additional dose 2 weeks later to boost liver stores. Parenteral dose (only if orally not possible) of 55 mg water-miscible retinol palmitate (*100,000 IU*) to replace the first dose.
- *Children aged 6–12 months:* Half of previously mentioned dose orally.
- *Children less than 6 months:* Quarter dosage is recommended.

Protein-energy malnutrition also needs to be simultaneously corrected in malnourished children. Children at high risk should receive repeated dosing at 4–6 months interval. Vitamin E can also impair vitamin A absorption and storage and needs correction.

Prevention is better than cure in this problem and vaccination against measles is imperative.

■ PEDIATRIC UVEITIS

Uveitis, or inflammation of uveal coat of eyeball including iris, ciliary body, and choroid, is not uncommon. Pediatric uveitis accounts for 12% of all uveitis cases. The most common etiologies of anterior uveitis are idiopathic and juvenile idiopathic arthritis (JIA). While the posterior uveitis and panuveitis group consists of a myriad of systemic conditions including infections (tuberculosis, syphilis, herpes, rubella, mumps, lyme to name a few), autoimmune (sarcoidosis, Behçet's disease, and granulomatosis with polyangiitis), and uveitis masquerade syndromes (retinoblastoma, leukemia, malignant melanoma, and juvenile xanthogranuloma).

Due to the vast spectrum of associated systemic conditions, there is a need for initial consultation with the pediatrician. An extensive history, thorough clinical examination and targeted laboratory investigation, is essential for diagnosis.

Clinical features depend on the etiology and can range from asymptomatic to severe pain, redness, blurring of vision, and watering. Even if they have no ocular complaints, children with the above conditions need an ophthalmic consultation (for a dilated fundus evaluation) to rule out any occult posterior segment pathology.

Corticosteroids (topical, periocular or systemic), and topical cycloplegics are the mainstay of treatment in the majority of cases that are idiopathic. Treating the cause is foremost where etiological diagnosis can be arrived. Recurrences are frequent and demands periodic follow-up for early detection and management of anticipated complications such as cataract, glaucoma and band-shaped keratopathy.

PEDIATRIC CATARACT

Pediatric cataract is the third most common cause of childhood blindness after refractive error and amblyopia. Its prevalence is about 1.03 per 10,000 children (0.32–22.9/10,000).

It can be congenital or acquired; unilateral or bilateral. The mode of inheritance in hereditary cataracts (usually bilateral) is autosomal dominant, mandating screening of family members. Conventionally, unilateral cataracts are idiopathic, and do not require systemic work-up. Trauma is one of the most common causes of unilateral cataract in developing countries. Bilateral cataracts, on the other hand, need systemic evaluation to rule out maternal infections (TORCH), metabolic disease (Galactosemia and Lowe syndrome) or genetic syndromes (Down syndrome and Nance-Horan syndrome).

Awareness among pediatricians is of paramount importance since they serve as the first point of contact with such children and hence play a crucial role in screening and referral. Parents usually present with complaint of white reflex in eye and on examination, absent or altered red reflex is noted. Immediate referral to a pediatric ophthalmologist for a thorough evaluation is warranted.

Not all cataracts require surgery. A visually significant cataract which is larger than 3 mm in diameter and obscures the visual axis is considered amblyogenic and qualifies for urgent surgical intervention.

The current surgical standard of care involves removal of lens and placement of intraocular lens (IOL) in children older than 2 years.

For infants less than 6 months of age, IOL implantation has been documented to be associated with more complications and higher reoperation rates, and hence, they may be left aphakic. Aphakic correction is achieved by spectacles or contact lens.

For children between 7 months and 2 years, IOL implantation is controversial, but recently published literature suggests a rising trend for IOL implantation with favorable outcome.

Rehabilitation in pediatric cataract can be a challenge. Owing to the loss of accommodation after the surgery, these children require near vision spectacles for lifetime. Rigorous postoperative follow-ups are essential to manage changing refractive status (due to growth of the eyeball), amblyopia, strabismus, and deal with anticipated surgical complications like glaucoma, uveitis, visual axis opacification (VAO) or retinal detachment. VAO due to inflammatory membrane or posterior capsular opacification (PCO) may need additional surgery or laser capsulotomy to clear the visual axis. Proper counseling of the parents about the disease, with emphasis on postoperative compliance, goes a long way in establishing a good physician-parent relationship and ensures higher probability of a favorable outcome for the child.

CONGENITAL NASOLACRIMAL DUCT OBSTRUCTION

Congenital nasolacrimal duct obstruction (CNLDO) is one of the most common ophthalmic conditions seen in newborns. It results from failure of canalization of nasolacrimal duct (NLD), mostly at the lower end.

The incidence of CNLDO in newborn has been reported to be approximately 6%. The obstruction can be unilateral or bilateral with no gender predilection.

Epiphora (watering due to obstruction of nasolacrimal outflow) is the presenting complaint of parents. Digital pressure over the lacrimal sac produces reflux of cloudy fluid through the punctum. Pediatricians are often among the first physicians to be consulted and should probe the parents for the history of photophobia. The combination of epiphora and photophobia should guide the clinician to alternative diagnosis such as congenital glaucoma, the confirmation of which requires a thorough examination under anesthesia by an ophthalmologist.

Initial management is conservative because up to 90% of infants improve within the first year of life. Crigler massage on the lacrimal sac uses hydrostatic pressure to open the NLD, and should be properly taught and demonstrated to the caregiver. In case of purulent discharge, broad-spectrum topical antibiotic like tobramycin is prescribed. Nonresponsive cases require surgical intervention by probing and syringing.

■ PRESEPTAL CELLULITIS AND ORBITAL CELLULITIS

Preseptal cellulitis refers to the inflammation of eyelid tissues anterior to the orbital septum, whereas orbital cellulitis involves eyelid tissues posterior to the orbital septum.

Preseptal cellulitis can occur secondary to insect bite (*Staphylococcus* and *Streptococcus*), contiguous severe conjunctivitis [adenovirus and methicillin-resistant *Staphylococcus aureus* (MRSA)] or upper respiratory tract infection (*Streptococcus*). Orbital cellulitis results due to paranasal sinusitis (ethmoid sinus most commonly affected), penetrating trauma or dental infections.

Eyelid edema that often extends to the forehead, full ocular motility, and absence of proptosis and pain on eye movement differentiates preseptal from orbital cellulitis. Presence of systemic features such as fever, lethargy, and headache suggest orbital cellulitis.

Orbital cellulitis is a medical emergency and requires hospital admission and treatment with broad-spectrum intravenous (IV) antibiotics. Computed tomography (CT) scan orbit should be done to look for presence of subperiosteal abscess. Frequent monitoring of vision and pupil is mandatory to look for signs of optic nerve compromise. If an orbital abscess forms, it has to be drained surgically.

■ PEDIATRIC GLAUCOMA

Primary congenital glaucoma (PCG) accounts for about 5% of irreversible blindness in children.

It can be present since birth and 1 month of age (newborn PCG), within 2 years (infantile PCG) or 2–4 years (late-onset PCG). Glaucoma between the age of 4 years and 35 years is termed juvenile-onset glaucoma and behaves similar to primary open angle glaucoma seen in adults.

The pathophysiology lies in abnormal development of the anterior chamber angle, leading to increased resistance to aqueous outflow through the trabecular meshwork.

Primary pediatric glaucoma can also be associated systemic diseases, such as chromosomal disorders (Down syndrome), connective tissue disorders (Marfan and Stickler syndromes), and the phakomatoses (Sturge-Weber syndrome).

Clinical manifestations include the classic triad of epiphora, photophobia, and blepharospasm. Until 3 years of age, elevated intraocular pressure (IOP) can cause the cornea to stretch, leading to increased corneal diameter, and globe enlargement (called buphthalmos or bull's eye). The corneal stretching produce breaks in the Descemet membrane (known as Haab striae), and may lead to corneal edema and corneal opacification. As the cornea swells, the child may become irritable and photophobic. Persistently, elevated IOP results in progressive optic nerve damage.

Management

Examination under anesthesia is mandatory to thoroughly evaluate the child and assess corneal diameters, optic disk, and to attempt refraction if there is no corneal haze. Large corneal diameters, optic disk cupping, characteristic corneal edema, and elevated IOP are the diagnostic clinchers.

Surgical treatment is the mainstay. Initially, raised IOP should be controlled medically by topical eye drops. Punctal occlusion for 3–5 minutes after applying eye drop is mandatory to prevent nasal absorption and avoid systemic side effects.

When target IOP is not achieved medically and is associated with objective evidence of ongoing ocular damage, then surgery is indicated. For PCG, angle surgery (goniotomy or trabeculotomy) is usually the procedure of choice due to its high rate of success, followed by trabeculectomy (with or without mitomycin-C augmentation), glaucoma drainage devices, and transscleral diode cycloablation (in intractable cases).

■ RETINOPATHY OF PREMATURITY

Retinopathy of prematurity (ROP) is a disorder of development of retinal blood vessels in premature infants. Normal retinal vascularization occurs centrifugally from the optic disk to ora serrata. Vascularization up to nasal ora is completed by 8 months (36 weeks) and temporal ora by 10 months (39–41 weeks). Preterm babies have avascular peripheral retina. The hyperoxic state, created in the neonatal intensive care unit (NICU), results in protective response of vasoconstriction of the retinal blood vessels. These babies, when removed from the oxygen-rich environment, develop relative retinal hypoxia, that triggers release of angiogenic factors [vascular endothelial growth factor (VEGF)], resulting in neovascularization at the junction of vascular and avascular retina.

Screening in Indian Scenario as Per the Retinopathy of Prematurity Operational Guidelines by Indian Institute of Public Health

- Birth weight (BW) <2,000 g.
- Preterm infant with gestational age (GA) at birth <34 weeks.
- Preterm infant with GA at birth 34–36 weeks with risk factors (prolonged exposure to oxygen >30 days, cardiorespiratory support, respiratory distress syndrome, sepsis, multiple blood transfusions, chronic lung disease, multiple births (twins/triplets), fetal hemorrhage, sepsis, apneic episodes, intraventricular hemorrhage, and poor postnatal weight gain.
- Other preterm infants based on the discretion of pediatrician or neonatologist.

The first screening should be done within 3–4 weeks after birth in infants with age >28 weeks of GA or BW >1,200 g. Screening should be done earlier (2–3 weeks after birth) if GA is <28 weeks or BW is <1,200 g.

A trained ophthalmologist, well versed with indirect ophthalmoscopy in ROP babies, should do the screening. The latest guidelines propose the use of wide-field fundus imaging (RetCam) screening by trained and competent nonophthalmologist health personnel.

Treatment

Laser photocoagulation using indirect ophthalmoscopy forms the mainstay of treatment. In recent times, intravitreal anti-VEGF injections have been used in severe ROP cases.

Follow-up

Long-term follow-up till 5 years of age is recommended in preterm infants treated for ROP, to detect anticipated complications of high myopia, strabismus, cortical visual impairment, and retinal detachment.

RETINOBLASTOMA

Retinoblastoma is the most common primary intraocular malignancy of childhood, with an incidence of 1:14,000–1:20,000 live births, and is fatal if left untreated. (AA)

It can be unilateral or bilateral (30–40%). Familial and bilateral cases are typically diagnosed during the first year, while sporadic unilateral cases present between 1 year and 3 years of age.

Clinical Features

Leukocoria, or white reflex in the pupil, is the most common mode of presentation, which is noticed by the parents or the pediatrician.

Other conditions such as cataract, Coat's disease, and toxocariasis may also present with a white reflex. Children may also present with a strabismus, and rarely hyphema, uveitis, etc.

Metastatic spread occurs along the optic nerve into the CNS, or through the vascular choroid (via hematogenous route) to bones, lungs, and abdominal solid organs.

Timely referral to an ophthalmologist is the key to effective treatment and survival.

Diagnosis is essentially clinical, based on the characteristic fundoscopic appearance. B-scan ultrasonography with intraocular calcification is typical.

Computed tomography or magnetic resonance imaging (MRI) is done to localize the spread of the tumor to the surrounding areas (Globe and Orbit) or extent of CNS involvement.

Genetic testing for RB1 gene is important to determine the risk of subsequent neoplasm (both retinoblastoma and other primary neoplasms) in the affected progeny and the risk of retinoblastoma in other family members, as it helps to differentiate between germline and somatic cases.

The treatment is multimodal. Chemotherapy, focal laser photocoagulation, cryotherapy, transpupillary thermotherapy, radiation therapy, and surgery, all play important roles. Intravenous chemotherapy, with vincristine, etoposide, and cisplatin, has been the mainstay of treatment since the past two decades. Intra-arterial chemotherapy has emerged as a novel alternative therapy, with promising results, for both advanced and refractory retinoblastoma.

ROD-CONE DYSTROPHIES (RETINITIS PIGMENTOSA)

Rod-cone dystrophies are a genetically diverse group of inherited diffuse retinal degenerative disorders characterized by history of night blindness (nyctalopia) and loss of peripheral field of vision (tunnel vision). Global prevalence of retinitis pigmentosa (RP) is approximately 1 in 5,000. It is a progressive condition that usually presents in 1st or 2nd decade and may cause complete blindness by 3rd or 4th decade.

It can show all types of inheritance, with autosomal dominant being the most common and X-linked recessive being the most severe one. It may be associated with systemic disease, e.g. hearing loss (Usher syndrome), malabsorption (Bassen-Kornzweig syndrome), and ichthyosis (Refsum disease).

The characteristic fundus appearance includes the triad of retinal arteriolar attenuation (often the earliest clinical manifestation), bony spicules in the midperipheral retina, and waxy optic disk pallor. Cystoid macular edema, which leads to decreased central vision, is not uncommon. Late complications include epiretinal membrane at the macula, posterior subcapsular cataract, and open angle glaucoma.

Full-field ERG (electroretinogram) is sensitive and shows reduced scotopic and combined responses in early stage and extinguished responses in advanced stage.

Till date no effective treatment is commercially available. Nutritional supplements in the form of high daily doses of vitamin A palmitate (15,000 IU/day), vitamin E, omega-3, and omega-6 fatty acid, have been tried with minimal success. The macular edema responds satisfactorily to oral acetazolamide.

Rehabilitative therapy with low vision aids (magnifiers and convex lenses) and UV-absorbing sunglasses are commonly employed.

Restorative artificial retina prosthesis device (Argus II Retinal Prosthesis System, by Second Sight Medical Products, Sylmar, California) is now commercially available but has yet to gain popularity in developing countries.

OPTIC ATROPHY

Optic atrophy is the end-stage of any pathology that causes ganglion cell axonal degeneration in the pathway between the retina and lateral geniculate nucleus.

Etiology in pediatric age group can be hereditary (Leber congenital amaurosis), perinatal hypoxic-ischemic injury, compression (hydrocephalus), chiasmal tumors (craniopharyngioma), traumatic, inflammatory (optic neuritis, meningitis, and encephalitis) or raised IOP (glaucoma).

Parents usually complain of child not maintaining eye contact with them. Objectively, a relative afferent pupillary defect (that can be easily demonstrable by simple torch light examination in an outpatient setting) may be the only demonstrable sign. Fundus examination shows a pale optic disk.

Unexplained optic atrophy must always be investigated with the following investigations to pinpoint the etiology: Color vision, visual fields, ultrasound/CT/MRI of brain and orbits. A thorough neurological examination of all cranial nerves is also essential to rule out associated pathology and aids in localizing the lesion.

As this is an irreversible process, it is imperative to detect and treat the underlying etiology before atrophy sets in. Prognosis is variable and depends upon the root cause.

PAPILLEDEMA

Optic nerve head edema secondary to elevated intracranial pressure (ICP). It is typically bilateral, and may develop over hours or weeks. Raised ICP increases the pressure in the subarachnoid space around the optic nerve, causing axoplasmic flow stasis, resulting in accumulation of toxic materials and eventually leads to the swelling of optic nerve head.

Elevated ICP in infants may not result in manifest papilledema, due to nonclosure of fontanelles, but can result in firmness and distension of the open fontanelles. Nausea, vomiting, and headache, along with sixth cranial nerve palsy (false localizing sign) are signs of elevated ICP.

Etiology

This includes a myriad of conditions such as hydrocephalus, intracranial mass lesions, encephalitis, meningitis, craniosynostosis, idiopathic intracranial hypertension, and use of drugs like tetracycline and corticosteroids.

Symptoms and Signs

Those specific to papilledema include transient obscurations of vision, which the older child may be able to describe. At the beginning, visual acuity, color vision, and pupillary reactions are all normal. However, chronic or severe papilledema results in visual dysfunction, constriction of visual field, and decreased color perception, when optic atrophy starts to set in. Fundus examination shows classic signs of optic disk hyperemia, obscuration of vessels at the disk margin, retinal hemorrhages, and exudates.

Management

A thorough evaluation, including perimetry, neuroimaging (CT, MRI, and MR venography), followed by lumbar puncture, is indicated to establish the diagnosis. Early detection of the condition, identification of the cause, and prompt initiation of treatment may be life-saving.

OCULAR TRAUMA

It is an important cause for visual morbidity and unilateral diminution of vision and amblyopia in children. Management includes both immediate care (to preserve vision) and long-term care (amblyopia treatment). An important factor in the assessment and management of pediatric traumatic disorders is obtaining a proper history and performing a detailed examination, which many a times is difficult due to poor cooperation, and risks further damage in case of forceful examination.

Accidental Trauma

This is commonly related to casual play and daily environmental injuries. Important predisposing factor is inadequate adult supervision in most cases. It is more commonly seen in younger boys than girls.

Extraocular foreign body (lid, conjunctival, and corneal), conjunctival and corneal abrasions, superficial ocular burns, and chemical injury (steam, household chemicals, and lime in whitewash) are common and can be treated in an outpatient department without much functional loss. Lid tear and canalicular tear are seen commonly and may require the child to be sedated for a surgical repair.

Penetrating and perforating injury may occur with household objects such as sharp pencil, scissors, etc. Cracker burst injuries are also a common mode of injury with both metallic and nonmetallic particles (such as sand) in developing countries. One of the important steps in management is to obtain a detailed and reliable history and to look for subtle signs of globe penetration (such as localized subconjunctival hemorrhage to look for localized scleral tear, irregular pupil and iris defects to rule out missile intraocular foreign bodies, localized circumcorneal congestion and hyphema to rule out anterior chamber foreign body and foreign body lodged in angles). Corneal tear, lenticular damage—traumatic cataract, intravitreal foreign body, retinal detachment, and open globe are serious injuries and require prompt and adequate treatment under sedation or general anesthesia.

Trauma can result in small and large hyphemas. It is important to rule out penetrating injury and localized foreign body in these cases. One other factor determining management of hyphema in pediatric patients is IOP and corneal blood staining. IOP measurement can be particularly difficult in pediatric population and may require sedation. Treatment is with bed rest/hospitalization after ruling out other serious injuries and topical steroids and cycloplegics. Detailed anterior and posterior segment evaluation is a must as soon as the media clears and may need to resort to ultrasound imaging in case of poor posterior segment visualization. Prevention of amblyopia and long-term secondary glaucoma is important in these cases.

TRAUMATIC OPTIC NEUROPATHY

One of the serious complications of blunt trauma orbit, head or globe injury, which can result in permanent vision loss. Clinical signs of vision loss, relative afferent pupillary defect, and defective color vision are classical. Imaging (MRI scan) can aid in diagnosis. Management is controversial and no effective treatment is available. High dose intravenous steroids with or without optic canal decompression is advocated.

Nonaccidental Trauma

Most injuries in childhood are accidental, however, a small subset involves injuries caused due to physical abuse in children. It is important to keep this in mind and look for such a cause when there are repeated injuries at the same site (at different stages of healing), inconsistent history from the caretakers, and when the history provided does not correlate with the nature of injury.

One of the unique combinations of injury involving eyes and cranium seen in infants can be caused due to violent shaking resulting in shaken baby syndrome (also known as abusive head trauma or inflicted childhood neurotrauma). It is commonly seen in children less than 5 years of age and mostly less than 12 months. The injuries include subdural hematoma (typically bilateral) and subarachnoid hemorrhage and results from the vigorous acceleration-deceleration injury due to violent shaking. Ocular features involve retinal, preretinal, and vitreous hemorrhage. In severe cases, traumatic retinoschisis and retinal detachment can also occur. It is a diagnosis of exclusion and it is essentially important to rule out all other possible causes before assumption of this as the causative factor.

SUGGESTED READING

1. All India Ophthalmological Society, National, Expert-based Consensus Statement Regarding Paediatric Eye Examination, Refraction and Amblyopia Management. New Delhi. AIOS Focus Group meeting; 2017.
2. Al-Shahwan S, Al-Tobak AA, Turkmani S. Side-effects of brimonidine tartrate in children. Ophthalmology. 2005;112 (12):2143.
3. Amblyopia. In: Hered RW, Archer SM, Braverman RS, Khan AO, Lee KA, Lueder GT, et al. (Eds). AAO BCSC Section 6: Pediatric Ophthalmology and Strabismus. San Francisco: AAO; 2018-19.
4. American Academy of Ophthalmology Preferred Practice Patterns Committee. Refractive Errors and Refractive Surgery Preferred Practice Pattern. Ophthalmology. 2018;125(1):1-104.
5. Beck A, Chang TCP, Freedman S. Definition, classification and differential diagnosis. In: Weinreb RN, Grajewski A, Papadopoulos M, Grigg J, Freedman S (Eds). Childhood Glaucoma. WGA Series-9. Amsterdam: Krugler Publications; 2013. pp. 3-10.

6. Bhuyan J. Management of pediatric cataract: a challenge. Int J Curr Med Applied Sci. 2014;5(1):11-13.

7. Bothun ED, Wilson ME, Traboulsi EI, et al.. Outcomes of unilateral cataracts in infants and toddlers 7 to 24 months of age. Toddler Aphakia and Pseudophakia Study (TAPS). Ophthalmology. 2019;126(8):1189-95.

8. Chia A, Lu QS, Tan D. Five-year clinical trial on atropine for the treatment of myopia 2: myopia control with atropine 0.01% eyedrops. Ophthalmology. 2016;123:391-9.

9. Childhood cataracts and other lens disorders. In: Hered RW, Archer SM, Braverman RS, Khan AO, Lee KA, Lueder GT, et al. (Eds). AAO BCSC Section 6: Pediatric Ophthalmology and Strabismus. San Francisco: AAO; 2018-19.

10. de Silva DJ, Khaw PT, Brookes JL. Long-term outcome of primary congenital glaucoma. J AAPOS. 2011;15(2):148-52.

11. Disorders of the Retina and Vitreous. In: Hered RW, Archer SM, Braverman RS, Khan AO, Lee KA, Lueder GT, et al. (Eds). AAO BCSC Section 6: Pediatric Ophthalmology and Strabismus. San Francisco: AAO; 2018-19.

12. External diseases of the eye. In: Hered RW, Archer SM, Braverman RS, Khan AO, Lee KA, Lueder GT, et al. (Eds). AAO BCSC Section 6: Pediatric Ophthalmology and Strabismus. San Francisco: AAO; 2018-19.

13. Eyelid disorders. In: Hered RW, Archer SM, Braverman RS, Khan AO, Lee KA, Lueder GT, et al. (Eds). AAO BCSC Section 6: Pediatric Ophthalmology and Strabismus. San Francisco: AAO; 2018-19.

14. Fierson WM. American Academy of Pediatrics Section on Ophthalmology, American Academy of Ophthalmology, American Association for Pediatric Ophthalmology and Strabismus, American Association of Certified Orthoptists. Screening examination of premature infants for retinopathy of prematurity. Pediatrics. 2018;142:2018-3061.

15. Hereditary fundus dystrophies. In: Bowling B (Ed). Kanski's Clinical Ophthalmology, 8th edition. New York: Elsevier; 2016. pp. 646-50.

16. Holden BA, Fricke TR, Wilson DA, et al. Global prevalence of myopia and high myopia and temporal trends from 2000 through 2050. Ophthalmology. 2016;123:1036-42.

17. Honavar SG. Do we need India-specific retinopathy of prematurity screening guidelines? Indian J Ophthalmol. 2019;67:711-6.

18. Honavar SG. Retinoblastoma: They live and see. AIOS CME Series no. 25, 2012.

19. Hong AR, Shute TS, Huang AJW. Bacterial Kerartitis. In: Mannis MJ, Holland EJ (Eds). Cornea, 4th edition. New York: Elsevier; 2017. pp. 875-901.

20. Infant Aphakia Treatment Study Group. A randomized clinical trial comparing contact lens with intraocular lens correction of monocular infancy: HOTV optotype acuity at age 4.5 years and clinical findings at age 5 years. JAMA Ophthalmol. 2014;132(6):676-82.

21. Khitri MR, Mills MD, Ying GS, et al. Visual acuity outcomes in pediatric glaucomas. J AAPOS. 2012;16(4):376-81.

22. Khokhar SK, Dhull C. Atlas of Pediatric Cataract. Singapore: Springer; 2019: pp. 1-5.

23. Lacrimal Drainage System Abnormalities. In: Hered RW, Archer SM, Braverman RS, Khan AO, Lee KA, Lueder GT, et al. (Eds). AAO BCSC Section 6: Pediatric Ophthalmology and Strabismus. San Francisco: AAO; 2018-19.

24. LaRoche GR. Examination, history and special tests in pediatric ophthalmology. In: Lambert SR, Lyon CJ (Eds). Taylor and Hoyts Pediatric Ophthalmology and Strabismus, 5th edition. New York: Elsevier; 2017. pp. 51-2.

25. Manjandavida FP, Stathopoulos C, Zhang J, et al. Intra-arterial chemotherapy in retinoblastoma: a paradigm change. Indian J Ophthalmol. 2019;67:740-54.

26. Mannis T, Mannis MJ, Paranjpe DR, et al. Nutritional Disorders. In: Mannis MJ, Holland EJ (Eds). Cornea, 4th edition. New York: Elsevier; 2017. pp. 676-84.

27. McKeown CA, Davidson SL. The Pediatric Eye Examination. In: Hunter DG, Mills MD (Eds). Albert and Jackobeic's Principles and Practice of Ophthalmology, 3rd edition. New York: Elsevier; 2008. p. 4134.

28. Neuro-ophthalmology. In: Bowling B (Ed). Kanski's Clinical Ophthalmology, 8th edition. New York: Elsevier; 2016. pp. 793-6.

29. Ocular trauma in childhood. In: Hered RW, Archer SM, Braverman RS, Khan AO, Lee KA, Lueder GT, et al. (Eds). AAO BCSC Section 6: Pediatric Ophthalmology and Strabismus. San Francisco: AAO; 2018-19.

30. Optic disc abnormalities. In: Hered RW, Archer SM, Braverman RS, Khan AO, Lee KA, Lueder GT, et al. (Eds). AAO BCSC Section 6: Pediatric Ophthalmology and Strabismus. San Francisco: AAO; 2018-19.

31. Orbital disorders. In: Hered RW, Archer SM, Braverman RS, Khan AO, Lee KA, Lueder GT, et al. (Eds). AAO BCSC Section 6: Pediatric Ophthalmology and Strabismus. San Francisco: AAO; 2018-19.

32. Parveen S, Chetan R, Nishant B. Retinopathy of prematurity: an update. Sci J Med and Vis Res Foun. 2015;33(2):93-6.

33. Project operational guidelines. Prevention of Blindness from Retinopathy of Prematurity in Neonatal Care Units. [online]. Available from: https://phfi. org/wp-content/uploads/2019/05/2018-ROP-operational-guidelines.pdf. [Last accessed on November 2019].

34. Ram J, Sukhija J. Pediatric Cataract Management. AIOS CME Series no. 26, 2012 December.

35. Sensory physiology and pathology. In: Hered RW, Archer SM, Braverman RS, Khan AO, Lee KA, Lueder GT, et al. (Eds). AAO BCSC Section 6: Pediatric Ophthalmology and Strabismus. San Francisco: AAO; 2018-19.

36. Sharma P. Strabismus Simplified, 2nd edition. New Delhi: CBS; 2015.

37. Shields JA, Shields CL (Eds). Intraocular Tumors: An Atlas and Textbook. 3rd edition. New York: Wolters Kluwer; 2016.

38. Swaminathan M. Progressive myopia: an update. Sci J Med and Vis Res Foun. 2015;33(3):122-5.

39. Trauma. In: Bowling B (Ed). Kanski's Clinical Ophthalmology, 8th edition. New York: Elsevier; 2016. pp. 862-85.

40. US Preventive Services Task Force. Vision Screening in Children Aged 6 months to 5 years: US Preventive Services Task Force Recommendation Statement. JAMA. 2017;318(9):836-44.

41. Uveitis in the Pediatric Age Group. In: Hered RW, Archer SM, Braverman RS, Khan AO, Lee KA, Lueder GT, et al. (Eds). AAO BCSC Section 6: Pediatric Ophthalmology and Strabismus. San Francisco: AAO; 2018-19.

42. Wu PC, Tsai CL, Wu HL, et al. Outdoor activity during class recess reduces myopia onset and progression in school children. Ophthalmology. 2013;120:1080-5.

43. Yam JC, Jiang Y, Tang SM, et al. Low-Concentration Atropine for Myopia Progression (LAMP) Study. Ophthalmology. 2019;126(1):113-24.

44. Yeung HH, Walton DS. Clinical classification of childhood glaucomas. Arch Ophthalmol. 2010;128(6):680-4.

Pediatric Dentistry in Tropics

Meet R Ramatri

INTRODUCTION

The World Health Organization defines oral health as "a state of being free from mouth and facial pain, oral and throat cancer, oral infection and sores, periodontal disease, tooth decay, tooth loss, and other diseases associated disorders that limit an individual's capability in biting, chewing, smiling, speaking, and psychosocial well-being." Some of the important functions of teeth are: speech, eating, smiling and socializing and therefore, healthy and efficiently functioning teeth are a prerequisite through each and every stage of life.

Permanent teeth occupy the space maintained by their healthy primary precedent teeth. Therefore, the premature loss of primary teeth either from dental caries or trauma, often results in loss of space which leads to crowding of the permanent teeth. This is where the role of pediatric dentist comes into picture. Pediatric dental specialty American Academy of Pediatric Dentistry (AAPD) is defined as "An age-defined specialty that provides both primary and comprehensive preventive and therapeutic oral healthcare for infants and children through adolescence, including those with special healthcare needs."

This chapter discusses the oral diseases affecting the children in tropics and also their treatment plan.

NATAL AND NEONATAL TEETH

Though tooth eruption follows a chronological process, sometimes the eruption time of the teeth undergoes small variation depending on the hereditary, endocrine, and environmental factors. Appearance of teeth in oral cavity at the time of birth is due to the significant alteration in the eruption time of primary teeth. These teeth are called "congenital teeth," "fetal teeth," "predeciduous teeth," and "precocious dentition." "Natal" teeth are the teeth present at birth and "neonatal teeth" are teeth that erupt within the first 30 days of birth **(Fig. 1)**.

Incidence of neonatal teeth is more frequent than natal teeth with no sex preference. Deciduous mandibular incisors are more common as natal or neonatal teeth. In most of the cases, these teeth are normal deciduous complement while the rest are supernumerary. The natal and/or neonatal teeth may be firmly fixed or just loosely attached to gum tissue.

Etiology

Literature states that the primary cause of natal or neonatal teeth are—fever (during or after birth), endocrine disorders, congenital syphilis, nutritional deficiencies, superficial positioning of tooth germ, family history and association with some syndromes such as chondroectodermal dysplasia, Ellis-van Creveld syndrome, Hallermann-Streiff syndrome, Pierre Robin

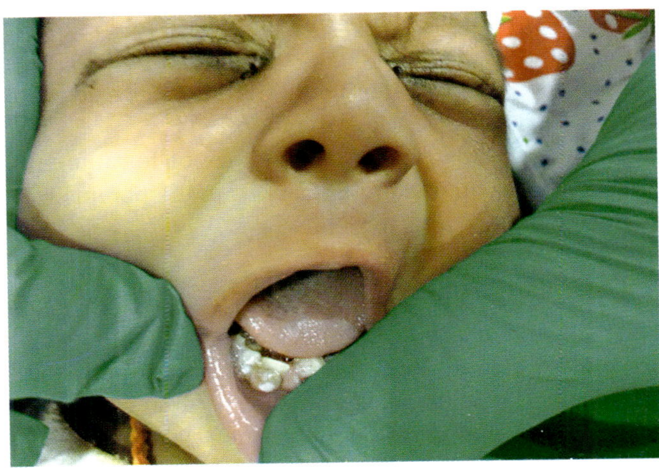

Fig. 1: Natal and neonatal teeth.

syndrome, Sotos syndrome, cyclopia, and CLCP. All these factors contribute to acceleration in the eruption process leading to appearance of teeth in oral cavity before their time.

Morphology and Clinical Features

Morphologically, natal teeth resemble normal teeth in size and shape; however, some might be smaller in size and conoid in shape with opaque yellow color. Generally, these teeth have absent or poorly developed roots. Natal or neonatal teeth can be:

- Mature, i.e. they are completely developed, have good prognosis, and should be maintained in oral cavity.
- Immature, i.e. structurally incomplete teeth having poor prognosis and may require their removal.

Complications

Riga–Fede disease is the appearance of a traumatic ulcer in the ventral surface of the tongue due to the trauma caused by presence of natal or neonatal teeth in oral cavity. This painful ulcer results in dehydration and difficulty in breastfeeding, besides increasing the likelihood of infections in the area. Rounding the incisal edge of these teeth using a finishing bur or a grinding disk is considered a conservative treatment.

Treatment

Proper evaluation and diagnosis are the two most important guidelines for the effective treatment planning of natal and neonatal teeth. Pediatricians are the ones, who usually first find these teeth and early consultation with dentist can prevent any major complications. Generally, the firmly attached natal or neonatal teeth should be kept in the oral cavity since their extraction may cause loss of space, causing hindrance in eruption of permanent teeth. Alternatively, smoothening the incisal edge is recommended for such teeth. Excessively mobile teeth should be extracted to prevent their swallowing or aspiration.

Periodic follow-up by dentists are of fundamental importance, as are recommendations to the parents with respect to home dental hygiene.

■ CLEFT LIP AND PALATE

Cleft lip and palate are congenital anomalies which are closely related embryologically, functionally, and genetically. These oral malformations occur in early stages of pregnancy, during the developmental stage of the child in utero. The process of formation of the lip and roof of the mouth (palate) starts between the 4th week and 7th

week of gestation. As a baby develops during pregnancy, frontonasal process and maxillary process of first brachial arch from each side of the head grow toward the center of the face and join together to make the lip and the palate. Failure of the tissue of the mesenchymal layer (that makes up the lip) to join completely before birth leads to the development of CLCP results from the failure of palatal shelves to approximate or fuse resulting in an opening in the upper lip and palate.

Incidence and Epidemiology

Cleft lip and/or palate have become frequent anomaly around the world with an average of about 1 in every 500–750 live births resulting in a cleft. Rate for cleft lip with or without cleft palate and cleft palate alone varies within different ethnic groups.

According to literature, the prevalence rate of this congenital anomaly is highest for Native Americans and Asians. Africans have the lowest prevalence rates.

Complications

- *Psychosocial problems*: Loss of hearing and speech abnormalities
- *Dental problems*: Difficulty in breastfeeding, multiple missing teeth, anterior and posterior cross-bite, ectopically erupted teeth, impacted teeth, supernumerary teeth, multiple carious teeth due to poor oral hygiene and reduced salivary gland function, and periodontal complications.

Treatment

Role of Pediatric Dentist in Cleft Lip and Palate Patient

A pediatric dentist is usually the first dental specialist whom the parents will encounter. The role of pediatric dental practitioner starts from first month of life right up to permanent dentition phase.

Fabrication of Feeding Obturator

Neonates with this congenital anomaly have problems in consuming food, which may lead to failure to thrive. The current scenario for the management involves reparative surgery within 12 months of life. Therefore, there is a need for the early intervention by conservative means to decrease complications by increasing body weight and decreasing risk of complications in surgery.

Feeding obturator blocks the defect and thereby prevents the tongue from entering into the defect which

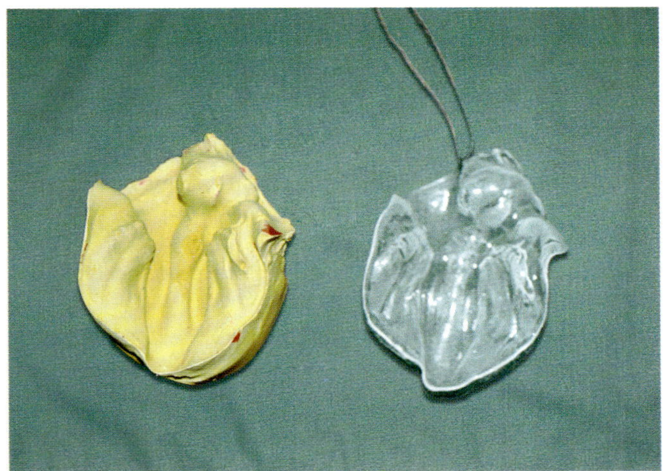

Fig. 2: Fabrication of feeding obturator.

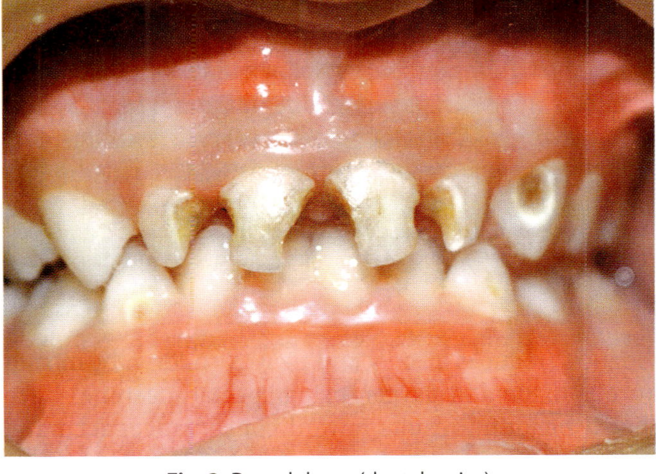

Fig. 3: Dental decay (dental caries).

would otherwise interfere with spontaneous growth of the palatal shelves. It also reduces nasal regurgitation and incidence of choking. Moreover, it also contributes to the development of the jaws and speech **(Fig. 2)**.

After the obturator has been made, parents need to take care of this appliance. After each feed, the plate should be removed and cleaned with running water and soaked once a day for 20 minutes in chlorhexidine solution.

Nasoalveolar Molding

The first presurgical nasoalveolar molding (PNAM) appliance was designed by Grayson et al. (1999). Nasoalveolar molding is a nonsurgical method of reshaping the gums, lip, and nostrils before CLCP surgery, thereby reducing the severity of the cleft. The objectives of PNAM are to:

- Guide the growth of maxillary segments and thereby reduce the cleft size
- Guide the cleft segments to achieve favorable alignment of the cleft segments within the first few months of infancy before cheiloplasty
- Facilitate surgical repair with minimal tension
- Reduce the protrusive position of the alveolar processes
- Prevent tongue from seating into cleft palatal region, thus facilitating transverse growth of palatal shelves
- Actively mold and reposition the deformed nasal cartilages
- Lengthen the columella
- Straighten the columella and correction of alar cartilage displacement
- Reduce the need for secondary alveolar bone grafting.

■ DENTAL DECAY (DENTAL CARIES)

One of the most widespread oral diseases worldwide affecting individuals of all age group is dental caries **(Fig. 3)**. Dental caries develops through a compounded interplay between acid-producing microorganisms and fermentable sugars, and many host factors such as teeth and saliva. Time plays a very vital role in development of caries. Children and young individuals of middle-income countries are majorly affected by dental caries, with about two-thirds of decay remaining untreated.

Cause and Development of Disease

Dental caries is a multifactorial disease. Factors like high numbers of cariogenic microorganism, inadequate flow from salivary glands, insufficient fluoride exposure, poor oral hygiene, inappropriate methods of feeding infants, and poverty lead to development of dental caries.

The dental decay can be diagnosed by visual or tactile methods. Many advanced techniques like using dyes, latest devices, digital radiographs, cone beam computed tomography (CBCT), DIAGNOdent, and other methods are used in detecting the depth of dental caries and extension of the infection.

Treatment of Dental Caries

Recently, many new technologies and advanced versions of old technologies have changed the method of treatments. The use of silver diamine fluoride (arrests dental caries), ICON (resin material which reverses the initial damage in enamel), zirconia crowns (esthetic crowns), chemo mechanical caries removing agents (for painless experience of dental caries removal), use of inhalation conscious

Table 1: Treatment of dental caries.

Primary preventive treatment	Topical fluoride application	Pit and fissure sealants for caries-prone teeth with deep pits and fissures	Diet counseling and anticipatory guidance
Secondary preventive treatment	In case of cavity involving enamel: Enameloplasty or conservative cavity preparation and restoration	In case of cavity involving enamel and dentin: Restoration	In case of cavity involving enamel and dentin and pulp: Pulpotomy/Pulpectomy followed by crown (stainless steel crown/zirconia/stripform crowns)
Tertiary preventive treatment	In case of grossly decayed tooth, extraction is needed	Post extraction of a primary tooth, space maintainer is advised to maintain the space for a succedaneous permanent tooth	In case of lost space of previous extraction space, space regainer is given to get the space back

sedation (reduces anxiety and pain in children by mixing nitrous oxide and oxygen using special machine) have shown beautiful results toward conservative, accurate, and preventive treatment results for all kids including kids with high anxiety rate, very young kids, and special need children **(Table 1)**.

PERIODONTAL DISEASES

Periodontium consists of the tissues that surround and support the teeth. Those tissues are gingiva, cementum, periodontal ligaments (PDLs), and alveolar bone **(Fig. 4)**.

The term "periodontal diseases" includes any genetic or noninheritable disorders of the tissues that are investing and supporting the teeth (gingiva, cementum, PDL, and alveolar bone).

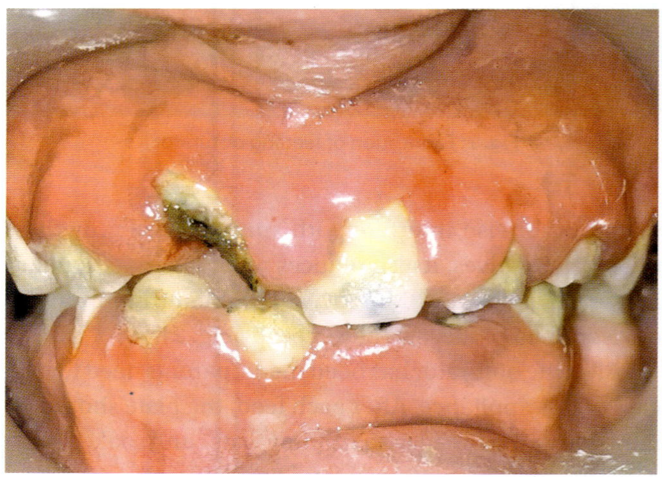

Fig. 4: Periodontal diseases.

Etiology

- Poor oral hygiene
- Trauma from occlusion
- Oral destructive habits like tobacco use
- Nutritional deficiency like vitamin C deficiency
- Endocrine disturbances like puberty, pregnancy, menopause, diabetes mellitus, hyperthyroidism, etc.
- Illiterate and poor patients with no access to good oral hygiene
- Immunological disorders like HIV, use of immuno-suppressant drugs, leukemia, etc.

Classification

Periodontal disease in children and adolescence is broadly classified as:

- Gingivitis
- Periodontitis.

Gingivitis is more common in children and its causes are as follows:

- Dental plaque
- Systemic disease
- Medication
- Malnutrition
- Trauma.

Periodontitis

Occurrence of periodontitis is less frequent in children and adolescence. However, following types of periodontitis can be seen:

- *Aggressive periodontitis in children (prepubertal periodontitis)*: It often begins at the age of 4–5 years. It may be localized or generalized.

  This condition causes rapid bone loss, which leads to premature loss of primary teeth. It is often associated with systemic problems like neutropenia, leukocyte adhesion or migration defect, hypophosphatasia, Papillon-Lefèvre syndrome, leukemia, and Langerhans cell histiocytosis.

- *Aggressive periodontitis in adolescents*: Localized aggressive periodontitis in adolescents is often characterized by rapid attachment loss, on at least two first molars and incisors. The causative organism is *Aggregatibacter* (*Actinobacillus*) bacteria.

  Generalized aggressive periodontitis occurs more in adolescents and young adults and is characterized by generalized interproximal bone loss, including three teeth that are not first molars and incisors.

- *Acute pericoronitis*: Acute inflammation of the flap of gingival covering that crown of partially erupted tooth is common in mandibular permanent molars. Accumulation of bacteria and debris between gingival flap and tooth precipitates inflammatory response. Severe pain and trismus is clinical feature of pericoronitis. Untreated cases can result in facial space infections and facial cellulitis.

  Treatment includes local debridement and irrigation, warm saline gargles, and antibiotic therapy **(Table 2)**.

- *Necrotizing periodontal disease*: Necrotizing periodontal disease, also known as "trench mouth" is a distinct periodontal disease associated with spirochetes and fusobacteria. It is generally a disease of developing countries where children have protein malnutrition.

  Clinical manifestations include necrosis and ulceration of interdental gingiva, oral malodor, cervical lymphadenopathy, malaise, and fever.

  Treatment is divided into acute management with local debridement, oxygenating agent (direct application of 10% carbamide peroxide in anhydrous glycerol qid), and analgesics. Dramatic resolution occurs within 48 hours. If the patient is febrile, adjunct antibiotic therapy will be helpful. A second phase of treatment may be necessary if the acute phase of the disease has caused irreversible damage to the periodontium **(Table 2)**.

■ MALOCCLUSION

Malocclusion has received a special focus by being the third most prevalent oral disease, outranked only by dental caries and periodontal disease. An unbalanced or incorrect relation between the teeth of the two dental arches when they come near each other as the jaws close is defined as malocclusion **(Fig. 5)**.

Etiology

The etiology of malocclusion is given in **Table 3**.

Classification

Malocclusion can be broadly classified based on the facial plane in which the malocclusion occurs **(Table 4)**.

Treatment

Treatment of malocclusion is divided into two active phases and one passive phase:

- *First active phase*: This phase of treatment occurs during mixed dentition period. Myofunctional appliances and habit breaking appliances are used in this phase to break abnormal habits of the child like tongue thrusting, thumb sucking, lip sucking, etc. Myofunctional appliances are used for narrow jaw and skeletal malocclusion. Examples of myofunctional appliances are—expansion plate and twin block appliance. The duration of this phase is about 6–15 months.

- *Second active phase*: Children undergo this phase of treatment when all the permanent teeth have erupted.

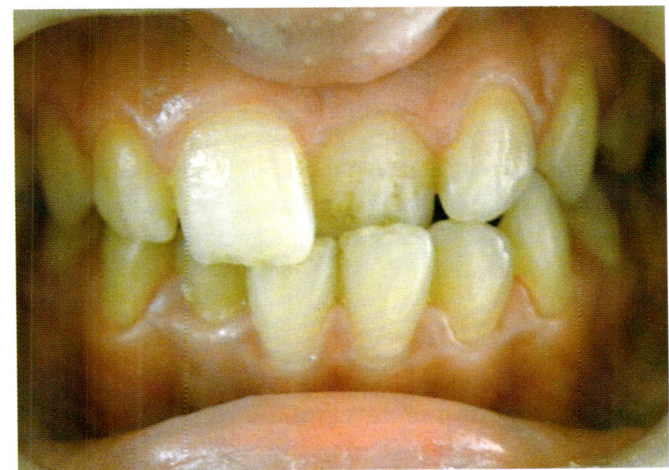

Fig. 5: Malocclusion.

Table 2: Treatment of periodontal disease.		
Medical interventions	*Nonmedical interventions*	*Other interventions*
• Oral prophylaxis • Oral and systemic antibiotics • Use of mouth washes • Gingival and periodontal surgery (Gingivoplasty, gingivectomy, flap surgery) Mucogingival surgeries, guided tissue regeneration, synthetic bones grafts, etc.)	• Oral health education • Nutrition and diet counseling • Proper methods of oral hygiene maintenance • Use of toothpaste and tooth brush • Use of interproximal cleaning. Devices such as interdental brushes, dental floss and waterpik, etc. • Regular dental check-up	• Make oral healthcare more accessible and affordable • Improve the socioeconomic and literacy level of the population • Include oral healthcare in general health insurance

Table 3: Etiology of malocclusion.

Direct	Indirect	Distant

• Hereditary/congenital
• Abnormal pressure habits and functional aberrations
  – Abnormal suckling
  – Mouth breathing
  – Thumb and finger sucking
  – Tongue thrusting and sucking
  – Abnormal swallowing habits
• Local factors—abnormalities of number (supernumerary teeth and missing teeth)
• Abnormalities of tooth size and shape
• Abnormal labial frenum and mucosal barriers
• Premature tooth loss
• Prolonged retention of deciduous teeth
• Delayed eruption of permanent teeth
	Environmental factors
	• Prenatal causes such as trauma, maternal diet and metabolism, German measles, certain drugs, and position in utero
	• Postnatal causes such as birth injury, cerebral palsy, and temporomandibular joint injury
		• Poor nutritional status, deficiencies of vitamin D, calcium and phosphates
		• Endocrine imbalance such as hypothyroidism
		• Metabolic disturbances and muscular dystrophies
		• Infectious diseases such as poliomyelitis
		• Functional aberrations

Table 4: Classification of malocclusion based on the facial plane.

Sagittal plane	Transverse plane	Vertical plane
Class II malocclusion • Division 1 • Division 2 Class III malocclusion • True class III • Pseudo class III	• Cross-bite: Anterior and posterior • Scissor bite • Midline shift	• Deep bite • Open bite

Final correction of tooth position, and functional and skeletal problems are undertaken during this phase. Braces and invisalign are the treatment options. Duration is between 18 months and 24 months.

- *Passive phase*: Between two active phase is the passive phase of 1 ½ to 3 years during which the growth of the child is evaluated.

DENTAL FLUOROSIS

Fluoride is trace element which has a caries-preventive effect. The optimum level of fluoride in drinking water is 0.75–1 ppm. Dental and skeletal fluorosis is caused by fluoride content higher than 1 ppm. Dental fluorosis appears as chalky white or yellowish-brownish discoloration of the teeth, sometimes with structural defects in the enamel such as pitting of the surface. Children during the mixed dentition phase are at higher risk for fluorosis because their permanent successors are still forming. Adults and children older than 8 years do not get fluorosis **(Fig. 6)**.

Causes of Dental Fluorosis

- Exposure to high level of fluoride either from water, industrial pollution, diet rich in fluoride (sea food, rock salt, green leafy vegetables, etc.)

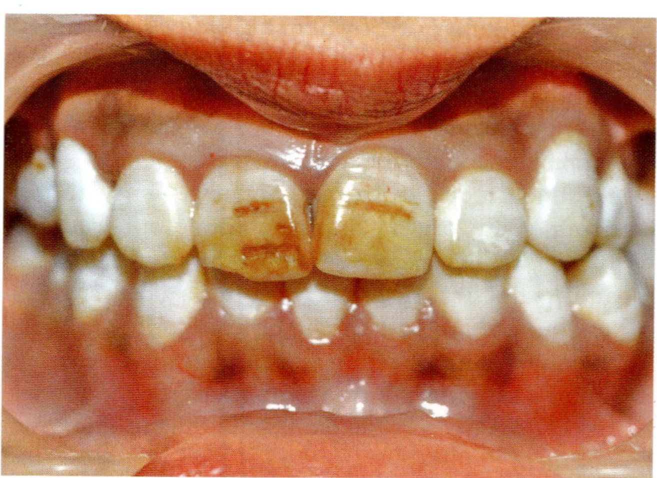

Fig. 6: Dental fluorosis.

- Patients having kidney disease and thyroid disease—affect the fluoride balance in body
- Deficiency of vitamin D, calcium, and phosphates.

Strategies for the Prevention of Dental Fluorosis

The strategies for the prevention of dental fluorosis is given in **Table 5**.

CHILDREN WITH SPECIAL HEALTHCARE NEEDS

Oral conditions like delayed tooth eruption, malocclusion, dental caries, dental anomalies, trauma, infections, and gingival enlargements are more frequent in infants or children with special healthcare needs. Children with special healthcare needs require different medications such as dilantin and phenobarbital (prescribed for

Table 5: Strategies for the prevention of dental fluorosis.

Primary prevention	Secondary prevention	Tertiary prevention
• Specific guidelines on the use and appropriate dose levels of fluoride supplements, and use of fluoride toothpaste for young children • In high fluoride areas • Provide an alternate supply of drinking water • Employ defluoridation techniques at the community level	• Improve the nutritional status, especially of expecting mothers, newborns and children up to the age 12 years • Treat other causes of fluoride toxicity such as kidney and thyroid diseases, etc.	Treat the discolored/disfigured dentition by appropriate esthetic treatment such as a bleaching, microabrasion, laminate veneers, etc.

epilepsy) which cause an array of dental problems and gingival enlargement. These medicines also cause dry mouth syndrome which increases the chances of dental caries. Regular dental referrals and follow-up is a prerequisite for these children. The children with special needs should visit the dentist within 6 months of eruption of the first tooth or at 12 months of age, just like normal children. Dental treatments may require additional time to accommodate the child's condition, medications, behavior, and complexity of care.

Preventive services include the following:

- Regular periodic examinations of the dentition and oral cavity, keeping into consideration the medical condition of the patient.
- Educating the patient and their family members about the importance of oral health and ways to maintain good oral hygiene.
- Providing counseling and guidance to age-appropriate children on nonnutritive habits, injury prevention, and tobacco use/substance abuse.
- Setting up periodic appointments for topical fluoride application based upon caries risk assessment and also prescribing dietary fluoride supplements in accordance with child's age, caries risk, and drinking water's fluoride level.
- Frequent oral prophylactic services on the basis of caries and periodontal risk factors.

ORAL MANIFESTATION OF NUTRITIONAL DEFICIENCY

Nutritional deficiencies develop when body metabolic requirements are not matched by intake and absorption. Factors causing the deficiency are many but often social, economic, medical, and even psychiatric factors play a major role. Vitamins and minerals are necessary for appropriate rapid cell turnover of the oral mucosa. The oral cavity manifests early signs of nutritional disorders and other systemic disease because of its unique anatomic

Table 6: Oral manifestation of nutritional deficiency.

Deficiency	Systemic effects	Oral effects
Vitamin A	Xerophthalmia	Leukoplakia, hyper-keratosis of oral epithelium
Thiamine B1	Neuritis, cardiac failure, and beriberi	None
Riboflavin B2	Dermatitis	Angular stomatitis, glossitis
Nicotinamide (Niacin B3)	Pellagra, central nervous system (CNS), diarrhea, and dementia	Glossitis, stomatitis, and gingivitis
Vitamin B12	Pernicious anemia	Glossitis and aphthae
Vitamin C	Scurvy	Gingival swelling and bleeding
Folic acid	Macrocytic anemia	Glossitis, aphthae, and atrophy of lingual papillae
Vitamin D	Rickets and osteomalacia	Hypocalcification of teeth and malformation

nature which in turn helps the practitioner to detect the nutritional disorder at an early stage and in turn initiate appropriate therapy **(Table 6)**.

ROLE OF PEDIATRIC DENTISTRY IN WORLDWIDE COMMON PROBLEMS

A pediatric dentist can help in various other problems such as oral habits and trauma cases. Variety of appliances and plates are given to the children with habits such as thumb sucking, mouth breathing, tongue thrusting, bruxism, or lip biting. These appliances can be removable or fixed. These habit of breaking appliances aids in discontinuing the harmful habit. Mostly the duration of using these appliances is 6–8 weeks depending on patient's cooperation and willingness to wear them.

In case of injury on tooth involving various structures can be treated by using various methods of repairs and splinting. Even avulsed tooth can be successfully replanted if it is brought urgently to the pediatric dentist in suitable medium such as saliva, milk, saline, coconut water, and lens solution. The preventive mouth guards can also help in case of aggressive sports activities.

■ SUGGESTED READING

1. American Academy of Pediatric Dentistry Foundation. Establishing a dental home: Using the American Academy of Pediatric Dentistry's Caries Risk Assessment Tool (CAT) as a first step. Chicago IL: American Academy of Pediatric Dentistry Foundation; 2007.
2. American Academy of Pediatric Dentistry, Council on Clinical Affairs. Definition of early childhood caries (ECC). Chicago IL: American Academy of Pediatric Dentistry; 2005-2006.
3. American Academy of Pediatric Dentistry. The use of a caries-risk assessment tool (CAT) for infants, children, and adolescents. Pediatr Dent. 2002;24(7):15-7.
4. American Academy of Pediatrics. Children's Health Topics. Elk Grove Village: American Academy of Pediatrics; 2007.
5. American Academy of Pediatrics. Oral Health Risk Assessment Training for Pediatricians and Other Child Health Professionals. Elk Grove Village, IL: American Academy of Pediatrics; 2005.
6. American Dental Council on Scientific Affairs. Professionally applied topical fluoride: Evidence-based clinical recommendations. JADA. 2006;137(8):1151-9.
7. Gardner DG. Some current concepts on the pathology of ameloblastomas. Oral Surg Oral Med Oral Path. 1996;82(6): 660-9.
8. Gerbase AC, Rowley JT, Mertens TE. Global epidemiology of sexually transmitted disease. Lancet. 1998;351(Suppl 3):2-4.
9. Glich M, Musyla B. Oral manifestations of AIDS related diseases as markers for immunosuppression. Oral Surg Oral Med Oral Pathol. 1994;77:344-50.
10. Wilson DF, Grappin G, Miquel JL. Oral Diseases in the Tropics. New York: Oxford University Press; 1989.

11

Accidents and Poisoning in the Tropics

Jaydeep Choudhury

SECTION

Animal Bites

Jaydeep Choudhury

INTRODUCTION

Rabies is a cause of serious encephalitis with fatal outcome. It is a zoonotic disease and transmission to humans occurs by bite or scratch of an infected animal. In India, the transmitting animal is dog in more than 95% cases.[1] Though rabies is fatal once symptoms of the disease develop, it is almost 100% preventable if prophylactic measures are instituted soon after the exposure.[2]

PROBLEMS OF RABIES INFECTION IN CHILDREN

In India and other developing countries, 50–60% of all rabies deaths occur in children less than 15 years of age. There are several reasons as to why children are more susceptible:[1,3]

- Children play in the streets and are more prone to dog bites. Because of their playful nature, they also tend to tease dogs and in consequence, dogs attack them.
- Because of their short stature, bites on heads and neck and upper part of the body are more common and bites tend to be severe. This results in greater risk for infection with relatively shorter incubation period. Because of their short stature, even bites on lower parts of the body may result in shorter incubation period.
- Many times, because of the fear of painful injections that may be given, they even tend to hide the fact that they were bitten.
- As children have soft skin even minor scratches and trivial bites may result in category III exposures.

Children at high risk or having pets at home need to be given pre-exposure prophylaxis to avoid painful rabies immunoglobulin infiltration if bitten in future whereas only wound care and booster vaccination would suffice.

ETIOLOGY

Causative Virus

Rabies virus is a bullet-shaped, single-stranded ribonucleic acid (RNA) virus, which belong to family Rhabdoviridae and genus *Lyssavirus*. It causes acute encephalitis in human being. The virus cannot penetrate intact skin but can penetrate intact mucosa. Rabies virus basically infects animals. Two cycles namely, sylvatic and urban cycles in the animals help this disease to exist in the world. Unless both these cycles are totally stopped, rabies will continue to stay.

Transmitting Animals

Apart from dogs, which are the main culprits, other warm-blooded animals like cat, fox, jackals, etc. transmit rabies. The domestic animals like cow, buffalo, goat, pig, and sheep also can transmit rabies when they are bitten and get infected by rabid animals. Raw milk from an infected cow can transmit rabies virus as rabies virus can penetrate intact mucus membrane. Boiling the milk kills the virus. Monkey can also transmit this disease if they are infected. Domestic rats do not transmit rabies virus but wild rodents do transmit.[4] Man-to-man transmission is rare, except in cases of cornea transplant from donors with undiagnosed rabies.

SIGNS OF RABIES IN ANIMALS

Animals suffering from usually have a nonspecific prodromal phase. Some animals develop aggressive behavior, irritability, and exaggerated reaction to external stimuli and increased salivation. This is typically described as furious rabies. This state is followed by paralytic phase characterized by weakness of one or more limbs and dribbling saliva from dropped lower jaw. The tongue or jaw may droop due to cranial nerve dysfunction and paralysis of muscles of the head and neck. Difficulty in making routine vocalizations leads to altered phonation. Death is due to cardiac and respiratory failure. Sometimes ataxia and primary paralysis may predominate with no overt aggressive signs, described as "dumb" rabies.

Incubation period: It usually ranges from 20 to 180 days, in most cases it is within 30–60 days. In extreme cases it might be as early as 9 days and as late as 1 year.[4,5] Incubation period is shorter if the bite is closer to brain. Since there are no symptoms during the incubation period, it is very difficult to diagnose early.

CLINICAL TYPES

Two types of clinical rabies are described. Furious type is seen in 80% and paralytic type in 20% (Dumb rabies). Both types are common for human and canine rabies.

The virus first multiplies in striated muscles, ascends along axons from periphery to spinal cord and eventually to neurons in the brain. There is neuronal destruction in the brainstem and medulla and severest changes in pons and IV ventricles but cortex are spared.

MODES OF TRANSMISSION

Common modes:
- Bite and scratch from infected animals.
- Lick—on broken skin and intact mucus membranes.

Rare:
- Aerosol transmission.
- Organ transplantation.

Bites by insectivorous bats can also transmit rabies and rabies can spread also by aerosol infection in bat-infested caves but these are not problems of India.

CLINICAL FEATURES

The furious type of rabies presents with acute neurological phase characterized by hydrophobia, aerophobia, photophobia, and dysphagia. No survival is so far reported in unvaccinated infected persons in the world literature. The difference of the presenting features in these two types is shown in the **Table 1**.

DIAGNOSIS

Diagnosis is mainly based on clinical signs of hydrophobia and aerophobia in the furious type of rabies. Confirmation of diagnosis is based on the following:
- Detection of Negri body in brain by Sellers stain
- Detection of virus antigen by immunofluorescence
- Mouse pathogenicity (biological test).

Table 1: Clinical features in furious and paralytic type of rabies.

Furious type (80%)	*Paralytic type (20%)*
• Tingling/numbness at bite site	• Tingling/numbness at bite site
• Nonspecific symptoms (Fever, malaise, headache, etc.)	• Nonspecific symptoms (Fever, malaise, headache, etc.)
• Hydrophobia and aerophobia	• Ascending paralysis
• Photophobia	• Coma
• Death in 3–5 days	• Death in 7–21 days
• (Cardiac and respiratory failure)	• (Cardiac and respiratory failure)

Detection of antibodies in cerebrospinal fluid or serum of unimmunized persons and detection of viral nucleic acid from infected tissue is also possible. Virus can be isolated from saliva.

MANAGEMENT

In rabies-endemic country like India, every animal bite is potentially suspected as a rabid animal bite, the treatment should be started immediately. Rabies has long incubation period. Prophylactic postexposure treatment should be started at the earliest to ensure that the individual will be immunized before the rabies virus reaches the nervous system. The classification of animal bite for postexposure prophylaxis (PEP) has been based on the World Health Organization (WHO) recommendations **(Table 2)**.[5]

Approach to Postexposure Prophylaxis

The PEP consists of the following three parameters and should be done simultaneously as per the category of the bites:
1. Management of animal bite wound(s)
2. *Passive immunization*: Rabies immunoglobulins (RIGs) and rabies monoclonal antibody (mAb)
3. *Active immunization*: Antirabies vaccines (ARV).

Management of Animal Bite Wound

Wound toilet: Since the rabies virus enters the human body through a bite or scratch, it is imperative to remove as much saliva as possible. Since the rabies virus can persist and even multiply at the site of bite for a long time, wound toilet must be performed even if the patient reports late **(Table 3)**.[1,5]

Prompt and gentle thorough washing with soap or detergent and flushing the wound with running water for 10 minutes can do this.

The application of irritants is unnecessary and damaging. In case irritants have been applied on the wound, enough gentle washing with soap or detergent to remove the extraneous material, especially oil should be

Table 2: Type of contact, exposure and recommended postexposure prophylaxis.

Category type of contact	Type of exposure	Recommended postexposure prophylaxis
I. Touching or feeding of animals Licks on intact skin	None	None, if reliable case history is available
II. Nibbling of uncovered skin Minor scratches or abrasions without bleeding	Minor	Wound management + Antirabies vaccine
III. Single or multiple transdermal bites or scratches, licks on broken skin Contamination of mucus membrane with saliva (i.e. licks)	Severe	Wound management + Rabies immunoglobulin/monoclonal antibody – Antirabies vaccine

Table 3: Principles of wound management.

Wound management	Purpose
Steps to be taken: Wash under running tap water for at least 10 minutes	Mechanical removal of virus from the wound
Washing the wound with soap and water, dry and apply disinfectant	Inactivation of the virus
Biological infiltration of immunoglobulins in the depth and around the wound in category III exposures	Neutralization of the virus
Avoid: Touching the wound with bare hand Applying irritants or corrosives like soil, chillies, oil, herbs, chalk, betel leaves, etc.	

done followed by flushing with copious amount of water for 10 minutes immediately.

Broken skin can be assessed by "Spirit test". If there is doubt then a spirit swab is applied on the affected area and if there is tingling/burning sensation, skin is broken and would require local RIG infiltration and vaccination after thorough wound wash and antiseptics.

Application of antiseptic: After thorough washing and drying the wound, any one of the available chemical agents should be applied, viz. povidone iodine (solution), Alcohol, chloroxylenol, chlorhexidine gluconate and cetrimide solution in appropriate recommended dilution.

Local infiltration of RIGs: In category III bites, RIG should be infiltrated in the depth and around the wound to inactivate the locally present virus.

Suturing of wound: It should be avoided as far as possible. If surgical intervention is unavoidable, minimum loose sutures should be applied after adequate local treatment along with proper infiltration of RIGs. Cauterization of wound is not recommended.

Tetanus toxoid injection (Antitetanus prophylaxis): This should be given to those children who had not received a booster dose. A properly immunized child can only take one dose of tetanus toxid, if there is a lapse of a period of 5 years from the last dose of tetanus toxoid.

To prevent sepsis in the wound, a suitable course of an antibiotic may be recommended.

Rabies Immunoglobulin

The RIG provides passive immunity to tide over the initial phase of the infection. It acts in the form of ready-made antibody to tide over initial phase of combating rabies infection. RIG has ability to bind to rabies virus, resulting in neutralization of the virus in the wound itself. As per WHO recommendation (2018), injecting RIG only into the wounds is required to neutralize the virus in the wounds, giving rest of RIG as intramuscular (IM) is of little or no value to the patient, rather this enhances the danger of reaction and also contradicts the effect of vaccine given concurrently.[5]

Two types of RIGs are available:
1. *Equine rabies immunoglobulin (ERIG):* ERIG is of heterologous origin raised by hyperimmunization of horses. The currently manufactured ERIGs are highly purified and enzyme refined, with these preparations, the occurrence of adverse reaction has been significantly reduced.
2. *Human rabies immunoglobulin (HRIG):* As it is homologous, HRIG is free from the side effects encountered in a serum of heterologous origin, and because of its longer half-life, it is given in half the dose of equine antirabies serum.

Dose of rabies RIGs: (1) The dose of ERIG is 40 IU per kg body weight of patient, up to a maximum of 3,000 IU. Skin testing for sensitivity is no longer recommended by WHO. The ERIG produced in India contains 300 IU/mL. (2) The dose of the HRIG is 20 IU per kg body weight (maximum 1,500 IU). HRIG preparation is available in concentration of 150 IU/mL.[2]

Administration of immunoglobulins: As much of the calculated dose of RIG as is anatomically feasible should be infiltrated into and around the wounds. Care should be taken to infiltrate each and every abrasion and scratch as even a single puncture wound left can cause rabies. The remaining RIG left in the vial, should not be injected at a distant site IM, but should be utilized to infiltrate wounds of other patient. RIG contains preservative. It can be stored for use subsequently under aseptic conditions. Only local wound infiltration of RIG also helps minimize the reaction. Sometimes the calculated dose of RIG may not be sufficient to infiltrate all wounds, particularly in severe and multiple wounds, especially in small children. In such situations, it is advisable to dilute the RIG in sterile normal saline to a volume sufficient for infiltration of all wounds. The total recommended dose of rabies immunoglobulin must not be exceeded as it may interfere and suppress the antibody production following antirabies vaccination in the child. If immunoglobulin was not administered when vaccination was begun, it can be administered up to the 7th day after the administration of the first dose of vaccine. RIG should never be administered in the same syringe of vaccine administration.

Rabies Monoclonal Antibody

Rabies mAb is the latest development in passive immunization against rabies. A single mAb product against rabies, was licensed in India in 2017. It is a human IgG1 mAb that binds to the ectodomain of the glycoprotein G. It has been demonstrated to be safe and effective in clinical trials. mAb neutralizes a broad panel of globally prevalent rabies virus isolates. The advantages of mAb products include large-scale production with standardized quality, greater effectiveness than RIG, elimination of the use of animals in the production process, and reduction in the risk of adverse events.

The recommended dose is 3.33 IU/kg. The available formulation contains 40 IU/mL. It is also given by local infiltration at bite wound. There is no contraindication for mAb use.[2,3]

In circumstances where no immunoglobulin or mAb are available, greater emphasis should be given to proper wound toileting followed by vaccination with double dose on day 0 at two different sites intramuscularly (0 day—two doses on left and right deltoid, following the single dose on each day, i.e. days 3, 7, 14, or 28). It is emphasized that doubling the first dose of cell culture vaccines (CCVs) is not a replacement to RIG. A full course of vaccine should follow thorough wound cleansing and passive immunization.

Antirabies Vaccines

Active immunization is achieved by administration of safe and potent ARV. The vaccines available at present are Modern CCV.[2]

- Cell culture vaccines
  - Human diploid cell vaccine (HDCV)
  - Purified chick embryo cell vaccine (PCECV)
  - Purified vero cell rabies vaccine (PVRV)
- Purified duck embryo vaccine (PDEV)

All these CCVs are safe for clinical use. The dosage schedules of these cell culture rabies vaccines are same, irrespective of the body weight or age of the child.

Storage and transportation: It is recommended that these vaccines should be kept and transported at a temperature range of 2–8°C. Vaccines should never be frozen.

Reconstitution and storage: The lyophilized vaccine should be reconstituted with the diluent provided with the vaccine immediately prior to use. In case of unforeseen delay, it should be used within 6–8 hours of reconstitution.

Adverse effects with CCVs/PDEV: The CCV and PDEV are safe and usually do not produce any side effects. Rarely, the local side effects are pain and tenderness at the injection site. Systemic side effects though rare may include fever, malaise, urticaria, and sometimes lymphadenopathy. Generally these side effects are self-limiting. In such cases Chick embryo vaccine should be replaced with vero cell-based vaccine and vice versa for doses next time to the patient.

Switch over from one brand or type of vaccine to the other: Switching from one brand or type of CCV/PDEV to other brand/type should not be encouraged in routine practice. However, under unavoidable circumstances, available brand/type of rabies vaccine may be used to complete PEP.

◼ STRATEGIES OF PREVENTION

The WHO recommends two main immunization strategies for the prevention of human rabies.

Postexposure Prophylaxis

It includes extensive and thorough wound washing at the site of exposure, RIG administration if indicated and administration of a course of rabies vaccine.

The indication and procedure for PEP depend on the type of contact with the suspected rabid animal and immunization status of the patient.[5]

- *Category I exposure*: No PEP is required.
- *Category II exposure*: Immediate vaccination is recommended.

- *Category III exposure*: Immediate vaccination and administration of RIG.

The first dose of rabies vaccine should be administered as soon as possible after exposure. Vaccine should always be administered when a category III exposure is recognized, even months or years after the contact. The probability of developing rabies declines progressively during the 12 months after the exposure with clinical rabies occurring rarely after 12 months.

If an individual has a repeat exposure <3 months after a previous exposure, and has already received a complete PEP, only wound treatment is required; neither vaccine nor RIG is needed. For repeat exposures occurring >3 months till years after the last PEP, the PEP schedule for previously immunized individuals should be followed. But RIG is not indicated in these situations. **Table 4** shows the PEP in categorywise exposure.[4,5]

Pre-exposure Prophylaxis

The process of administration of rabies vaccine before exposure to rabies.

Intradermal (ID) injection sites for any age is the deltoid region, anterolateral thigh, or suprascapular regions. The recommended site for IM administration is the deltoid area of the arm for adults and children aged ≥2 years, and the anterolateral area of the thigh for children aged <2 years. Rabies vaccine should not be administered IM in the gluteal area.

The WHO recommends two-site ID vaccine administered on days 0 and 7 or one-site IM vaccine administration on days 0 and 7.[5]

Guidelines for use of intradermal rabies vaccination (IDRV) are as follows:[2,4,5]

- Currently the following vaccines have been approved by Drugs Controller General of India (DCGI) for IDRV. However, WHO guidelines, 2018 mention that any vaccine for IM use can be used for ID route as well.
- Intradermal injections must be administered by trained staff.
- Vaccine vials must be stored at 2–8°C after reconstitution.
- The total content of reconstituted vial should be used as soon as possible, latest within 8 hours.
- Any leftover of reconstituted vaccine should be discarded after 8 hours of reconstitution/at the end of the day.
- Vaccine given ID should raise a visible and palpable bleb of 3–4 mm size on the skin.
- In the event that the dose is inadvertently given subcutaneously or intramuscularly or in the event of spillage, a new dose should be given ID in nearby site.
- If PEP is sought after discontinuation, it should be resumed and not restarted.
- There is no need for PEP in case of consumption of raw milk from a rabid cow.

Postexposure Prophylaxis in Immunocompromised Children

The best PEP options available should be used, regardless of the route of vaccine administration. Thorough wound cleaning as first aid to bite victims is of utmost importance in immunocompromised. When feasible, the rabies virus

Table 4: Postexposure prophylaxis (PEP) by category of exposure.			
	Category I exposure	*Category II exposure*	*Category III exposure*
Immunologically naive individuals of all age groups	Washing of exposed skin surfaces: No PEP required	Wound washing and immediate vaccination: • 2-sites ID on days 0, 3, and 7 *or* • 1-site IM on days 0, 3, 7, and between days 14 and 28 *or* • 2-sites IM on days 0 and one-site IM on days 7 and 21 RIG is not indicated	Wound washing and immediate vaccination: • 2-sites ID on days 0, 3, and 7 *or* • 1-site IM on days 0, 3, 7, and between days 14 and 28 *or* • 2-sites IM on days 0 and one-site IM on days 7 and 21 RIG administration is recommended
Previously immunized individuals of all age groups	Washing of exposed skin surfaces No PEP required	Wound washing and immediate vaccination • 1-site ID on days 0 and 3 *or* • At 4-sites ID on day 0 *or* • At 1-site IM on days 0 and 3 RIG is not indicated	Wound washing and immediate vaccination • 1-site ID on days 0 and 3 *or* • At 4-sites ID on day 0 *or* • At 1-site IM on days 0 and 3 RIG is not indicated

Source: World Health Organization. Rabies vaccines: WHO Position Paper, April 2018 Recommendations. Vaccine. 2018;36:5500-3.
(ID: intradermal; IM: intramuscular; RIG: rabies immunoglobulin)

neutralizing antibody response should be determined 2–4 weeks after vaccination to assess whether an additional dose of vaccine is required.

Coadministration

Rabies vaccines can be coadministered with other inactivated and live vaccines, using separate syringes and different injection sites.

SOME TYPICAL SITUATIONS

- *Vaccination status of the biting animal*: Vaccinated animals can transmit rabies if the vaccination of the biting animal was ineffective for any reason. Thus a history of rabies vaccination in an animal is not always a guarantee that the biting animal is not rabid.[4]
- *Provoked or unprovoked bite*: It should not be considered as criteria for denying vaccination. It can be difficult to understand what a dog considers provocation for an attack.
- *Observation of biting animal*: The postexposure vaccination may be modified if the biting animal remains healthy throughout an observation period of 10 days as by then three doses of vaccine due on days 0, 3, and 7 would have been given. Subsequently, PEP may be modified and made beneficial and effective for future. The observation period of 10 days is valid for dogs and cats only.[4]
- *Bite by wild animals*: Bites by all wild animals including foxes, wild dogs, jackals, mongooses, and others should be treated as category III exposure.
- *Bites by other domestic and peridomestic animals*: Bites by monkeys and squirrel should be given PEP depending on the category of exposure. Bites by other mammals such as horses, pigs, cattle, donkeys, and camels should be evaluated based on circumstances of bite. Bites by house rats and rabbits ordinarily do not require PEP, but when exposures occur in strange/peculiar/wild situations and when in doubt the physician may consider providing rabies PEP. The bites by snakes, lizards, birds, and insects do not require rabies PEP.
- *Bat rabies*: Bat rabies has not been conclusively proven in India and hence exposure to bats does not ordinarily warrant treatment.[4]
- *Human-to-human transmission*: There has never been a well-documented case of human-to-human transmission, other than the few cases resulting from organ transplant.[1]

REFERENCES

1. Association for Prevention and Control of Rabies in India. (2004). Assessing Burden of Rabies in India, WHO Sponsored National Multi-centric Rabies Survey, May 2004, KIMS, Bangalore, India. [online] Available from: http://www.apcri.org/pdf/WHO-APCRI%20Survey%20Report.pdf. [Last accessed on November, 2019].
2. Balasubramanian S, Shah A, Pemde HK, et al. Indian Academy of Pediatrics (IAP) Advisory Committee on Vaccines and Immunization Practices (ACVIP) Recommended Immunization Schedule (2018-19) and Update on Immunization for Children Aged 0 Through 18 Years. Indian Pediatr. 2018;55(12):1066-74.
3. Gogtay NJ, Munshi R, Ashwath Narayana DH, et al. Comparison of a Novel Human Rabies Monoclonal Antibody to Human Rabies Immunoglobulin for Postexposure Prophylaxis: A Phase 2/3, Randomized, Single-Blind, Noninferiority, Controlled Study. Clin Infect Dis. 2018;66(3):387-95.
4. Sudarshan MK. Rabies. In: Parthasarathy A, Kundu R, Agrawal R, et al. (Eds). Textbook of Pediatric Infectious Diseases, 1st edition. New Delhi: Jaypee Brothers Medical Publishers (P) Ltd.; 2013.
5. World Health Organization. Rabies vaccines: WHO Position Paper, April 2018 Recommendations. Vaccine. 2018;36:5500-3.

11.2 CHAPTER

Snakebite

Jaydeep Choudhury, Aniruddha Ghosh

INTRODUCTION

The World Health Organization (WHO) in 2009 included snakebite in the list of "neglected tropical diseases." The highest burden of snakebite is borne by south Asia, southeast Asia, and sub-Saharan Africa. India is at the top of the list among southeast Asian countries.[1] The four most common venomous snakes found in India are: The Indian cobra, *Naja naja*; the Indian krait, *Bungarus caeruleus*; Russell's viper, *Daboia russelii*; and the saw-scaled viper, *Echis carinatus*.[2]

There are three classes of poisonous snakes available in India:[2]

1. *Cardiotoxic and neurotoxic*: Cobra and krait. They are identified by hood-like head of cobra or small triangular head of krait, pit between eye and nostril, large belly scale, compressed tail, and characteristic bite mark of two fangs with or without other teeth.
2. *Hematotoxic*: Viper. They have a V-shaped mark on their head and white belly. They hiss loudly.
3. *Myotoxic*: Sea snakes.

CLINICAL EFFECTS[1]

- *Local tissue*: Pain, swelling, rhabdomyolysis, and lymphadenopathy.
- *Systemic*: Vomiting, nausea, abdominal pain, headache, tachycardia, and hypotension.
- *Neurological*: Blurred vision, bulbar/facial weakness, ptosis (may be an early sign of progressive muscle paralysis), lethargy, and loss of consciousness.
- *Hematological*: Defibrination, thrombocytopenia, and clinical bleeding (like hematemesis).
- *Others*:
  - *Respiratory*: Respiratory paralysis may occur due to neurotoxic component.
  - *Genitourinary*: Dark urine in hematuria may be due to myoglobinuria. Subsequently, acute renal failure develops.
  - *Musculoskeletal*: Generalized muscle pain due to muscle destruction from myotoxins. It is common with sea snake bites.
  - *Endocrinal*: Acute pituitary/adrenal crisis from infarction of anterior pituitary in cases of Russell's viper bite.

LABORATORY INVESTIGATIONS AND MONITORING

The decision to start snake antivenom (SAV) should be based on clinical judgement. The *20-minute whole blood clotting time (WBCT20)* is used to confirm hematotoxic snake bite:[3]

- Clean, dry, new, plain glass test tube is used.
- Few milliliters of blood from patient is put into it and kept undisturbed for 20 minutes.
- Then the tube is tilted to see if the blood has clotted.
- Absence of clotting confirms hematotoxic snakebite, especially viper.
- Only plain glass tubes are to be used. If the tube is made of other material or detergent is present on its wall, then surface activation of XII-Hageman factor may not result and the test will be invalid.

Blood should be drawn for following ancillary tests, if necessary, before antivenom is started:

- *Clotting factors*: Prothrombin time (PT) and partial thromboplastin time, fibrinogen, and platelet count.
- Full blood count, urea, and creatinine.
- Creatinine phosphokinase (CPK) and d-dimer (if facility available).

Urine examination (routine and microscopic), if available, should be done. Monitor HR, BP, and oxygen saturation. Gradual desaturation may be the indicator of respiratory muscle paralysis.[2]

MANAGEMENT

First Aid

- A wide crepe bandage should be applied from distal to proximal and cover the bitten area to occlude lymphatic spread. The wound should be cleaned with saline.
- Immobilization of the bitten extremity with a splint or sling.[3]
- Tetanus prophylaxis as indicated by immunization status. Consider tetanus immunoglobulin according to standard national recommendations.
- Do not apply suction, arterial tourniquet, or incise bitten area.
- The pressure immobilization bandage may be removed if there is no clinical or laboratory evidence of envenomation or once envenomation administration has been commenced.
- Even if there is no clinical evidence of envenomation and pressure immobilization bandage has been removed, the patient should be observed at least for 24 hours; then clinical and laboratory assessment should be repeated. The patient may be discharged if the second clinical and laboratory assessment shows no evidence of envenomation. Periods of observation may need to be longer in certain circumstances **(Flowchart 1)**.

Local Wound Management

- Wound should be cleaned and left open.
- If swelling or tenderness is present, the proximal edge and time of detection should be marked so that progression can be monitored.
- Similarly, the circumference of the limb at the level of edema should be recorded.
- Fasciotomy may be done to prevent compartment syndrome.
- Wound debridement may be required after 3–5 days.

  Table 1 summarizes the Do's and Don'ts of snakebite management.

Optimize ABC

Assisted ventilation and fluid resuscitation may be required and are important components even before specific treatment is started.

Specific Treatment

Polyvalent antivenin/SAV/anti-snake venom serum (AVS) with venoms of four common snakes, cobra, krait and two types of viper, are available. 1 mL of SAV neutralizes around 0.6 mg of cobra venom, 0.45 mg of saw-scaled viper venom, 0.6 mg of Russell's viper venom, and 0.45 mg of common krait venom.[2]

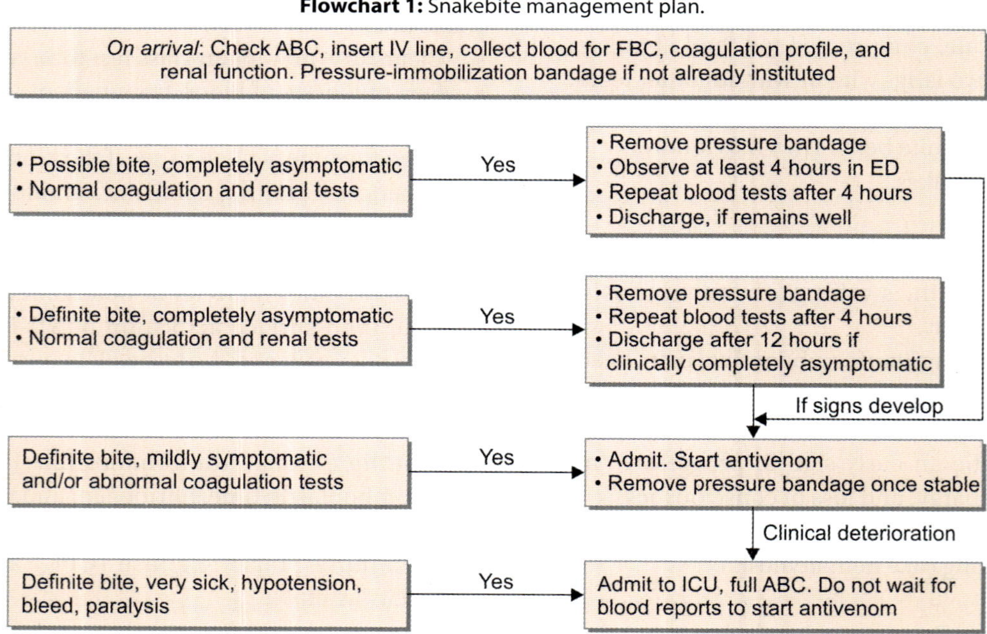

Flowchart 1: Snakebite management plan.

(ED: Emergency Department; FBC: full blood count; ICU: intensive care unit; IV: intravenous)

Table 1: Do's and Don'ts of snakebite management.

Do's	Don'ts
Do it R.I.G.H.T R = Reassure patient I = Immobilize properly, do not obstruct blood flow GH = Get to Hospital immediately T = Tell the physician about clinical symptoms such as ptosis	**Do not** • Use local incisions/puncture • Attempt to suck venom out • Use superstitious rituals such as black stone, etc. • Tie tight bands proximal to bitten area • Apply chemicals, herbs, etc.

Who should be given AVS?

Bite by any species may show no specific systemic effect due to presence of a "dry bite" where no venom is introduced. Some victims may not recall the bite as there may be minimal pain. Bite marks are not a good predictor of the degree of envenomation. Severe envenomations have occurred without obvious bite marks. These cause great dilemma in the management of snakebite.[1-4]

Severe envenomation: Clinical and laboratory pointers—
- Weakness includes ptosis, hypoventilation, oliguria, myoglobinuria, and altered consciousness.
- Collapse, shock, or convulsion after confirmed bite.
- Early spontaneous bleeding.
- Early tender lymph node swelling.
- Rapid spread of local features of snakebite.
- Positive nonclotting at WBCT20, INR (international normalized ratio) >1.2, or PT > 4–5 seconds longer than control, and thrombocytopenia.[1]

Anti-snake venom serum should not be started in those who only have minor headache, abdominal pain, nausea or vomiting, and lymphadenopathy.[3]

Anti-snake Venom Serum

Each vial contains 10 mL of antivenin. The total dose necessary in children ranges from 4 to 10 vials depending on the clinical progress and stability of the patient.

Two methods have been recommended by the WHO:[1]

1. *Intravenous "push" injection:* Reconstituted freeze-dried antivenom or neat liquid AVS is injected slowly (not more than 2 mL/min).
2. *Intravenous infusion:* Reconstituted or freeze-dried AVS is dissolved in isotonic intravenous fluids (5 mL/kg of isotonic fluids, i.e. normal saline/5% dextrose) and infused over 30–60 minutes at a constant rate.

Prediction of Reaction

Since the reactions of AVS are not IgE mediated and only lead to delay in initiation of therapy, skin tests are not recommended. If reaction to horse serum occurs, then prompt treatment has to be given.[1]

Reactions to anti-snake venom serum:
- Early anaphylactic reactions (within 1–180 minutes), IgG-mediated complement activation, or activation of mast cells and basophils causes reactions ranging from fever, rigor, and urticaria to severe circulatory collapse, bronchospasm, and angioedema.
- Pyrogenic reactions after 1–2 hours of AVS therapy initiation.
- *Late serum sickness type reactions* (1–12 days, mean 7 days after treatment): Fever, itching, rash, myalgia, arthralgia, lymphadenitis, mononeuritis multiplex, proteinuria, etc.[1-3]

Treatment of reactions: At the earliest signs of reactions, epinephrine (0.01 mg/kg; 1 in 10,000) should be administered. Corticosteroid (hydrocortisone 2 mg/kg/dose), antihistaminic (chlorpheniramine maleate 0.2 mg/kg intravenous infusion over few minutes), and ranitidine should be administered before starting antivenin as there is risk of anaphylaxis. Adrenaline, oxygen, fluid, and equipment for airway management should be kept ready for emergency.

For late reactions, chlorpheniramine (0.25 mg/kg/day) for 5 days along with prednisolone (0.7 mg/kg/day) is to be used.[1,2]

Prevention: A study from Sri Lanka showed that epinephrine (0.25 mg/mL of 0.1% solution subcutaneously) along with hydrocortisone (200 mg intravenously) and promethazine (25 mg intravenously) in adult patients prevented severe adverse reactions by 43% at 1 hour and by 38% up to 48 hours after AVS administration.[5,6]

Endpoint of anti-snake venom serum therapy: Early clinical signs of improvement are subsidence of nausea, headache, myalgia, etc.; spontaneous hemorrhage stops within 15–30 minutes; bradycardia and shock within 30–60 minutes; and coagulopathy within 3–9 hours. Postsynaptic blockade starts improving in 30 minutes but may take hours to days to recover fully.[4,6,7]

If neuroparalysis or cardiac involvement worsens after 1–2 hours, coagulopathy does not improve or recurs after 6 hours, or spontaneous bleeding ensues after 1–2 hours, then the same dose of AVS is to be repeated. Readministration of AVS may be guided by 6-hourly WBCT20 test results.[2,7]

The only scenario where intramuscular AVS therapy is indicated is in absence of anyone capable of giving an intravenous injection, i.e. on expedition, or in absence of peripheral first aid station.[1]

If indicated, antivenin should be started as soon as possible and should not be withheld due to late presentation.[7]

Neuroparalysis: Neurotoxin of cobra and krait may produce curare-like neuromuscular blockade. Both neuroparalysis and respiratory paralysis may develop. Neostigmine should be administered in all suspected neurotoxic snakebite cases (0.04 mg/kg intramuscularly, may be repeated 2–4 hourly).[1,4] Constant ECG (electrocardiogram) monitoring should be done.

The snakebite management plan algorithm is shown in **Flowchart 1**.

Supportive Treatment

- Pain relief. Tetanus toxoid is to be given if not received accordingly in the past.
- Broad-spectrum antibiotic should not be started prophylactically. If cellulitis, osteomyelitis, septicemia, or necrotizing fasciitis develops, then only it has to be started.
- Renal failure, if develops, should be managed appropriately. Sometimes, dialysis has to be commenced with caution in the context of coagulopathy.
- Bleeding manifestations and disseminated intravascular coagulation (DIC) are life-threatening and should be controlled with blood products and heparin. Fresh frozen plasma (FFP) and platelet will not help unless sufficient antivenom is also given.

- Myoglobinuria is diagnosed by red- or brown-colored urine, false positive for occult blood with absent RBC, and markedly elevated serum CPK. Forced alkaline diuresis should be instituted and/or early dialysis can be performed if rapid elevation of potassium and creatinine occurs.
- Surgical debridement is performed, if required, especially in case of compartment syndrome.

■ REFERENCES

1. Regional Office for the South-East Asia, World Health Organization (WHO) (2016). Guidelines for the management of snake-bites, 2nd edition. [online] Available from: http://apps. searo.who.int/PDS_DOCS/B5255.pdf?ua=1. [Last accessed on December, 2019].
2. Warrell DA. Snakebite: a neglected problem in twenty-first century India. Natl Med J India. 2011;24(6):321-4.
3. Indian National Snake Bite Protocols 2007. First aid and snake bite prevention. Snakebite treatment. Support concepts. www. whoindia.org.int/linkfiles/bct_snake_bite_guidelines.pdf [Last accessed on December, 2019].
4. Warrell DA. Snake bite. Lancet. 2010;375(9708):77-88.
5. de Silva HA, Pathmeswaran A, Ranasinha CD, et al. Low-dose adrenaline, promethazine, and hydrocortisone in the prevention of acute adverse reactions to antivenom following snakebite: a randomized, double-blind, placebo-controlled trial. PLoS Med. 2011;8(5):e1000435.
6. Ariaratnam CA, Sheriff MH, Arambepola C, et al. Syndromic approach to treatment of snakebite in Sri Lanka based on results of a prospective national hospital-based survey of patients envenomed by identified snakes. Am J Trop Med Hyg. 2009;81(4):725-31.
7. Kulkarni ML, Anees S. Snake venom poisoning: experience with 633 cases. Indian Pediatr. 1994;31(10):1239-43.

Scorpion Sting

Janani Sankar

INTRODUCTION

Scorpion stings are not uncommon. Around 99 species of scorpion have been identified in India, but only two, *Mesobuthus tamulus* (the common red scorpion) and *Palamnaeus swammerdami*, are poisonous. Cardiac manifestations are common in Indian red scorpion envenomation.

PATHOPHYSIOLOGY

Scorpion venom acts at the presynaptic nerve terminals by activating the sodium channel and blocking the calcium-activated potassium channel resulting in an autonomic storm where both the sympathetic and the parasympathetic systems are activated. The toxin induces a predominantly alpha receptor stimulatory effect, resulting in pulmonary edema, myocardial dysfunction, tachycardia, shock, hypertension, and excessive sweating. Scorpion venom also suppresses secretion of insulin which in turns leads to hyperglycemia, lipolysis, and increased free fatty acid concentrations. Increased free fatty acids is considered an important contributory factor to the occurrence of arrhythmias and heart failure in scorpion sting victims.

CLINICAL FEATURES

Clinical manifestations may be local or systemic. The symptoms may progress to maximal severity in 3–5 hours and subside within 1–2 days. The local manifestations include intense pain at the site of sting, swelling, and ecchymosis. The "autonomic storm" is the most important manifestation of scorpion envenomation. The initial cholinergic stimulation leads to vomiting, salivation, sweating, and cold extremities, priapism and bradycardia. Sweating and salivation may persist for 6–12 hours. Presence of priapism has been found to be associated with myocardial dysfunction.[1]

Sympathetic system activation leads to tachypnea, pulmonary edema, tachycardia, arrhythmias, hypertension, peripheral vasoconstriction, shock, and myocardial dysfunction. Hypotension occurs in the early cholinergic phase (1–2 hours) secondary to bradycardia and is usually a poor prognostic factor. Pulmonary edema, another life-threatening complication, may occur due to primary myocardial dysfunction (cardiogenic) or due to acute respiratory distress syndrome (noncardiogenic). Other rarer but fatal complications include encephalopathy, disseminated intravascular coagulation, hemolysis, hemiplegia, and pancreatitis.

Grading of Scorpion Sting

Grade 1: Severe excruciating local pain at the site of sting which radiates along the dermatomes with mild local edema and sweating at the sting site and no systemic symptoms.

Grade 2: Signs and symptoms of autonomic storm, parasympathetic and sympathetic symptoms (sweating, vomiting, hypersalivation, hypertension, and tachycardia).

Grade 3: Cold extremities, tachycardia, and features of pulmonary edema.

Grade 4: Hypotension, tachycardia, with or without pulmonary edema with warm shock.

MANAGEMENT

Local pain is managed with ice compression, paracetamol, and regional nerve block using low concentration of lidocaine (without epinephrine). Antiemetics may be needed if vomiting is severe. Profuse diaphoresis and vomiting can cause fluid loss which needs to be corrected by fluid replacement.

Prazosin

Prazosin suppresses the sympathetic outflow and activates venom-inhibited potassium channels. It blocks the postsynaptic alpha 1 receptors and also prevents prostaglandin production. It reduces cardiac preload, afterload, blood pressure (BP), and central nervous system (CNS) sympathetic stimulation without causing an increase in heart rate or cardiac output. It usually does not cause any stress on the heart.[2]

Prazosin is available as a 1 mg (scored) tablet. Sustained-release tablets are not recommended in this condition. The dose recommended is 30 µg/kg/dose.

Prazosin is administered only when features of autonomic storm exist. In hemodynamically unstable patients, the priority remains in stabilization of the Airway breathing and circulation. Prazosin is given only after stabilization of the hemodynamic status of the patient. The drug should not be given prophylactically in the absence of symptoms of autonomic shock. If the child is unable to swallow, it may be administered through a nasogastric tube. The mother should be instructed to keep the child in the supine to avoid first-dose hypotension due to prazosin.[3]

Rapid cardiopulmonary assessment should be performed every 30 minutes for next 6 hours and later every 4 hours till improvement. Prazosin is repeated in the same dose at the end of the 3 hours and later every 6 hours till extremities are warm and dry. Not more than four doses are usually required in a child.[4,5]

Management of Complications

If the cardiopulmonary assessment suggests shock, isotonic fluid bolus is given. Since the risk of myocardial dysfunction exists, it would be wise to correct with smaller boluses of 10 mL/kg up to a maximum of 30–40 mL/kg. If shock improves, further fluids may be stopped. If the shock does not improve, inotropes should be considered. Dobutamine is used if the BP is normal or high and should be avoided if the child is hypotensive. Severe myocardial dysfunction manifested by hypotension may be treated with epinephrine infusion.

In case of pulmonary edema or cardiogenic shock, early intubation is indicated for provision of PEEP (positive end-expiratory pressure). Vasodilators, such as sodium nitroprusside (0.3–1 mg/kg/min) infusion or nitroglycerin (5 µg/kg/min) infusate, have been used in patients with cold shock with high or normal BP. Close monitoring of central venous pressure (CVP) is needed to adjust fluid therapy. Prazosin should be given 1 hour before termination of sodium nitroprusside.

If sodium nitroprusside is not available, isosorbide dinitrate 10 mg may be used every 10 minutes sublingually as an emergency measure.

Signs of recovery are normal heart rate, appearance of warm peripheries, dilated peripheries veins, reappearance of pain, and recovery of mental status.

Scorpion Antivenom

Scorpion antivenom has been available for clinical use in India since 2002. Species-specific antivenom is needed to neutralize the circulating venom. Early administration of antivenom within 6 hours of sting in addition to prazosin is supposed to hasten the recovery. Rapid recovery in patients treated with antivenom is an advantage and the cost of 10 mL of antivenom is ₹ 350.

Initial dosage is three vials intravenously over 10 minutes. If needed, additional doses can be repeated. The most common adverse events are vomiting, pyrexia, rash, nausea, and pruritus.[6]

■ PROGNOSIS

Pain and age greater than 6 years are good prognostic signs. Delay in initiation of prazosin therapy, priapism pulmonary edema, arrhythmias, encephalopathy, and age less than 6 years indicate a bad prognosis.

■ CONCLUSION

Diagnosis of scorpion sting in children needs a high index of suspicion as clinical presentation is varied and definite history will usually not be present in most cases. Early initiation of Prazosin during autonomic storm will prevent complications. Administration of anti scorpion venom along with Prazosin will improve the outcome.

■ REFERENCES

1. Bawaskar HS. Diagnostic cardiac premonitory signs and symptoms of red scorpion sting. Lancet. 1982;1(8271):552-4.
2. Bawaskar HS, Bawaskar PH. Prazosin in management of cardiovascular manifestations of scorpion sting. Lancet. 1986; 1(8479):510-1.
3. Bawaskar HS, Bawaskar PH. Treatment of cardiovascular manifestations of human scorpion envenoming: is serotherapy essential? J Trop Med Hyg. 1991;94(3):156-8.
4. Bawaskar HS, Bawaskar PH. Envenoming by scorpions and snakes (Elapidae), their neurotoxins and therapeutics. Trop Doct. 2000;30(1):23-5.
5. Bawaskar HS, Bawaskar PH. Prazosin therapy and scorpion envenomation. J Assoc Physicians India. 2000;48(12):1175-80.
6. Bawaskar HS, Bawaskar PH. Utility of scorpion antivenin vs prazosin in the management of severe Mesobuthus tamulus (Indian red scorpion) envenoming at rural setting. J Assoc Physicians India. 2007;55:14-21.

Drowning

Lokesh Tiwari, Manish Kumar

INTRODUCTION

Drowning is a leading cause of accidental death, particularly in young. In recent years, scientific community has described drowning as a process and not as an event thus including terms like near drowning within its gamut. Management is stratified into prehospital, emergency room, and in-patient management with stress on early intervention for neurologically intact outcomes.

DEFINITION

Traditionally, multiple terms like drowning, near drowning, and immersion injury have existed. Near drowning has been described as nonfatal immersion injury with recovery (however transient), or death which occurs other than at the time of immersion while the term immersion injury was used to describe any compromise of physical function or mental status resulting from an immersion event, however, minor or transient, or secondary to other injury.[1] Confusion caused by multitude of terms prompted need for consensus in definition of drowning.[2] International Liaison Committee on Resuscitation (ILCOR) has adopted Utstein definition which refers to drowning as a process resulting in primary respiratory impairment from submersion or immersion in a liquid medium and its recent amendments.[3]

EPIDEMIOLOGY

Drowning accounted for about 360,000 deaths globally in 2015.[4] World Health Organization South-East Asia region along with Western Pacific region account for more than half of incidences of drowning while drowning deaths are maximum in African region.[4] Drowning is one of the most common causes of death in children, with a recent survey suggesting that it is the third most common cause of death in children aged 5–14 years in India.[5] Globally, most victims of drowning are less than 5 years of age.[4]

Lack of supervision, inquisitive or risk-taking behavior, drug or alcohol abuse, and comorbid diseases predispose children to drowning.

Risk factors associated with drowning are summarized in **Box 1**.

PATHOPHYSIOLOGY

A specific sequence of events orchestrates the pathophysiology of drowning **(Fig. 1)**.[6] Typically, the

Box 1: Risk factors for drowning.
• Lack of supervision • Risk taking behavior and overconfidence • Use of recreational drugs and alcohol • Associated trauma • Comorbidities such as seizure disorder or arrhythmia • Hypothermia-induced arrhythmia

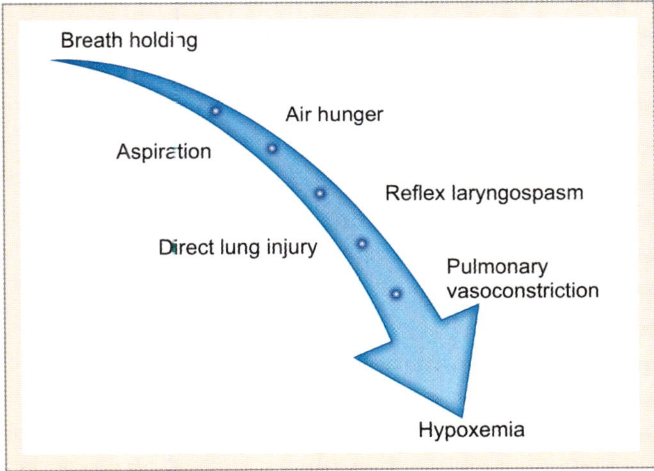

Fig. 1: Pathophysiology of drowning-induced hypoxemia.

panicked victim holds breath which produces air hunger. Eventually inspiratory effort takes place leading to reflex laryngospasm produced by contact of water with lower respiratory tract or direct lung injury due to aspiration. In event of prolonged laryngospasm, the victim may become hyporesponsive and may stop breathing resulting in what is referred to as *dry drowning* compared to *wet drowning* in which water is aspirated into lungs. In either mechanism, the resultant hypoxemia is further exacerbated by reflex pulmonary vasoconstriction, causing systemic end-organ damage.

Hypothermia is a significant contributor in pathophysiology of drowning, especially in cold water. Severe hypothermia with body temperature less than 30°C may lead to hypotension, loss of consciousness, arrhythmia, and cardiac arrest. It also decreases cerebral blood flow, metabolism, and oxygen requirement. This accidental hypothermia is neuroprotective and hence intact neurological survival even after prolonged resuscitative efforts is possible. Children who suffer from cold water drowning exhibit mammalian diving reflex with shunting of blood from nonessential organs toward cerebral and coronary circulation and manifesting as apnea and bradycardia.

End-organ damage resulting from drowning-induced hypoxemia affects all organ systems but majority of mortality and morbidity is due to cerebral hypoxia.

Pulmonary

Direct lung damage is caused due to aspiration of water into lungs. Debris and chemical present in it produce chemical pneumonitis. Significantly, surfactant is washed out causing atelectasis which may manifest as acute lung injury (ALI) or acute respiratory distress syndrome (ARDS). These pathologies lead to intrapulmonary shunting causing ventilation perfusion mismatch.

Neurologic

Hypoxic-ischemic cascade leads to neuronal damage which in turn produces cerebral edema. This neuronal damage leads to limited functional recovery in about 20% cases of nonfatal drowning.

Cardiovascular

Arrhythmia secondary to hypoxemia, hypothermia, and dyselectrolytemia is principal cardiovascular manifestation. Shock in a drowning victim may be multifactorial. It may be due to hypoxemia-induced cardiac dysfunction or cardiomyopathy, thus accounting for features of cardiogenic shock. Development of pulmonary edema also induces hypovolemia and hypotension. Another mechanism which brings about hypovolemia is diuresis due to decreased antidiuretic hormone release. This is in response to initial intense vasoconstriction which brings the blood to core, which the central volume receptors consider as hypervolemia.

Renal

Acute tubular necrosis may result from hypoxemia, shock, hemoglobinuria, or myoglobinuria.

Fluid—electrolytes

Dyselectrolytemia in form of fatal hyponatremia, hypernatremia, hypermagnesemia, etc. is relatively rare in drowning. Unlike previously believed, the difference of osmolality in fresh water compared to sea water is not significant in drowning as experimental studies have shown that about 22 mL/kg of water needs to be aspirated for fluid-electrolyte aberrations to occur.

Hematologic

Hemolysis and coagulopathy may occur rarely in nonfatal drowning. Again, it is not probable for victims to aspirate volumes sufficient to cause hemodilution.

■ MANAGEMENT

Management of drowning victim can be categorized into three distinct phases: Prehospital rescue by lay rescuer or first responders; emergency department stabilization; inpatient or intensive care management.

Prehospital Resuscitation

Bystander rescue and cardiopulmonary resuscitation (CPR) improve victim's chances of intact neurological survival. Principles of scene safety for rescuer as laid out in basic life support (BLS) guidelines should be adhered to. In drowning victims, ventilation takes precedence over chest compression and it is recommended that rescue breaths should be given as soon as rescuer reaches shallow water. The precedence of ventilation over compression is in deviation to usual CPR algorithm in adolescents and adults. Agonal gasps should not be confused with breathing. Chest compression should be initiated if victim remains unresponsive even after two rescue breaths which make the chest rise. Emphasis is on high quality CPR with compression rate of 30:2 in all single rescuer scenarios and 15:2 in case of two rescuer scenarios for an infant or child victim. Some other aspects of BLS in a drowning victim require special mention:[7]

- *Use of automated external defibrillator (AED)*: AED should be used as soon as it is available; however, care should be taken to remove the victim from water and chest should be dried before placement of AED pads for proper rhythm identification.
- *Cervical spine injury*: Contrary to previously held belief, cohort studies have now shown that incidence of cervical spine injury in drowning victims is apparently rare unless associated with circumstantial risks such as shallow water drowning, diving, alcohol intoxication, or signs of trauma. Hence, routine cervical spine immobilization is not recommended as such maneuvers interfere with initiation of rescue breaths.
- *Vomiting during resuscitation*: A drowning victim may vomit during CPR. If vomiting occurs, it is essential to turn the victim to side and remove vomitus using finger or cloth. In cases with suspected spinal trauma, it is important to turn the patient ensuring that head, neck, and torso rotate as a unit.
- *Heimlich maneuver*: Heimlich maneuver or any other positioning maneuver to drain water from lungs is not recommended. Heimlich maneuver or back slaps and chest thrusts (for infants) should only be used if there is clear evidence of airway obstruction due to solid debris.
- *Management of hypothermia*: Hypothermia correction should start from prehospital settings, if feasible. Wet clothes should be removed and passive warming by use of blankets, if available, should be started.

Emergency Department Stabilization

In Emergency Department (ED), ongoing cycles of evaluation, identification, and intervention for airway, breathing, and circulation physiology should continue. Some important aspects of ED management of drowning victims include the following:

- *Securing the airway*: Decision to intubate is guided by neurological status of patient and adequacy of oxygenation—ventilation. Indications of intubation include—victims with Glasgow coma scale (GCS) less than 8, inability to protect airway, hypoxemia manifested as PaO_2 less than 60 mm Hg despite oxygen supplementation through a high-flow device, and hypercarbia with $PaCO_2$ greater than 50 mm Hg. Prior to tracheal intubation, care should be taken regarding preoxygenation of victim and gastric decompression by using a nasogastric tube.
- *Respiratory support*: Drowning victims in whom immediate intubation is not indicated, should be given supplemental oxygen for as long as 72 hours by which surfactant may reconstitute. As noted in pathophysiology section, hypoxemia in a drowning victim stems from atelectasis and intrapulmonary shunting; which can be effectively alleviated by positive airway pressure. Noninvasive ventilation (NIV) modes such as continuous positive airway pressure (CPAP) or bilevel positive airway pressure (BiPAP) are extremely effective in reversing hypoxemia in a drowning victim. It is important to monitor patients on these NIV modes for hypotension resulting from increased intrathoracic pressure.
- *Trauma screening*: Drowning victims from suggestive circumstantial settings such as shallow water drowning, diving, and intoxication should undergo trauma screening in ED by appropriate clinical and imaging modalities.
- *Management of hypothermia*: Hypothermia management initiated in prehospital care should be augmented. External rewarming using heating pads, radiant heaters, or hot air blowers, etc. are used along with measures directed at internal rewarming by use of warmed intravenous fluids and warmed humidified oxygen. Guided by use of low reading thermometers, core body temperature is raised from 32°C to 35°C.
- *Ongoing assessment*: Continuous recording of vital signs along with frequent clinical reassessment are mandatory constituents of ED care in a case of drowning. End-tidal carbon dioxide ($ETCO_2$) measurement, if available, should be done. It is recommended that samples for lab monitoring of blood glucose, blood gas, renal functions, and coagulation profile should be sent from ED. In suggestive circumstances, especially in case of an adolescent, a toxicology screen for alcohol and recreational drugs may be considered.
- *Duration of resuscitation*: Neuroprotective effects of hypothermia have resulted intact neurological survival even after prolonged resuscitative efforts. Hence, it is recommended that resuscitation should be prolonged in drowning victims with hypothermia at least till core body temperature reaches 35°C.[7]
- *Triage and patient disposition*: Some studies have documented that symptoms in a drowning victim occur latest by 7 hours of event.[8] Based on this evidence, some guidelines recommend that asymptomatic patients should be observed for at least 8 hours and if any, clinical worsening is noted, they should be admitted. Given the possibility of fatal catastrophe,

all symptomatic patients should be admitted for stabilization of cardiorespiratory physiology and supportive management of organ dysfunction.

Inpatient Management

For drowning victims who achieve return of spontaneous circulation (ROSC), postresuscitation management is aimed at achievement of prevention of secondary organ dysfunction and optimization of metabolic derangements to achieve neurologically intact survival.[9]

- *Respiratory issues*: Ongoing clinical assessment for early identification of respiratory failure or its worsening is indicated. Bronchospasm is often seen in victims of nonfatal drowning and inhaled short-acting beta-agonists are indicated. Routine use of systemic glucocorticoids has been discouraged. Indication for initiating antibiotics is drowning in contaminated water or if there is evidence of pulmonary infection. In rare cases where drowning occurred in a water body with debris, bronchoscopy may be indicated if there is evidence of airway foreign body. Ventilatory strategies for drowning victims is similar to patient with ALI or ARDS due to any other etiology and if available extracorporeal membrane oxygenation may be considered in cases whose oxygenation is inadequate on traditional ventilatory strategies. There is anecdotal evidence, in form of case reports regarding use of surfactant in drowning victims; however, due to lack of high-quality scientific evidence, routine surfactant therapy in drowning is currently not recommended.
- *Cardiovascular issues*: As discussed in pathophysiology section, drowning victims may suffer from cardiogenic shock due to hypoxemia-induced cardiomyopathy or hypovolemic shock due to inappropriate diuresis. It is, therefore, pertinent that euvolemia is achieved through meticulous fluid management and optimal use of inotropes.
- *Neurological issues*: Favorable outcomes in drowning victims predominantly depend upon severity of cerebral hypoxia-mediated neuronal damage. Inpatient management aims to limit this damage to minimal. Raised intracranial pressure (ICP) due to hypoxia-induced neuronal damage requires astute clinical attention. Measures to reduce ICP such as head end elevation; hyperventilation in cases with imminent herniation; appropriate management of pain, fever, and seizure; ensuring normotension and euvolemia; and optimizing metabolic derangements to ensure euglycemia; should be taken. Controlled

> **Box 2:** Factors associated with poor prognosis in a drowning victim.
>
> - *Prehospital*:
>   - Submersion >25 minutes
>   - Time to effective BLS >10 minutes
>   - Age >14 years
> - *Emergency department*:
>   - Duration of CPR >25 minutes
>   - GCS <5
>   - Arterial pH <7.1 at presentation
>   - Persistent apnea
> - *Inpatient*:
>   - Features of raised ICP
>   - Secondary organ dysfunction

(BLS: basic life support; CPR: cardiopulmonary resuscitation; GCS: Glasgow coma scale; ICP: intracranial pressure)

hypothermia in drowning victims has not shown significant advantage, hence measures to achieve and maintain normothermia are recommended.

PROGNOSIS

Numerous studies have delineated factors associated with poor prognosis in drowning victims.[10] These poor prognostic markers relate to factors in prehospital, ED, and Pediatric Intensive Care Unit (PICU) settings. Prehospital factors such as duration of submersion and time to initiation of CPR are the most critical determinants of outcome. Prolonged CPR (>25 minutes), persistent apnea, and severe acidosis at presentation in ED also suggest poor chances of functional recovery. Features of raised ICP and other secondary organ dysfunction harbinger poor prognosis.

Poor prognostic factors have been summarized in **Box 2.**

PREVENTION

Majority of drowning deaths are preventable. Mass awareness regarding adult supervision of children near water bodies, use of protective flotation devices, desisting from swimming alone, and avoidance of alcohol and drugs can reduce incidence of drowning. On community level, fencing of inland water bodies and provision of lifeguards at pools and beaches can help in reducing incidence of drowning.

REFERENCES

1. Boffard KD, Bybee C, Sawyer B, et al. The management of near drowning. J R Army Med Corps. 2001;147(2):135-41.
2. Papa L, Hoelle R, Idris A. Systematic review of definitions for drowning incidents. Resuscitation. 2005;65(3):255-64.

3. Idris AH, Bierens JJLM, Perkins GD, et al. 2015 Revised Utstein-Style Recommended Guidelines for Uniform Reporting of Data From Drowning-Related Resuscitation: An ILCOR Advisory Statement. Circ Cardiovasc Qual Outcomes. 2017;10(7):e000024.

4. Drowning. [online] Available from: https://www.who.int/news-room/fact-sheets/detail/drowning. [Last accessed on November, 2019].

5. Fadel SA, Boschi-Pinto C, Yu S, et al. Trends in cause-specific mortality among children aged 5–14 years from 2005 to 2016 in India, China, Brazil, and Mexico: An analysis of nationally representative mortality studies. Lancet. 2019;393(10176): 1119-27.

6. Handley AJ. Drowning. BMJ. 2014;348.

7. Lavonas EJ, Drennan IR, Gabrielli A, et al. Part 10: Special Circumstances of Resuscitation: 2015 American Heart Association Guidelines Update for Cardiopulmonary Resuscitation and Emergency Cardiovascular Care. Circulation. 2015;132(18 Suppl 2):S501-18.

8. Noonan L, Howrey R, Ginsburg CM. Freshwater submersion injuries in children: a retrospective review of seventy-five hospitalized patients. Pediatrics. 1996;98(3 Pt 1):368-71.

9. Hazinski MF, Nolan JP, Aickin R, et al. Part 1: Executive Summary: 2015 International Consensus on Cardiopulmonary Resuscitation and Emergency Cardiovascular Care Science with Treatment Recommendations. Circulation. 2015;132 (16 Suppl 1):S2-39.

10. Quan L, Bierens JJ, Lis R, et al. Predicting outcome of drowning at the scene: a systematic review and meta-analyses. Resuscitation. 2016;104:63-75.

Burns

Aniruddha Ghosh, Rupa Banerjee

INTRODUCTION

Burns are a serious preventable public health problem. Burn is defined as injury to the skin or other organic tissue primarily due to heat or due to radiation, radioactivity, electricity, friction, or contact with chemicals. Thermal (heat) burns are some form of tissue or cellular injury due to hot liquids (scalds), hot solids (contact burns), or flames (flame burns).[1]

According to data published by World Health Organization (WHO), about 180,000 deaths occur annually across the globe from fire alone. Scalds, electricity, and other forms of burn cause more deaths for which appropriate data are not available. Almost half of these deaths occur in the WHO South-East Asia Region (SEAR). India being the most populated member of WHO SEAR, contributes over 10 million new cases of burn injuries every year.[2]

Out of five burn victims, four are women and children. Rate of child mortality due to burn injury is seven times higher in middle- and low-income countries.[2] Burns are 5th most common cause of nonfatal childhood injuries and 11th leading cause of death in children aged 1–9 years. Globally among all age groups affected by burn injuries, mortality is highest among infants.[1]

ETIOLOGY AND RISK FACTORS

Burn injuries can be commonly classified as thermal or inhalational based on the causative factor.[1]

Heat Burns

- *Scalds*: They are caused by hot liquids (water, oil), steam from boiling water, or heated food. Young children are mostly affected by scalds.
- *Contact burns*: Hot solid objects like ashes and coal, hot pressing irons, pots and utensils, light bulbs, etc. cause contact burns.
- *Flames*: Direct burn injuries by flames are mostly seen with leaking gas pipe or cylinder, stoves, crackers, etc.
- *Chemical burns*: Accidental contact with toilet cleaning agents, acids, etc.
- *Electrical burns*: Accidental contact with exposed "live" wires or short circuits. High tension wires near home, playground, etc. may also cause fatal electrical burn injuries.

Inhalational Burns

Inhalational burn injuries occur due to breathing in superheated gases, steam, hot liquids, or harmful products of incomplete combustion. They cause thermal injury to upper airways and irritation or chemical injury to lower respiratory tracts (from soot, asphyxia, carbon monoxide, and cyanide gases). Inhalational burns are often associated with skin burns.[1]

Inhalational burn injury is to be suspected if any of the following is present:[1]

- History of burns in closed space
- Deep burns to face, neck, or trunk
- Singed nasal hair, eyebrows, or eyelashes
- Carbonaceous sputum and carbon particles in oropharynx
- Change in voice with hoarseness or harsh cough
- Altered consciousness
- Tachypnea/dyspnea
- Expiratory rhonchi
- Dysphagia.

Depending upon severity burns can be classified as minor, moderate, or critical burns.[1]

Table 1: System-wise complications in burn injuries.[1,2]

System	Complications	Management
Lungs and airways	Airway edema CO toxicity ARDS Inhalation injury	O_2 inhalation Low threshold of intubation Lung-protective ventilation
Cardiovascular	Hypotension SIRS Myocardial depression	Aggressive fluid therapy Inotropes, if required Achieve resuscitation endpoints
Gastrointestinal (GI)	Gastric ulcer and bleeding Microbial translocation from gut and sepsis	GI prophylaxis Monitoring for gastric residues
Renal	AKI	Management of hypotension Avoidance of nephrotoxic drugs, renal adjustment, if required
Hepatic	Coagulopathy Altered drug metabolism	Monitoring of coagulation profiles and liver function on regular basis
Neuromuscular	Upregulation of acetylcholine receptors	Avoidance of succinylcholine in the initial PICU management
Immunological	Immunosuppression Decreased barrier function (gut and skin)	Monitoring for sepsis Appropriate antibiotic therapy

(AKI: acute kidney injury; ARDS: acute respiratory distress syndrome; CO: carbon monoxide; P CU: pediatric intensive care unit; SIRS: systemic inflammatory response syndrome)

- *Minor burns*: Burns affecting less than 10% body surface area (BSA) in children and less than 15% in adolescents and adults (chemical, electrical burns, and burns affecting face, hands or perineum are exceptions to this). Outpatient treatment is sufficient.[1]
- *Moderate burns*: Burns affecting between 10% and 15% BSA in children and 15% and 22% in adolescents and adults. Hospital management may be required.
- *Critical burns*: Burns above 5% BSA in newborn and infants, 15% in children, and 25% in adults; electrical, chemical, and respiratory burns; burns associated with orthopedic, chest, abdominal or head injury; often fatal, most of the time requires intensive care management.

Symptoms of burn injury depend on the depth of burn. Depending upon the depth, burn injuries are classified into the following:

- *First degree or superficial burns*: Only the upper part of skin involved leading to pain and erythema. Blister is absent. Found mostly in cases of solar radiation, contact burn, scald, etc. Healing is fast without any sequelae.
- *Second degree or partial thickness*: Affects deeper layers of skin and blisters are formed. Superficial second-degree burns classically take less than 3 weeks to heal and deeper second-degree burns take more than that with hypertrophic scar formation as sequelae.
- *Third degree or full thickness*: All skin layers are involved. Skin is white and due to complete destruction of nerves there is often no pain. Due to extensive damage to skin layers, this type of burn injury cannot regenerate on their own without skin grafting.

Most pediatric burn injuries are combination of superficial, partial, and full thickness burn.

- *Fourth degree*: Involves fascia, muscle, or bone. Pain occurs to deep pressure in the areas of fourth degree burn and surrounding areas of second-degree burn.[3]

There are several risk factors for burn injuries in children which are as follows:

- Floor cooking
- Open wood fire usage
- Overcrowding
- Young girls taking care of younger siblings and household works
- Inadequate safety measures for use of gas and stoves
- Underlying medical conditions like epilepsy, cognitive impairment, etc.[1]

PATHOGENESIS OF BURN INJURY: SPECIAL CONSIDERATIONS IN PEDIATRIC POPULATION

Pathogenesis of burn injury and its consequences are same in adults and children, only differences in size and metabolic rates make pediatric burn injury slightly more complicated.

- Respiratory tract injury, whether direct or indirect, is the most feared situation for emergency management.

The risk of airway obstruction and need for intubation is higher in children due to narrow airway opening and greater chances of complete obstruction due to edema. Risks of carbon monoxide poisoning and acute respiratory distress syndrome (ARDS) are also higher in pediatric population.[4]

- In response to burn injury, systemic inflammatory response syndrome (SIRS) occurs due to surge of several chemokines like catecholamines, vasoactive chemicals, inflammatory molecules leading to capillary leaks, protein loss, and interstitial edema. This leads to shock-like state and multiple organ dysfunction syndrome (MODS), i.e. cardiac depression, renal compromise, hepatic dysfunction, etc.[3] These inflammatory cascades of events are more pronounced in children than adults.[4]

- Pediatric patients are more susceptible to postburn hypermetabolic state caused by several inflammatory markers where loss of muscle and bone mineral density hamper the wound healing and this state can persist even for 6–9 months after the initial injury.[3,4] Nutritional support is of utmost importance to maintain lean body mass and help healing of wounds. But it has been noted that in spite of best nutritional management bone growth often lags behind for 2 years in children with severe burn injury.[3]

- As the dermal layer of skin is thinner in newborns, infants, and young children than adults, any given heat exposure leads to deeper burn injuries in them. Also, low subcutaneous fat stores in them make the assessment of depth of injury very difficult in comparison with adult patients (apart from geriatric patients).[5-7]

- In children, the surface area to mass ratio can be thrice that of adults leading to higher susceptibility to evaporative fluid loss and hypothermia.[7]

- Susceptibility to local infections and fulminant septicemia is also higher in pediatric population due to loss of the skin barrier and its armamentarium to fight against microorganisms.[6]

■ MANAGEMENT

Emergency room management of burn injuries is most crucial and sequential steps are needed to be followed in order to address all the injuries.

- *Primary survey*:

  A—airway: Maintenance of adequate airway along with cervical spine stabilization is very important. Stridor in a patient with burn injury is a very late sign of supraglottic airway injury. Intubation has to be done early if airway injury is apprehended otherwise later on patient may develop complete airway obstruction and intubation will become impossible. Cricothyrotomy or mini tracheostomy followed by formal tracheostomy is life-saving in these cases. In doubtful cases of airway injury, direct visualization of airways (direct laryngoscope and bronchoscopy) is often necessary. During intubation, all sizes of endotracheal tubes should be kept in hand apprehending partial airway blockage. Unnecessary intubation, sedative drugs used during intubation may deteriorate the condition of the patient. If the patient has history suggestive of reactive airways disease, laryngomalacia, adenoid, tonsillar hypertrophy, etc. chances of airway compromise increase.

  B—breathing: All burn patients are treated with 100% moist oxygen via nonrebreathing mask at the emergency room. Lower respiratory tract and lungs injury occurs due to several reasons in patients with burn injury (chemical pneumonitis, carbon monoxide poisoning, circumferential burns around torso causing restriction to chest movement, and pneumothorax in blast injury).

  C—circulation: Prompt initiation of fluid resuscitation through intravenous or intraosseous access (in case veins are not accessible) is of crucial impact. Crystalloids are preferred mostly over colloids. Central venous catheters are very useful where skin surface has been disfigured. Invasive arterial blood pressure monitoring should be done along with other vital parameters. Ultrasonogram of the inferior vena cava gives good idea regarding intravascular volume deficit.

  D—disability: Clinical assessment of higher function is very much necessary as any alteration in sensorium may indicate toward any or combination of the followings: Hypoxia, carbon monoxide toxicity, shock, or electrolyte imbalance.

  E—exposure: Full exposure after starting the aforementioned resuscitation steps is necessary for assessment of percentage of burn injury as well as identification of coexistent injuries. This should be meticulous and all measures to prevent or treat hypothermia should be available.

- *Secondary survey*: After primary survey is complete and appropriate resuscitation has been started, a secondary survey [allergy history, medications, medical problems, last meal time, and the event (AMPLE)] should be done along with a focused history taking regarding burn injury:

- Time and place of injury
- Type of burn injury (heat burn/scald/chemical/electrical, etc.)
- Risk factors for inhalational injuries (mentioned earlier)
- Whether any explosion or any other kind of added injury, i.e. fall from height, fall of heavy objects on head, etc. was there
- What initial treatments were done for initial cooling, first aid, etc.

Fluid Management

Fluid resuscitation is of paramount importance during the initial care of the child. During the initial phase of resuscitation, adequate vascular access must be obtained. Central venous access may be necessary in selected cases and does appear to be safe in children with burn injury.[8] The overall objective of resuscitation is to replace fluid losses and restore euvolemia, while avoiding the detrimental effects of fluid overload. Fluid resuscitation based on two major factors:

1. Total body surface area (TBSA) involved in second and third degree (Needs Lund and Browder chart or recently prepared modified Lund and Browder Chart for children, **Fig. 1**)
2. Patient's dry weight (in kg).

The fluid requirements may be calculated using several different formulae, all of which achieves good results. The Parkland formula provides a simple and easily remembered basis for resuscitation [4 mL Ringer's lactate (RL)/kg/percent BSA burned; one-half to be given during the first 8 hours after injury and the rest in the next 16 hours]. Other formula used is Galveston formula (estimated fluid requirements in first 24 hours = 5,000 mL/m^2 TBSA burn plus 2,000 mL/m^2 TBSA maintenance of which 50% infused in the first 8 hours postburn and 50% infused in the next 16 hours or in second 24 hours, 3,750 mL/m^2 plus 1,500 mL/m^2 TBSA maintenance). The type of fluid administered is generally an isotonic crystalloid, with the recommendation for the addition of dextrose to children under 20 kg to prevent the development of hypoglycemia. It is critical to monitor the endpoints of fluid resuscitation which includes the following:

- Hemodynamics
- Urine output with a goal of maintenance of 1–2 mL/kg/h for children <30 kg and 0.5–1 mL/kg/h for those ≥30 kg
- Mental status
- Lactate levels
- Base deficit.[9]

Urethral catheterization and hourly monitoring of urine volume and color is important. Patients with severe electrical burn injuries may have myoglobinuria or hemoglobinuria initially. As the children are prone to develop hypothermia, any fluid given for initial resuscitation should preferably be warmed.[10]

Sepsis and Septic Shock in Burn

Due to loss of barrier function of intact skin, loss of immunogenic proteins present in dermoepidermal layers and migration of commensal organisms of uninvolved skin children with burn injury are highly susceptible to wound sepsis. Prophylactic antibiotic therapy has no role in preventing wound infection except for very young infants.[11] Most common organisms implicated in burn wound sepsis are *Pseudomonas spp.*, *Staphylococcus aureus*, *Klebsiella spp.*, *Escherichia coli*, *Candida spp.*, etc. These microorganism isolates vary depending upon geographical location, seasonal factors, locally prevalent nosocomial pathogens, etc. *Pseudomonas spp.* and methicillin-resistant *Staphylococcus aureus (MRSA)* are notorious for biofilm formation in burn wounds and often it takes prolonged parenteral antibiotic regimens to clear sepsis. A high index of suspicion and regular assessment of wounds for superadded sepsis is the cornerstone of management. Clinically, increase in depth of involved skin, cellulitis surrounding the wounds, tissue necrosis, etc. should raise the suspicion of wound infection. These are the clinical stages of burn wound infection:

- *Wound colonization*: Presence of very low concentrations of microorganisms (less than 10^5 bacteria per gram tissue) without any tissue invasion and feature of local or systemic sepsis.
- *Noninvasive infection*: More than 10^5 bacteria per gram of tissues from the wound or eschar are found.
- *Invasive sepsis*: High concentrations of microorganisms at depth of the wounds leading to suppurative separation of eschar or appearance of systemic features of sepsis (high grade fever, progressive tachycardia, tachypnea, feed intolerance, bleeding tendency, etc.) or graft rejection from previously healthy wound denotes invasive sepsis. Local sepsis from wounds becomes fulminant septicemia and leads to septic shock very frequently.[12]

Complete blood count, blood and tissue (from wound) cultures, serum C-reactive proteins, procalcitonin levels, etc. are done as part of sepsis work-up. Patient with septic shock is to be treated in Pediatric Intensive Care Unit (PICU)-isolation wards with preferably empirical parenteral antibiotic combinations based upon local

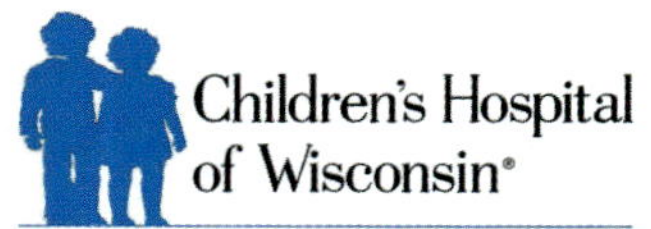
Children's Hospital of Wisconsin
A member of Children's Hospital and Health System.

Burn Estimate and Diagram

Date: _______________________

Age: ___________ Sex: ___________

Admit weight: _______________

Admit height: _______________

Mechanism of injury: _______________

Date of injury: _______________

Time of injury: _______________

KEY:

FT = Full thickness

PT = Partial thickness

Superficial/Partial thickness

Deep/Full thickness

Area	Percent of burn						Severity		Total percent	Donor areas
	Birth to 1 year	1–4 years	5–9 years	10–14 years	15 years	Adult	PT	FT		
Head	19	17	13	11	9	7				
Neck	2	2	2	2	2	2				
Ant. trunk	13	13	13	13	13	13				
Post. trunk	13	13	13	13	13	13				
R. buttock	2 1/2	2 1/2	2 1/2	2 1/2	2 1/2	2 1/2				
L. buttock	2 1/2	2 1/2	2 1/2	2 1/2	2 1/2	2 1/2				
Genitalia	1	1	1	1	1	1				
R.U. arm	4	4	4	4	4	4				
L.U. arm	4	4	4	4	4	4				
R.L. arm	3	3	3	3	3	3				
L.L. arm	3	3	3	3	3	3				
R. hand	2 1/2	2 1/2	2 1/2	2 1/2	2 1/2	2 1/2				
L. hand	2 1/2	2 1/2	2 1/2	2 1/2	2 1/2	2 1/2				
R. thigh	5 1/2	6 1/2	8	8 1/2	9	9 1/2				
L. thigh	5 1/2	6 1/2	8	8 1/2	9	9 1/2				
R. leg	5	5	5 1/2	6	6 1/2	7				
L. leg	5	5	5 1/2	6	6 1/2	7				
R. foot	3 1/2	3 1/2	3 1/2	3 1/2	3 1/2	3 1/2				
L. foot	3 1/2	3 1/2	3 1/2	3 1/2	3 1/2	3 1/2				

Diagram adapted from Lund-Browder burn assessment chart

Total

Signature/Title: _______________________   Date/Time: _______________

C7440N (3/06)

DT183

Fig. 1: Modified Lund and Browder chart.
Source: Adapted from Lund and Browder and courtesy of the Trauma Program, Division of Pediatric Surgery, Children's Hospital of Wisconsin.

microbiological data. Broad-spectrum antibiotics with coverage of *Pseudomonas* and *Staphylococcus* (like piperacillin-tazobactam/carbapenems and vancomycin) are first choice antibiotic combinations. If fungal sepsis is suspected especially in patients with long-term intravenous cannula, central venous catheters, etc. antifungals are added after sending fungal culture. Later on, antibiotic policy is guided by microorganisms isolated from tissue culture and blood culture. Unless local sepsis, especially with *Pseudomonas aeruginosa*, is controlled and bacterial concentration dips below acceptable level, skin grafting is put on hold. On regular basis, tissue cultures are done from wounds in search of any new local infection.[11,12]

Burn Wound Management

After stabilization of the critical care issues in the burn-injured child, attention is directed toward burn wound management. The key elements of burn wound management include the following:

- Cleansing
- Debridement
- Topical antimicrobial agents
- Dressing changes of the burned areas.

Cleansing allows better inspection of the wound surface, and debridement removes devitalized and necrotic tissue from the burn wound. Burn wounds are initially gently cleansed mild soap and water, and debridement is performed using gentle mechanical techniques, such as brushing or scraping.[13]

Treatment of burn wound depends on depth of burn injury. Definitive surgical management of the wound includes excision, grafting, and reconstruction. Burn reconstruction procedures have the ultimate goal of covering wounds, restoring function, and preserving aesthetics. In addition, the reconstruction is often completed in separate phases, depending on severity of burn and donor tissue availability.

- *Primary surgery*: The use of early excision and skin grafting allows initial acute coverage of burns; also, this reduces necrotic and infected tissues. In addition, it leads to decreased length of hospital stay, a reduced treatment cost, and a significant reduction in mortality.
- *Secondary surgery*: This option is availed when the burn injury leads to sepsis. After sepsis is controlled necrotic and unhealthy tissues are removed and autograft is placed under parenteral antibiotic coverage.
- *Reconstructions*: Free skin grafts with either full or split thickness are the conventional options for burn wound coverage after excision. Split thickness grafts allow the advantage of covering large surface areas with less donor skin, while full thick grafts allow the advantage of improved skin texture and aesthetics. As the child grows multiple surgeries may be needed.[3]

■ REHABILITATION

Children who suffer from burn injuries need to be rehabilitated. Well-planned physical therapy after surgery, early initiation of chest physiotherapy, etc. are extremely important for improvement of postoperative quality of life of the affected children.[7] Besides physical rehabilitation, psychological assessment and rehabilitation is also of crucial value as often these children suffer from anxiety disorders, depression, and post-trauma stress disorder (PTSD) after going through the accidents and subsequent prolonged treatment in the hospital wards, operation theatres, and intensive care units. Active involvement of parents, nursing staffs, nutritionists, physiotherapists, etc. in each and every step of treatment is necessary for a better outcome for children with extensive burn injuries.

■ REFERENCES

1. National Health Portal of India (2016). Burns. [online] Available from: https://www.nhp.gov.in/disease/skin/burns. [Last accessed on November, 2019].
2. World Health Organization (2018). Burns. [online] Available from: https://www.who.int/news-room/fact-sheets/detail/burns. [Last accessed on November, 2019].
3. Krishnamoorthy V, Ramaiah R, Bhananker SM. Pediatric burn injuries. Int J Crit Illn Inj Sci. 2012;2(3):128-34.
4. Lee J, Norbury W, Herndon DN. Special Considerations of age: The pediatric burned patient. In: Total Burn Care, 4th edition. Amsterdam, The Netherlands: Elsevier; 2012. pp. 405-14.
5. Fenlon S, Nene S. Burns in children. Contin Educ Anaesth Crit Care Pain. 2007;7(3):76-80.
6. Vallez LJ, Plourde BD, Wentz JE, et al. A review of scald burn injuries. Intern Med Rev. 2017;3:1-18.
7. Sharma RK. Parashar A. Special considerations in paediatric burn patients. Indian J Plast Surg. 2010;43:(Suppl)S43-50.
8. Sheridan RL, Weber JM. Mechanical and infectious complications of central venous cannulation in children: Lessons learned from a 10-year experience placing more than 1000 catheters. J Burn Care Res. 2006;27:713-8.
9. Fodor L, Fodor Ramon Y, et al. Controversies in fluid resuscitation for burn management: literature review and our experience. Injury. 2006;37(5):374-9.
10. Mitra B, Fitzgerald M, Cameron P, et al. Fluid resuscitation in major burns. ANZ J Surg. 2006;76(1-2):35-8.
11. Chavez–Bueno S, Stall TL. Antibacterial agents in pediatric. Infect Dis Clin North Am. 2009;23(4):865-80.
12. Greenhalgh DG, Saffle JR, Holmes JH, et al. American Burn Association concensus conference to define sepsis and infection in burns. J Burn Care Res. 2007;28(6):776-90.
13. Waisak J, Cleland H, Campbell F. Dressings for superficial and partial thickness burns. Cochrane Database Syst Rev. 2008:CD002106.

Accidental Hypothermia in Children

Sudip Dutta, Ashish Pradhan

DEFINITION

Hypothermia in children older than 1 month is defined as a core body temperature below 35°C. Core body temperature measurement is essential for accurate diagnosis and staging of hypothermia, although there are variability in the measurements. Accidental hypothermia is defined as an unintentional core body temperature of <35°C when heat loss to surroundings is greater than heat generation mostly due to cold environmental exposure. There are three stages of hypothermia defined by core temperature as given below:

1. *Mild*: Core temperature 32–35°C (90–95°F)
2. *Moderate*: Core temperature 28–32°C (82–90°F)
3. *Severe*: Core temperature below 28°C (below 82°F).

EPIDEMIOLOGY

Children especially younger children are vulnerable to hypothermia due to various factors like the larger ratio of surface area to body mass and lesser capacity to recognize, avoid, and escape hypothermic exposure. They have limited glycogen stores for nonshivering thermogenesis as well as shivering thermogenesis are less developed especially in younger children.

Accidental hypothermia in children can occur due to inadvertent prolonged exposure to a cold environment. These may occur in near drowning in cold water bodies like rivers, lakes, and immersion accidents in tubs and pools. They can experience hypothermia in accidents in mountainous regions, which may also cause frost bite and trench foot. The other situations include runaway or lost children and inebriated adolescents who become incapacitated outdoors. Mountain sport accidents are also an emerging cause of accidental hypothermia.

PATHOPHYSIOLOGY

We can lose heat from our body by radiation, convection, conduction, evaporation, and respiration. Wind exposure can increase heat loss by convection. Heat loss by both evaporation and conduction is increased on exposure to water, especially if cold. The physiologic response to cold is dependent on the stage of hypothermia. During mild hypothermia, there is increased metabolism and shivering to generate heat and peripheral vasoconstriction to reduce heat loss and increase in the heart rate. With moderate hypothermia, there is loss of compensatory shivering, decreased metabolism, and respiration becomes slow, shallow, and irregular. There is hypovolemia due to vascular leak and cold diuresis due to false internal sensing of blood volume and failure of renal concentration mechanism. There is decreased cerebral blood flow leading to altered mentation. In severe hypothermia, there is decreased heart rate and myocardial contractility and vasodilatation leading to circulatory collapse. There is suspended cerebral activity, the nerve conduction slows down, and the breathing stops. The muscles become rigid due to dysfunction of actin–myosin bundles.

The pathophysiologic changes seen especially in moderate-to-severe hypothermia are extravasation of blood due to vascular leak, sludging of blood, myocardial irritability leading to arrhythmogenicity of the heart, hypo- or hyperglycemia, hyperkalemia, metabolic acidosis or alkalosis, thrombocytopenia, and coagulopathy.

Severe hypothermia may provide cerebral protection against prolonged anoxia, especially among younger children. There are many reports of intact recovery of children who clinically appeared dead even after prolonged and delayed resuscitation. Hence, there is a need to recognize and treat such patients to the utmost possible.

CLINICAL FEATURES

The clinical manifestations of hypothermia depend on the stage of hypothermia, but some features may vary from patient to patient, especially mental status changes and the possibility of having cardiac arrhythmias.

During mild hypothermia, the child will be shivering, cold with goose bumps due to piloerection. The peripheries will be pale with prolonged capillary refill time and there will be presence of acrocyanosis. Paradoxically infants at this stage might have "rosy cheeks" giving a false healthy appearance.

In moderate hypothermia, the child stops shivering, has altered sensorium, lethargy, clumsy movements, delirium, incomprehensible speech, confusion, and behavior such as "paradoxical undressing" as the core body temperature further decreases.

With severe hypothermia, the child will have stupor progressing to coma with fixed and dilated pupils. There will be bradycardia and hypotension progressing to asystole or ventricular fibrillation (VF). The child will have irregular, slow respiration progressing to apnea.

Below 28°C, the child will have rigidity of the muscles described as "frozen stiff" with flushed skin, absent shivering, and vital signs resembling rigor mortis. Even in such children, efforts to resuscitate should be tried as some have recovered with good outcome.

DIAGNOSIS

The accurate measurement of core body temperature is essential for the diagnosis, staging, and management of hypothermia. The temperature should be measured with a low-reading thermometer. The methods include—deep rectal temperature measurements by rectal thermometers, indwelling bladder probes, esophageal temperature probes in the lower third of the esophagus are ideal and reflect cardiac temperature in children with secured airways, nasopharyngeal probes, and central venous catheter probes. Direct tympanic measurements are not so reliable but can be used if it is the only method feasible. In critically ill children, it is better to take measurements at two central sites.

INVESTIGATIONS

A 12-lead electrocardiogram needs to be recorded in all children with hypothermia along with continuous cardiac rhythm monitoring as they can develop VF, pulseless electrical activity (PEA), asystole, atrioventricular (AV) block, atrial fibrillation, and junctional rhythm. Hypothermia may produce a typical J or Osborn wave caused by J point elevation due to distortion of the earliest phase of membrane repolarization, although not always present. It also results in prolongation of all electrocardiography (ECG) intervals including RR, PR, QRS, and QT interval. There is a rhythmic irregularity of the ECG baseline and sometimes of the QRS complex caused by shivering.

Other investigations done for management of prolonged moderate or severe hypothermia include rapid serum glucose, serum electrolytes, serum blood urea nitrogen and creatinine, lipase, complete blood count, prothrombin time (PT), partial thromboplastin time (PTT), international normalized ratio (INR), arterial blood gas uncorrected for temperature, and blood type and crossmatch studies (if the need for extracorporeal warming is anticipated).

DIFFERENTIAL DIAGNOSIS

The other causes of hypothermia in children which need to be differentiated and considered in cases of accidental hypothermia in children are:

- Child abuse in the form of forced immersion in cold water, forceful bathing with cold water, and neglect of children. They are associated with signs of physical abuse or neglect in such cases.
- Sepsis especially among young infants and immuno-suppressed children.
- Accidental or intentional overdose of ethanol, opioids, benzodiazepines, beta-blockers, and clonidine. There will be other clinical findings of intoxication in such children.
- Medical problems like malnutrition, hypoglycemia, hypothyroidism, adrenal insufficiency, hypothalamic injury, etc.

TREATMENT

The treatment of hypothermia depends on the stage of hypothermia as defined by core body temperature. The moderate or severe hypothermia causes decreased metabolism which protects against hypoxia. There have been many reports of successful resuscitation with good outcome in pulseless, rigid children with severe hypothermia. Therefore in patients with cardiac arrest and absent vital signs with severe hypothermia, resuscitation should be attempted and continued for prolonged period before declaration of death. Hence, we should avoid premature declaration of death before accurate measurement of core body temperature. The treatment of hypothermic child includes initial stabilization of vitals, supportive care, treatment of other injuries, and medical conditions, supportive care, effective rewarming intervention, and ongoing monitoring and assessment.

Prehospital Management

The children with intact consciousness and shivering (mild hypothermia) should be removed from cold environment. They are encouraged mild muscle activity and warm drinks with calorie replacement should be provided. Passive rewarming involves removing cold or wet clothing and applying dry insulations such as blankets along with providing external heat in a warm environment is carried out. If the patient is having altered sensorium or unconscious (moderate-to-severe hypothermia), the child is transported to a nearby hospital with pediatric intensive care facility. The patient should be transported in a horizontal position with minimal rash handling and exertion to avoid arrhythmias. During transport steps to reduce heat loss should be carried out. This includes removal of wet clothing, gentle insulation of the patient with blanket or sleeping bags, warming of the transport vehicle, and pushing of warm intravenous fluids. Rewarming by application of external heat should be avoided in the initial stages. Prehospital declaration of death in hypothermic children should be done only when rescue is impossible or other injuries are clearly fatal.

Hospital Management

Initial Stabilization

The initial stabilization includes support of airway, breathing, and circulation along with accurate measurement of core body temperature.

Airway and breathing: Warm humidified 100% oxygen via a non-rebreather mask is given to all patients. If the child is having irregular shallow respiration or apnea, bag-valve mask ventilation is carried out till the child is intubated. Patients with compromised airway, hypotensive shock, or cardiac arrest are intubated in a gentle manner. In children with severe hypothermia, intubation may be difficult by direct laryngoscopy due to rigidity of jaw muscles hence advanced airway adjuncts such as fiberoptic bronchoscopy, and video laryngoscopy may be needed.

Circulation: A vascular access should be established at the earliest. If the peripheral access is difficult, an intraosseous needle or central line via femoral vein should be placed. A bolus of 20 mL/kg of heated (40–44°C) intravenous normal saline using high capacity warmers and tubings to deliver over 5–10 minutes and repeated as needed as per constant reassessments. An indwelling bladder catheter is placed to assess urine output as well as temperature probes can also

be inserted along with it to record core body temperature. Persistent hypotension and bradycardia after recovery is treated using vasopressors and inotropes.

In a child with perfusing bradycardic rhythms like sinus bradycardia, first-degree AV block, and atrial fibrillation with slow ventricular response reverts with rewarming. Medications like atropine, epinephrine, and cardiac pacing are used only if there is persistent bradycardia, despite rewarming to 32–35°C. Severely hypothermic children with nonperfusing rhythms should receive closed chest compression using standard rate and depth properly. The patients with VF or ventricular tachycardia without pulse should be defibrillated and appropriate medications given as per standard pediatric cardiac arrest algorithm with prompt active internal rewarming. Children with asystole and pulseless electrical activity (PEA) should receive airway support, prolonged chest compressions, epinephrine, and ideally extracorporeal rewarming. Resuscitation is discontinued if there is no return of spontaneous circulation (ROSC) despite appropriate interventions and the core body temperature has reached above 34–35°C.

Glucose (Dextrose) control: Intravenous dextrose (0.5 g/kg) should be administered to patients with hypoglycemia or suspected hypoglycemia, regardless of core body temperature. Whereas in hyperglycemia insulin is not administered as it is ineffective and may lead to hypoglycemia after rewarming.

Rewarming

The methods of rewarming in children are based on the degree of hypothermia and the status of circulation. The different methods of rewarming are:

- *Passive rewarming:* This involves removing cold or wet clothing and applying dry insulation such as blankets.
- *Active external rewarming:* In this, heat is applied externally in the form of forced heated air, radiant heat, application of heat packs, or water heating pads.
- *Active internal rewarming:* This method involves providing heat internally to the body which can be noninvasive, invasive, or extracorporeal.

Noninvasive: In this, we provide heated, humidified oxygen and warmed intravenous fluids.

Invasive: These include lavage of the pleura, bladder, stomach, or peritoneum with heated normal saline.

Extracorporeal: The techniques include cardiac bypass and extracorporeal membrane oxygenation (ECMO).

In moderate hypothermia, the child is given warm humidified oxygen and heated intravenous fluids. In addition, active external rewarming is done by forced air rewarming till core temperature reaches 35°C. The trunks are warmed first in this method. This forced air rewarming can cause severe shock, VF, and further core temperature cooling due to movement of cold and academic blood from peripheries into the central circulation. Hence, the child should receive a rapid infusion of 20 mL/kg of warmed normal saline at the start of rewarming and continuous cardiorespiratory monitoring.

In children with severe hypothermia and intact circulation, they are warmed by active internal rewarming. The methods include pleural lavage with heated (40–44°C), heated normal saline lavage of the stomach, bladder, peritoneum, and colon. The best approach is to use pleural lavage with heated normal saline using two chest tubes. In children with severe hypothermia with absent circulation, rapid rewarming is done with extracorporeal methods. This includes cardiac bypass or ECMO. If these techniques are not easily available, other methods are tried. These include active internal rewarming with cardiopulmonary resuscitation (CPR), active external rewarming with CPR, hemodialysis and hemofiltration systems, and endovascular rewarming.

Postresuscitation Care

The child is cared in a pediatric intensive care unit with continuous cardiorespiratory and core body temperature monitoring. The child undergoes serial biochemical testing and the electrolyte and coagulation abnormalities are managed vigorously. Pulmonary edema, acute kidney injury, and coagulopathy are treated till it resolves. The children with neurologic deficits are started on aggressive neurological rehabilitation till optimal recovery.

■ LOCAL INJURIES

Trench foot occurs due to exposure of feet to damp cold. The feet becomes cold, numb, pale, clammy, and edematous. It develops tissue maceration and autonomic disturbances. It is treated by drying the foot, gentle rewarming and control of pain, and autonomic disturbances.

Frost bite occurs due to exposure to dry cold weather. The exposed areas develop cold hard white anesthetic and numb areas with clear or hemorrhagic vesicles. There may be development of extensive tissue damage or even gangrene. The area should be rewarmed with warm (42°C) water. The injured regions should be dressed with sterility so as to keep the area dry and clean. Vasodilators agents like prazosin or phenoxybenzamine are helpful.

■ SUGGESTED READING

1. Antoon AY, Donovan MK. Cold injuries. In: Nelson's Textbook of Pediatrics, 20th edition. USA: Elsevier Saunders; 2016. pp. 577-9.
2. Aslam AF, Aslam AK, Vasavada BC, et al. Hypothermia: evolution, electrocardiographic manifestations, and management. Am J Med. 2006;119(4):297-302.
3. Brown DJ, Brugger H, Boyd J, et al. Accidental hypothermia. N Engl J Med. 2012;367(20):1930-8.
4. Corneli HM. Accidental hypothermia. J Pediatr. 1992;120: 671-8.
5. Danzl DF, Huecker MR. Accidental hypothermia. In: Auerbach PS, Cushing TA, Harris NS (Eds). Auerbach's Wilderness Medicine, 7th edition. Philadelphia: Elsevier; 2017. p. 135.
6. Giesbrecht GG. Cold stress, near drowning and accidental hypothermia: a review. Aviat Space Environ Med. 2000;71(7): 733-52.
7. Gustavson E, Levitt C. Physical abuse with severe hypothermia. Arch Pediatr Adolesc Med. 1996;150(1):111-2.
8. Mattu A, Brady WJ, Perron AD. Electrocardiographic manifestations of hypothermia. Am J Emerg Med. 2002;20(4): 314-26.
9. Maxton FJ, Justin L, Gilles D. Estimating core temperature in infants and children after cardiac surgery: a comparison of six methods. J Adv Nurs. 2004;45(2):214-22.
10. Tunnessen WW, Roberts KB. Hypothermia: Signs and Symptoms in Pediatrics, 3rd edition. Philadelphia: Lippincott, William and Wilkins; 1999. p. 8.
11. Zafren K, Giesbrecht GG, Danzl DF, et al. Wilderness Medical Society practice guidelines for the out-of-hospital evaluation and treatment of accidental hypothermia: 2014 update. Wilderness Environ Med. 2014;25(Suppl 4):S66-85.

General Management Principles and Approach to Unknown Poisonings

Ramachandran P, Shruthi TK

INTRODUCTION

Poisoning can be a diagnostic problem as the history may not be forthcoming in all situations. It is not unusual for young children and toddlers to consume lots of potentially harmful substances found in the household. Adolescents who intentionally consume toxic substances and become unconscious pose another diagnostic dilemma. The challenging scenario in many household poisons is the lack of information about the substance which was ingested due to the absence of a label on the container or pack. A set of symptoms and signs on presentation or later may point toward poisoning and the likely substance.

POINTERS TO SUSPECT POISONING

Poisoning should be considered in the differential diagnosis of children who present with acute onset of altered level of consciousness, respiratory depression, hypoglycemia, unexplained metabolic acidosis, seizures, arrhythmias, cyanosis, liver dysfunction, bleeding tendency, abnormal odor on skin or breath, multi-organ system dysfunction, or a puzzling clinical picture.

Situations suggesting poisoning are as follows:
- Sudden onset of symptoms and signs in a previously healthy child.
- Circumstantial evidences such as child left un-supervised, tablets kept within the reach of the child or tablets or chemicals found spilled. As per National Poisons Information Center, majority of poisoning in our children are accidental in the age group less than 6 years involving household products comprising pesticides, disinfectants, detergents, antiseptics, and corrosives.
- Appearance of symptoms and signs of specific poisons referred to as "toxidrome".

INITIAL STABILIZATION

Evaluation of a child with suspected poisoning always begins with assessment and stabilization of the airway, breathing, and circulation, and treatment of life-threatening trauma.

Airway, Breathing, and Circulation

Assess airway, breathing, and circulation (ABC) upfront in any child with suspected poisoning. If there is respiratory distress or shock, administer oxygen after ensuring that the airway is stable. Intubate and ventilate if the child has respiratory depression or impaired mental status with poor airway protective reflexes. Early intubation is recommended in poisoning as these children may develop respiratory failure rapidly. There should be a low threshold for intubation as a brief period of ventilatory support is enough in many cases. Intravenous (IV) access is recommended for any significant poisoning. Treat shock with fluid boluses of Ringer's Lactate or normal saline 20 mL/kg in about 20 minutes with reassessment after each bolus. Lesser boluses of 10 mL/kg over 30 minutes is recommended if the drug ingested has suspected cardiotoxicity, e.g. tricyclic antidepressant (TCA), calcium channel blockers. Continuous cardiorespiratory monitoring is necessary till the child stabilizes.

EVALUATION

After the initial stabilization, one should focus on identifying the agent(s) involved, predicting toxicity, and assessing the severity.

History

It is challenging to obtain history of toxin ingestion from an intoxicated patient or relatives, but is crucial. The relatives may be unable or unwilling to give the details of the history. Many times, the personnel accompanying the patient to hospital may not know the details of exposure. Whenever possible, efforts should be made to identify the agent, time, and volume of ingestion and immediate clinical effects.

The most common fatal drug ingestions in children include paracetamol, iron supplements, antidepressants, and cardiotoxic agents. The most common fatal nondrug ingestions include hydrocarbons, alcohol, cosmetics, button battery, cleaning products, rodenticides, and pesticides. Insect bites and envenomation also should be considered. It is important to collect information about recent illness and regular therapy with common medications. The overdose of common medications may result in acute as well as chronic poisoning. The circumstances surrounding the ingestion may provide useful information at times. It is important to ask about the possible exposure of young children to many potentially toxic substances stored at home such as drugs for chronic conditions (oral antidiabetics, cardiac drugs, and antidepressants), cosmetics, cleaning products, analgesics, cough and cold preparations, topical agents, plants, and pesticides. Unwitnessed, accidental ingestions in young children tend to occur at times of decreased parental supervision (e.g. when there are household visitors or holiday parties or when the parents are busy attending to another child or are themselves unwell).

Adolescents, particularly ones with intentional ingestion, may not give reliable history. They commonly present with ethanol or illicit drug intoxications or suicidal drug/chemical ingestion. It is important to ask other household members about all medications (prescription and over-the-counter), pesticides, and rodenticides that are present in the home. Social history helps in identifying the circumstances, intent, and/or agent of exposure.

Parents can provide important information about open containers, empty bottles, spilled contents, or suicide notes at the scene. If such items exist, ask parents to bring them to the hospital. Unknown pills or chemicals may be identified by consultation with a regional poison control center, computerized poison identification system, and product label on the container if available. Many insecticides and rodenticides are sold without any product information on the packets.

Information about the quantity and timing of ingestion is helpful in making decisions about decontamination or the use of antidotes. The common agents, estimated minimal fatal dose, and major effects are listed in **Table 1**.

Physical Examination

Rapid examination of mental status, vital signs, and pupils helps to classify the patient into:

- State of physiologic excitation [e.g. central nervous system (CNS) stimulation, hyperthermia, tachycardia, tachypnea, hypertension, and mydriasis]
- State of physiologic depression (depressed mental status, hypothermia, bradycardia, hypotension, bradypnea, and miosis)
- Mixed physiologic state.

In many situations of suspected poisoning, clinical monitoring should be supplemented with pulse oximetry and cardiac monitoring. The initial characterization helps to direct initial stabilization efforts and provides a clue to the etiologic agent. After the initial diagnostic evaluation and stabilization, other physical findings should be sought to further define a particular toxic syndrome (Toxidrome; **Table 2**), to narrow the potential etiologies of poisoning

Table 1: Minimum fatal dose and major effects of selected medications.

Drug	Minimal fatal dose	Major effects
Benzocaine	20 mg/kg	Methemoglobinemia and seizure
Camphor	50 mg/kg	Seizures and respiratory depression
Chloroquine	30 mg/kg	Seizures and arrhythmias
Clonidine	0.01 mg/kg	Bradycardia and CNS depression
Methyl salicylates	150–200 mg/kg	Acidosis and cardiovascular collapse
Phenothiazine	20 mg/kg	Seizures, arrhythmias and CNS depression
Sulfonylureas	1 mg/kg	Hypoglycemia
Theophylline	50 mg/kg	Seizure, arrhythmias
Tricyclic antidepressants	15 mg/kg	Seizure, arrhythmias, and hypotension
Toxic alcohols	0.3 mL/kg	CNS depression

(CNS: central nervous system)

Table 2: Common toxidrome with examples of toxic agents.

Toxidrome	Toxic agents
Sympathomimetic	Cocaine, amphetamines, ephedrine, pseudoephedrine, phenylpropanolamine, theophylline, caffeine
Anticholinergic	Antihistamines, tricyclic antidepressants, cyclobenzaprine, orphenadrine, antiparkinson agents, antispasmodics, phenothiazines, atropine, scopolamine, and belladonna alkaloids
Hallucinogenic	Phencyclidine, lysergic acid diethylamide, and designer amphetamines
Opioid	Heroin, morphine, methadone, oxycodone, hydromorphone
Sedative–hypnotic	Benzodiazepines, barbiturates, alcohols, and zolpidem
Cholinergic	Organophosphate and carbamate insecticides, nerve agents, nicotine, pilocarpine, physostigmine, edrophonium, bethanechol, and urecholine
Serotonin syndrome	Monoamine oxidase inhibitors alone or with selective serotonin reuptake inhibitors (SSRIs), meperidine, dextromethorphan, tricyclic antidepressants, and L-tryptophan

and to evaluate the possibility of child abuse. Periodic reevaluation of sensorium and vital signs should be done to determine the clinical course and the need for further intervention.

The diagnosis may be assisted by some important signs and symptoms as described in the following text.

Temperature Changes

- *Hyperthermia*: Neuroleptic malignant syndrome, nicotine, antihistamines, salicylates, sympathomimetics, anticholinergics, and antidepressants
- *Hypothermia*: Carbon monoxide, opiates, oral hypoglycemics, insulin, and sedative hypnotics.

Blood Pressure Alterations

- *Hypertension*: Cocaine, theophylline, sympathomimetics, caffeine, anticholinergics, amphetamines, and nicotine
- *Hypotension*: Clonidine, reserpine, antihypertensive agents, antidepressants, sedative hypnotics, opiates, and heroin.

Heart Rate Alterations

- *Tachycardia*: Cocaine, anticholinergics, antihistamines, amphetamines, sympathomimetics, and theophylline
- *Bradycardia*: Anticholinesterase drugs, beta blockers, clonidine, calcium channel blockers, ethanol, digoxin, and opiates.

Respiratory Variations

- *Tachypnea*: Sympathomimetics, central hallucinogens, anticholinergics, drug withdrawal states, salicylates, paracetamol, carbon monoxide, cyanide, methemoglobinemia, opioids, ethylene glycol, methanol, isoniazid, and iron

- *Bradypnea*: CNS depressants, opioids, sedative hypnotics, alcohol, antidepressants, antipsychotics, sympatholytics, volatile inhalants, cholinergics, muscle relaxants, antiepileptics, botulism, organophosphate poisoning, and carbamates.

Pupillary Changes

- *Mydriasis*: Antihistamines, antidepressants, anticholinergics, atropine, sympathomimetics such as cocaine, and amphetamine
- *Miosis*: Cholinergics, clonidine, opiates, organophosphate, phenothiazines, pilocarpine, pontine bleed, and sedative hypnotics.

Skin Changes

- *Red and flushed*: Atropine, TCA, antihistamines, belladonna alkaloids, phenothiazines, rifampicin, and carbon monoxide
- *Pale and diaphoretic*: Sympathomimetic, cholinergic agents, central hallucinogens, and salicylates
- *Cyanotic*: Methemoglobinemia, sulfhemoglobinemia, and hypoxemia
- *Desquamation*: Stevens–Johnson syndrome, toxic epidermal necrolysis, arsenic, and mercury.

Neurologic Changes

- *Seizures*: Propranolol, insecticides, lidocaine, sympathomimetics, drug withdrawal states, antidepressants, antipsychotics, salicylates, camphor, isoniazid, chemical nerve agents, lithium, and hypoglycemic agents
- *Tremors and myoclonus*: Antipsychotics, sympathomimetics, anticholinergics, drug withdrawal states, and heavy metals.

- *Rigidity and Parkinsonism*: Antipsychotics (neuroleptics), metoclopramide, carbon monoxide (delayed), methanol, ethylene glycol, monoamine oxidase inhibitors (MAOIs), serotonin syndrome, lithium, strychnine, cyanide, malignant hyperthermia, neuroleptic malignant syndrome, and postanoxic injury from any agent
- *Choreoathetosis*: Antihistamines, TCAs, phenytoin, and carbamazepine
- *Weakness and paralysis*: Barium, solvent abuse like toluene, gasoline, mercury, organophosphates, carbamates, botulism, neurotoxic snake envenomation, tick paralysis, and seafood poisoning.

Characteristic Odors

- *Fruity (acetone)*: Ethanol, isopropyl alcohol, chloroform, and salicylates
- *Bitter almonds*: Cyanide
- *Garlic*: Arsenic, organophosphates, phosphorus, thallium, and selenium
- *Mothball*: Naphthalene and paradichlorobenzene
- *Kerosene*: Petroleum distillate
- *Rotten eggs*: Hydrogen sulfide and sulfur dioxide.

Laboratory Evaluation

The laboratory evaluation of the child with an unknown ingestion is performed to detect metabolic effects of the poison that have both diagnostic and therapeutic implications.

Rapid Blood Glucose

It is indicated for any patient with altered mental status. Rapid assessment of blood glucose can be performed at the bedside with a glucose strip. Several drugs cause hypoglycemia (insulin, beta blocker, oral hypoglycemic agent, and ethanol) and hyperglycemia (beta-adrenergic agonist, calcium channel blockers, and iron).

Blood Gas

Arterial or venous blood gas measurement offers a rapid evaluation of acid–base status as well as assessment of oxygenation (arterial blood gas only) and ventilation. Co-oximetry can be used to rapidly establish the diagnosis of carbon monoxide toxicity or methemoglobinemia.

Electrolytes

Measurement of serum electrolytes provides information about renal function, which is essential for the elimination of some toxins, and further information about acid–base status. The electrolyte results can be used to calculate the anion gap ($Na - [Cl + HCO_3]$), which helps to differentiate metabolic acidosis (normal anion gap vs increased anion gap metabolic acidosis).

Urinalysis

Urinalysis is necessary for evaluation of rhabdomyolysis with myoglobinuria, the prompt treatment of which may prevent renal failure.

Examination of the urine can also be helpful in the diagnosis of ethylene glycol ingestion. Microscopic examination of the urine may reveal calcium oxalate crystals, although the absence of crystalluria does not preclude the presence of ethylene glycol ingestion. Urine examination by Wood's light (ultraviolet) may reveal fluorescence if the patient has ingested antifreeze solution, which contains fluorescein dye.

Electrocardiogram

Changes on electrocardiogram (ECG) suggest poisoning by certain agents and may indicate the need for specific intervention, e.g. a ventricular arrhythmia.

- *Bradycardia/atrioventricular (AV) blockade*: Beta blockers, calcium channel blockers, cardiac glycosides, alpha-adrenergic agonists, cholinergics, opioids, sedative hypnotics, and magnesium.
- *Supraventricular tachycardia*: Sympathomimetics, anticholinergics, thyroid hormones, carbon monoxide, and drug withdrawal states.
- *Ventricular tachycardia*: Sympathomimetics, antidepressants, antipsychotics, cardiac glycosides, potassium, fluorides, and chlorinated hydrocarbons.
- *QRS and QT interval prolongation*: Antidepressants, antipsychotics, antihistamines, antiarrhythmics, antimicrobials such as macrolides, arsenic, and lithium.

Toxicology Screen

Toxicology screening is rarely necessary in children who have an unintentional ingestion and are asymptomatic or have clinical findings that are consistent with the history. It is indicated in whom the diagnosis of poisoning is uncertain, who have coma of unknown etiology, where there is suspicion of child abuse or Munchausen syndrome by proxy, and in whom the administration of an antidote depends upon the rapid identification of the toxic agent. Unfortunately, it is neither available in most places nor the results arrive in time to help in clinical decision-making.

Urine screens provide qualitative data about the recent use of substances included in the screen. Urine screens usually test for a limited number of substances (typically drugs of abuse, e.g. amphetamines, cocaine, marijuana, opiates, and phencyclidines). Positive and negative immunoassay screens for drugs do not absolutely confirm or refute poisoning diagnoses and may need confirmation by gas chromatography–mass spectrophotometry (GC–MS). False positives may occur if structurally similar substances cross-react with the assay. On the other hand, a negative screen may reflect a drug concentration below the threshold limit of detection because the specimen was obtained before or after peak concentration. Furthermore, the newer synthetic illicit drugs (such as cannabinoids, cathinones, synthetic opioids, and many others) will not be detected by routine drug abuse screens.

Serum testing provides quantitative data and is important in the diagnosis and management of ingestion of several drugs and medications **(Table 3)**. Screening for paracetamol and salicylates is strongly recommended for patients with an uncertain history or intentional poisoning; few early signs may be present following lethal doses of these agents, and specific treatments are available and highly effective if implemented early. Quantitative testing may also be considered for agents that have delayed clinical effects. Serial testing might be necessary for agents with delayed absorption.

The interpretation of a single drug concentration for any drug must be made with caution because poisoning is a dynamic and rapidly changing process. Intervention may be required despite serum concentrations in the therapeutic range. Results of these tests should be considered in conjunction with the time of exposure. Levels that are obtained early in the course, while the drug is still distributing throughout the body, are difficult to interpret properly. On the other hand, levels drawn very late after an exposure may be deceptively low.

Comprehensive qualitative toxic screening of urine, blood, or other body fluids is expensive and usually requires 6 hours or longer for results. Such testing rarely leads to changes in patient management and is unlikely to affect patient outcome. Nonetheless, such a comprehensive panel may be useful in patients who are critically ill or in whom the clinical picture does not fit the stated history.

Radiologic Evaluation

Plain radiographs of the chest should be obtained in children and adolescents with inhalation exposures and in those with respiratory symptoms and signs. In addition, certain radiopaque toxins (e.g. chloral hydrate, heavy metals such as iron, iodinated compounds, and TCAs) may be visualized by plain film radiographs.

■ MANAGEMENT

Supportive care is the mainstay of therapy, which involves decontamination, antidote administration, and enhanced elimination techniques. Optimal management of the poisoned child depends upon the specific poison(s) involved, the presenting and predicted severity of illness, and elapsed time between exposure and presentation.

Supportive Care

Supportive care for toxic exposures is similar to that provided for other problems, but certain issues are managed slightly differently. In many poisonings, supportive therapy alone can be life-saving, despite failure to identify specific poison.

Airway protection by endotracheal intubation should be performed early in the poisoned patient (a) with depressed mental status because of the high risk for aspiration and its associated complications, particularly when gastric decontamination is necessary, (b) with severe acid–base disturbances or acute respiratory failure, and (c) in patients who require sedation and/or paralysis to limit the extent of complications such as hyperthermia, acidosis, and rhabdomyolysis.

Hypotension should be managed initially with isotonic IV fluid boluses. Vasopressors are required when hypotension does not resolve with volume expansion. Direct-acting vasopressors, such as norepinephrine, have been shown to be more effective.

Hypertension in agitated patients is best treated initially with nonspecific sedatives such as benzodiazepine. When hypertension necessitates specific therapy because of

Table 3: Serum quantitative levels suggestive of toxicity.	
Drug or toxin	*Toxic level*
Paracetamol	>150 mg/L at 4 hours (if later plot on nomogram)
Salicylate	>30 mg/dL
Phenytoin	>20 mg/L
Phenobarbital	>50 mg/L
Valproic acid	>150 mg/L
Theophylline	>20 mmol/L
Digoxin	>2 ng/L
Ethanol	>100 mg/dL
Carboxyhemoglobin	>10%
Methemoglobin	>15%
Iron	>500 µg/dL
Lead	>25 mg/dL

associated end-organ dysfunction, preferred treatments are nitroprusside, esmolol, or phentolamine. The use of beta blockers alone for patients with sympathetic hyperactivity (e.g. cocaine intoxication) is not recommended because it may result in unopposed alpha-adrenergic stimulation and intensified vasoconstriction. Short-acting agents are generally preferred because they are easily titrated.

Ventricular tachycardias are usually treated with standard Pediatric Advanced Life Support (PALS) recommendations: Lidocaine, procainamide, amiodarone, and cardioversion or defibrillation. However, when ventricular tachycardias occurs in the context of intoxication with TCA, sodium bicarbonate infusion is the first-line therapy. Treatment with magnesium sulfate, overdrive pacing with isoproterenol or a temporary pacemaker may be effective in patients with drug-induced torsades de pointes and prolonged QT intervals on ECG. Digoxin-poisoned patients with life-threatening tachyarrhythmias or bradyarrhythmias should be treated with specific Fab fragments (Digibind).

Bradyarrhythmias associated with hypotension should be treated in the standard fashion with atropine or temporary pacing. However, in patients with calcium channel blocker or beta blocker intoxication, the administration of calcium and glucagon may bring a rapid improvement. In the more severe cases, and in consultation with the poison center or clinical toxicologist, high-dose insulin and dextrose (also known as hyperinsulinemia/euglycemia therapy) or lipid infusions can be used.

Seizures are typically treated with benzodiazepines followed by barbiturates if necessary. Phenytoin may be effective in controlling seizures caused by agents that stabilize neuronal membranes (e.g. propranolol), but is not indicated in most poisonings and is potentially harmful in seizures resulting from theophylline. Seizures caused by certain agents may require specific antidotes for their successful termination (e.g. pyridoxine for isoniazid toxicity, glucose for hypoglycemic agents). If hypoglycemia is present or suspected, administer 2–4 mL/kg of 25% dextrose or 5–10 mL/kg of 10% dextrose.

Drug-associated agitation is usually treated with benzodiazepines, carefully supplemented with high-potency neuroleptics (e.g. haloperidol) as needed. Agitation associated with certain toxidromes may be best treated with specific agents (e.g. physostigmine for the anticholinergic syndrome).

Decontamination

Following initial patient stabilization, patient decontamination is a priority. The sooner decontamination is performed, the more effective it is at preventing poison absorption. Activated charcoal (AC) has become the preferred method of gastrointestinal (GI) decontamination in children.

Activated Charcoal

The use of AC is controversial in the asymptomatic patient and probably unnecessary in most cases.

Activated charcoal can be tried for most of the drugs and chemicals except in iron, lithium, strong acids or alkalis, kerosene, and organophosphorus compounds. It is given orally or through nasogastric (NG) tube in a dose of 1 g/kg for children up to 6 years. For adolescent and adults 25–100 g; the doses may be repeated 2–4 hourly if indicated. It is available as tablets or powder. It is mixed with water and given as a slurry (muddy liquid mixture). It can be administered orally (mixed with fruit juice) or through NG tube.

Gastric Lavage

Gastric lavage is found to be useful only when it is done within 1 hour of ingestion. It is contraindicated in patient with unprotected airway, corrosive poisoning, and hydrocarbon ingestion. Patient should have intact airway protective reflexes, i.e. cough and gag reflex when gastric lavage is attempted. If the child is comatose and cannot protect his airway, intubation should be done first. Child is kept in right lateral position. Largest possible sized orogastric tube (OGT) should be passed and position should be confirmed. Then normal saline should be administered through OGT in the aliquots of 15 mL/kg (maximum 300 mL) by syringe or with infusion set. Returning fluid is drained by gravity or by suction. Procedure is repeated till the returns are clear. First NG aspirate is preserved for possible analysis. At the end of the procedure, AC should be administered and left in the stomach.

The clinical benefit of gastric lavage has not been confirmed in controlled studies and hence is not routinely recommended.

Whole Bowel Irrigation

Whole bowel irrigation is another technique that may be used for patients who have ingested large amounts of substances such as iron and lithium and sustained release preparations that are not well bound to AC.

For whole bowel irrigation, colonic cathartic solution such as polyethylene glycol with electrolytes is administered rapidly through a NG tube at 500 mL/hr for preschool children and 1–2 L/hr for teenagers. It is continued till rectal effluent is clear; usually for about 4–6 hours. It is contraindicated if the child has ileus, GI obstruction and significant GI bleed.

Antidotes

Antidote administration is appropriate when there is a poisoning for which an antidote exists, the actual or predicted severity of poisoning warrants its use, expected benefits of therapy outweigh its associated risk, and there are no contraindications. Antidotes may prevent absorption, bind and neutralize poisons directly, antagonize end-organ effects, or inhibit conversion to more toxic metabolites. The pediatric doses for antidotes recommended for stocking in hospitals that accept emergency admissions are provided in **Table 4**.

The pharmacokinetics of the intoxicant and the antidote must be considered because the toxidrome may recur if the antidote is eliminated more rapidly than the ingested substance. Somnolence and respiratory depression due to ingested opiates acutely reverse with the administration of naloxone, but recur in approximately one-third of cases because the elimination half-life of naloxone is only 60–90 minutes. Thus, in certain situations antidotes may require repeated administration or continuous infusion.

The risks and benefits of antidote administration also must be carefully weighed in the setting of multiple drug ingestion.

Diagnostic Trial

In some cases, the clinical response to an antidote may suggest the etiology of poisoning. This can be attempted by an experienced clinician or after consultation with a regional poison center. Examples include improved alertness in response to flumazenil for benzodiazepine ingestion; flumazenil is contraindicated in drug ingestions that may precipitate seizures and in patients with a known seizure disorder. It also may precipitate withdrawal in patients with benzodiazepine dependence; improved alertness in response to glucose for insulin or oral hypoglycemic agent ingestion; improved alertness in response to physostigmine for anticholinergic agent ingestion. Physostigmine is contraindicated in TCA overdoses. Physostigmine should not be administered to patients who have a widened QRS interval on ECG; improved alertness in response to naloxone for opiate/opioid ingestion; improved clotting in response to protamine for heparin overdoses; abatement of dystonia in response to diphenhydramine for phenothiazine ingestion; temporary reduction of muscarinic effects after one dose of atropine administration in suspected organophosphate poisoning.

Enhanced Elimination

- Enhanced elimination techniques can be used for several drugs and toxins.
- *Ion trapping*: Aspirin, phenobarbital
- *Multidose AC*: Multiple doses of AC, given every 4–6 hourly, in the dose of 1 g/kg are proven to be useful in carbamazepine, dapsone, quinine, phenobarbitone, and theophylline ingestion. It is supposed to interrupt enterohepatic and enteroenteric recirculation and act like enteral dialysis. AC may cause mild constipation. If planned to give repeated doses of AC, give a dose of laxative with the first dose of AC.
- *Hemodialysis*: Ethylene glycol, methanol, ethanol, aspirin, salicylates, and lithium.
- *Hemoperfusion*: Theophylline.
- *Chelation*: Iron, mercury, lead, and arsenic.

Table 4: Recommended antidotes in pediatric poisoning.	
Toxin	*Antidote*
Organophosphate, carbamate	Atropine
Calcium channel blocker	Calcium
Cyanide, nail polish remover, amygdaline, and nitroprusside	Amyl nitrite, sodium nitrite, and sodium thiosulfate
Iron	Deferoxamine
Digoxin	Digibind
Benzodiazepines	Flumazenil
Ethylene glycol and methanol	Fomepizole
Beta blocker, calcium channel blocker	Glucagon
Insulin	Glucose
Cyanide, amygdaline, and nitroprusside	Hydroxocobalamin (Vitamin B$_{12}$)
Beta blocker and calcium channel blocker	Insulin (high dose)
Methemoglobinemia	Methylene blue
Paracetamol and carbon tetrachloride	N-acetyl cysteine
Opioid toxicity	Naloxone
Antimuscarinic delirium	Physostigmine
Sulfonylurea toxicity	Octreotide
Organophosphate poisoning	Pralidoxime
Heparin	Protamine sulfate
Isoniazid	Pyridoxine
Salicylates and tricyclic antidepressants	Sodium bicarbonate

- *Urinary alkalinization with sodium bicarbonate*: Salicylate, phenobarbital, chlorpropamide, and methotrexate.

Discharge

Following initial evaluation, treatment and a short period of observation, discharge of the patient is based upon the observed and predicted severity of toxicity. Patients who develop only mild toxicity and who have only a low predicted severity can be observed in the emergency department until they are asymptomatic. An observation period of 6 hours is usually adequate for this purpose. All patients with intentional overdose require psychiatric assessment prior to discharge.

Other factors to consider in the disposition include whether the child's caregivers understand the potential for delayed consequences of poisoning, have a means of transportation to return if necessary and are able to provide adequate observation at home.

Hospitalization is necessary for patients who are thought to have ingested substances with delayed effects or sustained release preparations; multiple agents or when caregivers cannot be relied for assessment. The duration of observation varies depending upon the expected time of onset and duration of symptoms. The half-lives of drugs are calculated based upon therapeutic dosing; in the overdose setting, the calculated half-life may be inaccurate and the duration of symptoms prolonged.

The toxicity of agents varies depending upon whether the ingestion is acute or chronic, whether other substances have been coingested, the time between ingestion and presentation, and the child's baseline health status. Thus, decisions regarding admission should be based both on drug levels and the clinical scenario.

Patients with moderate observed toxicity or those who are at risk for such on the basis of history or initial laboratory data should be admitted for appropriate observation, continued monitoring, and treatment. Patients with significant toxicity should be admitted to an intensive care unit (ICU) **(Box 1)**.

■ PREVENTION

Infants and toddlers are at maximum risk of nonintentional poisoning because of their innate inquisitiveness, increased mobility, and attraction toward the bright packaging or smell of many chemical products. Measures such as keeping the drugs and chemical substances in locked cabinets, storing household products in original containers or clearly labeled bottles with the product

---

Box 1: Criteria for ICU admission of poisoned patient.

- CNS depression, including significant lethargy, and coma
- Agitation requiring chemical or physical restraint
- Respiratory depression ($PCO_2 > 45$ mm Hg), hypoxia or respiratory failure (ARDS), and/or endotracheal intubation required
- Hypotension (SBP ≤ 80 mm Hg)
- Seizures that are prolonged or recurring
- Second or third degree AV block on ECG
- Non-sinus cardiac rhythm on ECG
- Significant acid–base disturbances (e.g. metabolic acidosis with pH ≤ 7.2)
- Significant metabolic abnormalities requiring close monitoring or aggressive correction
- Extremes of temperature (T) (e.g. hyperthermia with T > 104°F)
- Ingested drug packets, sustained-release preparations
- Quantitative level of drug which predicts unfavorable outcome
- Need for invasive hemodynamic monitoring (e.g. pulmonary artery catheter or arterial line) or cardiac pacing
- Need for whole bowel irrigation to enhance GI elimination of poison
- Need for emergency hemodialysis, hemoperfusion, and hemofiltration
- Need for emergency antidote which requires close monitoring (e.g. N-acetyl cysteine infusion, atropine/pralidoxime, digibind, physostigmine, and naloxone drip)
- Ischemic chest pain from toxin (e.g. cocaine and carbon monoxide)
- TCA or other drug exposure with QRS > 120 ms or QTc > 500 ms

(AV: atrioventricular; CNS: central nervous system; ECG: electrocardiogram; GI: gastrointestinal; ICU: intensive care unit; SBP: systolic blood pressure; TCA: tricyclic antidepressant; ARDS: acute respiratory distress syndrome)

---

information, and safe disposal of toxic substances and unused or outdated drugs will help in preventing this catastrophe.

Adolescents with emotional problems and suicidal ideas should be recognized and counseled.

National Poison Information Center (Toll Free No.: 1800-116-117; Tel No.: 26589391, 26593677) is functioning round the clock from All India Institute of Medical Sciences, New Delhi, for any enquiry related to poisoning.

■ SUGGESTED READING

1. Bar-Oz B, Levichek Z, Koren G. Medications that can be fatal for a toddler with one tablet or teaspoonful: a 2004 update. Paediatr Drugs. 2004;6(2):123-6.
2. Barrueto F Jr, Gattu R, Mazer-Amirshahi M. Updates in the general approach to the pediatric poisoned patient. Pediatr Clin North Am. 2013;60(5):1203-20.
3. Calello DP, Henretig FM. Pediatric toxicology: specialized approach to the poisoned child. Emerg Med Clin North Am. 2014;32(1):29-52.
4. Dart RC, Borron SW, Caravati EM, et al. Expert consensus guidelines for stocking of antidotes in hospitals that provide emergency care. Ann Emerg Med. 2009;54(3):386-94.

5. Gummin DD, Mowry JB. 2017. Annual Report of the American Association of Poison Control Centers' National Poison Data System (NPDS): 35th Annual Report. Clin Toxicol (Phila). 2018; 56(12):1213-415.

6. Henry J, Wiseman H. Management of poisoning: A handbook for health care workers. World Health Organization; 1997.

7. Litovitz TL, Klein-Schwartz W, Rodgers GC Jr, et al. 2001 Annual report of the American Association of Poison Control Centers Toxic Exposure Surveillance System. Am J Emerg Med. 2002;20:391.

8. Matteucci MJ. One pill can kill: assessing the potential for fatal poisonings in children. Pediatr Ann. 2005;34(12):964-8.

9. Michael JB, Sztajnkrycer MD. Deadly pediatric poisons: nine common agents that kill at low doses. Emerg Med Clin North Am. 2004;22(4):1019-50.

10. Peshin SS, Srivastava A, Gupta YK. Poisoning in children: a helpline experience. J Clin Toxicol. 2014;4:51.

11. Schabelman E, Kuo D. Glucose before thiamine for Wernicke encephalopathy: a literature review. J Emerg Med. 2012;42(4): 488-94.

12. Thangavelu S, Ramachandran P, Mahender E. Handbook on Poisoning in children, IJPP Series 6. Chennai: Alamu Printers; 2013.

13. Woolf AD. Poisoning by unknown agents. Pediatr Rev. 1999; 20:166.

Chemical Pollution: A Man-made Disaster

Bhaskar Shenoy, Sanjay Deshpande

INTRODUCTION

Chemical pollution is a process, which introduces certain compounds in our environment or increases the levels of certain hazardous elements. Majority of the man-made pollutants in the environment have resulted from the various activities, which give rise to these toxic chemicals.

Chemical *contaminants* can be stratified based on their chemical composition into two broad categories, i.e. "man-made" or "natural." They can further be classified based on the carbon content into organic or nonorganic.

Humans come into direct contact with these pollutants via either the inhalation, ingestion, or contact with skin or mucosal surfaces.[1]

Chemical compounds are organic or inorganic compounds that cause pollution. The most common compounds are the ones that are used in agriculture and industries.

Exposure to these compounds causes small-term or long-term health effects which encompass the term *chemical intoxication*.[1]

EFFECTS OF CHEMICAL POLLUTION

The catastrophic effects of chemical pollution can cause a variety of health effects ranging from simple digestive problems to sudden death. The effects are directly proportional to the quantity and the time of exposure to elevated levels of these compounds. The point of contact is either by ingesting contaminated food, drinking pollutant-laden water, or inhaling air, which contains fine particulates causing contamination.

The time frame of clinical outcomes of exposure to pollutants varies with the nature of pollutants (inhalation and ingestion) and the time frame to which one is exposed which ranges from days to months or sometimes years. For example, our earth is made up of 70% water, and various man-made compounds that accumulate in these water bodies over a large frame of time could cause a direct effect on the marine life and indirectly cause a potential health hazard to humans when they consume fish or sea food[1] which could cause immediate symptoms such as mercury poisoning or delayed effects secondary to lead poisoning.[1]

CHILDREN'S UNIQUE SUSCEPTIBILITY TO SYNTHETIC CHEMICALS

Children are particularly vulnerable to toxicities secondary to chemical pollutants for the following reasons:

- The per kilogram weight consumption of air, water, and food in children is higher than adults; hence, the frequency of exposures is higher too. Children also engage in play which includes frequent touching of mucosal to skin contact such as hand to mouth by themselves and to other children which leads to transference.
- In some cases, children can cope with environmental toxicants better than adults; because of their immature metabolic pathways of homeostasis, they are unable to convert them into their active form or not able to adequately eliminate them effectively from their body.
- Complex developmental processes and an evolving neurological system in infants and young children are susceptible to insults secondary to these man-made toxins. Smallest exposure to toxic chemicals during this period of growth has been shown to cause a wide spectrum of childhood diseases and an increased risk for long-term neurological impairment.
- As children have the potential to grow and evolve into normal adults, smaller insults during the early developmental stage can cascade into larger catastrophic outcomes.

Table 1: Effects of selected chemical pollutants on infants and children.

Chemical pollutant	Effect
Air pollution	Asthma, other respiratory diseases, and sudden infant death syndrome
Asbestos	Mesothelioma and lung cancer
Benzene, nitrosamine, vinyl chloride, and ionizing radiation	Cancer
Diethylstilbestrol	Adenocarcinoma of the vagina after intrauterine exposure
Environmental tobacco smoke	Increased risk of sudden infant death syndrome and asthma
Ethyl alcohol	Fetal alcohol syndrome after intrauterine exposure
Lead	Neurobehavioral toxicity from low-dose exposure
Methyl mercury	Developmental neurotoxicity
Organophosphate insecticides Polychlorinated biphenyls Polybrominated diphenyl ether	Developmental neurotoxicity
Phthalates	Developmental neurotoxicity and reproductive impairment
Thalidomide	Phocomelia after intrauterine exposure
Trichloroethylene	Elevated risk of leukemia after intrauterine exposure

Although there are many synthetic chemicals causing toxicity to children, for the ease of discussion for this text, we have summarized the various types of synthetic pollutants and their harmful side effects **(Table 1)**.

HEAVY METAL POISONING

The World Health Organization (WHO) has labeled lead, mercury, arsenic, and cadmium as the top priority of the "10 chemicals of greatest public health concern," posing the greatest threats to humans. Human consumption of heavy metals leads to impairment of cellular homeostasis leading to end-organ failure. A careful history of relevant clinical encounter with environmental pollutants is important to correctly identify heavy metals as the source of the protean manifestations associated with such exposure.

The scope of discussion for this text will be limited only to Lead, Arsenic, and Mercury, as their toxicity is common in children as well as adults.

LEAD POISONING

Environmental lead exists in four isotopic forms. Till date, there is no life form on earth that needs lead to sustain

Box 1: Sources of exposure.

Paint chips
- Dust
- Soil
- Parent's or older child's occupational exposure (auto repair, battery manufacturing or recycling, smelting, construction, mining, remodeling, plumbing, gun/bullet exposure, indoor firing ranges, and painting)
- Glazed ceramics
- Herbal remedies (e.g. Ayurvedic medications)
- Home remedies, including antiperspirants, and deodorants (e.g. litargirio)
- Jewellery (as toys or belonging to parents)
- Stored battery casings (or living near a battery smelter)
- Lead-based gasoline
- Moonshine alcohol
- Contaminated foods (e.g. Mexican candies, Ecuadorian chocolates, and imported rice)
- Indoor firing ranges
- Imported spices (svanuri marili, saffron, and kuzhambu)
- Cosmetics (kohl, surma, kajal, tiro, and lipstick)
- Lead plumbing (water)
- Imported foods in lead-containing cans
- Imported toys
- Home renovations
- Antique toys or furniture

cellular vitality. Lead is a stable compound, which makes it favorable to be used in commercial manufacturing processes leading to widespread contamination of lead in the ecosystem and subsequent human contact. **Box 1** lists the common sources of lead poisoning.

In children, the most common pathway for lead to enter the body is oral ingestion due to frequent mucosal skin contact such as hand to mouth. In nearly all cases, ingestion of solids or dissolution in liquids is the most common mode of lead intoxication.

The proportion of lead absorbed from the intestines varies on several parameters:
- Size of the particle size
- *pH*: Acidic or alkaline
- Presence of other elements in the gut
- Nutritional status.

Luckily, larger chunks of paint pieces are not digestible and are mainly eliminated from the body as they are, as a single chip may contain a lethal dose of lead. Finer particles, which are termed "lead dust," are easily dissolved in an acidic medium; hence, absorption is better on an empty stomach than when the stomach is full. Elemental calcium and iron retard the absorption by direct competition for attachment sites and hence, their relative deficiencies may lead to enhanced absorption and toxicity.

Lead is preferentially retained in the bone, for a very long time (years). It binds selectively to red blood cells

(RBCs). *Blood lead levels (BLLs) are the gold standard for diagnosis and starting treatment.*

Intracellular Effects of Lead in Cells (RBCs)

Lead binds to the enzymes, which have sulfur groups, which alter the contour thus depleting their function. The last enzyme in the heme synthesis pathway is ferrochelatase that enables protoporphyrin to chelate iron, thus forming heme that is essential for multiple metabolic pathways and not merely as a component of hemoglobin. Selective inhibition of these enzymes by lead results in accumulation of various heme precursors, which causes cellular abnormality and toxicity. For example, RBC protoporphyrin levels higher than 35 µg/dL are above the reference range and are probably indicative of lead poisoning or other clinical conditions such as iron deficiency anemia or recent inflammatory disease.

Published literature on cellular metabolism says that lead is a competitive inhibitor of calcium. Most of the calcium-binding proteins have more binding capacity for lead than for ionic calcium, which may alter cellular function, leading to abnormal intracellular and intercellular processing of neurotransmitter release.

The most important action of lead is that it halts *development of the central nervous system (CNS) and is potentially irreversible.* Lead inhibits the multiple intercellular brain connections of the developing mammalian brain, thus interrupting the normal neuronal pruning process leading to failure to construct the appropriate tertiary brain structure during infancy and childhood, which culminates in a permanent abnormality. Published literature of childhood lead poisoning that followed a cohort from birth and into their 2nd decade performed MRI and functional MRI. Phosphorus magnetic resonance spectroscopy assessments confirmed the association of early childhood lead exposure and subsequent decreased gray and white matter volume and neuronal function and concluded that early lead exposure in life causes a persistent reorganization of brain architecture and diminished function.

Clinical Symptoms

Gastrointestinal (GI) symptoms of lead poisoning include loss of appetite, nonspecific abdominal pain, vomiting, and constipation, which occur over a period of weeks. *Children with BLLs higher than 20 µg/dL are twice as likely to have GI complaints as those with lower BLLs.*

Central nervous system symptoms are due to cerebral edema and raised intracranial pressure. Headaches, change in mentation, lethargy, papilledema, seizures, and coma leading to death are rarely seen at levels lower than 100 µg/dL but have been documented in children with a BLL as low as 70 µg/dL. There is no clear cutoff BLL value for the appearance of hyperactivity, but it is more likely to be observed in children who have levels higher than 20 µg/dL. Adults develop a peripheral neuropathy leading to wrist and foot drop.

Other organs systems may be affected by lead toxicity, but symptoms usually are not apparent in children. At high levels (>100 µg/dL), a reversible Fanconi syndrome and renal tubular dysfunction are observed.

Hemolytic anemias are due to shortened RBC survival although most iron deficiency anemia and hemoglobinopathies are commonly seen in the hemtological system. A summary of the lead toxicity in different systems is given in **Table 2**.

Diagnosis

Screening procedures are by far the most common tool to identify children with lead poisoning rather than clinical symptoms.[2] Owing to the irreversible action of lead on the nervous system, the main aim of management of lead poisoning is to prevent further absorption and to take efforts to eliminate it outside the body.

The following points are the broad principles of management of lead poisoning:

- *Identification and elimination of environmental sources of lead exposure*
- *Behavioral modification to reduce nonnutritive hand-to-mouth activity*
- *Dietary counseling to ensure sufficient intake of the essential elements such as calcium and iron.*

For the proportion of children with more severe lead poisoning, chelation therapy is necessary as it enhances lead excretion.

Drug Therapy (Chelation)

The current guidelines for chelation are based on the BLL. *A venous BLL of 45 µg/dL or higher needs chelation therapy.* Currently, the following four drugs are licensed to treat lead poisoning (**Table 3** contains the therapeutic profile):

- 2,3-dimercaptosuccinic acid (DMSA) (*Succimer*)
- CaNa$_2$EDTA (Calcium disodium ethylenediamine tetra acetic acid)
- British anti-lewisite (BAL) (*Dimercaprol*)
- Penicillamine.

Table 2: Clinical symptoms of lead—symptom-wise.

Gastrointestinal system	Anorexia, abdominal pain, vomiting, and constipation
Central nervous system	Headaches, change in mentation, lethargy, papilledema, seizures and coma worsening cerebral edema, hyperactivity, peripheral neuropathy, wrist drop and foot drops
Renal system (levels > 100 µg/dL)	Tubular dysfunction Fanconi syndrome
Hematological system	Shortened RBC (red blood cell) survival Hemolytic anemia, iron deficiency Hemoglobinopathies

Table 3: Summary of pharmacotherapeutics of chelation agents.

Drug and route	Synonym	Dose	Toxicity
Succimer (oral)	Chemet, 2,3-dimercaptosuccinic acid (DMSA)	350 mg/m² body surface area/dose (not 10 mg/kg) q 8 hours, PO for 5 days, then q 12 hours for 14 days	Gastrointestinal distress, rashes; elevated LFTs, depressed white blood cell count
Edetate (parenteral)	CaNa₂EDTA (calcium disodium edetate), versenate	1,000–1,500 mg/m² body surface area/day; IV infusion—continuous or intermittent; IM divided q 6 hours or q 12 hours for 5 days	• Proteinuria, pyuria, rising blood urea nitrogen/creatinine—all rare • Hypercalcemia if too rapid an infusion • Tissue inflammation if infusion infiltrates
British anti-lewisite (BAL) (parenteral)	Dimercaprol	300–500 mg/m² body surface area/day; IM only divided q 4 hours for 3–5 days. Only for BLL ≥ 70 µg/dL	Gastrointestinal distress, altered mentation; elevated LFTs, hemolysis if glucose-6-phosphate dehydrogenase deficiency; no concomitant iron treatment
D-pen (oral)	Penicillamine	10 mg/kg/day for 2 weeks increasing to 25–40 mg/kg/day; oral, divided q 12 hours. For 12–20 weeks	• Rashes, fever, blood dyscrasias, elevated LFTs, proteinuria • Allergic cross-reactivity with penicillin

(BLL: blood lead levels; IM: intramuscular; IV: intravenous; LFT: liver function test)

Monotherapy versus Combination Chelation

Children with BLLs of *44–70 µg/dL* may be treated with a *single* drug, preferably DMSA. Those with BLLs of *70 µg/dL* or greater require *two-drug* treatment (**Table 4**).

Acute drug-related toxicities, including *GI distress, transient elevations in transaminases, active urinary sediment,* and *neutropenia,* are usually transient and reversible. These types of events are more common for BAL and penicillamine and least common for CaNa₂EDTA and DMSA. All of the chelating agents are effective in reducing lead levels. Some authorities also recommend the concomitant catharsis to eliminate any lead already in the gut. None of these therapeutic agents described in the preceding text completely eliminates bound and unbound lead from the body. Within days to weeks after completion of a course of therapy, there is a "*rebound phenomenon.*" *The source of this rebound in the BLL is the release of lead into the blood by from the bone.* Serial examinations of bone lead content have shown that chelation with CaNa₂EDTA is associated with a decline in bone lead levels, but that residual bone lead remains detectable even after multiple courses of treatment.

Table 4: Dual-therapy regimens.

Children with encephalopathy	CaNa₂EDTA and BAL for those with encephalopathy
Children without encephalopathy	CaNa₂EDTA in combination with either DMSA or BAL

(BAL: British anti-lewisite; DMSA: 2,3-dimercaptosuccinic acid; CaNa₂EDTA: calcium disodium ethylenediaminetetraacetic acid)

Repeat chelation is indicated if the BLL rebounds to 45 µg/dL or higher. Children with initial BLLs higher than 70 µg/dL are likely to require more than one course. A minimum of 3 days between courses is recommended to prevent treatment-related toxicities, especially in the kidney.

The indication for chelation therapy for children with BLLs < 45 µg/dL is less defined. Use of these chelation agents in children with BLLs from 20 to 44 µg/dL results in transiently lowered BLLs and, in some cases, reversal of lead-induced enzyme inhibition.

With successful intervention (with or without chelation), BLLs decline with the greatest fall in BLL occurring in the *first 2 months* after therapy is initiated. Subsequently, the rate of change in BLL declines slowly so that by 6–12 months after identification, the BLL of the average child with moderate lead poisoning (BLL > 20 µg/dL) will be 50% lower. Children with more markedly elevated BLLs may take years to reach the CDC (Centers for Disease Control and Prevention) reference level, 5 µg/dL, even if all sources of lead exposure have been eliminated, behavior has been modified, and nutrition has been maximized.

Prevention

Early screening remains the best way of avoiding and therefore obviating the need for the treatment of lead poisoning.

◼ ARSENIC

Arsenic is a metalloid that exists in four forms:
1. Elemental arsenic
2. Arsine gas
3. Inorganic arsenic salts (pentavalent arsenate form or trivalent arsenite form)
4. Organic arsenic compounds.

The most toxic form of all the arsenic compounds is arsine gas.

Data from India

Over a million Indians have been exposed to high levels of arsenic with more than 2 lakh documented cases of arsenicosis. Published data from adult studies from 18 years to 65 years showed the incidence of arsenicosis to be around 19%. Within this cohort, 7% of the patients developed neuropsychiatric manifestation as compared to an average 7% prevalence of mental disorders in India. The participants in this study were from seven different villages, 90% of which had arsenic levels ranging from 25 to 900 µg/L. The incidence was higher in males with low socioeconomic status (SES) and a 25% rate of unemployment. In India, patients with arsenic toxicity exhibited anxiety and depression as the most common neuropsychiatric manifestations.[3]

Mechanisms of Action

Long-term exposures to arsenic are likely compounded with exposures to pollution, non-nut diet, and low SES. Basic scientific research is aimed at controlling these confounding factors, including extent and timing of exposure. This data shows the various pathophysiologic mechanisms of arsenic[3,4] (**Box 2**) and its CNS effects (**Box 3**).

Box 2: Mechanisms of toxicity of arsenic.

- Depletion of methyl groups affecting epigenetic profiles
- Uncoupling of oxidative phosphorylation and increased reactive oxygen species
- The inhibition of thiol-containing enzymes and proteins (including the depletion of glutathione)
- Altered signal transduction and cell proliferation
- Reduced DNA repair thereby inducing genotoxicity

Box 3: Structural changes in the central nervous system (CNS) as a result of arsenic toxicity.

- Hippocampal dysfunction
- Glutamatergic, glucocorticoid, cholinergic, and monoaminergic signaling
- Pathways associated with Alzheimer's disease
- Synaptic plasticity, particularly neurogenesis

Pathophysiology

After exposure to arsenic compounds, the absorbed arsine is taken up by the erythrocytes and is converted to dihydride compounds and native arsenic. This couples with red cell sulfhydryl groups leading to cell membrane instability and a large-scale hemolysis. The inorganic arsenic salts poison enzymatic processes vital to cellular metabolism. Trivalent arsenic binds to sulfhydryl groups, resulting in reduction of adenosine triphosphate synthesis through the inhibition of enzyme systems such as the pyruvate dehydrogenase and α-ketoglutarate complexes. Pentavalent arsenic may be biotransformed to trivalent arsenic or substituted for phosphate in the glycolytic pathway leading to uncoupling of oxidative phosphorylation.[5]

Clinical Manifestations

Arsine gas is colorless, odorless, nonirritating, and highly toxic. Inhalation causes no immediate symptoms. After a latent period of 2–24 hours, exposed individuals present with multisystemic involvement such as massive hemolysis, malaise, headache, weakness, dyspnea, nausea, vomiting, abdominal pain, hepatomegaly, pallor, jaundice, hemoglobinuria, and renal failure.

Acute ingestion of arsenic (early sequelae) produces certain effects which are given in **Table 5**.

Lethal doses of arsenates are 5–50 mg/kg; lethal doses of arsenites are <5 mg/kg.

The delayed effects of arsenic toxicity (sequelae) are given in **Table 6**.

Adult survivors of infant arsenic poisoning experience higher mortality from disorders of the nervous system compared to adults without such exposure.

Table 5: Early sequelae of acute Arsenic poisoning.

Gastrointestinal toxicity	Nausea, vomiting, abdominal pain, and diarrhea, hemorrhagic gastroenteritis with extensive fluid loss and third spacing may result in hypovolemic shock
Cardiovascular toxicity	QT interval prolongation, polymorphous ventricular tachycardia, congestive cardiomyopathy, pulmonary edema, and cardiogenic shock
Neurological toxicity	Delirium, seizures, cerebral edema, encephalopathy, and coma

Table 6: Late sequelae of arsenic poisoning.

Kidneys	Hematuria, proteinuria, and acute tubular necrosis
Neurological system	A delayed sensorimotor peripheral neuropathy secondary to axonal degeneration manifesting as painful dysesthesias followed by diminished vibratory, pain, touch, and temperature sensation; decreased deep tendon reflexes; and, in the most severe cases, an ascending paralysis with respiratory failure mimicking Guillain-Barré syndrome

Subacute toxicity is heralded by prolonged fatigue, malaise, weight loss, headache, chronic encephalopathy, peripheral sensorimotor neuropathy, leukopenia, anemia, thrombocytopenia, chronic cough, and gastroenteritis. Approximately 5% of patients demonstrate the classical *Mees' lines* in the nails usually after 1–2 months after the exposure. Dermatologic findings include alopecia, oral ulceration, peripheral edema, pruritic macular rash, and desquamation.

Chronic arsenic toxicity results in skin lesions, lung disease, and diminished intellectual function. Chronic low level exposure is usually from environmental or occupational sources. Over the course of years, dermatologic lesions develop, including hyperpigmentation, hypopigmentation, hyperkeratoses (especially on the palms and soles), squamous and basal cell carcinomas, and Bowen's disease (cutaneous squamous cell carcinoma in situ).

Encephalopathy and peripheral neuropathy may be the presenting neurological manifestations. The GI manifestations include hepatomegaly, hypersplenism, noncirrhotic portal fibrosis, and portal hypertension. Blackfoot disease is an obliterative arterial disease of the lower extremities associated with chronic arsenic exposure that has been described in published literature from Taiwan. Malignancies secondary to chronic arsenic exposure are reflected in increased rates of cancers of the *skin, lung, liver, bladder, and kidney as well as of angiosarcomas.* The effects of prenatal exposure to arsenic are uncertain but may include intrauterine growth retardation.

Laboratory Findings

The diagnosis of arsenic intoxication is based on characteristic clinical findings, a history of exposure, and elevated urinary arsenic values. A spot urine arsenic level should be determined for symptomatic patients before chelation, although initially the result may be negative. Because urinary excretion of arsenic is intermittent, definitive diagnosis depends on a 24-hour urine collection. *Concentrations greater than 50 µg/L in a 24-hour urine specimen are consistent with arsenic intoxication.*

Urine specimens must be collected in metal-free containers. Ingestion of seafood containing nontoxic arsenobetaine and arsenocholine can cause elevations of urinary arsenic. *Blood arsenic levels rarely are helpful because of their high variability and the rapid clearance of arsenic from the blood in acute poisonings.* Elevated arsenic values in the hair or nails must be interpreted cautiously because of the possibility of external contamination. Abdominal radiographs may demonstrate ingested radiopaque arsenic.

Later in the course of illness, a complete blood cell count may show anemia, thrombocytopenia, and leukocytosis, followed by leukopenia, karyorrhexis, and basophilic stippling of RBCs. The serum concentrations of creatinine, bilirubin, and transaminases may be elevated; urinalysis may show proteinuria, pyuria, and hematuria; and examination of the cerebrospinal fluid may show protein elevations.

Treatment

The principles of management for arsenic intoxication include prompt removal from the source of poisoning, aggressive stabilization and supportive care, decontamination, and chelation therapy when appropriate similar to lines of treatment of lead toxicity. Once the diagnosis is suspected, the local poison control facility should be contacted, and a multidisciplinary team comprising physicians who are familiar with the management of heavy metal poisoning is essential for successful treatment.

Supportive care for patients exposed to arsine gas requires close monitoring for signs of hemolysis, including evaluation of the peripheral blood smear and urinalysis. Transfusion of packed RBCs may be necessary, as may administration of intravenous fluids, sodium bicarbonate, and mannitol to prevent renal failure secondary to the deposition of hemoglobin in the kidneys. After inhalation of elemental mercury vapor, patients require careful monitoring of respiratory status, which may include pulse oximetry, arterial blood gas analysis, and chest radiography. Supportive care involves administration of supplemental oxygen and, in severe cases, intubation and mechanical ventilation.

Acute ingestion of inorganic arsenic salts results in *hemorrhagic gastroenteritis, cardiovascular collapse, and multiorgan dysfunction*. Fluid resuscitation, inotrope, and transfusion of blood products may be required for management of cardiovascular instability. Severe respiratory distress, coma with loss of airway reflexes, intractable seizures, and respiratory paralysis are indications for intubation and mechanical ventilation. Renal function must be monitored carefully for signs of renal failure and the need for hemodialysis.

Gastrointestinal decontamination after ingestion of the inorganic arsenic and mercury salts has not been well studied. Due to the corrosive effects of these compounds, induced emesis is not recommended, and endoscopy may be considered before gastric lavage. Arsenic and mercury are not well adsorbed to activated charcoal, but its use may be helpful if coingestants are suspected. Whole-bowel irrigation is used to remove any radiopaque material remaining in the GI tract.

Chelation for acute arsenic poisoning is most effective when administered as soon as possible after the exposure. *Chelation should be continued until 24-hour urinary arsenic (<50 μg/L for arsenic)*, the patient is symptom-free, or the remaining toxic effects are believed to be irreversible. The efficacy of chelation in long-term exposures is decreased as heavy metals in the tissue compartment are relatively unexchangeable and some degree of irreversible toxicity has already occurred.

Dimercaprol, also known as 2,3-dimercaptopropanol or BAL, is the chelator of choice for a patient who cannot tolerate oral therapy, as often is true for critically ill patients and after ingestion of the corrosive inorganic arsenic and mercury salts. BAL is available suspended in peanut oil and benzyl benzoate in 3 mL ampules at a concentration of 100 mg/mL for deep intramuscular (IM) injection.

Box 4: Dose of BAL for acute arsenic poisoning.

- 2.5 mg/kg IM q 6 hours for the 1st 2 days
- 2.5 mg/kg IM q 12 hours on the 3rd day
- 2.5 mg/kg/day IM for 10 days

(BAL: British anti-lewisite; IM: intramuscular)

Box 5: Dose of BAL for severe acute arsenic poisoning.

- 3 mg/kg IM q 4 hours for 2 days
- 3 mg/ kg IM q 6 hours on day
- 3 mg/kg IM q 12 hours for 10 days.

(BAL: British anti-lewisite; IM: intramuscular)

For arsenic poisoning, the recommended regimen of BAL is 2.5 mg/kg IM q6h for the 1st 2 days, 2.5 mg/kg IM q12h on the 3rd day, and then 2.5 mg/kg/day IM for 10 days **(Box 4)**.

For severe arsenic poisoning, the dose of BAL is increased to 3 mg/kg IM q4h for 2 days, 3 mg/kg IM q6h on day 3, and then 3 mg/kg IM q12h for 10 days **(Box 5)**. BAL–heavy metal complex is excreted in the urine and bile. A period of 5 days between courses of chelation is recommended. Oral chelating agents are used to replace the painful BAL injections when the patient is stable enough to tolerate oral therapy and prolonged chelation is necessary. Succimer, also known as 2,3-dimercaptosuccinic acid (DMSA), is an orally administered water-soluble derivative of BAL. DMSA is available in 100 mg capsules. The recommended regimen of DMSA is 10 mg/kg orally every 8 hours for 5 days. The DMSA–heavy metal complex is excreted in the urine and bile. A period of 2 weeks between courses of chelation is recommended. Mild adverse effects include nausea, vomiting, diarrhea, loss of appetite, and transient elevations in liver enzyme levels. DMSA also may cause hemolysis in glucose-6-phosphate dehydrogenase-deficient patients.

■ MERCURY POISONING

Mercury exists in three forms: (1) Elemental mercury, (2) inorganic mercury salts, and (3) organic mercury. Elemental mercury is present in thermometers, sphygmomanometers, barometers, batteries, and some latex paints produced before 1991. Workers in industries producing these products may expose their children to the toxin when mercury is brought home on contaminated clothing. Vacuuming of carpets contaminated with mercury and breaking of mercury fluorescent light bulbs may result in elemental mercury vapor exposure. Severe inhalation poisonings have resulted from attempts to separate gold from gold ore by heating mercury and forming a gold–mercury amalgam. Elemental mercury has been used in folk remedies by Asians and Dental amalgams containing elemental mercury release trace amounts of mercury. Published data from the WHO panel decided to put a permanent ban on the use of dental amalgams that pose a serious health concern to public health. However, this committee recommended that alternatives to amalgam should be sought as part of a phaseout of the use of mercury-containing products.[2]

Inorganic mercury salts are found in most of the commercial products, such as pesticides, disinfectants, antiseptics, pigments, dry batteries, and explosives, and as preservatives in some medicinal preparations. The most common source of mercury poisoning was found via consumption of contaminated fish. Mercury compounds in the environment are methylated to methyl mercury by soil and water microorganisms that rapidly accumulate in fish (swordfish, king mackerel, fresh tuna, tile fish, and shark) and other aquatic organisms, which are in turn consumed by humans. To address concerns that maternal consumption of large quantities of fish during pregnancy may expose the fetus to concentrations of mercury with adverse consequences, multiple studies were carried out and showed a positive association between exposure and its after effects. Historically, marked prominent large outbreaks of methyl mercury intoxication include the incidents in Japan in the 1950s (Minamata disease, from consumption of contaminated seafood) and in Iraq in 1971 (from consumption of grain treated with a methyl mercury fungicide).[2]

Thiomersal is a mercury-containing preservative used in some vaccines. Thiomersal contains 49.6% mercury by weight and is metabolized to ethyl mercury and thiosalicylate. During an ongoing review of biologic products in response to the US Food and Drug Administration (FDA) Modernization Act of 1997, the FDA determined that infants who received thiomersal-containing vaccines at multiple visits might have been exposed to more mercury than recommended by federal guidelines. The larger risks of not vaccinating children far outweigh any known risk of exposure to thiomersal-containing vaccines. Studies do not demonstrate a link between thiomersal-containing vaccines and autistic spectrum disorders, and no evidence supports a change in the standard of practice with regard to administration of thiomersal-containing vaccines in areas of the world where they are used. A rise in blood mercury levels following a single dose of hepatitis vaccine was seen in preterm infants, but the clinical significance is unknown.[2]

Pharmacokinetics

Inhaled elemental mercury vapor is highly lipid soluble of which 80% absorbed by the lungs and is distributed rapidly to the CNS. The elemental mercury is oxidized by catalase to the mercuric ion, which is the reactive form that causes cellular toxicity. Elemental mercury liquid is poorly absorbed from the GI tract, with less than 0.1% being absorbed. The half-life of elemental mercury in the tissues is approximately 60 days, most of the excretion occurring in the urine.

Inorganic mercury salts are approximately 10% absorbed from the GI tract and cross the blood–brain barrier to a lesser extent than elemental mercury. Mercuric salts are more soluble than mercurous salts and, therefore, produce greater toxicity. Elimination occurs primarily in the urine, with a half-life of approximately 40 days.

Methyl mercury is the most avidly absorbed of the organic mercury compounds, with most of the absorption occurring from the GI tract (90%). The lipophilic, short-chain alkyl structure of methyl mercury allows it to be distributed rapidly across the blood–brain barrier and placenta. Methyl mercury is approximately 90% excreted in the bile, with the remainder being excreted in the urine. The half-life is 70 days.[2]

Pathophysiology

After absorption, mercury is distributed to all tissues, particularly the CNS and the kidneys. Mercury reacts with sulfhydryl, phosphoryl, carboxyl, and amide groups, resulting in:

- Disruption of enzymes
- Transport mechanisms
- Disruption of cell membranes and structural proteins
- Widespread cellular dysfunction or necrosis which results in the multiorgan toxicity, characteristic of mercury poisoning.[2]

Clinical Manifestations

Five syndromes describe the clinical presentation of mercury poisoning. *Acute inhalation* of elemental mercury vapor results in rapid onset of cough, dyspnea, chest pain, fever, chills, headaches, and visual disturbances.

Gastrointestinal findings include metallic taste, salivation, nausea, vomiting, and diarrhea. Depending on the severity of the exposure, the illness may be self-limited or may progress to respiratory symptoms of *necrotizing bronchiolitis, interstitial pneumonitis, pulmonary edema, and death from respiratory failure.* Younger children are more susceptible *to pulmonary toxicity. Survivors may demonstrate restrictive lung disease.*

Renal dysfunction and neurologic disturbances (ataxia, persistent weakness, and emotional lability) may develop over a period of time. Chronic exposure to volatilized elemental mercury in dental amalgams has not been found to be of any clinical significance.[2]

Acute ingestion of inorganic mercury salts (typically secondary to ingestion of a button battery) can occur in a few hours as corrosive gastroenteritis, signified by metallic taste, oropharyngeal burns, nausea, hematemesis, severe abdominal pain, hematochezia, acute tubular necrosis, cardiovascular collapse, and death.[2]

Chronic inorganic mercury intoxication produces the syndromic manifestations of *tremor, neuropsychiatric disturbances, and gingivostomatitis.* The syndrome results from long-term exposure to certain organic mercury compounds, elemental mercury, and inorganic mercury salts, which may be processed to ionic mercury. The fine intention tremor of the distal extremities (fingers) later progresses to the face, evolving as involuntary movements such as *choreoathetosis* and spasmodic *ballismus. Mixed sensorimotor neuropathy* and visual disturbances are the other neurological manifestations, such as emotional lability, delirium, headaches, memory loss, insomnia, anorexia, and fatigue, which are the neuropsychiatric manifestations. Renal dysfunction ranges from asymptomatic proteinuria to nephrotic syndrome.[2]

A rare idiosyncratic hypersensitivity reaction to mercury that occurs predominantly in children exposed to mercurous powders (*Acrodynia or pink disease*) that includes a generalized pain, paresthesias, and an acral (hands, feet) rash, which progressively involves the face. The rash is a characteristic red-pink, papular, pruritic, and painful; it may progress to desquamation and ulceration. Other variants of rash such as morbilliform, vesicular, and hemorrhagic variants are not uncommon. Other clinical features include anorexia, apathy, photophobia, and hypotonia, especially of the pectoral and pelvic girdles. Irritability, tremors, diaphoresis, insomnia, hypertension, and tachycardia may be present. Some cases were initially diagnosed as pheochromocytoma. Source reduction usually results in a favorable outcome.[2]

Methyl mercury intoxication (also known as *Minamata disease* after the widespread mercury poisoning that occurred at Minamata Bay in Japan in people who had ingested contaminated fish) manifests as delayed *neurotoxicity* that appears after a latent period of weeks to months that is characterized by ataxia; dysarthria; paresthesias; tremors; movement disorders; impairment of vision, hearing, smell, and taste; memory loss; progressive dementia; and death.

Infants exposed in utero are the most severely affected, with low birth weight, microcephaly, profound developmental delay, cerebral palsy, deafness, blindness, and seizures. Although there is significant residual morbidity from methyl mercury neurotoxicity, observations on long-term follow-up of children exposed in Iraq reveal complete or partial resolution in most cases.[2]

Laboratory Findings

The diagnosis of mercury intoxication is based on characteristic clinical findings, a history of exposure, and elevation of whole blood or urine mercury values, the last of which confirms the exposure. *Thin-layer and gas chromatographic techniques* are helpful fatigue organic from inorganic mercury. Blood should be collected in special tubes for trace elements from laboratories that are capable of performing those tests.

Levels <10 µg/L in whole blood and <20 µg/L in a 24-hour urine specimen are considered normal. Although blood mercury levels may reflect acute exposure, they decrease as mercury redistributes into the tissues. Urine mercury levels are most useful for identifying long-term exposures, except in the case of methyl mercury, which undergoes minimal urinary excretion. Urinary mercury levels are used in monitoring efficacy of chelation therapy, whereas blood levels are used primarily in monitoring organic mercury poisonings. Hair analysis for mercury is not reliable because hair reflects both endogenous and exogenous mercury exposure (hair avidly binds mercury from the environment). Abdominal radiographs may demonstrate ingested radiopaque mercury.[2]

Urinary markers of early nephrotoxicity include micro-albuminuria, retinol-binding protein, β2-microglobulin, and N-acetyl-β-d-glucosaminidase. Early neurotoxicity may be detected with neuropsychiatric testing and nerve conduction studies, whereas severe CNS toxicity is apparent on CT or MRI.[2]

Treatment

The principles of management for mercury intoxication follow the same lines of arsenic, which include:

- Prompt removal from the source of poisoning
- Aggressive stabilization and supportive care
- Decontamination
- Chelation therapy (when appropriate).

Box 6: Dose of BAL in mercury poisoning.

- 5 mg/kg IM on the 1st day
- Followed by 2.5 mg/kg IM q 12–24 hours for 10 days

(BAL: British anti-lewisite; IM: intramuscular)

Chelation for acute mercury poisoning is most effective when given as early as possible after identification of potential exposures. Chelation should be continued until 24-hour urinary mercury levels are within permissible levels (<20 µg/L for mercury) and the patient is symptom-free, or the remaining toxic effects are believed to be irreversible. The efficacy of chelation in long-term exposures is low as heavy metal in the tissue compartment is relatively unexchangeable and some degree of irreversible toxicity has already occurred.[2]

Dimercaprol, also known as 2,3-dimercaptopropanol or BAL, is the chelator of choice for a patient who cannot tolerate oral therapy, as often is true for critically ill patients and after ingestion of the corrosive inorganic mercury salts. BAL is available suspended in peanut oil and benzyl benzoate in 3 mL ampules at a concentration of 100 mg/mL for deep IM injection. The BAL–heavy metal complex is excreted in the urine and bile. A period of 5 days between courses of chelation is recommended.[2]

*The dose of BAL for inorganic mercury poisoning is given in **Box 6**.*

CONCLUSION

Pediatricians have always played pivotal roles in the identification of "Toxidromes." Every pediatrician needs to be an "alert clinician" and keep an open mind for identifying new diseases in children caused by exposures in the environment. With the current environmental changes such as global warming, use of synthetic lifestyle, and origins of noninfectious disease, it is important to enquire details about biome of surrounding environment, occupational exposures, and neighborhood factories. A cluster of cases occurring in large numbers at a single point of time is a valuable clinical clue.

Index of suspicion, which is elicited via a focused history and a sound clinical assessment, is the key parameter for detection of children environmental exposures. Data about travel is an important aspect of the questionnaire. Trends in patterns of exposure, a new onset of an emerging pattern is an important that needs to be elicited and pursued.

REFERENCES

1. Environmental Pollution Centers. Chemical Pollution. [online] Available from: https://www.environmentalpollutioncenters.org/chemical/. [Last accessed on December, 2019].
2. Kliegman RM, St Geme III JW. Nelson Textbook of Pediatrics, 20th edition. Philadelphia, USA: Elsevier; 2016.
3. Hughes MF, Beck BD, Chen Y, et al. Arsenic exposure and toxicology: a historical perspective. Toxicol Sci. 2011;123(2): 305-32.
4. Watanabe T, Hirano S. Metabolism of arsenic and its toxicological relevance. Arch Toxicol. 2013;87(6):969-79.
5. Tyler CR, Allan AM. The Effects of Arsenic Exposure on Neurological and Cognitive Dysfunction in Human and Rodent Studies: A review. Curr Environ Health Rep. 2014;1:132-47.

Herbal Medicine and Plant Poisoning

Narmada S

INTRODUCTION

Herbal medicines have been in usage in India since the Vedas. Usage of herbal medicines dates back to 3,000 BC where a Sloka in Rig Veda says "Let all the medicinal plants become sweet, let all the trees become sweet." Apart from that Indians have been traditionally using many herbal medicines at home. Our forests are home to countless medicinal plants.[1] Herbal medicines are also used extensively in West and many people use it in their home.[2]

The total sale and the value of commercial herbal medicines are increasing day by day. In China, the sale of herbal medicine reached US $5 billion and in India, 100 metric tonnes of 178 high-volume herbal products are being used. The total annual world sale of herbal medicines has approached US $60 billion paralleling or exceeding allopathic medicine sales.[3] Over 40% of Americans and 20–60% of Europeans utilize some form of complementary and herbal medicines.[4] Despite their wide use, no controlled trials are there to assess their safety and efficacy. One of the main reasons is that the dosage and chemically active ingredients cannot be specifically determined and comparative trials are lacking.[5]

In this era of government introducing AYUSH healthcare providers and patients relying more on herbal medicines, it is important that we as healthcare providers should have a knowledge about the herbal medicines and its effects. We also need to adopt a nonjudgmental approach while evaluating children who have been given these medicines. This chapter aims to provide an idea about the common herbal medicines used in our Indian homes and also about the effects of these plant products in normal and toxic doses.

COMMON MEDICINES USED IN INDIA

Herbal medicines are processed and taken in various forms—paste, distilled concoction, powders, small tablets, natural supplements, teas, essential oils, ointments, salves, rubs, and capsules **(Table 1 and Fig. 1)**.

REASONS FOR USING HERBAL MEDICINES IN CHILDREN

There has been a significant increase in the use of herbal medicines. As compared to 34% using herbal medicine in 1990, statistics report that around 42% of people were using in 1997. Though recent data are not available this number is bound to increase.

The reasons for the increase use of herbal medicines are:

- Lack of satisfaction with conventional medicine
- Previous good experiences with herbal medicines
- Family traditions and influence of family
- Herbal medicine is considered healthier and natural
- Herbal medicines have fewer side effects and good tolerability
- Having knowledge of the content of medicines[5]
- It is more affordable
- Allays concerns over the chemical products
- Gives an impression of more personalized healthcare
- More public access to health care[3]
- Claims on their effectiveness in social media
- Change in consumer attitude to preferring natural remedies
- False belief that they have less side effects
- High cost of conventional medicines and becoming unaffordable for a large section of the society
- A movement toward self-medication and treatment

Table 1: Herbal medicines used in India.

Name of the herbal medicine used in India	Compositions	Uses
Ajwain (*Trachyspermum ammi*)	Powder, raw seed	Relief of acidity and flatulence, prevents premature graying of hair
Adhatoda Vasica	Syrup Adhatoda	Expectorant and bronchodilator, for all LRTI
Betel nut (*Areca catechu*)	To be given with other herbal products	Prevents flatulence, reduces bad odor of mouth
Bhringraj (*Eclipta prostrata*)	Various forms	Liver cirrhosis, infectious hepatitis, hair and skin problems
Chitharathai (*Alpinia officinarum*)	Powder	Digestive problems
Common madder/Manjistha (*Rubia cordifolia*)	Roots or powder mixed in coconut oil	Chronic wounds, diabetic ulcers and nonhealing varicose ulcers
Camellia sinensis (Green tea)	Decoction	Antioxidant, improves brain function
Gale of the wind (*Phyllanthus niruri*)	Capsule, tea or powder form	Liver-related disorders
Garlic (*Allium sativum*)	Raw form and mixed with other ingredients	Antioxidant, antihypertensive, improves cholesterol levels
Green chireta/kirayat (*Andrographis paniculata*)	Powder Anvir syrup	Antiviral properties
Glycyrrhiza glabra (licorice)–Adhimathuram/Mulethi	Powder	Cough and liver abnormalities
Karunjeeragam (*Nigella sativa*)	Raw seed	Soaked in hot water and used for cholesterol and blood sugar
Papaya extract	Syrup Pop E, Syrup Caripill	Viral fever. Supposed to increase the platelets
Pepper (*Piper nigrum*), long pepper (*Piper longum*), dry ginger (*Zingiber officinale*)	Mixture—powder/syrup	Digestive problems
Silymarin (milk thistle)	Powder	Appetizer, hepatic cirrhosis, and dyspepsia
St. John's wort (*Hypericum perforatum*)		Treating mild-to-moderate depression
Tulsi (*Ocimum tenuiflorum*), betel leaf (*Piper betel*), Camphor	Powder soaked in hot water	Increases the immunity and antiviral property
Talisathi mixture–Abies webbiana (Talispatra or Indian Silver Fir), Black pepper (*Piper nigrum*), Sonth (*Zingiber officinale*), Pippali (Long pepper–*Piper longum*), Green cardamom (Elaichi)	Herbal powder	Bronchodilator, antitussive, expectorant, anti-inflammatory, antiviral, antibacterial, carminative
Thai nightshade (*Solanum procumbens*)		Relieves stomach irritation, spasms and pain
Vasambu (*Acorus calamus* root)	Burnt powder	Stomach ulcer, infant flatulence

(LRTI: lower respiratory tract infection)

- The methodology of conventional physicians gives a feeling to patient that he/she has not been given adequate attention.[7]

CONDITIONS WHERE HERBAL MEDICINES ARE USED

Numerous Indian medicinal plants have been used globally. Lot of historical documents have documented the effects and also have been believed by people to cure various ailments. There has been concept of reverse pharmacology on these selected plants which have given novel targets and drugs. The very famous discovery is the discovery of digoxin from digitalis plant after it was observed that the plant healed dropsy.

The conditions where herbal medicines are used are as follows:

- *Immunomodulation*: This is one of the most common usage in India according to a study conducted in rural north India. About 20% of people using herbal medicines believed the medicines can help in improving their children's immune status.
- *Gastrointestinal disorders and antispasmodic*: About 18% of people used herbal medicines to relieve their gastrointestinal disturbances. They have also been widely used as antispasmodics for newborns.

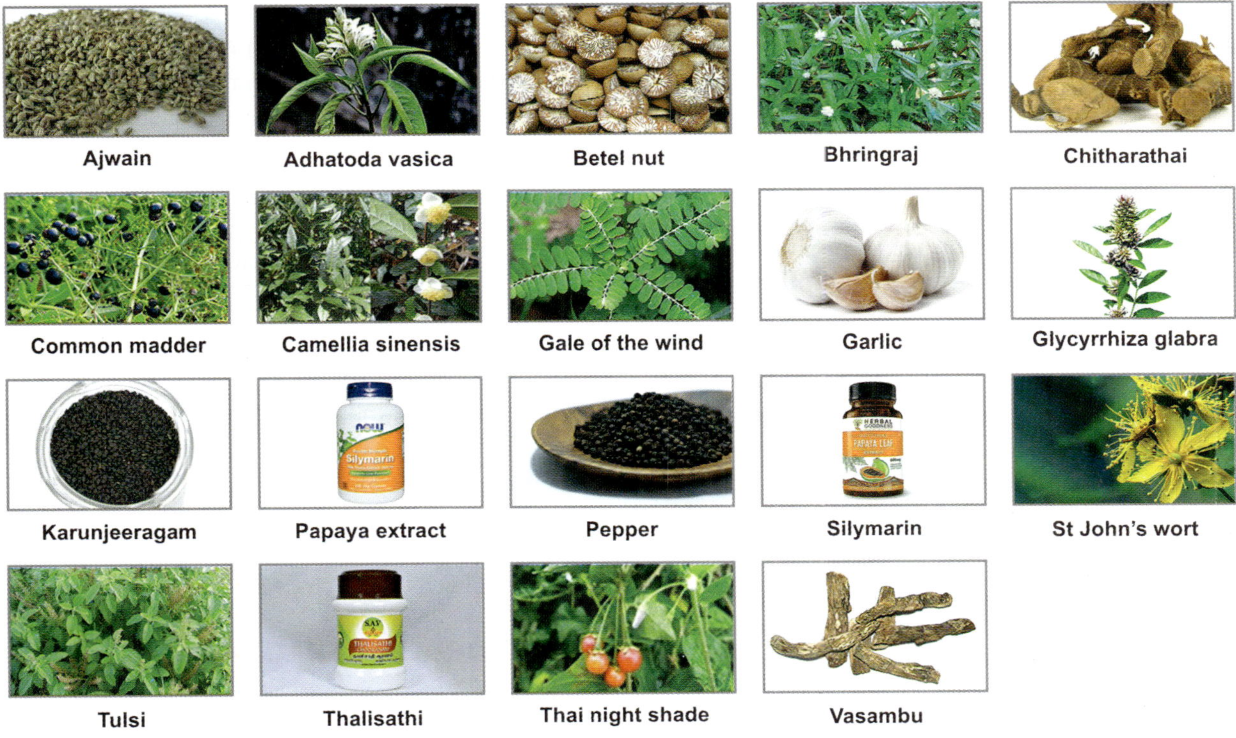

Fig. 1: Common herbal medicines used in India.

- *Blood purifier*: About 15% of people considered herbal medicines to purify their blood of harmful chemicals. Several of the medicines are now being used in anti-aging preparations and are considered as antioxidant.[8]
- *Nootropic and aphrodisiac preparations*: In adults, herbal medicines are used in nootropic and aphrodisiac preparations.
- *Anticold preparations*: This is another common usage (10%) especially for children.
- Skin diseases and burns.
- *For liver-related disorders and jaundice*: Among the users, around 10% of them used it for liver-related disorders. Many consider herbal medicines to be curative for jaundice.
- Memory enhancing preparations are commonly used by adolescents during exam times and also for children with developmental delays.
- Antiobesity drug.
- *Antidiabetic*: With advent of media publicity many adults try these preparations to control their sugars.[8,9]

INCIDENCE AND REASONS FOR TOXICITY OF HERBAL MEDICINES

India is the country with the greatest reported use of traditional herbal medicine. About 11.7% of population

have reported that their most frequent source of care is only traditional medicine.[10] This is the highest among South East Asian countries. Lower socioeconomic status, unemployment, and low health status were the main reason for usage. Besides being a part of tradition and culture, it is widely believed that it can cure almost all ailments. Added to that, there is lot of patronizing by the government and community in terms of policies and funding.[10] However, natural is not always "safe" and now lot of studies have brought out the toxicity of medicinal plants which led to the World Health Organization (WHO) releasing guidelines on safely monitoring of herbal medicines in pharmacovigilance systems.[11]

One of the main problems is that the pharmacokinetics or toxicokinetics of herbal medicines is very difficult to be studied. The active ingredient is often not known in these products. Most of the products are crude/partially processed. Also within a herbal product, there are large number of potentially interfering components that either enhance or reduce the toxicity.[12]

The reasons for the toxicity of herbal medicines are due to:
- Overingestion without the knowledge of the medicine
- Adulteration of herbal products with other undeclared medicines and potent pharmaceutical substances such as steroids and nonsteroidal anti-inflammatory

agents. Some herbal products were found to contain 0.1–0.3 mg of betamethasone.[13]

- Wrong species of closely related medicinal plants.
- Misidentification of the medicinal plant species. There was also renal failure when plant materials containing aristolochic acid was used for manufacturing herbal products.[13]
- Errors in the prescription by healthcare providers.
- Use of products potentially contaminated with hazardous substance like toxic metals, pathogenic microorganisms, and fertilizer residues. There is evidence that Indian herbal products like Karela tablets and churna powders produced by popular companies had high levels of lead, mercury, and arsenic in analysis done at Canadian markets.[11,13,14]

Toxic Effects of Herbal Medicine

Gastrointestinal disturbances: These are predominant side effects of taking the herbal medicines, mostly due to improper usage and large quantity present in the gastrointestinal tract causing abdominal distension, tenderness, and vomiting. Medicinal plants like Vasaka (*Justicia adhatoda*), Vasambu (*Acorus calamus*) are known to produce these complications.[15,16] Silymarin is known to cause abdominal pain, bloating, diarrhea, and indigestion.

Central nervous system (CNS) toxicity: There has been evidence of CNS toxicity in the form of seizures or anticholinergic toxicity. Acorus causing seizures is very well known in the South.[16] St John's wort (*Hypericum perforatum*) is a serotonin agonist and also a monoamine oxidase inhibitor and has been documented to interact with other drugs to produce severe serotonin syndrome causing hallucinations, tremors, and anxiety.[17]

Cardiovascular toxicity: Certain herbal medicines can produce cardiotoxicity. Number of herbs contain potent cardioactive glycosides that can produce palpitations, arrhythmias, and heart block either due to overdosage, potent interaction with other medications, or intentional poisoning.[18] Ephedrine popularly used for respiratory conditions has been known to produce cardiac stimulation, hypertension, vasoconstriction, chest pain, and hemorrhage. It was banned in India but still available as combination products in over-the-counter products.[17]

Hepatotoxicity: Hepatotoxicity of the herbal drugs has been reported frequently. It is predominantly due to the contamination with heavy metals when used as a preparation. There is a growing body of evidence to prove that hepatic injury and fibrosis probably due to contamination and presence of high volatile compounds have been documented.[19] Hepatic encephalopathy has been reported with high dosages of herbal medicines used for treatment of viral hepatitis.

Carcinogenic effects: Number of traditionally used medicinal plants have been suspected to have carcinogens. For example *Gingko biloba* has been implicated in hepatocellular carcinomas both in humans and rodents.[20]

Other systems:
- Severe dermatitis has been reported.
- Garlic, chamomile tea, and capsicum may produce contact dermatitis.
- Echinacea and chamomile tea has been known to produce anaphylaxis.[17]
- Nephrotoxicity has been reported with prolonged usage of herbal medicines for skin disorders.

■ HERB-DRUG INTERACTIONS

As herbal medicines are used very frequently, they can cause reactions when used along with other allopathic medicines. *Ginkgo biloba* when taken with sodium valproate can produce seizures within 2 weeks; *Zingiber officinale* along with metronidazole can cause reduction in the clearance of the drug and increase the drug toxicity. Interaction of protein and vitamin supplements derived from plant sources can lead interactions with other drugs particularly to anticoagulants if the child is on anticoagulants. Hence, knowledge about the herb drug interaction is required when both are coadministered.[17,21]

Allergic Reactions

Herbal drugs can also cause serious allergic reactions including anaphylactic shock. Itching, pruritus, and rashes of skin are very common manifestations of topical application. Herbal products can increase the existing skin diseases like fissures and dryness. Garlic (*Allium sativum*) and onion (*Allium cepa*) used along with medicines can cause irritation. Tea tree oil used as a disinfectant can cause allergic reactions.[17]

Reliable information on the allergy of the food supplements is scarce and more its components. Both food supplements and medicinal products can have fragrance components which can induce allergic reactions. Cross-reactivity with components of plant products and various allergic syndromes due to that have been documented.[12]

CHALLENGES IN MONITORING OF ADVERSE EVENTS AND TOXICITY

- Herbal medicines come from all traditions from various countries. Basically, there is no uniform method of herb naming system.
- Naming issues or adulterations do not fit into the existing software of pharmacovigilance and data systems.
- Unlike synthetic compounds, herbal medicines are complex and no single compound. Thus, the qualitative and quantitative chemical profile can vary.
- There are lots of over the counter products and self-prescription habits which are difficult to monitor and not reported to their doctor by the patients. The patients feel reluctant to admit that they have used herbal medicines.
- There is a lot of cumulative, chronic or delayed toxicity which often takes months or years after starting or stopping the herbs to appear. Their correlation tend to be missed by the patient and the doctors.[22]
- *Lack of regulatory guidelines*: There is a lack of clear guidelines on quality, good agricultural and collection practices, and good storage practices. There is also a need for more elaborate regulatory guidelines in terms of raw material standardization and quality during production. As such India does not require a safety and efficacy study for approval of herbal product.[23]

METHODS TO REDUCE TOXICITY

- *Standardization of the products*: The likelihood of side effects increases when herbal medicine dosages are not regulated. Hence, regulatory controls are necessary to safeguard the dosage and drug interactions.
- Improper dosage/usage should be avoided by education and effective communication.[24]
- Establishment of pharmacovigilance for herbal products, which will include education of healthcare professionals, providers of herbal medicine, and patients/consumers about the misuse of herbal medicine.[11]
- *Recording and coding of herbal medicines*: It is desirable to have a directory which has structured/classified information like allopathic medicines.[11]
- Naming of herbal medicines needs to be consistent. International drug monitoring had insisted on using binomial names for herbs used in medicine. This would ensure compatibility of reporting from international pharmacovigilance databases.[13]

- Healthcare professionals should remain vigilant for potential interactions with various prescription medicines.[13]

WAY FORWARD

Herbal medicines are here to stay and their use only seems to be increasing as days go by. We need to modify our systems to increase and harmonize our reporting of adverse events for herbal medicines. A good initiative by WHO is the starting of Uppsala Monitoring Center (UMC). They are doing pioneering work in pharmacovigilance. They are an independent, nonprofit foundation started in Uppsala, Sweden in 1978 as the WHO Collaborating Centre for International Drug Monitoring. They have recorded reports from over 100 countries and their databases contain approximately 21,000 reports of adverse reports of herbal or natural products, which is incorporated in a single database. The expansion of such pharmacovigilance networks and forming our own national pharmacovigilance committee will definitely help our patients to make their decisions better and reduce herbal toxicity.[22,25] There is a need for development of monographs and reference standards for medicinal herbal preparations along with the need for elaborate guidelines on the quality control of herbal medicines.[23]

CONCLUSION

Herbal medicines are gaining popularity. It is imperative that we as treating pediatricians have an idea about the common herbal medicine used in our community both for legal purpose and also to manage in case of adverse events due to the usage of herbal medicines. It is also imperative that strict guidelines are made for the usage of these products. A national pharmacovigilance committee needs to be formed to record the adverse events that occurs with their usage.

REFERENCES

1. Mitra A. Science reveals the magic in herbal cures. [online] Available from: https://www.downtoearth.org.in/coverage/science-reveals-the-magic-in-herbal-cures-31793. [Last accessed on November, 2019].
2. Choonara I. Safety of herbal medicines in children. Arch Dis Child. 2003;88(12):1032-3.
3. Wachtel-Galor S, Benzie IFF. Herbal medicine: an introduction to its history, usage, regulation, current trends, and research needs. In: Benzie IFF, Wachtel-Galor S (Eds). Herbal Medicine: Biomolecular and Clinical Aspects, 2nd edition. Boca Raton (FL): CRC Press/Taylor & Francis; 2011.
4. Adhikari PP, Paul SB. History of Indian traditional medicine: A medical inheritance. Asian J Pharmaceut Clin Res. 2018;421-6.

5. Du Y, Wolf IK, Zhuang W, et al. Use of herbal medicinal products among children and adolescents in Germany. BMC Complement Altern Med. 2014;14:218.

6. Welz AN, Emberger-Klein A, Menrad K. Why people use herbal medicine: insights from a focus-group study in Germany. BMC Complement Altern Med. 2018;18(1):92.

7. Ekor M. The growing use of herbal medicines: issues relating to adverse reactions and challenges in monitoring safety. Front Pharmacol. 2014;4:177.

8. Vaidya ADB, Devasagayam TPA. Current status of herbal drugs in India: An overview. J Clin Biochem Nutr. 2007;41(1):1-11.

9. Imran M. The prevalence and patterns of usage of Ayurveda, Unani and home remedies in younger adults of rural North India. Int J Green Pharmacy. 2017;11(02).

10. Oyebode O, Kandala NB, Chilton PJ, et al. Use of traditional medicine in middle-income countries: a WHO-SAGE study. Health Policy Plan. 2016;31(8):984-91.

11. World Health Organization. WHO guidelines on safety monitoring of herbal medicines in pharmacovigilance systems, 2004. [online] Available from: http://apps.who.int/medicinedocs/documents/s7148e/s7148e.pdf. [Last accessed on November, 2019].

12. Pelkonen O, Duez P, Vuorela PM, et al. Toxicology of Herbal Products. Switzerland: Springer International Publishing; 2017.

13. Wal P, Wal A, Gupta S, et al. Pharmacovigilance of herbal products in India. J Young Pharm. 2011;3(3):256-8.

14. Sakharkar P. Lead poisoning due to herbal medications. Indian J Clin Biochem. 2017;32(4):500-1.

15. Singh J. Adhatoda vasica: Vasaka—benefits, uses, dosage and safety profile. Ayur Times; 2017. [online]. Available from: https://www.ayurtimes.com/adhatoda-vasica-vasaka/. [Last accessed on November, 2019].

16. Tanigasalam V, Vishnu Bhat B, Adhisivam B, et al. Vasambu (*Acorus calamus*) administration: A harmful infant rearing practice in South India. Indian J Pediatr. 2017;84(10):802-3.

17. Abdul MIM, Siddique S, Rahman SAU, et al. A critical insight of modern herbal drugs therapy under the purview of toxicity and authenticity. Biomed Res. 2018;29(16).

18. Mashour NH, Lin GI, Frishman WH. Herbal medicine for the treatment of cardiovascular disease: clinical considerations. Arch Intern Med. 1998;158(20):2225-34.

19. Devarbhavi H. Ayurvedic and herbal medicine-induced liver injury: It is time to wake up and take notice. Indian J Gastroenterol. 2018;37(1):5-7.

20. Moreira D de L, Teixeira SS, Monteiro MHD, et al. Traditional use and safety of herbal medicines. Revista Brasileira de Farmacognosia. 2014;24(2):248-57.

21. Fatima N, Nayeem N. Toxic effects as a result of herbal medicine intake. Toxicology - New Aspects to This Scientific Conundrum; 2016. [online] Available from: https://www.intechopen.com/books/toxicology-new-aspects-to-this-scientific-conundrum/toxic-effects-as-a-result-of-herbal-medicine-intake. [Last accessed on November, 2019].

22. Shaw D, Graeme L, Pierre D, et al. Pharmacovigilance of herbal medicine. J Ethnopharmacol. 2012;140(3):513-8.

23. Sahoo N, Manchikanti P. Herbal drug regulation and commercialization: An Indian industry perspective. J. Altern. Complement Med. 2013;19(12):957-63.

24. George P. Concerns regarding the safety and toxicity of medicinal plants: an overview. J Appl Pharmaceut Sci. 2011;5:40-44.

25. UMC (Uppsala Monitoring Centre). [online] Available from: https://www.who-umc.org/. [Last accessed on November, 2019].

12

Emergencies and Intensive Care in the Tropics

Abhay K Shah

Intensive Care in Tropics: Current Status

Swathi Rao, Santosh Soans

INTRODUCTION

The tropical countries face a large burden of critical illnesses which is steadily increasing with growing population, urbanization, and emerging epidemics. The development of intensive care, however, is not at par with demand because of the high cost of trained healthcare workers, infrastructure, and limited supplies, especially in low middle-income countries (LMICs). Also, the priority is given to other significant community health problems, e.g. malnutrition.[1] An efficient health system planning is essential, which requires data on critical care capacity, i.e. physical resources and healthcare professionals. Intensive care in pediatrics was a neglected subspecialty in the tropical countries; however, it has started gaining momentum since the last decade. The need for a well-equipped pediatric intensive care unit (PICU) run by a team specialized in handling critically ill children is paramount.

THE BURDEN OF CRITICAL ILLNESSES IN THE TROPICS

The epidemiological patterns of medical problems seen in tropical intensive care units (ICUs) are dissimilar to those seen elsewhere. There is a higher rate of nosocomial infections in LMICs and a high prevalence of multidrug-resistant bacteria such as methicillin-resistant *Staphylococcus aureus* (MRSA).[2] Unlike in the high-income countries (HICs) where the causes of severe sepsis are mainly bacterial, in LMICs, nonbacterial infections like protozoal diseases such as malaria and viral diseases such as dengue and viral hemorrhagic fevers (HFs) also cause sepsis. There is also a large burden of critical illness due to trauma, which disproportionately affects low-income countries. A number of tropical infections such as measles, respiratory syncytial virus, malaria, leptospirosis, tuberculosis, salmonellosis, etc. form a significant proportion of the patients. Polytrauma also ranks high in the occupancy charts. Trauma-related cases constitute a sizeable proportion of admissions into the PICUs and were made up of road traffic accidents (3.5%), head injuries (2.6%), burns (1.5%), and other forms of trauma (1.5%).

On reviewing reports from various ICUs in tropical countries, it is noticed that infectious diseases are the most common cause of ICU admission as well as mortality. According to World Health Organization (WHO), the majority (99%) of childhood deaths are occurring in developing countries, highest in sub-Saharan Africa and major causes are preventable and curable diseases. It was found that the presence of infection increases the mortality when compared to noninfected patients in a study of ICUs in 75 countries from varied resource levels. The mortality from infections specific to the tropics are decreasing but still high when compared to HICs. The Global Burden of Disease Study estimated that there were still over 700,000 deaths from malaria and over 1.6 million deaths from diarrheal illnesses.[3] In a study done in tertiary referral hospital in Ethiopia, most of the patients had respiratory and central nervous system (CNS) infections.[4] Mortality analysis showed that meningitis, cardiogenic shock followed by pneumonia were major contributors to death. Similar epidemiology is seen in most of the referral hospitals in sub-Saharan Africa, India, Brazil, and China.[5,6] The mortality rates vary from 2.1% to 41%.[7-11] The reported mortality rate in Ethiopian ICU was 8.5% which was lower than the mortality in sub-Saharan countries (40–42%) while in India and China, it was reported to be 2.1% and 6.5%, respectively, and 15% mortality rate was documented in Brazil by Costa et al.[12,13] This value is in consonance with the mortality rate (2.6%) documented

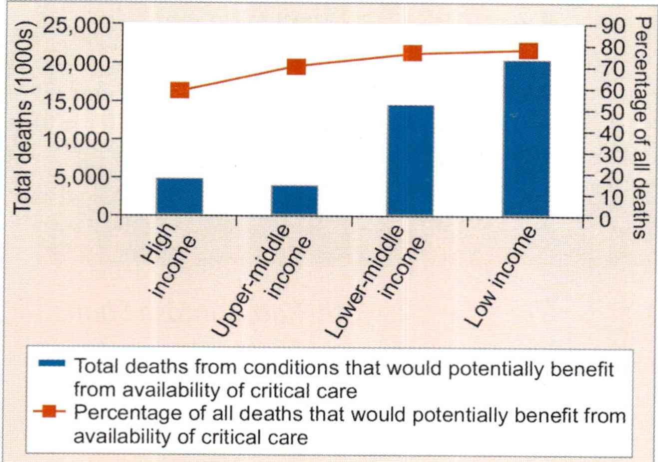

Fig. 1: Deaths potentially preventable with critical care, by country income.[15]

by Choi et al. for a five-bed PICU in a general hospital in Hong Kong.[9]

With this background, when the infrastructure available to handle this burden of critical illnesses was looked into, the data was lacking in many LMICs. In a recent systematic review about the capacity of the intensive care facilities in 15 LMICs, it was noticed that most of the ICUs were concentrated in the major cities with median size of 8 beds. Most of the pediatric beds were within the adult ICU with the mean ratio of adult and PICU beds to hospital beds being 1.5%. Nepal and Uganda had 16.7 and 1.0 ICU beds per million population, respectively. National data from other countries were not available. Low-income countries lack ICU beds, and more than 50% of these countries lack any published data on ICU capacity. Among the 36 ICUs, 77% had mechanical ventilators and there were few data on physician staffing (1 of 36 ICUs), nurse:patient ratios (2 of 36 ICUs), or the presence of an educational mandate (10 of 36 ICUs).[14] Also, there is difference in the disease characteristics and mortality rates of patients admitted to ICUs from one population to another. The sick children from regional hospitals are sent to referral hospitals for ICU care.[16]

Many studies done in the tropics in the last decade have found that if sick children are cared in a well-equipped ICU with trained staff, the mortality rates could be reduced by 15–60%.[15] The various factors which helped in reducing the mortality **(Fig. 1)** were the presence of isolated PICU, (many centers use common ICU for adults and children) and separate burn unit (burns contribute to high case fatality rate for those who have common ICU for all cases).[16] ICU mortality rate varies depending on the case mix, age, and organizational aspects of the unit.

Also, the mortality may go up in ICUs, which also cater to surgical and trauma patients.

■ DEVELOPMENT OF PEDIATRIC CRITICAL CARE MEDICINE IN HICS

The importance of continuous monitoring of the vital signs of a patient was emphasized when respiratory failure due to poliomyelitis increased during the epidemic in 1920–1950s. The epidemic was associated with high case fatality rates and required respiratory support in the form of artificial ventilation. The concept of intensive care emerged when specialized care was given to these patients by a team of physicians and nurses. However, pediatric intensive care was confined to few beds allotted to children in adult ICU. It took few more decades for an exclusive pediatric critical care center to start functioning in Toronto, Canada. The guidelines for establishment of pediatric critical care units were published by the American Academy of Pediatrics and the Pediatric Section of the Society for Critical Care Medicine. Since then, there has been a steady increase in the number of ICUs and trained physicians and nurses. Nowadays, most of the centers follow protocolized treatment and run accredited fellowship programs.

■ DEVELOPMENT OF PEDIATRIC CRITICAL CARE MEDICINE IN LMICS

While this was the scenario in most of the countries in the temperate zone, the tropical zone which consists mainly of low middle-income countries (LMICs) had their own challenges. It was a few decades later, PICUs were established and functioned in these countries. However, this development was slower, since intensive care was an area which was down the priority list when compared to HICs because of various factors.

The challenges faced by the tropical countries are several. The following are the few to mention: (1) The geography is such that the climatic conditions are favorable for several organisms responsible for deadly communicable diseases to thrive; (2) the poor economic status hinders access to optimal nutrition, preventive medicines such as vaccination, and hygienic living, which puts the children at increased risk of infections requiring intensive care; (3) the lack of awareness leads to delay in seeking medical attention; (4) delay in reaching the appropriate facility, less number of well-equipped medical facilities, and poor transport system; and (5) delay in receiving quality care at the facility due to lack of trained personnel.

In spite of all these challenges, in the last two decades there has been rapid development in the emergency and intensive care services, especially in the large cities throughout China, India, South Africa, South America, and the Middle East, which are at par with HIC.[2] In the initial stages, the critically ill children were taken care by general pediatricians who had limited expertise in the field and the nurses were mostly untrained. The majority of hospitals did not have a designated space and pediatric critical care services were provided in mixed adult-pediatric ICU. It was when the native pediatricians who started undergoing training within the country or from good centers in the HIC started setting up PICUs and making protocolized treatment that the quality of care improved and became more streamlined. In India, by early 2000s there were already more than a 100 centers with the pioneering institutions placed in Chandigarh, Delhi, Mumbai, and Chennai.[17] Initially, these centers were equipped with limited gadgets and equipment, gradually moved on to have the latest technology.[4]

CURRENT STATE OF PEDIATRIC CRITICAL CARE SERVICES IN THE TROPICS

The burden of pediatric mortality remains high in the tropics contributed mainly by infections, such as sepsis, pneumonia, malaria, and diarrheal diseases which are actually preventable. Among the noninfectious causes, 90% of childhood trauma deaths occur in LMICs. Poorest countries contribute nearly 90% of the global under-five mortality each year. Most of the urban intensive care settings are giving high-quality services but there is still a huge gap between the pediatric critical care services available in most HIC settings and added to the inadequate pediatric critical care services available in the rural areas. This regional disparity in the availability of critical care is alarming and contribute majorly to the mortality due delayed treatment and/or improper transport to the higher center.

The focus in the developing countries has been on improving the hygiene and nutritional status by promoting breastfeeding and immunizations, rather than on developing intensive care facilities.[5] The Integrated Management of Childhood Illness program was established by the UNICEF and WHO to screen and recognize sick children. According to this program, 20% of children attending the outpatient department require special care and referral to higher centers with PICU. Despite this, the recognition of a sick child, triage, and ability to provide rapid interventions before referral still remains largely absent in many LMIC settings. There is a steady decrease in case mortality rates in many hospitals in the urban areas, however it still remains high in

rural settings which lack higher levels of intensive care, highlighting the need for improved facilities in these settings. The optimal care of the sickest hospitalized children includes triage, emergency, and critical care services.[3] The Emergency Triage, Assessment, and Treatment (ETAT) guidelines were developed by WHO, which focuses on early recognition of children who need immediate care and hospitalization.[18] The WHO also published and updated the clinical guidelines for nurses and physicians caring for hospitalized children in these settings stressing on the importance of appropriate triage and rapid treatment using relatively inexpensive modalities, such as fluids, oxygen, and antibiotics.[20] The mortality rate was reported to be reduced by half (10–18 to 6–8%) in 6 years after implementation of these guidelines in a hospital in Malawi.[3] The authors in several tertiary institutions have published standardized individual guidelines which are followed by other government and private tertiary hospitals in these countries.

The current practice of critical care in India is diverse and varies between regions. There are three types of hospitals in India, namely, the government hospitals which essentially result in no cost to the patients, the private teaching hospitals which give affordable healthcare, and lastly the corporate hospitals which are too expensive. Critical care is a technology-dependent branch and therefore involves high expenditure. Hence, the government community hospitals contribute less to the field of critical care. Some of the rural hospitals and clinics in are not equipped with even the basic resources, such as oxygen, resuscitation equipment, and medication to provide pediatric emergency care, and appropriately trained staffs are rarely available. Most of the teaching hospitals have well-equipped PICUs but lack trained staff. Private tertiary care hospitals have trained personnel and ICUs with latest technology backup and they form the most major contributor to the critical care facilities in the country. The facilities are on the upswing however, manpower development of the specialists has been a major issue.

Training and Research

In order to standardize the care given to critically ill patients, a formal pediatric critical care training, curriculum, or certification process is necessary. Most of the tropical countries now run certified fellowships for both physicians and nurses with standard curriculum designed by the national academic groups.

Pediatric intensive care certificate course is running since 2000s; nearly 100 units all over India are accredited for training. Other courses are Fellowship of National Board of Examination in Pediatric Critical Care since 2007 and DM in Pediatric Critical Care since 2009 at Chandigarh, now also at AIIMS, Delhi, and JIPMER, Puducherry. The Intensive Care Chapter under Indian Academy of Pediatrics (IAP), and Indian Society of Critical Care Medicine (ISCCM) are active in the organization of these academic training activities. The training of nurses is also happening under the same academic group. The ICUs are running in three levels suggested by international taskforce—a level 1 ICU is capable of providing oxygen and noninvasive monitoring, whereas a level 2 ICU can provide invasive monitoring and basic life support including mechanical ventilation for a short period. A full spectrum of monitoring and life support technologies such as dialysis and extracorporeal membrane oxygenation (ECMO) must be available in level 3 ICU.[5]

The interest toward research in the field of intensive care has picked up enormously and Indian pediatric intensivists have contributed many original papers addressing the common issues. Notable among these are papers on fluid therapy, fluid overload, dengue, pneumonia, CNS infections, use of latest gadgets in ICU, and so on. The guidelines for management of various tropical infections has been consolidated and locally relevant issues has been addressed under the aegis of Indian Society of Critical Care Medicine (ISCCM) by a multicenter collaboration. The Journal of Pediatric Intensive Care and the Indian Journal of Critical Care Medicine are the official journals of Pediatric Intensive Care Chapter in IAP and the ISCCM, respectively. These journals are successful in the past few years in publishing ICU-related statistics and recent updates. The ISCCM and the IAP have taken the lead in the development of a number of other related issues. The cardiopulmonary resuscitation (CPR) Training Project and the IAP Advanced Life Support Program are very successful in training the physicians and nurses in emergency management of life-threatening conditions and team concepts. These academic groups along with other like-minded bodies are also organizing critical care-related conferences, updates, continuing medical education programs, and workshops for interested physicians can update their knowledge through participation.[12,19]

THE SPECTRUM OF DISEASES IN THE TROPICAL ICU

The tropical infections usually are of acute onset and form a large portion of ICU admissions. The diagnosis has to be timely and interventions prompt to make a world of change and ensure good recovery. The clinical presentations of these illnesses are syndromic like bleeding, respiratory distress, hypotension, shock, alteration of consciousness, etc. In the scenario of late presentation, multiple organ systems can be involved at admission, e.g. leptospirosis, dengue, and malaria. The following are the few clinical syndromes we face in our ICU:

- *Fever with bleeding disorders*: In the tropics, thrombocytopenia-associated infections are the most common in this category. The symptoms which mandate intensive care are massive gastrointestinal, pulmonary, or intracranial bleed. Massive bleeding can also present with shock and acute kidney injury. Other complications of these diseases are disseminated intravascular coagulopathy (DIC), hemolytic uremic syndrome (HUS), thrombotic thrombocytopenic purpura (TTP), or vasculitis. The infections such as dengue fever, leptospirosis, malaria, rickettsial infections and some of the viral infections such as herpes simplex, yellow fever, Ebola, Marburg, Lassa, hantavirus, Crimean-Congo HF, and Omsk fevers can present with bleeding manifestations. Severe sepsis with vasculitis (gram-negative sepsis and meningococcemia) may also cause hemorrhage.

- *Fever with respiratory distress*: Respiratory distress and failure are the most common indications for ICU admission. The various causes for respiratory distress include pneumonia and acute respiratory distress syndrome (ARDS) due direct or indirect lung injury. The common organisms which cause pneumonia include *Streptococcus pneumoniae*, *Chlamydia*, *Mycoplasma*, *Legionella*, and less commonly *S. aureus* and *Klebsiella pneumoniae* which are common to all regions. The organisms which are endemic to the tropics are influenza, parainfluenza, adenovirus, respiratory syncytial viruses (RSV), influenza A H1N1, avian influenza viruses (H5N1 and H7N9), severe acute respiratory syndrome-associated coronavirus (SARS-CoV), the Middle East respiratory syndrome coronavirus (MERS-CoV) and the hantavirus. Melioidosis caused by a gram-negative pathogen *Burkholderia pseudomallei* is endemic to southeast Asia, northern Australia, India, south China, and Taiwan and cases have been documented in Brazil and elsewhere in South America, Papua New Guinea, Fiji, and New Caledonia. It is one of the most common causes of fatal community-acquired bacteremic pneumonia in Northeast Thailand and Darwin.[20]

Fever with shock: Many tropical infections (leptospirosis, dengue fever, chikungunya fever, malaria, and diarrheal diseases) are associated with hypovolemia, hypotension and shock. Sepsis caused by various gram-negative organisms leads to regional changes in oxygen demand and regional alteration in blood flow of various organs due to peripheral vasodilation and development of increased systemic microvascular permeability.

- *Fever with hepatorenal involvement*: In many parts of India and the tropics, leptospirosis, malaria, scrub typhus, and fulminant hepatitis present with hepatic/renal failure. The various manifestations include oliguria, jaundice, hematuria, altered consciousness, irritability, and presence of visible hemorrhages in the skin and mucus membranes.
- *Fever with CNS involvement*: The common tropical infectious diseases under this category are cerebral malaria, Japanese encephalitis (JE), typhoid fever, and viral meningoencephalitides. Many tropical infections may present with postinfective demyelination presenting as weakness or sensory disturbances. In JE, neurologic invasion develops, possibly by growth of the virus across vascular endothelial cells, leading to involvement of large areas of the brain, including the thalamus, basal ganglia, brainstem, cerebellum, hippocampus, and cerebral cortex. The intensive care admission is required when they present with poor sensorium compromising the airway, raised intracranial pressure or refractory seizures. Cerebral abscesses can form part of the differential diagnosis of encephalitis and these generally present with focal neurological deficits.[21] Viral encephalitis is mainly caused by arboviruses. Three genera of arboviruses are seen in the tropics namely flavivirus (Zika virus, yellow fever virus, dengue virus, Japanese encephalitis virus, and Rocio virus), alphavirus (Chikungunya), and bunyavirus (Oropouche).[22-25]
- *Fever with diarrhea*: In addition, many diseases are spread by contaminated water and food sources, since clean water and sanitary conditions are often a luxury in developing countries. Diarrhea remains one of the most common diseases that also affects children under 5 years of age, leading to a considerable mortality in childhood. Rotavirus remains the most common cause of severe diarrheal illness, albeit a myriad of countries (such as Bangladesh, Somalia, Rwanda, Zaire, and Nepal) have seen serious epidemics due to the multiple resistant bacterium *Shigella dysenteriae* that causes dysentery:
  - *Rotavirus:* Rotaviral infection is waterborne and causes watery diarrhea and vomiting, primarily in young children. The majority of infections are self-limiting, but infant mortality is higher in developing countries and is generally associated with severe dehydration requiring replacement of lost fluids and electrolytes followed by monitoring in the ICU. Cholera is a diarrheal disease caused by infection with *Vibrio cholerae*, a bacterium most often found in contaminated water and shellfish, which produces a toxin that upsets the biochemical balance of cells lining the intestine and makes them secrete copious amounts of water and electrolytes.
  - *Ebola virus*: Ebola virus causes fever, severe headache, backache, vomiting, diarrhea, and severe hemorrhaging.

Other important tropical infections significantly contributing to ICU admissions are mentioned below:

- *Malaria*: Severe malaria presenting as coma, seizures, acute kidney injury, liver dysfunction, thrombocytopenia, DIC and ARDS is common cause of ICU admission in tropical countries in Africa, Asia, Oceania and south and central America.[26] *Plasmodium falciparum* accounts for most cases, although *P. vivax* is increasingly found to cause severe malaria in Asia. Cerebral malaria has a high morbidity and mortality.[27] The WHO has estimated that 70% of deaths worldwide occur in children <5 years of age and majority in sub-Saharan Africa. In 2015, 212 million new cases of malaria worldwide of which 90% were in the African Region, 7% in southeast Asia, and 2% in the Eastern Mediterranean region, with about 429,000 deaths.[27]
- *Human immunodeficiency virus*: The human immunodeficiency viruses (HIVs) associated with the Acquired Immunodeficiency Syndrome (AIDS) have become widespread in developing nations. In 2018, 23.3 million people were accessing antiretroviral therapy (ART) and 770,000 (570,000–1.1 million) people died from AIDS-related illnesses worldwide. The number of infected individuals in Asia is also rapidly rising; it is currently estimated that over 5 million people are living with HIV/AIDS in south and southeast Asia. The various reasons for which HIV patients may be admitted to ICU are acute respiratory failure as a result of opportunistic infections (25–50% of admissions) secondary to *Pneumocystis jiroveci* pneumonia (PJP), and bacterial and fungal pneumonia. Other common indications for ICU admission are sepsis and CNS dysfunction and complications due to various encephalitis. The spectrum of diseases requiring ICU admission is changing in the setting of ART. In highly active ART (HAART) era, hospitalization of HIV-infected patients has significantly decreased, but the rate of ICU admissions are same as before because the

number of patients living with HIV has increased, as overall survival has improved. The infected patients are being admitted to ICU for medical and surgical causes unrelated to their HIV infection such as trauma, postoperative care, asthma, renal failure, liver diseases, and surgical causes.[28]

- *Tuberculosis*: The incidence of tuberculosis (TB) is on the rise in tropical areas due to the interaction between tuberculosis and HIV epidemics and is the leading cause of death due to increasing resistance to antitubercular drugs. The prevalence of TB in India is 2.79 million cases in 2016 with a mortality of 423,000.[29] Patients with TB can be admitted to an ICU for a variety of reasons, including respiratory failure, multiorgan failure and decreased consciousness associated with central nervous system disease.

■ SUMMARY AND WAY FORWARD

Tropical countries face a large burden of critical illnesses due to preventable diseases like infections and trauma in the setting of limited critical care facilities. Despite various challenges, there has been a steady improvement in the intensive care facilities and more trained personnel in the field. With more institutions following standardized protocols, the quality of care has improved contributing to lesser mortality and morbidity. However, the discrepancy in the standard of care persists in rural areas. The need of the hour is more uniform, affordable intensive care facilities throughout these countries. Establishing well-equipped PICUs with a backup of trained physicians and nurses in rural areas is essential. Critical care depends on a team of dedicated, well-trained, and compensated medical and nursing staff. The training has to be focused and team based aimed at early recognition and treatment of critical illnesses. There is an urgent need for greater policy focus and research efforts in the field.

Nurses who work in PICUs should receive pediatric-specific training focused on how to care for critically ill infants and children. They should have knowledge of age-dependent vital signs and the key differences in resuscitation of pediatric patients. The training of physicians handling sick children include goal-directed therapy, procedural skills for safe tracheal intubation, mechanical ventilation, use of vasopressors, and placement of central lines. The importance of team work can be reinforced by regular mock codes, critical cases review, and simulation. The field of intensive care is dynamic and full of challenges. The efforts to be put for a humane, scientific, and meaningful service for the multitude of critically ill patients.

India is running a well-organized training program in Pediatric Critical Care with a curriculum designed by experts in the field. The physicians from other developing countries are seeking training in India. The PICUs in most of the in metropolitan cities are "State of the Art" with facilities including ECMO. Many of the institutions also offer a trained transport team with ambulance with ventilators and oximetry-enabling safe transport of unstable children from one center to a higher one. However, such facilities are still lacking in tier two and three cities. We need to find ways of supporting the development of pediatric critical care facilitating the growth and development of research in pediatric critical care and supporting the work and development of all people who work in the setting of pediatric critical care.

■ REFERENCES

1. Slusher TM, Kiragu AW, Day LT, et al. Pediatric critical care in resource-limited settings: overview and lessons learned. Front Pediatr. 2018;6:49.
2. Abhulimhen-Iyoha BI, Pooboni SK, Vuppali NKK. Morbidity pattern and outcome of patients admitted into a pediatric intensive care unit in India. Indian J Clin Med. 2014;5:IJCM. S13902.
3. Baker T. Pediatric emergency and critical care in low-income countries. Paediatr Anaesth. 2009;19(1):23-7.
4. Turner EL, Nielsen KR, Jamal SM, et al. A review of pediatric critical care in resource-limited settings: a look at past, present, and future directions. Front Pediatr. 2016;4:5.
5. Riviello ED, Letchford S, Achieng L, et al. Critical care in resource-poor settings: lessons learned and future directions: Crit Care Med. 2011;39(4):860-7.
6. Abebe T, Girmay M, Michael G, et al. The epidemiological profile of pediatric patients admitted to the general intensive care unit in an Ethiopian university hospital. Int J Gen Med. 2015;8:63-7.
7. Shah GS, Shah BK, Thapa A, et al. Admission patterns and outcome in a pediatric intensive care unit in Nepal. In 2014.
8. El Halal MG dos S, Barbieri E, Filho RM, et al. Admission source and mortality in a pediatric intensive care unit. Indian J Crit Care Med Peer-Rev Off Publ Indian Soc Crit Care Med. 2012;16(2):81-6.
9. Kapoor K, Jain S, Jajoo M, et al. Risk factors and predictors of mortality in critically ill children with extensively-drug resistant Acinetobacter baumannii infection in a pediatric intensive care unit. Iran J Pediatr. 2014;24(5):569-74.
10. Mevstrović J, Polić B, Mevstrović M, et al. Functional outcome of children treated in intensive care unit. J Pediatr (Rio J). 2008;84(3):232-6.
11. Srinivas M, Hannah W. Clinical review: international comparisons in critical care, USA, 2012. BMC Crit Care. 2012;16:218.
12. Barbosa AP. Neonatal and pediatric intensive care in Brazil: the ideal, the real, and the possible. J Pediatr (Rio J). 2004;80(6):437-8.
13. Simon R, Gilyoma JM, Dass RM, et al. Paediatric injuries at Bugando Medical Centre in Northwestern Tanzania: a prospective review of 150 cases. J Trauma Manag Outcomes. 2013;7:10.

14. Murthy S, Leligdowicz A, Adhikari NKJ. Intensive care unit capacity in low-income countries: a systematic review. Azevedo LCP (Ed). PLOS ONE. 2015;10(1):e0116949.

15. Mathers C, Fat DM, Boerma JT. World Health Organization (Eds). The global burden of disease: 2004 update. Geneva, Switzerland: World Health Organization;2008. p. 146.

16. Haftu H, Hailu T, Medhaniye A, et al. Assessment of pattern and treatment outcome of patients admitted to pediatric intensive care unit, Ayder Referral Hospital, Tigray, Ethiopia, 2015. BMC Res Notes. 2018;11(1):339.

17. History of PICU in India–World Federation of Pediatric Intensive and Critical Care [Internet]. [cited 2019 Dec 17]. Available from: http://www.wfpiccs.org/history-of-picu-in-india/

18. World Health Organization. Pocketbook of Hospital Care for Children Guidelines for the Management of Common Illnesses with Limited Resources. Geneva: World Health Organization (2013).

19. Murthy S, Wunsch H. Clinical review: international comparisons in critical care: lessons learned. Crit Care. 2012;16(2):218.

20. Nor MBM, Richards GA, McGloughlin S, et al. Council of the World Federation of Societies of Intensive and Critical Care Medicine. Pneumonia in the tropics: report from the task force on tropical diseases by the World Federation of Societies of Intensive and Critical Care Medicine. J Crit Care. 2017;42:360-5.

21. Silva GS, Richards GA, Baker T, et al. Council of the World Federation of Societies of Intensive and Critical Care Medicine. Encephalitis and myelitis in tropical countries: report from the task force on tropical diseases by the World Federation of Societies of Intensive and Critical Care Medicine. J Crit Care. 2017;42:355-9.

22. Christo PP. Encephalitis by dengue virus and other arboviruses. Arq Neuropsiquiatr. 2015;73(8):641-3.

23. Jmor F, Emsley HCA, Fischer M, et al. The incidence of acute encephalitis syndrome in Western industrialised and tropical countries. Virol J. 2008;5:134.

24. Carteaux G, Maquart M, Bedet A, et al. Zika virus associated with meningoencephalitis. N Engl J Med. 2016;374(16):1595-6.

25. Figueiredo LT. Saint Louis encephalitis virus and other arboviruses in the differential diagnosis for dengue. Rev Soc Bras Med Trop. 2014;47(5):541-2.

26. Karnad DR, Nor MBM, Richards GA, et al. Council of the World Federation of Societies of Intensive and Critical Care Medicine. Intensive care in severe malaria: report from the task force on tropical diseases by the World Federation of Societies of Intensive and Critical Care Medicine. J Crit Care. 2018;43:356-60.

27. World malaria report 2016. 2016.

28. Global HIV and AIDS statistics—2019 fact sheet | UNAIDS [Internet]. [cited 2019 Dec 17]. Available from: https://www.unaids.org/en/resources/fact-sheet

29. TB Statistics India–latest 2018 figures–TBFacts [Internet]. [cited 2019 Dec 17]. Available from: https://tbfacts.org/tb-statistics-india/

Septic Shock

Mahesh A Mohite

INTRODUCTION

Septic shock is a common emergency in pediatric practice may be in office or in intensive care units (ICUs). It is one of the common causes of death in pediatric age. Late recognition, poor resuscitation, inappropriate coverage of antibiotics lead to multiorgan failure and death in most of such failed management cases.

DEFINITION

Severe infection with systemic inflammatory response syndrome (SIRS) leading to dysregulated immune response, microcirculatory failure and organ dysfunction is called septic shock.[1] Thus, there are five components in the definition and all are essential to define the condition. Adult septic shock has moved ahead with revised definition of severe infection with sequential organ failure assessment (SOFA) score of two or more than two. We in pediatric patient group have not accepted it so far due to limitations in categorizing the tissue damage specific to various age groups in pediatric spectrum. A combined summit of four apex pediatric intensive care unit (PICU) research bodies are having multiple meetings to form new definition for sepsis and septic shock. Till then we have to follow the present existing definition.

There are further severity categories in sepsis and septic shock.

- *Sepsis*: It is severe infection with SIRS, where SIRS is defined two of the four criteria, and of the two at least one of leukocyte number or temperature abnormality being present.[2] The four criteria are:
  1. Temperature abnormality: >38.5°C or <36.0°C
  2. WBC count: >15,000/ mm^3 or <5,000/mm^3
  3. Tachycardia or bradycardia for the age
  4. Tachypnea or bradypnea for the age.

- *Severe sepsis*: Sepsis with two or more than two organ dysfunction.
- *Septic shock*: Sepsis with cardiocirculatory failure not recovering with 40 mL/kg isotonic fluid bolus, needing inotropes, decreased urine output and other system hypoperfusion.
- *Refractory septic shock*: Septic shock needing more than 60 mL/kg (fluid refractory) and an inotropes (catecholamine refractory) still not recovering, or becoming inotrope dependent.
- *Multiorgan dysfunction syndrome (MODS)*: Mainly six organs are considered here:
  1. *Neurological*: Falling Glasgow coma scale (GCS) 11–15 with altered sensorium, seizures and other clinical features of acquired new onset neurological dysfunction.
  2. *Circulatory*: Hypotension, inotrope dependency, clinical and laboratory manifestation of under-perfusion of tissue.
  3. *Respiratory*: Tachypnea or bradypnea for the age group, PaO_2/FiO_2 (P/F) ratio < 300, $PaCO_2$ > 65 or 20 more than normal, needs more than 50% FiO_2 to maintain 92% SPO_2.
  4. *Hematological*: Features of disseminated intra-vascular coagulation (DIC) or platelet count < 80,000/mm^3 or drop by 50%.
  5. *Hepatological*: Bilirubin > 4 mg% for more than one month age, serum glutamic-pyruvic transaminase (SGPT) rising by > 2 times.
  6. *Renal*: Creatinine increasing by double the number, or glomerular filtration rate (GFR)dropping by > 50% for the age.

Adult definition of septic shock is severe infection with two or more tissue dysfunction (SOFA > 2) as mentioned above. The dysfunction criteria for pediatric age are not validated yet and lactate is not a reliable parameter in children yet so this adult definition is not validated yet for pediatrics.[3]

PATHOLOGY

As the definition mentions, its infection induced severe SIRS leading to cytokine storm.[4] The infection may be in one tissue in body but effects of cytokines observed at distant tissue. The cytokines injuring capillary microcirculatory channels leading to:

- Capillary leak leading to intravascular hypovolemia, third spacing, increased fluid in interstitial compartment, increased tissue pressure compromising blood supply further, the best example is being acute kidney injury (AKI).
- Endothelial glycocalyx injury contributing to more capillary leak and vascular and tissue injury.
- Vasoplegia in all size vessels creating relative hypovolemia.
- Opening of arteriovenous capillary shunts, shunting blood away from tissue, leading to anaerobic metabolism, lactic acidemia.
- Sluggish circulation leading to higher extraction of oxygen (O_2) by tissue.
- Myocardial dysfunction due to toxins and cytokines leading to poor inotropism and contributing to shock.
- Septic tissue dysfunction directly due to cytokine storm.

CLINICAL FEATURES

Septic shock is typical maldistributive shock. In classical hypovolemic shock, decreasing intravascular volume is compensated by autonomic stimulation and increased peripheral vasoconstriction serially redistributing the blood flow to vital organs compromising the flow to not so vital organs. This body protective mechanism is possible due to physiological distribution of vasoconstrictive receptors in higher density in not so vital organ, thus blood is serially withdrawn initially from skin, then gastrointestinal (GI), renal, liver, lungs, heart and finally brain. This allows brain to function till late in shock victim in hypovolemic or cardiogenic shock. But in septic shock, due to cytokine-mediated injury, there is vasoplegia, preventing the protective diversion of blood flow to vital organs. Thus, vital tissue perfusion may be compromised far before or along with skin, GI or kidney.[5,6] This will also make clinical diagnosis slightly difficult. Clinical features of shock are:[7]

- Tachycardia

- Increased core-toe temperature difference > 3°C, with line of demarcation of temperature—the peripheries being cold and core being warm. This line shifting up toward trunk defines deteriorating shock and shifting toward periphery defines improving shock.
- Peripheral pulses being weaker than central pulses.
- Features of serial loss of perfusion of tissue:
  - *Skin underperfusion*: Delayed capillary refilling time more than 3 seconds.
  - *Renal underperfusion*: Decreasing hourly urine output less than 1 mL/kg/h.
  - *Brain underperfusion*: Deteriorating GCS or AVPU score (alert, responsive to voice, responsive to pain, unresponsive).
- *Hypotension*: Drop of mean arterial pressure below 3rd percentile for the age.

In septic maldistributive shock, you may see drowsy child with capillary refill time (CRT) < 2 seconds, or tachypneic hypoxic child with good urine output.

While defining septic shock, we look for evidence of severe infective focus with clinical evidence of tissue hypoperfusion and laboratory evidence of systemic hypoperfusion.

Laboratory Evidence[8-10]

- *Tests to locate or define infection*: This can be obvious infective focus like cellulitis, or you may have to look for hidden focus or its evidence in laboratory reports, like neutrophilic leukocytosis, raised acute-phase reactants. To locate infection site, urine test, X-ray chest, cerebrospinal fluid (CSF), etc. may help.
- *Microbiological diagnosis*: It is desirable to have detection of etiological agent. In a given case, possible source of infection needs to be evaluated. We need to send culture samples of blood in all cases of septic shock and urine, CSF, pus, pleural, peritoneal, pericardial fluids, etc. as per case. Standard norms of blood culture sample collection need to be followed to get best yield. One set of sample for blood culture gives approximately 30% yield. Three sets in antibiotic naive patient can have positive result in as many as 94% samples.
- *Indirect markers of infection in culture negative sepsis*: C-reactive protein (CRP) as marker of infection especially its trend in a given patient may guide the management and progress of patient. Serum procalcitonin level is a new infection marker available, more specific for infection than other acute-phase reactants like erythrocyte sedimentation rate (ESR) or CRP with higher specificity and sensitivity.[11]

- *Tests to define tissue underperfusion*: Various tests represent tissue underperfusion and anaerobic metabolism:
  - Arterial blood gas (ABG): Metabolic acidemia
  - Increased plasma lactate > 2[12]
  - Mix venous O_2 < 70%.
- *Test to define system dysfunction or failure*: Various system screens are performed to know the tissue well-being: Hemogram with hemoglobin (Hb)-red blood cell (RBC) count and platelet count, serum creatinine, alanine aminotransferase/aspartate aminotransferase (ALT/AST), prothrombin time (PT), and partial thromboplastin time (PTT).
- *Tests to avoid confounders in management*: Electrolytes, calcium, magnesium, hypoglycemia or hyperglycemia, etc. Blood sugar monitoring and controlling the level in narrow spectrum has been studied aggressively with little evidence in favor of tight glucose level control.

One may go for radiological evaluation when needed, like X-ray chest, USG abdomen and various scans to define the infection and its extent.

MANAGEMENT OF SEPTIC SHOCK

Septic shock is a critical emergency. Delay in recognition or resuscitation of shock exponentially increases morbidity and mortality with every passing minute. Strictly following Advanced Life Support (ALS) guidelines will help early recognition and management in field practice and improve survival.

Surviving sepsis guidelines designed for adult and extrapolated to pediatrics are in use since 2002 and since then it has been revised four times till 2016 based on newer evidence. The algorithmic time bound management of septic shock was a popular protocol a decade ago and basic principles are still followed, but there have been some major changes in understanding and hence in management of septic shock.

Immediate steps after recognizing septic shock:
- Give 100% O_2 by nonrebreathing mask.
- Ensure patent airway and adequate breathing. A patient with abnormal or insufficient breathing efforts may need alternative airway like laryngeal mask airway or endotracheal (ET) tube intubation. If breathing efforts are insufficient, mechanical ventilatory support may be needed. Sometimes spontaneous ventilation may be adequate but shock does not respond to primary modality; here patient is electively intubated and ventilated to secure airway and reduce respiratory workload on cardiocirculatory system. ET intubation

in septic shock patient is highly skillful and risky procedure and should be done by senior intensivist with safe rapid sequence intubation (RSI) method, avoiding drugs compromising hemodynamic status of the patient.
- Put two big bore needle and collect blood cultures and relevant cultures appropriate for the case.
- Collect blood sugar and serum calcium samples.
- Give first dose antibiotic specific to the case or broad spectrum if focus is not defined. Delay in antibiotic delivery after 1 hour, increases mortality by 7.6% for every 1-hour delay.[13] Antibiotics are chosen according to source of infection if known at initial diagnosis. Since exact organism is not known at the beginning, broad-spectrum antibiotics are started and later de-escalated according to clinical response and microbiological reports if positive. For community acquired septic hypotensive shock without exact clinical focus (source), carbapenem is the most efficacious agent today which can be de-escalated later. For health care-associated infection, the choice of antibiotic is determined by antibiogram of the local unit. When source is known, e.g. pneumonia, urinary tract infection (UTI), dysentery, cellulitis, etc. the antibiotics are selected appropriately. In nosocomial, spectrum antifungal agents may be indicated. Immunological status of the patient may also guide one in choosing appropriate antibiotic. Rarely an antiviral may be needed in suspected viral sepsis like H1N1.
- Initially the emphasis was more on rapid isotonic fluid replacement with 20 mL/kg NS repeated boluses to total 60 mL/kg in first 1 hour, followed by inotropes and optimizing and titrating their effects. With more evidence against excess fluids, present guidelines suggest minimal optimum fluid.[14] While managing shock, fluid excess (positive balance) is continuously observed and as soon as shock is resuscitated, surplus above 10% is actively removed.
- In early sepsis guidelines (2003), dopamine was the first-line inotrope followed by adrenaline, noradrenaline (NA), dobutamine, milrinone, vasopressin in various sequence and combinations customized for individual patient. With more evidence and experience, adrenaline is replacing dopamine as first-line vasoactive agent in pediatric septic shock. Adult septic shock being warm vasoplegic shock has already established NA as first-line vasoactive drug.[15] Pediatric evidence is still recommending adrenaline as first-line agent though debate is on between adrenaline and NA as first-line agent. Adrenaline is uptitrated from 0.1 μg/kg/minute

to 0.5 µg/kg/minute while optimizing the intravascular fluid volume. If shock persists, it is labeled as fluid refractory and catecholamine-resistant shock. At this point in potentially steroid-deficient patient (e.g. nephrotic syndrome on long-term steroids, connective tissue disorders or autoimmune disorders), stress dose steroid is given. If shock is still not recovered, other vasoactive drugs are added and titrated to the effect.

Colloids versus Crystalloids

Various trials failed to show advantage of colloids over crystalloids in fluid resuscitation of shock, thus after initial crystalloid bolus occasional colloids with gelatin or 5% albumin can be tried. Starch is not recommended due to its nephrotoxicity. Balanced salt solution (Plasmalyte) has limited advantage over crystalloids (NS) as rare hyperchloremic acidosis can be prevented by its use.[16]

The early goal-directed therapy (EGDT) proposed by evidence[17] was planned with 1-hour goal to improve microcirculation with:

- Equal central and peripheral pulsations
- Improved sensorium
- Improved urine output > 1 mL/kg/h
- Warm limbs.

And 6-hour goal of:
- Mean arterial pressure 65 mm Hg
- Central venous pressure (CVP) 5–9 cm
- Mix venous O_2 saturation > 70%
- Plasma lactate < 2.

Early goal-directed therapy initially showed survival benefit of 50% (mortality dropped from 45% to 30%). But further review reported excess use of fluids to achieve targets which increased tissue injury and lead to poor outcome. ARISE trail conducted in adults[18] showed poor outcome with time-bound EGDT; thus, EGDT was challenged and not followed aggressively now.

FEAST trial conducted in sub-Saharan Africa showed higher mortality with liberal use of fluids in initial resuscitation; thus, the new surviving sepsis guidelines have proposed minimal optimal fluids during early resuscitation and after stabilization for 6–12 hours, quickly remove the surplus fluids that have been pushed. Calculation of fluid balance and removing the surplus volumes by diuresis or by continuous renal replacement therapy (CRRT) has shown improved survival and less complication following septic shock management. The new SS guidelines recommend *first 3-hour bundle* as:

- Recognition of shock (as soon as possible)
- Collection of blood culture and other necessary culture samples (immediately after securing IV line)
- Giving first dose of antibiotics (within 1 hour)
- Minimal 30 mL/kg NS fluid (within 3 hours)
- Lactates to be checked.

SUPPORTIVE CARE

Mechanical ventilation: Timely support with ventilatory care is crucial in management. Once fluid refractory, with one or two inotropes, it is desirable to offload patient's effort of breathing on to mechanical ventilator. Continue it till patient stabilizes hemodynamically.

Blood components: Anemia and reduced O_2-carrying capacity of blood increases cardiac workload. In septic shock, it is desirable to maintain Hb above 9 g/dL. Platelet transfusion is needed if platelets are less than 50,000/mm^3 with active bleeding. Plasma is needed only for actively bleeding child in DIC.

Blood sugar targets: There has been huge debate about risk with hyperglycemia leading to diuresis and dyselectrolytemia and hyperosmosis. Target sugar suggested was 100–140 mg/dL (tight glycemic control). But this has not given added benefits and occasional hypoglycemia in the stringent management is far more dangerous than hyperglycemia, thus such stringent control is not recommended.

Role of steroids: Apart from steroids for fluid refractory and inotrope-resistant shock, there is no other indication for steroid. In this condition, hydrocortisone is recommended 50 mg/m^2 divided doses daily for 2 days.

Role of H_2 *antagonist* for prevention of GI bleed is controversial.

MONITORING SEPTIC SHOCK

It needs intense clinical monitoring in pediatric septic shock. Hemodynamic parameters can be best monitored continuously by invasive and noninvasive monitors. Electrocardiogram (ECG) and pulse oximetry are basic needs in ICU monitoring but have serious limitations in critical shock. In cold pulseless patient, SPO_2 may not be detected. Noninvasive blood pressure is not reliable in hypotensive patient. In patients on multiple vasoactive drugs, monitoring with invasive blood pressure monitors is standard of care. One hourly urine output needs to be monitored. Functional echo and lung sonography are becoming more popular and reliable monitors for titrating intravascular volume and deciding proper inotropic combination. Modern ultrasound-guided cardiac output monitors (USCOMs) are being tested world over and need some time to reach the level of graded recommendation in all PICU septic patients.

Apart from routine laboratory parameters of critical child in PICU, we monitor downstream parameters of tissue perfusion. These parameters indirectly reflect tissue delivery and uptake of O_2. Plasma lactate is increased in case of tissue underperfusion leading to anaerobic metabolism. If liver is injured as part of multiorgan dysfunction, lactates lose its utility as marker of shock status. Metabolic acidemia on background of shock suggests tissue underperfusion. Mix venous or central venous O_2 levels also indicate tissue perfusion status. Levels less than 70% suggest sluggish circulation (shock) leading to higher extraction of O_2. Thus, during management, central or mix venous O_2 saturation is targeted above 70%.

More advanced modalities are invented by biomedical technology... one such being near-infrared spectroscopy (NIRS). This determines capillary flow in monitored tissue. One can determine muscle, intestine, liver, renal tissue, brain capillary perfusion at individual tissue level. Multiple devices used simultaneously and reports interpreted collectively along with clinical parameters give the best outcome.

■ REFERENCES

1. Biban P, Gaffuri M, Spaggiari S, et al. Early recognition and management of septic shock in children. Pediatr Rep. 2012;4:e13.
2. Goldstein B, Giroir B, Randolph A, et al. International Pediatric Sepsis Consensus Conference: definitions for sepsis and organ dysfunction in pediatrics. Pediatr Crit Care Med. 2005;6:2-8.
3. Singer M, Deutschman CS, Seymour CW, et al. The Third International Consensus Definitions for Sepsis and Septic Shock (Sepsis-3). JAMA. 2016;315:801-10.
4. Remick DG. Pathophysiology of sepsis. Am J Pathol. 2007;170: 1435-44.
5. Kawasaki T. Update on pediatric sepsis: a review. J Intensive Care. 2017;5:47.
6. NICE. (2016). Sepsis: recognition, diagnosis and early management. NICE guideline [NG51]. [online] Available from https://www.nice.org.uk/guidance/ng51 [Last accessed November, 2019].
7. PALS Algorithms 2017. [online] Available from https://www. acls-pals-bls.com/algorithms/pals/#shock [Last accessed November, 2019].
8. Randolph AG, McCulloh RJ. Pediatric sepsis: important considerations for diagnosing and managing severe infections in infants, children, and adolescents. Virulence. 2014;5: 179-89.
9. Dellinger RP, Levy MM, Rhodes A, et al. Surviving sepsis campaign: international guidelines for management of severe sepsis and septic shock: 2012. Crit Care Med. 2013;41: 580-637.
10. Faustino EV, Bogue CW. Relationship between hypoglycemia and mortality in critically ill children. Pediatr Crit Care Med. 2010;11:690-8.
11. Jacobs DM, Holsen M, Chen S, et al. Procalcitonin to detect bacterial infections in critically ill pediatric patients. Clin Pediatr (Phila). 2017;56:821-7.
12. Bai Z, Zhu X, Li M, et al. Effectiveness of predicting in-hospital mortality in critically ill children by assessing blood lactate levels at admission. BMC Pediatr. 2014;14:83.
13. Kumar A, Roberts D, Wood KE, et al. Duration of hypotension before initiation of effective antimicrobial therapy is the critical determinant of survival in human septic shock. Crit Care Med. 2006;34(6):1589-96.
14. Maitland K, Kiguli S, Opoka RO, et al. Mortality after fluid bolus in African children with severe infection. N Engl J Med. 2011;364(26):2483-95.
15. Avni T, Lador A, Lev S, et al. Vasopressors for the treatment of septic shock: systematic review and meta-analysis. PLoS One. 2015;10(8):e0129305.
16. Avila AA, Kinberg EC, Sherwin NK. The use of fluids in sepsis. Cureus. 2016;8(3):e528.
17. Angus DC. Early, goal-directed therapy for septic shock—a patient-level meta-analysis. N Engl J Med. 2017;377:994-5.
18. ARISE, ProCESS, ProMISe. Osborn TM. Severe sepsis and septic shock trials (ProCESS, ARISE, ProMISe): What is optimal resuscitation? Crit Care Clin. 2017;33(2):323-44.

Toxic Shock Syndrome

Rahul Patil, Mahesh A Mohite

INTRODUCTION

Toxic shock syndrome (TSS) is severely fatal but rare disease, caused by disproportionate immune response to infection caused by toxin-producing strains of *Staphylococcus aureus* (more common) and *Streptococcus pyogenes*. *S. aureus*, even after minor infection, produces TSS toxin-1 (TSST-1), which acts as a superantigen, which leads to immune response with cytokine release and produces spectrum of clinical manifestations resembling septic shock.

PATHOPHYSIOLOGY

Staphylococcus aureus produces staphylococcal enterotoxin, TSST-1 and staphylococcal enterotoxin like toxin which acts as superantigen [which leads to excessive and nonconventional T-cell activation by unprocessed binding to T-cell receptor (TCR) and MHC type 2 molecule in combination and leads to catastrophic overamplification of cytokine cascade].[1] These superantigens are capable of more than 20% stimulation of T cell as compared to conventional antigens with more potency.[2] After T-cell activation by superantigen, there is biphasic release of proinflammatory cytokines, first interleukin (IL)-2, IL-6, tumor necrosis factor-alpha (TNF-α) followed by slow release of IL-12 and interferon-gamma (IFN-γ).[3] Among all *S. aureus*, only 50–80% of isolates can produce superantigens.[4]

Streptococcal enterotoxins, SPES [a, b, c, f (mitogenic factor), g, h, and j] and superantigen are the major toxins associated with streptococcal TSS.[5-7] The portals of entry for group A streptococcus (GAS) infection include the vagina, pharynx, mucosa, and skin, and frequently at sites of minimal local trauma due to infections with viruses such as varicella and influenza.[5,8]

CLINICAL FEATURES

Toxic shock syndrome is characterized by acute-onset fever, rapid-progressive hypotension, and multiorgan involvement. Clinical case definitions are presented in **Tables 1 and 2**.

Staphylococcal TSS develops with abrupt rise of fever with flu-like symptoms without clinical evidence of septic focus. Within next 6–12 hours progresses to hypotension, behaves like septic shock, may progress to disseminated intravascular coagulation (DIC) and multiorgan involvement.[9] The disease may last 1–2 weeks with desquamation in 2nd week followed by normalization of laboratory parameters. In TSS, associated with postoperative cases, signs of inflammation are not present at surgical wound, since TNF-α inhibits neutrophil mobilization;[9] hence, diagnosis by high index of suspicion is very important. Blood cultures are positive in < 5% of patients that to only from sites of infection are usually positive.[10]

Differential diagnoses (in addition to conventional septic shock) include streptococcal toxic shock, meningococcal septicemia, scarlet fever, Rocky Mountain spotted fever and leptospirosis.

Streptococcal TSS lacks specific flu-like symptoms initially, more often have nonspecific symptoms (like localize skin or soft tissue pain and tenderness) to begin with.[12] However, in children below 10 years with invasive streptococcal disease, presentation is like bacteremia without focus blood culture, specifically from site of infection is positive in 60% case.[6]

MANAGEMENT

Diagnosis is usually made on the basis of clinical features with or without evidence of infection. Polymerase chain reaction (PCR)-based detection of superantigen genes

Table 1: Staphylococcal toxic shock syndrome: clinical case definition.[11]

- *Fever*: Temperature >38.9°C (102.0°F)
- *Rash*: Diffuse macular erythroderma
- *Desquamation*: 1–2 weeks after onset, particularly palms and soles
- *Hypotension*: Systolic blood pressure (SBP) < 90 mm Hg for adults; lower than fifth percentile for age in children aged < 16 years
- Orthostatic drop in diastolic blood pressure of >15 mm Hg from lying to sitting; orthostatic syncope or orthostatic dizziness
- Multisystem involvement (three or more of the following):
    - *Gastrointestinal*: Vomiting or diarrhea at onset of illness
    - *Muscular*: Severe myalgia or creatinine phosphokinase level greater than twice the upper limit of normal
    - *Mucous membrane*: Vaginal, oropharyngeal, or conjunctival hyperemia
    - *Renal*: Serum urea nitrogen or serum creatinine level greater than twice the upper limit of normal or urinary sediment with > 5 WBC cells per high-power field in the absence of a urinary tract infection
    - *Hepatic*: Total bilirubin, aspartate aminotransferase (AST), or alanine aminotransferase (ALT) level greater than twice the upper limit of normal
    - *Hematologic*: Platelet count < 100,000
    - *Central nervous system (CNS)*: Disorientation or alterations in consciousness without focal neurologic signs when fever and hypotension are absent

Negative results on the following tests, if obtained:
- Blood, throat, or cerebrospinal fluid cultures; blood culture may be positive for *S. aureus*
- Serologic tests for Rocky Mountain spotted fever, leptospirosis, or measles

Case classification:
- *Probable*: A case with five of the six aforementioned clinical findings
- *Confirmed*: A case with all six of the clinical findings, including desquamation. If the patient dies before desquamation could have occurred, the other five criteria constitute a definitive case

Table 2: Streptococcal toxic shock syndrome: clinical case definition.[13]

1. Isolation of group A β-hemolytic streptococci:
    (a) From a normally sterile site (e.g. blood, cerebrospinal fluid, peritoneal fluid, tissue biopsy specimen)
    (b) From a nonsterile site (e.g. throat, sputum, vagina)
2. Clinical signs of severity:
    (a) *Hypotension*: SBP < 90 mm Hg in adults or lower than the fifth percentile for age in children
    (b) Two or more of the following signs:
        - *Renal impairment*: Creatinine level > 177 µmol/L (≥2 mg/dL) for adults or two times or more the upper limit of normal for age
        - *Coagulopathy*: Platelet count < 100×10^9/L (≤100×10^3/µL) or DIC
        - *Hepatic involvement*: ALT, AST, or total bilirubin levels two times or more the upper limit of normal for age
        - Acute respiratory distress syndrome (ARDS)
        - A generalized erythematous macular rash that may desquamate
        - Soft tissue necrosis, including necrotizing fasciitis or myositis, or gangrene

An illness fulfilling criteria 1(a), 2(a), and 2(b) can be defined as a definite case. An illness fulfilling criteria 1(b), 2(a), and 2(b) can be defined as a probable case if no other cause for the illness is identified

may provide prompt support for the diagnosis.[14] Anti-TSST-1 antibody assays may also provide supportive data.[15] Flow cytometric analysis of T-cell populations provides corroborative diagnostic information, and this can help to differentiate TSS from septic shock.[16]

Investigations are used to exclude alternative diagnoses, to identify and track progression of organ dysfunction, and to provide supportive evidence for a diagnosis of TSS.

Fluid Resuscitation

Mainstay of management is early suspicion and recognition of TSS with initial hemodynamic stabilization and early institution of antibiotics[10] covering staphylococcus and streptococcus.

Shock needs to be treated with optimal fluid boluses. In nonresponders, vasopressors are also required to correct shock. Ongoing evaluation with intermittent fluid boluses is required most of times. Blood cultures should be sent from all possible sites of infection.

After initial hemodynamic stabilization, it may need to support other organ injuries, like renal replacement therapy (RRT) for renal failure, and proper ARDS management if required. For hematological impairment, transfusion with packed cell volume (PCV) for anemia,

Table 3: Antimicrobial choice for staphylococcal toxic shock syndrome (TSS).

Organism	Option A	Option B Beta-lactam intolerant	Option C
Methicillin-sensitive *S. aureus* (MSSA)	Nafcillin or cloxacillin or flucloxacillin, and clindamycin	Clindamycin	Linezolid or daptomycin or tigecycline ± rifampicin
Methicillin-resistant *S. aureus* (MRSA)	Vancomycin or teicoplanin, and clindamycin	N/A	Linezolid or daptomycin or tigecycline ± rifampicin
Glycopeptide resistant or intermediate-sensitive *S. aureus*	Linezolid ± clindamycin, or daptomycin	N/A	Tigecycline

platelet and/or fresh frozen plasma (FFP) for bleeding if required in few cases.

Antimicrobial Therapy

Initial empirical therapy for TSS should cover both GAS and *S. aureus* because of their similar clinical appearance.[10] Empirically ceftriaxone with or without vancomycin is to be started, which can be modified as per the culture sensitivity pattern.

For TSS, along with antibiotics source reduction is very important to remove the preformed toxin and prevent further production of toxin. Even in absence of signs of inflammation, surgical wounds need to be reopened for debridement, abscesses need to be drained, removal of foreign bodies from site of infection is very important.

Total duration of therapy should be continued for at least 10–14 days, depending upon underlying focus of infection.[10] It helps in reducing bacteremia load and prevent relapse, but acute duration of illness remains same since it is cytokine mediated.[9,17]

Antimicrobial choice for staphylococcal TSS has been shown in **Table 3**.

Intravenous penicillin G (200,000–400,000 units/kg/day) in four to six divided doses is the drug of choice for GAS infection. Along with that surgical intervention for debridement and fasciotomy are must if required. Despite of susceptibility, inoculum effects make it ineffective for penicillin to act, hence for suspected GAS infections, penicillin along with clindamycin (25–40 mg/kg/day) in divided doses is recommended. However, clindamycin alone should not be a choice to begin with.[10]

Intravenous Immunoglobulin

Intravenous immunoglobulin (1–2 g/kg) in single dose in addition to antimicrobial therapy inhibits cell activation by blocking superantigens and thereby reducing production of inflammatory cytokines.[18,19]

Adjuvant Therapy

Use of recombinant-activated protein C has currently being studied in pediatric patients,[20] it has got direct anti-inflammatory property by inhibiting cytokine production.

The role of steroid was studied in adults, there was no survival benefit.

■ REFERENCES

1. Sperber SJ, Francis JB. Toxic shock syndrome during an influenza outbreak. JAMA. 1987;257:1086-7.
2. Centers for Disease Control (CDC). Toxic shock syndrome following influenza—Oregon; update on influenza activity—United States. MMWR Morb Mortal Wkly Rep. 1987;36(5):64-5.
3. McCarthy VP, Peoples WM. Toxic shock syndrome after ear piercing. Pediatr Infect Dis J. 1988;7:741-2.
4. Chau TA, McCully ML, Brintnell W, et al. Toll-like receptor 2 ligands on the staphylococcal cell wall downregulate superantigen-induced T-cell activation and prevent toxic shock syndrome. Nat Med. 2009;15:641-9.
5. Stevens DL. The flesh-eating bacterium: what's next? J Infect Dis. 1999;179(Suppl 2):S366-74.
6. Stevens DL. Streptococcal toxic-shock syndrome: spectrum of disease, pathogenesis, and new concepts in treatment. Emerg Infect Dis. 1995;1:69-78.
7. McCormick JK, Pragman AA, Stolpa JC, et al. Functional characterization of streptococcal pyrogenic exotoxin J, a novel superantigen. Infect Immun. 2001;69:1381-8.
8. Stevens DL. Toxic shock syndromes. Infect Dis Clin North Am. 1996;10(4):727-46.
9. Chesney JP, Davis JP. Toxic shock syndrome. In: Feigin RD, Cherry JD (Eds). Textbook of Pediatric Infectious Diseases, 4th edition. Philadelphia, PA: WB Saunders; 1998. pp. 830-52.
10. American Academy of Pediatrics. Toxic shock syndrome. In: Pickering LK (Ed). 2000 Red Book: Report of the Committee on Infectious Diseases, 25th edition. Elk Grove Village, IL: American Academy of Pediatrics; 2000. pp. 576-81.
11. Wharton M, Chorba TL, Vogt RL, et al. Case definitions for public surveillance. MMWR Recomm Rep. 1990;39(RR-13):1-43.
12. American Academy of Pediatrics. Committee on Infectious Diseases. Severe invasive group A streptococcal infections: a subject review. Pediatrics. 1998;101:136-40.

13. The Working Group on Severe Streptococcal Infections. Defining the group A streptococcal toxic shock syndrome. Rationale and consensus definition. JAMA. 1993;269:390-1.

14. Granger K, Rundell MS, Pingle MR, et al. Multiplex PCR-ligation detection reaction assay for simultaneous detection of drug resistance and toxin genes from Staphylococcus aureus, Enterococcus faecalis, and Enterococcus faecium. J Clin Microbiol. 2010;48:277-80.

15. Javid Khojasteh V, Rogan MT, Edwards-Jones V, et al. Detection of antibodies to Staphylococcus aureus toxic shock syndrome toxin-1 using a competitive agglutination inhibition assay. Lett Appl Microbiol. 2003;36:372-6.

16. Ferry T, Thomas D, Perpoint T, et al. Analysis of superantigenic toxin Vbeta T-cell signatures produced during cases of staphylococcal toxic shock syndrome and septic shock. Clin Microbiol Infect. 2008;14:546-54.

17. Andrews MM, Parent EM, Barry M, et al. Recurrent nonmenstrual toxic shock syndrome: clinical manifestations, diagnosis, and treatment. Clin Infect Dis. 2001;32:1470-9.

18. Schlievert PM. Use of intravenous immunoglobulin in the treatment of staphylococcal and streptococcal toxic shock syndromes and related illnesses. J Allergy Clin Immunol. 2001;108:S107-10.

19. Barry W, Hudgins L, Donta ST, et al. Intravenous immunoglobulin therapy for toxic shock syndrome. JAMA. 1992;267:3315-6.

20. Dalton HJ. Recombinant activated protein C in pediatric sepsis. Pediatr Infect Dis J. 2003;22(8):743-5.

Foreign Body

Pallab Chatterjee

INTRODUCTION

As kids have a tendency to introduce various materials in the nose, ears, and gut, foreign bodies are one of the most common emergencies seen by pediatricians in their daily practice and also have a significant medicolegal implication. Foreign bodies in other places, like retained surgical foreign bodies and eyes (corneal, conjunctival, and intraorbital) are uncommon and is beyond the scope of this discussion.

FOREIGN BODIES IN THE AIRWAYS

Introduction

One of the most common foreign bodies encountered by pediatricians are the nasal ones, and are usually removed easily in the OPD. A foreign body lower down in the tracheobronchial airway can be life-threatening, especially if the central airways are blocked leading to impaired ventilation and oxygenation.

Epidemiology

Nasal foreign bodies are the most common around 3 years of age, and are usually asymptomatic or may present as a foul-smelling discharge from the nose, usually unilateral. Seeds are the most common, followed by batteries and rubber; and more than half are usually in the right nostril.

Tracheobronchial foreign bodies are a common cause of morbidity and mortality in young children, and account for around 1 death in 1 lakh children below 4 years of age. Mortality due to aspiration of foreign bodies accounted for around 24% mortality in the early 20th century. The incidence is much less now, thanks to improved bronchoscopy instruments, expertise, and technique. Majority (80%) of foreign body aspirations occur below the age of 3 years, the peak incidence being between 1 year and 2 years, as at this age most children can stand and explore their world by putting small things in the mouth, while lacking the molars necessary for adequate chewing. The tendency to engage in various playful activities during feeding, and the presence of older siblings who tend to insert food into their mouth also increase the prevalence of foreign body aspirations at this age; while the small size of their airways make them more vulnerable. In older children and adolescents, it is seen more commonly in neurologic disorders, altered sensorium, and sedative or alcohol overdose. There is a male preponderance of approximately 2:1 on an average in various studies.

The features of foreign bodies that make them dangerous are round, smooth and slippery surface, and compressibility. While older children tend to aspirate nonfood items like coins, button batteries, pins, caps of pens, clips, etc., vegetable foreign bodies, like groundnuts and Bengal gram (approximately 50%), other nuts, seeds (like watermelon seeds), popcorn, and other food items are commonly aspirated by toddlers. Aspiration of balloon-like materials (such as gloves or condoms) are commonly fatal. Certain drugs, like iron and potassium, cause severe inflammation and stenosis by tending to dissolve in the airways, and hence early diagnosis and definitive treatment is essential.

The majority of the aspirated foreign bodies tend to locate in the right lung (60%), of which 52% is in the bronchus intermedius; followed by the left lung (23%), trachea (13%), larynx (3%), and bilateral (2%). The laryngotracheal foreign bodies are usually irregular or large, and are associated with increased mortality than those that lodge in the bronchi.

Presentation

Nasal foreign bodies are usually a late presentation with only around one-third of the children presenting within 24 hours.

Foreign body aspirations present within 24 hours of the episode in 50–75% of children. The signs and symptoms depend on the age of the child, nature of the foreign body, location and degree of blockage of the airways, and time elapsed. Only about half of the children present with a history of choking, which is defined as a sudden onset of cough, with or without dyspnea or cyanosis, in a previously healthy child.

If there is a complete airway obstruction or reflex laryngospasm following an acute choking episode, there can be immediate death due to suffocation. However, most children enter a temporary symptom-free period after the acute episode, which may last for seconds to minutes, followed by persistent symptoms in the form of unexplained dyspnea, recurrent wheeze and cough; or may come back later with suppurative complications like pneumonia (acute or recurrent), lung abscess, and bronchiectasis. A minority can expectorate the foreign body after a bout of violent cough following the choking episode. The classic triad of cough, localized wheeze, and decreased breath sounds, present in about 57% of children, have a high specificity but a low sensitivity.

Signs and symptoms vary according to the site of the foreign body. In the central airways, they are usually life-threatening and present with stridor, difficulty in breathing, hoarseness, and sometimes dysphagia (in case of large penetrating foreign bodies). The foreign bodies in the large bronchi present with cough, wheeze, dyspnea, cyanosis, and decreased breath sounds. Foreign bodies in the lower airways are usually the ones that present with a delayed diagnosis with fever and chest infiltrates on the X-ray that do not resolve or recur.

Management

In around 5% of children, the nasal foreign bodies can be dislodged spontaneously. Majority of nasal foreign bodies can be removed in the outpatient department using a Magill forceps. However, old foreign bodies with granulations and dangerous foreign bodies like button batteries and penetrating foreign bodies should be handled by a specialist in the operating room under general anesthesia.

In a life-threatening foreign body aspiration where the child has a complete obstruction of the airway, dislodgement should be attempted. In infants below 1 year, 5 slaps on the back in the head low position with 5 chest thrusts; while in kids above 1 year, 5 abdominal thrusts (Heimlich maneuver), is recommended. After each such series the airway obstruction is to be reviewed. However, such procedures, including "blind finger-sweep," should be avoided in children who are able to cough or speak, as they may convert a partial obstruction to a complete obstruction.

If the foreign body is still not dislodged, a direct laryngoscopy and an attempt to removal by a Magill forceps should be done. If it is still not removed and the foreign body is above the vocal cords, a cricothyroidotomy should be done either surgically or with a needle. If the foreign body is below the vocal cords, the patient should be intubated intentionally to the right side to push the foreign body into the right main bronchus, and then to withdraw the endotracheal tube (ET) tube and ventilate the left lung with the right side down, while proceeding for definitive removal by a rigid bronchoscopy under vision.

In cases of a suspected foreign body aspiration and an asymptomatic child, a plain chest X-ray is performed, preferably in both inspiration and expiration (or left lateral decubitus, if expiratory film is not possible). The usual findings are hyperinflation, atelectasis, mediastinal shift away from the foreign body, and consolidation. Late manifestations include bronchiectatic changes and abscess. However, if this is normal (approximately in 30% of cases), and the suspicion is very high, a flexible bronchoscopy or a CT scan of the chest is performed, the former being more definitive **(Fig. 1)**.

Once detected, the definitive management is usually removal with the help of a rigid bronchoscope. Though the American Thoracic Society recommends only rigid bronchoscopy, some centers with high expertise use the flexible bronchoscope for removal of foreign bodies, the main advantages being avoidance of general anesthesia and the ability to reach deeper, with the disadvantage of dislodging the foreign body and leading to a further compromise.

In case of a prolonged retained foreign body, it may be difficult to remove it at one sitting and may require a second bronchoscopy after a course of antibiotics and steroids.

Prevention

The American Academy of Pediatrics suggests some guidance to be provided to all caregivers at 6 months of age

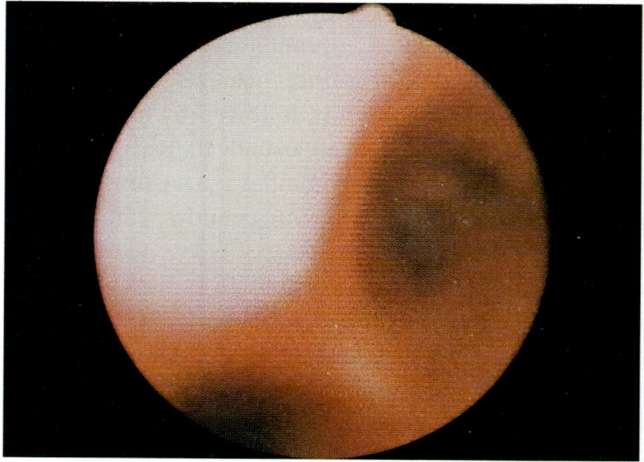

Fig. 1: Prolonged retained cap of a pen in the right middle lobe bronchus.

regarding foreign body aspiration. Some of these include avoidance of marbles, balloons, coins, and toys with small parts; feeding of solid food in infants only by adults, and supervised feeding in older children sitting only in the upright position, and not during other activities like playing, running, crying or laughing; chewable medications after 3 years of age and hard round foods above 4 years of age. All child caregivers, teachers, and parents should take a course in basic life support. The Indian Academy of Pediatrics has taken a lead role in spreading the mass awareness of basic life support to the caregivers through various activities.

■ FOREIGN BODIES IN THE GASTROINTESTINAL TRACT

Introduction

The most common foreign bodies in children are the ingested foreign bodies. They are usually not life-threatening and majority tends to pass spontaneously.

Epidemiology

The majority of ingestions of foreign objects are seen between 6 months to 3 years **(Fig. 2)**. Of these, only about 10% need endoscopic removal. The most common foreign bodies ingested are coins, followed by button batteries, small toys or parts thereof, safety pins, marbles, magnets, etc.

Of these, button batteries are wrought with danger as they tend of cause pressure necrosis and a high risk of perforation as a result of contact of esophageal walls with both poles of the battery. In the recent times, ingestion of magnets has increased due to their increased usage in various toys and household items. They are known to cause intestinal obstruction when they stick together from two different sites in the small intestine. Lead items present in certain household materials like toys, curtain weights, rifle pellets, etc. are known to cause lead toxicity and fatalities.

Foreign bodies in the gastrointestinal tract tend to get stuck in physiological narrow areas, like upper esophageal sphincter, at the level of the arch of the aorta and at the lower esophageal sphincter.

Presentation

In about half of the children, ingested foreign bodies are asymptomatic and brought by parents or caregivers who have noticed the episode. Symptoms, when present, are according to the site of the foreign body. Esophageal foreign bodies may be associated with dysphagia, drooling, stridor, wheeze, and retrosternal pain. More serious complications like perforation into the trachea to

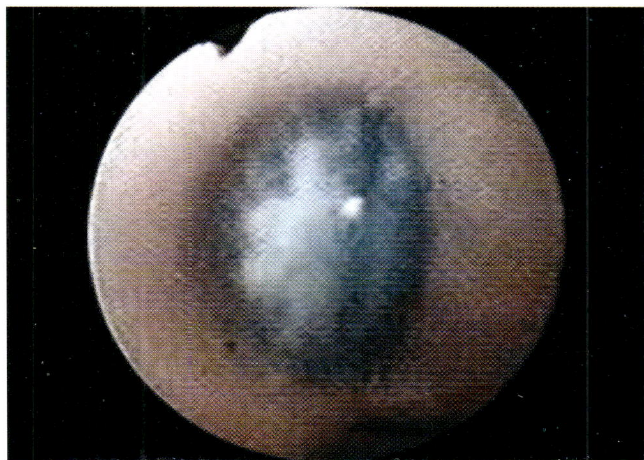

Fig. 2: Bronchoscopic view of a foreign body (shirt button) in the right main bronchus of a 3-year-old boy.

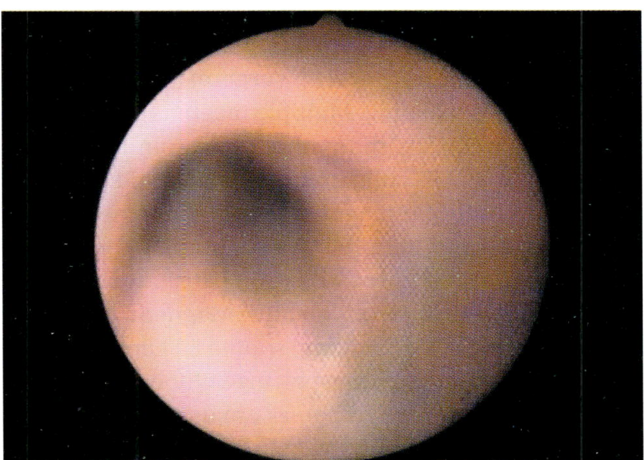

Fig. 3: Bronchoscopic view of an acquired tracheoesophageal fistula caused by aspirated button battery in an 18-month-old child.

cause a fistula **(Fig. 3)**, or into the mediastinum to cause pneumomediastinum, or into the aorta to cause severe gastrointestinal hemorrhage has also been reported.

Foreign bodies that reach the stomach are usually asymptomatic. However, occasionally foreign bodies may lead to gastric outlet obstruction or distal obstruction mimicking appendicitis.

Management

Initial evaluation of swallowed foreign bodies should be an X-ray of the neck, chest, and abdomen. CT scan is done if the patient is symptomatic, or the foreign body is either long (>5 cm length) or large (>2 cm width) or sharp, or is unknown.

In case of a blunt radiopaque object in the esophagus, watchful expectancy is advocated. Foreign bodies that are small and crossover into the stomach are most likely to pass out by 12 weeks. Hence, serial radiographs at weekly intervals is recommended. If it is still in the esophagus after 24 hours, or in the stomach by 4 weeks, or in case of other warning signs suggestive of obstruction or distress, retrieval by endoscopy is advocated. Urgent endoscopic removal is advised in cases of a long or sharp object, magnets, disk battery, and in cases of esophageal obstruction, airway compression, or intestinal obstruction.

Of the various ingested foreign bodies, disk batteries and magnet ingestions have increased in the recent times and they deserve special mention. Batteries can cause very early ulceration, and perforation by 8 hours, due either to the electrical discharge from the negative pole, release of various caustic substances or pressure necrosis. They can be differentiated from coins on the X-ray by their double-ring and scalloped edge. In an asymptomatic child, they should be removed as early as possible endoscopically. A symptomatic child usually signifies perforation, and should be removed in the operation theater by a pediatric surgeon or a cardiothoracic surgeon, depending on whether there is bleeding. Multiple magnets have a higher risk of complications than single ones, and thus both anteroposterior (AP) and lateral views should be taken to differentiate multiple magnets sticking together leading to a misdiagnosis. Multiple magnets in the intestine may attract layers of the gut leading to obstruction, necrosis and perforation, fistula, or volvulus. Magnetic or metallic objects (like buckles or buttons) should be kept away from the child and an attempt must be made for early removal.

Gastrointestinal foreign bodies are usually removed by flexible endoscopy, while Magill's forceps, rigid endoscopy, or surgery may sometimes be used depending on the site and nature of the foreign body.

Prevention

Caregivers should be counseled about keeping small objects away from the reach of children. Battery compartment of household items and toys should preferably be secured with extra tapes.

■ FOREIGN BODIES IN THE EAR

Introduction

Commonly seen foreign bodies in the ear in children are in the external auditory canal and pinna.

Epidemiology

Most foreign bodies in the external auditory canal are seen in children below the age of 6 years. Common objects are beads, seeds, stones, paper, small toy parts, button batteries, and insects. Foreign bodies in the pinna are from embedded earrings, and are seen in older children and adolescents.

Presentation

Usually the caregiver gives a history of introduction of a foreign body being observed. Rarely children may present with decreased hearing or pain in the ears, excessive crying in young children, and unilateral purulent ear discharge of incidentally found on otoscopy.

Management

Button batteries can cause extensive damage as a result of electrical discharges leading to damage to the skin, tympanic membrane and ossicles, and may even cause permanent deafness; and hence early removal is required. Live insects, like cockroaches, may cause severe discomfort and should be first killed with mineral oil and then removed. Penetrating foreign bodies like pins, cotton ear buds, pencil tips, etc. can damage the middle ear and needs urgent ENT referral.

■ CONCLUSION

Diagnosis of foreign bodies in children requires a high index of suspicion. It should be thought of in kids who have a sudden onset of symptoms that do not respond to the standard management of other suspected causes. Suggestive histories like choking should be evaluated even if they occur weeks before the presentation. An asymptomatic presentation is very common with foreign bodies other than airways, like gastrointestinal, ears, vaginal, etc. An early evaluation and treatment can go a long way in preventing serious long-term complications. Prevention is of utmost importance and can be achieved by education of the caregiver, product surveillance and to some extent by legislation.

■ SUGGESTED READING

1. Centers for Disease Control and Prevention (CDC). Nonfatal choking-related episodes among children—United States, 2001. MMWR Morb Mortal Wkly Rep. 2002;51:945.
2. Hitter A, Hullo E, Durand C, et al. Diagnostic Value of various investigations in children with suspected foreign body aspiration. Eur Ann Otorhinolaryngol. 2011;128:248-52.
3. Jatana KR, Litoritz T, Reilly JS, et al. Pediatric button battery injuries: 2013 task force update. Int J Ped Otolaryngol. 2013;77: 1392-99.
4. Kramer TA, Riding KH, Salkeld LJ. Tracheobronchial and esophageal foreign bodies in the pediatric population. J Otolaryngol. 1986;15:355.

13

Environmental Issues

Piyush Gupta

Vector Control in Tropics

Alok Gupta, Mohit Vohra

INTRODUCTION

The *tropics* are a haven for innumerous arthropods like mosquitoes, ticks, bugs, mites and flies. Being cold-blooded they breed and survive easily in warm and humid climates. The tropical habitat is well suited to them to complete their entire life cycle. Some of these arthropods affect the human life by harboring disease causing organisms and then transmitting them to humans and other animals causing morbidity and mortality. When this morbidity and mortality reaches an alarming stage, they become a cause of concern. Control, elimination and eradication of these vector-borne diseases make it essential that these arthropods (vectors) are controlled, eliminated or eradicated in addition to other measures.

DEFINITIONS

- *Vector*: It is an agent (living organism), typically a biting insect or a tick which can transmit infectious diseases from humans, animal, or plants to others.
- *Vector-borne diseases*: These are human illnesses caused by bacteria, viruses or parasites transmitted by mosquitos, ticks, etc.
- *Tropics*: It is a region of the Earth covered between Tropic of Cancer in the north and the Tropic of Capricorn in the south. It is also called Tropical Region. This includes South East Asia, Africa (Central, East and West), America (Central and South) and Caribbean.
- *Control*: It is defined as reduction in newer infections and also reduction in the number of patients who become diseased or acquire death due to a disease in local area. This can be accomplished through efforts including vaccines and other public health interventions.

Vector-borne diseases contribute in majority to the total worldwide burden of disease. According to the latest WHO data, vector-borne diseases contribute nearly 20% of all infectious diseases, resulting in more than 700,000 deaths per year. Nearly 4 billion people in around 130 countries are in probable risk of getting dengue, with more than 90 million cases occurring per year. Malaria alone is responsible for more than 400,000 deaths every year globally; with maximum contribution to under-5 mortality. Many other diseases such as leishmaniasis and Chagas disease have an impact on many people around the world. It is also an important obstacle to socioeconomic development in resource-poor countries. Vector control being an important tool can save lives not only by preventing but also by reducing or eliminating transmission. The strategies applied all over the world for integrated vector control (IVC) provide a basis for strengthening vector control programs in such a manner that goes hand in hand with national health systems and local community needs. To make the program successful and to be continued for long, IVC balances the use of human, financial resources and government organizations for the control of vector-borne disease with involvement of local people. The program insists on a two-way control approach, which includes various disease control measures and various interventions in a systematic manner. To make the efforts successful and program fruitful, there should be a strong political will, healthy and firm collaboration of the health sector with various other sectors together with public and private agencies and institutions. For effective control, WHO's strong commitment will require effective public health regulation policy to be implemented by respective countries. Similarly, the habitats which are more important epidemiologically and in terms of productivity constitute to be the important target for success of IVC. The various stepwise approaches also require detailed knowledge and facts regarding the habits of the residents and the knowledge regarding vector breeding and transmission in that place depending on the environmental conditions.[1,2]

The common vector-borne diseases in tropics are as follows:

- Malaria
- Dengue
- Chikungunya
- Japanese encephalitis
- Schistosomiasis
- Onchocerciasis
- Lymphatic filariasis
- Leishmaniasis
- Chagas disease
- Human African trypanosomiasis.

Common vectors transmitting the disease in the tropics are as follows:

- *Anopheles*
  - Malaria
  - Lymphatic filariasis
- *Culex*
  - West Nile fever
  - Lymphatic filariasis
  - Japanese encephalitis
- *Aedes*
  - Dengue fever
  - Chikungunya
  - Lymphatic filariasis
  - Yellow fever
  - Zika
  - Rift Valley fever
- Fleas
  - Plague (Flea-borne)
  - *Rickettsia* infection
- Black flies
  - Onchocerciasis (river blindness)
- Sandflies
  - Leishmanial infection
- Tsetse flies
  - Sandfly fever (Phlebotomus fever)
  - Sleeping sickness (African trypanosomiasis)
- Triatomine bugs
  - Chagas disease
- Aquatic snails
  - Schistosomiasis (bilharziasis)
- Ticks
  - Relapsing fever
  - Rocky Mountain spotted fever and Q fever (rickettsial disease)

- Lyme disease
- Crimean-Congo hemorrhagic fever
- Tularemia
- Lice
  - Typhus and louse-borne fever.

CONTROLLING VECTORS; CONTROLLING DISEASES

Environmental Management

Changes are needed in the environment to minimize or prevent vector propagation and related activities. This includes reduction of larval habitats by alteration, removal and recycling of the larval habitats which may be in the form of containers or collection of nonessential water in tires or broken utensils.

Three types of environmental management are defined:

1. *Physical changes in the environment*: Long-lasting and permanent physical changes to decrease the habitats of vector larvae such as of adoption of closed pipe system for water supply to communities, including household connections are needed.
2. *Changes in vector habitat*: Changes to vector habitats which include the treatment of "essential" containers such as:
   - Frequent cleaning by throwing the residual water and scrubbing of water-storage vessels
   - Changing of water in flower pots, room coolers, etc.
   - Treatment of drains and sewage system
   - Destruction or covering of stored tires, pots, etc. before rainfall
   - Disposal in a proper manner and recycling of discarded containers
   - Removal and safe disposal or discarded vehicles lying on the deserted roadside or junkyards
   - Removal of wild plants such as wild bromeliads that is commonly found in the axils of leaf in the residential areas.
3. *Alteration in human behavior*: Actions to reduce human-vector contact. This includes such as:
   - Use of mosquito screens on doors, windows and other probable entry sites of the house
   - Installation of mosquito nets at night during sleeping
   - Wearing full clothes
   - Good hygiene habits.

Since large vector population is often affected with scanty supply of water, nonessential water collection, poor sanitation and waste disposal, improvement in essential basic services like piped water, proper waste disposal and good urban infrastructure would contribute to reduction in the habitats of larvae.

Improvement in Water-related Issues

- One of the key methods in controlling vectors is the improvement in the water supply. The water which is drawn from wells is inferior to the water which is supplied by the pipeline to the households. Emphasis should be laid on regular supply of potable water by pipelines directly to the households so that drums open tanks and jars are not required. Such steps would decrease the storage practices which have been followed traditionally since years.
- Designs of the water containers should be made in such a manner so that laying of the eggs by mosquitoes can be prevented. Lid-fitted vessels can be used. In case of rain filled collection of water, rainwater harvested from roofs should be covered with a tight-fitted mesh screens. These covers should be replaced every time water is removed. Physical barrier such as expanded polystyrene beads is also of some help.
- Reduction in solid waste from household and industries would also benefit in vector control. The concept of proper storage, collection and disposal of waste from community plays important role in the protection of public health. The important rule of reduce, reuse, recycle is gold standard and should be followed. Discarded tires, containers undergoing recycling can contribute to economic improvement besides their impact on vector population.
- Regular cleaning of roads and streets to clean the drains and discard the water-bearing containers. To reduce potential larval habitats, the construction sites of new buildings or renovation of old buildings should also follow the strict rules to be imposed by the government.

Chemical Control: Larvicides

Larvicides are commonly and widely used method of chemical control and are environmentally friendly too. Their major limitation is their use in indoor habitats. The ideal properties of larvicide are that it:

- Does not change the taste of water
- Does not change the color of water
- Does not change the odor of water.

The commonly used chemicals are:

- Temephos
- Pyriproxyfen

- Methoprene:
  - This method is used only if others (environmental control methods or nonpharmacological method) are not accessible or costly. Power operated or manually driven methods to spray the chemical in a perifocal manner are being used. This will kill not only the larval infestations in containers but also the adult mosquitoes that visit such sites. The spray of these chemicals coats the internal, external walls and extends up to 60 cm from the containers.
  - For potable drinking water Temephos and methoprene can be used in the range of up to 1 mg/L (1 ppm), pyriproxyfen can be used at a dosage up to 0.01 mg/L (0.01 ppm) and *Bacillus thuringiensis israelensis* (Bti) can be applied at 1–5 mg/L.[3]
  - The following methods are adopted for application of insecticides:
    - Pipette and syringe for indoor flower vases
    - Manual operated liquid sprayers for the larger habitat
    - Knapsack sprayers for spraying wettable powders
    - Granule and solid preparations should be used with a standard measure like spoon.
  - Two or three rounds of spray per year in a timely manner depending upon the species of mosquito, season, and pattern of rainfall. Efficacy of larvicides is enough in a short transmission season.
  - Extreme care to check drinking water to keep chemicals well below the upper safe levels.

Chemical Control: Adulticides

Chemical control methods that would affect adult vectors have large impact on:

- Population density of the mosquito
- Transmission of the mosquito
- Life cycle and sustainability.

The *adulticides* are applied in two ways:

1. Residual surface treatments
2. Space treatments:
   - Residual treatment in form of perifocal spraying has both adulticide and larvicide effects. Hand-operated compression sprayers are being used for application of insecticides whereas the power sprayers can be used to treat large accumulations of discarded containers (e.g. tire dumps) rapidly.
   - To treat and prevent epidemic, space spraying is recommended since it is vast and results in rapid destruction of the adult vector population. It

remains a matter of debate whether the impact of space treatment is transient or epidemiologically long term in reducing the virus transmission. The control methods applied are successful in decreasing the number of adult mosquitos' population which is infective. There is no well-documented literature in the past of the effectiveness of this approach in interrupting an epidemic. There is sufficient data to support that if space spraying is used early in an epidemic and on a sufficiently large scale, the intensity of transmission may be decreased and which in turn would buy time for the application of other vector control measures that provide benefit in terms of longer-term control, including larvicide and community-based source reduction.

- The size of droplet, indoor coverage, susceptibility of the insecticide and the rate of application are important to the successful reduction or elimination of the vector density. In the extensive areas where ground equipment is difficult and require rapid treatment low flying aircraft using release space sprays may be of utility to suppress vector to cover large areas. Indoor penetration of insecticide droplets is the most important deciding factor for effectiveness of insecticide in this method. In applying space sprays from the air, factors modifying the success include environmental conditions, especially speed of the air or wind at spray height and at ground level and also the size of the droplet at the flying speed of the aircraft. For all these aerial spraying operations, prior clearance from civil aviation office must be sought. Twin-engine aircraft can be used in the populated areas with safety. Populated areas must usually be sprayed from twin-engine aircraft with prior information and safety precautions needed if any, to the public. The aircraft now used contains the system for accurate positioning which is a global variety and also uses the precise application, which can be recorded accurately.
- Space spraying should cover the areas which are heavily populated (e.g. high-density housing, schools, hospitals) and where the chances of vector being high or where vectors are found abundant. Perifocal spraying up to 400 m in the neighboring area in and around the houses where dengue cases occur is commonly practiced.[4,5]
- For space spraying in and around houses, the insecticide formulation should be based on (1) immediate impact on the surroundings, (2) the environment and (3) the acceptability of the community. Only insecticide products which are marked with high propensity of high utility index with safety and with high flashpoints should be considered for thermal fogging. The oil carrier present in oil-based space-spraying formulations prevents evaporation of small fog droplets. For thermal fogging agents, diesel fuel has been used as a carrier. The disadvantage associated with it includes thick smoke, strong smell and oily deposits, which may lead to the denial of its use in the community. Water-based formulations are also available, some of which contain substances that prevent rapid evaporation are also available. The golden rule to be strictly followed while using insecticides is the label instructions should always be taken care of.

- Space sprays can be used in two forms:
  1. Thermal fogs at 10–50 L/ha
  2. Ultra-low-volume applications of insecticide which may be slightly diluted or undiluted.

It includes cold aerosol of droplets of controlled size (15–25 µm) at a rate of 0.5–2.0 L/ha. For ground application, portable or vehicle-mounted cold fog or thermal generators can be used. Application rates depend upon the susceptibility of the target species and environmental considerations and may vary depending upon them. Wind speed plays a major role on droplet distribution and contact with insects. Large-wing aircraft at approximately 240 km/h and 60 m above the ground, with swath spacing of 180 m is being used for the cold fog applications. Smaller, fixed-wing aircraft with slower speeds usually at 160 km/h, 30 m above the ground, with a swath width of 50–100 m is used at the lower altitudes. In emergencies, agricultural spraying aircraft fitted with rotary atomizers or other suitable nozzles with specific formulations are being used.

- For a rapid reduction of the adult vector population the space treatment should ideally be worked out in almost every 2–3 days for 7–10 days with frequent repetition once or twice a week. To determine the effectiveness of these strategies of application, continuous epidemiological and entomological surveillance should be done which would also determine the application schedule.

Safe Use of Insecticides

A safety guideline for insecticide application is as follows:

- All instructions on the labels of pesticides should be read and understood thoroughly and followed meticulously.

- Apron or full uniform along with gloves, goggles and masks should be used for any pesticide-related activities.
- All clothes worn at work should be washed regularly, preferably daily as soon as possible after use.
- Spray operators should not be exposed to toxic material for the longer periods of recommendation.
- Safe disposal of used insecticide containers and unused pesticide.
- Blood cholinesterase level is an important parameter and should be monitored in use organophosphate insecticides.
- There should be clear instructions for the householders and pets to remain outside the dwelling. During and immediately after indoor space spray operations, householders and pets must remain outside the dwelling.

The WHO has published specific guidelines on use of insecticides and safety procedures.[3-7]

Monitoring of Insecticide-resistant Population

A significant level of resistance to organophosphates, carbamates pyrethroids, and organochlorines especially with *Aedes aegypti* has been documented in controlling vector population and is considered a serious potential threat in chemical control of vectors. The program which monitors the susceptibility of vectors to the insecticides should be the integral part in monitoring insecticide-resistant population.

In the countries where there is the history of extensive use of dichlorodiphenyltrichloroethane (DDT), resistance may be widespread. Since DDT and pyrethroid have same target site, i.e. the voltage-gated sodium channel, resistance to DDT goes hand in hand predisposing to pyrethroid resistance. As proved in *A. aegypti*, both the insecticides DDT and pyrethroid have been associated with mutations in the *KDR* gene. Similarly, in the countries where pyrethroids have been extensively used—including deltamethrin, cypermethrin and permethrin—for space spraying, the mosquitoes with this mutation are likely to develop resistance sooner. Thailand with the use of pyrethroids has been a recent example of this phenomenon. These evidences clearly depict the importance of routine susceptibility testing which is done regularly during such control program which may save time and money both.

The many kits for conducting the tests for the susceptibility of adult and larval mosquitoes are available but only those issued by WHO remain the standard methods for determining the susceptibility status as are being used for *Aedes* populations. The various instructions and guidelines laid by WHO concerned laboratories for kits containing chemicals and instruments for testing including test papers solutions are being readily available.[1]

Personal Protection

- Clothing which covers the most of the exposed areas provides less chances of biting and contributes to the protection from the bites of vectors.
- Skin which is uncovered and the clothing of the residents applied with repellents that contain DEET (N,N-diethyl-3-methyl-benzamide), IR3535 [3-(N-butyl-N-acetyl)-aminopropionic acid, ethyl ester] or icaridin [1-piperidinecarboxylic acid, 2-(2-hydroxyethyl)-1-methylpropyl ester]. These repellents do not allow mosquitoes to come in contact with skin and clothes and play an indirect role in protecting from bites of mosquitoes.
- Mosquito nets impregnated with insecticide afford good protection. There are also other insecticide-treated materials (ITMs) like curtains, doorway, etc. which also prove to protect from bites of mosquitoes.
- The biting activity of the indoor mosquitos can be reduced with the use of mosquito coils, insecticide vaporizers or household insecticide aerosol products. The chances of biting can also be reduced with the use of air-conditioning and window and door screens.

Biological Control

Biological control involves the introduction of living organism to compete for sustainability of vector. It includes introduction of an organism that harbors and compete with the vector and would result into reduction of the population of target species. In small water-containing habitats especially water containers, some species of larvivorous fish and small freshwater crustaceans like predatory copepods are effective.

The utility of biological control organisms is mainly for the vector in the container habitats which are hardly cleaned or emptied and also large water storage tanks and wells.

The limitations of the biological methods include:

- Effective only against the immature stages vector
- Temperature and PH of water may not be suitable for the organism in the larval habitats
- Operational limitations—expense involving large scale rearing and distribution
- Difficulty in applying, distribution, monitoring and restocking the containers with the fish or copepods.

Fish: Poecilia reticulata, which is the viviparous variety of fish, is found to be effective in eliminating the mosquitoes in the water bodies.[8] A variety of fish species have been deployed for this job. The limitation with this method is the use of native and larvivorous fish lest it may endanger the natural fauna of the place along with reintroduction at regular intervals.

Predatory copepods:[9] Freshwater crustaceans, copepods species have also been proved to be effective against vectors. The advantage of copepod species over fish is the survival for a longer period. The reintroduction of fish for a sustained control is a limitation as compared with crustaceans.

The practical experience of using copepods in large water-storage tanks under vector program control in North Vietnam has successfully eliminated *A. aegypti* in many communities.

Improved Tools for Vector Control

For the use under public health intervention, some new promising vector control tools have emerged. These tool needs to be field tested on a wide scale for their use and recommendations as public health measures depending on the operational research. Such tools are found to be more promising in dengue vector control management. The WHO in the year 2006 has identified and recommended the use of such promising new tools in the area of vector control especially based on researches on dengue.

Insecticide-treated materials: Insecticide-treated materials commonly used as insecticide-treated bed nets, curtains and other material used in houses have come out to be an effective tool in prevention of mosquito-transmitted diseases especially those which show activity in late evenings and night. Many researches done on the efficacy and safety in use of ITMs and its positive impact in reducing vector load have encouraged the use of ITM especially for controlling mosquito like *A. Aegypti* which is active both in day as well as night. There is enough evidence that insecticide-treated window, door curtains and insecticide-treated cloth covers used for household water-storage containers are highly effective in reducing the vector load particularly in terms for reducing dengue transmission risk. Still many more studies for different methods are required to prove worth of such interventions to declare it as a personal and public health protection tool. ITMs appear to be proven for especially for dengue prevention and control.

The use of ITM need not be limited to bed nets or curtains at home lest it can also be used as a window curtains, screens, wardrobe curtains, etc. The location is not only at home but also at schools, offices, hospitals, workplaces and other locations. If the application of these interventions is shown to be safe, cost effective and efficacious, this will prove to be one of the most appropriate interventions to be used by communities.[10]

Ovitraps: These are devices which are lined with medicine that traps the ova which can be modified to render it lethal. Ovitraps or oviposition traps collect the laid by mosquitoes that will further grow into larva pupa and then into adults. The further be improvised as:
- *Lethal ovitraps*: In this trap, the chemical in form of insecticide is present on the oviposition of the substance used.
- *Autocidal ovitraps*: In this trap, oviposition is allowed but the adult mosquitoes are not allowed to emerge.
- *Sticky ovitraps*: In this variety, mosquito is trapped where it lands.

Studies have shown that population densities can be reduced with the use of traps. The benefits of ovitraps include decreased number of infective vectors by decreasing the life expectancy of the vector. Secondly the sensitivity and specificity of ovitraps against vectors is high. Its effectiveness against container breeders has proven to be better when used in integration with other chemical and biological control methods.[11,12]

■ NATIONAL VECTOR BORNE DISEASE CONTROL PROGRAMME[13]

The National Vector Borne Disease Control Programme (NVBDCP) was launched in 2003–2004 in India for safeguard and elimination of the major vector-borne diseases. It includes:
- National Anti-Malaria Control Programme
- Dengue Control Programme
- National Filaria Control Programme
- Kala-Azar Control Programme
- Japanese Encephalitis Control Programme
  The objectives of the above program are:
- Interruption of transmission by reducing vector population
- Strengthening early diagnosis and prompt management
- Information, education and communication (IEC) activities to increase awareness in the community to encourage personal protection and case reporting
- Vector control measures
- Development of safe and acceptable vaccine.

RECENT DEVELOPMENT IN VECTOR CONTROL STRATEGIES: REAR-AND-RELEASE STRATEGIES

Rear-and-release Methods

Using male mosquitoes to control the vector-borne disease.

This includes a unique formula in developing the sterile insect technique (SIT) in which there occurs irradiation and sterilization of the male flies. There is mating with wild females which results in infertility of eggs and reduction followed by elimination of potent mosquito. SIT is currently being used in agricultural field where it has been proved a boon to control many agricultural pests. Methods of male sterilization include:

- *Physical method*: Radiation technique for the pupae.
- *Chemical methods*: Double-stranded RNA of particular species interferes with the production of sperm.
- *Genetic modification*: Sperm production genes dropped out.
- *Microbiological methods*: For male sterility, induction the *Wolbachia* bacteria can be used.

WHO GLOBAL VECTOR CONTROL RESPONSE STRATEGY (2017–2030)

The WHO took up the Global Vector Control Response globally in May 2017 for the time period of 2017-2030 to limit the spread and minimize the catastrophes caused by vector-borne disease worldwide. The Global Vector Control Response primarily focuses on the various human-related activities and integrated approach for vector management to fight back the disease strategically. This is the basis for making the integrated effective, locally adapted and sustainable vector control strategies worldwide, with the aim reducing the load and also ill impact of vector-borne diseases.

Integrating vector control includes:

- Integration of interventions
- Integration of disease entomology
- Integration of existing resources for vector management.

Global Goals with Vector Control

- To control poverty, since the vector-borne diseases disproportionately affect the poorest who are more vulnerable in a cycle of illness, suffering and poverty.
- Decreasing the prevalence of vector-borne diseases helps in achieving universal health coverage and reducing maternal and neonatal mortality rates.
- Control of vector-borne diseases decreases the school absenteeism which would have occurred in resulted during high transmission season. Infections also affect the overall physical, social and mental development of children.
- Improved water supply and sanitation is necessary for vector control to be successful.
- Successful vector control will lead to cleaner safer and most sustainable places to live in.
- Involvement of partners like health agencies and various environmental agencies across countries to have fruitful association and commitment in successful vector control.

VECTOR INDICES[13]

The vector indices have been classified as:

- Indirect and direct estimates
- Factors related to eradication era
- Vector indices.

Indirect Estimates

Environmental

- Temperature
- Humidity
- Rainfall
- Altitude.

All the above environmental factors affect the life cycle and life span including sporogony and survival.

Entomological

- These indices provide vector per person night and also denote infective mosquito bites per person night.
- This includes human landing rate, sporozoite rate, and entomological inoculation rate.

Clinical

This includes estimation of level of antibodies to various antigenic proteins example immunoglobulin M (IgM), immunoglobulin G (IgG) antibodies, merozoite surface antigen (MSA), etc. It also includes crude estimation like child spleen rate in children more specific for malaria in the age group of 2–10 years. It is calculated as:

Number of children with enlarged spleen/total number of children estimated × 100.

Direct Estimates

Active Surveillance

- Active case detection
- Active case survey
- Period prevalence
- Attack rate/cumulative incidence.

Passive Surveillance

- Annual parasite incidence (API)
- Annual blood examination rate (ABER)
- Passive case detection (PCD) rate

Vector Indices

- Mosquito density rate
- Human blood index
- Human biting rate
- Inoculation rate.

Trends of vector-borne diseases in India can be well understood based on the above parameters. Control measures at community level along with individual active participation with government inter-sectorial commitment and involvement can save us from epidemics and huge financial and life loss which is predictable.

■ REFERENCES

1. A toolkit for integrated vector management in sub-Saharan Africa. Geneva: World Health Organization; 2016.
2. Global vector control response 2017–2030. Geneva: World Health Organization; 2017.
3. WHO-supported collaborative research projects in India: the facts. WHO Chron. 1976;30(4):131-9.
4. McNaughton D, Duong TT. Designing a community engagement framework for a new dengue control method: a case study from central Vietnam. PLoS Negl Trop Dis. 2014;8(5):e2794.
5. Ramsey JM, Bond JG, Macotela ME, et al. A regulatory structure for working with genetically modified mosquitoes: lessons from Mexico. PLoS Negl Trop Dis. 2014;8(3):e2623.
6. Kolopack PA, Lavery JV. Informed consent in field trials of gene-drive mosquitoes. Gates Open Res. 2017;1:14.
7. James S, Collins FH, Welkhoff PA, et al. Pathway to deployment of gene drive mosquitoes as a potential biocontrol tool for elimination of malaria in sub-Saharan Africa: recommendations of a Scientific Working Group. Am J Trop Med Hyg. 2018;98(Suppl 6):1-49.
8. Bartumeus F, Oltra A, Palmer JR. Citizen science: a gateway for innovation in disease-carrying mosquito management? Trends Parasitol. 2018;34(9):727-9.
9. Institute for Science, Innovation and Society (University of Oxford) and Department of Global Health and Social Medicine (King's College London). Community participation in the control of disease vectors: old questions, new approaches. [online] Available from: https://insis.web.ox.ac.uk/event/community-participation-control-disease-vectors-old-questions-new-approaches. [Last accessed on November, 2019].
10. Curtis CF. Appropriate technology in vector control. Boca Raton, Florida: CRC Press; 1990.
11. Vaughan M. A research enclave in 1940s Nigeria: The Rockefeller Foundation Yellow Fever Research Institute at Yaba, Lagos, 1943–49. Bull Hist Med. 2018;92(1):172-205.
12. Gubler DJ, Clark GG. Community involvement in the control of Aedes aegypti. Acta Trop. 1996;61(2):169-79.
13. Park K. Measurement of malaria. Park's Textbook of Preventive and Social Medicine, 23th edition. Jabalpur, India: Banarsidas Bhanot Publishers; 2013. pp. 261-3.

Heat-related Illness in Tropics

Niranjan Mohanty, Jyoti Ranjan Behera

■ INTRODUCTION

As the Earth is getting warmer, the incidence of heat-related illness (HRI) and injury is on the rise. Among those suffering from HRI, children comprise almost half (47.6%) as per US data.[1] In the pediatric population, the most common form of HRI occurs in adolescent athletes and in children at risk, exposed to excessively warm environment.

Heat-related illnesses in children constitute a wide spectrum of presentations ranging from minor conditions such as heat rash and heat cramp to fatal thermoregulatory emergencies like heatstroke. Physiological differences in children in comparison to adults make them particularly vulnerable to HRI. Appropriate precautionary measures can prevent pediatric HRI, and early diagnosis and management of heatstroke in children can drastically reduce life-threatening complications related to multi-organ dysfunction. Management of heatstroke rests primarily on prompt initiation of rapid cooling measures, evaluation and appropriate treatment for organ dysfunction.

Even though significant number of deaths occur due to HRI in India, the exact data is not available. Therefore, the magnitude of morbidity and mortality is not known. Considering the global climatic changes, India is likely to experience increase in number, intensity, and duration of heat waves over due course of time which may result in rise of HRI in future. In view of morbidity and mortality due to HRI are largely preventable, the public information system and the healthcare facilities should be activated for early reporting, timely diagnosis, and appropriate treatment which are expected to substantially reduce HRI-related deaths.

■ PROBLEM STATEMENT

As per reports from US, approximately 668 HRI deaths occurred annually among people of all ages from 2006 to 2010. Of these, 7% were children below 4 years out of which 2.5% were infants and 4.5% were between 1 year and 4 years. These figures have remained relatively constant over the last decade.[2] Adolescents are particularly at risk for HRI and in them heatstroke is the third leading cause of death after trauma and cardiac causes. Heatstroke has a mortality rate ranging from 6.4% to 33% spreading over all ages.[3] Annual report of Indian Meteorological Department (IMD) on "Disastrous Events" documented 1,539 deaths in 2003 from all over India.[4] Death due to heatstroke rose to more than 2,500 in 2015—five times greater than 2001. Odisha, Telangana, Andhra Pradesh, Punjab, Uttar Pradesh, and West Bengal were most affected by heatstroke.[5]

■ PATHOPHYSIOLOGY

Human body temperature is maintained within a range of 36.5–37.5°C chiefly by thermoregulatory center situated in anterior hypothalamus. As the core temperature increases due to either metabolic derangement or environmental changes, the hypothalamus primarily acts on the autonomic nervous system to engage in mechanisms of heat dissipation.[6] Evaporation of sweat is believed to be the mechanism of heat dissipation in humans. However, it becomes less effective when humidity rises above 75%.[7]

There is a complex interaction between the higher environmental temperature and the human body system. Heat stress is the burden or load of heat that must be dissipated if the body is to remain in thermal equilibrium. The factors which influence heat stress are metabolic rate, air temperature, humidity, air movement, and radiant temperature. The amount of heat gained by the body must be equaled by the amount of heat lost from it. In this context, many heat stress indices have been devised out of which the "heat index" is important where the air temperature and relative humidity are considered to predict different HRI including heat exhaustion and heatstroke.[8]

As the core body temperature increases, vasodilation leads to increased heart rate, stroke volume and cardiac output. Warmer blood moves peripherally to the skin, allowing for sweat production and evaporation. As blood circulation shifts from the center to the periphery, visceral perfusion is compromised making kidneys and gut mostly affected. If exposure to heat is excessive or prolonged, the body fails to adapt resulting in HRI.

The critical thermal maximum (CTM) is the core body temperature and duration of heat exposure that is lethal to an animal. In humans, the CTM is estimated to be 106.9–107.6°F (41.6–42°C) for 1–8 hours. Prolonged hyperthermia exceeding the CTM can lead to a dangerous cascade of ischemia, end organ damage, multi-organ failure, and potentially death.

As the body attempts to cool, high demand on the heart can lead to high-output cardiac failure and cardiogenic shock. Hypotension can occur due to multiple factors like vasodilation (as part of the thermoregulatory process) and hypovolemia (secondary to profuse sweating and insensible losses). In extreme cases, hypovolemia can also be due to cardiogenic shock. Prolonged hypotension will ultimately lead to poor perfusion, ischemic injury, and end-organ damage. In addition, the vascular endothelium is sensitive to heat and excessive exposure may result in disseminated intravascular coagulation (DIC). Cerebral and gut edema develop due to altered vascular and mucosal permeability.

At cellular level, the resulting stress from hyperthermia can directly injure cells, leading to cytokine storm and endothelial injury. Heat can cause proteins to denature and cells to undergo apoptosis.

PHYSIOLOGICAL DIFFERENCE OF THERMOREGULATION IN CHILDREN

Thermoregulation in children is unique in contrast to adults both in terms of physiological and developmental parameters as follows:

- Immaturity of hypothalamus in infancy compromises their ability to use adaptive mechanisms to dissipate heat.[9]
- Blunted sweating capacity of infant and young children makes evaporative cooling less effective.[10]
- Endogenous heat generation per body weight in children is more than adults by virtue of their higher basal metabolic rate.
- Low blood volume than adults restricts the ability to transfer warm blood to the periphery to decrease the core temperature.[11]

- Higher surface area-to-body mass ratio in children leads to increased heat absorption.
- Children lack developmental capabilities to change their behavior in response to overheating (e.g. to drink water, remove seat belts or clothing, and change the place).

ETIOLOGY AND RISK FACTORS

Several risk factors predispose children to HRIs.

- *Heat wave condition*: It is defined as any increase in temperature above normal. An increase of 5–6°C is moderate and >7°C or atmospheric temperature > 45°C for more than 2 days is severe heat wave, potentially leading to heatstroke.[12]
- *Physical:* Dehydration, being unacclimatized, unusual exertion, inappropriate clothing, sleep deprivation, sunburn, sweat gland dysfunction, and obesity.
- *Infants who are overdressed or left in a hot car* are particularly at risk for HRIs.[13]
- *Pregnant women* are more susceptible to heatstroke and exhaustion because fluid volume depletion and electrolyte imbalance also get affected. Raised maternal core body temperature affect development of fetus (neural tube defects).
- Children with chronic medical conditions are less likely to sense and respond to changes in temperature. Hence, conditions such as sickle cell disease and trait, cystic fibrosis and diabetes (mellitus and insipidus), dermatological conditions with decreased sweating, epilepsy, febrile illness, gastroenteritis, spinal injuries and thyrotoxicosis predispose to higher incidence of HRI.
- *Medications*: Medications may worsen the impact of extreme heat. Important examples are beta-blockers, diuretics, alcohol, anticholinergic, alpha-adrenergic, tricyclic antidepressants, selective serotonin reuptake inhibitors (SSRIs), phenothiazines, etc.[14]
- *Outdoor workers*: Child laborers and migrants engaged in outdoor works in hot humid climate are at risk of getting dehydrated and more likely to get HRI.
- *People who exert in hot environment*: Athletes or people who exercise vigorously in hot environment.

CLASSIFICATION OF HEAT-RELATED ILLNESSES

The effects of exposure to heat can be directly heat related (HRI) or can contribute to worsening of respiratory, cardiovascular diseases, electrolyte disorders, and kidney problems. HRI occurs as a continuum from mild illnesses to fatalities. Different types of HRI are listed below:

- *Minor HRI*:
  - Heat rash
  - Heat edema
  - Heat tetany
  - Heat cramp
  - Heat syncope.
- *Major HRI*:
  - Heat exhaustion
  - Heatstroke.

Minor Heat-related Illnesses

Miliaria Rubra

Miliaria rubra, also known as heat rash or prickly heat is a common, benign manifestation of heat exposure in infants and young children. A combination of heat exposure and blocked sweat glands leads to a pruritic, erythematous rash with papules and pustules. This is often seen in areas of friction from skin rubbing against skin or clothing.[15] It is usually self-limiting. Treatment is supportive and includes wearing light, loose garments and avoiding overheating.

Heat Edema

A mild form of HRI manifested as swelling of the feet, hands, and other dependent areas. It occurs due to vasodilatation as the body attempts to shunt warm blood to the periphery.[16] This is more common in adults than in children. The body temperature of the individual is normal and there is no underlying systemic cause like cardiac or renal disease. Treatment is supportive like elevation of the affected limbs, compressive stockings, and moving to a cooler environment.

Heat Cramp

It is a state of involuntary contractions of skeletal muscle that occur during or after exercise. The term heat cramp is a misnomer because the heat does not directly trigger cramping, and high-intensity exercise in cold environments can also cause such cramps. A more appropriate term is exercise-associated muscle cramp. The spasm is painful and usually affects the muscle groups actively involved in exercise. It typically occurs in dehydrated and poorly acclimatized athletes. Risk factors include previous occurrence of muscle cramp or injury to the muscle, tendon or ligament, heavy sweating, poor salt intake before, or during exercise. Treatment is supportive including rest, hydration, and static stretching.

Heat Syncope

It is mostly related to vasodilatation and venous pooling. It is an orthostatic event resulting in brief loss of consciousness and is found in an individual standing for a prolonged period or changing positions rapidly in warm environment. Heat exposure is not the causative factor but contributes to the event. Like heat edema, body temperature is found to be normal.[16] Treatment is also similar. Patient should be moved to a cooler environment and remain supine until light-headedness has resolved and vital signs have normalized. Enough oral and intravenous (IV) fluids to be supplemented for hydration.

Heat Stress

It is a mild form of HRI with perceived discomfort and physical strain that result from exposure to heat or a warm environment. Symptoms are typically mild, and core temperature remains within the normal range. It is managed by adequate hydration and removing the individual to a cooler environment.

Major Heat-related Illnesses

Heat Exhaustion (Heat Injury)

Heat exhaustion occurs in patients with a known heat exposure and is characterized by raised body temperature up to 104°F. Heat exhaustion is manifested by nonspecific symptoms such as sweating, nausea, vomiting, weakness, fatigue, headache and mild confusion. Dehydration often plays vital role in heat exhaustion. Heat exhaustion should be carefully differentiated from heatstroke as the treatment modalities differ significantly. In contrast to heatstroke, sensorium usually remains normal or there may be transient mild confusion in heat exhaustion.[17]

Prehospital treatment: Though heat exhaustion is usually the forerunner of heatstroke, it is not true in all cases. Sepsis being the most common differential diagnosis should be ruled out by relevant investigations. Children with symptoms of heat exhaustion should stop exercising immediately and should be moved to a cooler environment. Excess clothing should be removed and the patient should be given chilled salt-containing liquids. Most patients with mild heat exhaustion respond to these measures and do not require further care.

Hospital management: Patients not responding to prehospital measures or initially presenting with dehydration or altered mental status, warrant hospitalization and further evaluation. Recording of rectal temperature and complete neurological examination should be done on admission.[17] In addition to providing a cool ambient environment, the following measures should be ensured:

- Measurement of rectal temperature every 15–30 minutes till improvement
- Bolus of normal saline (20 mL/kg; maximum initial infusion 1 L)
- Measurement of serum electrolytes and treatment focus on sodium abnormalities.

All patients recovering from heat exhaustation are carefully monitored for any deterioration.

Heatstroke

Heatstroke occurs in patients with high environmental heat exposure and is defined as a core body temperature $\geq$40–40.5°C (104–105°F) accompanied by central nervous system (CNS) dysfunction.[16] This is due to failure of the body's capacity to maintain thermoregulatory homeostasis. Heatstroke is further classified as follows:

- *Classic (nonexertional) heatstroke*: Classic heatstroke results from environmental exposure to heat and is more common in younger children who are unable to escape from hot environment or with underlying chronic medical conditions impairing thermoregulation.
- *Exertional heatstroke*: Exertional heatstroke generally occurs in young otherwise healthy individuals who engage in heavy exercise during periods of high environmental temperature and humidity. Typical patients are athletes.

Clinical features: Body temperature > 104°F along with CNS manifestations is the hallmark of heatstroke. CNS symptoms vary from subtle deceptive symptoms to significant neuromorbidity. There are overlapping features between heat exhaustion and heatstroke **(Table 1)**. Whenever distinction between heat exhaustion and heatstroke is unclear, children with elevated body temperature and CNS abnormalities should be treated as heatstroke, considering the significant morbidity and mortality associated with this condition.

Children commonly present with altered mentation or inappropriate behavior to more severe neurologic symptoms such as seizure, delirium, hallucination, ataxia, dysarthria or coma. Typical finding on general examination includes tachycardia and tachypnea. In terms of skin findings, patients with classic or nonexertional heatstroke will have hot, dry skin secondary to prolonged thermoregulatory dysfunction. In contrast, patients with exertional heatstroke may have cool, clammy skin or may be warm and diaphoretic if they were engaged in exercise or strenuous activity prior to presentation. Vomiting and

Table 1: Comparative clinical features of heatstroke and heat exhaustion.

	Heatstroke	Heat exhaustion
CNS status	Abnormal mental status (e.g. obtunded, coma, delirium, hallucinations, seizures, ataxia, and slurred speech)	Normal mental status, dizziness, or mild confusion that rapidly normalizes within 30 minutes of treatment
Airway and breathing	May be compromised due to altered mental status, tachypneic	Clear airway, may be tachypneic
Circulation	Tachycardia with hypotension, moderate to severe dehydration	Tachycardia with normal blood pressure, mild-to-moderate dehydration
Skin findings	Dry skin (classic heatstroke) or sweating (exertional heatstroke)	Sweating
Other clinical features	• Vomiting • Diarrhea • Clinical and laboratory findings of DIC, rhabdomyolysis, acute renal failure, cardiogenic shock and liver failure	• Nausea • Vomiting • Headache • Fatigue and weakness • Hyponatremia or hypernatremia

(CNS: central nervous system; DIC: disseminated intravascular coagulation)

diarrhea are also common due to ischemic effect of heat on gastrointestinal mucosa. Heat-induced tissue damage resulting in systemic inflammatory response leads to multiorgan dysfunction.[18] Since the pediatric brain is particularly sensitive to extremes of temperature, cerebral edema, and herniation are potential complications of heatstroke.[19] Damage to myocardial tissue coupled with dehydration and systemic vasodilation results in hypotension and poor systemic perfusion.[20] Muscle breakdown causes rhabdomyolysis that can lead to kidney failure and hepatic injury. Degradation of clotting factors disrupts the clotting system and can cause DIC.[21] Damage to the mucosal lining of the intestine may result in ischemia and massive hematochezia.[22]

History: Key questions to be asked by the treating physician in the emergency room should include:

- Has the patient been involved in exertional activities in a hot or humid environment?
- Is the patient new to the physical activity?
- Is the patient taking any type of stimulant medication, either prescribed or recreational?
- How long has the patient been exposed to heat?

Physical examination: The clinician should focus on vital signs to urgently address any abnormality. The rectal or esophageal temperature should ideally be recorded to estimate the core temperature as recording of temperatures elsewhere could be inaccurate to predict core temperature. Poor prognosis is likely if the patient's core temperature is >42°C (107.6°F). Either profuse sweating or lack of sweating can be the presenting symptom of heatstroke. Neurologic examination and Glasgow Coma Scale (GCS) scoring shall help the emergency clinician to address the severity of heatstroke and to decide for immediate intervention and resuscitation. Cardiovascular assessment should aim at detecting tachycardia and/or dysrhythmias along with adequacy of perfusion. Abnormal pattern of respiration can also be a manifestation of the heatstroke.

Laboratory evaluation: The primary diagnosis of heatstroke is chiefly based on clinical symptoms and does not require any laboratory investigations. Since heatstroke often leads to various fatal complications, the specific laboratory investigations as warranted may be asked for as follows:

- Random blood glucose to identify hypoglycemia[23]
- Arterial blood gas to evaluate the presence and severity of metabolic acidosis (especially in patients with exertional heatstroke) and/or respiratory alkalosis[24]
- Complete blood count, prothrombin time and international normalized ratio, partial thromboplastin time to detect anemia and DIC.[25]
- Serum electrolytes to check for sodium and potassium levels[23]
- Liver enzymes to assess for liver injury
- Renal function tests to identify prerenal azotemia or renal failure resulting from myoglobinuria
- Creatine phosphokinase, ionized calcium and phosphate to detect hypocalcemia and hyperphosphatemia in presence of rhabdomyolysis
- Urinalysis to diagnose myoglobinuria
- Toxicologic screening as side effects of prescribed medications or drug abuse
- Chest radiograph to detect pulmonary edema
- Electrocardiogram for electrolyte abnormalities
- *Computed tomography* scan of brain in a child having persistently altered mental status despite cooling or showing signs suggestive of cerebral edema or intracranial hemorrhage.

Differential diagnosis: As the chief manifestation of heatstroke is hyperthermia with significant neurological features in presence of very hot environment, the treating physician should make all efforts to differentiate heatstroke from any other disease having similar manifestations and if heatstroke is associated with any potential pre-existing conditions like chronic medical disease or use of offending drugs.

- *Sepsis:* In association with meningitis, it can cause high fever and abnormal mental status. But usually the height of the fever does not exceed 41°C (105.8°F) and a focus for infection (e.g. pneumonia, cellulitis, and meningitis) or an infectious prodrome (e.g. upper respiratory infection and gastrointestinal complaints) is frequently present.
- *Central nervous system conditions:* CNS pathology involving hypothalamus has to be differentiated from heatstroke.[26] Common etiologies being CNS infection, cerebrovascular accident, hemorrhage, traumatic brain injury, and congenital anomalies of brain. In all of these conditions, the CNS abnormality precedes temperature elevation.
- *Status epilepticus:* The most common cause of status epilepticus in young children is prolonged febrile seizures or underlying epilepsy, which can result in hyperthermia simulating heatstroke.
- *Toxic overdose:* Drugs and toxic overdose can cause seizures and hyperthermia. Overdose of cocaine, amphetamine, salicylates and anticholinergic agents is important consideration in the hyperthermic child. Even therapeutic levels of amphetamines and anticholinergic agents may impair thermoregulation.
- *Hemorrhagic shock and encephalopathy syndrome:* This rare condition, primarily seen in previously healthy infant, is associated with hyperpyrexia, altered mental status, shock, disseminated intravascular coagulopathy, diarrhea, renal insufficiency, and liver failure.[27] Although the etiology is unknown, this syndrome is very similar to heatstroke and is treated with supportive care and rapid cooling.
- *Neuroleptic malignant syndrome:* This is an idiosyncratic reaction to antipsychotic agents characterized by hyperthermia with "lead pipe" muscle rigidity, altered mental status, choreoathetosis, tremors, and evidence of autonomic dysfunction. The history of antipsychotic drug exposure is a key component of the diagnosis.

Prehospital management: The patient is moved to a cooler place. Local emergency medical service to be informed urgently. Till the ambulance arrives, patient's clothing to be removed and the body is drenched with cool water. Ice packs are placed on armpits and groin area. Cold fluid is offered to drink in conscious patients. Airway, breathing, and pulse are monitored periodically. The patient is transferred to the nearest healthcare facility for emergency care. While transferring, the above cooling measures need to be continued.

Lowering of core body temperature (cooling): Cooling is the most vital part of management of heatstroke. Cooling causes redistribution of blood flow from periphery to the core and decreases hypermetabolic state. Thus, it should be started as early as heatstroke is suspected since morbidity and mortality correlates directly to duration of hyperthermia.[28] The importance of cooling in the first golden hour should be emphasized in all possible ways for a better prognosis.

The target of cooling is to reduce the temperature by at least 0.2°C/minute to approximately 39°C. Decrease in core temperature as measured by rectal probe lags behind actual core temperature at the hypothalamus.[29] Hence, core temperature continuously monitored by a flexible indwelling thermistor rectally or an esophageal probe. The recommended threshold to stop cooling varies in the literature and ranges from 101.5 to 102°F (38.6–38.9°C).[30]

Cooling can be achieved by two types of method: (1) Immersion and (2) evaporative cooling.

- *Immersion cooling*: It is mostly used in older children and athletes. Immersion in an ice bath or cooling blankets used in conjunction with ice packs to the axilla, groin, neck, and head may be the most rapid methods of cooling. Ice-water immersion by virtue of its high thermal conductivity has the advantage of rapidly reducing core body temperature to less than 39°C in approximately 20–40 minutes. The disadvantages of ice-water immersion include discomfort to conscious patients and subcutaneous vasoconstriction. Recent guidelines recommend ice-water immersion as the superior method for rapidly lowering core body temperature below the critical level for those with exertional heatstroke.

- *Evaporative cooling*: It is preferred in smaller children and infants. The patient's skin is exposed to warm air at 40°C (104°F) passing over the body while a mist of cool water at 15°C (59°F) speeds heat dissipation. Cooling rates with this technique have been measured at 0.31°C/minute (0.5°F/minute). This type of evaporative and convective cooling is effective for classic heatstroke. Other methods useful for all children may include application of cold, wet towels, continuously resoaked, and reapplied or placing the patient under a cold shower. Ice packs to the axilla or groin have is only marginally effective and should be used only when alternatives are unavailable.

Hospital-based management: The main aim of hospital management should include: (1) Urgent and appropriate clinical assessment to rule out other differential diagnosis, (2) initiation of life saving measures, and (3) detection of complications and further management.

Airway and breathing: Children with heatstroke frequently require basic or advanced airway management to maintain oxygenation and ventilation because of CNS involvement.

Circulation: All patients with heatstroke need circulatory access, ideally with two large-bore IV catheters or a central venous catheter. Fluid resuscitation depends on the type of heatstroke and should replenish intravascular volume while avoiding fluid overload. Children with classic (nonexertional) heatstroke tend to be only mild to moderate hypovolemic, while those with exertional heatstroke may have higher degree of hypovolemia. The resuscitation fluid requirement can be 20–40 mL/kg of isotonic crystalloid in classic heatstroke, in contrast to a higher requirement of 60 mL/kg or more in exertional type. Patients with shock, unresponsive or minimally responsive to fluid resuscitation should undergo central venous pressure monitoring and may require vasopressor therapy.

Disability: Altered mental status usually resolves with oxygenation, adequate tissue perfusion, and normothermia. Seizures, if any can be managed with benzodiazepines.

Rapid cooling: The methods of cooling, as enumerated above need to be continued and properly monitored to achieve desired core temperature.

Medications: There are no specific medications indicated in the treatment of heatstroke. Antipyretics are not useful in lowering core temperature as HRI may exacerbate hepatic, gastrointestinal, clotting and renal dysfunction. Similarly, dantrolene, which is used to treat malignant hyperthermia, has no role in the management of heatstroke. Benzodiazepines and anticonvulsants should be used to control shivering and seizures. In refractory seizures, thiopentone infusion 1% and even nondepolarizing muscle relaxants may be required along with intubation and positive pressure ventilation.

Treatment of end-organ dysfunction: The child with heatstroke always remains at high risk for multi-organ failure, electrolyte abnormalities, and disorders of coagulation. The clinician should carefully evaluate for the following abnormalities and treat as warranted: (1) Rhabdomyolysis with hyperkalemia, hypocalcemia, and hyperphosphatemia, (2) DIC, (3) acute kidney injury, (4) hyponatremic dehydration, (5) cardiogenic shock with low systemic vascular resistance, (6) cardiogenic and noncardiogenic pulmonary edema, (7) liver failure, and (8) cerebral edema.

Prognosis: Severity of heatstroke is related to the degree and duration of hyperthermia. Thus, the outcome is directly related to quick initiation and maintenance of cooling. Poor prognostic signs include hemoptysis, hematuria, conjunctival hemorrhage, and gastrointestinal (GI) bleeds. Patients with higher initial temperatures, hypotension or low GCS scores (<12) are more likely to die and death is usually from cardiovascular collapse. Patients with mild heatstroke usually experience complete recovery with normal neurologic function. But severe heatstroke (>42°C) patients may end in fatality (10%) or survive with permanent neurologic sequelae. The common neurologic morbidities consist of spasticity, ataxia, dysarthria, poor coordination, impaired memory and behavioral changes.[30]

PREVENTION OF HEAT-RELATED ILLNESS

As HRI is largely avoidable, appropriate preventive strategies are crucial in protecting susceptible children. Family counseling for awareness of weather changes, dangers of heat exposure, necessary clothing, and coverage for infants and children are of paramount importance. The preventive steps include:

- *Plenty of fluid intake*: Drink water to the point where your urine is light yellow color. Rehydration is best with water and not with carbonated drinks. Avoid alcohol and caffeinated drinks during exercise as it increases the risk of hyperthermia.
- Avoiding exercising/strenuous outdoor activities in the heat.
- *Acclimatization*: Athletes should acclimatize to warm weather and increase activity over 1–2 weeks. The intensity and duration of physical activity should increase gradually during this period.[31] During acclimatization the body becomes more efficient in work production as well as heat dissipation through various mechanisms, including changes in sweat rate, volume, and composition.
- *Light clothing*: To help evaporation of sweat, wear lightweight, light-colored, loose, porous clothes and a wide-brimmed hat/umbrella.
- *Keep cool indoors*: Keep your home cool with curtains, shutters, or awnings on the sunny sides and leave windows open at night.
- *Schedule outdoor activities carefully:* Try to restrict your outdoor activities to cooler parts of the day.
- *Do not leave children alone in parked cars*: Look before you lock.[32]

- *Precooling* either by cold water immersion and cold drinks or the application of cooling garments for those who are going to exercise in hot environments. It has been shown to be effective for lowering pre-exercise core temperature, increasing heat storage capacity and improving exercise performance in the heat.

CONCLUSION

- The essential criteria to diagnose heatstroke are exposure to hot climate with a core body temperature ≥40–40.5°C accompanied by CNS dysfunction.
- The diagnosis of heatstroke is mostly clinical. It should be carefully differentiated from other causes in each patient.
- Whenever the distinction between heat exhaustion and heatstroke is unclear, children with elevated body temperature and CNS abnormalities should be treated as victims of heatstroke.
- Rectal temperature is the most commonly obtained core temperature measurement, although esophageal or bladder probe temperatures are alternatives.
- Prehospital cooling measures should be initiated prior to/or simultaneously with activation of emergency medical services.
- The clinician should anticipate and aggressively manage dehydration, rhabdomyolysis, DIC, high-output cardiac insufficiency, renal failure, and hepatic failure.
- Children who have recovered from heatstroke are at greater risk for repeated HRI. They should be counseled properly to avoid heat exposure.

REFERENCES

1. Nelson NG, Collins CL, Comstock RD, et al. Exertional heat-related injuries treated in emergency departments in the U.S., 1997-2006. Am J Prev Med. 2011;40(1):54-60.
2. Berko J, Ingram DD, Saha S, et al. Deaths attributed to heat, cold, and other weather events in the United States, 2006-2010. National health statistics reports; no 76. Hyattsville, MD: National Center for Health Statistics; 2014.
3. Zeller L, Novack V, Barski L, et al. Exertional heatstroke: clinical characteristics, diagnostic and therapeutic considerations. Eur J Intern Med. 2011;22(3):296-9.
4. Bal NC, Pant M, Maurya SK, et al. Increased incidence of heatstroke in India: Is there a genetic predisposition? GERF Bull Biosci. 2012;3(1):7-17.
5. Paul S, Bhatia V. Heat stroke—Emerging as one of the biggest natural calamity in India. Int J Med Res Prof. 2016;2:15 20.
6. Romanovsky AA. Thermoregulation: some concepts have changed. Functional architecture of the thermoregulatory system. Am J Physiol Regul Integr Comp Physiol. 2007;292(1): R37-46.
7. Smith CJ, Johnson, JM. Responses to hyperthermia. Optimizing heat dissipation by convection and evaporation: Neural control

of skin blood flow and sweating in humans. Auton Neurosci. 2016;196:25-36.

8. Park K. Park's textbook of preventive and social medicine, 23rd edition. Jabalpur: Banarsidas Bhanot; 2015. pp. 745-50.

9. Aggarwal Y, Karan BM, Das BN, et al. Prediction of heat-illness symptoms with the prediction of human vascular response in hot environment under resting condition. J Med Syst. 2008;32(2):167-76.

10. Charkoudian N. Human hermoregulation from the autonomic perspective. Auton Neurosci. 2016;196:1-2.

11. Falk B, Dotan R. Children's thermoregulation during exercise in the heat: a revisit. Appl Physiol Nutr Metab. 2008;33(2):420-7.

12. Jain Y, Srivastan R, Kollannur A, et al. Heatstroke: Causes, consequences and clinical guidelines. Natl Med J India. 2018;31(4);224-7.

13. Booth JN 3rd, Davis GG, Waterbor J, et al. Hyperthermia deaths among children in parked vehicles: an analysis of 231 fatalities in the United States, 1999-2007. Forensic Sci Med Pathol. 2010;6(2):99-105.

14. Levine M, LoVecchio F, Ruha AM, et al. Influence of drug use on morbidity and mortality in heatstroke. J Med Toxicol. 2012;8(3):252-7.

15. O'Connor NR, McLaughlin MR, Ham P. Newborn skin: Part I. Common rashes. Am Fam Physician. 2008;77(1):47-52.

16. Howe AS, Boden BP. Heat-related illness in athletes. Am J Sports Med. 2007;35(8):1384-95.

17. Glazer JL. Management of heatstroke and heat exhaustion. Am Fam Physician. 2005;71(11):2133-40.

18. Leon LR, Helwig BG. Heat stroke: role of the systemic inflammatory response. J Appl Physiol. 2010;109(6):1980-8.

19. Sharma HS. Methods to produce hyperthermia-induced brain dysfunction. Prog Brain. Res. 2007;162:173-99.

20. Wilson TE, Crandall CG. Effect of thermal stress on cardiac function. Exerc Sport Sci Rev. 2011;39(1):12-7.

21. Chapin JC, Hajjar KA. Fibrinolysis and the control of blood coagulation. Blood Rev. 2015;29(1):17-24.

22. Lambert GP. Intestinal barrier dysfunction, endotoxemia, and gastrointestinal symptoms: the 'canary in the coal mine' during exercise-heat stress? Med Sport Sci. 2008;53:61-73.

23. Bouchama A, Dehbi M, Chaves-Carballo E. Cooling and hemodynamic management in heatstroke: practical recommendations. Crit Care. 2007;11(3):R54.

24. Bouchama A, De Vol EB. Acid-base alterations in heatstroke. Intensive Care Med. 2001;27(4):680-5.

25. Mustafa KY, Omer O, Khogali M, et al. Blood coagulation and fibrinolysis in heat stroke. Br J Haematol. 1985;61(3): 517-23.

26. Thompson HJ, Pinto-Martin J, Bullock MR. Neurogenic fever after traumatic brain injury: an epidemiological study. J Neurol Neurosurg Psychiatry. 2003;74(5):614-9.

27. Gefen R, Eshel G, Abu-Kishk I, et al. Hemorrhagic shock and encephalopathy syndrome: clinical course and neurological outcome. J Child Neurol. 2008;23:589-92.

28. Vicario SJ, Okabajue R, Haltom T. Rapid cooling in classic heatstroke: effect on mortality rates. Am J Emerg Med. 1986; 4(5): 394-8.

29. Jardine DS. Heat illness and heat stroke. Pediatr Rev. 2007;28(7): 249-58.

30. Mangus CW, Canares TL. Heat-related illness in children in an era of extreme temperatures. Pediatr Rev. 2019;40(3): 97-107.

31. Casa DJ, DeMartini JK, Bergeron MF, et al. National Athletic Trainers's Association Position Statement: Exertional heat illnesses. J Athl Train. 2015;50(9):986-1000.

32. Guard A, Gallagher SS. Heat related deaths to young children in parked cars: an analysis of 171 fatalities in the United States, 1995-2002. Inj Prev. 2005;11:33-7.

Environmental Pollution and Child Health

Piyali Bhattacharya

INTRODUCTION

Environmental pollution has become a public health crisis globally. The number of people who die prematurely every year due to increasing air pollution levels is steadily rising. The burden of disease, attributable to particulate matter (PM) in air, is highest in low- and middle-income countries (LMICs). Air-polluting agents such as black carbon and ozone are also responsible for atmospheric warming in addition to environmental pollution. Interventions aimed at reducing their emission would be beneficial not only for child health but also for ushering in climatic changes for the better. Pollutant exposure through ingestion, inhalation, or in utero may lead to health hazards in children that leave footprints for a lifetime. Children are especially vulnerable to air pollution due to the following causes:

- Their lungs, brains, and other vital organs are still maturing and therefore have greater vulnerability to inflammation and damage.
- Compared to adults, children breathe faster thereby inhaling more pollutants.
- Kids spend much time playing outside in the polluted atmosphere.
- Newborn and infants mostly spend time indoor and become more susceptible to household air pollution (HAP).
- Younger children stay near their mothers or in their mother's lap while cooking and are thereby exposed to pollutant fuel and smoke.
- Latent disease gets a longer time to affect health where children are concerned.
- Preconception exposure of a mother to pollutants will also carry a latent risk for the unborn fetus.

Ambient air pollution (AAP) and HAP are attributable to a large proportion of childhood morbidity and mortality caused by environmental pollution. Scientific knowledge regarding the adverse effects of exposure to air pollution on child health requires urgent attention due to its long term and damaging effect and the greater vulnerability of children.

National Air Quality Monitoring Programme (NAMP) instituted by The Central Pollution Control Board comprises 621 monitoring stations in 262 cities/towns in 29 states and 5 union territories of India. Under the program, three air pollutants, namely, sulfur dioxide (SO_2), nitrogen dioxide (NO_2), and particulate matter (PM10) have been identified for regular monitoring. Available data till date show that the PM10 levels have been hazardous all throughout the year for 2015–2016 in most cities of India.

EPIDEMIOLOGY

Exposure to fine particles in the environment and household results in approximately 7 million premature deaths each year.[1,2] A regional and global research program (Global Burden of Disease), including researchers ($n = 500$) from 300 institutions and 50 countries, estimated that 11.98 lakh (3,283/day) Indians died of outdoor air pollution in 2015. World Bank estimates that approximately 3% of India's GDP (Gross Domestic Product) is lost due to air pollution.

Childhood Burden

93% of all children live in conditions with air pollution levels exceeding the World Health Organization (WHO) guidelines globally. One in every four deaths of children <5 years is directly or indirectly related to environmental risks:[3]

- In children less than 5 years, AAP and HAP resulted in 543,000 deaths while 52,000 deaths were reported in the ages between 5 years and 15 years in 2016.[1]

- Combined childhood death due to AAP and HAP accounts for 9% of the total deaths worldwide.
- HAP from cooking alone with AAP is responsible for >50% of acute lower respiratory infections (ALRI) in children <5 years in LMICs.

Ambient Air Pollution

An estimated 286,000 deaths of children under 15 years due to AAP exposure has been reported in 2016.

Sources of Ambient Air Pollution

Urban: Fossil fuel combustion for cooking, transport, energy production, heating, and waste incineration.
Rural: Kerosene burning, biomass, and coal used in cooking, heating, and lighting; waste incineration in agriculture; and some agroforestry activity.

The fossil fuel processes produce complex mixtures which include pollutants such as carbon monoxide (CO), nitrogen oxide (NO), sulfur dioxide (SO_2), lead, mercury, arsenic, PM, and aromatic hydrocarbons (HC). In fact, PM which is used broadly as an indicator of air pollution has more adverse effects than other air pollutants.

Adulteration of diesel and gasoline with low-priced fuel is common in Asian countries such as India. Adulterated fuel increases the tailpipe emissions of CO, HCs, oxides of nitrogen and PM, of which polyaromatic hydrocarbons (PAHs) and benzene and are known carcinogens. The high sulfur level of kerosene is also one of the major issues.

As per statistics, most Indian cities violate world air quality PM10 targets. As of 2017, India remains the third largest emitter of CO_2 at 6.82% after China (27.21%) and United States (14.58%). Transport, coal, oil-fired or natural gas-fired thermal power plants, and engines are significant sources of greenhouse gas emission in India.

Table 1: Top seven cities in India with high particulate matter (PM) 2.5 in 2018.

City	PM 2.5 levels
Delhi, Gurugram	135.8
Ghaziabad	135.2
Faridabad	129.1
Bhiwadi	128.4
Noida	123.6
Patna	119.7
Lucknow	115.7

Source: Greenpeace and AirVisual.

Emphasis on cleaner transport and industrial technologies, clean cooking and heating fuels, urban planning and energy-efficient housing, low power generation, and better municipal waste management are the ultimate solutions to this disastrous situation.

Household Air Pollution

Household air pollution is an important source of AAP and produced due to incomplete combustion of fuels used for cooking, heating, and lighting. Traditional fuel such as fuel wood, crop residue, and dung cakes are still dominating the domestic energy use in rural India. Biomass cakes and wood are being used for daily cooking and meeting day-to-day heating needs. It is evident that smoke from burning coal, biomass, and kerosene for the purpose of cooking, lighting, and heating are the primary contributors to HAP. According to WHO, use of "chullahs" kills 300,000–400,000 people in India as they cause indoor air pollution and CO poisoning.

Tobacco smoke from *bidi*, cigarette, and hookah is a significant source of indoor air pollution as well. Other indoor pollutants are volatile organic compounds from household supplies, pesticides, mosquito repellents and spray, mercury (e.g. from broken thermometers), radon, etc.

In rural houses, some compounding factors such as poor ventilation and emission of fine PM from stoves further enhance air pollution to 100 times greater than the recommended safe levels. Poverty correlates with exposure to air pollution as poor people often resort to use of polluting sources for their basic energy needs.

WHO estimates that in LMICs, 3 billion people or roughly 41% of the global population use cooking sources that are pollutants. Of an estimated 3.8 million premature deaths due to HAP in 2016 (6.7% of global mortality), 403,000 were among children under 5 years of age. This mortality is estimated to be greater than combined total deaths from tuberculosis, AIDS (acquired immune deficiency syndrome), and malaria.

Discouraging use of household kerosene and unprocessed coal and implementing wider use of solar stoves or high-performing biomass stoves, liquefied petroleum gas (LPG), biogas, and electricity are probable solutions to this emerging crisis.

Health Effects

Exposure to AAP and HAP adversely affects birth outcomes and infant mortality. The evidence of association between exposure to air pollution and adverse health outcomes is compelling us to take necessary steps for harm reduction. Studies over the past decade have shown beyond doubt that air pollution causes neurodevelopmental disorders, childhood obesity, deterioration of lung function, ALRI, asthma, otitis media, and cancers in children.

Mothers when exposed to air pollution, particularly to fine PM, have increased risk of preterm birth and infant mortality There is also strong evidence that exposure to PM, SO_2, NO, O_3, and CO is associated with low birth weight (LBW), small for gestational age (SGA), and stillbirths.

Prenatal or postnatal exposure to AAP or HAP leads to lower cognitive outcomes and may be responsible for attention deficit hyperactivity disorder and autism spectrum disorders. Thus, AAP has a negative neurodevelopmental effect on children's mental and motor development.

Association has also been reported between insulin resistance in children and traffic-related air pollution. Some studies also establish a positive correlation between postnatal weight gain and obesity in children and their exposure to air pollution in utero.

Even at lower levels of exposure, air pollution damages children's lung. Prenatal exposure to air pollution impairs lung development as well as lung function in children. It has been proved beyond doubt that children living in areas with ambient air quality experience a better lung function.

AAP and HAP increase the risk of ALRI in children. NO_2, O_3, and especially PM2.5 are associated with respiratory infections and pneumonia in <5-year-old children. Both AAP and HAP increase the risk of developing asthma in children. Research also shows that AAP and HAP exacerbate asthma in children exposed to pollutants in respired air.

Few studies have suggested that combustion-derived HAP may increase the risk of otitis media in children.

Traffic-related air pollution has been found to have an association with increased risk of childhood leukemia and higher risk of retinoblastomas.

ROLE OF THE PEDIATRICIAN

The Agenda for Sustainable Development 2030 offers a unique opportunity to relook into environmental hazards damaging to child health. For all health professionals, the call for action is to reduce exposure to air pollution globally.

A pediatrician must conduct health assessments, monitor child health in his/her own localities, emphasize the health burden of air pollution to caretakers, and convey the need to protect children at risk to decision-makers. He/she also plays a pivotal role in communicating and educating families and public at large about the risks of air pollution and finding possible solutions.

Pediatricians can also provide evidence through research publications and partner with government agencies for effective health policies to reduce exposure to air pollution in children. Training other colleagues regarding health hazards of air pollution and preventive strategies to reduce exposure can increase the reach of their messages at large.

Preventing burning of biomass and firewood will not stop unless electricity or clean burning fuel and combustion technologies become reliably available and widely adopted in rural and urban India. Simple protective measures such as solar stoves for cooking may significantly reduce HAP and improve the health of the whole family. Moving toward rooftop solar panels, increasing use of public transport or carpooling, cycling and walking, using energy-efficient appliances, waste minimization, segregation, and recycling are efficient measures for reducing the burden of environmental pollution.

REFERENCES

1. World Health Organization. Ambient Air Pollution: A Global Assessment of Exposure and Burden of Disease, 2nd edition. Geneva: World Health Organization. (in press).
2. World Health Organization (2018). Burden of disease from the joint effects of household and ambient air pollution for 2016, Version 2, May 2018. Summary of results. [online] Available from: http://www.who.int/airpollution/data/cities/en/ [Last accessed on November, 2019].
3. Prüss-Ustün A, Wolf J, Corvalán C, et al. Preventing disease through healthy environments: a global assessment of the burden of disease from environment risks. Geneva: World Health Organization; 2016. [online] Available from: http://www.who.int/iris/handle/10665/204585 [Last accessed on November, 2019].

Miscellaneous Issues

Ashok Gupta

Pretravel Preparedness: Travel to Tropics

Digant D Shastri, Kamlesh Agarwal

With the advancement of the travel modalities and easy availability of travel facilities, it is estimated that annually more than 900 million international journeys are undertaken over the globe. Global travel on this scale exposes person to a range of health risks including infections and injuries. Over 2.5 million children travel internationally each year, including adolescents traveling abroad with school groups. Tourists including children traveling internationally are increasing every year in both high- and low-income countries and tourism is the first or second largest source of revenue in 20 of the 48 least developed countries.[1]

Pretravel consultation is necessary to the travelers to prevent them from infection and other environmental hazards, but it was found in a study that pretravel consultation was received only in 36% of international travelers in which 60% consulted a primary care clinician, 10% a travel subspecialist, and 30% turn to friends and family.[2] The European Travel Health Advisory Board conducted a cross-sectional pilot survey to evaluate current travel health knowledge, attitudes, and practices (KAP) and to determine where travelers going to developing countries obtain travel health information, what information they receive, and what preventive travel health measures they employ. The results showed that only 52.1% of responders had sought travel health advice.[3]

In a 10-year study from Germany, it was found that age was a significant determinant of morbidity among 890 children and adolescents returning from the tropical countries with an infectious disease. Adolescents developed dengue significantly more as compared to the young pediatric group (6.6% compared to 0.3%, respectively).[4] In another study from the GeoSentinel Surveillance Network, it was found that international travelers of 12–17 years age had a significantly higher proportionate morbidity rate for systemic febrile illness, but a lower for respiratory illnesses or diarrhea following a trip to Asia, sub-Saharan Africa, or Latin America.[5]

Children traveling internationally are at increased risk of acquiring diseases such as malaria, diarrhea, enteric fever, dengue fever, and various dermatoses. According to an analysis of posttravel data from a large multicenter study, children were less likely to receive pretravel advice and more likely to require inpatient care than adults.[5]

■ COMPONENTS OF PRETRAVEL PREPARATION

For effective pretravel preparation, first to enquire about the health background of the traveler and travel itinerary, trip duration, travel purpose, and activities, all of which determine health risks. Pretravel consultation also includes discussion about availability and efficacy of chemoprophylaxis or vaccination. Sometimes, physical examination is not included in pretravel health consultation so a separate visit to primary care physician is required, as travel medicine clinics are not always available. Travel health advice should be personalized with special attention to likely exposures and also reminding the traveler of risks, such as injury, foodborne and waterborne infections, vector-borne disease, respiratory tract infections, and blood-borne and sexually transmitted infections.

The pretravel consultation is the major opportunity to educate the traveler about health risks at the destination and how to prevent from them.

Information required for a risk assessment during pretravel consultations:

- *Travel history*: Travel itinerary (countries/regions traveling including order of countries if >one country), travel duration, and style of travel, rural or urban, and timing of travel (season of travel).

- Past medical history including underlying conditions, allergies (especially to any vaccines, eggs, or latex), medications, breastfeeding, disability or handicap, immunocompromising conditions, psychiatric condition, seizure disorder, recent surgery, and history of Guillain-Barré syndrome.
- *Immunization history*: Routine vaccines, travel-specific vaccines
- Dietary habits
- *Prior travel experience*: Malaria chemoprophylaxis in previous travel and its complication, experience with altitude, and sickness related to prior travel
- Sex practices
- Sun protection practices.

Based on these factors, traveler's individual risk is to be assessed and accordingly the healthcare professional has to decide about need for immunizations and/or preventive medication (prophylaxis) and provide advice.[6,7]

Regardless of administration of vaccine/medications, traveler should always follow all possible precautions against infection for avoiding disease.

While planning the vaccination strategies for travelers, following points are to be considered:

- *Timing of vaccination*: Since the immune response in the vaccinated individual will varies with the type of vaccine, the number of doses required and whether the individual has been vaccinated previously against the same disease, ideally the traveler should consult his healthcare provider or physician 4–8 weeks before departure in order to allow sufficient time for optimal immunization schedules to be completed. For the traveler who needs more than one doses of vaccines, slight variation in the time intervals for administration of vaccines can be made to accommodate the needs of travelers who otherwise may not be able to complete the schedule. In situations where imminent departure is must, still the traveler should be advised about the immunization and should be provided with at least some vaccines.
- *Multiple vaccines*: As per the basic principle of immunology, most live vaccines should be given simultaneously provided that they are administered at different anatomical sites. If it is not possible to inject two live virus vaccines on the same day, the two injections should be separated by an interval of at least 4 weeks. Combination vaccines offer important advantages of compliance because of reduced number of injection and visits.
- *Vaccination schedule*: There cannot be single schedule for the administration of immunizing agents which

may be applicable to all travelers. With considering individual traveler's immunization history, the countries to be visited, the type and duration of travel, and the availability of time for vaccination before departure, a tailored made schedule should be suggested to travelers.

Pretravel vaccination details should be documented in International Certificate of Vaccination or Prophylaxis as approved by the World Health Organization **(Fig. 1)**.[8]

CHOICE OF VACCINES FOR TRAVEL

In deciding which vaccines should be offered to the traveler, following points are to be considered:
- Risk of exposure to the disease
- Age, health status, and vaccination history of traveler
- Reactions to previous vaccine doses, allergies
- Risk of infecting others
- Cost.

Vaccines for travelers include:
- Basic vaccines used in national routine immunization programs, particularly but not only restricted to pediatric age group
- Others that may be advised before travel to countries or areas at risk of these diseases
- Those that, in some situations, are required by the International Health Regulations.

The vaccines that may be recommended or considered for travelers are summarized in **Table 1**.

Travel specific vaccination, indications, and doses are summarized in **Table 2**.

Vaccination for Immunocompromised Travelers

An increasing number of children with conditions that reduce immune competence, including organ transplantation, human immunodeficiency virus (HIV) infection, and treatment with corticosteroids or immunosuppressive agents for a variety of indications often have to travel. HIV-infected traveler degree of immune compromise can be quantified with modest precision by measuring CD4 lymphocytes and there is abundance of recommendations. There is little evidence and fewer recommendations with respect to transplant patients. There is very little information relating to other forms of immune suppression[9,10] and no well-validated laboratory measures to quantify the degree of immune suppression in most of these patients. The travelers, who has been on corticosteroid therapy for >2 weeks at a dose equivalent to

This is to certify that (name) ....

Date of birth .... Sex ....

Nationality ....

National identification document, if applicable ....

Whose signature follows ....

Has on the date indicated been vaccinated or received prophylaxis against (name of disease or condition) ....

.... in accordance with the International Health Regulations.

Vaccine or prophylaxis	Date	Signature and professional status of supervising clinician	Manufacturer and batch number of vaccine or prophylaxis	Certificate valid from................. until.................	Official stamp of administering center
1					
2					

Fig. 1: Model international certificate of vaccination or prophylaxis.

Source: Adapted from World Health Organization (WHO) (2005). International certificate of vaccination or prophylaxis. [online] Available from: https://www.who.int/ihr/ports_airports/icvp/en/. [Last accessed on November, 2019].

Table 1: Vaccines for travelers.

Routine vaccination	• Diphtheria • Hepatitis B • *Haemophilus influenzae* type b • Seasonal influenza • Measles • Mumps • Pertussis • Rubella • Pneumococcal disease • Poliomyelitis (polio) • Rotavirus • Tuberculosis (TB) • Tetanus • Varicella
Selective use for travelers	• Hepatitis A • Typhoid fever • Rabies • Cholera • Japanese encephalitis • Tick-borne encephalitis • Meningococcal disease • Yellow fever
Required vaccination	• Yellow fever • Meningococcal disease (against serogroups A, C, Y, and W135) and polio (required by Saudi Arabia for pilgrims)

>20 mg/day of prednisone, should be considered analogous to patients with HIV infection with a CD4+ cell count <200 cells/mm^3 and decision of administration of live vaccines should be taken accordingly. Patients receiving other immunosuppressive drugs should be advised on a case-by-case basis depending on the degree of immune suppression as judged by the prescribing physician.

Splenic patients and persons with terminal complement deficiencies are susceptible to overwhelming sepsis with encapsulated bacterial pathogens. These groups of people should be immunized with the meningococcal A/C/Y/W-135 conjugate vaccine.[11]

Patients with limited immune deficits or asymptomatic HIV going to yellow fever endemic areas may be offered yellow fever vaccine and monitored closely for possible adverse effects. As vaccine response may be suboptimal, such vaccines are candidates for serologic testing 1 month after vaccination. Travelers with severe immune compromise should not be vaccinated with yellow fever vaccine and should be strongly discouraged from travel to destinations that put them at risk for yellow fever.

Table 2: Travel-specific immunization.

Vaccines	Indications	Doses
Yellow fever	• Travelers to endemic areas (tropical Africa and tropical South America) • Age ≥ 9 months	Previously recommended one dose every 10 years; now the CDC and the Prevention Advisory Committee on Immunization Practices recommended a single dose, it has long-lasting protection, and is adequate for most travelers
Typhoid fever	Consider for all travelers to low-income nations, higher priority for high-risk destinations, rural travel, or duration of travel more than 1 month	• *IM (inactivated)*: Boosters required every 2 years • *Oral (live)*: Four tablets, one taken every other day; provides protection for 5 years
Japanese encephalitis	Travel to endemic areas in Asia and Western Pacific; higher priority ≥1 month and rural travel (risk is very low with urban, short-term travel)	Two IM doses at days 0 and 28, booster administered at 1 year for those at ongoing risk
Meningococcal	Travelers to the meningitis belt of Africa and if crowded living conditions (dormitory) are anticipated	• One dose of MenACWY—those 2–55 years of age • One dose of MPSV4—those 56 years or older who have never received meningococcal vaccine • A booster dose is advised 5 years after the previous dose of vaccine for those who received their previous dose at ≥7 years of age
Cholera	Adults 18–64 years of age traveling to cholera affected areas, specially persons at high risk of cholera (e.g. healthcare workers who will be caring for patients during cholera epidemics); not indicated for most travelers	Single oral dose of Vaxchora
Poliovirus	• Travelers to a country with ongoing transmission of polio • Long-term (more than 4 weeks) travelers to Afghanistan and Pakistan • Vaccine—should be received 4 weeks to 12 months before departure from polio endemic countries	In addition to four childhood dose adult travelers to polio-endemic destinations, single dose of the inactivated poliovirus vaccine is recommended
Rabies	Travelers visiting countries where rabies is enzootic, higher priority for longer duration of stay, and rural or remote travels	• Three IM doses at days 0, 7, and 21 or 28; boosters not advised for those at low risk • In high-risk cases (e.g. cavers, wildlife workers in endemic areas), serology should be tested every 2 years and a booster is administered if antibodies are below protective levels

(CDC: Centers for Disease Control and Prevention; IM: intramuscular)

Protection against Malaria and Arthropod-borne Diseases

Travelers and physician should note the five principles—the *ABCDE*—of malaria protection:

- *Aware* about the risk, the incubation period, the possibility of delayed onset, and the main symptoms.
- *Biting* by mosquitoes should be avoided, especially between dusk and dawn areas.
- *Chemoprophylaxis*—use antimalarial chemoprophylaxis when appropriate, at regular intervals to prevent acute malaria attacks.
- *Diagnosis* and treatment should be immediate if a fever develops 1 week or more after entering an area where there is a malaria risk and up to 3 months (or, rarely, later) after departure from a risk area.
- *Environments* that are mosquito breeding places should be avoided, such as swamps or marshy areas, especially in late evenings and at night.

- *Protection against mosquito bite*: Taking antimalarials does not nullify the need for personal protective measures that prevent from malaria and other arthropod-borne diseases like dengue fever, scrub typhus, and common illness in most tropical countries.[12,13] Insect bites can be prevented by following measures:
  - *Insect repellents*:
    - Insect repellent should be applied to exposed part of body. The most effective insect repellents are N,N-diethyl-meta-toluamide (DEET) which contains 20–50% diethyltoluamide or 20% picaridin.
    - Other insect repellents are oil of lemon eucalyptus [p-menthane-3,8-diol (PMD)] and IR3535. IR3535 does not provide adequate protection against *Anopheles* mosquitoes and should not be used in malaria-endemic areas.

- - Insect repellent should not be applied onto or under clothing and regular reapplication is required.
    - Permethrin can be applied to clothing, it will increases protection against insect bites.[14,15]
    - In malaria-endemic regions, bed net impregnated with permethrin can be used.
- Wearing full sleeves shirts and pants provides additional protection.
- Minimizing outdoors time during dusk, nighttime, and dawn hours, when mosquitoes are more active that will reduce risk of bite.
- Travelers should inspect their bodies and cloths after outdoor activity at the end of the day with the help of a mirror or companion to prevent from tick bite.
- Air-conditioning is also highly effective means of keeping mosquitoes and other insects out of a room as long as the room has no gaps around windows or doors. In air-conditioned hotels, other precautions are not necessary in indoors.
- *Antimalarial prophylaxis*: Travelers visiting malaria-endemic region should be given antimalarial prophylaxis based on travel characteristics and local resistance patterns. The choice of antimalarial prophylactic drug should be based on various factors including whether the traveler is going to an area with chloroquine-sensitive or chloroquine-resistant malaria, whether there could be potential side effects or interactions with the patient's medical conditions or other medications, the convenience of dosing schedule, the cost, and age of traveler. Medications for antimalarial prophylaxis, doses and contraindications are summarized in **Table 3**.[16,17]

In chloroquine-sensitive areas like Mexico and Central America and the island of Hispaniola, chloroquine and hydroxychloroquine can be used as chemoprophylaxis. In chloroquine-resistant areas including most of South America, Asia, and Africa, doxycycline, atovaquone-proguanil, and mefloquine are drugs of choice for chemoprophylaxis.

TRAVELER'S DIARRHEA

Traveler's diarrhea (TD) is another most common infection in international travelers, with a rate of 30–70% depending on destination and season of travel. The risk of infection is highest in the first 2 weeks of travel and slowly declines thereafter.[18] Risk factors that increased the risk of TD are medications that reduce gastric acidity, including proton pump inhibitors and antacids, younger age, diabetes, and immunosuppression.

Bacterial pathogens are main cause up to 80–90% of TD. Intestinal viruses may account for at least 5–15% of illnesses. Protozoal infections are gradual onset symptoms and account for about 10% of cases in longer-term travelers. The most common pathogen is enterotoxigenic *Escherichia coli (E. coli)*, followed by *Campylobacter jejuni*, *Shigella* spp., and *Salmonella* spp. Enteroaggregative and other *E. coli* pathotypes are also commonly found in cases of TD. Viral diarrhea can be caused by norovirus, rotavirus, and astrovirus. *Giardia* is the main protozoal pathogen causing TD. *Entamoeba histolytica* and *Cryptosporidium* are relatively uncommon cause of TD.[19]

Preventive steps like avoiding food from street stands, tap water, raw foods, and ice have not been shown to reduce the incidence of TD.[20] Handwashing may reduce risk by 30% and alcohol-based hand sanitizer also significantly reduces risk.[21] Prophylactic antibiotics are not routinely recommended in TD. For patients who are at high risk, bismuth subsalicylate (two tablets four times daily for the duration of the trip) reduces risk of TD by 50–65%.[22] Side effects of bismuth subsalicylate include a black tongue and dark stool, and contraindications include aspirin allergy, renal insufficiency, breastfeeding, and concurrent use of anticoagulants. There is not sufficient evidence for the use of probiotics to prevent TD.

ZIKA VIRUS INFECTION

Zika virus infection is primarily transmitted by mosquito (*Aedes aegypti* and *Aedes albopictus*), but it can also be sexually transmitted. Since May of 2015, Zika virus has been spread to Mexico and essentially every country in Central and South America and the Caribbean. Risk of microcephaly in the newborn if a woman is infected during first trimester of pregnancy has been estimated at 1–13%. Zika virus infection can be prevented by avoidance of mosquito bites. Continue to protect against mosquito bites for 3 weeks after returning home as mosquitoes back home could bite and get infected, and then spread Zika to other people. Pregnant women should avoid travel to areas with Zika virus outbreak. Men who live in or visit a Zika-endemic area should use a condom or abstain from sex with a pregnant partner for the remainder of the pregnancy. If a woman traveling without male partner, wait 2 months after return before becoming pregnant. If a man traveling with partner planning pregnancy, use condoms or do not have sex for at least 3 months after return.[23,24]

Table 3: Medications used for antimalarial chemoprophylaxis.

Medications	Doses	Comments
Atovaquone-proguanil	Pediatric tablets contain 62.5 mg atovaquone and 25 mg proguanil hydrochloride • *5–8 kg*: One-half pediatric tablet daily • *>8–10 kg*: Three-fourths pediatric tablet daily • *>10–20 kg*: One pediatric tablet daily • *>20–30 kg*: Two pediatric tablets daily • *>30–40 kg*: Three pediatric tablets daily • *>40 kg*: One adult tablet daily (250 mg atovaquone and 100 mg proguanil)	• Prophylaxis in all areas • Start 1–2 days before travel to malaria-endemic areas. Take daily at the same time each day and continue for 7 days after leaving such areas • It should be taken with food or a milky drink • Contraindications—severe renal impairment (creatinine clearance < 30 mL/min). Not recommended for prophylaxis for children weighing <5 kg, pregnant women, and women breastfeeding infants weighing <5 kg
Chloroquine	5 mg/kg base (8.3 mg/kg salt) orally, once/week, and up to maximum adult dose of 300 mg base	• In areas with chloroquine-sensitive malaria • Begin 1–2 weeks before travel. Take weekly on the same day of the week while in the malaria-endemic area and for 4 weeks after leaving such areas • May exacerbate psoriasis • For short trips—some people would rather not take medication for 4 weeks after travel • Not a good choice for last-minute travelers, because it needs to be started 1–2 weeks before travel
Doxycycline	≥8 years of age: 2.2 mg/kg up to adult dose of 100 mg/day	• Can be given in all areas • Begin 1–2 days before travel to malaria-endemic areas. Take daily at the same time each day while in the malaria-endemic area and for 4 weeks after leaving such areas • Contraindicated in children <8 years of age and pregnant women • Least expensive antimalarial
Hydroxychloroquine	5 mg/kg base (6.5 mg/kg salt) orally, once/week, and up to a maximum adult dose of 310 mg base	• An alternative to chloroquine for prophylaxis only in areas with chloroquine-sensitive malaria • Begin 1–2 weeks before travel to 4 weeks after leaving malaria-endemic areas
Mefloquine	• *9 kg*: 4.6 mg/kg base (5 mg/kg salt) orally, once/week • *>9–19 kg*: One-fourth tablet once/week • *>19–30 kg*: One-half tablet once/week • *>30–45 kg*: Three-fourths tablet once/week • *>45 kg*: One tablet once/week.	• In areas with mefloquine-sensitive malaria • Start ≥2 weeks before travel to malaria-endemic areas and continue for 4 weeks after leaving such areas • Cannot be used in patients with certain psychiatric conditions, seizure disorders, and cardiac conduction abnormalities
Primaquine	0.5 mg/kg base (0.8 mg/kg salt) up to adult dose 30 mg base (52.6 mg salt) orally, daily	• For short duration, travel to areas with principally *Plasmodium vivax* • Start 1–2 days before travel to malaria-endemic areas and for 7 days after leaving such areas
Tafenoquine	200 mg orally	• Prophylaxis in all areas • Not indicated in children <16 years old • Start taking daily for 3 days prior to 1 week after leaving the malaria-endemic areas

Source: Adapted from World Health Organization (WHO)(2017). International Travel and Health: Malaria. [online] Available from: http://www.who.int/ith/2017-ith-chapter7.pdf?ua=1. [Last accessed on November, 2019]; Tan KR, Arguin PM, Centers for Disease Control and Prevention (CDC)(2019). Travel-Related Infectious Diseases: Malaria. [online] Available from: https://wwwnc.cdc.gov/travel/yellowbook/2020/travel-related-infectious diseases/malaria. [Last accessed on November, 2019].

◼ NONINFECTIOUS TRAVEL-RELATED HAZARDS

Traffic-related accidents, drowning, accidents related to water activities, and violence constitute the most common causes of injuries in travelers, including adolescents. Natural hazards during outdoor and wildlife activities are other causes of injuries. Travelers are 10 times more likely to die from injury than from infection during treveling.[25,26] Motor vehicle accidents are also leading cause of death among pediatric and adolescent international travelers and it accounts for more 50% fatal events. Drowning is the second most common cause of death.[27] It has been found that United States pediatric traveler's age 0–14 years are more than two times as likely to die from a motor vehicle accident and 3.7 times as likely to die as a result of drowning as compared with nontravelers.[27]

Families should be firmly advised to supervise their children around the streets and roads. Travelers should "look both ways" before crossing roads in countries with driving habits different from their country. Children should always supervised near water, and when playing in the water by an adult. Risk factors which lead to boating injuries such as alcohol consumption by drivers and propellers left running while people are still swimming or climbing in or out of the boat should be avoided. Parents and adolescents planning to use a boat during travel should be well informed about good boating safety practices.[28]

Animal bites are also a common cause of injury and it can be prevented by avoiding playing around unknown animals, and viewing of animal from a safe distance. Animal bites should be treated promptly by a health professional in view of injury, bacterial contamination, and rabies. International travelers to rabies-endemic regions like Asia and Africa should be informed about the potential risk of rabies exposure and the efficacy and safety of pretravel vaccination against rabies.[28]

Alcohol and other substance abuse are also a significant problem for adolescents while travel. In a study, it was found that two-thirds of young traveler including adolescents, visiting Mediterranean destinations, reported having been drunk on holiday, and over 10% using illicit drugs. Pretravel consultations should include advice to avoid the unsafe use of alcohol and other illicit substances during traveling. Adolescents should be advised that monogamous sex with a stable and uninfected partner or sexual abstinence are the only effective ways to protect against sexually transmitted infections (STIs).

Body piercing and tattooing are well-known sources of transmission of hepatitis B, hepatitis C, HIV, and syphilis in highly endemic countries.[29] Adolescents frequently engage in such activities, therefore, piercing, tattooing, and acupuncture should be avoided in a settings with low or poor hygiene standards.

Jet lag is also a common problem develop after crossing multiple time zones. Children with jet lag may find difficulty falling asleep at night and may wake up earlier than usual. These children become irritable and tired during the day. Long daytime sleep may worsen jet lag as there is difficulty in falling asleep at night. Encourage short daytime naps and exposure to sunlight and following the local time zone schedule can help to minimize jet lag.

■ LAST-MINUTE TRAVELERS

All travelers should be encouraged to seek pretravel consultation at least 1 month before departure, but sometime pretravel consultation can be asked by traveler who is leaving on short notice even within days or sometimes hours of departure. Providing complete pretravel services to last-minute travelers can be challenging.

- *Vaccination*:
  - Routine vaccinations—most travelers have received standard routine vaccinations. If the traveler is not received routine vaccines, provide the first or additional doses of routine vaccines, including a seasonal influenza vaccination.
  - Recommended single-dose vaccines—even when a traveler has limited time before travel, research supports the use of certain single-dose vaccines, if indicated, to initiate protection. These include hepatitis A (monovalent), typhoid (injectable), polio (inactivated), cholera, and quadrivalent (ACWY) meningococcal meningitis vaccines.
  - Recommended multiple-doses vaccine—these travelers often cannot complete the full course of vaccines before departure to induce full protection. If a traveler requires protection against hepatitis B, Japanese encephalitis, or rabies, the physician can consider approved accelerated schedules or information on resources for vaccination at the destination.
    - Hepatitis B—the accelerated monovalent hepatitis B schedule is 0, 1, and 2 months, plus a 12-month booster or the super-accelerated schedule for combination hepatitis A/B (Twinrix) is 0, 7, and 21–30 days, plus a 12-month booster. If an accelerated schedule cannot be completed before starting travel, vaccination series can be started and schedule a follow-up visit to complete it or, for extended-stay travelers, help them identify resources at the destination to complete the series.
    - Rabies—multiple doses of rabies immunizations required to complete a primary rabies vaccine series (0 and 7 days), last-minute travelers may not be able to complete the series before departure. If vaccination started but does not complete a primary series and is exposed should receive the same postexposure prophylaxis as a completely unimmunized person. Counseling on animal avoidance and the need for urgent care after an exposure are required.

- ◆ Japanese encephalitis vaccine—administered as two doses on days 0 and 7–28 and if traveler receives only a single dose may have a suboptimal response and may not be protected. If the primary vaccine series cannot be completed ≥1 week before travel, he should be counseled to adhere rigidly to mosquito precautions if they will be at risk for Japanese encephalitis or the physician can help them identify resources for vaccination that may be available at their destination, particularly if they will be long-stay travelers.

- *Malaria*: The choice of malaria prophylaxis for last-minute travelers (<2 weeks) are doxycycline, atovaquone-proguanil, or primaquine.[30]

TRAVELERS EDUCATION

Traveler should be educated about their fitness, important precautions, health insurance coverage for hospitalization and the availability of healthcare facility in the planned destination, and the importance of a follow-up visit, particularly for long-term stays in developing countries.

Emphasis should be given on personal hygiene like handwashing. Food and water precautions include the use of bottled water, eating food that is cooked hot, and cold food when it is cold. All fresh fruit should be eaten after peeling. Unpasteurized dairy products should be avoided unless it was prepared from bottled water.

CONCLUSION

The pretravel preparation is an important opportunity for children to update routine immunization and provide travel specific vaccines and prophylaxis. Pretravel consultation also includes education and screening for intended international travel during routine pediatric health examinations by primary care providers. If immunization or prophylaxis could not given, children should advised about other methods to reduce the risk such as avoidance of animal bite, prevention from insect bite, safe sex practices, and hand and food hygiene. Healthcare physician should identify the barriers in pretravel care and try to address them appropriately.

REFERENCES

1. United Nations World Tourism Organization (UNWTO) (2010). Tourism and Poverty Alleviation. [online] Available from: http://step.unwto.org/content/tourism-and-poverty-alleviation-1. [Last accessed on November, 2019].
2. Hamer DH, Connor BA. Travel health knowledge, attitudes and practices among United States travelers. J Travel Med. 2004;11(1):23-6.
3. Van Herck K, Van Damme P, Castelli F, et al. Knowledge, attitudes and practices in travel-related infectious diseases: the European airport survey. J Travel Med. 2004;11(1):3-8.
4. Herbinger KH, Drerup L, Alberer M, et al. Spectrum of imported infectious diseases among children and adolescents returning from the tropics and subtropics. J Travel Med. 2012;19(3):150-7.
5. Hagmann S, Neugebauer R, Schwartz E, et al. Illness in children after international travel: analysis from the GeoSentinel Surveillance Network. Pediatrics. 2010;125(5):e1072-80.
6. Steffen R, Dupont HL, Wilder-Smith A. Manual of Travel Medicine and Health, 2nd edition. London: BC Decker; 2003.
7. Steffen R, Connor BA. Vaccines in travel health: from risk assessment to priorities. J Travel Med. 2005;12(1):26-35.
8. World Health Organization (WHO) (2005). International certificate of vaccination or prophylaxis. [online] Available from: https://www.who.int/ihr/ports_airports/icvp/en/. [Last accessed on November, 2019].
9. Kotton CN, Ryan ET, Fishman JA. Prevention of infection in adult travellers after solid organ transplantation. Am J Transplant. 2005;5(1):8-14.
10. Avery RK. Vaccination of the immunosuppressed adult patient with rheumatologic disease. Rheum Dis Clin North Am. 1999;25(3):567-84.
11. Centers for Disease Control and Prevention (CDC) (2009). Vaccination of Persons with Primary and Secondary Immune Deficiencies. [online] Available from: http://www.cdc.gov/vaccines/pubs/pinkbook/downloads/appendices/A/immuno-table.pdf. [Last accessed on November, 2019].
12. Alpern JD, Dunlop SJ, Dolan BJ, et al. Personal Protection Measures Against Mosquitoes, Ticks, and Other Arthropods. Med Clin North Am. 2016;100(2):303-16.
13. Hill DR, Ericsson CD, Pearson RD, et al. The practice of travel medicine: guidelines by the Infectious Diseases Society of America. Clin Infect Dis. 2006;43(12):1499-539.
14. Banks SD, Murray N, Wilder-Smith A, et al. Insecticide-treated clothes for the control of vector-borne diseases: a review on effectiveness and safety. Med Vet Entomol. 2014;28 Suppl 1:14-25.
15. Rowland M, Durrani N, Hewitt S, et al. Permethrin-treated chaddars and top-sheets. Trans R Soc Trop Med Hyg. 1999;93(5):465-72.
16. World Health Organization (WHO) (2017). International Travel and Health: Malaria. [online] Available from: http://www.who.int/ith/2017-ith-chapter7.pdf?ua=1. [Last accessed on November, 2019].
17. Tan KR, Arguin PM, Centers for Disease Control and Prevention (CDC) (2019). Travel-Related Infectious Diseases: Malaria. [online] Available from: https://wwwnc.cdc.gov/travel/yellowbook/2020/travel-related-infectious diseases/malaria. [Last accessed on November, 2019].
18. Kollaritsch H, Paulke-Korinek M, Wiedermann U. Traveler's diarrhea. Infect Dis Clin North Am. 2012;26(3):691-706.
19. Connor BA, Centers for Disease Control and Prevention (CDC) (2019). Preparing International Travelers: Traveler's Diarrhea. [online] Available from: https://wwwnc.cdc.gov/travel/yellowbook/2020/preparing-international-travelers/travelers-diarrhea. [Last accessed on November, 2019].
20. Steffen R, Tornieporth N, Clemens SA, et al. Epidemiology of travelers' diarrhea: details of a global survey. J Travel Med. 2004;11(4):231-7.

21. Henriey D, Delmont J, Gautret P. Does the use of alcohol-based hand gel sanitizer reduce travellers' diarrhea and gastrointestinal upset?: A preliminary survey. Travel Med Infect Dis. 2014;12(5):494-8.

22. Ericsson CD. Nonantimicrobial agents in the prevention and treatment of traveler's diarrhea. Clin Infect Dis. 2005;41(Suppl 8): S557-63.

23. Johansson MA, Mier-y-Teran-Romero L, Reefhuis J, et al. Zika and the Risk of Microcephaly. N Engl J Med. 2016;375(1):1-4.

24. Centers for Disease Control and Prevention (CDC) (2016). Zika Travel Information. [online] Available from: https://wwwnc. cdc.gov/travel/page/zika-information. [Last accessed on November, 2019].

25. Hargarten SW, Baker TD, Guptill K. Overseas fatalities of United States citizen travelers: an analysis of deaths related to international travel. Ann Emerg Med. 1991;20(6):622-6.

26. Stewart BT, Yankson IK, Afukaar F, et al. Road Traffic and Other Unintentional Injuries Among Travelers to Developing Countries. Med Clin North Am. 2016;100(2):331-43.

27. Guse CE, Cortes LM, Hargarten SW, et al. Fatal injuries of US citizens abroad. J Travel Med. 2007;14(5):279-87.

28. Summer AP, Fischer PR. The pediatric and adolescent traveler. In: Keystone J (Ed). Travel Medicine. United States: Elsevier; 2013. pp. 231-40.

29. Han P, Balaban V, Marano C. Travel characteristics and risk-taking attitudes in youths traveling to nonindustrialized countries. J Travel Med. 2010;17(5):316-21.

30. Rosselot GA, Centers for Disease Control and Prevention (CDC). (2019). Preparing International Travelers: Last-Minute Travelers. [online] Available from: https://wwwnc.cdc.gov/travel/yellowbook/2020/preparing-international-travelers/last-minute-travelers. [Last accessed on November, 2019].

Approach to Fever in a Returning Child Traveler

Ashok Gupta

INTRODUCTION

The number of travelers is increasing day by day in almost all parts of the world. In 2018, international tourist organizations reported 1.4 billion overseas trips with an increase of 6% from the previous year.[1] According to the World Tourism Organization (UNWTO), the number of international travelers will increase to 1.8 billion by the year 2030.[2] There are various reasons of international travel that include education, tourism, research, business, and travel to friends and relatives. Fever was more commonly reported in children who traveled to their friend and relatives than other groups of travelers, especially in travel areas such as India, sub-Saharan Africa, South-Central Asia, Oceania, and Latin America.[3] Due to Ebola epidemics in western Africa and emergence of Middle East respiratory corona virus, chikungunya, these should also considered as a causative agent for fever in a returning traveler.

Fever is a common clinical problem in children returning from a travel, and sometimes it is the only symptom of a serious life-threatening condition and requires hospitalization.[4] Travelers who returned commonly suffer from problems related to traveling which can be minor self-limiting illnesses or life-threatening infections. Nonspecific viral illness, respiratory illness, diarrhea, malaria, dengue, and salmonella infections including typhoid are the most common causes of fever among returned travelers.

The physician should focus initially to identify the causes that are treatable, severe life-threatening, and communicable during assessment of a child with fever after traveling. But in 25% or more children with fever after traveling, the specific cause may not be identified even after detailed history and examinations.[5]

DEMOGRAPHIC FACTORS

In GeoSentinel research (1997–2006), it was found that fever after travel was more common in male travelers (32%) than in female travelers (24%). Female travelers are generally less prone to febrile illnesses and vector-borne diseases such as malaria, dengue, or rickettsia. Age difference was also not seen in travelers presenting with fever and those without fever in the survey.[6] In GeoSentinel Surveillance Network analysis 2009, it was seen that in children after international travels, malaria was the most common cause of fever followed by viral infections (28%), unspecified febrile illnesses (11%), dengue fever, and enteric fever (6% each).[7] In another study done by Herbinger et al., it was found that causes of fever after travel were mainly malaria, infectious mononucleosis and dengue fever. In children, the most common cause of fever varied in different age groups. In children of age group 0–4 years, acute diarrhea was significantly a more frequent cause; among children aged between 10 years and 14 years, dengue fever was more frequently diagnosed; and in adolescents aged between 15 years and 19 years, infectious mononucleosis was the more common cause of fever after travel.[8] Common causes of fever in different geographical areas are summarized in **Table 1**.

HOST RISK FACTORS

The risk factors that make the children more susceptible to serious infections are given in the following text, and a physician should carefully evaluate these children:
- Unimmunized or children with incomplete immunization
- Immunocompromised children
- Undernutrition or severe acute malnutrition
- Children less than 1 month of age.

Table 1: Common causes of fever in different geographical areas.

Geographical areas	Common infections	Infections cause outbreaks
Caribbean	Chikungunya, dengue, malaria, Zika virus	Acute histoplasmosis, leptospirosis
Central America	Chikungunya, dengue, malaria (primarily *Plasmodium vivax*), Zika virus, enteric fever	Leptospirosis, histoplasmosis, coccidioidomycosis, leishmaniasis
South America	Chikungunya, dengue, malaria (primarily *P. vivax*), Zika virus	Bartonellosis, leptospirosis, enteric fever, histoplasmosis
South Central Asia	Dengue, enteric fever, malaria (primarily nonfalciparum)	Chikungunya, scrub typhus
Southeast Asia	Dengue, malaria (primarily nonfalciparum)	Chikungunya, leptospirosis
Sub-Saharan Africa	Malaria (primarily *P. falciparum*), tick-borne rickettsiae (main cause of fever in southern Africa), acute schistosomiasis (Katayama fever), dengue	African trypanosomiasis, chikungunya, enteric fever, meningococcal meningitis

The initial assessment of children who returned after travel and have fever includes detailed history and physical examination, which will help to narrow down the long list of investigations to more specific investigations and hence less time consuming and less costly. As causes of fever vary with geographical areas, travel duration, and different exposures, investigations should be chosen according to this history.

TRAVEL HISTORY

The type of infections varies according to the area of travel. It is important to take a detailed history regarding travel, including areas visited, duration of stay, activities undertaken, and potential exposures, in particular bites by insects or animals, injuries, exposures to open water (rivers, lakes, ponds, or sea), animals, unpasteurized milk, and sick contacts. It is crucial to frame an accurate timeline that includes the travel itinerary, likely exposures, symptom onset and progression, precautionary measures taken (if any), and treatment received. Comparing this information with the known incubation periods of different infections may help to identify or exclude specific illnesses.

CHEMOPROPHYLAXIS AND IMMUNIZATIONS

Children usually travel with their families to visit friends and relatives to their native country. In these children, there are low rates of malaria prophylaxis and pre-travel vaccine uptake. This group is also at more risk of acquisition of infections as they are more likely to travel to rural areas, travel for longer periods, and eat and drink local food and water.[9,10] The clinician also consider the fact that malaria prophylaxis may delay the onset of symptoms of malaria. The common vaccine-preventable diseases found in children with fever after travel are typhoid fever (typhoid and paratyphoid), measles, influenza, and viral hepatitis. Child travelers may also have incomplete routine childhood immunizations so they may be at risk of vaccine-preventable infections. Preventive strategies for travel-associated infection are summarized in **Table 2**.

TIMING OF FEVER IN RELATION TO TRAVEL

Infections such as those with short incubation periods usually present within 1 month of return from their travel. However, schistosomiasis, malaria leishmaniasis, or tuberculosis can present months or even years later after travel **(Table 3)**.

UNDERLYING MEDICAL ILLNESS

Children with comorbid conditions and immunocompromised state are more susceptible for infection and they may have more severe illness.

SEVERITY OF ILLNESS

Some potentially life-threatening infections such as malaria, severe respiratory syndrome or hemorrhagic fever, and encephalitis may necessitate prompt involvement of public health authorities. The initial assessment of a child with fever after travel should be done similarly as that for any ill child suspected of infection. A complete history should be taken including exposure risks, risks related to particular geographic areas, and incubation periods. Detailed physical examination should be done, including assessment for signs of severity, rash, eschar, and focus of infection such as a chest infection or icterus indicating hepatitis. The Third International Consensus Definitions for Sepsis and Septic Shock (Sepsis-3) recommended quick Sepsis-Related Organ Failure Assessment (qSOFA) score for rapid clinical assessment of patients to identify the patients who are at risk for severe sepsis and in need of immediate and high levels of care.[11]

Table 2: Preventive strategies for common travel-associated infections.

Infections	Immunization and chemoprophylaxis	Other preventive methods
Meningococcal	• Quadrivalent meningococcal A, C, W135, Y vaccine for children >9 months of age • Vaccine compulsory for travel to Saudi Arabia for Hajj or Umra, especially recommended for travel to sub-Saharan Africa (meningitis belt)	Avoid contact with ill individuals
Tuberculosis	• *Chemoprophylaxis*: Not indicated pretravel; consider in vulnerable young children (<5 years) if documented TB exposure or infection (in the absence of disease; adult pulmonary TB cases are the most infectious) • *Immunization*: BCG recommended (ideally 3 months prior to travel) for children aged <5 years traveling for extended periods to countries with high prevalence of TB	Avoid close contact with known TB cases and individuals with suggestive symptoms
Hepatitis A	*Immunization >1 year of age*: • Immunization recommended for travel to areas of moderate or high endemicity (all developing countries)	• Boiling and cooking of food • Pay close attention to hand hygiene • Use bottled water for drinking and tooth brushing • Avoid ice cubes in drinks
Japanese encephalitis	Immunization >1 year of age, recommended for travel for over a month in rural areas in high-risk endemic regions	• Use topical insect repellents (e.g. DEET) • Wear long-sleeved clothing during bushwalking or hiking
Yellow fever	Immunization >9 months of age, recommended for travel to endemic areas, required for travel to or from certain countries	• Use topical insect repellents (e.g. DEET) • Wear long-sleeved clothing, especially during bushwalking or hiking
Malaria	• *Chloroquine-sensitive areas*: Chloroquine, once weekly from 1 week prior until 4 weeks after travel • *Chloroquine-resistant areas*: Atovaquone + proguanil daily from 1 day to 2 days prior to 7 days after travel, or doxycycline (children >8 years) daily from 1 day to 2 days prior to 4 weeks after travel, or mefloquine once weekly from 2 weeks to 3 weeks prior to 4 weeks after travel	• Use topical insect repellents (e.g. DEET) • Wear long-sleeved clothing • Avoid outdoor activities at night

(DEET: N,N-diethyl-meta-toluamide)

ACUTE FEVER WITH RASH OR ULCER

Maculopapular: Arboviral infections (dengue, chikungunya), measles, rubella, parvovirus, drug rash, fungal infections (histoplasmosis, penicilliosis), rickettsial infections (tick typhus), viral hemorrhagic fever, syphilis, infectious mononucleosis group (Epstein-Barr virus, cytomegalovirus), HIV (human immunodeficiency virus) seroconversion, lepra reaction.

Vesicular: Herpes simplex, herpes zoster, chickenpox, monkeypox, rickettsialpox.

Purpuric: Dengue hemorrhagic fever, viral hemorrhagic fevers (Lassa, Ebola, Crimean-Congo hemorrhagic fever, rift valley fever), meningococcal infection, severe rickettsial infection, severe sepsis with disseminated intravascular coagulation, plague, hemorrhagic herpes zoster.

Erythroderma: Early dengue, Kawasaki disease, toxic shock syndrome, Scarlet fever, sunburn.

Ulcer

Chancre: Trypanosoma infection, Yersinia pestis (bubonic plague).

Eschar: Tick typhus, scrub typhus, anthrax disease.

Genital ulcer: Syphilis, herpes simplex virus.

Skin ulcer: Fungal infection, infected bacterial ulcer, Buruli's ulcer, anthrax disease, diphtheria. Clinical features in a child with fever after travel are summarized in **Table 4**.

DIFFERENTIAL DIAGNOSIS

Malaria, traveler's diarrhea, and enteric fever are the most important causes of fever after travel. Malaria with onset within 6 months of return from travel accounts for 20–30% of cases, traveler's diarrhea for 10–20% cases, enteric fever (onset within 60 days of return) for 2–7% of cases, and dengue (within 14 days of return) for 5% of cases.[12,13] Respiratory tract infections are also a common cause and occur worldwide. Infections that are life-threatening or highly contagious should be excluded initially.

PRIMARY INVESTIGATIONS FOR RETURNED TRAVELERS WITH FEVER

A febrile traveler to a malaria-endemic area should be considered to have malaria until proven otherwise.

Table 3: Incubation period of different infections causing fever in returning travelers.

Infections	Incubation period (range)	Distribution
Incubation <14 days		
Chikungunya	2–4 days (1–14 days)	Tropical, subtropical areas
Dengue	4–8 days (3–14 days)	Tropical, subtropical areas
Encephalitis, arboviral (Japanese encephalitis, tick-borne encephalitis, West Nile virus and others)	3–14 days (1–20 days)	Specific agents vary by region
Enteric fever	7–18 days (3–60 days)	Especially in the Indian subcontinent
Acute HIV	10–28 days (10 days to 6 weeks)	Worldwide
Influenza	1–3 days	Worldwide
Legionellosis	5–6 days (2–10 days)	Widespread
Leptospirosis	7–12 days (2–26 days)	Widespread, most common in tropical areas
Malaria (*Plasmodium falciparum*)	6–30 days (98% onset within 3 months of travel)	Tropical, subtropical areas
Malaria (*P. vivax*)	8 days to 12 months (almost half have onset >30 days after completion of travel)	Widespread in tropics and subtropics
Spotted-fever rickettsiae	Few days to 2–3 weeks	Causative species vary by region
Zika virus infection	3–14 days	Widespread in Latin America, endemic in Africa, Southeast Asia, and Pacific Islands
Incubation 14 days to 6 weeks		
Encephalitis, arboviral; enteric fever; acute HIV; leptospirosis; malaria	See above incubation periods for relevant diseases	See above distribution for relevant diseases
Amebic liver abscess	Weeks to months	Most common in resource-poor countries
Hepatitis A	28–30 days (15–50 days)	Most common in resource-poor countries
Hepatitis E	26–42 days (2–9 weeks)	Widespread
Acute schistosomiasis (Katayama syndrome)	4–8 weeks	Most common in sub-Saharan Africa
Incubation >6 weeks		
Amebic liver abscess, hepatitis E, malaria, acute schistosomiasis	See above incubation periods for relevant diseases	See above distribution for relevant diseases
Hepatitis B	90 days (60–150 days)	Widespread
Leishmaniasis	2–10 months (10 days to years)	Asia, Africa, Latin America, southern Europe, and the Middle East
Tuberculosis	• *Primary*: Weeks • *Reactivation*: Years	Global distribution

Travel history should be cited on all laboratory requisitions.

- *Complete blood count with differential*: Lymphopenia in viral infections and typhoid, eosinophilia indicate parasitic or fungal infections, acute HIV, and severe sepsis.
- Malaria smears (thick and thin smear) ± dipstick antigen detection for at least three times over 24–48 hours (first sample should be taken immediately and second subsequent samples over 24–48 hours).
- Liver enzymes, serum urea, creatinine, electrolytes.
- Blood cultures (*Salmonella typhi* or *paratyphi*, and meningococcus are common agents of bacteremia).
- Urine routine and microscopic examination ± urine culture for proteinuria, hematuria in leptospirosis, and hemoglobinuria in malaria.

■ SPECIFIC TESTS BASED ON HISTORY AND EPIDEMIOLOGY

- Chest X-ray
- Ultrasonography of abdomen (hepatosplenomegaly)
- Stool culture (for *S. typhi* and *paratyphi*, Yersinia, Shigella, *Campylobacter jejuni*, *Escherichia coli*)
- Stool examination for ova and parasites (*Giardia*, *Cyclospora*, *E. histolytica*, and *Cryptosporidium*)

Table 4: Physical examination of the returned traveler with fever.

Physical examination	Diagnostic evaluation
Pulse rate	A pulse rate that is slow for the degree of fever (pulse-temperature dissociation) may suggest typhoid fever or a rickettsial disease
Rash	Skin rash may be present in many travel-related infections. The type of rash, its distribution, and time of appearance and disappearance are important in differentiating the cause of fever. Dengue, typhoid, rickettsia, measles, leptospirosis • *Rose spots* (clusters of 2–3 mm pink macules, usually on the trunk)—typhoid • *Maculopapular rash*—leptospirosis and many rickettsial diseases • *Petechiae* followed by purpura—dengue fever, meningococcemia, and viral hemorrhagic fevers
Eyes	Conjunctivitis (leptospirosis)

Lymphadenopathy	• *Generalized*:
	  – *Bacterial*: Brucellosis, leptospirosis, melioidosis, secondary syphilis, tuberculosis, enteric fever
	  – *Protozoal*: Toxoplasmosis
	  – *Viral*: Epstein-Barr virus, acute HIV cytomegalovirus, rubella, hepatitis B, measles, Lassa fever, dengue fever
	  – *Fungal*: Histoplasmosis, blastomycosis, coccidioidomycosis
	  – *Parasitic*: Visceral leishmaniasis
	  – *Noninfectious*: Malignancy, SLE, rheumatoid arthritis, sarcoidosis
	  – Drugs
	• *Localized*:
	  – *Bacterial*: Bartonellosis (cat scratch disease), plague, *Staphylococcus*, *Streptococcus*, tuberculosis, typhus, tularemia
	  – *Parasitic*: African trypanosomiasis, American trypanosomiasis, filariasis, and toxoplasmosis

Jaundice	Hepatitis A, B, E viral hemorrhagic fever (VHF), typhoid fever, leptospirosis, malaria
Abdominal pain	Enteric fever, amebic or pyogenic liver abscess
Hepatomegaly	Malaria, typhoid, dengue, viral hepatitis
Splenomegaly	Malaria, typhoid, mononucleosis, visceral leishmaniasis, brucellosis
Neurological finding	Altered mental status is a medical emergency and may occur in cerebral malaria or shock associated with hemorrhagic disease

- Dengue serology [NS1 antigen, immunoglobulin M (IgM), IgG]
- Polymerase chain reaction if viral hemorrhagic fever/arboviral disease is suspected
- Sample should be saved and paired with convalescent sera if no diagnosis is reached in the initial 10–14 days. Brucellosis, arboviral infection, and HIV serology can be done.

■ MANAGEMENT

Empirical treatment of a child with fever after travel should be started immediately without waiting for lab reports that includes broad-spectrum antibiotics and antimalarial for *Plasmodium falciparum* malaria if there is history of travel in a malaria-endemic area. Supportive therapies such as fluid resuscitation for severe diarrhea, inotropic support, and oxygen therapy should be initiated promptly.

Children with *Plasmodium falciparum* malaria who were initially well can deteriorate quickly and there may be coinfection with pneumonia or bacteremia, so treatment should be started without much delay.[14] As drug-resistant malaria is also a common problem, recent treatment guidelines or advice should be followed.

If the condition of a critically ill child deteriorates, immediate consultation with an infectious diseases specialist is indicated. After excluding malaria and septicemia in a well-appearing, clinically stable child, targeted therapy should be initiated according to his history, physical exam, and results of investigations.

Treatment of many of these infections will require a combined opinion from infectious disease physicians and microbiologists.

If enteric fever is suspected, antibiotic treatment should be started immediately with either oral azithromycin, cefixime fluoroquinolones, or intravenous ceftriaxone until antibiotic sensitivities are known. In Africa, most of the cases of enteric fever are fluoroquinolone (ciprofloxacin) sensitive but not in Asia.[15]

For rickettsial infections like scrub typhus, doxycycline or azithromycin is advised. Treatment of dengue fever is supportive including paracetamol and judicious fluid replacement. Public health services should be notified about travel-related infections so that epidemiological data can be collected and preventive and control measures can be started immediately. Approach to a child with fever after travel is summarized in **Flowchart 1**.

Flowchart 1: Approach to fever in a returning child traveler.[16]

Fever in returning traveler

- Initial risk assessment
- Assess qSOFA score (altered mentation, tachypnea' hypotension)
- Assess for signs of severe disease (cyanosis, meningism, peritonism, digital gangrene)
- Possible highly transmissible infection? If yes, isolate patient as appropriate

Possible severe disease, qSOFA score ≥2
- Resuscitate if patient in shock
- Perform blood cultures
- Obtain malaria films or RDT, if appropriate; treat severe malaria with parenteral artesunate, followed by ACT
- Consider empirical antibiotic treatment, taking into account possible pathogens and likely AMR patterns
- History, examination, and investigations (as for qSOFA score <2)
- Consider causes of life-threatening tropical infections, as well as cosmopolitan causes of sepsis
- Assess risk of highly transmissible infection

Uncomplicated disease (qSOFA score <2 and no signs of severe disease)
- *History*: Travel, fever onset, symptoms, possible exposures
- *Examination*: Rash, jaundice, altered mentation, neck stiffness, cellulitis, abdominal tenderness, pulmonary consolidation, eschar, lymphadenopathy, genital sores, eye signs
- *Risk assessment*:
  - Suspected life-threatening tropical infection?
  - Suspected highly transmissible infection?
  - Isolate patient as appropriate
- *Investigations*: CBC, biochemical studies (e.g. LFTs and creatinine), C-reactive protein, blood cultures, chest film, urine microscopy and culture, baseline serologic tests, whole-blood EDTA sample for PCR, saving of serum for later testing, and specific investigations for focal disease; RDTs for diseases endemic in the visited areas (e.g. dengue, leptospirosis, and rickettsioses for Southeast Asia)

Urgent hospitalization
If qSOFA score ≥2, consider ICU care, If highly transmissible disease suspected, isolate patient as appropriate

A. Fever with respiratory symptoms

Fever within 4 days after returned from community where an outbreak of influenza occurred
- Test for influenza with rapid test or PCR
- Treat with neuraminidase inhibitor
- Isolate at home (or in hospital, if avian influenza suspected)

Consolidation on X-ray or clinical pneumonia
- If bacterial pneumonia suspected, treat as community-acquired pneumonia
- Consider highly transmissible infections (influenza, tuberculosis, MERS CoV, measles)
- Consider unusual infections with pulmonary involvement (Q fever, psittacosis, leptospirosis, Katayama fever, scrub typhus, melioidosis)
- If eosinophilia, consider filariasis, strongyloidiasis, fungal infections

B. Suspected malaria

Obtain thick and thin blood films or RDT

Plasmodium falciparum malaria

P. vivax, P. ovale, P. malariae, or *P. knowlesi* malaria

- Uncomplicated falciparum malaria
- Treat with ACT
- Consider hospitalization for 24 hours

- Uncomplicated nonfalciparum malaria
- Treat with ACT or chloroquine, with or without primaquine

C. Fever with jaundice
- Rule out possible life-threatening infections (leptospirosis, severe malaria, viral hemorrhage fevers, yellow fever, severe dengue, Carrión's disease)
- Consider acute viral hepatitis (hepatitis A, B, C, E), CMV, EBV (serologic tests)
- Consider acute cholangitis—stones, liver flukes (ultrasound, blood cultures, stool examination)

D. Fever with abdominal pain/tenderness (without diarrhea)
- *Consider*: Cosmopolitan causes (e.g. appendicitis, urinary tract infection, cholecystitis, pancreatitis)
- Enteric fever (blood culture) giardiasis (stool microscopy, Ag detection, PCR); treat with tinidazole or metronidazole
- Acute cholangitis—stones, liver flukes (ultrasound, blood cultures, stool examination)
- Liver abscess—pyogenic or amebic (blood cultures, ultrasound, serologic tests)

F. Undifferentiated nonmalarial fever
- *Consider*: Cosmopolitan causes (e.g. urinary tract infection, EBV, viral URTI, cellulitis, abscesses)
- Common tropical or subtropical causes [e.g. dengue, rickettsial infections, leptospirosis, chikungunya, Zika virus (all diagnosed on serologic tests, Ag detection, or PCR) and enteric fever (blood cultures)]
- Consider empirical antibiotics (doxycycline or azithromycin) to cover rickettsia and leptospirosis

Contd...

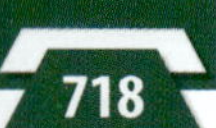

Contd...

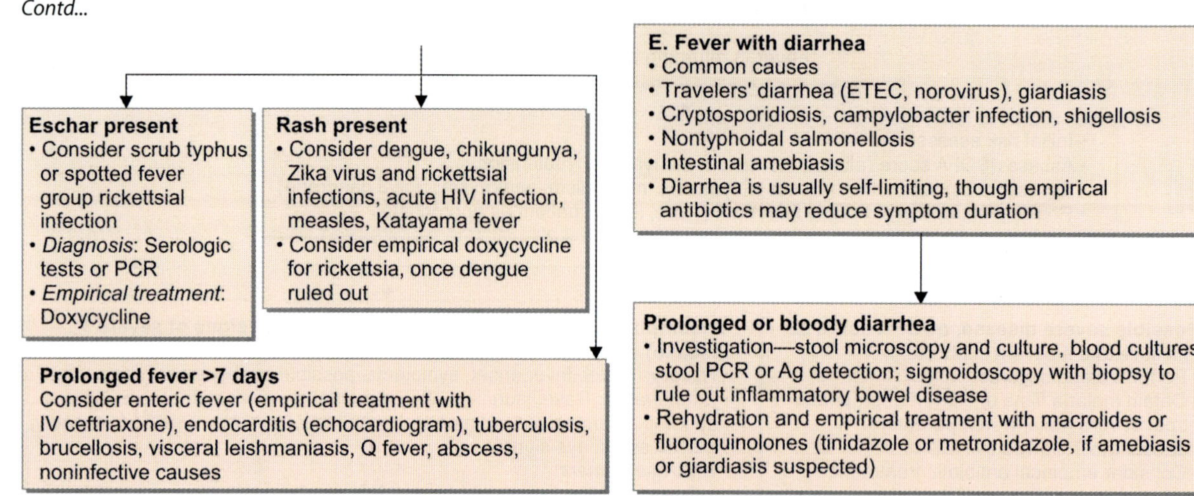

(ACT: artemisinin-based combination treatment; AMR: antimicrobial resistance; CBC: complete blood count; CMV: cytomegalovirus; EBV: Epstein-Barr virus; EDTA: ethylenediaminetetraacetic acid; ETEC: enteropathogenic *Escherichia coli*; HIV: human immunodeficiency virus; LFT: liver function test; MERS-CoV: Middle-East respiratory syndrome-coronavirus; PCR: polymerase chain reaction; qSOFA: quick Sepsis-related Organ Failure Assessment; RDT: rapid diagnostic test; URTI: upper respiratory tract infection)

Source: Adapted from Thwaites GE, Day PJ. Approach to fever in the returning traveler. N Engl J Med. 2017;376:548-60.

Parents and adolescent travelers should be educated about all the available measures to prevent ill health on future travel. Education should include advise related to food and drink hygiene, safe sex, available vaccines, malaria prophylaxis, importance of compliance, and avoidance of mosquito/insect bites.

■ REFERENCES

1. United Nations World Tourism Organization. World tourism barometer and statistical annex (2019). [online] Available from: http://www2.unwto.org/publication/unwto-world-tourism-barometer-and-statistical-annex-january-2019. [Last accessed on November, 2019].

2. World Tourism Organization. UNWTO Tourism Towards 2030: Global Overview. Republic of Korea.

3. Wilson ME, Freedman DO. Etiology of travel-related fever. Curr Opin Infect Dis. 2007;20:449-53.

4. Boggild AK, Geduld J, Libman M, et al. Travel-acquired infections and illnesses in Canadians: surveillance report from CanTravNet surveillance data, 2009–2011. Open Med. 2014; 8:e20-e32.

5. Brunette GW, Nemh JB. CDC Yellow Book 2020: Health Information for International Travel. UK: Oxford University Press; 2019.

6. Wilson ME, Weld LH, Boggild A, et al. GeoSentinel Surveillance Network. Fever in returned travelers: results from GeoSentinel surveillance network. Clin Infect Dis. 2007;44:1560-8.

7. Hagmann S, Neugebauer R, Schwartz E, et al. Illness in children after international travel: analysis from the GeoSentinel Surveillance Network 2009. Pediatrics. 2010;125:e1072-80.

8. Herbinger KH, Drerup L, Alberer M, et al. Spectrum of imported infectious diseases among children and adolescents returning from the tropics and subtropics. J Trav Med. 2012;19:150-7.

9. Angell SY, Cetron MS. Health disparities among travelers visiting friends and relatives abroad. Ann Intern Med. 2005; 142:67-72.

10. Bacaner N, Stauffer B, Boulware DR, et al. Travel medicine considerations for North American immigrants visiting friends and relatives. JAMA. 2004;291:2856-64.

11. Singer M, Deutschman CS, Seymour CW, et al. The third international consensus definitions for sepsis and septic shock (Sepsis-3). JAMA. 2016;315:801-10.

12. Public Health Agency of Canada, Committee to Advise on Tropical Medicine and Travel (CATMAT). Fever in the returning international traveller: Initial assessment guidelines. Can Commun Dis Rep 2011;37(ACS-3). [online] Available from: https://www.canada.ca/content/dam/phac-aspc/migration/phacaspc/publicat/ccdrrmtc/11vol37/acs-3/pdf/returningtravellerfever-fievrevoyageurderetour-eng.pdf. [Last accessed on April, 2018].

13. West NS, Riordan FA. Fever in returned travellers: a prospective review of hospital admissions for a 2(1/2) year period. Arch Dis Child. 2003;88(5):432-4.

14. Public Health Agency of Canada. Committee to Advise on Tropical Medicine and Travel (CATMAT). Canadian Recommendations for the Prevention and Treatment of Malaria: An Advisory Committee Statement, 2014. [online] Available from: http://publications.gc.ca/collections/collection_2014/aspc-phac/HP40-102-2014-eng.pdf. [Last accessed on April, 2019].

15. Bell DJ. Fever in the returning traveller. JR Coll Physicians Edinb. 2012;42(1):43-6.

16. Thwaites GE, Day PJ. Approach to fever in the returning traveler. N Engl J Med. 2017;376:548-60.

Legal Issues in Medical Tourism

Satish Tiwari, Mukul Tiwari

■ INTRODUCTION

Medical tourism is "Traveling by patients/medical service recipients from one institution, jurisdiction or country to another institution, jurisdiction or country where they can obtain, without legal hindrances, the kind of medical procedures and innovative treatments they desire; mostly, at a lower cost but, in some cases, at a higher cost, for better results."

The medical tourist gets doubly benefited as they can enjoy the holiday and sightseeing in the visiting country. The three basic aspects of medical tourism consist of—hospital/health services, hotels, and travel/leisure. The attractive policies and/or the correct marketing strategies give this emerging industry significant opportunity for economic growth and infrastructure development for involved countries and nations.

■ INCIDENCE OF MEDICAL TOURISM

Around 11 million US citizens in 2016 visited other countries in search of economic healthcare.[1] In the next decade, this figure will grow by up to 25% every year according to report by Visa and Oxford Economics. Presently, there are about 50 countries offering these kinds of services.

■ HOW MEDICAL TOURISM EVOLVED?

Medical tourism concept is not new to the society or community. People have traveled to other countries or destinations since ancient times for various reasons to seek medical treatments and health-related purposes. The ancient Greeks and Egyptians traveled to health resorts in the Mediterranean for purification and spiritual healing.[2] The first recorded case of medical tourism describes Greek pilgrims traveling from the Mediterranean Sea to Epidaurus, a territory in the Sardonic Gulf also known as sanctuary of Asclepius, i.e. the healing God.

Since 15th and 16th centuries, India has enjoyed a rich history of providing yoga instruction so also Ayurveda healing to patients from different parts of the world. Roman British patients traveled to a reservoir around hot springs at Bath for healing and rejuvenation. Europeans traveled to spas at the end of 18th century in Germany and the Nile in Africa, in the hope that they would obtain relief from their disabling conditions, such as tuberculosis, gouts, bronchitis, or liver diseases. Especially in Europe, over the years, well-to-do people have traveled to spas to "take the waters" for cure of various illnesses.[3]

The 20th century is known for patients beginning to travel in search for alternative forms of treatment, e.g. Hoxsey Clinic, Tijuana, Mexico; Bumrungrad International Hospital and Bangkok International Hospital, Asia.

Internationally promoted centers of excellence by the US in 21st century include world-renowned Cleveland Clinic, Mayo Clinic, University of Pittsburgh Transplant Center, MD Anderson Cancer Centers, etc. This attracted "cash paying" patients from around the world. Recently, less-developed countries have also developed expertise, infrastructure, and facilities for management of complicated medical disorders to a level comparable with that of developed countries. Now, these countries also have attractive programs and policies at their place and have implemented unique marketing strategies that encourage the patients to avail the facilities of medical tourism.

■ TYPES OF MEDICAL TOURISM[4]

Many specialty markets are recognized within medical tourism so also there are many specialties which are emerging as significant businesses. One of the subspecialties is travel (Health tourism) to a recuperative climate with natural therapeutic resources. This tourism business mainly provides yoga, massages and traditional Ayurvedic medicine and spa resorts.

Another common specialty is Fertility tourism. The main reasons for this specialty are legal regulation in the home country and lower price. Treatment procedures in this specialty are in vitro fertilization and donor insemination. There may be other legal regulations which contribute for the increasing trend in this field. The residents of People's Republic of China seek fertility tourism to circumvent the one-child norm policy in their own country. Many countries have unrestricted numbers of embryos transferred. India is one of the main destinations for surrogacy. Indian surrogates are popular worldwide because of the relatively low cost and easier regulatory norms for those who are seeking infertility treatments. The standards of Indian infertility clinics have gradually improved and almost match with those of the west. They have become more competitive, as far as pricing is concerned, and in the availability of surrogate mothers. Indian hospitals charge approximately between $10,000 and $28,000 for the complete package including fertilization, the surrogate's fee, and delivery of the baby at a hospital. The total costs including that of flight tickets, medical procedures, and hotels come to roughly a third of the price compared with the similar procedure in the UK. Thus, surrogacy treatment in India is economical along with added advantages of flexible rules and regulations. In 2008, the Supreme Court of India, in the Manji's case, has held that commercial surrogacy is permitted and accepted in India. This has increased international confidence in Indian infertility treatments worldwide.

Russian legislations make Russia an attractive destination for "reproductive tourists." These countries lack many advanced techniques. Couples interested visit these countries for oocyte donation, because of advanced age or marital status, and for facilities of surrogacy. In Russia, commercial surrogacy service is not unlawful or illegal.

Surrogate mothers in the US are sought by couples seeking Green Card. The child born by such procedure can get citizenship in the US, and at 21 years of age can apply for Green Cards for the parents.

Suicide tourism, although at a very small scale, is yet another branch of medical tourism. Only a few countries are providing this service, mainly Netherlands, Switzerland, etc. This practice, much more so than the others, is tightly structured by policy.

■ INDIA'S MEDICAL TOURISM

Indian medical tourism industry has currently (in 2019) grown by nearly 18% of the global medical tourism market share which is expected to be 20% by 2020 and worth 9 billion. It is growing year on year.[5]

India is ranked as one of the low-cost, top medical tourism destinations in the world. The annual growth rate of India's medical tourism sector is about 25–30%. The main advantages are widespread use of English, economic packages, the state-of-the-art technologies, and an increasing compliance to international quality standards. Poor infrastructure of the country is still a big hurdle in the growth of medical tourism. The Indian government is trying to deal with these issues. The treatment packages in India cost around a fifth of the price of comparable treatment in America or Britain. The main treatments for which tourists come to India are alternative medicine, cardiac bypass, bone marrow transplant, hip replacement, eye surgery, etc.

Patients from many surrounding countries such as Pakistan, Bangladesh, Myanmar, and central Asia having less-developed healthcare systems are visiting India for medical facilities. Some come even from further afield countries such as Africa and the Middle East. India is also becoming popular with Americans, Canadians, and Europeans for the cost-effective medical treatment.

In India, the popular treatments include those for fertility, organ transplants, orthopedic, cardiac and oncology problems, etc. According to the Medical Tourism Resource Guide, a heart valve is worth about $15,000 versus $150,000 in the US. Hospitals such as Apollo and Fortis Healthcare have made their mark for medical tourism in international markets. The city of Chennai getting about 45% of health tourists from abroad and 30–40% of domestic health tourists is unofficially India's Health Capital.

The Ministry of Tourism (MoT), India is planning schemes to cover Joint Commission International (JCI) and extend its Market Development Assistance (MDA) and National Accreditation Board of Hospitals (NABH)-certified hospitals. A policy decision to this effect is likely to be soon in near future.

The Paradox in India

India is supposed to be one of the best medical tourism destinations for many developing Third World countries. But, unfortunately many senior politicians, sports, and film personalities probably have no faith in Indian health services. Paradoxically, they are running after the medical services in western countries and thus bringing bad name, defamation, or feeling of inferiority in the minds of people of India. We feel that good sense shall prevail in the minds of these role models, so that the medical professionals practicing in India will get due respect, credibility, and recognition. It is high time that we start promoting the world-class medical care facilities and services available in India.

RISKS IN MEDICAL TOURISM[6]

Medical tourism carries the following risks:

- Communication may be a problem. In destination country, because of language barriers, the visitor and care givers may not be able to communicate effectively leading to errors and misunderstanding.
- Southeastern countries such as India, Malaysia, or Thailand may impose upon the tourist from western hemisphere some infections not experienced by them in their host country, and the tourists may not have enough immunity in their body system to deal with such infections, e.g. gastrointestinal diseases such as Hepatitis A, amoebic dysentery, paratyphoid, mosquito-transmitted diseases, influenza, and tuberculosis. These can be contracted by tourists, resulting in complicated prognosis while they are availing of the treatment. However, at the same time, doctors in southeastern countries may be more open to recognizing and diagnosing these infections.
- There is also concern that medical tourists are at risk of exposure to blood-borne infection due to inadequate blood collection, screening, and storage protocols in destination countries. Persons visiting for organ transplantation specially may face higher rates of severe infections, and there may be complications because of less stringent screening protocols in destination countries.
- The concern that medical tourists may transmit infections to their home countries. An example is the spread of New Delhi metallo-beta-lactamase 1 (NDM 1) to the home countries of patients who had been treated abroad.
- The quality of medical treatment and postoperative care may vary between the developing and the developed world, between the hospitals and countries, and may be different from US or European standards. The WHO acknowledged that there are differences in healthcare provider standards around the world; and in 2004, it launched the World Alliance for Patient Safety. This body helps hospitals and governments around the world set up patient safety policies and practices which can be very useful when providing medical tourism services.
- Traveling long distances can increase the risk of postoperative complications. Decreased mobility in long-distance flights with cramped seating is a risk factor for venous thrombosis or pulmonary embolus. This phenomenon is also known as "economy class syndrome."
- The quality of medication is also an issue. In many countries where corruption is rampant and regulations are lax, medicines may be of poor quality and counterfeit.
- Post-treatment complications are another issue; researchers found that in Oman at least 15% patients who had taken treatment abroad experienced post-treatment complications. About 37% of members had encountered patients with complications in a survey of the British Association of Plastic, Reconstructive and Aesthetic Surgery.

LEGAL ISSUES IN MEDICAL TOURISM

- In the evolving stage of medical tourism, many issues are not addressed adequately. Health facilities in a country may lack an adequate complaints policy. Hence, many complaints made by dissatisfied patients may not be appropriately and fairly dealt with.
- In developing countries, the limited and uncertain nature of litigation cover may be responsible for slow uptake of medical tourism there. Some countries have established and attractive medical tourism destinations. These countries provide some form of legal remedies for medical malpractice. These remedies may be insufficient for the issues related to medical tourists. There may not be covered sufficiently by personal insurance. Malpractice lawsuits might be unable to cover compensation in many cases.
- Hospitals and/or doctors in many countries may not be able to pay the financial damages awarded by a court to a patient as they may not possess appropriate medical indemnity or insurance cover. Newer insurance policies are now available for the patient in such situation or circumstances.
- The other issues and gray area include the illegal purchase of organs and tissues for donation or transplantation in some countries such as India and China. What is the liability of the medical tourists in cases of any such racket apprehended by police, who have received organ donation from a health facility which has been involved?

ETHICAL ISSUES IN MEDICAL TOURISM

- There are many ethical issues with medical tourism. It is debated that the medical tourism is only for rich people and will lead to a divide between haves and have nots. In 2008, it was observed in Thailand that doctors have become so preoccupied with foreigners that their own patients are neglected. In India also, the industry's tremendous growth may not be a positive development for the poor who do not directly benefit from it. Should the Indian government create policies when thousands of Indians die every year from preventable illnesses? Should the government use public funds to assist private hospitals that are serving or catering predominantly to the demands of the rich and foreign patients? A concept of cosmopolitan nationalism must guide solutions to these dilemmas. In India, if basic health is improved and provided to all then only medical tourism will truly become an ethical success.

- A striking example of "health for rich" India is a leading hospital in New Delhi. The hospital was built in 1996 on 15 acres of land leased by the Delhi government. Millions were invested in the construction of the hospital. Tax waiver and duty waivers were provided on import of equipment. The agreement was there that the hospital would reserve one-third of its beds for the treatment of poor patients free of cost. Only 2% patients in this hospital in 1999–2000 were treated free, but most of these were staff, bureaucrats, and politicians or their relatives.
- Stem cell treatments facilities or services are often criticized for misinformation, fraud, lack of scientific rationale, and patient safety. There is an urgent need to harness these technologies which are costly and are of unproven benefits. There is a need to differentiate medical innovations which are acceptable to most of us so as to prevent patient exploitation.
- There is a need for systematic legal frameworks for medical tourism. There may be different regulations in different countries but in some countries the legal cover is very deficient. The countries which are taking more risks with healthcare liability are attracting more medical tourists. Many developed countries, such as United States, have not been able to provide services of medical tourism because of increased legal responsibility and policy.
- There are many ethical issues in reproductive (abortions and *in vitro* fertilization) and suicide tourism. Consumers often travel to another jurisdiction for reproductive tourism to receive a low-cost service that cannot be provided at home. Abortions and in vitro fertilization can be two specific practices that can have many ethical objections. This is also true for suicide tourism. These issues are surrounding the rights of the individual as well as accompanying consumer.
- A consumer's rights are important issues in reproductive and suicide tourism. Consumers must consider their rights, and they may seek treatment in alternative locations. This could be true for practices or procedures such as abortions, in vitro fertilization, as well as euthanasia. Thus, a consumer's rights may play a part in decisions made for the medical tourism product.
- There have been allegations of illegal purchase of organs and tissues for transplantation in many countries including India and China prior to 2007.

INTERNATIONAL HEALTHCARE ACCREDITATIONS[7]

As far as healthcare is concerned, the standards are important; there are many parallel issues around medical tourism, international healthcare innovations, accreditation, technical advances, evidence-based medicine, and quality assurance.

The best known accreditation group in USA is the JCI. Their role is to inspect and accredit medical tourism facilities outside USA. They are known veritable source for American medical tourists. Many international medical tourism facilities seek JCI accreditation to attract American patients.

The Trent International Accreditation Scheme is operational in the UK and Hong Kong in this field. The different international healthcare accreditation schemes vary in quality, size, cost, intent and the skill and intensity of their marketing. They also vary in terms of cost to the hospitals and healthcare institutions making use of them. Many hospitals are trying for dual accreditation, JCI to cover US patients and Trent for British and European clientele.

Other relevant organizations include:
- The "SOFIHA" (Society for International Healthcare Accreditation)
- A US-based nonprofit organization: HealthCare Tourism International accredits the nonclinical aspects of health tourism such as language issues, business practices, and prevention of false or misleading advertising
- The "UKAF" (United Kingdom Accreditation Forum)
- The "IMTA" (International Medical Travel Association is based in Singapore)
- Medical Tourism Association is the second nonprofit association in the industry which focuses on transparency in quality and pricing.

CONCLUSION

The medical tourism is a relatively new kind of medical business that is becoming more and more popular worldwide. There is possibility of exponential increase in this business in future. It helps in increasing a country's prosperity in many ways. These services have a very competitive field and the competition is likely to increase many a folds in future. India also has an emerging medical tourism industry. But at present the volume of business coming to India is less as compared to some other countries. India will have to make its medical and tourism infrastructure and marketing better if we have to really benefit from this phenomenon. The services should be cost effective and time saving and the policies more tourists friendly. The countries which continually analyze in this field and those who adapt better policies will prosper in this emerging medical tourism industry.

■ REFERENCES

1. Stephano RM. Top 10 Medical Tourism Destinations in the World. www.medicaltourismmag.com/article/top-10-medical-tourism-destinations-world. [Last accessed on November, 2019].
2. Kazen T. Purification and spiritual healing. https://www.academia.edu/34900085/13_Purification_Ritual_in_the_Ancient_Mediterranean_World._ [Last accessed on November, 2019].
3. Tiwari M. Legal issues in Medical Tourism. J of Indian Med Legal and Ethics Asso. 2014;2(4):124-7.
4. Pocock NS, Phua KH. Medical tourism and policy implications for health systems: a conceptual framework from a comparative study of Thailand, Singapore and Malaysia. Global Health. 2011;7:12.
5. Sultana S, Haque A, Momen A, et al. Factors affecting the attractiveness of medical tourism destination: an empirical study on India. Iran J Public Health. 2014;43(7):867-76.
6. Crooks VA, Turner L, Cohen IG, et al. Ethical and legal implications of the risks of medical tourism for patients: a qualitative study of Canadian health and safety. BMJ Open. 2013;3(2):e002302.
7. Wikipedia. List of International Healthcare Accreditation Organizations. https://en.wikipedia.org/wiki/List_of_international_healthcare_accreditation_organizations. [Last accessed on November, 2019].

Swati Kalra, Bakul Jayant Parekh

BACKGROUND

Rational use of drugs is one of the key factors which determines the efficiency of a good healthcare delivery system. Various governing bodies worldwide have been putting in a lot of efforts to keep this drug prescribing practice as much rational and scientific as possible, for which they have adopted National Medicine Policies and Essential drug programs. Despite these efforts, irrational drug prescription practices are becoming a global threat for individuals and society worldwide.[1] The World Health Organization (WHO) data suggests that governing bodies in tropical countries have not been able to develop strict guidelines and methods to keep a check on prescription behavior of practitioners in their regions; therefore, more than half of all medicines prescribed, dispensed, or sold in these regions are inappropriate.[2] This irrational behavior and lack of organized drug policy ultimately imposes a huge financial burden on developing countries because of the limited resources and poor socioeconomic status.[3] Since a family physician is the one who prescribes medications in a healthcare system and pharmacist is the one who dispenses these medications, prescription behavior of physicians and pharmacists becomes the key factor in determining the healthcare expenditure of the users.

INTRODUCTION

Prescription is a paper or electronic document issued by a licensed medical practitioner detailing the medicine or medicines to be dispensed for an individually named patient. Prescription writing is a science, an art, and a basic skill that every prescriber needs to learn as it is an essential prerequisite of a good healthcare delivery system. **Table 1** elaborates upon the core parts of prescription.

Inappropriate and unethical prescription practices may lead to ineffective treatment, an increased risk of adverse effects, prolongation of treatment, and prolonged hospital stay, thereby increasing the overall cost of healthcare expenditure. This also creates a sense of distrust among patients. It has been observed that among the prescribed medications, almost half are prescribed, dispensed, or sold inappropriately and out of those prescribed appropriately, only 50% take them correctly. Polypharmacy, overuse of antibiotics, prescription of

	Table 1: Core components of prescription.	
1.	Prescriber information	Name, address, qualification, telephone number, and license number
2.	Patient information	Full name, address, weight, and age
3.	Date	Necessary for record keeping
4.	Superscription	Contains the heading Rx
5.	Subscription	Gives specific directions for the pharmacist (right) on how to compound the medication
6.	Inscription	Body of the prescription which provides the names and quantities of the main ingredients of the prescription along with the dose and dosage form, such as tablet, suspension, capsule, syrup
7.	Signatura	Gives instructions to the patients on how, how much, how long, and when the medicine is to be taken
8.	Prescriber signature	It is the legal requirement of prescription that it should contain signature of the prescriber

unnecessary injectables, inadequate doses of prescribed medications, nonadherence to clinical guidelines, and self-medications are some of the commonly observed irrational prescription behaviors.[4] Such malpractice may result in serious morbidity and mortality in addition to increasing the expenditure on healthcare services. This increased economic burden leads to reduction in the quality of drug therapy, wastage of resources, increased treatment cost, increased risk for adverse drug reactions, and emergence of drug resistance.

Although there are no strict guidelines, the WHO has advocated a six-step approach to prescription writing which suggests that a physician should evaluate and clearly define the patient's problem; specify the therapeutic objective; select the appropriate drug therapy; initiate therapy with appropriate details; give information, instructions, and warnings; and evaluate therapy regularly by monitoring outcomes following initiation of treatment. A physician should also consider the cost of therapy and try to use electronic prescriptions in order to avoid prescription errors.[5] It is mandatory for the physicians to follow the guidelines for prescription writing to maintain a good-quality prescription for patient benefit.[5,6] The WHO has suggested certain indicators to assess the quality of an ideal prescription as shown in **Table 2**.[7] Several other indicators have now been added in the last 10 years; however, there is no consensus on the standard for prescription quality indicators worldwide.

There is a lot of data to suggest that many a times, patients are not prescribed appropriate treatment indicated for their condition. There are many reasons which have been identified behind such irrational practice including the level of knowledge, personal interests of

Table 2: The WHO prescribing indicators and recommended reference values.

The WHO prescribing indicator	Reference value
Average number of medicines per encounter	<2
Percentage of medicines prescribed by generic name	100%
Percentage of encounters with an antibiotic prescribed	<30%
Percentage of encounters with an injection prescribed	<20%
Percentage of medicines prescribed from an essential medicines list or formulary	100%

Source: Harvard Medical School and Harvard Pilgrim Health, World Health Organization. (2006). Using indicators to measure country pharmaceutical situations Fact Book on WHO Level I and Level II monitoring indicators. [online] Available from: http://apps.who.int/medicinedocs/index/assoc/s14101e/s14101e.pdf. [Last accessed on December, 2019].

physicians, and hospital drug policies. This may also lead to overuse and misuse of pharmaceutical products. The overall impact of this is ultimately the loss of health and quality of life of patients and society and the increase of healthcare expenditure. Thus, for health and economic reasons, it is important to follow the recommended optimal and established drug prescription guidelines.[8]

Other important issue to be addressed while analyzing the quality of prescription is related to the various errors identified while writing a prescription. These errors are classified into two types—error of omission and error of commission. Error of omission is the missing of essential information and error of commission involves wrongly written information on prescription. Omission errors are seen in the government sector prescriptions which could be attributed to huge patient load and scarcity of manpower, whereas commission errors are commonly seen in the private hospital prescriptions, the reason of which could be quackery and lack of knowledge.

Such errors may certainly lead to major consequences more so in pediatric patients as pediatric age group is among the most vulnerable population prone to adverse effects of medications due to different pharmacodynamic and pharmacokinetics, making them more susceptible to various adverse drug reactions.[9]

■ FACTORS INFLUENCING PRESCRIPTION BEHAVIOR

Physicians are the primary decision makers on healthcare resources. They serve as a common link between the healthcare-providing facilities and consumers. Therefore, it is very important to have an understanding of factors which influences their decision-making. Therefore, researchers are trying to analyze and understand the factors which influence physician prescribing decisions and practice. It has been observed that a physician's prescribing pattern is a result of a series of complex factors.[10] Some of the factors are fixed as they cannot be modified that include the age and sex of the treating doctor or the patient, the socioeconomic characteristics of the practicing area, or the reimbursement status of therapy. On the other hand, there are factors which can be influenced and can affect the prescribing behavior of physicians. These include the level of qualification of physician, i.e. an undergraduate, a postgraduate, or a consultant, and the experience of the physician, various social factors, influence of pharmaceutical marketing of drugs, the number of practitioners in a practice, and others such as the healthcare sector in which they are working and patient requirements.[11] The prescribing decision is therefore a result of a multitude of intertwined factors. Factors influencing prescribers' decisions are the most important input to develop practice guidelines, healthcare policy, and to devise a regulation for the pharmaceutical market.

Pharmaceutical marketing of drugs is an important factor which influences the choice of drugs to be prescribed among the armamentarium of available brands. The prescription behavior of physicians may be affected by factors such as promotional tools and drug samples. Although the government has provided a list of certain essential drugs which should be prescribed by generic names in government sector but in private sector, this brand selection depends on how the salesperson promote their brands. Physician prescription behavior is the real thought for all the pharmaceutical organizations. Drug advertising methodologies are outlined and executed on the premise of the physician prescription behavior toward the drug. Even though the products are being bought by the patients for treating an infected situation, the choice of what item that individual should take is guided by the physician.[12]

The variation in physician practice brings about a difference in expenditure in the health sector and patient outcomes.[13] Pharmaceutical companies usually do face-to-face detailing, provide medicine samples, provide written evidence, organize meetings, organize medicine launches, sponsor continuous medical education, and provide gifts. Physicians' involvement in the hospital decision-making process and development of hospital-specific guidelines influence their prescribing decision.

While prescribing medications, prescribers decide the indication of the medicine based on the certain criteria such as patients' condition including the sign and symptoms, comorbid conditions, need for hospitalization, and surrounding environment of workplace. In developing countries, the choice of medications is also affected by the financial condition of the patient.[14,15]

Incomplete clinical pictures influence prescribers to change their prescribing decision. The clinical effectiveness and safety of pharmaceuticals are often considered to achieve the goal of therapy and enhance the patient compliance. Previous exposure of prescribers to the medicine and its past clinical success have a big role in altering prescribing decision. It was shown that the use of diagnostic procedures for identification of the clinical condition and valid clinical guidelines fosters the rational prescribing effectively.[14]

A number of factors associated with the working and external environment influence prescribing decision of physicians. It is a well-known fact that learning organizations and organizational structures increase the performance of employees.[16] Availability of diagnostic and pharmaceutical resources in the organization could also influence the prescribing decision of physicians. Pharmaceutical companies try to influence the prescribing decision of prescribers by creating a mutual benefit-based relationship such as funding for CME (continuing medical education), personal gifts, and certain travel allowances.[17]

The physicians' attributes which include the clinical experience, speciality, continuous professional development, and practice decision is another important factor which affects the prescription writing behavior of prescriber. The exposure of physicians for different class of medicines and patient outcome are expected to increase with increased clinical experience and years of service.[18,19] Although medical reference books and scientific literatures have a large theoretical importance, colleagues, clinical meetings, and medical representatives are key sources of information used to prescribe new medicines. Information from pharmaceutical companies increases awareness on available medicines in the market. However, this information may turn physicians to high cost prescribers with low prescription quality practitioners. Physicians' interest in a particular area and involvement in clinical trial are also important factors for new medicine prescribing.[20]

Patient/caregiver-related factors include the sociodemographic status, knowledge of patient about medicines, expectation, and request to a particular treatment. The patient's sociodemographics such as age, sex, and social status have to be considered for better quality of care. The knowledge of the patient on pharmaceutical products makes the patient request for a specific medication and alters patient expectations.[21] A patient's pressure on physicians may lead to unnecessary prescribing and referral; but the transition from the old paternalistic care to engagement of patients in decision-making has increased the role of patients in decision-making. Moreover, self-medication practice toward antibiotics has made physicians to let the patient continue the unnecessary antibiotics to prevent resistance or to change the regimen to the more potent medicine due to the perception of resistance.[22]

Socioeconomic factors such as cost, insurance, and financial incentives also affect the decision-making of prescribers. Insurance has been found to influence the selection of type and quantity of healthcare utilization and also improve health as insured patients consume more healthcare service than uninsured patients with a lower expenditure.[23] The financial incentives for the prescriber are motives that influence the prescribing behavior and could increase induced demand.[22]

Overall, a physician's personal characteristics and choices, pharmaceutical industries' marketing and promotion strategies for a specific drug are certainly few of the most important factors which influence the prescribing decision of practitioners. Unfortunately, prescription by a physician is geared not only for a patient's benefit, but also toward a physician's interest. There is a need to formulate guidelines which are valid and reliable so as to keep a check on the factors which are influencing the healthcare providers negatively and restricting them from providing appropriate treatment to the consumers.

■ CONCLUSION

In this era of global poor prescription habits, prescription pattern-monitoring studies (PPMS) may be considered as a good resort to keep a check on extent and profile of drug use, trends, quality of drugs, and compliance with regional, state, or national guidelines such as standard treatment guidelines, usage of drugs from essential medicine list, and use of generic drugs. These PPM studies can provide a bridge between areas such as rational use of drugs, pharmacovigilance, evidence-based medicine, pharmacoeconomics, and pharmacogenetics.[24] The state-level data generated from such studies can serve to keep a check on the prescription behavior of physicians and thereby can help to promote rational use of drugs in developing countries.

■ REFERENCES

1. Sadigh-Rad L, Majdi L, Javaezi M, et al. Comparison of prescribing indicators of academic versus non-academic specialist physicians in Urmia, Iran. J Res Pharm Pract. 2015;4(2):45-50.
2. World Health Organization. World medicines situation report 2011. [online] Available from: http://apps.who.int/medicinedocs/documents/s20054en/s20054en.pdf. [Last accessed on December, 2019].
3. Kshirsagar MJ, Langade D, Patil S, et al. Prescribing patterns among medical practitioners in Pune, India. Bull World Health Organ. 1998;76(3):271-5.
4. Mohammad IS, Khan HMS, Akhtar N, et al. Significance of prescription elements and reasons of prescription errors in South Punjab, Pakistan. World Applied Sciences Journal. 2015; 33(4):668-72.
5. Pollock M, Bazaldua OV, Dobbie AE. Appropriate prescribing of medications: an eight-step approach. Am Fam Phys. 2007; 75(2):231-6.
6. Meyer TA. Improving the quality of the order-writing process for inpatient orders and outpatient prescriptions. Am J Health Syst Pharm. 2000;57(Suppl 4):S18-22.
7. Harvard Medical School and Harvard Pilgrim Health, World Health Organization (2006). Using indicators to measure country pharmaceutical situations Fact Book on WHO Level I and Level II monitoring indicators. [online] Available from: http://apps.who.int/medicinedocs/index/assoc/s14101e/s14101e.pdf. [Last accessed on December, 2019].
8. O'Mahony D, Gallagher PF. Inappropriate prescribing in the older population: need for new criteria. Age Ageing. 2008;37(2): 138-41.
9. Ginsberg G, Hattis D, Sonawane B, et al. Evaluation of child/adult pharmacokinetic differences from a database derived from the therapeutic drug literature. Toxicol Sci. 2002;66(2): 185-200.
10. Davari M, Khorasani E, Tigabu BM. Factors influencing prescribing decisions of physicians: a review. Ethiop J Health Sci. 2018;28(6):795-804.
11. Khael EM, Alhilali DN. Gift acceptance and its effect on prescribing behavior among Iraqi specialist physicians. Pharma Pharmacol. 2014;5(7):705-15.
12. Theodorou M, Tsiantou V, Pavlakis A, et al. Factors influencing prescribing behaviour of physicians in Greece and Cyprus: results from a questionnaire based survey. BMC Health Serv Res. 2009;9:150.
13. Jain S, Elon LK, Johnson BA, et al. Physician practice variation in the pediatric emergency department and its impact on resource use and quality of care. Pediatr Emerg Care. 2010; 26(12):902-8.
14. van Buul LW, van der Steen JT, Doncker SM, et al. Factors influencing antibiotic prescribing in long-term care facilities: a qualitative in-depth study. BMC Geriatr. 2014;14:136.
15. Ljungberg C, Lindblad AK, Tully MP. Hospital doctors' views of factors influencing their prescribing. J Eval Clin Pract. 2007;13(5):765-71.
16. LePore P, Tooker J. The influence of organizational structure on physician satisfaction: findings from a national survey. Eff Clin Pract. 2000;3(2):62-8.
17. Anderson BL, Silverman GK, Loewenstein GF, et al. Factors associated with physicians' reliance on pharmaceutical sales representatives. Acad Med. 2009;84(8):994-1002.
18. Al-Areefi MA, Hassali MA, Mohamed Ibrahim MI. The role of pharmaceutical marketing and other factors in prescribing decisions: the Yemeni experience. Res Social Adm Pharm. 2013;9(6):981-8.
19. Enato E, Mohammed A, Dayom D, et al. Medication prescribing practices of healthcare professionals in primary health centres in Niger State, Nigeria. J Pharm Bioresources. 2013;10(1):1-7.
20. Lublóy Á. Factors affecting the uptake of new medicines: a systematic literature review. BMC Health Serv Rese. 2014;14: 469.
21. Choi KH, Park SM, Lee JH, et al. Factors affecting the prescribing patterns of antibiotics and injections. J Korean Med Sci. 2012;27(2):120-7.
22. Reynolds L, McKee M. Factors influencing antibiotic prescribing in China: an exploratory analysis. Health Policy. 2009; 90(1):32-6.
23. Al-Mohamadi A, Al-Harbi AM, Manshi AM, et al. Medications prescribing pattern toward insured patients. Saudi Pharmaceutical Journal. 2014;22(1):27-31.
24. Strom BL, Stephan EK. Pharmacoepidemiology, 4th edition. Philadelphia, USA: Wiley-Blackwell: John Wiley and Sons; 2005.

Index

Page numbers followed by *b* refer to box, *f* refer to figure, *fc* refer to flowchart, and *t* refer to table.